UNIVERSAL PRECAUTIONS

Universal precautions is an approach to infection control whereby all blood and certain body fluids are treated as potentially infectious for human immunodeficiency virus (HIV), hepatitis B virus (HBV), and certain other blood-borne pathogens. The following precautions are required under federal law, as established by the Occupational Safety and Health Act, and are based on the Centers for Disease Control guidelines for the prevention of HIV and HBV exposure.

Occupational exposure means reasonably anticipated skin, eye, mucous membrane, or parenteral contact with blood or other potentially infectious materials that may result from the performance of an employee's duties. In this definition, parenteral refers to piercing mucous membranes or the skin barrier through such events as needle sticks, human bites, cuts, and abrasions.

Other potentially infectious materials means

1 The following human body fluids: semen, vaginal secretions, cerebrospinal fluid, synovial fluid, pleural fluid, pericardial fluid, peritoneal fluid, amniotic fluid, saliva in dental procedures, any body fluid that is visibly contaminated with blood, and all body fluids in situations in which it is difficult or impossible to differentiate between body fluids.

2 Any unfixed tissue or organ (other than intact skin) from a human (living or dead).

3 HIV-containing cell or tissue cultures, organ cultures, and HIV- or HBV-containing culture media or other solutions.

Health care personnel at risk for exposure to potentially infectious materials shall use **personal protective equipment** such as—but not limited to—gloves, gowns, laboratory coats, face shields or masks, and eye protection, as well as mouthpieces, resuscitation bags, pocket masks, or other ventilation devices. Personal protective equipment will be considered *appropriate* only if it does not permit blood or other potentially infectious materials to pass through to reach the employee's work clothes, street clothes, undergarments, skin, eyes, mouth, or other mucous membranes. Masks, eye protection (such as goggles or glasses with solid side shields), and face shields shall be worn whenever there is risk of splashing, spraying, spattering, or generation of droplets of blood or other infectious materials. Employers shall ensure that appropriate personal protective equipment in the appropriate sizes is readily accessible at the worksite.

Hands and other skin surfaces shall be washed immediately and thoroughly if contaminated with blood or other fluids and after removal of gloves or other personal protective equipment. Personnel wash hands for at least 10 seconds when the hands are soiled, before each new client contact, and after gloves are removed (wearing gloves does not eliminate the need to wash hands).

Contaminated needles and other contaminated sharps shall not be bent, recapped, or removed except as noted. Sharing or breaking of contaminated needles is prohibited. Contaminated needles and other sharps shall not be recapped or removed unless the employer can demonstrate that no alternative is feasible or that such action is required by a specific medical procedure. Such recapping or needle removal must be done through the use of a mechanical device or a one-handed technique. Immediately or as soon as possible after use, contaminated reusable sharps shall be placed in appropriate containers until properly reprocessed. These containers shall be puncture resistant, labeled or color coded, and leakproof on the sides and bottom.

Eating, drinking, smoking, applying cosmetics or lip balm, and handling contact lenses are prohibited in work areas where there is reasonable likelihood of occupational exposure. Food and drink shall not be kept in refrigerators, freezers, or cabinets, or on shelves, countertops, or benchtops where blood or other potentially infectious materials are present.

All procedures involving blood or other potentially infectious materials shall be performed in such a manner as to minimize splashing, spraying, spattering, and generation of droplets of these substances. Specimens of blood or other potentially infectious materials shall be placed in a container that prevents leakage during collection, handling, processing, storage, transport, or shipping.

Regulated waste means liquid or semiliquid blood or other potentially infectious materials, such as contaminated items that if compressed would release blood or other potentially infectious materials in a liquid or semiliquid state. Items that are caked with dried blood or infectious materials are included. Contaminated sharps are considered regulated waste. Regulated waste shall be placed in closable receptacles constructed to contain all materials and prevent leakage of fluids during handling, storage, or transporting. The containers shall be color coded for ease of identification and closed before removal to prevent spillage or protrusion of contents. If the outside of a container is contaminated, it shall be placed in a second container that is closed before removal.

An employer shall make available the hepatitis B vaccine and vaccination series to all employees who have occupational exposure; postexposure evaluation and follow-up shall be available to all employees who have had an exposure incident. This service shall be made available at no cost to the employee.

Body substance isolation (BSI) is an approach to infection control whereby all body fluids, mucous membranes, and nonintact skin are treated as potentially infectious. In many institutions the terms *body substance isolation* or *BSI* have been interchanged with the term *universal precautions*. The procedures and skills within this textbook conform to body substance isolation principles. It is the belief of the authors that all health care personnel should exercise extreme caution when contacting any form of body fluid.

Ingalls & Salerno's

MATERNAL AND CHILD HEALTH NURSING

Ingalls & Salerno's

MATERNAL AND CHILD HEALTH NURSING

EIGHTH EDITION

JULIE C. NOVAK, DNSc, RN, CPNP
Director, Family Nurse Practitioner Programs, School of Nursing
Professor, Department of Pediatrics, School of Medicine
University of Virginia
Charlottesville, Virginia

BETTY L. BROOM, PhD, RN
Associate Professor
Coordinator, Nursing Care of the Childbearing Family
School of Nursing, San Diego State University
San Diego, California

415 Illustrations

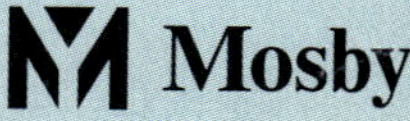

St. Louis Baltimore Berlin Boston Carlsbad Chicago London Madrid
Naples New York Philadelphia Sydney Tokyo Toronto

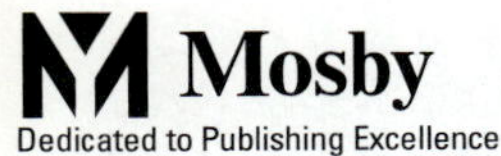

Publisher: Nancy L. Coon
Editor: Susan Epstein
Senior Developmental Editor: Beverly J. Copland
Project Manager: Carol Sullivan Weis
Production Editor: Jennifer J. Byington, Rick Dudley
Design: Theresa Breckwoldt, Sheilah Barrett
Project Supervisor: Kathy Grone

EIGHTH EDITION

Printed in the United States of America
Composition by Graphic World, Inc.
Printing/binding by Von Hoffman Press, Inc.

Mosby–Year Book, Inc.
11830 Westline Industrial Drive
St. Louis, MO 63146

Library of Congress Cataloging-in-Publication Data

Novak, Julie C.
Ingalls and Salerno's maternal and child health nursing. /Julie C. Novak, Betty L. Broom.—8th ed.
p. cm.
Rev. ed. of: Maternal and child health nursing / A. Joy Ingalls, M. Constance Salerno. 7th ed. 1991.
Includes bibliographical references and index.
ISBN 0-8151-6448-3
1. Maternity nursing. 2. Pediatric nursing. I. Ingalls, A. Joy.
Maternal and child health nursing. II. Broom, Betty L. III. Title.
IV. Title: Maternal and child health nursing.
[DNLM: 1. Maternal-Child Nursing.]
RG951.I5 1995
610.73′62--dc20
DNLM/DLC
for Library of Congress

94-33454
CIP

To my parents Caryl and Robert Fort Cowan
for their strong sense of the importance
of the family and community.
To my husband Bob and sons Christopher,
Nicholas, and Andrew for their love,
support, and humor.
To Drs. June Triplett, Sara Arneson, Fran Lewis,
and June Lowenberg
for their mentoring and friendship.
J.C.N.

To my parents Dena and Ray Bollinger
and my brother Art for providing a warm and
loving family.
To my husband Glen, my mentor and
best friend, for his love, encouragement,
and support.
To Drs. Marjorie White and Ted Huston for
instilling a strong belief in the importance
of focusing on the family in nursing care and
in research.
B.L.B.

In Memorium
Sherrian L. Simpson
1994

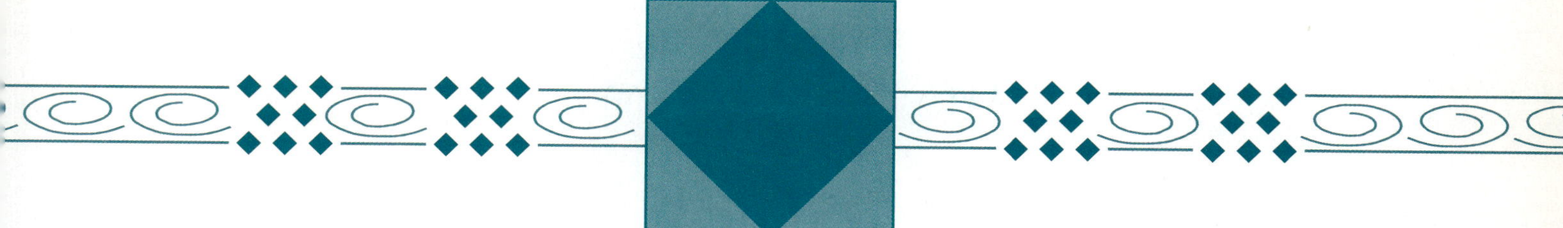

Contributors

CAROLYN B. COLWELL, RN, MA
Lecturer, Child Health Nursing
San Diego State University
San Diego, California

WILLIAM GRISWOLD, MD
Professor, School of Medicine
University of California-San Diego
La Jolla, California

A. JOY INGALLS, RN, MS
Former Instructor, Maternal and Child Health Nursing
Grossmont Vocational Nursing Program
Grossmont Health Occupations Center
Santee, California

MARGUERITE M. JACKSON, RN, MS, CIC
Director, Medical Center Epidemiology Unit and Assistant Clinical Professor of Community and Family Medicine
University of California-San Diego Medical Center
San Diego, California

VICKY NEWMAN, MS, RD
Perinatal Nutritionist, Wellstart International
Assistant Clinical Professor
Departments of Reproductive Medicine and Preventive Medicine
University of California, San Diego
San Diego, California

ROBERT E. NOVAK, PhD, CCC
Director, Department of Communication Disorders
University of Virginia
Charlottesville, Virginia

ALEX PUE, MD
Director of Anesthesia
Mary Birch Hospital for Women
San Diego, California

M. CONSTANCE SALERNO, RN, MS, PNP
Professor Emeritus of Child Health Nursing
San Diego State University
San Diego, California

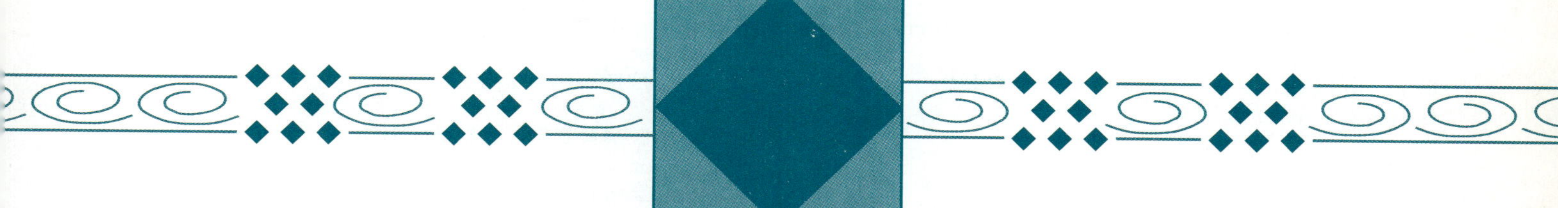

Reviewers

DAWN BLEAU, RN, BSN
Director, Practical Nurse Education
Knoedler School of Practical Nursing
Jefferson, Ohio

CATHY BOLTON, RN, BSN, MSN
Director of Nursing
Vernon Regional Junior College
Vernon, Texas

ARLINE BORELLA, RN, BSN, CIC
Infection Control Coordinator
St. Mary's Health Center
St. Louis, Missouri

ROBERT G. BURKE, SR., RN, BA, BSN, MA
Instructor
Central Carolina Technical College
Sumter, South Carolina

CATHERINE BURKE, RN, BSN, MS
Nursing Instructor
Kankakee Community College
Kankakee, Illinois

MARTI BURTON, RN, BS
Instructor, Practical Nursing
Metrotech Vocational-Technical Center
Oklahoma City, Oklahoma

BARBARA A. BYRD, RN, BS, BSN, MEd, MS
Instructor
Hocking College
Nelsonville, Ohio

MARY ANN COSGAREA, RN, BA, BSN
Coordinator
W. Howard Nicol School of Practical Nursing
Portage Lakes Career Center
Greensburg, Ohio

CYNTHIA M. DAVIS, RN, BA, BSN, MEd
Associate Professor of Nursing
Bainbridge College
Bainbridge, Georgia

CAROLYN DEAN, RN, BSN
Instructor, Allied Health
North Central Missouri College
Trenton, Missouri

KATHLEEN REILLY DOLIN, RN, BSN
Instructor
Monroe County Area Vocational-Technical School
Bartonsville, Pennsylvania

CATHY FRANKLIN, RN, BSN, MA
Dean of Nursing and Allied Health
Rockingham Community College
Wentworth, North Carolina

MARY-PAT HAMM, RN, BA, BSN, MSN
Assistant Professor
St. Charles County Community College
St. Peters, Missouri

BETTE B. HAMMOND, RN, BSN, MSN
Assistant Professor of Nursing
St. Charles County Community College
St. Peters, Missouri

PATRICIA M. JACOBSON, RN, BSN, MSN
Nursing Instructor
Bullard Havens Regional Vocational-Technical School
Bridgeport, Connecticut

NANCY K. MAEBIUS, RN, BSN, MSN, PhD
Instructor
The Health Institute of San Antonio
San Antonio, Texas

ELIZABETH K. MICHEL, RNC, BSN, MSN
Assistant Dean of Instruction, Health Occupations Division
Galveston College
Galveston, Texas

LINDA NORTH, RN, BSN, MSN
Instructor, ADN Program
Athens Area Technical Institute
Athens, Georgia

ANITA NORTON, RN, BSN, MSN
Instructor & Chairperson, Department of Nursing
Jefferson State Community College
Birmingham, Alabama

SHARON A. ROBERTS, RN, MSN, ARNP
Director
The Health Institute of Tampa Bay
St. Petersburg, Florida

PAMALA ST. CYR, RN, BSN
Instructor
The Health Institute of Louisville
Louisville, Kentucky

JOANNA SCALABRINI, RNC, BSN, MA
Associate Professor of Nursing
Westchester Community College
Valhalla, New York

YVONNE VAN DYKE, RN, BSN, MSN
Instructor
Austin Community College
Austin, Texas

WENDY WILSON WESLOWSKI, RN, BSN, MSN, NHA
Nursing Home Administrator
St. Luke Hospital
Ft. Thomas, Kentucky

ROSE WILCOX, RN, BSN, MEd
Instructor, School of Practical Nursing
Columbus Public Schools
Columbus, Ohio

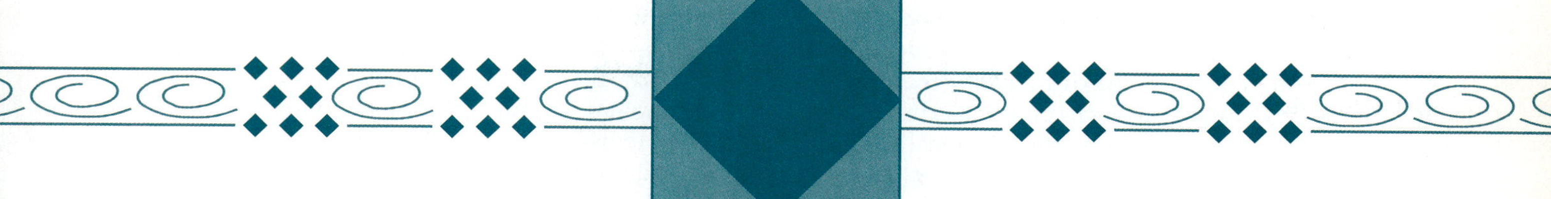

Preface

As we move through the final years of the twentieth century and look ahead, it does not require a crystal ball to see that the future will bring tremendous change in health care. Practical and vocational nursing in the twenty-first century promises to open up new opportunities and challenges. These coming changes in nursing practice require changes now in nursing education, as well as in nursing textbooks.

For nearly three decades, Ingalls and Salerno's *Maternal and Child Health Nursing* has been the book of choice for preparing practical and vocational nurses to care for maternity and pediatric patients. Both students and faculty have trusted this text to provide comprehensive, accurate, and timely information that reflects current practice. In this eighth edition, we have responded to dramatic changes in practice with an aggressive revision that truly reflects the scope and depth of nursing, both today and in the future.

As new authors for this text, we have retained the superb approach and organization of previous editions and continued to focus on the learning needs of the student. We have addressed current issues and trends in practice, updated and expanded content, added new student-oriented learning aids, and enhanced the teaching-learning package.

Current Issues and Trends

We begin the eighth edition with a new unit, "Perspectives in Maternal and Child Health Nursing," that addresses both the health care system and nursing practice. Current trends in delivery of health care focus on national goals for the year 2000 and include cost-containment and increased emphasis on community-based care. The practice of nursing in the 1990s and beyond will provide continually expanding roles for the practical and vocational nurse. This new unit explores those roles, as well as discussing essential concepts that provide the basis for contemporary practice. These concepts include legal and ethical considerations, the nursing process, and health promotion.

A new chapter on "The Family in a Multicultural Society" stresses the importance of including all family members and addressing the cultural preferences of today's patients when planning nursing care. This chapter introduces these topics, which are highlighted and emphasized throughout the text.

Updated and Expanded Content

Every chapter has been extensively reviewed and carefully revised to ensure accuracy and currency. New chapters on "Fertility Management" and pediatric "Hemotological Problems" address the expanding responsibilities of nurses in these areas. Other areas of expansion include increased coverage of psychosocial aspects, parent-infant attachment, HIV and AIDS, adolescent pregnancy and pregnancy in the older woman, and new guidelines for childhood immunizations, universal precautions, nutrition, and induction and augmentation of labor. We have also responded to the increased focus on health promotion and disease prevention with additional discussions throughout the text that address the nurse's role in assessment and patient teaching.

Learning Aids

Recognizing that today's student must learn more than ever before, we have endeavored to provide a wide variety of learning aids that address various types of learners. The basic design of the text incorporates a contemporary, visually attractive format that invites the student to learn. Bold headings and clear print make the text easy to read and follow. Tables and boxes highlight and summarize important information, while numerous photographs and illustrations provide both clarification and interest.

To guide the student in identifying important content, each chapter begins with learning objectives and ends with key concepts. To promote the development of the strong decision-making skills required of the successful nurse, each chapter includes Critical Thought Questions that ask the student to apply factual knowledge in a clinical context. A glossary at the end of the text allows students quick access to important nursing and medical terminology.

Practical information is clearly presented and highlighted for emphasis and ease of location. Boxed Nursing Care Plans provide detailed examples of how to plan and implement care to meet identified client goals and expected outcomes. Step-by-step guidelines for commonly-performed procedures are pulled out of the narrative and boxed for easy location. New Nursing Alerts provide practical tips for students new to the clinical area.

Teaching and Learning Package

We recognize that educators today have limited time in which to prepare classroom and clinical activities. We have therefore provided an expanded Instructor's Resource Manual, which includes numerous suggested activities, guidelines for discussion of the Critical Thought Questions in the book, and a comprehensive Test Bank keyed chapter-by-chapter to the text. In addition, we have added a set of 54 two-color transparency acetates designed to supplement and enhance lectures.

To help students make maximum use of their study time and reinforce learning, we again offer a comprehensive Study Guide. This workbook includes a wide variety of questions and activities to promote understanding and retention of key content. Both the Instructor's Resource Manual and the Study Guide focus on reinforcing and evaluating achievement of the learning objectives in the text.

We are pleased to note the growing number of men currently involved in maternal and child nursing, and acknowledge their dedication, skill, and professionalism. We have, therefore, made every effort to eliminate any gender-specific pronouns. It is only to avoid the awkward, repetitive grammatical patterns of "his or her" and "she or he" that, in some instances, the feminine pronoun has been used to refer to the nurse and the masculine pronoun to refer to the infant or child.

ACKNOWLEDGMENTS

We have had the benefit of several contributors, reviewers, and consultants. We wish to acknowledge them for sharing their experience and expertise. For this edition we welcomed a new contributor, Vicky Newman, MS, RD, who assisted with extensive revision of the sections on maternal and newborn nutrition in Chapters 9 and 17. Former contributors also returned to assist us. Alex Pue, MD, an anesthesiologist, once again ably assisted with updating Chapter 12 content on pharmacological pain management of labor and birth. Connie Salerno, RN, MS, PNP, remained to update the childhood immunization section of Chapter 22, and revise Chapter 31 on infectious disease. Marguerite Jackson, MS, RN, CIC, nationally known infection control specialist, supplied information to aid in the revision of portions of Chapter 31. Carolyn Colwell, RN, MA, updated pediatric orthopedic content in Chapters 32 and 33. William Griswold, MD, revised pediatric genitourinary content in Chapter 36. Robert Novak, MA, PhD, assisted with updating content on pediatric otitis media and hearing in Chapters 32 and 34. A special thanks is due Joy Ingalls, RN, MS, who carefully scrutinized the maternity chapters and provided many thoughtful suggestions.

We would like to extend our special thanks to the former authors of this text, Joy Ingalls and Connie Salerno, for trusting us to carry on their tradition of commitment to excellence and continued expansion of the knowledge in maternal and child health nursing. They recognize the need for the book to grow and develop, reflecting the current rapid changes in health care.

Others who deserve special recognition in the preparation of this revision include Katie Doyle, director of the ultrasound department at Kaiser Permanente Hospital, San Diego, California, who helped find just the right film to provide an excellent illustration of a fetal ultrasound. When deadlines were tight, Karmen Jones, a senior nursing student, provided valuable computer skills. We would also like to thank the many families who gave permission for photos to modernize illustrations, and the artistic contributions of Robert Novak and Jack Reuter. A special thanks to Patricia M. Jacobson, RN, MSN, and Anita Norton, RN, MSN, for the many hours spent reading the entire manuscript to assist the authors in a final check for content accuracy and readability. Their professional comments and suggestions were greatly valued.

From planning through manuscript development Susan Epstein, Editor, and Beverly Copland, Senior Developmental Editor, provided these new authors with the valuable assistance necessary for a smooth transition. Jennifer Byington, Production Editor, guided the book through production and was always patient and helpful.

J.C. Novak
B.L. Broom

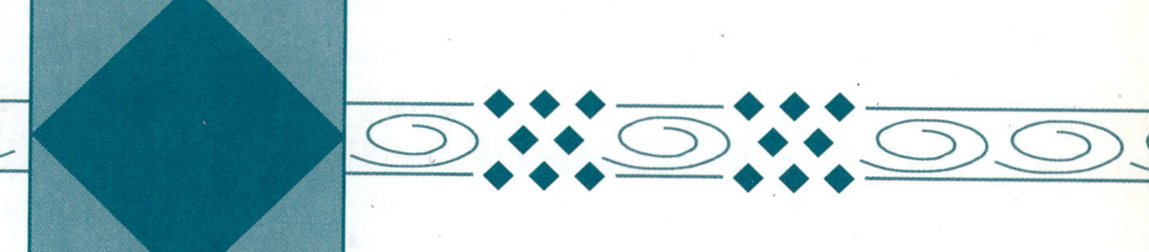

Contents

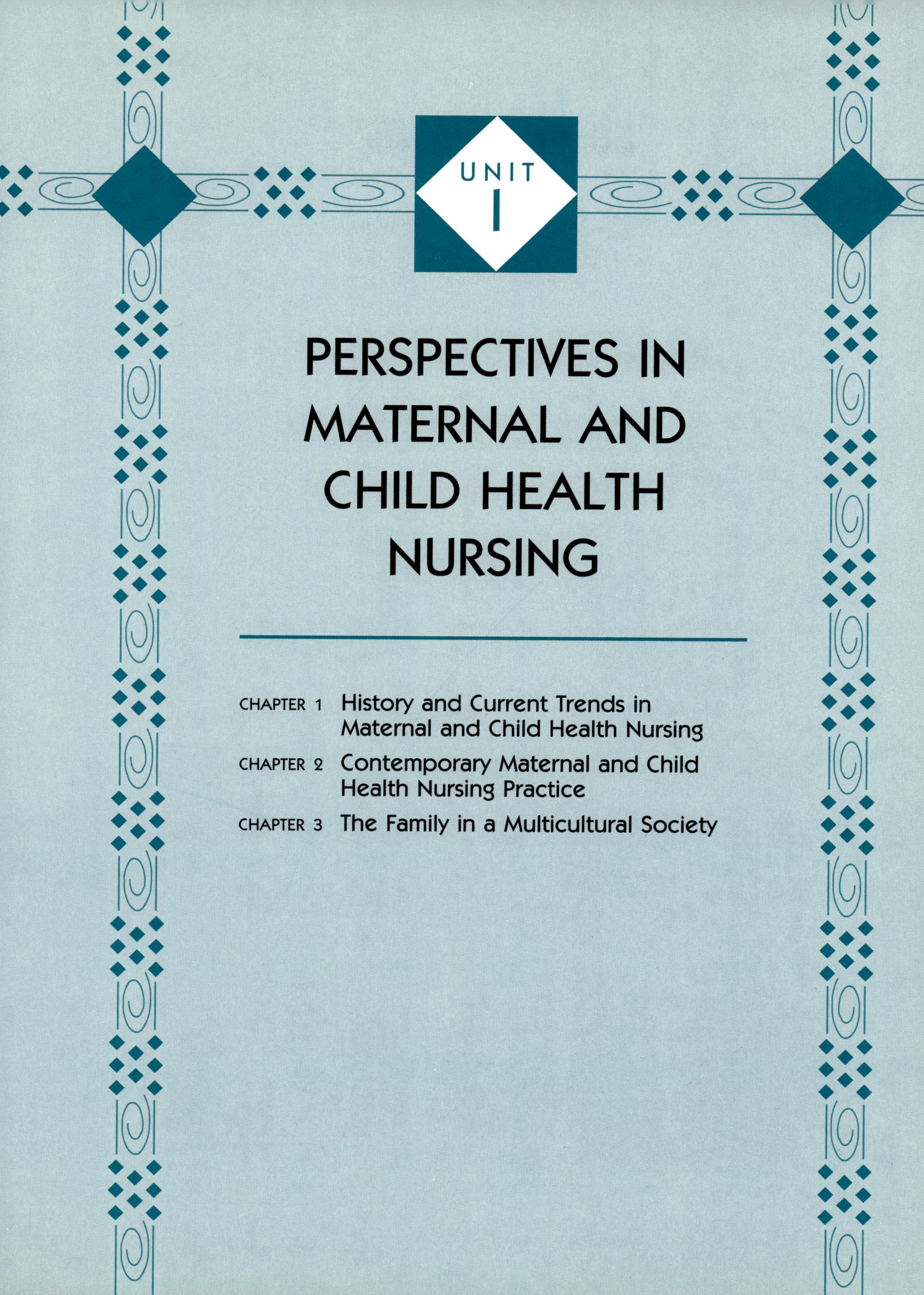

UNIT I

PERSPECTIVES IN MATERNAL AND CHILD HEALTH NURSING

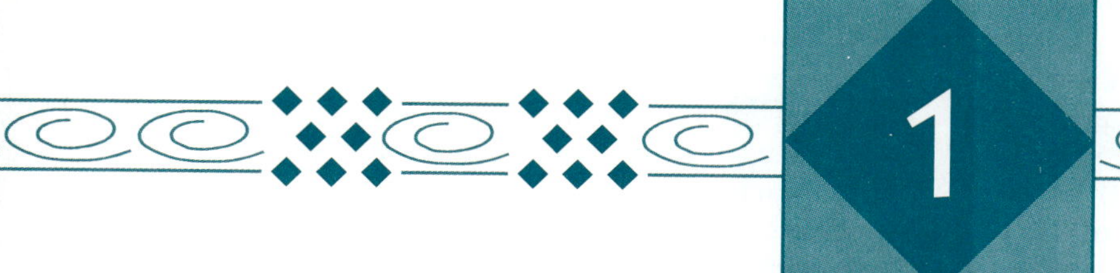

History and Current Trends in Maternal and Child Health Nursing

CHAPTER OBJECTIVES

After studying this chapter, the student should be able to:

1. Discuss contributions to maternal and child health made by medical pioneers Ignaz Semmelweis, Louis Pasteur, and Joseph Lister.
2. Cite the factors that contributed to the shift from home births to hospital births.
3. Discuss nursing's historical contributions to maternal and child health care.
4. Describe ways that federal governmental agencies, conferences, and legislation historically have assisted in meeting the needs of mothers, children, and youth.
5. Discuss the current trends in maternal and child health care, noting the implications for nursing practice.
6. Cite the 1990 infant mortality rate in the United States.
7. Discuss the possible reasons for the United States' infant mortality ranking among developed nations.
8. List three major causes of infant mortality in the United States.
9. List the four leading causes of maternal mortality in the United States.
10. Cite the leading cause of childhood deaths in the United States.
11. Cite four national maternal and child health objectives for the year 2000.

The ultimate goal of maternal and child health nursing is to help children and parents attain and maintain optimum health. To achieve that goal, nurses engaged in maternal and child health care must be aware of historical and current developments and goals in these specialties.

This chapter reviews the history of maternal and child health care and presents current trends, with implications for nursing practice. National goals for the year 2000 are outlined.

HISTORY OF MATERNAL AND CHILD HEALTH NURSING

In North America during the 1700s and 1800s, childbearing women were primarily attended by midwives in their own homes. These midwives had no formal training but learned their skills from each other and from their own birth experiences. Some colonies required civil licensing of midwives to ensure that they would attend the poor as well as the rich, not give medicine to induce miscarriage, and be honest in record keeping (Wertz and Wertz, 1989).

After 1750, physicians trained in Europe brought scientific advances back to North America and were eager to establish midwifery as a medical specialty. Their efforts were successful and marked the beginning of male physicians supplanting female midwives as birth attendants. Physician practice moved away from reliance on nature toward reliance on "artful intervention," including the use of forceps to shorten the time in labor (Wertz and Wertz, 1989). In 1828, physician midwives chose to rename themselves "obstetricians," marking their view of themselves as professionals (Wertz and Wertz, 1989).

Until the 1800s there was little formalized recognition of the special needs of children, the medical and surgical problems peculiar to childhood, and the different ways in which infants and children, in contrast to adults, respond to disease. In 1802 the first children's hospital was founded in Paris. The first children's hospital in the United States was not established until 1855 in Philadelphia. But in most regions, sick, hospitalized children were often quartered with ill adults, sometimes in the same bed. Gradually pediatrics was established as a separate area of study in medical schools. Nursing schools followed, offering special classes in pediatric nursing. General hospitals established pediatric departments, and separate treatment centers for children were initiated. An early leader in the recognition of the special needs of children was Abraham Jacobi, the first president of the American Pediatric Society (1888) and founder of the first clinic operated exclusively for children (Kalisch and Kalisch, 1986).

Scientific Advances

In the mid-1800s, infection was such a common companion of childbirth, notably among hospitalized patients in Europe, that it was termed *childbed* or *puerperal fever* (referring to the puerperium, the approximate 6-week period after birth). Standards of cleanliness in most nineteenth century hospitals were nonexistent. Ignaz Semmelweis' (1818-1865) suggestion in 1847 that puerperal fever was contagious and spread by the unwashed hands of physicians and medical students was met with opposition and scorn. At about the same time in America, Oliver Wendel Holmes observed that physicians and midwives were responsible for the spread of puerperal infections because of unsanitary conditions. His ideas were also ignored. In 1861, Louis Pasteur (1822-1895), a French chemist, confirmed that childbed or puerperal fever was caused by bacteria and was contagious (Wertz and Wertz, 1989).

With the acceptance of the germ theory, new methods of care evolved and were imported to North America. Britain's Joseph Lister (1827-1912), the Father of Antisepsis, began to combat infection by chemical means and new wound-dressing techniques. New tools, such as improved obstetric forceps, sutures, and syringes; antibiotic medications; laboratory clinical tests; transfusions; and anesthesia were developed. Hospitalization of the childbearing woman and her child was no longer considered dangerous (Wertz and Wertz, 1989).

Significant reduction in the high mortality rate of children resulted from the discovery that contaminated water and food supplies, including milk, resulted in digestive or diarrheal diseases. This discovery led to the pasteurization of milk and helped raise dairy industry standards (Cone, 1976; Kalisch and Kalisch, 1986).

The Shift to Hospital Births

By the 1900s in North America the gradual shift to physician-attended births by the middle and upper classes, improved hospital conditions, improved nurse training programs, and the increased popularity of analgesia and anesthesia for childbirth ushered in the shift from home births to hospital births. By the 1970s, most births were in hospitals and attended by physicians (Wertz and Wertz, 1989).

Consumerism

In the late 1960s, as hospital-based childbirth became more technological and less family-oriented, a growing number of expectant parents, health care professionals, and childbirth educators demanded changes in obstetric practice and hospital policies. The natural childbirth movement, as it came to be known, developed as women of child-bearing age realized that physicians had turned a natural process into a depersonalized medical procedure in which women had little voice (Mathews and Zadak, 1991). Routine use of analgesia and anesthesia for childbirth and the exclusion of fathers and other family members from childbirth units were challenged. Families became educated in care options and patient rights and sought more active participation in the process of pregnancy and childbirth. The Pregnant Patient's Bill of Rights (see Appendix A), developed by the International Childbirth Education Association, was the result of consumers' concerns about practices surrounding childbirth. The consumer movement toward more natural childbirth was responsible for many changes in hospital policies and in obstetric and nursing practices. This movement underlies the current trend toward family-centered care.

Nursing's Contribution to Maternal and Child Health

Florence Nightingale, the founder of modern nursing, was called to the Crimean War in 1854 by the British Secretary of War. Her task was to improve the conditions of the British soldier. Within 6 months, Nightingale and her group of nurses lowered the hospital mortality rate from 42% to 2%. Her establishment of sanitary measures, nutrition guidelines, and exercise programs formed the historical basis for nursing's current role in health promotion (Novak, 1988). She emphasized putting the soldier in the best possible condition for nature to act on him. Nightingale's success during the Crimean War gave her further credibility; she used this credibility in developing programs for mothers and children. She emphasized the importance of teaching mothers in the home and discussed accurate characteristics of child development decades before the field had been established (Novak, 1988).

In the United States, nurses have a strong history of influencing the health of families and children. Visiting nursing (later known as public health nursing) began its development in Philadelphia in 1839. The same year, two nurses, Lillian Wald and Mary Brewster, established the Women's Branch of the New York City Mission to care for indigent families. In 1892, demand for their services resulted in a move to larger quarters, which became known as the Henry Street Settlement House. By 1902 the Henry Street staff numbered 37 nurses who conducted infant immunization clinics, performed case finding, and provided health promotion education to families. In 1912, at Wald's suggestion, the American Red Cross established a rural nursing service to provide nurses to care for the sick and to give instruction in sanitation and hygiene in the homes of people living in rural areas (Kalisch and Kalisch, 1986).

Lillian Wald was also instrumental in the development of school nursing. In 1902, concerned about the extensive absenteeism of children because of illness, she offered one of the Henry Street nurses to serve as a school nurse for 1 month. The experiment was a success, and the New York Board of Health soon appointed dozens of school nurses to assist in schools (Kalisch and Kalisch, 1986).

In 1910, nurse Margaret Sanger began her fight for the right of families to limit their size, the rights of women to health care and personal choice, and the rights of children to be loved and wanted (Sanger, 1922). In 1916, Sanger organized the Planned Parenthood Foundation of America, which established hundreds of family planning centers throughout the United States.

Nurse midwifery began in the United States in the 1930s. In 1925, Mary Breckenridge, a nurse midwife, organized the Frontier Nursing Service in rural southeastern Kentucky. Because no quality nurse midwifery programs were available in the United States until the 1930s, the early nurse midwives received their training in England and Scotland. The Frontier Nursing Service began training nurse midwives shortly before World War I. The Maternity Center Association in New York City began training public health nurses in midwifery in 1932. Nurse midwives from these programs gave prenatal, labor and delivery, and postpartum care and provided child-health visits to the urban and rural poor (Varney, 1987). Nurse midwives continue to provide such care to low-income families throughout the United States. Over the last decade a growing number of health maintenance organizations (HMOs) have established nurse midwifery services that provide care to childbearing families.

Federal Involvement in Promoting Maternal and Child Health

The greatest improvement in maternal health in the early 1900s was the recognition of the importance of prenatal care. Medical and nursing care delivered by prenatal clinics and public health nurses resulted in the reduction of morbidity and mortality (Kalisch and Kalisch, 1986).

The new demands of the industrial revolution, often untempered by regard for the individual—child or adult—caused sudden urban congestion and worker exploitation that further resulted in public health problems. Some of the laborers working in the mills, factories, and mines were children (Kalisch and Kalisch, 1986). The inauguration of the White House Conferences and the establishment of the Children's Bureau led to the promotion of a better life for all children.

White House Conferences

Influenced by public health reformers, such as Lillian Wald, President Theodore Roosevelt called the first White House Conference on Children. From 1909 through 1971, near the beginning of each decade, the national White House Conferences were held. These conferences focused attention on the prominent needs of children and youth. Delegates of private and local, state, and federal governmental agencies concerned with maternal and child health care, as well as selected youth representatives, convened to evaluate these needs and consider how they could be met (Lesser, 1985). The 1980 White House Conferences were cancelled, but funds were made available for state-level conferences.

Children's Bureau

The Children's Bureau was founded in 1912, principally because of the problem of child labor and the support of the first White House Conference. Lillian Wald was instrumental in its development. It was initially placed under the jurisdiction of the Department of Labor and was later moved to the Department of Health, Education and Welfare (DHEW), created in 1953. The Children's Bureau was entrusted with investigating and reporting on all matters pertaining to the welfare of children in the United States; to conduct research, demonstration, and training; to help coordinate programs for children and parents in the DHEW (today known as the Department of Health and Human Services); to promote programs for youth; and to identify areas requiring the development of new projects (Lesser, 1985).

A Children's Bureau study revealed high maternal and infant mortality rates among the poor, which led to the Maternal and Infant Act, also known as the Sheppard-Towner Act of 1921. This act granted federal funds, matched by state funds, to provide state-managed services to improve and promote maternal and child health. Despite evidence that these programs helped to significantly reduce infant and maternal mortality, the Sheppard-Towner Act was opposed by many who thought it a socialist movement, including the American Medical Association (AMA), and was not renewed in 1929. During this period the country was suffering under the Great Depression, which further reduced the budgets of programs for mothers and children (Kalisch and Kalisch, 1986).

Social Security legislation

The 1930 White House Conference urged public support for a comprehensive program of medical and health care, including services for maternal and child health and for crippled children. The Children's Bureau prepared a plan that later served as the basis for Title V legislation. Signed into law in 1935, the Social Security Act (SSA) provided for a federal-state partnership to promote maternal and child health. Under the SSA, Title V programs authorized federal grants to states, which were matched by state funds, to provide maternal and child health (MCH) services, crippled children's services (CCS), and child welfare services. In 1985 the name of the CCS was changed to the Program for Children with Special Health Needs (CSHN), reflecting its broadened services. The federal responsibility for administering the Title V programs was given to the Children's Bureau until 1969, when it became the responsibility of the Public Health Service (Lesser, 1985). Title VI of the Social Security Act provided funds for educating public health personnel. During the first year of the Social Security program, 1000 nurses received stipends to study at universities offering public health nursing programs (Kalisch and Kalisch, 1986).

In 1965, under Title XIX of the Social Security Act, Medicaid was authorized in an effort to reduce financial barriers to health care for the poor. A 1972 extension of Title XIX provides preventive child health services to all Medicaid recipients under age 21 through the Early and Periodic Screening, Diagnosis, and Treatment (EPSDT) program. Whether a child is eligible for such aid depends on the problem or diagnosis and the financial status of the family. Financial eligibility varies considerably from state to state.

In 1975 a wide variety of social services was authorized under Title XX of the Social Security Act. Funds were allocated to each state to provide family planning and child care services, including foster care.

Project Head Start

Organized public concern for the health and welfare of children in poverty resulted in the 1965 establishment of Project Head Start. Project Head Start is a comprehensive program launched by the Office of Economic Opportunity and delegated to the DHEW (now the Department of Health and Human Services) in 1969. It is designed to help preschool children from disadvantaged backgrounds to develop their full potential and social competence. The program provides a daily program of learning activities, nutritious meals, medical and dental care, and psychologic, social, and economic services for these children and their families. This very successful program requires parental participation.

Special supplemental food program

In 1966 a special supplemental food program for Women, Infants, and Children (WIC) was established to provide nutritious food and education to low-income pregnant, postpartum, and breast-feeding women, and to infants and children up to age 5. This program has been very successful in improving the health of childbearing women, infants, and children.

Education for All Handicapped Children Act

In 1975 the Education for All Handicapped Children Act was passed to provide a free, public education to all handicapped children from ages 3 to 21. Supportive services, such as speech therapy, were authorized to facilitate necessary special education. Amendments to the act were passed in 1986, expanding services to infants and toddlers and their families.

National Center on Child Abuse

In 1978 the Child Abuse Prevention and Treatment Act Amendments and Reform Act was enacted. Federal funds provided for the National Center on Child Abuse, which has the legislative mandate to receive reports of child abuse and to disseminate information on activities and research on abuse and neglect. Federal funds provide for demonstration projects that provide preventive, social, and medical services, including treatment services for families and children at risk.

Missing Children's Act

In 1982 the Missing Children's Act authorized a national clearing-house for information about missing children. Names of children under 17 years of age, who have been missing for 48 hours and have no history of running away, are entered into the Federal Bureau of Investigation's National Crime Information Computer.

Administration for Children, Youth, and Families

The Administration for Children, Youth, and Families (ACYF) administers all programs formerly carried out by the Office of Child Development, which it replaced. The ACYF includes three major divisions: the Head Start Bureau, the Children's Bureau, and the Youth Development Bureau, which has responsibility for the runaway youth program and other youth activities. The ACYF coordinates all children's programs throughout the federal government.

Omnibus Budget Reconciliation Act

Major legislative changes in 1980 reduced federal expenditures for a wide variety of health and welfare services. The Omnibus Budget Reconciliation Act of 1981 consolidated seven existing categories of programs under the Maternal and Child Health Services Block Grant, allowing for the continuation of Title V programs by individual states. The Maternal and Child Health Block Grant is administered under the Maternal and Child Health Bureau of the DHHS.

Private Voluntary Organizations

Numerous private volunteer organizations are interested in specific diseases or conditions and provide considerable funds for research, diagnosis, and treatment. The March of Dimes Birth Defects Foundation is particularly interested in preventing birth defects and reducing infant mortality. The Cystic Fibrosis Research Foundation, the American Heart Association, the Epilepsy Association of America, the Muscular Dystrophy Association, and the National Association for Retarded Children are examples of other such private, voluntary groups. The Children's Defense Fund is a privately financed fund that publishes child health and welfare reports and works to build diverse support for children's issues. Other private, social agencies provide essential community services, such as adoption, care of single mothers, counseling and psychiatric services, homemaking, and recreational facilities. The Teen Outreach Program (TOP) is an example of one such private agency. Established in St. Louis in 1981 and sponsored by the Association of Junior Leagues, the organization works to build self-esteem through mentoring and voluntarism with at-risk teenagers. The 350 participating schools have reported a significant reduction in teen pregnancy, dropout rates, and school failure.

International Organizations

Two organizations under the auspices of the United Nations provide maternal and child services. The first is the United Nations International Children's Emergency Fund, called the United Nations Children's Fund since 1950, although the former initials, UNICEF, have been retained. This organization, supported entirely by voluntary contributions, was established in 1946 to relieve the children's distress caused by war. It has since greatly expanded its scope. It currently includes not only distribution of food, clothing, and medicine but also provisions for education and training of national health care workers. It is the world's largest international agency devoted to children and has received the Nobel Peace Prize for its efforts on behalf of children.

The second United Nations-sponsored agency is the World Health Organization (WHO), formed in 1948. It helps coordinate efforts for disease control, provides a mechanism for sharing new information in the fight against disease, and cooperates with UNICEF in promoting maternal and child health. (See Appendix B for the United Nations Declaration of the Rights of the Child.)

CURRENT TRENDS IN MATERNAL AND CHILD HEALTH CARE

National trends in health care naturally influence the specialties of maternal and child health care (see box on p. 8). Nurses need to be aware of these trends and their implications for Maternal and Child Health nursing practice.

CURRENT TRENDS IN MATERNAL AND CHILD HEALTH CARE

Family-centered care
High technology care
Cost containment
Prevention and health promotion
Changing demographics

Family-Centered Care

The consumer movement, which began in the 1960s, continues to influence maternal and child health care. Family-centered care is based on the philosophy that quality care can be provided in an environment that supports family integrity and promotes the psychological and physiological health of the individual and the family. It assumes that the family, given adequate information and professional support, is capable of making health care decisions (McKay and Phillips, 1984). Examples of family-centered care include father participation in birth and sibling visitation during the postpartum period. Nurses will be challenged more than ever to make family-centered care a reality in the increasingly high technology hospital environment.

High Technology Care

Scientific developments in maternal and child health care include laboratory methods of assessing fetal maturity and health, the wide use of ultrasonic and electronic fetal monitoring, and more aggressive techniques in treating the immature or sick newborn. Such advanced technology and the demand for computer skills in the workplace will challenge nurses to continually update their knowledge and adapt their practice. High technology care may also present ethical dilemmas for nurses and other health care providers. Technological developments, such as fetal surgery, have often outpaced society's ability to determine the ethical implications of their use.

Cost Containment

Although high technology care has resulted in reductions in maternal and child deaths and illnesses, it has also resulted in concerns about the high cost of such care. For example, 1 day of care for a premature infant in a neonatal intensive care unit (NICU) can cost as much as $3000. Advanced technology, however, is not the only contributor to rising health care costs. As health care costs rise, the trend toward cost containment has become a national priority. A number of current trends in health care are attempts to control the *cost* of care, yet preserve the *quality.*

Regionalization

Regionalized services for high-risk childbearing mothers and their newborns was one of the early attempts to improve care to women and children. This trend involves arranging for their care at tertiary (large, centrally located) medical centers. These centers also engage in outreach education for smaller, rural communities. Regionalization is also viewed as a way to reduce costs by reducing duplication of high-cost services and equipment, such as neonatal intensive care units and magnetic resonance imaging machines. Although regionalization of care results in lowered infant death rates, it creates challenges for nurses committed to family-centered care. Because of the distances involved, adult family members are sometimes separated during birth and after discharge must travel long distances to visit a newborn in the NICU.

Shortened length of hospital stay

Shortened hospital stays are another outgrowth of the desire to control health care costs. Within the last decade, postpartum hospital stays have been reduced from 3 to 4 days for a normal vaginal birth to 24 hours or less. Stays following cesarean births have been reduced from 5 to 7 days to 4 days or less. The establishment of a prospective (pretreatment) payment system based on diagnostic-related groups (DRGs) has contributed to shortened maternity stays. These groups assign a predetermined number of days for treatment of a particular condition. The guidelines for DRGs were developed by the federal government and are often adopted by private insurance companies. Some women are well prepared and request early discharge, but others may be slated for discharge before they are ready. The future impact of DRGs on pediatric hospital stays is less certain. Nursing is being challenged to develop new methods of care to ensure that families are ready for discharge. Printed materials reinforcing discharge teaching and providing important phone numbers is one way nurses are preparing families for discharge. Whatever the setting, early discharge is creating a demand for home care and other community-based services.

Home care

As more health care has shifted from acute care settings to the home, nurses are being asked to become more independent and skilled in giving maternal and child health care in the home setting. Early discharge has spurred many health care facilities to provide home care follow-up for adolescent parents and those with medical or psychosocial complications. Few facilities, however, provide home care for families without such complications. Nurse entrepreneurs have begun to establish home care services to fill the gap.

Managed care and case management

Two newer methods aimed at controlling costs while maintaining quality of care are managed care and case management. Managed care is instituted at the unit level. It coordinates the activities of health professionals to meet the patient's needs. It then relies on managed care paths to evaluate how the patient is progressing (Giuliano and Poirier, 1991). Nurses, in collaboration with other health professionals, are usually responsible for developing managed care paths. Case management is a broader system in which a case manager, frequently a nurse, plans and coordinates patient care for the entire stay. In both methods the primary goal is to meet patient care needs, using appropriate resources, within a reasonable length of time. As with other cost-containment measures, nurses will be challenged to devise methods of care that control costs while maintaining quality of care.

Prevention and Health Promotion

In maternal health care the focus is shifting from high technology care toward prevention, chiefly involving prenatal care. This change is a way to limit costly treatment for conditions that can be avoided with adequate monitoring during pregnancy. Likewise, pediatric health care is shifting the focus from treatment of disease to promotion of health. These shifts challenge nurses to assume a greater role in ambulatory (outpatient) care, emphasizing health teaching as a means of achieving optimum health and preventing disease. Nursing, with its strong history of health promotion, is well suited to take up the challenges of health promotion in the 1990s (Novak, 1988).

Changing Demographics

An increasing number of women are waiting longer to have their first babies. Between 1986 and 1990 the greatest increase in pregnancies was for women aged 35 to 44 years (US Department of Health and Human Services, 1992). The second greatest increase was for adolescents aged 15 to 17 years. By the year 2000, children under 18 will comprise a smaller proportion of the population than they did in 1990. There will be more older children than younger children, a decrease in the Caucasian population, and an increase in the non-Caucasian population (Evans, 1989). These changes will challenge maternal and child health nurses to be knowledgeable about the effects of pregnancy on older women. They must also determine strategies to reduce the incidence of adolescent pregnancy, keep abreast of changes in adolescent medicine, and be sensitive to cultural differences in their practice.

VITAL STATISTICS DEFINITIONS

Birth rate refers to the number of live births per 1000 population.

Maternal mortality refers to the number of maternal deaths per 100,000 live births.

Infant mortality refers to the number of deaths in the first year of life per 1000 live births (includes neonatal and postneonatal deaths).

Neonatal mortality refers to the number of deaths under 28 days of life per 1000 live births.

Postneonatal mortality refers to the number of deaths from 28 days of life to the first birthday per 1000 live births.

Childhood mortality refers to the number of deaths from birth to 19 years of age per 100,000 population for that age group.

INDICATORS OF MATERNAL, INFANT, AND CHILD HEALTH

Statistical information regarding mortality (death) and morbidity (illness) for childbearing women, infants, and children helps health care professionals evaluate the effectiveness of the health care system in the United States. Such information also helps professionals identify trends and groups at high risk for specific conditions. Awareness of this information enables nurses and other health care professionals to plan improvements in care and target areas in need of new strategies and resources. (See box above for selected definitions used in gathering vital statistics.)

Birth Rate

The birth rate in the United States steadily declined from a high of 25.0 per 1000 population in 1955 to a low of 14.6 in 1975. There have been small yearly increases in the rate since then, with 16.3 live births per 1000 reported in 1990 (National Center for Health Statistics, 1992).

Maternal Mortality

In the United States, maternal deaths during pregnancy or within 42 days of the end of pregnancy have steadily declined from 37.1 per 100,000 live births in 1960 to 7.3 in 1990 (National Center for Health Statistics, 1992). Pulmonary embolism, pregnancy-induced hypertension, hemorrhage, and ectopic pregnancy are the four leading causes of maternal death (Atrash et al, 1990). A high proportion of these deaths are preventable.

There is a racial difference in maternal mortality rates. African-American women died at more than three times the rate of Caucasian women in 1990 (18.6 compared with 5.4). Socioeconomic factors affect access to health care, nutrition, and a myriad of other factors that affect maternal health. In 1989, 34% of families living at or below the poverty level were African-American. Improved socioeconomic conditions are likely to reduce the risk factors associated with pregnancy and birth for all racial and ethnic groups.

◆ TABLE 1-1
Low birth-weight Percentages, United States, 1990

Race/Ethnic Background	Percent of Live Births
All races	6.97
Caucasian	5.7
African-American	13.25
American Indian	6.11
Asian	6.45
Chinese	4.69
Japanese	6.16
Filipino	7.3
Other Asian and Pacific Islander	6.69

From *Health: United States and healthy people 2000 review 1992,* US Department of Health and Human Services, 1993.

Birth Weight

The average birth weight for infants born in the United States in 1990 was 3368 gm. (7 lb 7 oz). Of particular concern for health care professionals is the incidence of infants born with low birth weights (under 2500 gm or 5 lb 8 oz). Low-birth-weight infants are 40 times more likely to die in their first month of life. Those who survive are two to three times more likely to suffer from short- and long-term disabilities. The percent of all newborns born with a low birth weight between 1980 and 1990 has remained generally stable at 7%, placing the United States behind 30 other nations (US Department of Health and Human Services, 1993). The percentage of very-low-birth-weight newborns (under 1500 gm or 3.5 lb) increased during this period to 1.3% of all births.

The percentage of low-birth-weight and very-low-birth-weight newborns is greater for minority groups, particularly African-Americans. In 1990 the percentage of African-American babies born with a low birth weight was more than double the rate for Caucasians (13.2% compared with 5.7%) (Table 1-1). The percentage of very-low-birth-weight African-American newborns was three times that of Caucasian babies (2.92% compared with 0.95%).

Risk factors for low birth weight are largely preventable. They include poor maternal nutrition, adolescent pregnancy, use of alcohol and other drugs, premature birth, smoking, and sexually transmitted diseases (Institute of Medicine, 1985; US Department of Health and Human Services, Public Health Service, 1992). Poor families are at the greatest risk for all of these factors, and children from minority groups make up a disproportionate share of poor children (National Commission to Prevent Infant Mortality, 1992).

Infant Mortality

In 1990 the infant mortality rate in the United States was 9.2 per 1000 births, a record low. While the United States' rate of infant mortality has steadily declined over the years, the rate of decrease slowed dramatically in the 1980s, lagging behind the reductions in other countries. The United States currently ranks twenty-second among other nations, suggesting that other nations are doing a better job of meeting the needs of childbearing families (Fig. 1-1). The United States' poor ranking may be due, in part, to the lack of universal access to prenatal care and to the high rate of adolescent pregnancy (National Commission to Prevent Infant Mortality, 1992).

The leading causes of infant mortality are low birth weight, disorders related to prematurity (birth before 38 weeks' gestation), congenital anomalies (birth defects), and Sudden Infant Death Syndrome (SIDS). Approximately two thirds of infant deaths occur in the neonatal period (the first 28 days of life). Another one third occurs in the postneonatal period (from 28 days of life to the first birthday). Much of the reduction in infant mortality in the United States to date has been due to technological advances, which save the lives of infants who previously would not have survived. Future reductions are likely to depend on improved prevention (National Commission to Prevent Infant Mortality, 1992).

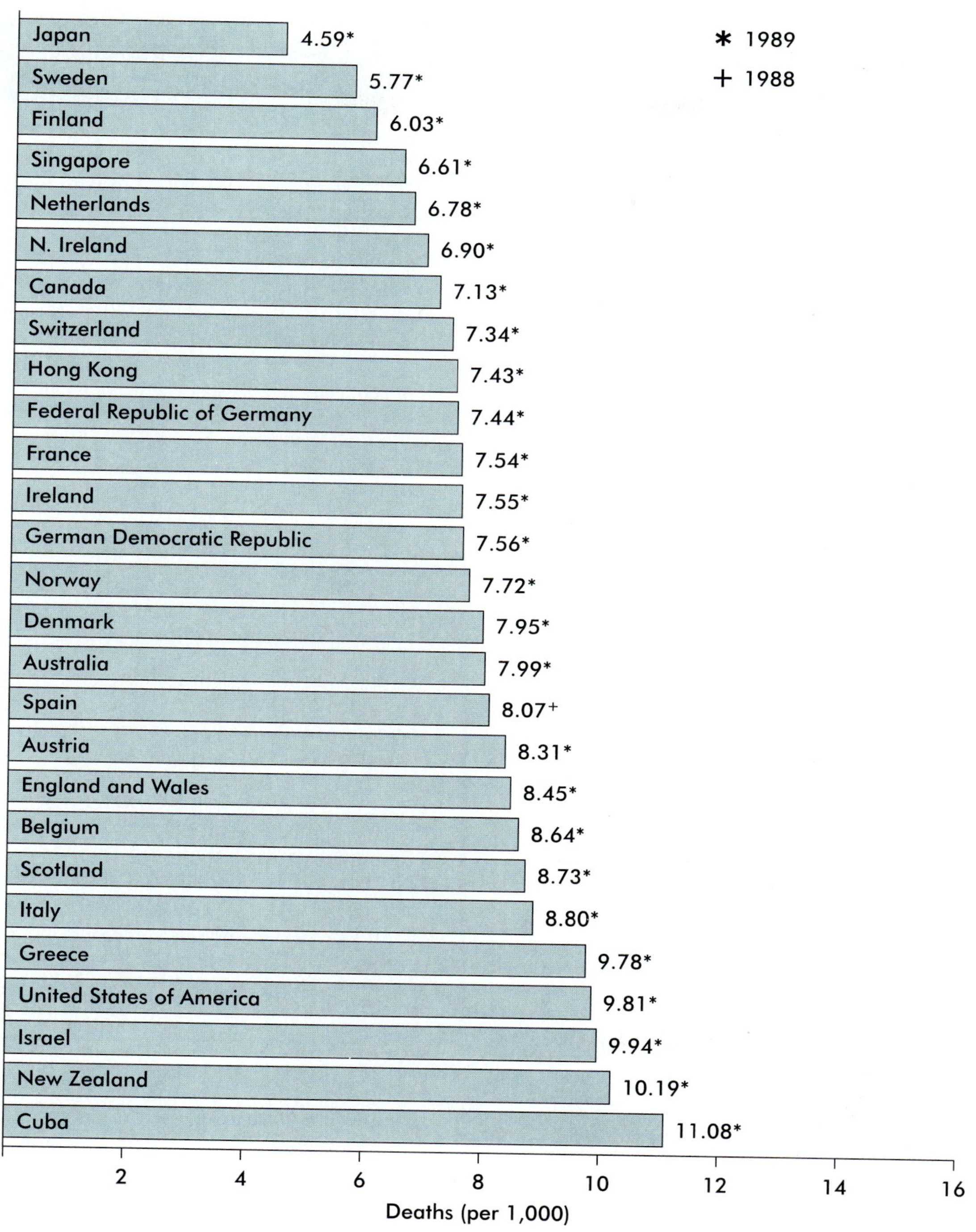

Fig. 1-1 International infant mortality 1989. Data from Health: United States and healthy people 2000 review, *Department of Health and Human Services,* August 1993, DHHS Publication No. 93-1230, 1992.

A wide gap exists between the rates of infant mortality for African-Americans and Caucasians in the United States (Table 1-2). Research indicates that this gap is primarily due to the higher rate of low-birth-weight babies born to African-American women (Binkin et al, 1988).

Childhood Mortality

Mortality rates during childhood vary according to the age of the child (Table 1- 3). The school-age years have the lowest rate of death, followed by a sharp rise in later adolescence, primarily from injuries, homicide,

♦ TABLE 1-2
Infant Mortality Rates by Race, 1990 (per 1000 live births)

	Infant Mortality	Neonatal Mortality	Postneonatal Mortality
All races	9.2	5.8	3.4
White	7.7	4.9	2.8
African-American	17.0	10.9	6.1

From *Health: United States and healthy people 2000 review 1992,* US Department of Health and Human Services, 1993.

♦ TABLE 1-3
1990 Childhood Mortality Rates According to Age and Race (per 100,000 children)

Age (years)	All Races	White	African-American
1-4	44.2	40.0	66.9
5-14	24.1	23.1	30.8
15-24	104.1	95.1	161.8

From *Health: United States and healthy people 2000 review 1992,* US Department of Health and Human Services, 1993.

and suicide. After 1 year of age injuries are the leading cause of death throughout childhood. The trend in racial differences regarding infant mortality occurs in childhood deaths for all ages and for both genders (US Department of Health and Human Services, 1993).

National Maternal and Child Health Objectives for the Year 2000

The government set national health objectives for the year 1990. Although progress was made, few of these objectives were met and, in 1990, several troubling trends persisted (see box at right). New health objectives were established for the year 2000 (US Department of Health and Human Services, 1992). The following three broad goals were proposed: (1) increase the span of healthy life for Americans, (2) reduce health disparities among Americans, and (3) achieve access to preventive services for all Americans. (Selected goals specific to MCH are shown in the box above.) Nurses will play a major role in helping achieve universal access to care, developing strategies to improve that care, and emphasizing health promotion.

TROUBLING TRENDS IN MATERNAL AND CHILD HEALTH

Reductions in infant mortality continue to be minimal.

The percentage of infants born with low birth weights has grown.

The number of high-risk pregnant women and children has increased.

Fewer women are receiving early, prenatal care.

Epidemics of preventable, childhood diseases have reappeared.

From National Commission to Prevent Infant Mortality: *Troubling trends persist: shortchanging America's next generation,* Washington DC, 1992, The Commission.

SELECTED NATIONAL MATERNAL AND CHILD HEALTH OBJECTIVES FOR THE YEAR 2000

Reduce the maternal mortality to no more than 3.3 per 100,000 live births.

Reduce low birth weight to no more than 5% of live births and very low birth weight to no more than 1% of live births.

Reduce the infant mortality rate to no more than 7 per 1000 live births.

Reduce the death rate for children to no more than 28 per 100,000 children aged 1 through 14.

From US Department of Health and Human Services: *Healthy people 2000: national health promotion and disease prevention objectives,* Boston, 1992, Jones and Bartlett.

KEY CONCEPTS

1 Acceptance of the germ theory revolutionized maternal and child health care in Europe and in the United States.

2 The gradual shift to physician-attended births; improved hospital conditions, especially the presence of well trained nurses; and the consumer demand for painless childbirth ushered in the move from home births to hospital births in the 1900s.

3 Nursing has a strong history of improving the health of childbearing women and children in the United States. From the 1830s through the 1930s, nursing pioneers established public health nursing, school nursing, and nurse midwifery. During the same period a nurse founded Planned Parenthood. Nurses were also instrumental in establishing the first federal programs to improve the health and lives of pregnant women, children, and families.

4 The Maternal and Child Health Block Grant helps fund seven categories of programs that improve the health of pregnant women, children, and families.

5 National trends in health care and the consumer movement have profoundly influenced maternal and child health care and nursing practice in these specialties. Technological advances have saved lives and improved the quality of lives. These advances, however, have also given rise to concerns about cost containment. Nurses are challenged by the need to cut costs, yet preserve or improve the quality of care. Nurses are also challenged to give family-centered care in increasingly technological settings.

6 The national trend toward prevention and health promotion presents additional opportunities and challenges for maternal and child health nurses who have a strong foundation in patient teaching and health promotion.

7 The following three broad objectives must be accomplished if the United States is to meet national health objectives for the year 2000: (1) increase the span of healthy life for Americans, (2) reduce health disparities among Americans, and (3) achieve access to preventive services for all Americans.

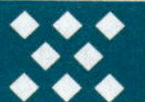

CRITICAL THOUGHT QUESTIONS

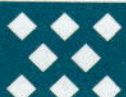

1 A 30-year-old, married woman delivered her first baby 10 hours ago. Although the mother's physical status is good, her healthy, full-term infant is having great difficulty breast-feeding. The obstetrician, unaware of the breast-feeding problems, evaluates the mother's physical health and writes an order for early discharge at 12 hours postpartum. What is the nurse's responsibility in this situation? Why? How would you handle it?

2 Recall your most recent experience in the health care system. Did your health care provider take advantage of the opportunity for health promotion teaching? As a consumer, did you ask for health information? What do you think is the responsibility of the provider and the consumer in these situations?

3 One of the goals for health care in the next decade is to provide access to preventive services for all Americans. Do nurses have a responsibility to help accomplish this goal? If so, what are some ways that maternal and child health nurses can help? How can student nurses help?

REFERENCES

Atrash HK, Koonin LM, Lawson HW, et al: Maternal mortality in the United States, 1979-1986, *Obstet Gynecol* 76(6):1055-1060, 1990.

Binkin N, Rust K, Williams R: Racial differences in neonatal mortality: what causes of death explain the gap? *Am J Dis Child* 142:434-440, 1988.

Cone TE: Highlights of two centuries of American pediatrics, 1776-1976, *Am J Dis Child* 130:762-775, 1976.

Evans V: Sociodemographic trends toward the 21st century. In Feeg VI, editor: *Pediatric nursing: forum on the future: looking toward the 21st century,* Pitman, NJ, 1989, Anthony J. Jannetti.

Giuliano K, Poirier C: Nursing case management: Critical

pathways to desirable outcomes, *Nsg Management* 22:52-58, 1991.

Institute of Medicine: *Preventing low birthweight,* Washington, DC, 1985, National Academy Press.

Kalisch PA, Kalisch BJ: *The advance of American nursing,* ed 2, Boston, MA, 1986, Little, Brown and Co.

Lesser AJ: The origin and development of maternal and child health programs in the United States, *Am J Public Health* 75(6):590, 1985.

Mathews JJ, Zadak K: The alternative birth movement in the United States: history and current status, *Women Health* 17(1):39-56, 1991.

McKay S, Phillips C: *Family-centered maternity care,* Rockville, MD, 1984, Aspen Publishing.

National Center for Health Statistics: Advance report of final natality statistics, 1989, June 1992, *Monthly Vital Statistics Report.*

National Commission to Prevent Infant Mortality: *Troubling trends persist: shortchanging America's next generation,* Washington, DC, 1992, The Commission.

Novak J: The social mandate and historical basis for nursing's role in health promotion, *J Prof Nurs* 4(2): 80-87, 1988.

Sanger M: *The new motherhood,* London, 1922, Jonathan Cape.

US Department of Health and Human Services: *Health: United States and healthy people 2000 review,* DHHS Pub. No. (PHS) 93-1232, Hyattsville, MD, 1993, The Department.

US Department of Health and Human Services: *Healthy people 2000: national health promotion and disease prevention objectives,* Boston, MA, 1992, Jones & Bartlett.

Varney H: *Nurse midwifery,* ed 2, Boston, MA, 1987, Blackwell.

Wertz RW, Wertz DC: *Lying-in: a history of childbirth in America,* New Haven, CT, 1989, Yale University Press.

BIBLIOGRAPHY

Aumann GM-E: New chances, new choices: problems with perinatal technology, *J Perinat Neonatal Nurs 1(3):11-23, 1988.*

Bishop BE: Is it managed care or managed costs? *MCN* 18(1):7, 1993.

Center for the Study of Social Policy: *Kids count data book: state profiles of child well-being,* Washington, DC, 1992, The Center.

Cohen E: Nursing case management: does it pay? *J Nurs Adm* 21(4):20-26, 1991.

Grad RK: Why do I have to work so hard? *MCN* 18(1):9-10, 1993.

Klerman L: Perinatal health care policy: how it will affect the family in the 21st century. *J Obstet Gynecol Neonatal Nurs* 23(2):124-128, 1994.

McClanahan P: Improving access to and use of prenatal care, *J Obstet Gynecol Neonatal Nurs* 21(4):280-283, 1992.

Merkatz IR, Thompson JE, Mullen PD, et al: *New perspectives on prenatal care,* New York, NY, 1990, Elsevier.

National Perinatal Information Center: *Perinatal health: strategies for the 21st century,* Providence, RI, 1992, The Center.

Styles MM: Challenges for nursing in this new decade, *MCN* 15(6):347, 1990.

Williams LR, Cooper MK: Nurse-managed postpartum home care, *J Obstet Gynecol Neonatal Nurs* 22(1):25-31, 1993.

Contemporary Maternal and Child Health Nursing Practice

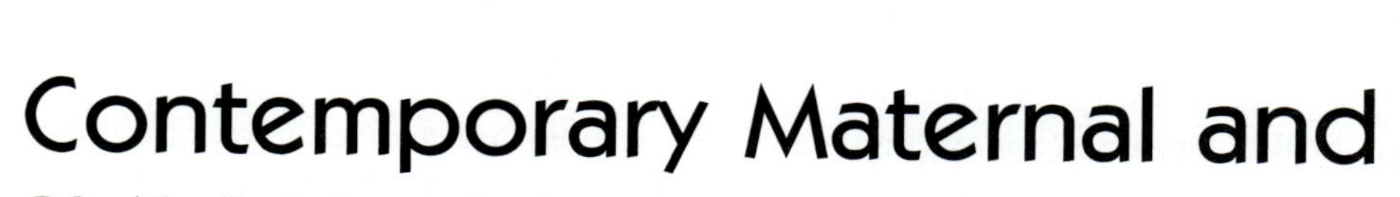

CHAPTER OBJECTIVES

After studying this chapter, the student should be able to:

1. Describe the nature of maternal and child health nursing.
2. Discuss the advantages of using a nursing conceptual model in clinical practice.
3. Describe the educational preparation and professional responsibilities of the clinical nurse specialist, the nurse practitioner, and the certified nurse midwife.
4. Identify the two major nursing specialty organizations in maternal and/or child health nursing.
5. Describe the five steps of the nursing process.
6. Define "standard of care."
7. Discuss the legal implications of the American Nurses Association (ANA) Standards of Maternal and Child Health Practice.
8. Identify three ways the nurse can reduce the risk of committing an error that may violate the standard of care.
9. Discuss the ethical implications of the ANA Code for Nurses.

NATURE AND SCOPE OF MATERNAL AND CHILD HEALTH NURSING PRACTICE

According to the American Nurses Association (ANA), "Maternal and child health nursing is a specialized area of nursing focused on the health needs and identifiable responses of women, their partners, and families to real or potential health problems associated with childbearing and childrearing. It includes concern for the developing fetus from conception to birth and the child from birth through adolescence (ANA, 1983a)." Because parents and children are generally healthy and childbearing is usually a normal, healthy event, the practice of maternal and child health nursing emphasizes health promotion and prevention of disease. Specifically, maternal and child health nurses work to enhance the developmental potential of individuals, increase the health knowledge of individuals, and serve as family and child health advocates. In addition, maternal and child health nurses develop health care resources and provide conditions that promote, maintain, and restore the health of children through adolescence and the health of the adults who are responsible for them (ANA, 1983b).

Maternal and child health nurses practice at all levels of care and in a variety of settings, from homes, schools, and outpatient clinics to the most sophisticated intensive care units. Specialization has developed within nursing, as it has in medicine. The primary specialties in maternal and child health nursing are maternity and pediatric nursing. The term *perinatal nursing* is increasingly used instead of maternity nursing or obstetric nursing. (The term *perinatal* refers to the period from 28 weeks of pregnancy through the first 28 days after birth.) Two newer specialties in medicine, perinatology and neonatology, have also led to expanding specialization and responsibilities in nursing practice. Perinatology is the medical practice specializing in the care of the mother and fetus experiencing complications before and during childbirth. Neonatology is the medical care of high-risk newborns.

Expanded Nursing Roles

Maternal and child health nurses have a variety of educational backgrounds: licensed vocational nursing programs and registered nursing programs at the diploma, associate degree, and baccalaureate degree levels. Nurses with advanced preparation (certification and/or master's degree) assume correspondingly more advanced and independent responsibilities for patient and family care. A brief overview of the preparation and responsibilities of nurses with advanced preparation follows.

Clinical nurse specialist

A clinical nurse specialist has usually completed a master's degree in the specialty and has considerable clinical experience. The clinical nurse specialist typically provides expert care to individuals, participates in educating health care professionals and paraprofessionals, and is involved in research.

Nurse practitioner

A nurse practitioner has completed either a certification program or a master's degree in the specialty and is also certified by the appropriate specialty organization. The nurse practitioner typically performs independent health assessments and diagnoses, treats, and counsels clients and families. Clients with complicated conditions are referred to physicians or are managed in collaboration with physicians.

Certified nurse midwife

A certified nurse midwife (CNM) is a registered nurse who has completed either a certification program or a master's degree program in the specialty and has taken the certification examination administered by the American College of Nurse Midwives. Certified nurse midwives provide relatively independent pregnancy, childbirth, postpartum, and gynecological care. Clients with high-risk problems are referred to physicians or are managed in collaboration with physicians. Nurse practitioners and nurse midwives have a history of delivering care within the scope of their practice, that is comparable to or higher in quality and at a lower cost than that of physicians (Jacox, 1987; Safriet, 1992).

Specialty Organizations

There are two primary specialty organizations in maternal and child health nursing: (1) the Division on Maternal and Child Health Nursing Practice within the American Nurses Association, and (2) the Association of Women's Health, Obstetric, and Neonatal Nurses (AWHONN), formerly the Nurses Association of the American College of Obstetricians and Gynecologists (NAACOG). Specialty organizations specifically for pediatric nurses include the Society of Pediatric Nurses and the National Association of Pediatric Nurse Associates/Practitioners (NAPNAP). These organizations set standards for practice, develop and administer certification examinations, participate in the legislative process to affect laws that affect practitioners and clients, and disseminate information to members.

Nursing Knowledge and Its Application in Clinical Practice

The knowledge base that guides nursing practice is still developing. It is organized around the following four major concepts or ideas: *person, health, environment,* and *nursing*. *Person* refers to the individual, family, community, or group that is the recipient of nursing care (the client). *Health* refers to the client's state of wellness or illness. *Environment* refers to the client's significant others, as well as their physical surroundings. *Nursing* refers to the nurse's actions taken on behalf of or in conjunction with the client (Fawcett, 1989).

The way nurses view these concepts and the relationships among them guides their practice and provides direction for nursing research. This view of the concepts and the relationships among them is called a conceptual model or framework. Conceptual models provide a structure for thinking, for assessments, and for interpreting assessment findings (Fawcett, 1989). Many hospitals and clinics are adopting nursing conceptual models to provide a distinctive nursing framework for nursing care and documentation. The following is a brief overview of the most common frameworks encountered in maternal and child health nursing.

Orem's self-care model

The self-care model of nursing practice focuses on activities that adult individuals perform on their own behalf to maintain life, health, and well-being. The child, however, is viewed as a dependent who must be cared for or guided by a responsible adult (Orem, 1986). A person's health and environment are factors that influence the individual's ability to perform self-care activities. Nursing interventions are needed when the person is unable to perform the necessary self-care activities. This model has a strong health-promotion and maintenance focus.

Roy's adaptation model

The adaptation model of nursing practice focuses on the ability of individuals, families, communities, or societies ability to adapt to change. The degree of internal or external environmental change and the person's ability to cope with that change are likely to determine the person's health status. Nursing interventions are aimed at promoting physiological, psychological, and social functioning or adaptation (Roy, 1984).

Rogers' holistic model

Rogers' holistic model of nursing practice views the person as a unified whole—more than just the sum of the individual's parts. It assumes that the individual is constantly interacting with the environment and that the life process, although constantly changing, has a wholeness and a continuity. Nursing interventions seek to promote harmonious interaction between persons and their environments, strengthen the wholeness of the individual, and redirect human and environmental patterns or organization to achieve maximum health (Rogers, 1980).

Leininger's transcultural model

Leininger's transcultural model of nursing practice focuses on the fact that different cultures have different caring behaviors, as well as different health and illness values, beliefs, and patterns of behavior (Leininger, 1985). Awareness of these differences allows nurses to design culture-specific nursing interventions.

Watson's human care model

Watson's human care model of nursing practice is based on a deep respect for the individual's spirituality and ability to grow and change. Nurses are viewed as participating with the client in the human care process. Nursing interventions seek to facilitate the person's growth toward gaining increased self-knowledge, self-control, and self-healing within health and illness (Hill and Smith, 1990).

Nursing has not adopted any single nursing model. Nurses frequently blend elements of several models as they care for families and children.

Nursing Process

Nursing process is the application of a systematic problem-solving approach to clinical nursing care. This process involves critical thinking at each step and allows the nurse to individualize care. The nursing process has the following five steps: assessment, nursing diagnosis, planning, implementation, and evaluation. The circular nature of the nursing process is illustrated in Fig. 2-1.

Assessment phase

The assessment phase is the first step in the nursing process. The nurse collects information from a variety of sources to identify current and potential health problems. Examples of information that the nurse gathers include health history; health assessment, including vital signs and other physiological indi-

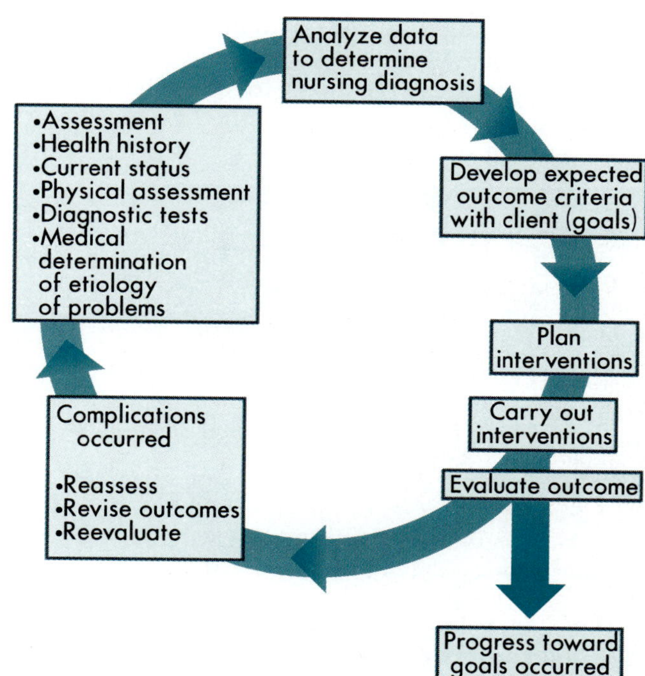

Fig. 2-1 The circular nature of the nursing process. From Dickason EJ, Silverman BL, Schult MO: *Maternal-infant nursing care,* St. Louis, 1994, Mosby.

cators; and the client record, including the results of diagnostic tests.

Nursing diagnosis

The nurse then analyzes the collected information and identifies client actual or potential problems that are amenable to nursing intervention. Nursing diagnoses are made using the categories established by the North American Nursing Diagnosis Association (NANDA). See the box below for examples of nursing diagnoses related to maternal and child health nursing.

Planning

The nurse must decide which problems have priority and which can be dealt with at a later time. For example, a woman who is hemorrhaging must be stabilized before other less-pressing problems are considered. Once priorities are set, the nurse formulates a plan of care. The plan of care includes designating expected outcomes or goals, which specify what will be accomplished within a particular time frame, and nursing interventions likely to help the client attain these goals. To increase cooperation and compliance, the client and the family should be involved in the planning process as much as possible.

Implementation

The plan of care is carried out in the implementation phase. The nurse may implement the plan or may delegate certain interventions to other health care providers.

EXAMPLES OF NURSING DIAGNOSES RELATED TO MATERNAL AND CHILD HEALTH NURSING

Fatigue related to physiological changes during the first trimester of pregnancy.

Knowledge deficit related to lack of experience in caring for a newborn.

Constipation related to physiological changes of pregnancy and iron supplementation.

Altered nutrition: high risk for less than body requirements related to increased metabolic demands of pregnancy, nausea, and poor appetite.

Pain related to cervical dilatation in labor.

High risk for infection related to cervical laceration and blood loss.

Fear related to threatened loss of a premature newborn.

Evaluation

In evaluation the nurse considers how the client has responded to nursing interventions and how much progress has been made toward meeting the stated outcomes. If outcomes were not met, the plan of care may need to be revised.

LEGAL AND ETHICAL ASPECTS OF MATERNAL AND CHILD HEALTH NURSING

Standards of Nursing Practice

The standard of care is the average degree of skill and care exhibited by a nurse with comparable education while in similar circumstances. State boards of nursing governing licensure define the scope of nursing practice in each state. In addition, specialty organizations have established standards specific to maternal and child health nursing. The box on p. 19 lists the ANA Standards of Maternal and Child Health Practice. The AWHONN standards are specific to women's health and perinatal nursing (see box on p. 19). Hospitals and other health care agencies have policies and procedures related to nursing practice in their facilities. These policies are also considered standards of practice. Nurses must be familiar with the standards and scope of practice for their profession, as well as for their facility. If a nurse causes injury to a patient because he or she fails to meet the standard of care, the nurse may be guilty of professional malpractice. Failing to meet the standard of care includes failing to do something that should have been done, doing something incorrectly, or doing something outside the scope of nursing practice.

Nurses can reduce the risk of committing an error that violates the standard of care in a number of ways; for example, carefully documenting care in the patient record, obtaining informed consent before performing any procedure on a patient, and pursuing continuing education to ensure that professional knowledge is up-to-date.

Documentation provides a record of the client's status with regard to the illness or condition and documents the plan of care. The record also serves as an important avenue of communication for all persons involved in the client's care. Therefore documentation should be accurate, objective, and complete. Errors should be corrected by drawing a single line through the erroneous information and writing "Error" over it. All documentation should be signed with your full professional name and title.

Clients have the legal right to refuse or consent to

AMERICAN NURSES ASSOCIATION STANDARDS OF MATERNAL AND CHILD HEALTH NURSING

STANDARD I
The nurse helps children and parents attain and maintain optimum health.

STANDARD II
The nurse assists families in achieving and maintaining a balance between the personal growth needs of individual family members and optimum family functioning.

STANDARD III
The nurse intervenes with vulnerable clients and families at-risk to prevent potential developmental and health problems.

STANDARD IV
The nurse promotes an environment free of hazards to reproduction, growth and development, wellness, and recovery from illness.

STANDARD V
The nurse detects changes in health status and deviations from optimum development.

STANDARD VI
The nurse carries out appropriate interventions and treatments to facilitate survival and recovery from illness.

STANDARD VII
The nurse assists clients and families in understanding and coping with developmental and traumatic situations during illness, childbearing, childrearing, and childhood.

STANDARD VIII
The nurse actively pursues strategies to enhance the client's access to and use of adequate health care services.

STANDARD IX
The nurse improves maternal and child health nursing through evaluation of their practice, education, and research.

From American Nurses Association: *Standards of maternal and child health nursing practice,* Washington, DC, 1983, The Association. Reprinted with permission.

SELECTED AWHONN STANDARDS FOR THE NURSING CARE OF WOMEN AND NEWBORNS

STANDARD I: NURSING PRACTICE
Comprehensive nursing care for women and newborns focuses on helping individuals, families, and communities achieve their optimum health potential. This is best achieved within the framework of the nursing process.

STANDARD II: HEALTH EDUCATION AND COUNSELING
Health education for the individual, family, and community is an integral part of comprehensive nursing care. Such education encourages participation in and shared responsibility for health promotion, maintenance, and restoration.

STANDARD III: POLICIES, PROCEDURES AND PROTOCOLS
Written policies, procedures, and protocols clarify the scope of the nursing practice and delineate the qualifications of personnel authorized to provide care to women and newborns within the health care setting.

STANDARD IV: PROFESSIONAL RESPONSIBILITY AND ACCOUNTABILITY
Comprehensive nursing care for women and newborns is provided by nurses who are clinically competent and accountable for their professional actions and the legal responsibilities inherent to the nursing role.

STANDARD V: UTILIZATION OF NURSING PERSONNEL
Nursing care for women and newborns is conducted in practice settings that have qualified nursing staff in sufficient numbers to meet patient-care needs.

STANDARD VI: ETHICS
Ethical principles guide the process of decision-making for nurses caring for women and newborns at all times. These principles are especially important when personal or professional values conflict with those of the patient, family, colleagues, or practice setting.

From *NAACOG* standards for the nursing care of women and newborns,* ed 4, Washington, DC, 1991, The Association. Reprinted with permission of the Association of Women's Health, Obstetric, and Neonatal Nurses.
*Now AWHONN

diagnostic and treatment procedures. It is usually the responsibility of the person performing the procedure to obtain informed consent. The client should be informed about the procedure, the risks involved, the anticipated results, and the alternatives. Consent or refusal must be documented in the client's record. Although the health care provider may be responsible for getting the informed consent, the nurse may assist in the process by providing background information or witnessing the signature (Sweeney, 1991).

The nurse is responsible for maintaining professional competency. Some states require continuing education to renew licensure but many do not. It is the nurse's individual responsibility to continually update professional knowledge.

Litigation has become more common in recent years, particularly in perinatal health care (Fiesta, 1991). This is due in part to the expectation of a "perfect" outcome of childbirth. Many health care providers have responded to litigation concerns by practicing "defensive" health care, which contributes to the problem of escalating costs. For example, ultrasound examinations are becoming more frequent during pregnancy, even in the absence of problems. Professional liability insurance protects nurses and other health care professionals from significant financial losses in the event of legal judgments against them.

Ethical Dilemmas

Ethical dilemmas occur in maternal and child health nursing as they do in other areas of nursing. Rapid technological advances, such as genetic diagnosis and fetal surgery, are affecting health care before health care professionals can assess the risks and benefits of a

CODE FOR NURSES

1 The nurse provides services with respect for human dignity and the uniqueness of the client unrestricted by considerations of social or economic status, personal attributes, or the nature of health problems.
2 The nurse safeguards the client's right to privacy by judiciously protecting information of a confidential nature.
3 The nurse acts to safeguard the client and the public when health care and safety are affected by the incompetent, unethical, or illegal practice of any person.
4 The nurse assumes responsibility and accountability for individual nursing judgments and actions.
5 The nurse maintains competence in nursing.
6 The nurse exercises informed judgment and uses individual competence and qualifications as criteria in seeking consultation, accepting responsibilities, and delegating nursing activities to others.
7 The nurse participates in activities that contribute to the ongoing development of the profession's body of knowledge.
8 The nurse participates in the profession's efforts to implement and improve standards of nursing.
9 The nurse participates in the profession's efforts to establish and maintain conditions of employment conducive to high-quality nursing care.
10 The nurse participates in the profession's effort to protect the public from misinformation and misrepresentation and to maintain the integrity of nursing.
11 The nurse collaborates with members of the health professions and other citizens in promoting community and national efforts to meet the health care needs of the public.

From American Nurses Association: *Code for nurses with interpretive statements,* Washington, DC, 1985, The Association. Reprinted with permission.

BIOETHICAL DECISION-MAKING MODEL

Review the situation to determine the patient's health problems, the decisions that must be made, the ethical dilemmas, and the key individuals involved.

Gather any additional information or obtain consultation that may clarify the clinical situation.

Identify the ethical issues of the case.

Define the personal and professional moral positions or responsibilities.

Identify the moral values of key individuals involved.

Identify value conflicts, if any.

Determine who should be responsible for making decisions.

Identify a range of actions, with anticipated outcomes for each.

Decide on a course of action and carry it out.

Evaluate and review the results of decisions and actions.

From Thompson JE, Thompson HO: *Bioethical decision making for nurses,* Norwalk, CT, 1985, Appleton-Century-Crofts.

procedure to individuals and families. Difficult questions often arise, such as What treatment is in the best interest of the patient? Who decides? What is the role of the nurse as patient advocate? What is the legal liability of the hospital ethics committee regarding these decisions? (Novak, 1988).

All nurses have individual values arising from their personal backgrounds. They also have professional values developed during their educational preparation and subsequent practice. These values influence how they view themselves and others and how they respond in clinical situations. Ethical dilemmas for the nurse occur when personal values conflict with professional values. In health care situations, several individuals, each with their own set of values, are involved—physicians, nurses, patients, family members—and emotions may be high.

Nurses should be familiar with the following basic ethical principles in health care: beneficence (do good), nonmalfeasance (do no harm), confidentiality (patient's right to privacy), self-determination (patient's right to decide what happens to his or her body); and justice (fair allocation of resources) (Dalby, 1993). The ANA Code for Nurses (see box on p. 20) incorporates these principles and emphasizes that the nurse's primary commitment is to the patient's care and safety.

Frameworks or procedures for analysis and evaluation of ethical dilemmas are similar to those for the nursing process. They both involve problem solving and critical thinking. The box on p. 20 presents an example of a framework that provides guidelines for moral decision making in nursing practice. As technology increases, maternal and child health nurses can expect to be more involved in ethical decision making. Familiarity with the professional code for nurses and with frameworks for ethical decision making will provide some guidance in this difficult task.

KEY CONCEPTS

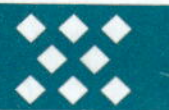

1 Because parents and children are generally healthy and childbearing is usually a normal, healthy event, the practice of maternal and child health nursing emphasizes health promotion and disease prevention.
2 Nursing conceptual models or frameworks provide a way to structure thinking, assessments, and interpretation of assessment findings. There is no single framework for nursing practice. Nurses typically blend elements from a variety of models to guide their care of families and children.
3 The nursing process is the application of a systematic problem solving approach to clinical nursing care. It involves critical thinking at each step and allows the nurse to individualize care.
4 Standards of nursing practice provide legal guidelines for maternal and child health nurses. Client injury that results from a nurse's failure to meet the professional or agency standard of care may result in a malpractice judgment.
5 Nurses can reduce the risk of malpractice judgments against them by carefully documenting care, obtaining or assisting in obtaining informed consent, and maintaining professional competency.
6 The ANA Code for Nurses incorporates basic ethical principles and provides ethical guidelines for maternal and child health nursing practice. Nurses should be aware of the way in which their personal and professional values influence their ability to adhere to the Code.
7 Advances in technology often present difficult ethical questions concerning risks and benefits, what is in the best interest of the patient, and who will make the decisions. As technological developments increase, maternal and child health nurses can expect to be more involved in ethical decision- making.

CRITICAL THOUGHT QUESTIONS

1 A friend with multiple medical problems has just discovered that she is pregnant. She wants a "natural childbirth" and has heard that nurse midwives are more likely to accommodate requests for natural birth procedures than are obstetricians. She asks if you can recommend a nurse midwife. How would you advise her? Why?
2 A 23-year-old Asian woman is pregnant with her first child. She is receiving prenatal care at a community clinic where you are a nurse. Choose one of the nursing conceptual frameworks presented in this chapter. Consider how that framework would affect the emphasis of your care. Now, choose another framework. Would the emphasis be different? If so, why? If not, why not?
3 Careful documentation of care reduces the nurse's

risk of a malpractice judgment against him or her. How can you improve the accuracy, objectivity, and completeness of your charting?

4 Mrs. Garcia, a Spanish-speaking woman, has been in labor for many hours with little progress. The obstetrician notes that the fetus is showing signs of distress and decides that a cesarean delivery is necessary. The obstetrician talks with the couple, who agree to the procedure. The physician, however, does not speak Spanish and you do not think the couple fully understands the information. As the nurse, what is your responsibility? What would you do?

5 A doctor who helps the terminally ill commit suicide has sparked debate on the ethical and legal issues surrounding a person's right to die when he or she chooses, and whether health care providers should assist. Compare and contrast your personal and professional values about this issue. What do you think are the ethical issues for other health care personnel? What are the ethical issues for patients and family members?

REFERENCES

American Nurses Association: *ANA code for nurses,* Washington, DC, 1985, The Association.

American Nurses Association, Division on Maternal and Child Health Nursing Practice: *A statement on the scope of maternal and child health nursing practice,* Washington, DC, 1983a, The Association.

American Nurses Association, Division on Maternal and Child Health Nursing Practice: *Standards of maternal and child health nursing practice,* Washington, DC, 1983b, The Association.

Dalby J: Nurse participation in ethical decision making in the clinical setting, *AWHONN's Clin Issues Perinat Women's Health Nurs* 4(4):606-610, 1993.

Dickason EJ, Silverman BL, Schult MO: *Maternal-infant nursing care,* St. Louis, 1994, Mosby.

Fawcett J: Analysis and evaluation of conceptual models of nursing: analysis and application, ed 2, Philadelphia, 1989, FA Davis.

Fiesta J: Obstetric liability, *Nurs Manage* 22(5):17, 1991.

Hill L, Smith N: *Self-care nursing: promotion of health,* ed 2, Norwalk, CT, 1990, Appleton & Lange.

Jacox A: The OTA report: a policy analysis, *Nurs Outlook* 35(6):262-268, 1987.

Leininger M: Transcultural care diversity and universality: a theory of nursing, *Nurs Health Care* 6:209-212, 1985.

North American Nursing Diagnosis Association: *Classification of nursing diagnoses: proceedings of the tenth conference,* Philadelphia, 1993, JB Lippincott.

Novak J: An ethical decision-making model for the neonatal intensive care unit, *J Perinat Neonatal Nurs* 1(3):57-67, 1988.

Nurses Association of the American College of Obstetricians and Gynecologists: *NAACOG standards for the nursing care of women and newborns,* ed 4, Washington, DC, 1991, The Association.

Orem DE, Taylor SG: Orem's general theory of nursing. In Winstead-Fry P, editor: *Case studies in nursing theory,* New York, 1986, National League for Nursing.

Rogers ME: Nursing: a science of unitary man. In Riehl JP, Roy C, editors: *Conceptual models for nursing practice,* ed 2, New York, 1980, Appleton-Century-Crofts.

Roy C: *Introduction to nursing: an adaptation model,* ed 2, Englewood Cliffs, NJ, 1984, Prentice-Hall.

Safriet BJ: Health care dollars and regulatory sense: the role of advanced practice nursing, *Yale Journal on Regulation* 9(2):417-487, 1992.

Sweeney RN: Your role in informed consent, *RN* 55, Aug. 1991.

Thompson JE, Thompson HO: *Bioethical decision making for nurses,* Norwalk, CT, 1985, Appleton-Century-Crofts.

BIBLIOGRAPHY

American Nurses Association: *Nursing's agenda for health care reform,* Washington, DC, 1991, The Association.

Chaska NL: *The nursing profession: turning points,* St. Louis, 1990, Mosby.

Corley MC, Raines DA: Environments that support ethical nursing practice, *AWHONN's Clin Issues Perinat Women's Health Nurs* 4(4):611-619, 1993.

Davis AJ, Aroskar MA: *Ethical dilemmas and nursing practice,* ed 3, Norwalk, CT, 1993, Appleton & Lange.

Henrikson M, Wall G, Lethbridge D, et al: Nursing diagnosis and obstetric, gynecologic, and neonatal nursing: breastfeeding as an example, *J Obstet Gynecol Neonatal Nurs* 21(6):446-456, 1992.

Johnson SA: Ethical dilemma: a patient refuses a life-saving cesarean, *MCN* 17(3):121-125, 1992.

McFarland GK, Mcfarlane EA: *Nursing diagnosis and intervention: planning for patient care,* ed 2, St. Louis, 1993, Mosby.

Nurses Association of the American College of Obstetricians and Gynecologists: *The obstetric-gynecologic women's health nurse practitioner: role definition, competence, and educational guidelines,* ed 3, Washington, DC, 1990, The Association.

Patch FB, Holaday SD: Effects of changes in professional liability insurance on certified nurse midwives, *J Nurse Midwifery* 34(3):131-135, 1989.

Pearson J: 1990-91 update: how each state stands on legislative issues affecting advanced nursing practice, *Nurse Pract* 16(1):11-17, 1992.

Rogers A, Batterson J, Shurak E: User-friendly forms for mother-baby nursing, *MCN* (18(6):297-301, 1993.

Zukowsky K, Coburn CE: Neonatal nurse practitioners—who are they? *J Obstet Gynecol Neonatal Nurs* 20(2):128-132, 1990.

3

The Family in a Multicultural Society

CHAPTER OBJECTIVES

After studying this chapter, the student should be able to:

1. Define the family.
2. Differentiate among the varying types of families.
3. Discuss the influences that have led to changes in contemporary family structure and function.
4. Explain the functions of the family.
5. Discuss the developmental stages of the family and their associated developmental tasks.
6. Explain the relationship between the individual's psychosocial developmental tasks and the family's developmental tasks.
7. Define culture and acculturation.
8. Define ethnicity and ethnocentrism.
9. Explain how cultural values differ for: time, activity, interpersonal relationships, person-environment relationships, and human nature.
10. List the major points to be determined in a cultural assessment.
11. Discuss the value of doing a cultural assessment.

Perinatal and pediatric nurses have a unique opportunity to influence the health and well being of families. Problems affecting any one family member tend to affect other members and the family as a whole. For example, the birth of a new member, developmental setbacks, or illness or injury to a child requires adaptation on the part of other family members. The extent to which they are able to adapt influences the health and well being of each family member and the family as a whole. Nurses therefore need to appreciate the variety of family forms and develop some understanding of how families function and adapt to change.

Families do not exist in isolation but shape and are shaped by the larger society. In an increasingly multicultural society, it is essential that nurses understand how culture and ethnicity influence a family's values and beliefs about health and illness, childbearing and childrearing, appropriate ways of communicating, and expectations of health care providers. To be effective the nurse must be aware that others may not share similar health beliefs and practices and must be willing to look at a situation from the other person's perspective.

This chapter introduces basic family concepts and discusses the impact of the family's culture on family relationships and health values and beliefs.

THE FAMILY AS A UNIT OF CARE

Definition of Family

There is no single accepted definition of family. Some definitions focus on family structure, others on family function, and still others on the emotional ties that bind members. Friedman's (1992) definition is broad enough to cover most of the varying family forms represented in contemporary America. She defines family as "two or more persons who are joined together by bonds of sharing and emotional closeness and who identify themselves as being part of the family." In obtaining consent for a procedure, nurses must also be aware of the legal definition of family—members bound together by the civil or religious bonds of marriage and adoption.

The Contemporary American Family

Since the 1950s, rapid social changes have resulted in a major shift in attitudes and expectations about family life. These changes include increased acceptance of the single lifestyle (marriage is no longer viewed as essential for a healthy and satisfying life or for childrearing), increased acceptance of women's employment outside the home, more tolerance of divorce, and more tolerance of homosexual relationships between consenting adults. This shift in attitudes and expectations is in part responsible for some of the following changes in contemporary family configurations and lifestyles: a steady reduction in family size, an increase in the divorce rate, an increase in the rate of remarriage, an increase in first births to older women and to single women, and more employed mothers.

Family structure

The "typical" family of the 1950s was the nuclear family, comprised of the husband provider, the wife homemaker, and their children. According to the US Census Bureau, that traditional nuclear family now accounts for only 26% of all households (US Bureau of the Census, 1991). The most dramatic change in the nuclear family has been the increase in employment among married women and particularly the increase in employment of married women with young children (more than 60% of women with children under 6 years of age and more than 50% of women with infants). The majority of nuclear families have both parents employed in jobs or careers. These units are often referred to as "dual worker" or "dual career" families. The distinction between job and career is based on the belief that a job is a position that is not a major life interest, whereas a career is a position that is a source of considerable satisfaction and personal identity.

When mothers are employed, fathers are more likely to assume a greater share of household tasks and child care (Fig. 3-1). In spite of the tendency for fathers to be more involved, employed mothers still assume the major responsibility for domestic tasks. As a result, women often experience stress in trying to balance the demands of the work place, child care, homemaking, and the marital relationship. Employed women often manage these multiple responsibilities at the expense of their own well being. Walker and Best (1991) reported that the majority of employed mothers rarely

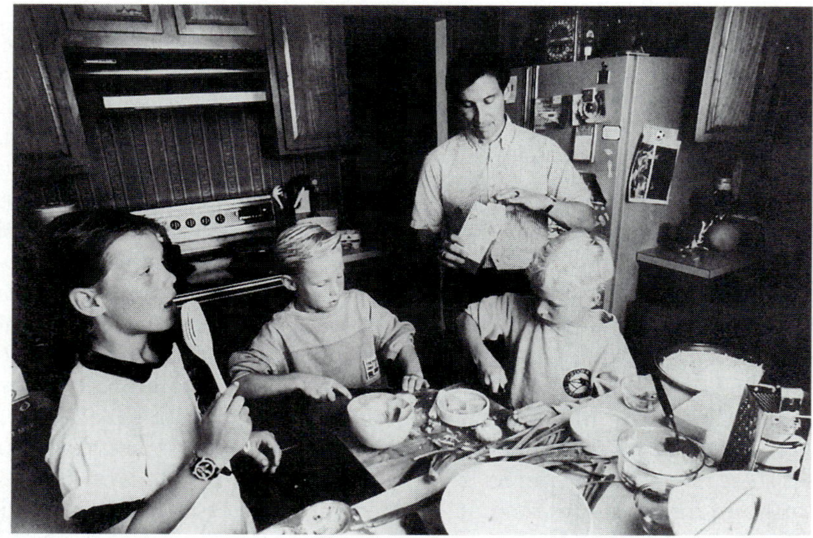

Fig. 3-1 Changing family roles make nutrition a family affair.

FAMILY FORMS

1 **Nuclear family**—husband, wife, and dependent children living in the same household, separate from their families of origin
   a. First marriage families
   b. Blended or step-parent families
2 **Nuclear dyad**—husband and wife alone
   a. Married couples who do not have children
   b. Married couples who have adult children not living at home
3 **Unmarried couples with dependent children**—often a common-law marriage
4 **Single-parent family**—an adult head of household living with one or more dependent children
   a. Single parent as a result of divorce, abandonment, separation, or death of a spouse
   b. Single parent, never married—usually comprised of a mother and a child
5 **Three-generation extended family**—nuclear family, nuclear dyad, or single-parent family living with one or more parents in the same household
6 **Extended kin network**—two or more nuclear family households (parents and/or siblings of spouses) living in close proximity and providing mutual support
7 **Single adult** living alone
8 **Cohabiting couple**—unmarried couple living together
9 **Gay/lesbian family**—persons of the same gender living together as marital partners
10 **Commune family**—household of more than one couple with children sharing common facilities, resources, and responsibilities

Adapted from Friedman (1992).

took time to relax, seldom ate three meals a day, and seldom engaged in exercise. Broom (1992) found that in households where both parents were employed, mothers and fathers alike had less time to engage in such health-promoting behaviors.

The increase in the divorce rate, births to single women, and cohabitation have resulted in a variety of family forms other than the nuclear family (Friedman, 1992) (see box above) (Fig. 3-2). The fastest growing family form is the single-parent family (26%). Although single-parent families have strengths, as a group they are disadvantaged when compared with other family forms. They are economically poorer, more mobile, parented by individuals who are less educated, and disproportionately from minority groups.

The majority (56.5%) of single-parent families are headed by women, and a disproportionate number of them live at or below the poverty level ($10,860 for a family of three, $13,924 for a family of four). Between 1989 and 1991, the poverty rate for female-headed households with children under 18 years of age increased from 43% to 47%. Minority groups once again made up a disproportionate share of this group (see box on p. 26). Lack of earning power, cutbacks in social welfare programs, and lack of financial support from the absent parent are the major causes of poverty in single-parent families (National Center for Children in Poverty, 1993). The health consequences of poverty for parents and children are substantial because of inadequate funds for basic needs such as food, shelter, and often, health insurance.

Family functions

The family carries out functions or tasks essential for the survival and development of individual members, as well as for the larger society. Social institutions have assumed some of the responsibility for functions once considered the exclusive domain of families. For example, schools have taken on much of the responsibility for educating children, and churches have assumed responsibility for much religious teaching. The box on p. 26 indicates family functions that continue to be major family responsibilities.

Theoretical Frameworks for Understanding the Family

Just as nursing conceptual frameworks can help guide nursing practice, family frameworks can help perinatal and pediatric nurses more effectively care for families. Family frameworks are tools to help us understand and analyze families. There are a number of family frameworks but perhaps the most useful in working with childbearing families and children is the developmental framework. Just as individuals go through stages of growth and development, the family unit is viewed as going through predictable stages of growth and development over the life cycle (Duvall, 1977; Duvall and Miller, 1985). See the box on p. 27 for Duvall's stages of the life cycle.

Individuals have developmental tasks that they must accomplish during each stage of development to proceed to the next stage (see box on p. 28 for a list of the stages of individual psychosocial development). Families also have specific developmental tasks that they must accomplish during each stage of family

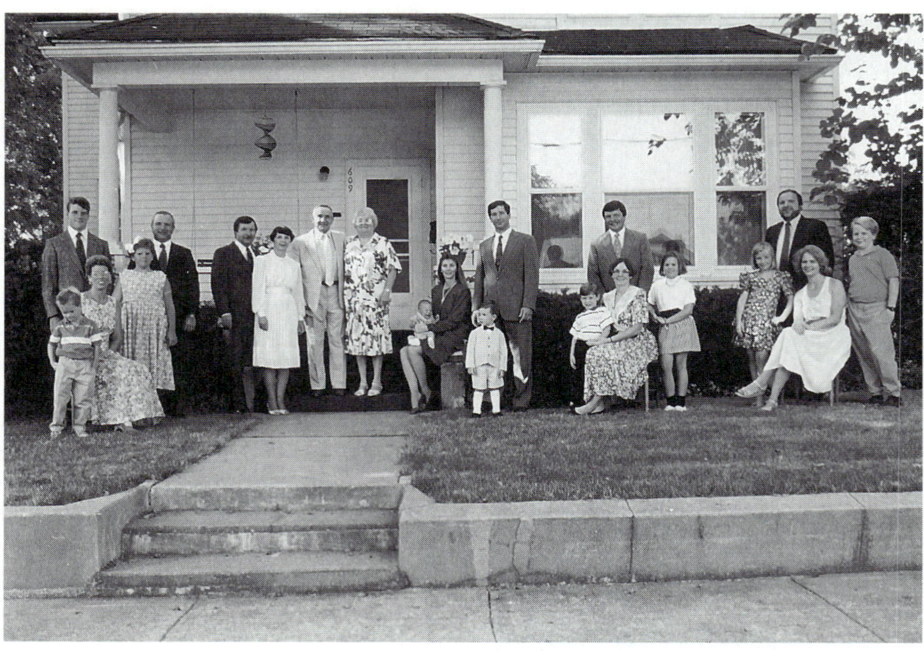

Fig. 3-2 Extended family gathers to celebrate fiftieth anniversary.

PERCENTAGE OF FEMALE-HEADED HOUSEHOLDS, WHICH INCLUDE CHILDREN UNDER 18, LIVING BELOW THE POVERTY LEVEL, 1991

All races	47%
Caucasian	40%
African-American	61%
Hispanic	60%

From US Department of Commerce Economics and Statistics Administration, Bureau of the Census: *1990 Census of population and housing: summary of social, economic, and housing characteristics, United States, CPH-5-1, 1990.*

MAJOR FAMILY FUNCTIONS

Affective is defined as meeting emotional needs.

Reproductive is defined as ensuring survival of the family.

Socialization of children is defined as teaching children their roles in the family and in society.

Health care is defined as providing or securing health care, food, shelter, clothing, and warmth.

Economic support is defined as securing economic resources for essential products and services.

Adapted from Friedman (1992).

development to proceed to the next stage (see box on p. 29 for family life cycle stages and corresponding family developmental tasks). At times the individual's developmental tasks and the family's developmental tasks may coincide. For example, an individual's need to establish and guide the next generation (stage of generativity versus stagnation) leads to the childbearing family's need to integrate a new baby into the family and subsequently to socialize the child. An important goal for nurses who work with families is to help them achieve a balance between the personal growth needs of individual members and optimal family functioning (ANA Division on Maternal and Child Health Nursing Practice, 1983).

At each family stage, nurses should anticipate health concerns. For example, the childbearing family is likely to need family-centered maternity education and care; well-baby care, including immunizations; teaching about child development, family planning, and family interaction; and general health-promotion counseling (Friedman, 1992). Although the family developmental framework presents a somewhat middle-class view of

STAGES IN THE LIFE CYCLE OF THE FAMILY

STAGE I
Married couples/beginning families begin with marriage and end with the birth or adoption of the first child.

STAGE II
Childbearing families exist from the birth of the first child until that child is 30-months-old.

STAGE III
Families with preschool children exist from the first child's 2½-year birthday until that child is 6-years-old.

STAGE IV
Families with school children exist from the first child's sixth birthday until that child is 13-years-old.

STAGE V
Families with teenagers exist from the first child's thirteenth birthday until that child is 20-years-old.

STAGE VI
Families launching young adults exist from the first child leaving home until the last child leaves home.

STAGE VII
Middle-aged parents exist from the departure of the last child to retirement or death of one of the spouses.

STAGE VIII
Families in retirement and old age exist from retirement to death of both spouses.

Adapted from Duvall (1977); Duvall, Miller (1985).

the family, it can help health care professionals anticipate what to expect at different stages of family life. The framework can also give nurses ideas about what teaching and anticipatory guidance may be useful for health promotion and maintenance. In the case of serious illness or disability the nurse can assess the impact of the illness or disability by comparing the "ideal" family's accomplishment of developmental tasks with the actual behavior of the client family (Friedman, 1992).

CULTURAL BACKGROUND AND ITS RELATIONSHIP TO HEALTH

Understanding an individual's or a family's cultural background may be the key to effective nursing care, particularly when the client's culture differs from that of the nurse. Cultural differences between care givers and clients, as well as a lack of sensitivity to those differences, often lead to poor communication, avoidance of working with certain clients, and an inaccurate or poor assessment of health problems and treatments (Friedman, 1992). For example, a nurse who believes that lack of eye contact indicates dishonesty may have difficulty dealing with an Asian client who believes that direct eye contact conveys disrespect.

Culture and Ethnicity

Culture refers to the learned patterns of behavior shared by a particular group. It is the sum of beliefs, customs, values, communication patterns, and norms that we learn from our families during our socialization. Consequently, much of what we believe, think, and do is determined by our cultural background (Spector, 1991). All individuals grow up under the influence of at least one cultural group. As people develop, they may become part of other cultural sub-groups that also influence their beliefs and behaviors. For example, the educational process of becoming a nurse socializes the care giver to the professional values and beliefs of nursing and the health care system.

Ethnicity refers to a sense of community or belonging to a particular ethnic group. Ethnicity, therefore, refers to membership, usually through birth, in a cultural group based on traits such as religion, language, or racial characteristics (Spector, 1991). Culture is a basic component of ethnic background and together these factors determine individual and family values and belief systems. *Ethnocentrism* refers to the belief that the values and practices of one's own culture are superior to those of other cultural groups (Spector, 1991). There are more than 100 ethnic groups currently residing in the United States.

Cultural Values and Health Behavior

Values are rules or standards that people use to assess themselves and others. Cultural groups can be distinguished by their common values in five different areas. These value orientations can deter clients from seeking health care, using health care resources, complying with treatment recommendations, and engaging in health-promoting behavior (Lantz, 1989). A

STAGES AND DEVELOPMENTAL TASKS OF THE INDIVIDUAL'S PSYCHOSOCIAL DEVELOPMENT

1 Infancy (0 to 1 year)—Basic trust versus basic mistrust.

As infants grow older, they acquire increasing awareness of themselves as individuals. When they sense they are loved and their needs are gratified they are happy and content. They begin to develop a sense of trust. Discontinuities in care bring frustration and pain and subsequent mistrust. Significant persons: mother or primary caretaker.

2 Toddler (1 to 3 years)—Autonomy (self-esteem) versus shame (self-consciousness) and doubt.

Energies center around asserting that they are individuals with their own minds and wills. They need the right to choose; they want to do more and more for themselves. Feelings of pride and independence develop as they learn to make decisions and become more self-reliant. Those who guide them must avoid shaming them and causing them to doubt their sense of worth. Significant persons: parents and child care providers.

3 Preschool (3 to 6 years)—Initiative versus guilt.

There is enjoyment of motor and mental power. They imagine what it is like to be a grown-up. They imitate parents and yearn to share in their activities. Conscience has developed. They have avid curiosity and consuming fantasies, which lead to feelings of guilt and anxiety. Initiative should be fostered and care taken that young children do not feel guilty about their dreams and fantasies. Significant persons: family members, preschool teacher, and classmates.

4 School age (6 to 10 years)—Industry versus inferiority.

Preoccupation with fantasy subsides. Children want to be engaged in real tasks that they can carry through, to learn to accept instruction, and to win recognition by producing "things." Through this activity, they develop a sense of adequacy and accomplishment. When children do not receive recognition for their efforts, they develop a sense of inadequacy and inferiority. Significant persons: school and neighborhood friends and teachers.

5 Preadolescence (10 to 12 years) and early adolescence (12 to 16 years)—Identity versus diffusion (role confusion).

Adolescents seek to establish a sense of identity. If a good foundation has been laid (trust, autonomy, sexual identification, initiative, and learning), they will be able to integrate childhood identifications, basic biological drives, native endowment, and opportunities offered in social roles to feel secure with their part in society. Self-diffusion or lack of a feeling of identity may be temporarily unavoidable because of physiological changes and psychological upheavals. Significant persons: peer group, parents, teachers, and clergy.

6 Late adolescence (16 to 19 years)—Intimacy versus isolation.

When young persons feel secure in their identity, they are able to establish warm, meaningful, constructive relationships with others and eventually a love-based, mutually satisfying, sexual relationship. When they are unable to relate to others, they may develop a deep sense of isolation and consequent self-absorption. Significant persons: opposite sex partner, peer group, teachers, and parents.

7 Adulthood—Generativity versus stagnation.

Adults become concerned with establishing and guiding the next generation. During this period, they start their own families or meet this need in other ways, such as teaching. When they are unable to meet this need, they may experience a sense of stagnation or personal impoverishment.

8 Maturity—Ego integrity versus despair.

The older adult eventually develops a sense of the world order and an acceptance of the inevitability of one's own life cycle. If adults do not develop this "comfort" with life and what they have accomplished, they may experience despair—a feeling that no time is left to start over.

Adapted from Erikson (1963).

FAMILY LIFE CYCLE STAGES AND CORRESPONDING FAMILY DEVELOPMENTAL TASKS

STAGE		FAMILY DEVELOPMENTAL TASKS
I	**Married couples/beginning families**	1 Establishing a mutually satisfying marriage. 2 Relating harmoniously with kin network. 3 Making decisions about parenthood.
II	**Childbearing families**	1 Integrating a new baby into the family. 2 Reconciling conflicting developmental tasks and the needs of individual family members. 3 Maintaining a satisfying marital relationship. 4 Expanding relationships with extended family (parents, grandparents, etc).
III	**Families with preschool children**	1 Meeting family members' needs for adequate housing, space, privacy, and safety. 2 Socializing children. 3 Integrating new child members into the family, while still meeting needs of older children. 4 Maintaining healthy relationships with marital partner, children, extended family, and community members.
IV	**Families with school children**	1 Socializing children, fostering school achievement and healthy peer relationships. 2 Maintaining a satisfying marital relationship. 3 Meeting the physical health needs of family members.
V	**Families with teenagers**	1 Balancing freedom with responsibility, as teenagers mature and become increasingly independent. 2 Focusing more attention on the marital relationship. 3 Communicating openly among family members.
VI	**Families launching young adults**	1 Expanding the family circle to include new family members acquired by marriage of children. 2 Continuing to renew and readjust in the marital relationship. 3 Assisting aging and ill parents of the husband and wife.
VII	**Middle-aged parents**	1 Providing a health-promoting environment. 2 Sustaining satisfying and meaningful relationships with aging parents and children. 3 Strengthening the marital relationship.
VIII	**Families in retirement and old age**	1 Maintaining satisfying living arrangements. 2 Adjusting to a reduced income. 3 Maintaining a satisfying marital relationship. 4 Adjusting to the loss of a spouse. 5 Maintaining intergenerational family ties. 6 Continuing to make sense out of one's life.

Adapted from Friedman (1992).

brief summary of each of these value orientations follows, with selected examples of how these value orientations may affect health behavior.

Time

Attitudes about time can be *past-oriented* (valuing tradition), *present-oriented* (valuing "now"), or *future-oriented* (valuing planning for the future, being on time, saving time, youth, and novelty). Those who are future-oriented are more likely to engage in health promotion activities than are those who are present-oriented.

Activity

Attitudes about activity center on "doing," "being," or "being-becoming." Someone who values "doing" enjoys personal accomplishments and getting the job done. Those who value "being" enjoy self-expression and spontaneity. Those who value "being-becoming" enjoy pursuing personal development in many areas. Those who are "doing"-oriented are likely to assess their own health status and develop a health promotion action plan that they will follow.

Interpersonal relationships

Values about ways of relating to others cause persons to prefer authoritarian, egalitarian, or individualistic patterns of interpersonal relations. Those who prefer an *authoritarian* style value someone in authority and expect obedience from those who are lower in the hierarchy. Those who prefer an *egalitarian* style value consensus and a more democratic distribution of power. The person who prefers an *individualistic* style values autonomy over responsibility and is primarily interested in how the relationship will be self-benefiting. The nurse-client relationship will be affected by the preferred style. For example, clients who prefer an individualistic style will only cooperate with the nurse if they see the relationship as self-benefiting.

Person-environment relationships

Attitudes about the person's relationship with the environment may be interpreted as a person mastering, submitting to, or in harmony with the environment. Those who value *mastery* view personal power and technology as able to solve most problems. Those who value *submitting* see human passivity and endurance as the best way to cope with difficult situations. Those who view the person as in *harmony* with nature value a balance between human actions and earthly and heavenly forces. The person who values mastery is likely to become actively involved in health promotion activities to prevent disease. The person who values submitting, on the other hand, is likely to accept illness as inevitable and be less motivated to engage in health-promoting behaviors.

Human nature

Attitudes about the basic good or evil in humans also vary. Some believe that a person is born neither good nor evil but is thereafter influenced by parents, school, community, and nation. Others believe that a person is born *evil* but, with the proper discipline, rules, and regulations, is capable of becoming a good person. Still others believe that a person is born *good* but is corruptible and must avoid temptation. Those who view people as basically evil may see illness as a punishment for unacceptable behavior.

In this multicultural society the nurse needs to be aware of ethnic and cultural differences yet avoid stereotyping individuals. It is useful to be able to discuss things that are generally characteristic of a cultural group to learn about the culture. We must, however, remember that in doing so we are only talking about group, not individual, characteristics. There is a great deal of variation between ethnic and cultural groups. However, there is also a great deal of variation *within* groups. Unfortunately, there is a tendency to simplify things by stereotyping or labeling people. With that caution in mind, the boxes on pp. 31-32 present brief overviews of cultural values concerning family relationships and cultural values related to health care for specific cultural groups.

Cultural Assessment

A set of values and beliefs constitute the dominant culture in the United States. The extent to which a member of an ethnic group has been *acculturated* (adopted the values of the dominant culture) is not always easy to determine. To avoid stereotyping individuals because of their racial characteristics, religion, or language, the nurse should try to determine the beliefs, values, and practices of the client. A variety of culturally focused assessment guidelines have been developed to assist health care providers. Most guidelines suggest gathering the information indicated in the box on p. 33. Although a complete cultural assessment is not necessary for every client, it is very helpful to know how the person identifies with his or her ethnic background, the degree to which the person

CULTURAL VALUES CONCERNING FAMILY RELATIONSHIPS

ASIAN-AMERICANS

Chinese

Extended family pattern common; strong concept of loyalty of young to old, with respect for elders taught at early age, emphasizing acceptance without questioning or talking back

Children's behavior a reflection on family; family and individual honor and "face" important

Self-reliance and self-restraint highly valued; self-expression repressed

Males valued more highly than females; women submissive to men in family

Japanese

Close intergenerational relationships; family provides anchor; family also tends to keep problems to self

Value self-control and self-sufficiency

Concept of *haji* (shame) imposes strong control; unacceptable behavior of children reflects on family

Many adopt practices of contemporary middle class; concern over child missing school may result in sending them to school before they are fully recovered from illness

Vietnamese

Family is revered institution; many families are multigenerational; family is chief social network, with needs and interests of individual subordinate to those of family unit

Children highly valued; father is main decision maker, women taught submission to men, and parents expect respect and obedience from children

Filipino

Family is highly valued with strong family ties; multigenerational family structure common, often with collateral members as well; personal interests subordinated to family interests and needs

Members avoid behaviors that would bring shame on family

AFRICAN AMERICAN

Strong kinship bonds in extended family; members come to aid of others in crisis; augmented families common (unrelated persons living in same household)

Less likely to view illness as a burden

Place strong emphasis on work and ambition

Gender-role sharing among parents

HAITIAN

Maintenance of family reputation is paramount

Linear authority supreme, with children in subordinate position in family hierarchy; children valued for parental social security in old age and expected to contribute to family welfare at an early age; children often viewed as gifts from God and treated with indulgence and affection

HISPANIC AMERICAN

Mexican-American (Latino, Chicano, Raza-Latino)

Traditionally men seen as breadwinners, women as homemakers; males considered big and strong (macho)

Strong kinship; extended families include *compadres* (godparents) established by ritual kinship

Children valued highly and desired, taken everywhere with family

Many homes contain shrines with pictures and statues of saints

Puerto Rican

Family usually large and home-centered (the core of existence), with father in complete authority as family provider and decision maker; wife and children in subordinate roles

Children valued as gift from God; taught to obey and respect parents; corporeal punishment used to ensure obedience

Cuban-American

Strong family ties with mother and father kinships; elderly cared for at home

Children supported and assisted by parents long after becoming adults

NATIVE AMERICAN (NUMEROUS TRIBES)

Extended family structure that usually includes relatives from both sides of family; elder members assume leadership role

Modified from Whaley LF, Wong DL: *Nursing care of infants and children,* ed 4, St. Louis, 1991, Mosby; from Schrefer S (editor): *Quick reference to cultural assessment,* St. Louis, 1994, Mosby.

CULTURAL BELIEFS RELATED TO HEALTH CARE

ASIAN-AMERICANS

Chinese

A healthy body viewed as gift from parents and ancestors and must be cared for; health is one of results of balance between the forces of *yin* (cold) and *yang* (hot), the energy forces that rule the world; illness is caused by imbalance

Chi is innate energy and blood is source of life that is not regenerated; lack of *chi* and blood results in deficiency that produces fatigue, poor constitution, and long illness

Japanese

Three major belief systems are *shinto* (religious influence stating that humans are inherently good, evil caused by outside spirits, and illness caused by contact with polluting agents, e.g., blood, corpses, skin diseases); Chinese and Korean influence (health is achieved through harmony and balance between self and society with disease caused by disharmony and society and not caring for body); Portuguese influence (upholds germ theory of disease)

Vietnamese

Good health a balance between *yin* (cold) and *yang* (hot); health results from harmony with existing universal order, attained by pleasing good spirits and avoiding evil ones; practice some restrictions to prevent incurring wrath of evil spirits; many use rituals to prevent illness

Believe person's life predisposed toward certain phenomena by cosmic forces; belief in *am duc,* the amount of good deeds accumulated by ancestors

Filipino

Believe God's will and supernatural forces govern universe; illness, accidents, and other misfortunes are God's punishment for violations of God's will

Widely accept hot and cold balance and imbalance as causes of health and illness

AFRICAN AMERICAN

Illness either natural (because of forces of nature when not adequately protected, e.g., cold air, pollution, food, and water) or unnatural (because of evil influences, e.g., witchcraft, voodoo, hoodoo, hex, fix, rootwork, symptoms often associated with eating)

Serious illness sent by God as punishment (e.g., parents punished by illness or death of child; can be avoided); may resist health care because illness is will of God

HAITIAN

Illnesses either natural or supernatural; supernatural caused by angry voodoo spirits, enemies, or the dead, especially deceased relatives; natural because of irregularities of blood volume, flow, purity, viscosity, color, and/or temperature (hot/cold), gas, movement and consistency of mother's milk, hot/cold imbalance of body, bone displacement, movement of diseases

Health maintained by good dietary and hygienic practices

HISPANIC AMERICAN

Mexican-American (Latino, Chicano, Raza-Latino)

Health belief strongly associated with religion; some maintain good health is the result of good luck or a reward for good behavior and illness is a punishment from God for wrongdoing, or is caused by forces of nature or the supernatural

Some believe in a body imbalance causing illness, especially imbalance between *caliente* (hot) and *frio* (cold) or wet and dry

Illness prevented by performing properly, eating proper foods, working proper amount of time, praying, wearing religious medals or amulets, and sleeping with relics in the home

Puerto Rican

Subscribe to the hot-cold theory of disease causation

Also believe some illness caused by evil spirits and forces

Cuban-American

Prevention and good nutrition related to good health

NATIVE AMERICAN (NUMEROUS TRIBES)

Believe health is state of harmony with nature and universe; all disorders believed to have aspects of supernatural, such as violation of restriction or prohibition causing illness, fear of witchcraft, and carrying objects believed to guard against witchcraft

Respect of body through proper management

Theology and medicine strongly interwoven

Modified from Whaley LF, Wong DL: *Nursing care of infants and children,* ed 4, St. Louis, 1991, Mosby; from Schrefer S (editor): *Quick reference to cultural assessment,* St. Louis, 1994, Mosby.

CULTURAL ASSESSMENT

1 Ethnic/racial identity (how does the person or family identify itself?).
2 Language(s) spoken at home and with outsiders.
3 Place of birth (if not US, how long in the US?).
4 Religion.
5 Ethnic affiliation (are person's or family's friends and associates from the same ethnic group?).
6 Neighborhood characteristics (ethnically similar or mixed?).
7 Dietary habits and food preferences.
8 Ethnic health care practices (folk healing, etc).
9 Community acceptance (to what extent is the family affected by discrimination?).

Adapted from Friedman (1992).

identifies with the dominant culture versus the traditional culture, and the person's religious preference and practices (Friedman, 1992).

As a nurse, you must be aware of your own cultural values and develop sensitivity toward those of your client. The ability to recognize when these values differ will enable you to avoid ethnocentric responses and give care that is truly individualized.

KEY CONCEPTS

1 Problems affecting any one family member tend to affect other family members and the functioning of the family as a whole.
2 Family may be broadly defined as two or more persons who are joined together by bonds of sharing and emotional closeness and who identify themselves as being part of a family.
3 The legal definition of the family is necessary when obtaining consent for a procedure.
4 Significant social changes since the 1950s have resulted in a major shift in attitudes and expectations about family life. As a result of this shift, many varying family forms exist in contemporary America.
5 The biggest change in the nuclear family is the increase in mothers employed outside the home. The fastest growing family form is the single-parent family.
6 The majority of single-parent families are headed by women. A disproportionate number of these families are poor and from minority groups. Lack of earning power, cutbacks in social welfare programs, and lack of financial support from the absent parent are the major causes of poverty in single-parent families.
7 Institutions have in part assumed some of the functions once considered the domain of families. Meeting the emotional needs of members is the primary family function in contemporary America.
8 The family developmental framework views the family unit as going through predictable stages of growth and development over the life cycle. Each stage has specific developmental tasks that the family must accomplish to proceed to the next stage.
9 At any given point, individual developmental tasks may coincide with or create the need for family developmental tasks.
10 Much of what we believe, think, and do is determined by our cultural and ethnic background. If individuals are not sensitive to cultural backgrounds that differ from their own, they are likely to engage in ethnocentric behavior.
11 Value orientations about time, activity, interpersonal relationships, person-environment relationships, and human nature can determine whether or not people seek health care, use health care resources, comply with treatment recommendations, and engage in health-promoting behavior.
12 In this multicultural society the nurse needs to be aware of ethnic and cultural differences yet avoid stereotyping individuals.
13 Self-awareness of one's own beliefs, values, and practices is the first step in developing cultural sensitivity to the different ways of others.

14 Assessing how the client identifies his or her ethnic/racial background, the degree to which the client identifies with the dominant culture versus the traditional culture, and the client's religious preference and practices helps the nurse recognize when the client's cultural values differ from their own. Recognition of these differences can help the nurse avoid ethnocentric behavior and provide individualized care.

CRITICAL THOUGHT QUESTIONS

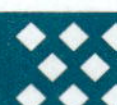

1 Mr. and Mrs. Bork have two children, ages 6 and 8. What health promotion teaching and health care needs should the nurse anticipate for this generally healthy family?

2 Andrew is 15-years-old and quite rebellious. His parents have always been very strict. They have come to you for counsel because his behavior is causing problems for the whole family. How would you go about assessing the situation? How would you advise them?

3 John and Jake are a monogamous, gay couple who have been together for many years. John has been in a serious accident and needs emergency surgery. However, he is unable to sign the consent form. Who can sign the consent for him?

4 Examine your own values about time, activity, interpersonal relationships, person-environment relationships, and human nature. How do you think they compare with those of the dominant culture? How has your nursing education influenced those values?

5 A Chinese family has just given birth to their first child—a girl. Both parents seem subdued. Neither parent wishes to hold the baby, even after the urging of the labor-delivery room nurse. Given this information, what is your initial analysis of the situation? Why? How would you proceed if you were the nurse?

6 Mrs. Valdez is frequently late for her prenatal appointments. When confronted about her behavior, she seems surprised that the nurse is upset. What cultural value orientation may be causing this tardiness? If you were the clinic nurse, how would you handle this problem?

REFERENCES

American Nurses Association Division on Maternal and Child Health Nursing Practice: *Standards of maternal and child health nursing practice,* Kansas City, MO, 1983, The Association.

Broom BL: Impact of marital quality and psychological well-being on parental sensitivity: second phase of a panel study, unpublished manuscript, 1992.

Duvall EM: *Marriage and family development,* ed 5, New York, 1977, JB Lippincott.

Duvall EM, Miller BL: *Marriage and family development,* ed 6, New York, 1985, Harper & Row.

Erikson EH: *Childhood and society,* ed 2, New York, 1963, WW Norton.

Friedman MM: *Family nursing: theory and practice,* Norwalk, CT, 1992, Appleton & Lange.

Lantz JM: Family culture and ethnicity. In Bomar PJ, editor: *Nurses and family health promotion,* Philadelphia, 1989, WB Saunders.

National Center for Children in Poverty: Study shows effect of 1990-1991 recession on children under 6 living in poverty, *News and Issues* 3(3):1-2, 1993.

Spector RE: *Cultural diversity in health and illness,* ed 3, Norwalk, CT, 1991, Appleton & Lange.

US Bureau of the Census: *Census and you,* 26(4). Washington, DC, 1991, US Government Printing Office.

Walker LO, Best MA: Well being of mothers with infant children: a preliminary comparison of employed women and homemakers, *Women Health* 17(1):71-89, 1991.

BIBLIOGRAPHY

Carter EA, McGoldrick M (Eds.): *The changing family life cycle: a framework for family therapists,* ed 2, New York, 1988, Gardner.

Mallinger KM: The American family: history and development. In Bomar PJ, editor: *Nurses and family health promotion,* Philadelphia, 1989, WB Saunders.

Pakizegi B: Emerging family forms: single mothers by choice—demographic and psychosocial variables, *Matern Child Nurs J* 19(1):1-19, 1990.

Ramer L: *Culturally sensitive caregiving and childbearing families,* Series 4, Module 1, White Plains, NY, 1992, March of Dimes Birth Defects Foundation.

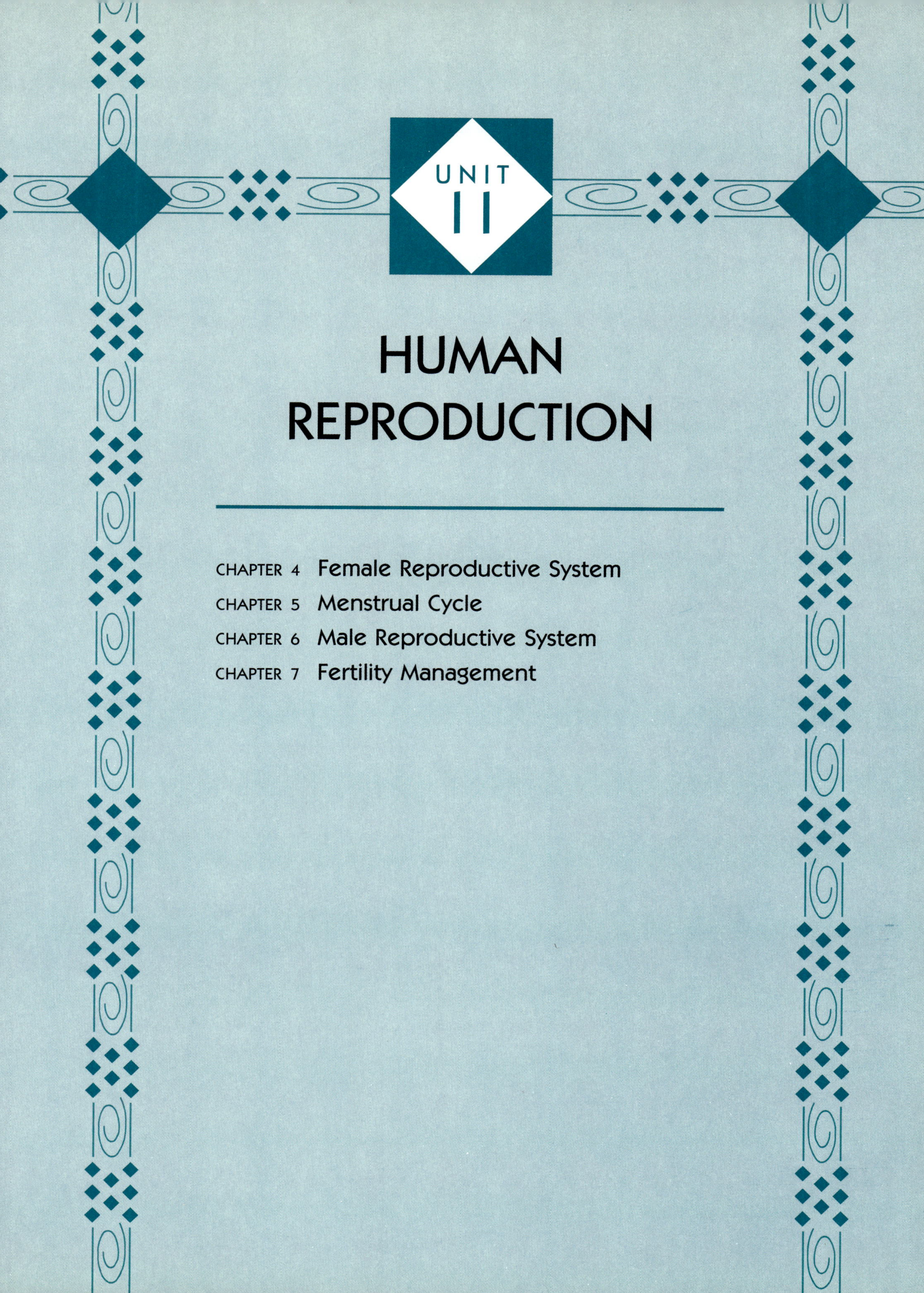

UNIT II

HUMAN REPRODUCTION

Female Reproductive System

CHAPTER OBJECTIVES

After studying this chapter, the student should be able to:

1. Identify the female external genitalia structures.
2. Identify the female internal reproductive structures.
3. Describe the functions of the ovaries, fallopian tubes, uterus, and vagina.
4. Draw a pear-shaped uterus, indicating its three main anatomical parts.
5. Name and describe the three main tissue layers that form the uterine wall.
6. Name the main or largest muscle group that helps form the female pelvic floor.
7. Identify the location of all pelvic bones, landmarks, and joints.
8. Point out differences in the shape of the pelvic canal at its inlet, midpelvis, and outlet, and explain how they affect the mechanism of an infant's birth.
9. Indicate the practical significance of such measurements as the diagonal conjugate (CD), the distance between the ischial tuberosities (Bi-Ischial or TI), and the angle of the pubic arch.
10. List four causes of abnormal pelvic structure.
11. Enumerate three instances in which assessment of the size and shape of the pelvic canal would be especially important.
12. Describe four ways in which pelvic size, shape, and contents may be evaluated.

To understand the events of childbearing the nurse needs knowledge of female and male reproductive anatomy and physiology. Such understanding allows the nurse to more effectively plan, implement, and evaluate nursing care for the childbearing family. This chapter reviews the female reproductive system.

EXTERNAL REPRODUCTIVE STRUCTURES

The female external genitalia, or vulva, include the mons veneris, labia majora, labia minora, clitoris, vestibule, urethral opening, hymen, Bartholin's glands, fourchette, and perineum. When the woman is lying on her back with knees flexed the external genitalia, or vulva, can be visually assessed (Fig. 4-1).

Mons Pubis

The mons pubis, or mons veneris, is a fatty pad over the symphysis pubis. After puberty, this structure is covered with pubic hair.

Labia Majora

The labia majora (larger lips; singular, labium majus) are two fleshy, hair-covered, protective folds, extending on each side of the midline from the mons pubis to

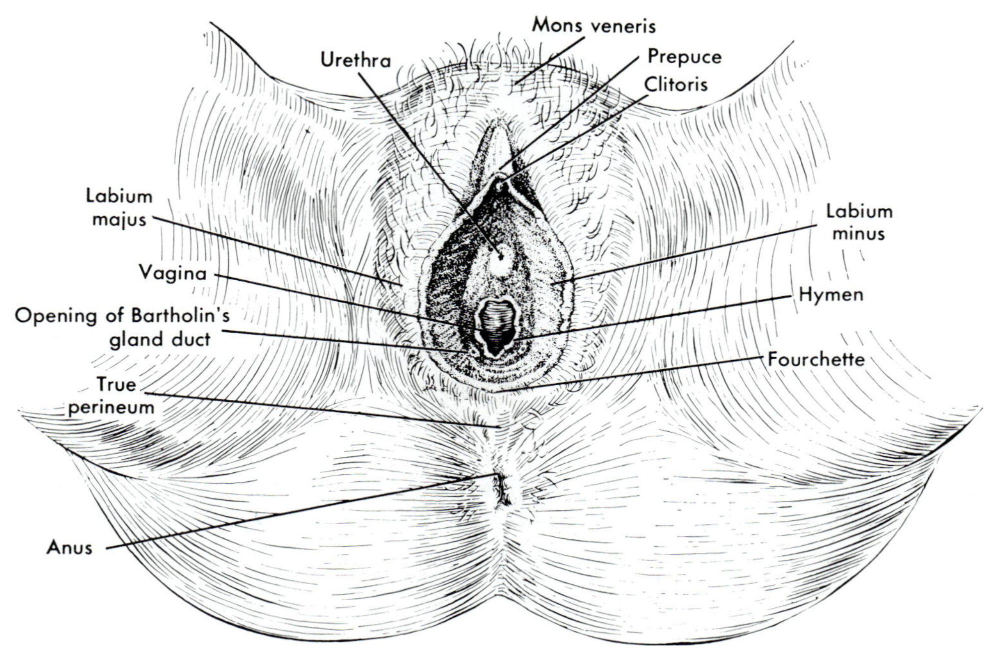

Fig. 4-1 External female genitalia.

the perineum. In a child or woman who has not borne a child, these folds almost completely cover the structures between them. The labia majora correspond to the two halves of the scrotum in the man. They are highly vascular and their inner surfaces are rich in oil and sweat glands.

Labia Minora

The labia minora (smaller lips; singular, labium minus) are two smaller, hairless folds of tissue, extending from the clitoris to the fourchette. These small folds are very vascular and sensitive to stimulation. Glands within the labia minora lubricate the vulva.

Clitoris

The clitoris is a small, sensitive, erectile structure at the anterior junction of the labia minora. Folds of the labia minora surround the clitoris; the top fold forms a fleshy hood, or *prepuce,* and the lower fold forms the *frenulum.* The clitoris corresponds to the penis as the primary anatomical center of sexual arousal.

Vestibule

The vestibule is the oval-shaped space bounded by the labia minora, clitoris, and fourchette. It contains the openings of the urethra, the paraurethral (Skene's) glands, the vagina, and the paravaginal (Bartholin's) glands.

Urethral opening*

The urethra, a tissue tube about 1 to 1½ inches (2.5 to 3.5 cm) in length, leads from the urinary bladder to the exterior and opens in the midline between the clitoris and the vagina. This opening usually appears as a dimple or slit and, after childbirth, may be slightly displaced or more difficult to locate because of local swelling. On the floor of the urethra, two ductal openings lead to *Skene's glands* (also called the *lesser vestibular glands*), which produce lubricating, alkaline mucus.

Hymen

In virgins the vaginal opening is usually partially covered by an elastic membrane called the hymen. However, an intact hymen is not necessarily proof of virginity. This membrane can be quite elastic and can fail to tear during intercourse. The hymen may be torn during physical activity, tampon use, intercourse, or childbirth, leaving irregular tags of tissue. In rare cases the hymen completely covers the vaginal opening,

* The urethral opening is not part of the female reproductive system but is included here because of its strategic location.

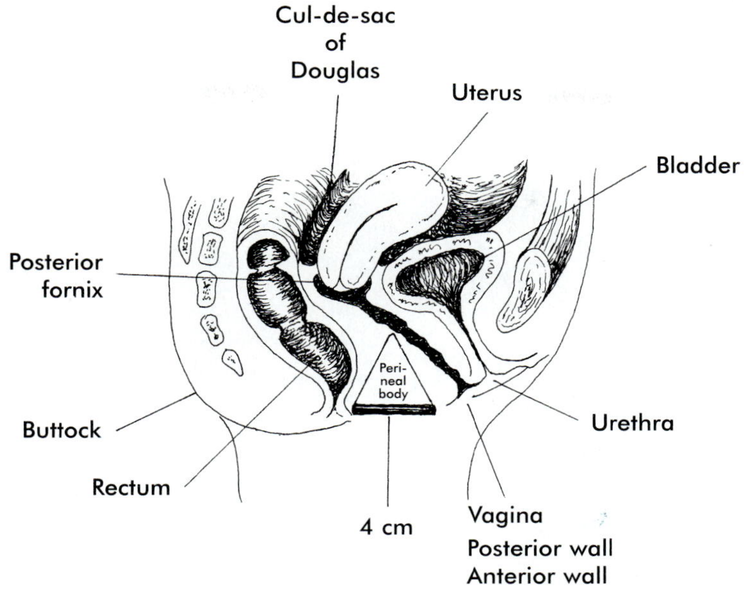

Fig. 4-2 Perineal body and surrounding organs and tissues, woman sitting.

interfering with menstrual flow, the use of tampons, and intercourse. This condition is termed *imperforate hymen* and is corrected by a hymenectomy.

Bartholin's glands

Bartholin's glands are also known as the greater vestibular glands. They are located at the base of each of the labia majora but are not usually visible. These two glands produce a mucoid substance during sexual stimulation, which drains into the vestibule on either side of the vagina by way of two ducts. The alkaline nature of the mucus from Bartholin's glands supports sperm and provides lubrication for intercourse.

Fourchette

The fourchette is a tissue fold below the vaginal opening, formed by the fusion of the posterior edges of the labia minora. It is often lacerated in childbirth.

Perineum

The true or obstetrical perineum is the muscular tissue between the posterior edge of the vagina and the anus or rectal opening. It contains the perineal body, a mass of connective tissue that forms the point of attachment for the muscles and fascia of the pelvic floor. This area is frequently the site of episiotomy or laceration during childbirth. The true perineum is a critical area of pelvic support. Pelvic organs such as the vagina, uterus, bladder, and rectum may be affected by injury or inadequate repair of the perineum. Fig. 4-2 shows these internal pelvic organs and clarifies their relationships and the need for pelvic support.

INTERNAL REPRODUCTIVE STRUCTURES

The internal organs of reproduction include the ovaries, fallopian tubes, uterus, and vagina (Figs. 4-3 and 4-4). They are usually assessed by a combination of palpation during manual vaginal examination and visualization with a vaginal speculum.

Ovaries

The ovaries (female gonads) are two sex glands sized and shaped like almonds. They are located on each side of the uterus beneath the open-ended oviducts. They are supported by the ovarian ligaments and the mesovarian portion of the broad ligament. Ovaries produce the female hormones estrogen and progesterone, as well as the female sex cells (eggs or ova; singular, ovum). At birth an infant's ovaries contain the same number of eggs that she will possess as an adult—a lifetime supply. However, the eggs are immature. During childbearing years, a woman's ovaries usually release only one mature ovum per month.

Fallopian Tubes

Fallopian tubes, or oviducts, are paired slender, hollow tubes about 4 inches (10 cm) in length. They

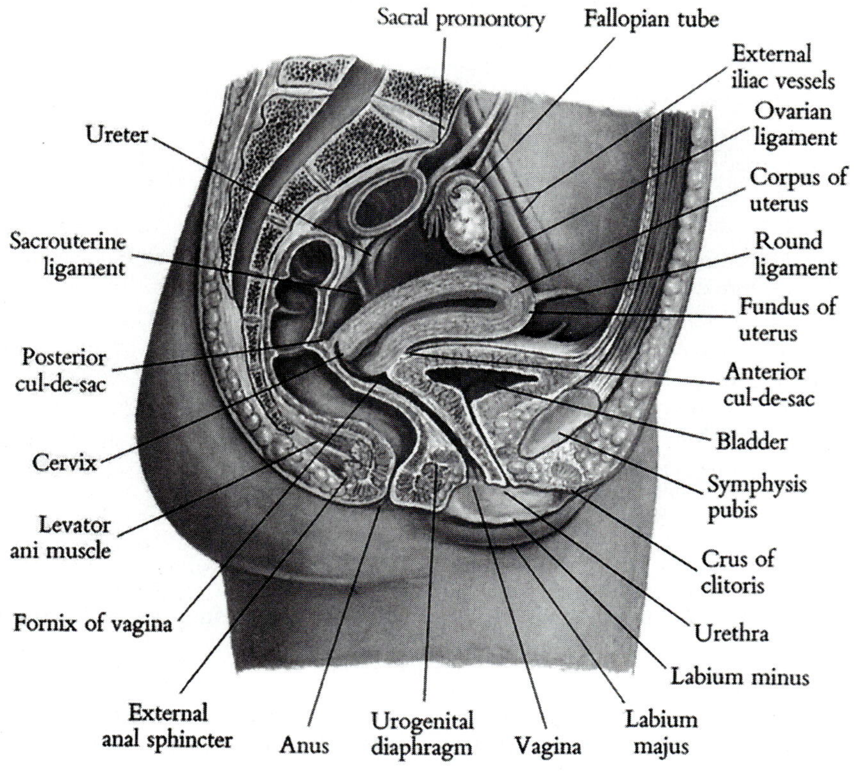

Fig. 4-3 Midsagittal view of female pelvic organs. (From Seidel HM, et al, eds: *Mosby's guide to physical examination,* ed 2, St. Louis, 1991, Mosby.)

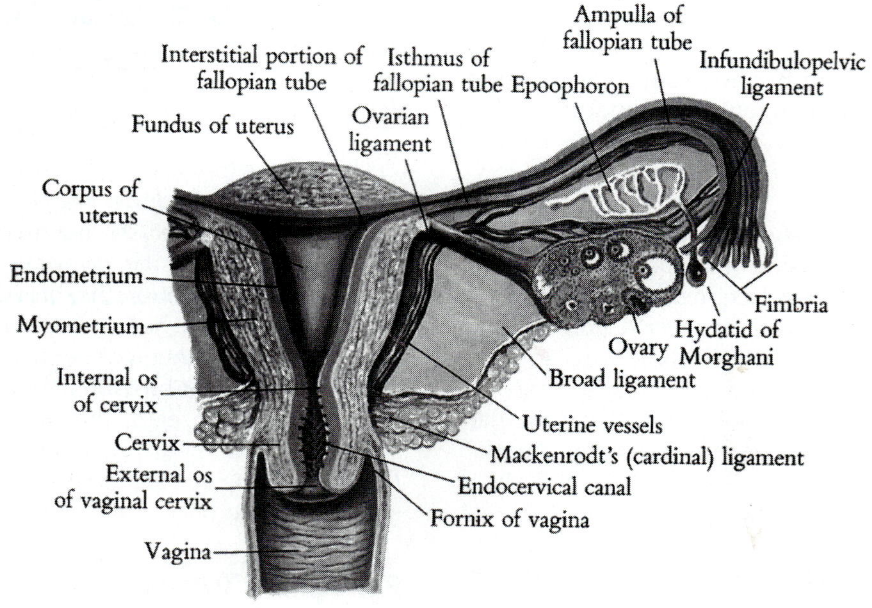

Fig. 4-4 Cross section of uterus, adnexa, and upper vagina. (From Seidel HM, et al, eds: *Mosby's guide to physical examination,* ed 2, St. Louis, 1991, Mosby.)

originate from opposite sides of the uterine cavity just below the fundus and terminate outside the uterine wall near each ovary. Each tube has three parts (Fig. 4-4): the *infundibulum* is the most distal to the uterus and is covered with fringelike tissues called fimbriae, the *ampulla* is the middle portion, and the *isthmus* is the narrower portion closest to the uterus. When the mature egg is released (ovulation), it is characteristically swept up into a fallopian tube by the fimbriae that have hovered over the productive ovary during the maturation of the ovum. The ovum then travels through the uterine tube toward the uterus. If the ovum unites with a male sex cell (sperm) causing fertilization or conception, the event normally occurs within the ampulla portion of the oviduct. The oviducts and ovaries are often referred to as *adnexa* and are adjacent to the uterus.

Uterus

In a nonpregnant adult the uterus, or womb, is a flattened, pear-shaped, and hollow muscular organ about 3 inches (7.6 cm) long, 2 inches (5 cm) wide, and 1 inch (2.5 cm) thick. It protects and nourishes the developing fetus and aids in the child's birth. The uterine wall is composed of three layers (see Fig. 4-4).

Perimetrium

The outermost layer of the uterine wall is the perimetrium, which with the enfolding pelvic peritoneum forms a strong connective tissue covering.

Myometrium

The middle layer, the myometrium, is made up of smooth muscle fibers that provide forceful, efficient contractions of the uterine wall during and after birth.

Endometrium

The vascular, mucus-producing innermost uterine lining is the endometrium, which fluctuates in depth and character during the menstrual cycle. In pregnancy the endometrial layer responds to hormonal stimulation in preparation for receiving the fertilized ovum.

The three main parts of the uterus are the corpus, ithmus, and cervix.

Corpus (or body)

The main portion of the uterus, the corpus, is also the main contractile portion. The upper, rounded portion of the corpus, located between and above the oviducts, is the fundus.

Isthmus

The isthmus is the slightly narrower portion of the uterus that joins the corpus to the cervix. During pregnancy, it is called the *lower uterine segment.*

Cervix (or narrow neck)

The cervix forms the main opening of the uterus. It is composed primarily of fibrous connective tissue, which allows it to stretch while accommodating the fetal head and then return to the closed position after birth. The cervical canal connects the uterine cavity with the vagina; the internal os separates the cervix from the uterine cavity; and the external os separates the cervix from the vagina. See the box below for a listing of the risk factors for cervical cancer. See also the Nursing Alert below.

Normally the corpus of the uterus is tipped toward the front of a woman's body (anteverted) and slightly flexed forward (anteflexed), lying above the urinary bladder. The uterine cervix dips down into the posterior portion of the vagina from above. Although less common, other uterine positions are midposition, tipped backward (retroverted), significantly flexed forward (anteflexed), or significantly flexed backward (retroflexed) (Fig. 4-5). Regardless of position, however, vaginal and cervical tissue ultimately join, forming two pouches: the anterior and the posterior fornices (singular, fornix). The posterior fornix is adjacent to a fold in the peritoneal lining of the pelvic cavity, termed

RISK FACTORS FOR CERVICAL CANCER

Early age of first coitus (under 20 years of age).
Multiple sex partners.
History of sexually transmitted diseases.
Smoking.
History of abnormal Pap smear with subsequent treatment.
Daughter of a woman who received diethylstilbestrol (DES) during early fetal development.

Nursing Alert

Papanicolaou (Pap) smear is an effective screening tool for cervical cancer. Both the American College of Obstetricians and Gynecologists and the American Cancer Society recommend that all sexually active women and those women who are 18 years of age and over receive annual Pap smears.

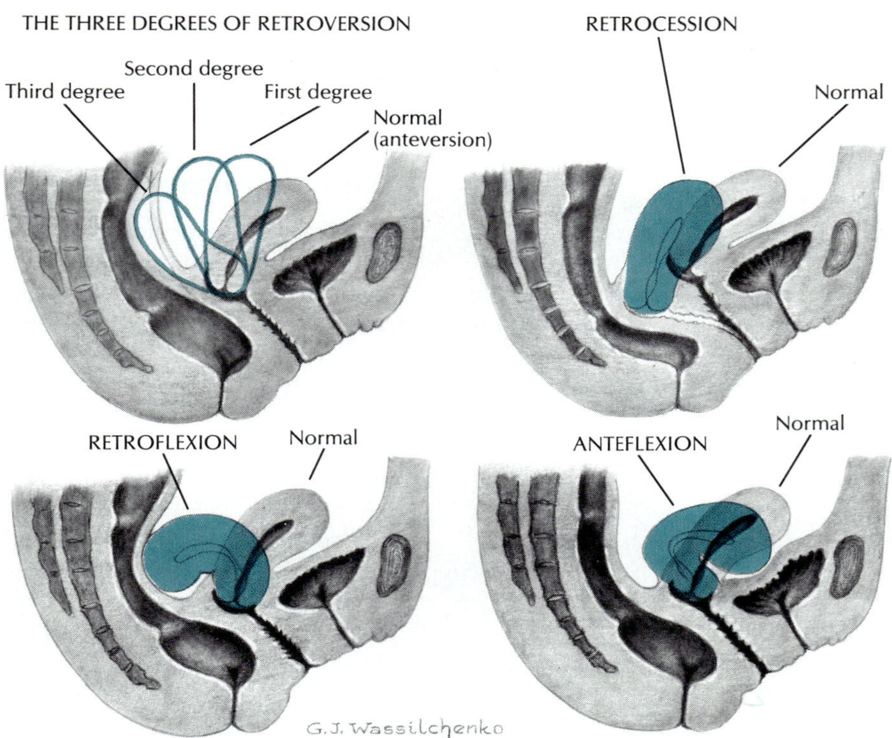

Fig. 4-5 Uterine positions. (From Bobak IM, Jensen MD: *Maternity and gynecologic care,* ed 5, St. Louis, 1993, Mosby.)

the *pouch of Douglas* or the *cul-de-sac*. Occasionally, because of infection or bleeding in the pelvis or abdomen, pus or blood drains into this cul-de-sac and may be aspirated vaginally or rectally by the health care provider.

Uterine blood supply

Together the paired uterine and ovarian arteries form an elaborate and rich vascular network over the cervix and body of the uterus (Fig. 4-6). Muscular uterine contractions are involuntary, guided by hormonal controls rather than motor nerves. Painful sensations that accompany contractions of the uterus and dilation of the cervix during labor and childbirth are transmitted by sympathetic nerve fibers passing through the tenth, eleventh, and twelfth thoracic and possibly the first lumbar spinal nerves. As labor progresses and the baby descends in the birth canal, discomfort is also caused by pressure on pelvic and perineal structures outside the uterus. These sensations are transmitted by nerve fibers leading to sacral nerve pathways.

Vagina

The vagina, a large distensible tube or sheath about 3 to 4 inches (7.5 to 10 cm) long, leads down and back to the uterine cervix. The mucous membrane of its interior surface is arranged in transverse folds (rugae) that allow considerable stretching. It is the exit point for menstrual flow, the female organ of intercourse or coitus, and the soft tissue birth canal. Vaginal fluid is normally acidic (pH 4.0 to 5.0) and provides protection from infection. See the Nursing Alert on p. 43.

Support for the Pelvic Contents

The fetus must pass through the pelvis, in which there are many soft tissue structures vital to normal body function. These structures are supported by layers of muscle, fibrous coverings called *fasciae,* ligaments, and tendons. The fasciae help cushion the passage of the fetus through the hard, bony canal and direct its descent. Occasionally, they impede the infant's progress, and the child may sustain damage at the time of birth.

Ligaments

Not only is the uterus indirectly supported by the true perineum, it is enfolded in layers of the broad ligaments (see Fig. 4-4). These ligaments are portions of the abdominal peritoneal lining. The lower portions of the broad ligaments, sometimes called cardinal liga-

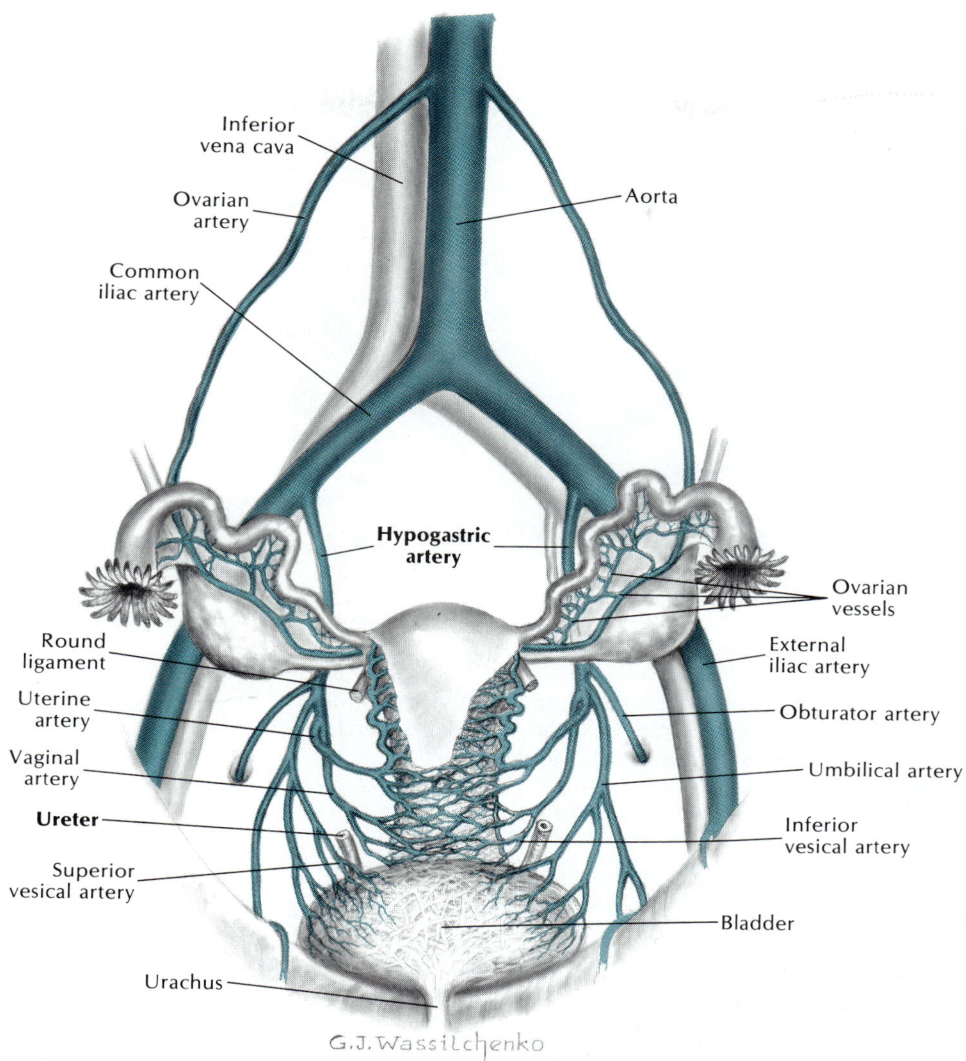

Fig. 4-6 Pelvic blood supply. (From Bobak IM, Jensen MD: *Maternity and gynecologic care,* ed 5, St. Louis, 1993, Mosby.)

ments, are thicker than the broad ligaments. The uterus is also positioned and stabilized by other fibrous attachments, such as the round ligaments (Fig. 4-7). They lead from the uterine walls toward the front, just below the fallopian tubes, and down the inguinal canals to the labia majora. The round ligaments help hold the uterus in its forward position. The uterosacral ligaments connect the posterior cervical portion of the uterus to the sacrum. The ovaries are supported principally by the ovarian and broad ligaments.

Muscles

The deep muscles of the pelvic floor form a type of hammock, pierced only by the urethra, vagina, and rectum. This muscle grouping, sometimes called the upper pelvic diaphragm, is formed by the three branches of the large levator ani muscle (paired pubococcygeus, iliococcygeus, and puborectalis muscles) and the coccygeus muscles (Fig. 4-7).

The superficial muscles, including the bulbocavernosus muscles, the transverse muscles, and the anal sphincter, converge in the area at the point of the true

> **Nursing Alert**
>
> Antibiotic therapy, frequent douching, and use of deodorant tampons alters the pH of vaginal secretions, making women more prone to vaginal infections.

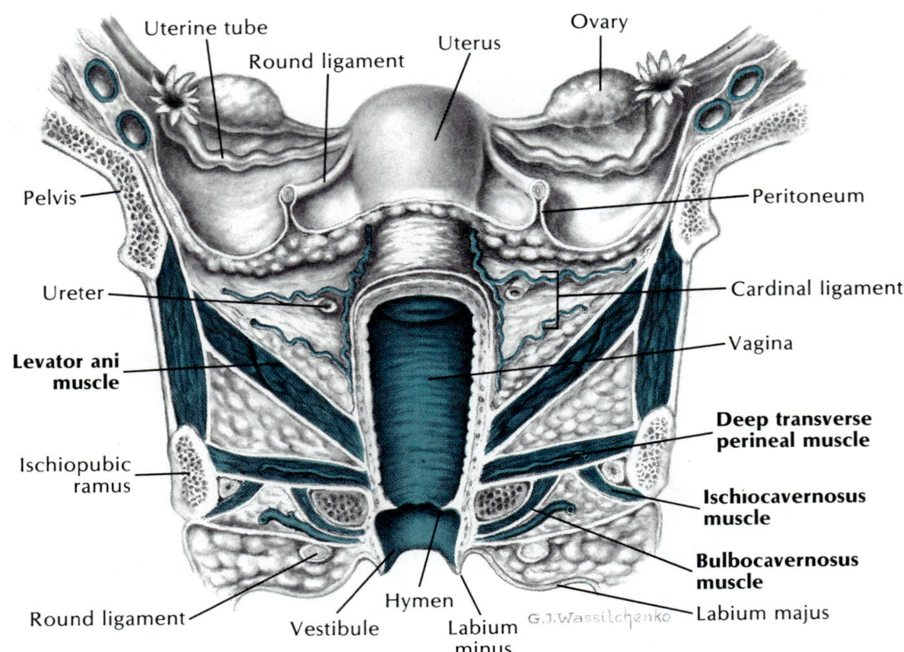

Fig. 4-7 Ligaments and muscles of upper pelvic diaphragm and urogenital (lower pelvic diaphragm), anterior view. (From Bobak IM, Jensen MD: *Maternity and gynecologic care,* ed 5, St. Louis, 1993, Mosby.)

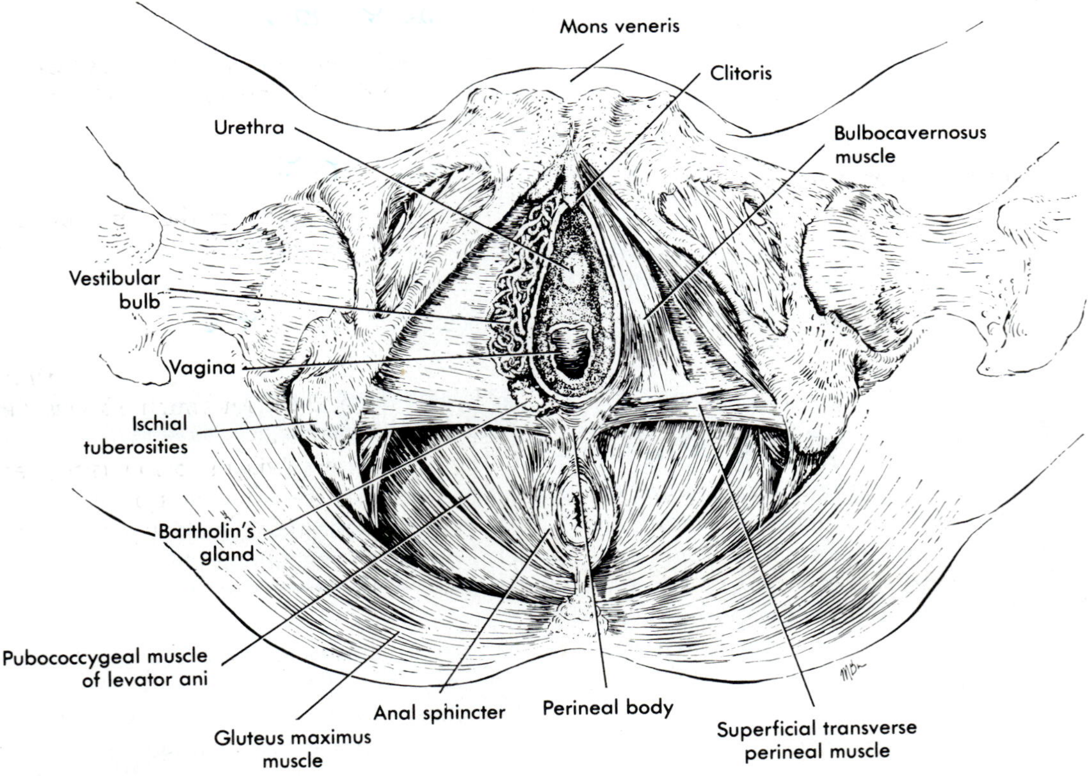

Fig. 4-8 Muscles of the pelvic floor. Coccygeus muscle is obscured by the gluteus maximus muscle.

> **Nursing Alert**
>
> Regular, conscious exercise of the musculature of the perineal floor (particularly the pubococcygeal muscle) improves pelvic relaxation during childbirth, helps avoid and treat urinary incontinence, and enhances sexual response. See Chapter 9 for a discussion of Kegel exercises.

perineum and reinforce the levator ani (Fig. 4-8). See the Nursing Alert, above.

PELVIS: THE BONY PASSAGEWAY

The bony pelvis supports and protects pelvic structures, including the growing fetus. To understand the events of labor and birth the nurse must be acquainted with the first journey the fetus takes—that of a few inches through the mother's birth canal. This canal is shaped largely by the bones of the pelvis.

Anatomy: Bones, Landmarks, and Joints

The pelvis is formed by the two innominate bones, the sacrum and the coccyx (Fig. 4-9). Each innominate bone is the end result of the fusion of three distinct bones: the ilium, ischium, and pubis.

Iliac crests

The iliac crests form the upper margin of the ilium (Fig. 4-9, **A**).

Anterosuperior iliac spines

The anterosuperior iliac spines form the lower front end of the iliac crest line (Fig. 4-10).

Iliopectineal line (linea terminalis, brim)

The iliopectineal line forms the bony ridge on the inner surface of the ilium and pubic bones. This line divides the upper or false pelvis from the lower or true pelvis (Fig. 4-10).

Sacral promontory

The sacral promontory is the internal junction of the last lumbar vertebra and the sacrum (Figs. 4-9, **A** and 4-10). It is an important landmark in obtaining an internal obstetric measurement, known as the diagonal conjugate (CD) of the pelvic inlet.

Ischial spines

Ischial spines are bony projections at the posterior border of the ischium, which may feel sharp or blunt to palpation. They are important landmarks in estimating the transverse diameter of the midpelvis (Figs. 4-9, **A** and Fig. 4-11).

Ischial tuberosities

Ischial tuberosities are rounded protuberances of the ischium that provide sitting support. They are important landmarks in measuring the transverse diameter of the pelvic outlet (Fig. 4-9, **A** and Fig. 4-11).

Pubic arch

The pubic arch is formed by the lower border of the symphysis pubis and the ischial bones (Fig. 4-9, **A**).

Sacrococcygeal joint

The sacrococcygeal joint is located between the sacrum and coccyx. It retains limited mobility, which allows additional room for the passage of the fetus because it pushes the coccyx slightly backward as much as 1 inch (2.54 cm) (Fig. 4-12).

Sacroiliac joints

Sacroiliac joints are found at either side of the sacrum joining with the iliac bones (Fig. 4-9, **A**).

Symphysis pubis

The symphysis pubis is the junction of the pubic bones (Figs. 4-10 and 4-11).

True and false pelvis

The false pelvis, formed chiefly by flaring wings of the iliac portions of the innominate bones, helps guide the fetus into the true obstetrical canal (Fig. 4-12); however, the true pelvis just below is the real concern of the health care provider. In its journey the fetus must adapt to the different diameters and shapes of the relatively rigid true pelvis to successfully reach the outside world.

Inlet, midpelvis, and outlet

The entrance to the true pelvis is the inlet (Fig. 4-13, **A**). Its shape is traced in part by the iliopectineal line. It is wider from side to side than from front to back. Therefore, the head usually enters the true pelvis with its longest diameter (front to back) pointed from side

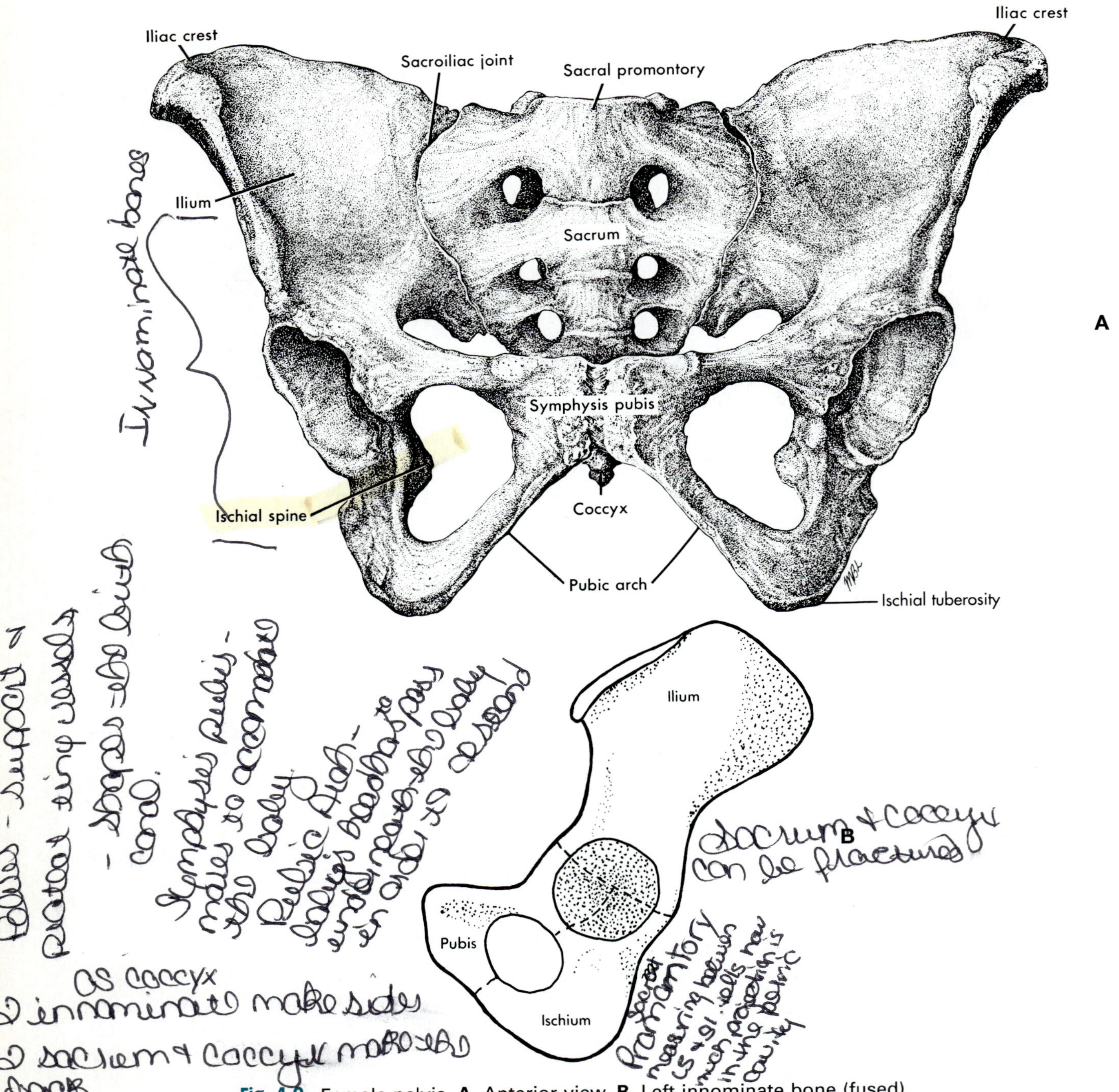

Fig. 4-9 Female pelvis. **A,** Anterior view. **B,** Left innominate bone (fused).

to side, or in transverse position. The midpelvis is an irregularly curved cavity between the inlet and the outlet. The midpelvis is wider from front to back than it is from side to side (Fig. 4-13, **A**).

The exit of the true pelvis is the outlet and is wider from front to back than from side to side (Fig. 4-13, **A**). To pass through the midpelvis and outlet the head usually must turn to accommodate its longest diameter to the longest diameters of the midpelvis and outlet. This turning is called *internal rotation*. The canal formed by the true pelvis curves slightly near the outlet and has been likened in shape to the letter J (Fig. 4-13, **B**).

Pelvic Differences

Classification

Although pelvic dimensions vary widely among humans, pelves are most commonly classified accord-

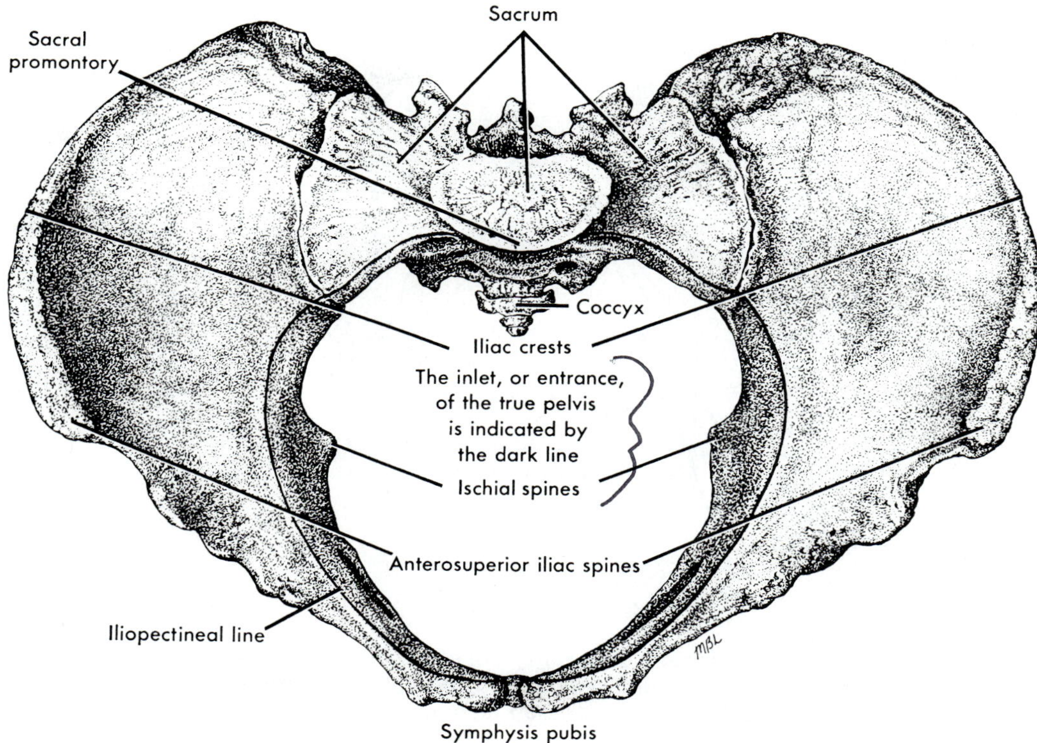

Fig. 4-10 Pelvic inlet, traced by dark iliopectineal line, viewed from above.

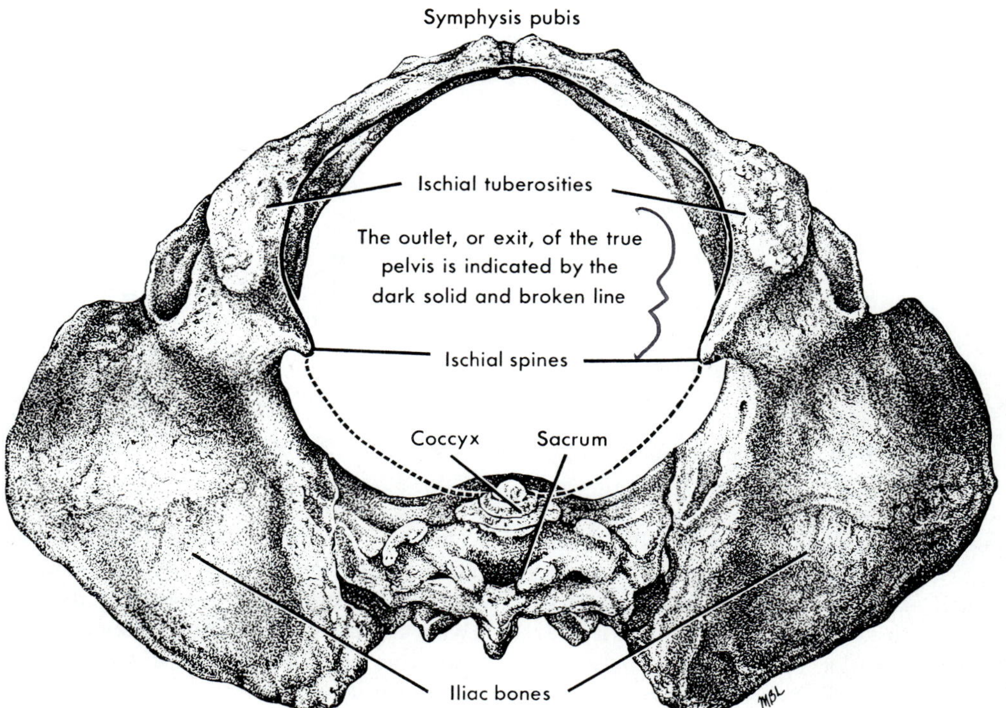

Fig. 4-11 Pelvic outlet, traced by solid and broken dark lines, viewed from below.

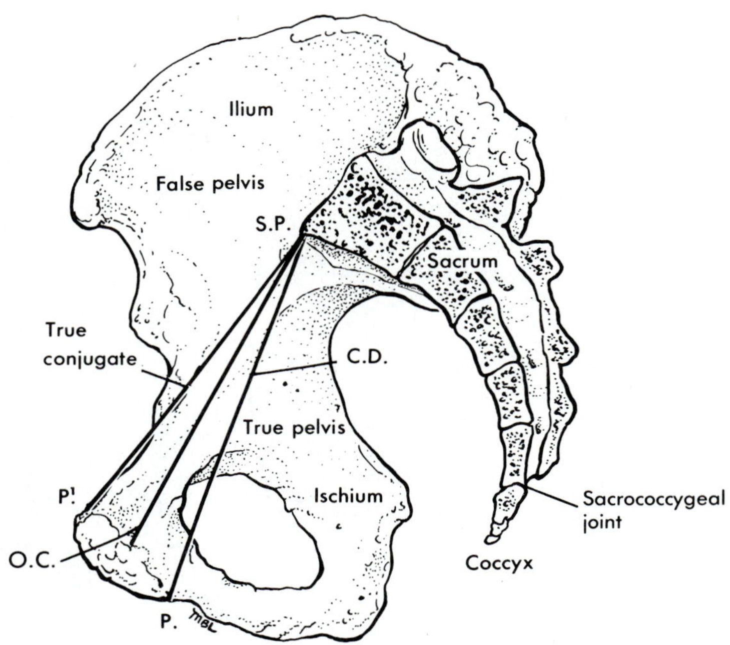

Fig. 4-12 Female pelvis, sagittal section: *P¹*, inner superior border of pubis; P, outer inferior border of pubis; *SP*, sacral promontory. Diameters of the pelvic inlet: *CD*, diagonal conjugate, true conjugate; *OC*, obstetrical conjugate.

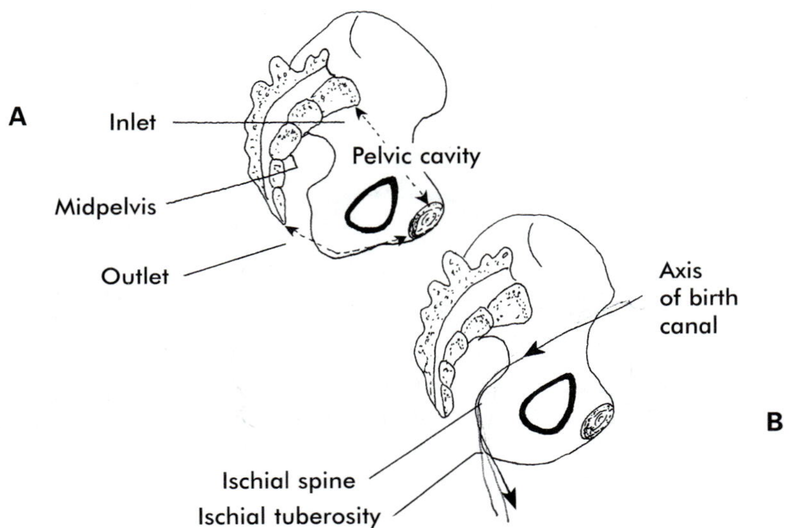

Fig. 4-13 Female pelvis. **A**, Inlet, midpelvis, outlet. **B,** Axis of birth canal.

ing to the shape and dimensions of the inlet (Fig. 4-14). The typical female pelvic inlet is *gynecoid*. The typical male inlet is *android*. A look at a male pelvis offers at least one reason why the human male could not bear children. Typically the inlet of the male pelvis is heart-shaped and angular. The whole pelvic structure is heavier and more shallow than that of the female and has a steep and narrow pubic arch. In contrast a typical woman's pelvis is relatively light and commodious. The pubic arch is shallow and wide. Occasionally a woman's pelvic inlet is abnormally flat, or *platypelloid,* with a decreased anteroposterior diameter. It is also possible that it may have an *anthropoid* or ape like configuration with an enlarged anteroposterior measurement and a restricted transverse diameter. These problems may necessitate a cesarean birth (abdominal

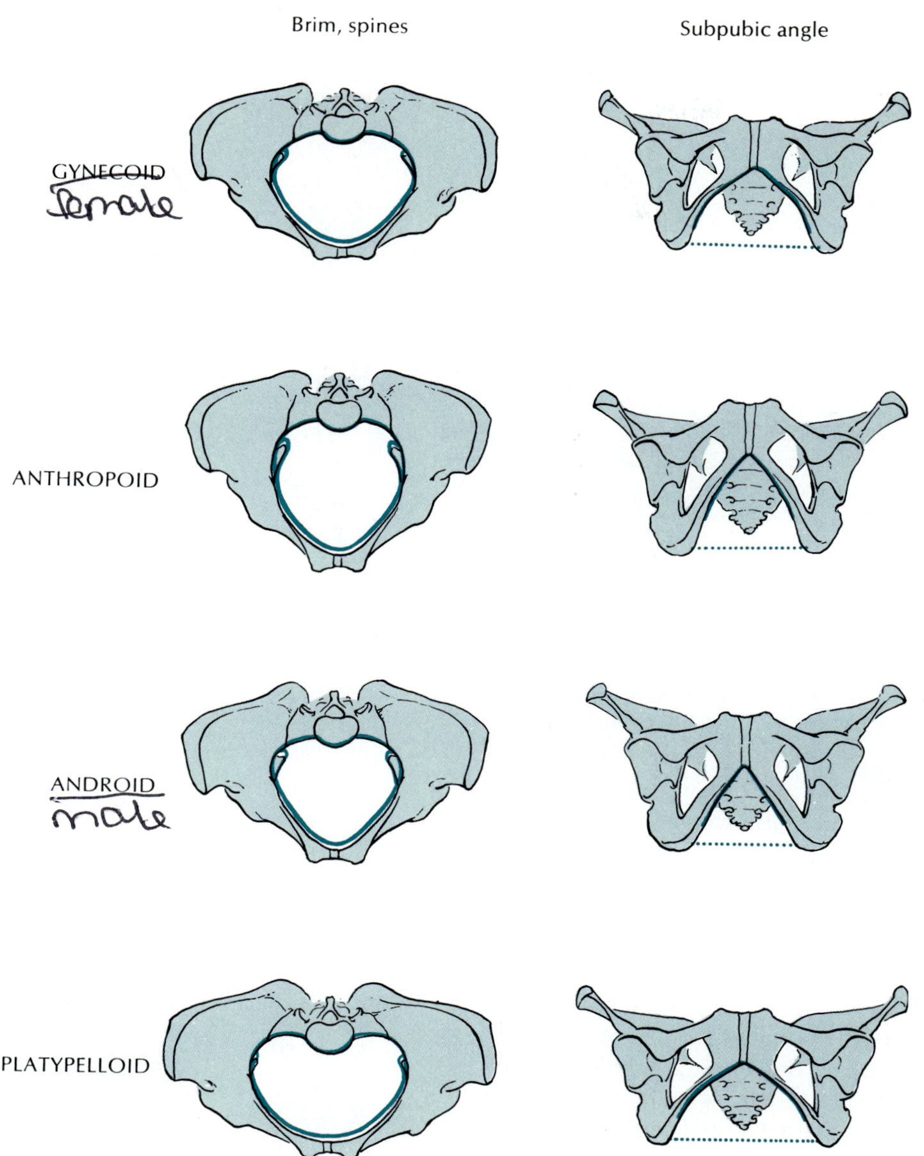

Fig. 4-14 Classification of pelvic types. (Adapted from Barkauskas VH, Stoltenberg-Allen K, Baumann LC, Darling-Fisher C: *Health and physical assessment,* St. Louis, 1994, Mosby.)

delivery). Whether a birth is abdominal or vaginal depends on several factors. These include the type of passageway; the size, position, and well-being of the fetus; the strength of the uterine contractions; and the condition of the laboring mother.

Causes of abnormalities

A history of certain conditions may alert the health care provider to expect difficulties because of pelvic structural variations. The six main causes of abnormal pelvic measurements are heredity (characteristic familial problems, dwarfism), infections (poliomyelitis, osteomyelitis, tuberculosis of the bone), poor nutrition (rickets), accidents (fractured pelves), paralysis of one or both extremities, and poor posture and exercise habits.

Methods of Pelvic Evaluation

Pelvic size, contour, and adequacy may be assessed by the following methods.

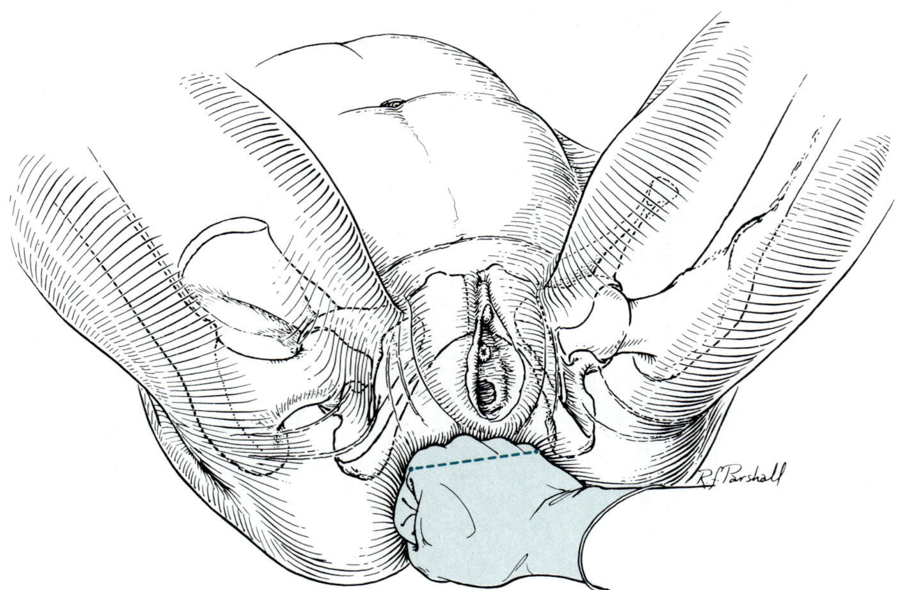

Fig. 4-15 Estimating the transverse diameter of the pelvic outlet. (From Barkauskas VH, Stoltenberg-Allen K, Baumann LC, Darling-Fisher C: *Health and physical assessment,* St. Louis, 1994, Mosby.)

External palpation

With the woman in the lithotomy position, the transverse diameter of the pelvic outlet and the angle of the pubic arch can be estimated by external palpation. To measure the transverse diameter of the outlet the examiner places a closed fist or uses a pelvimeter to judge the distance between the ischial tuberosities (Bi-ischial or TI, averaging 10 to 11 cm) (Fig. 4-15). The angle of the pubic arch (subpubic angle) is estimated by palpating the bony angle with the thumbs of each hand (Fig. 4-16). A wide pubic arch (90°) is the most favorable for vaginal delivery.

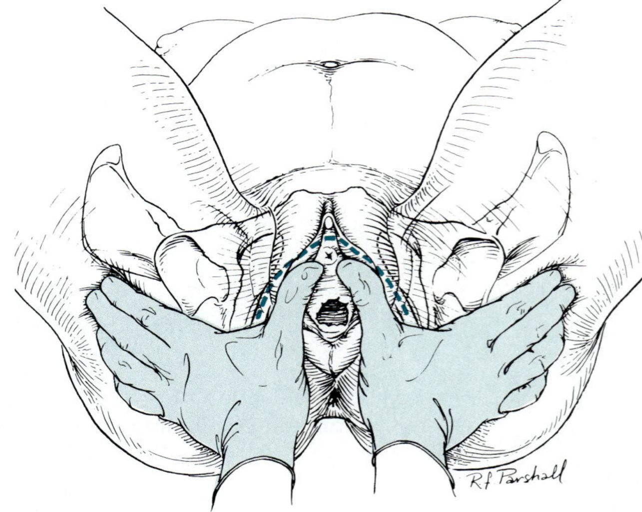

Fig. 4-16 Estimating the angle of the pubic arch. (From Barkauskas VH, Stoltenberg-Allen K, Baumann LC, Darling-Fisher C: *Health and physical assessment,* St. Louis, 1994, Mosby.)

Internal palpation

The anteroposterior diameters of the pelvic inlet (three conjugates), adequacy of the midpelvis, and the anteroposterior diameters of the outlet are estimated by internal palpation. The examiner uses a lubricated, gloved, middle finger to determine the distance between the sacral promontory and the inferior border of the pubis—the inlet diameter known as the *diagonal conjugate* (CD, averages 12.5 cm) (Figs. 4-12 and 4-17). From this measurement a closer estimate of the second, anteroposterior diameter of the inlet, the *true conjugate* (conjugata vera or CV, averages 11 cm) is made. To do this, subtract 1 cm from the diagonal conjugate to compensate for the thickness and tilt of the pubic bone. This measure has little obstetrical significance. The shortest distance, and therefore the most important anteroposterior diameter of the inlet, is the *obstetric conjugate* (OC, averages 10.5 cm). It is the distance between the posterior (inner) surface of the symphysis pubis and the sacral promontory. Like the true conju-

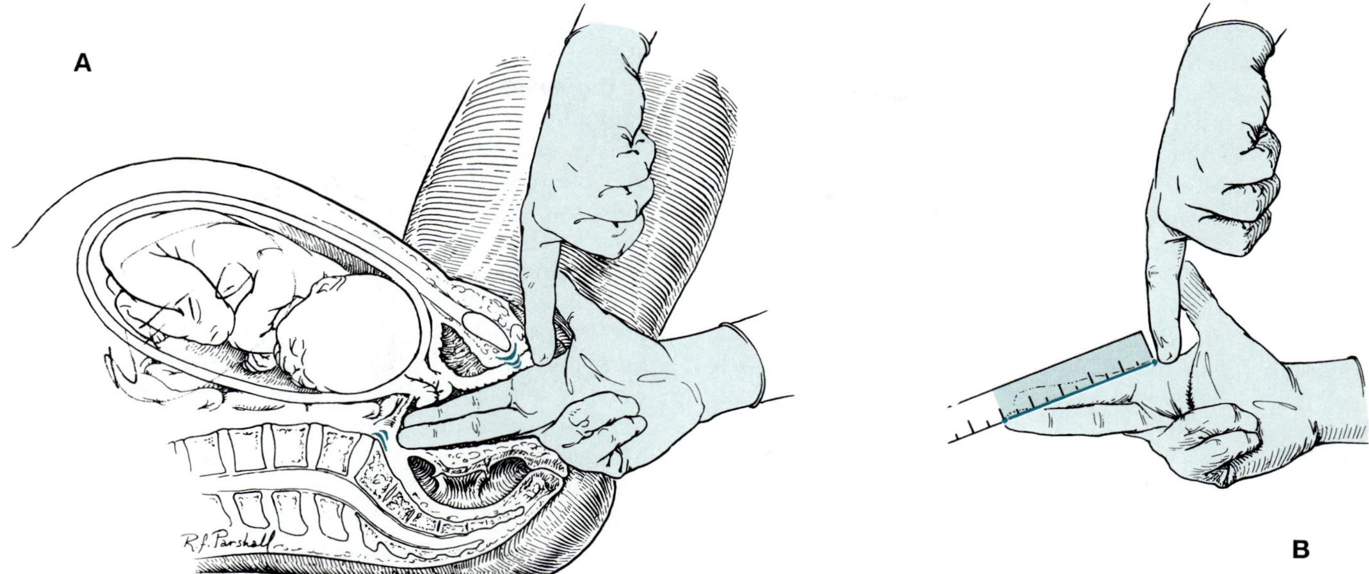

Fig. 4-17 Measurement of the diagonal conjugate. **A**, Internal palpation. **B**, Use of a ruler to specify estimation in centimeters. (From Barkauskas VH, Stoltenberg-Allen K, Baumann LC, Darling-Fisher C: *Health and physical assessment,* St. Louis, 1994, Mosby.)

gate, it is only clinically estimated by subtracting 1.5 to 2 cm from the length of the diagonal conjugate.

Although the diameters of the midpelvis cannot be accurately measured clinically, an assessment of adequacy is made by internal palpation. The examiner determines whether the ischial spines feel blunt or prominent (Fig. 4-18). Prominent spines indicate a narrower transverse diameter. The adequacy of the cavity is also assessed by sweeping the fingers down the pelvic side walls to determine how close together they are.

To measure the anteroposterior diameter of the outlet the examiner measures from the inferior border of the pubis to the tip of the sacrum (averages 9.5 to 11 cm). The mobility of the coccyx can be determined by pressing down on it with the forefinger and middle finger.

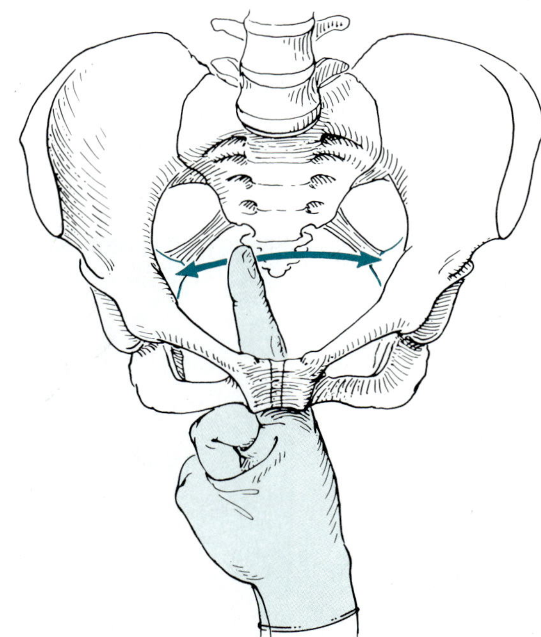

Fig. 4-18 Estimation of interspinous diameter of the midpelvis. (From Barkauskas VH, Stoltenberg-Allen K, Baumann LC, Darling-Fisher C: *Health and physical assessment,* St. Louis, 1994, Mosby.)

Pelvimetry

Once an important diagnostic tool, x-ray pelvimetry is rarely used in most maternity settings today. This change is due, in part, to the fact that the reason for lack of progress in labor is not often demonstrated by x-ray. More often the lack of progress is due to a large baby (rather than a contracted pelvis) or an inefficient uterine contraction pattern. Careful clinical evaluation of the pelvis and a trial of labor are the most likely means of determining pelvic adequacy; however, evaluation of the pelvis by pelvimetry plays a role in determining the safest method of delivery for a woman in labor at term with a breech presentation. Because x-ray pelvimetry has the disadvantage of exposing the fetus to ionizing radiation, other methods of pelvic evaluation are being investigated. Computed tomography (CT) also involves ionizing radiation but much less (about 20% to 30%) than that required by conventional x-ray pelvimetry. Magnetic resonance imaging (MRI) is accurate, shows soft-tissue structures as well as bone, and does not involve radiation. Cost and availability of the CT and MRI are the major disadvantages (Friedman, Rosenfield, 1992; Wright, et al, 1992).

Ultrasonography

Ultrasonography detects differences in tissue density by directing high-frequency sound waves into tissue and electrically measuring the reflected echoes from internal structures (Fig. 4-19). It is increasingly used in modern obstetrics because it helps evaluate the condition of and clarify many potential problems affecting a mother and her unborn child (see Chapter 8). Although ultrasonography cannot effectively provide traditional pelvic measurements, it does assist in the evaluation of a mother's ability to give birth vaginally. It reveals multiple pregnancies, fetal positions, and abnormalities of the mother or fetus that may complicate the pregnancy or delivery. An ultrasound can indicate the position and size of the baby's head (biparietal diameter) as well as the approximate fetal weight. This information, along with internal and external estimates of the mother's pelvic size, a knowledge of her reproductive history, her progress during labor, and the well-being of her unborn infant, facilitates more informed decision making concerning obstetrical care (Thurnan, Scates, Morgan, 1991).

During the approximately 20 years in which diagnostic ultrasound has been used, no injuries to a mother or fetus have been recorded; however, routine screening of all pregnancies is still controversial (Chervenak, McCullough, Chervenak, 1989). The cost-effectiveness of such screening in the United States has not as yet been demonstrated.

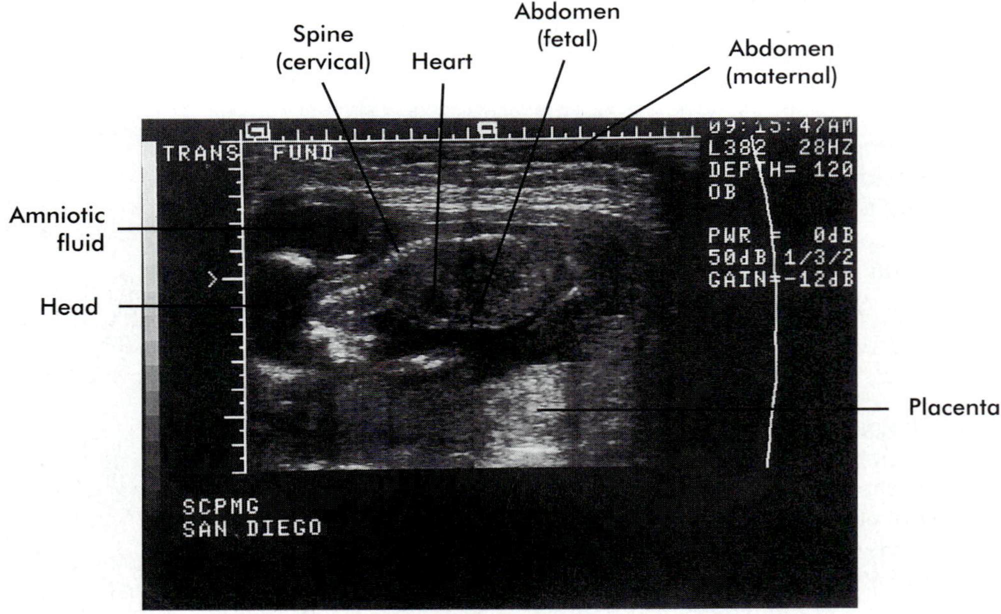

Fig. 4-19 View of fetus taken using ultrasound. Fetus is facing maternal spine. (Courtesy Kaiser Foundation Hospital, San Diego.)

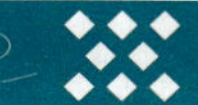

KEY CONCEPTS

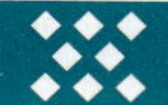

1. The structures of the female external genitalia are the mons pubis, labia majora, labia minora, clitoris, vestibule, urethral opening, hymen, Bartholin's glands, fourchette, and perineum.
2. The female internal reproductive structures are the ovaries, fallopian tubes, uterus, and vagina.
3. The uterine wall is composed of three layers: the perimetrium, the myometrium, and the endometrium. The uterus is composed of three main parts: the corpus, the isthmus, and the cervix.
4. The uterus is enfolded in layers of broad ligaments and is positioned and stabilized by other fibrous attachments, such as the round ligaments.
5. The pelvic floor is formed mainly by the three branches of the large levator ani muscle (paired pubococcygeus, iliococcygeus, and puborectalis muscles) and the coccygeus muscles.
6. The pelvis is formed by the sacrum, coccyx, and the two innominate bones that are the end result of the fusion of the ilium, ischium, and pubis.
7. The entrance to the true pelvis (inlet) is wider from side to side than from front to back; the midpelvis is wider from front to back than from side to side; the exit (outlet) is wider from front to back than from side to side. Internal rotation enables the fetus to adapt to these differences in diameter.
8. The typical female pelvis is gynecoid. Pelvic abnormalities may make vaginal delivery difficult or impossible. The six main causes of abnormal pelvic measurements are heredity, infections, poor nutrition, accidents, paralysis of one or both extremities, and poor posture and exercise habits.
9. Pelvic size, shape, and contents may be measured or evaluated by the following methods: external palpation, internal palpation, pelvimetry, and ultrasonography.

CRITICAL THOUGHT QUESTIONS

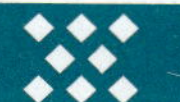

1. Many women are not well educated about their reproductive structures and their body functions. How would you increase their knowledge and understanding? What sort of teaching aids would you use?
2. Note the recommendations for frequency of Pap smears. How would you advise a 30-year-old woman whose mother was given DES during early pregnancy? Why? How would you advise a 40-year-old woman who has never been sexually active? Why? How would you advise a 68-year-old woman who is postmenopausal? Why?
3. Identify the most common diagnostic tests related to the pelvis and reproductive organs. Is it safe to perform these tests if pregnancy is suspected?

REFERENCES

Barkauskas V, Stoltenberg-Allen K, Baumann LC, Darling-Fisher C: *Health and physical assessment*, St. Louis, 1994, Mosby.

Chervenak FA, McCullough LB, Chervenak JL: Prenatal informed consent for sonogram: an indication for obstetric ultrasonography, *Am J Obstet Gynecol* 61(4):857-860, 1989.

Friedman WN, Rosenfield AT: Computed tomography in obstetrics and gynecology, *J Reprod Med* 37(1):3-18, 1992.

Seidel HM, Ball JW, Dains JE, Benedict GW: *Mosby's guide to physical examination*, ed 2, St. Louis, 1991, Mosby.

Thurnan GR, Scates DH, Morgan MA: The fetal-pelvic index: a method of identifying fetal-pelvic disproportion in women attempting vaginal birth after previous cesarean section, *Am J Obstet Gynecol* 165(2):353-358, 1991.

Wright AR, English, PT, Cameron, HM, Wilsdon JB: MR pelvimetry—a practical alternative, *Acta-Radiol* 33(6):582-587, 1992.

Ginsberg CK: Exfoliative cytologic screening: the papanicolaou test, *J Obstet Gynecol Neonatal Nurs* 20(1):39-46, 1991.

Masters W, and Johnson V: *Human sexual response*, Boston, 1966, Little, Brown & Co.

Modica MM, Timor-Tritsch IE: Transvaginal sonography provides a sharper view into the pelvis, *J Obstet Gynecol Neonatal Nurs* 17(2):89-95, 1988.

Oxorn H: *Human labor and birth*, ed 5, New York, 1986, Appleton-Century-Crofts.

Thibodeau G, Patton K: *Anatomy and physiology*, ed 2, St. Louis, 1993, Mosby.

Van-Loon AJ, Mantingh A, Thijn CJ, Mooyaart EL: Pelvimetry by magnetic resonance imaging in breech presentation, *Am J Obstet Gynecol* 163 (4 Pt.1):1256-1260, 1990.

Wiesen EJ, Crass JR, Bellon EM, et al: Improvement in CT pelvimetry, *Radiology* 178(1):259-262, 1991.

BIBLIOGRAPHY

Creasy RK, Resnik R: *Maternal-fetal medicine*, ed 3, Philadelphia, 1994, WB Saunders.

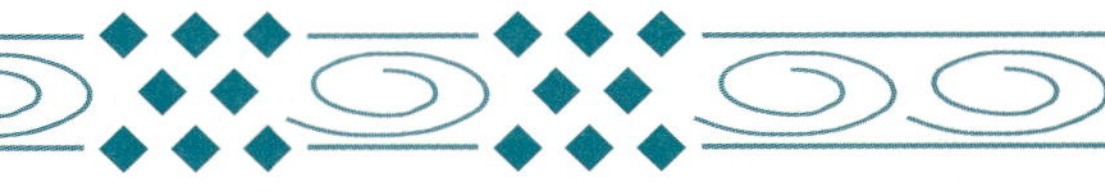

The Menstrual Cycle

CHAPTER OBJECTIVES

After studying this chapter, the student should be able to:

1. Define the following terms: menstruation, menarche, ovum, ovulation, graafian follicle, corpus luteum, menorrhagia, metrorrhagia, and dysmenorrhea.
2. Describe the two primary endocrine glands involved with regulation of the menstrual cycle.
3. State the origins and actions of FSH, LH, estrogen, and progesterone in relation to the menstrual cycle.
4. List three possible indications of ovulation, and explain the practical use of these indications.
5. State when the following phases occur during the menstrual cycle: follicular phase, luteal phase, menstrual phase, proliferative phase, secretory phase, and ischemic phase.
6. Discuss three ways to treat the symptoms of premenstrual syndrome.
7. Discuss three ways to prevent or treat the symptoms of primary dysmenorrhea.
8. Name four possible causes of secondary dysmenorrhea.

MENSTRUATION

Menstruation is the monthly shedding of the uterine lining. This lining has been prepared to protect and nurture a fertilized egg in the event of pregnancy. Menstruation is also called *menses,* and, more commonly, a *period* or *monthly flow.* Menstruation is not an illness but an expected and necessary part of healthy, mature womanhood. A woman's attitude toward menstruation depends a great deal on her social and cultural background, as well as her knowledge about her body. The nurse can help women develop healthy attitudes toward menstruation by educating them about their bodies and the menstrual cycle. See the Nursing Alert at right.

The advent of a woman's menstrual cycle is a signal of impending physical maturity. The first menses is called *menarche.* Menstruation occurs periodically throughout the childbearing years, except during pregnancy and lactation or breast-feeding. The ages of onset and termination differ from person to person but seem to be affected by heredity, racial background, and nutrition.

In the United States the average age of menarche is 12½ years of age. Menarche is preceded by other bodily changes, such as the development of breasts, widening of the hips, fat deposits in the buttocks and mons pubis, and the appearance of axillary and pubic hair.

Nursing Alert

Teaching teenagers and adults about reproductive functioning can help them develop appropriate sexual self-care behaviors and practice responsible sexual activity.

THE MENSTRUAL CYCLE

In most women, menstruation occurs approximately every 28 days and lasts about 5 days. The time between the beginning of one period and the beginning of the next is called the *menstrual cycle.* It generally repeats itself every 4 weeks, although variations of several days in the cycles of different women or even in the cycles of the same woman are normal (Fig. 5-1). Day 1 is distinguished by the appearance of the menstrual flow.

Hormonal Regulation

It is important that the nurse have a basic understanding of the physiology of the menstrual cycle. The menstrual cycle consists of two overlapping cycles: the ovarian cycle and the endometrial cycle. These cycles are regulated by hormones produced by endocrine glands. *Endocrine glands* are those that empty their manufactured products directly into the blood circulation. Their products are called *hormones.*

The endocrine gland outside the pelvis that is especially important in ovarian and uterine function is the *pituitary,* located at the base of the brain. It is regulated in part by that portion of the brain called the *hypothalamus.* At the beginning of the menstrual cycle, low levels of estrogen and progesterone in the bloodstream cause the hypothalamus to stimulate the anterior pituitary gland to release a follicle-stimulating hormone (FSH) and a lutenizing hormone (LH). These hormones help govern the ovarian and, more indirectly, the endometrial cycles. Blood levels of FSH during the normal cycle have a moderate early elevation, followed by a slight decline until the peak at midcycle (see Fig. 5-1). This peak is followed by a gradual decrease until just before the next menses. Follicle-stimulating hormone, as its name implies, is responsible for the initiation of the ovarian follicle's growth. It works, however, in conjunction with LH to continue the follicle's maturation and produce the characteristic increase in estrogen production. The blood level of LH peaks at midcycle. This surge of LH is responsible for ovulation.

The *ovaries* are endocrine glands that produce estrogen and progesterone, which also help to regulate the menstrual cycle. As mentioned, low levels of these hormones trigger the pituitary's release of FSH and LH in the ovarian cycle. These ovarian hormones also play an important role in the endometrial cycle because they are responsible for the build up of the uterine endometrial lining in preparation for implantation of a fertilized ovum.

Pituitary and ovarian hormonal levels inhibit and stimulate each other's hormonal secretions, using negative and positive feedback systems. Special neurohormones produced by the hypothalamus are also involved in these functions.

Prostaglandins, a special group of fatty acids also classified as hormones, are produced by many organs of the body. The endometrium, however, is especially rich in prostaglandins, which are thought to be involved in such diverse reproductive activities as ovulation, the reception and transport of ova and sperm, and the onset of menstruation. They also appear to be associated with episodes of uterine hyperirritability, contraction, and may be a triggering factor in the onset of labor.

There appears to be a wide variation in normal hormonal patterns among women. Disturbances of other endocrine glands, such as the thyroid and adrenals, or nutritional and psychological factors may also influence menstrual function.

Ovarian Cycle

The ovaries have two basic functions. The first is the production of the hormones estrogen and progesterone. These products regulate the activities of the uterus and the pituitary gland, bringing about the many body changes in the maturing female. The second basic function of the ovaries is the maturation of microscopic eggs or ova that contain maternal hereditary material. The ovarian portion of the menstrual cycle has two phases: the follicular phase and the luteal phase.

Follicular phase

The eggs or ova are stored according to varying degrees of immaturity in the underlying tissues of both ovaries. Under the influence of FSH and LH, usually only one egg in the body develops to maturity, growing within a protective tissue envelope called a *follicle.* This maturing follicle is called the *graafian follicle.* This follicle and other ovarian tissue are filled with estrogenic fluid, which is secreted in relatively large amounts into the blood. One of the functions of estrogen at this time is to build up or thicken the lining of the uterus. As the follicle enlarges, it pushes to the surface of the ovary to create a blisterlike bulge that may be clearly seen if the ovary is observed directly. Finally, with the peak in LH at midcycle, the follicular envelope breaks open, releasing its tiny ovum from the ovary. This expulsion of the egg is termed *ovulation.* Some women experience abdominal pain (*mittelschmerz*) at the time of ovulation. Mittelschmerz is thought to be related to peritoneal irritation caused by minor bleeding from the follicle. Midcycle spotting may also indicate that ovulation has occurred. Ovulation characteristically occurs on the fourteenth day of a 28-day menstrual cycle.

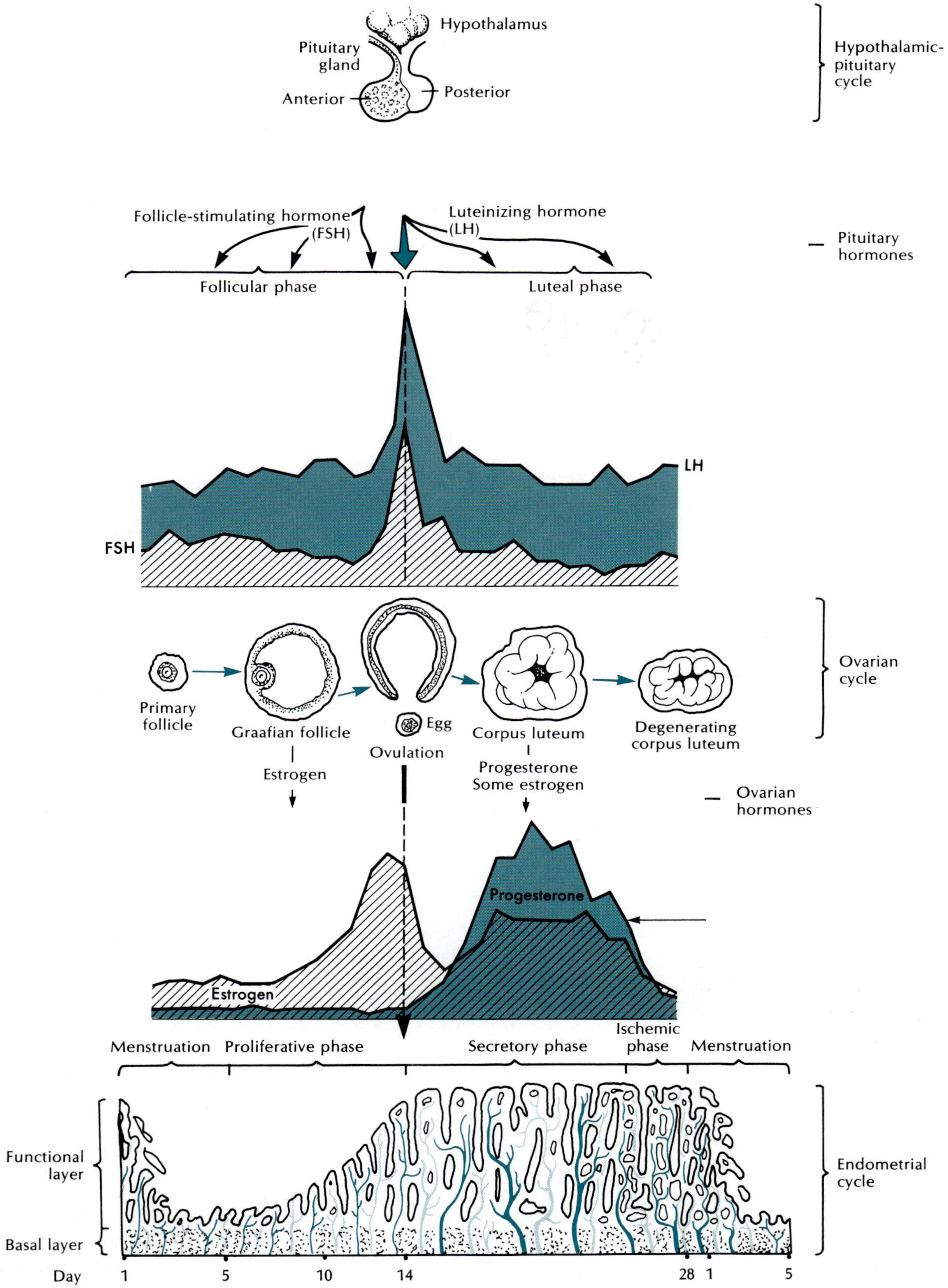

Fig. 5-1 Normal menstrual cycle: hormone production, ovulation, ovarian, and endometrial response. (From Bobak IM, Jensen MD: *Maternity and gynecologic care*, ed 5, St. Louis, 1993, Mosby.)

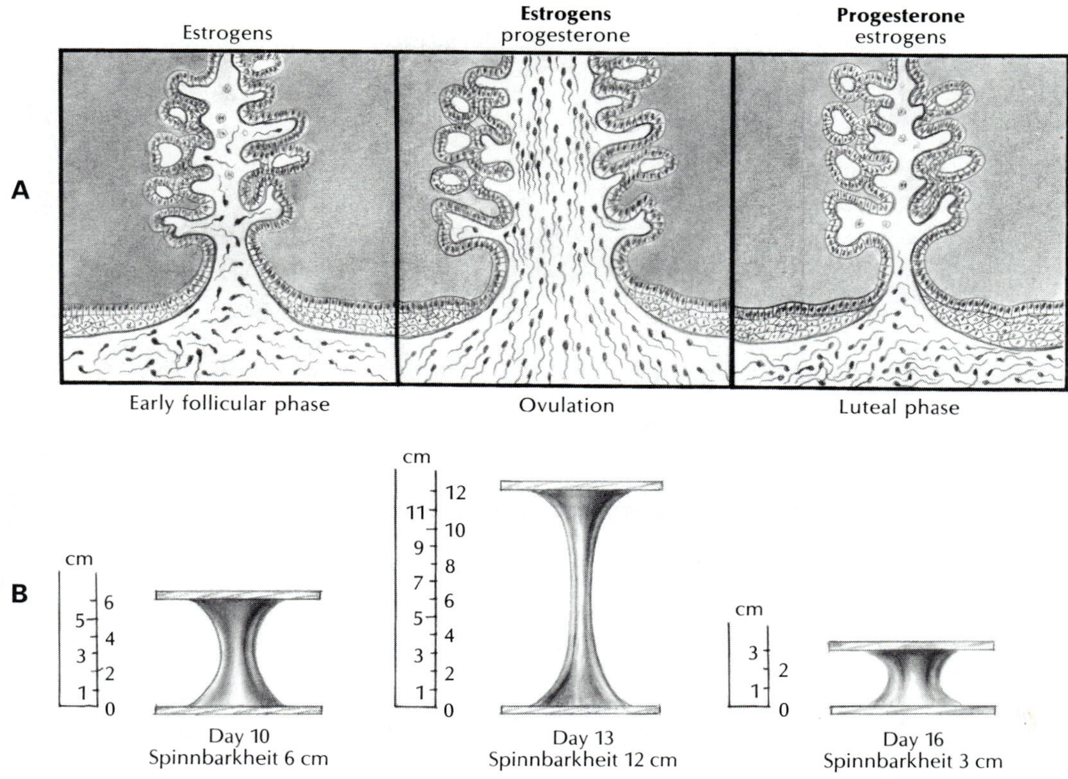

Fig. 5-2 Changes in cervix and cervical mucus during menstrual cycle. **A**, Changes in the opening of the cervix that facilitates sperm migration. **B**, Characteristic stretchable quality of cervical mucus demonstrated between two glass slides. (From Bobak IM, Jensen MD: *Maternity and gynecologic care,* ed 5, St. Louis, 1993, Mosby.)

Luteal phase

After ovulation the mature egg is normally swept up into the Fallopian tube to begin its journey to the uterus. The empty follicle then alters its function. The walls of the follicle begin to thicken and form a yellow deposit about the size of a lima bean called the *corpus luteum* (yellow body). The name graafian follicle is no longer used. The corpus luteum continues to produce estrogen but, in addition, manufactures the hormone progesterone, which further prepares the uterus for pregnancy.

Endometrial Cycle

The uterine or endometrial cycle consists of four phases: the menstrual phase, the proliferative phase, the secretory phase, and the ischemic phase.

Menstrual phase

When pregnancy does not occur, progesterone and estrogen levels fall. Disintegration of the uterine lining that was prepared to receive a fertilized ovum (functional layer) follows. The menstrual phase begins and the functional layer of the uterine lining is shed. The first day of menses marks the beginning of another menstrual cycle.

Proliferative phase

The effect of estrogen in building up the uterine endometrium has caused the interval between menses and ovulation to be labeled the *proliferative phase.* In addition to these changes in the uterine lining, alterations occur in the amount and type of mucus formed by the glands of the cervix. During the proliferative

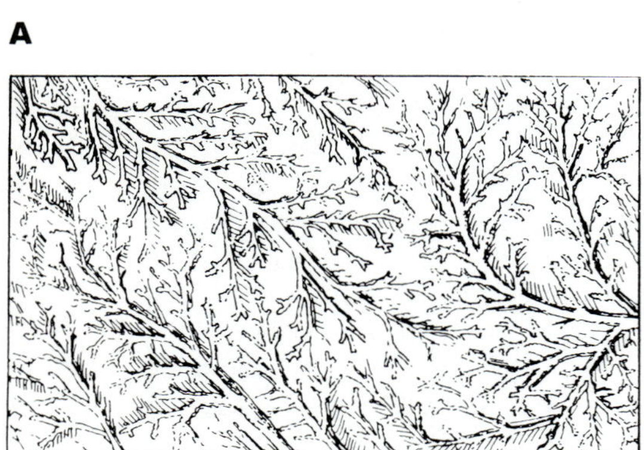

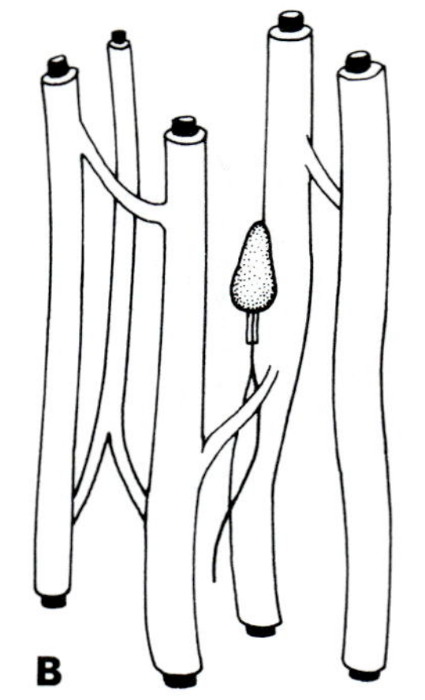

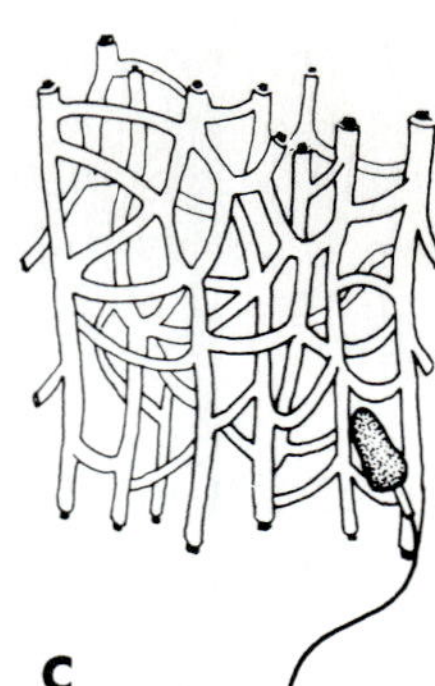

Fig. 5-3 Cervical mucus changes during menstrual cycle. **A**, Fern pattern under estrogen influence; **B**, mucus receptive to sperm passage under estrogen influence; **C**, mucus nonreceptive to sperm passage under progesterone influence. (From Fogel CI, Woods NF: *Health care of women: a nursing perspective*, St. Louis, 1981, Mosby.)

phase of the menstrual cycle, cervical mucus typically becomes profuse and thin. Around the time of ovulation, it can be pulled into long strands and suspended, for example, between two glass slides. This distensible quality is called *spinnbarkheit* (Fig. 5-2). These changes in cervical mucus enhance the entry of sperm into the cervix.

Microscopic changes are also seen when the mucus is placed on a slide and dried. As the time of ovulation nears, under the influence of estrogen, special *ferning* patterns may be detected (Fig. 5-3). When progesterone is secreted in the secretory phase of the menstrual cycle, these ferning patterns disappear. If ovulation does not occur, ferning persists because little progesterone is produced. Knowledge of spinnbarkheit and ferning has been used in treating infertility and has been incorporated into natural family planning techniques (see Chapter 7).

Secretory phase

The second half of the cycle is frequently called the *secretory phase* because of the secretion or storage of nutrients, glycogen, and mucin in the thickening uterine wall. This storage is in response to the formation of progesterone produced by the corpus luteum. *Progesterone* (which means a hormone designed to promote pregnancy) helps maintain the soft, nutritious wall long enough to receive a fertilized egg and nourish it until the developing fetus is able to establish its life-sustaining placenta and umbilical cord.

Ischemic phase

On the twenty-sixth day of the menstrual cycle, if pregnancy has not occurred, the corpus luteum begins to degenerate. Approximately 2 days later the thickened lining of the uterus starts to disintegrate, having lost its progesterone and estrogen support. Menstrual bleeding marks the end of the ischemic phase and the beginning of a new menstrual cycle.

MENSES AND OVULATION

The menstrual flow consists of a varying mixture of cellular debris, mucus, and blood. The average amount of blood lost per cycle approximates 30 to 50 ml. The average daily loss of iron is 0.5 to 1 mg. Losses of more than 80 ml of blood during a single menses are considered excessive, depleting the body's iron supplies and resulting in the need for iron supplementation.

Ovulation may not occur each time the menstrual cycle repeats and is not dependent on menstruation. For example, ovulation does not always occur in the early menstrual cycles around menarche. Ovulation also does not always occur in cycles near menopause. In these anovulatory cycles a graafian follicle matures and estrogen is produced. Progesterone, however, is lacking to trigger the onset of menses. This can result in light, irregular menses or in heavy, prolonged menstrual flow if uterine lining has built up over several cycles. The latter can result in anemia.

In the absence of a disease causing alterations in

body temperature, ovulation can be detected by recording temperatures taken before rising from sleep. Just before ovulation the body's temperature usually drops to its lowest level found in the menstrual cycle. This drop is followed by an abrupt rise of up to 1° F, indicating that ovulation has taken place. This information, along with the knowledge of cervical mucus changes, can be used in planning pregnancies (see Chapter 7).

Alteration of Ovulation

Pregnancy and lactation

When pregnancy occurs the human chorionic gonadotropin (hCG) hormone is released by the developing fertilized egg. This hormone interrupts the normal menstrual cycle by maintaining the higher level of estrogen and progesterone, thus inhibiting ovulation. The detection of hCG is the basis of pregnancy tests. After the birth of an infant the hormone prolactin, produced by the anterior pituitary gland, stimulates maternal milk production and may inhibit (but not stop) ovulation during breast-feeding.

Artificial hormonal control

Oral contraceptives, such as "the pill," containing estrogen and progesterone-like compounds, simulate some degree of the changes in the uterine lining and the regulation of ovarian and pituitary activity that occur during pregnancy. Ovulation is then artificially suppressed (see Chapter 7).

In some instances, ovulation is induced by the administration of hormones. For example, fertility drugs such as menotropins (Pergonal) and clomiphene (Clomid) may be used to stimulate ovulation in women who do not consistently ovulate. These drugs can cause multiple follicles to mature, resulting in twins, triplets, or even larger "instant families."

PROBLEMS IN MENSTRUATION

Dysmenorrhea

The most common menstrual disturbance is *dysmenorrhea*, or painful menstruation. Although most women experience some discomfort (e.g., pelvic congestion, fatigue, or irritability), severe cramping and incapacitation should not be the rule. *Primary dysmenorrhea* is discomfort in the absence of an underlying disease. It occurs most often in younger women and is the result of prostaglandins, which produce painful uterine contractions. Prostaglandin-synthetase inhibitors and oral contraceptives are both effective means of treatment. Prostaglandin-synthetase inhibitors are nonsteroidal, antiinflammatory, and work by reducing uterine muscle contractions. They include such medications as aspirin, ibuprofen (Motrin, Advil, Nuprin), naproxen (Naprosyn, Anaprox), and mefenamic acid (Ponstel). See the Nursing Alert below. Oral contraceptives work by inhibiting ovulation and reducing the amount of endometrium. The use of rest, heat, massage, exercise, and a dietary reduction of sodium are often helpful in reducing discomfort.

Secondary dysmenorrhea has an underlying physical pathology, such as endometriosis (colonization of endometrial tissue outside the uterus), pelvic inflammatory disease, adhesions, genital tract obstruction, poor uterine positioning, presence of pelvic tumors, or a possible hormonal imbalance. Treatment of secondary dysmenorrhea depends on the cause.

Premenstrual Syndrome

Premenstrual syndrome (PMS) is a group of symptoms, both physical and psychological, that occur in the latter half of the menstrual cycle. Since no laboratory tests exist to diagnose PMS, diagnosis is based on history—PMS patients suffer their symptoms *only* during the luteal phase of the menstrual cycle. Common symptoms include abdominal bloating, breast tenderness, edema of the lower extremities, weight gain, headache, depression, crying, and loss of concentration. These symptoms may interfere with work and personal relationships. The cause of PMS is unknown. Treatment is also controversial. Counseling, prostaglandin inhibitors, diuretics for edema, exercise, a well-balanced diet low in caffeine and sodium, and vitamin supplementation with vitamin B^6 have all been prescribed with varying success. See the Nursing Alert on p. 60.

Nursing Alert

Prostaglandin-synthetase inhibitors (PGSIs) should not be given to patients who have shown a previous sensitivity to these drugs. They are also contraindicated for women with a history of (1) nasal polyps, angioedema, and bronchospasm related to aspirin or nonsteroidal antiinflammatory agents; (2) chronic ulceration or inflammatory disease of the upper or lower gastrointestinal tract; and (3) chronic renal disease.

> **Nursing Alert**
>
> PMS patients should be encouraged to exercise 3 to 4 times each week, particularly during the luteal phase.

Disturbances in Flow

A variety of menstrual irregularities are possible. *Amenorrhea* is the absence of menses resulting from pregnancy or from a pathological condition. Primary amenorrhea is defined as the absence of established menses by the age of 16½. Secondary amenorrhea is the cessation of menstruation in a woman who has previously established menses. *Menorrhagia* refers to an excessive (more than 80 ml) or prolonged (more than 7 days) menstrual flow. See Chapter 13 for a discussion of estimating blood loss. *Metrorrhagia* is uterine bleeding occurring between menses. Variations in menstrual flow that are not explained by pregnancy should be investigated by a health care provider. Treatment depends on the underlying cause of each disturbance (Herbst et al, 1992).

KEY CONCEPTS

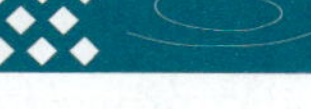

1 Menstruation, also known as *menses,* a *period,* or *monthly flow,* is the monthly shedding of the functional layer of the uterine lining.

2 The age of menarche, the first menses, seems to be affected by heredity, racial background, and nutrition.

3 Menstruation usually occurs approximately every 28 days and lasts about 5 days.

4 Two primary endocrine glands are involved in menstruation: the pituitary gland and the ovaries.

5 The ovaries have two basic functions: the production of the hormones, estrogen and progesterone and the maturation of microscopic eggs or ova.

6 Two anterior pituitary hormones, the follicle-stimulating hormone (FSH) and the luteinizing hormone (LH), help govern the *ovarian* and, more indirectly, the *endometrial* or *uterine* cycles. FSH initiates the ovarian follicle's growth and works with LH to continue the follicle's maturation and produce the characteristic increase in estrogen production.

7 Estrogen causes the build up of the uterine endometrium during the *proliferative phase* between menses and ovulation.

8 Progesterone production results in the secretion or storage of nutrients, glycogen, and mucin in the thickening uterine wall during the second half of the cycle, known as the *secretory phase.*

9 Possible indications of ovulation include cervical mucus changes (spinnbarkheit and ferning patterns) and an abrupt rise in morning body temperature. Less consistent indicators are abdominal pain (mittelschmerz) and midcycle spotting. Knowledge of these changes can be used in treating infertility and implementing natural family planning.

10 The cause of premenstrual syndrome (PMS) is unknown. Counseling, prostaglandin inhibitors, diuretics, exercise, diet, and vitamin B^6 supplementation have been used to treat PMS symptoms with varying success.

11 When no physical cause has been determined, dysmenorrhea can be prevented or treated with moderate exercise, rest, massage, applying heat to the pelvis, dietary reduction of sodium, oral contraceptives, or medications that inhibit the activity of prostaglandins.

12 Secondary dysmenorrhea may be caused by endometriosis, pelvic inflammatory disease, adhesions, pelvic tumors, genital tract obstructions, poor uterine positioning, or a hormonal imbalance.

CRITICAL THOUGHT QUESTIONS

1. Many women have little accurate knowledge about the menstrual cycle and its role in reproduction. How would you assess the knowledge level of a 16-year-old woman? A 40-year-old woman? Would your teaching strategies differ for each of these women? If so, why? If not, why not?
2. Many myths and superstitions about PMS exist. How can nurses correct this misinformation? What points do you think should be stressed?
3. A friend confides that her menstrual cycle has become irregular and that she is experiencing increased discomfort during menstruation. What advice would you give her? On what principles would you base this advice?
4. A 30-year-old woman is concerned because her menstrual flow is much heavier than in the past. How would you determine that menstrual blood loss is excessive? What advice would you give her? Why?

REFERENCES

Fogel CI, Woods NF: *Health care of women: a nursing perspective*, St. Louis, 1981, Mosby.

Herbst AL, Mishell DR, Stenchever MA, et al: *Comprehensive gynecology*, ed 8, St. Louis, 1992, Mosby.

BIBLIOGRAPHY

Berman MK, Taylor ML, Freeman E: Vitamin B^6 in premenstrual syndrome, *J Am Diet Assoc* 90(6):859-861, 1990.

Clark-Caller T: Dysfunctional uterine bleeding and amenorrhea: differential diagnosis and management, *J Nurse Midwifery* 36(1):49-62, 1991.

Estok PJ, Rudy EB, Kerr ME, et al: Menstrual response to running: nursing implications, *Nurs Res* 42(3):158-165, 1993.

Galle PC, McRae MA: Amenorrhea and chronic anovulation: finding and addressing the underlying cause, *Postgrad Med* 92(2):255-260, 1992.

Lindow KB: Premenstrual syndrome: family impact and nursing implications, *J Obstet Gynecol Neonatal Nurs* 20(2):135-138, 1991.

Murata JM: Abnormal genital bleeding and secondary amenorrhea: common gynecological problems, *J Obstet Gynecol Neonatal Nurs* 19(1):26-36, 1990.

Polaneczky MM, Slapp GB: Menstrual disorders in the adolescent: amenorrhea, *Pediatri Rev* 13(3):83-87, 1992.

Male Reproductive System

CHAPTER OBJECTIVES

After studying this chapter, the student should be able to:

1 Define puberty.
2 List four signs of the onset of male puberty.
3 Identify the external structures of the male reproductive system.
4 Identify the internal structures of the male reproductive system.
5 Explain the functions of the penis, scrotum, testis, epididymis, vas deferens, and the male hormone testosterone.
6 Name three paired glands that add secretions to spermatozoa to form semen.

Puberty, or the maturation of the reproductive system, usually occurs late in the male (average age, 14 years) when compared with that of the female. On the average the development of the male sex organs and secondary sex characteristics takes place 2 years later than that of the female. It involves changes such as the enlargement of the larynx and deepening of the voice; the appearance of axillary, pubic, and facial hair; the development of increased musculature; the production of semen; and the normal occurrence of nocturnal emissions (wet dreams). Nurses can educate young men about their changing bodies and provide accurate information about reproductive function.

EXTERNAL REPRODUCTIVE STRUCTURES

The male external genitalia include the mons pubis, the penis, and the scrotum (Figs. 6-1 and 6-2).

Mons Pubis

As in the female the area over the symphysis pubis is called the mons pubis. In the mature male, long, dense, curly pubic hair forms a diamond-shaped pattern from the umbilicus to the anus, covering the mons pubis.

Penis

The penis is the organ of copulation and urination. It consists of the shaft or body, the glans penis, urethra, and prepuce or foreskin. The shaft or body is composed of three columns of erectile tissue that include two corpora cavernosa and the corpus spongiosum (Fig. 6-1). The corpus spongiosum contains the urethra, which is the passageway for both urine and sperm. These three columns of erectile tissue are bound together by fibrous tissue and are covered by a thin, hairless outer layer of skin. With sexual stimulation the blood vessels of the penis become engorged, causing the penis to become erect.

The glans penis is similar in function to the female clitoris. It is smooth and sensitive to touch, pressure, and temperature. The urethral opening is at the tip of the glans. In uncircumcised men the glans is hooded by a retractable fold of skin called the *prepuce*, or *foreskin*. The prepuce is often surgically removed by circumci-

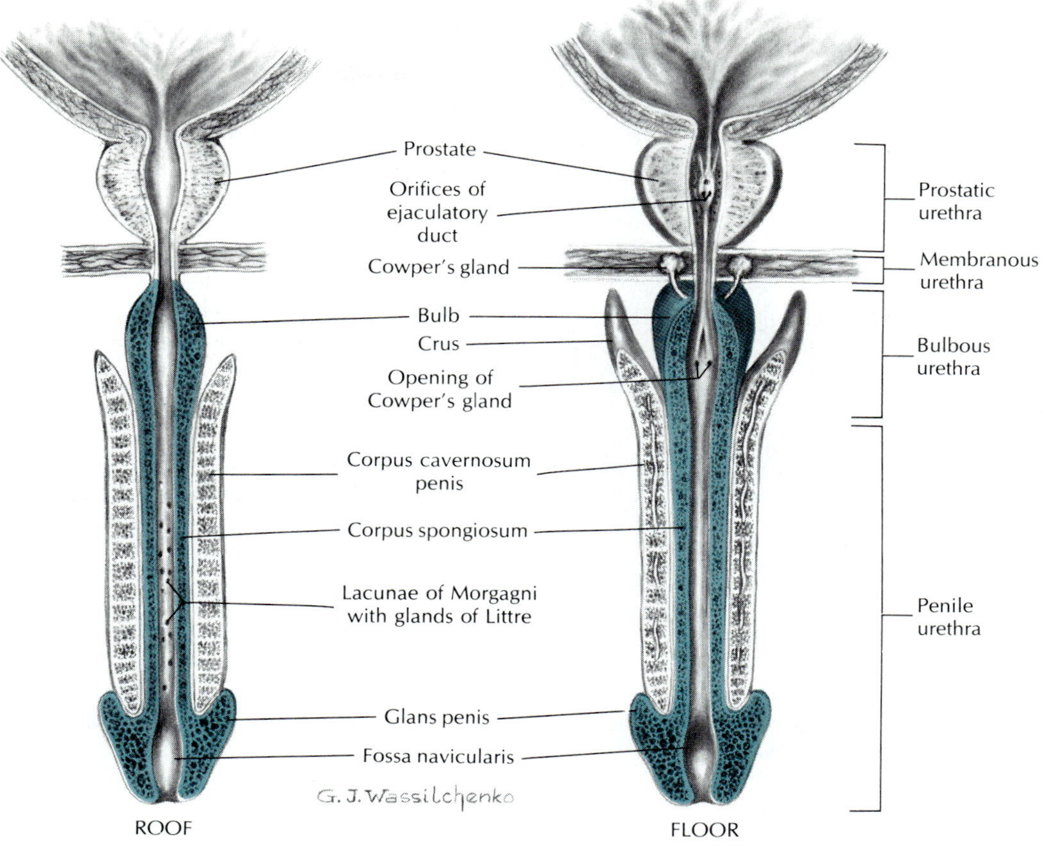

Fig. 6-1 Anatomy of the urethra and penis. (From Bobak IM, Jensen MD: *Maternity and gynecologic care,* ed 5, St. Louis, 1993, Mosby.)

sion, a procedure usually performed within a few days of birth.

Scrotum

The scrotum is a deeply pigmented pouch formed by an outer layer of thin, wrinkled skin covering a tight muscle layer (cremaster muscle). Internally the scrotum is divided into two compartments separated by a midline septum. Each compartment contains a testis, its epididymis, and part of the spermatic cord (vas deferens). The left side of the scrotum is often lower than the right, since the left spermatic cord is usually longer. The scrotum protects the testes from trauma and temperature changes that would jeopardize sperm and their development. With exposure to cold the cremaster muscle of the scrotum contracts to draw the testes closer to the body. With exposure to heat (environmental or fever) it relaxes to move the testes further from the body.

INTERNAL REPRODUCTIVE STRUCTURES

The male internal structures include the testes, the ducts of the testes (e.g., epididymis, vas deferens, and ejaculatory duct), and accessory glands (e.g., seminal vesicles, prostate gland, and bulbourethral glands). See Figs. 6-1 and 6-2.

Testes

The male sex glands, or gonads, are two smooth, oval, and mobile endocrine organs called testes (singular, testis), or testicles, which are located within the scrotum. During part of fetal development the testes are located in the abdominal cavity, but they migrate to the scrotal sac by way of the inguinal canal before birth. Occasionally, this migration does not occur and a condition known as *undescended testicles,* or *cryptorchidism,* exists. If this condition persists, sterility may occur, since the higher temperature of the abdominal cavity

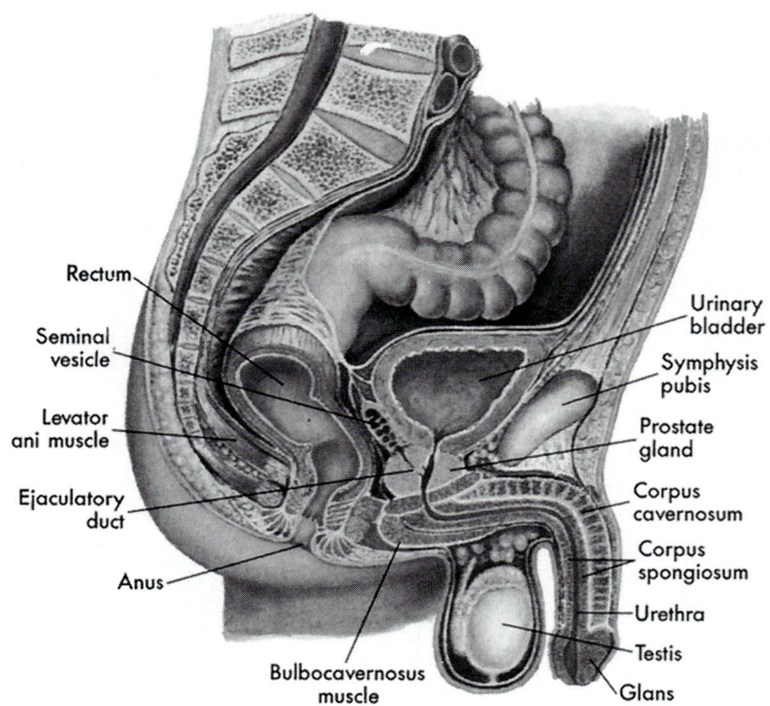

Fig. 6-2 Male genitourinary tract. (From Dickason EJ, Silverman BL, Schult MO: *Maternal-infant nursing care,* ed 2, St. Louis, 1994, Mosby.)

RISK FACTORS FOR TESTICULAR CANCER

Family history.
Undescended testicle (10 to 40 times higher risk).
Early puberty.
Female family members with breast cancer.
Mononucleosis.
Overweight.
Mother exposed to diethylstilbestrol (DES) during early fetal development.

Nursing Alert

Testicular cancer is the leading cause of death in men aged 15 to 35 years of age. The American Cancer Society recommends that young men be instructed in monthly testicular self-examinations starting at age 14.

tends to interfere with the manufacture of sperm (see Chapter 36 for a discussion of the treatment for cryptorchidism). If the condition continues, malignant changes can occur. See the box above for additional risk factors for testicular cancer (Bell, 1990). (See the Nursing Alert above right.)

The testes, which correspond in function to ovaries in the female, perform two main actions: the manufacture of male sex cells (gametes), or spermatozoa, and the production of several steroid hormones, primarily testosterone. Each testis contains seminiferous tubules, which house sperm cells at all stages of development, and interstitial cells (Leydig's cells), which produce testosterone. This hormone is responsible for the appearance of male characteristics, just as estrogen in the woman controls female characteristics. Testosterone also increases sperm production in the seminiferous tubules and stimulates production of seminal fluid.

Hormonal Regulation

The male pituitary and nearby hypothalamus help regulate events of male reproductive physiology, just as these organs in women assist in the control of female reproductive function. The male pituitary secretes follicle-stimulating hormone (FSH) and luteinizing hormone (LH). These hormones in a man, however, perform different tasks than they do in a woman. FSH is responsible for promoting the maturation of spermatozoa, whereas LH, also known as *interstitial cell-stimulating hormone* (ICSH) in the male, is involved in the production of testosterone.

Ducts of the Testes

To exit the body, sperm must travel through a series of ducts. Attached to the top of each testis is a coiled structure called an *epididymis*. This organ is actually an extension of the seminiferous tubules of the testis in which sperm are formed. In the epididymides (plural of epididymis) the male sex cells mature. In turn, each epididymis is attached to a long tube called the *ductus deferens*, or vas deferens. With associated nerves and blood vessels the ductus deferens travels up the inguinal canal as the spermatic cord. The ductus deferens eventually loops downward in back of the urinary bladder. The ductus deferens carries sperm from the scrotum to a small pouch called the *seminal vesicle*. This small pouch secretes a fluid that is added to the spermatozoa and aids in the motility of the sex cell. The tube leading forward from the point of attachment of the seminal vesicle is called the *ejaculatory duct*. This duct allows the sperm to enter the urethra and then exit the body. The duct then joins the long urethra after passing through the tissue of the prostate gland.

Accessory Glands

Three paired glands add secretions to the spermatozoa traveling from the testes to the body's exterior to form semen, or seminal fluid. These glands are the seminal vesicle, the prostate, and the bulbourethral, or Cowper's gland, which opens directly into the urethra. These secretions regulate the acidity of the semen and influence the sperm's motility and life span. As a result of sexual excitement and subsequent ejaculation of 2 to 6 ml of semen, approximately 250 to 500 million sperm at a time are released from the penis through the urethral meatus.

KEY CONCEPTS

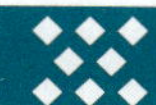

1. Male puberty, the maturation of the reproductive system, involves changes such as the enlargement of the larynx and the deepening of the voice; the appearance of axillary, pubic, and facial hair; the development of increased musculature; the production of semen; and the occurrence of nocturnal emissions.
2. The penis is the male organ of copulation or intercourse. When not sexually stimulated, it serves as the excretory organ of the urinary system.
3. The scrotum protects the testes and sperm from trauma and from fluctuations in environmental and body temperature.
4. The two oval endocrine organs called testes perform two main functions: the manufacture of spermatozoa and the production of several steroid hormones, primarily testosterone.
5. Testosterone is responsible for the appearance of male characteristics, for increasing sperm production in the seminiferous tubules, and for stimulating the production of seminal fluid.
6. The epididymides are extensions of the seminiferous tubules of the testes. The male sex cells mature within the epididymides.
7. The vas deferens, or ductus deferens, travels from the epididymis and up the inguinal canal as part of the spermatic cord. It carries sperm from the scrotum to the seminal vesicle.
8. The seminal vesicle, the prostate, and the bulbourethral, or Cowper's gland, add secretions to spermatozoa to form semen, or seminal fluid.

CRITICAL THOUGHT QUESTIONS

1. Your clinical group has been asked to conduct a sex education class for a local high school group. What information about the male reproductive system would you include in your teaching outline?
2. A female nurse must teach a young man how to do a testicular self-examination. What strategies could she use to increase her own comfort and that of the young man? What teaching tools could she use?
3. Surveys of high school and college males indicate that few know about or have ever been taught how to do a testicular self-examination. How can nurses increase the public's awareness of this important examination?

REFERENCES

Bell I: Testicular self-examination, *Nurs Times* 86(9):38-40, 1990.

Bobak IM, Jensen MD: *Maternity and gynecologic care,* ed 5, St. Louis, 1993, Mosby.

Dickason EJ, Silverman BL, Schult MO: *Maternal-infant nursing care,* ed 2, St. Louis, 1994, Mosby.

BIBLIOGRAPHY

Barkauskas V, Stoltenberg-Allen K, Baumann LC, et al: *Health and physical assessment*, St. Louis, 1994, Mosby.

Goldenring JM: A lifesaving exam for young men, *Contemp Nurs* 10(4):63-68, 1992.

Thibodeau G, Patton K: *Anatomy and physiology*, ed 2, St. Louis, 1993, Mosby.

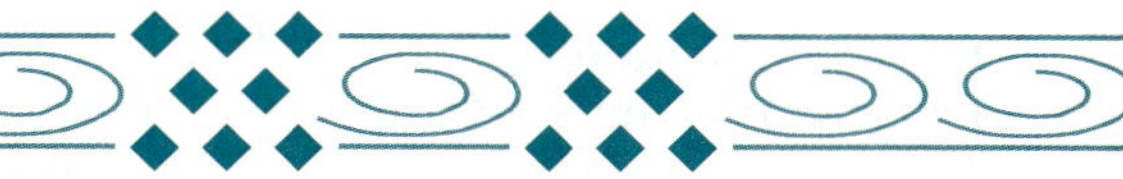

7 Fertility Management

CHAPTER OBJECTIVES

After studying this chapter, the student should be able to:

1. Define fertility.
2. List the components of a comprehensive family planning program.
3. Discuss philosophical considerations that may influence a person's attitude toward contraceptive options.
4. State three main types of contraception and discuss the ways they prevent the formation or early development of a fertilized ovum.
5. Explain what is meant by "natural family planning."
6. Explain the advantages, disadvantages, and effectiveness of five methods of preventing fertilization.
7. Identify three side effects of oral contraceptives.
8. List the three most effective methods of (temporary) contraception.
9. Discuss three aspects of the 1973 US Supreme Court decision regarding abortion: permissions necessary, conditions under which the procedure may be performed, and the age of the fetus.
10. Identify the possible impact of the decision rendered by the US Supreme Court in *Webster v. Reproductive Health Services* in 1989.
11. Describe the four surgical interventions performed to limit childbearing through sterilization.
12. Define infertility and discuss what may be done if failure to conceive is due to blocked fallopian tubes.

Fertility refers to the ability of the body to reproduce—to create and sustain new life. Family planning is the conscious effort to manage fertility by a variety of methods: contraceptive education, genetic counseling, infertility counseling and methods of fertility enhancement, alternative birth technologies, and adoption.

The ability to conceive and bear children and one's views toward planning the number and spacing of children are associated with many social, religious, and cultural values for both men and women. Not all persons accept the same explanation of the origin and meaning of life, nor do they agree on the order of life's priorities. Philosophical differences in viewpoint cause various groups or individuals to endorse, tolerate, or condemn certain methods of family planning. These philosophical considerations include convictions regarding the following: (1) the ultimate purpose and potential of the individual and mankind as a whole, (2) how the developmental state of the unborn child affects his or her status as a person or soul, (3) the rights of the unborn versus those of the parents and society, (4) the purposes of the marriage relationship and sexual intercourse, (5) the responsibility and ability of the individual to make and implement decisions involving personal conduct, and (6) the role of a deity in the affairs of human beings. Nurses must be sensitive to these differing values and viewpoints.

CONTRACEPTION

From a public health point of view the primary goal of family planning is to reduce the number of unintended births (unwanted or earlier than planned). (See the box below for the related national health objective for the year 2000.) Pregnancies that are planned and spaced with regard to physical health and family resources are likely to have better outcomes than those that are not. Pregnancies spaced too closely (within one year of a previous birth), teenage pregnancies, and pregnancies occurring in families with financial and other problems have been associated with low birth weight, child abuse, and infant morbidity and mortality (Institute of Medicine, 1985; US Department of Health and Human Services, 1992).

Nurses have many opportunities to provide patients with information about contraception. The nurse's role includes providing accurate, unbiased information about the various contraceptive methods and correcting any misinformation that the patient may have (NAACOG, 1991). Teaching should include information about the advantages and disadvantages, effectiveness, correct use, and contraindications of each of the methods. The nurse can help the patient weigh the risks and benefits of each method and determine which method will best fit his or her lifestyle. In addition to the prevention of pregnancy, contraceptive education should include information about protection against the human immunodeficiency virus (HIV), hepatitis B, and other sexually transmitted diseases (STDs). Each set of potential parents should consciously make the decision of whether or not to have children and which contraceptive method they will use. This decision should be appropriate for them and in accordance with their personal, societal, and religious values and beliefs.

Contraceptive methods that are used to temporarily prevent conception fall into three main categories: those that prevent fertilization, those that prevent ovulation, and those that prevent implantation. Scientifically speaking, the last is not a method of contraception, since the egg may be fertilized but unable to embed itself into the uterine lining to maintain life. A brief description of these methods follows.

NATIONAL HEALTH OBJECTIVE FOR THE YEAR 2000

Reduce unintended pregnancies to no more than 30% of all pregnancies.

Methods That Prevent Fertilization

Abstinence

Refraining from sexual intercourse is becoming a more accepted contraceptive measure. The woman who chooses this method must be confident that she can avoid or control situations where there is pressure to engage in sexual intercourse. Those who choose abstinence should consider having a backup method of contraception readily available.

Coitus interruptus

Coitus interruptus is probably the oldest type of birth control practiced. This method involves premature withdrawal of the penis from the vagina before ejaculation. Although this method is used by many couples, its reliability is low because sperm are emitted in varying quantities in the lubricating fluid secreted before and during intercourse. It may also be difficult for the man to anticipate and control the timing of ejaculation. The failure rate of this method among typical users is 19%* (Hatcher, et al, 1994). This method provides no protection from STDs or HIV.

Periodic abstinence (natural family planning)

Four methods use abstinence during the fertile period of the menstrual cycle: calendar, temperature, mucus, and symptothermal. These methods are known as "natural family planning" and are based on the following principles: (1) ovulation occurs approximately 14 days before the onset of the next menses, (2) the human ovum is susceptible to fertilization for approximately 18 to 24 hours after ovulation, and (3) sperm deposited in the vagina are ordinarily capable of fertilizing the ovum for no more than 72 hours. The effectiveness of these methods depends on the ability of the individual to accurately predict ovulation and on the couple's willingness to abstain from intercourse during the fertile period. The failure rate for these methods of periodic abstinence among typical users is 20%.

Calendar Also known as the rhythm method, the calendar method uses mathematical calculations to predict the probable fertile period. Because menstrual cycles can vary considerably for any woman, the woman must record the length of menstrual cycles for about a year to determine the shortest and longest cycle. Subtracting 18 days from the length of the shortest cycle determines the first day of the fertile

* Failure rates refer to the percentage of couples who have an accidental pregnancy during the first year of using the method in a typical manner (occasionally inconsistently or incorrectly).

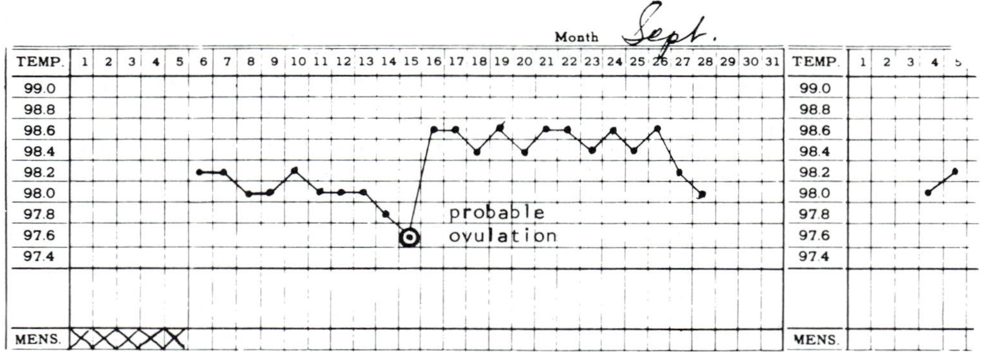

Fig. 7-1 Basal body temperature (BBT) graph. Ovulation may be signaled by a drop in basal body temperature 12 to 24 hours before the postovulation rise of about 0.4° to 0.8° F. However, not all women demonstrate this initial dip in temperature readings. The BBT elevation usually continues until about 2 days before menstrual flow reappears. If pregnancy occurs, temperature remains within a relatively high range. Basal body temperatures must be taken consistently, either orally, rectally, or vaginally before any activity, on awakening each morning.

period. Subtracting 11 days from the length of the longest cycle determines the last day of the fertile period. For example, if a woman's cycle lasts from 28 to 32 days, the fertile phase would be calculated as day 10 through day 21. This method is more reliable if used along with the temperature and cervical mucus methods described below.

Temperature The temperature method relies on slight changes in basal body temperature (BBT) that begin just before ovulation. The woman takes her temperature every morning before rising. The temperature usually drops just before ovulation and then rises (usually from .4° to .8° F) in response to increased progesterone, remaining elevated for several days (Fig. 7-1). A careful calendar history of menses and daily basal body temperature patterns help to identify the "safe" luteal phase of the menstrual cycle, when intercourse would be least likely to produce a pregnancy. To prevent conception, the couple should avoid intercourse on the day of the temperature rise and for the next three days. Potential problems with this technique stem from the fact that basal body temperature may vary with sleeplessness, illness, digestive disturbances, immunizations, alcohol ingestion, fever, emotional upset, and medications to induce sleep.

Cervical mucus The cervical mucus method (also called "Billings" or "ferning" method) depends on identifying fertile periods through awareness of the "dryness" and "wetness" in the vagina. These changes result from alterations in the amount and kind of cervical mucus formed at different times in the menstrual cycle (see Chapter 5). Right before ovulation the vagina's watery, thin mucus increases in amount and thickness and can be stretched (spinnbarkheit). This type of cervical mucus marks the most fertile period.

Symptothermal The symptothermal method effectiveness depends on periodic abstinence during fertile periods identified by a combination of factors. Records are kept of the length of menstrual cycles, basal temperature, changes in cervical mucus, libido, and many other factors (spotting, breast tenderness, abdominal cramping, cervical softening, and other secondary signs). The symptothermal method is the most effective of the natural family planning methods.

In recent years, several devices have been developed to aid in fertility awareness. They include computerized basal body temperature thermometers, electronic fertility monitors, and chemical and hormonal ovulation detection kits.

These four methods of natural family planning may be acceptable to those who have religious objections to other methods of contraception. Another advantage is that women who use these methods become more knowledgeable about their bodies. None of these methods, however, provides protection from STDs or HIV. Although natural family planning (NFP) is characterized by avoidance of intercourse during fertile periods, the "fertility awareness method" (FAM) uses a barrier method of birth control during fertile intervals.

Local barrier methods

Barrier methods prevent sperm from entering the reproductive system. Spermicides that immobilize and kill sperm are often used with these methods. Used in conjunction with barrier methods, they provide enhanced protection against STDs and increased protection against pregnancy.

Condom The most widely used birth control device in the world, the male condom was probably first used to prevent the spread of sexually transmitted diseases. Largely because of the fear of acquired immune deficiency syndrome (AIDS), the public acceptance of condoms has increased markedly. The transmission of herpes, chlamydia, gonorrhea, and syphilis, however, is also reduced by condom use. Condoms offer the best protection against STDs and HIV. The most protective condoms are those made of latex. (See the Nursing Alert below.) Natural skin condoms do not protect against STDs and HIV. Condoms are available in a lubricated or unlubricated form and with or without spermicide. Shaped like a finger cot the condom is applied over the erect penis before intercourse. A half-inch space or "pocket" should be left at the end to collect the ejaculate and to prevent the condom from tearing during ejaculation. To prevent spilling sperm into the vagina after intercourse the man should hold onto the condom as the penis is removed. Petroleum jelly should never be applied to a condom. It weakens the fiber of the latex, thus increasing the risk of tearing. Additional spermicide or water soluble jellies can be used if additional lubrication is desired. Condoms should be stored away from heat and should never be reused. The failure rate among typical users of this method is 12%.

> **Nursing Alert**
>
> Patients should be questioned about their sensitivity to latex or latex-containing products when discussing condom use. Sensitivity to latex can cause serious anaphylactic reactions.

The Food and Drug Administration (FDA) recently gave provisional approval for a female condom, which is a soft, polyurethane pouch with two flexible rings at opposite ends. One ring is inside the closed end of the pouch and surrounds the cervix whereas the other ring remains outside the vagina. The woman can insert the device as early as a few hours before intercourse and should remove it before standing. It is prelubricated, disposable, and intended for only one sex act. Studies indicate that when used correctly, the failure rate of the female condom is equivalent to that of the male condom (12%).

Cervical caps and diaphragms Diaphragms are latex domes with spring rims (Fig. 7-2). They are positioned over the cervix between the pubic bone and the posterior vaginal wall (Fig. 7-3). Diaphragm use is associated with increased incidence of bladder infections in some women, most likely because of the rim's pressure against the urethra or neck of the bladder. The failure rate among typical users of the diaphragm is 18%.

Long popular in Europe, cervical caps fit closely over the cervix. In 1988 the FDA approved the importation and use of the Prentif cavity-rim soft latex cervical cap

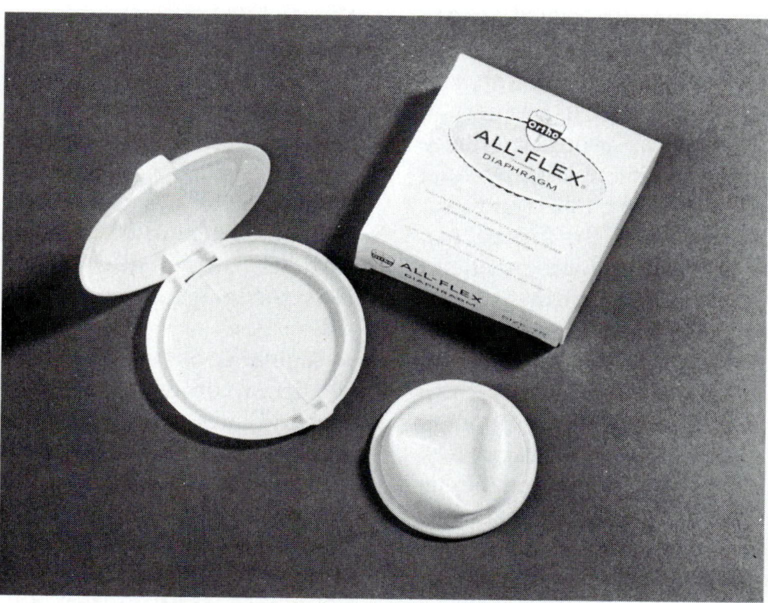

Fig. 7-2 Rubber-spring diaphragm with case.

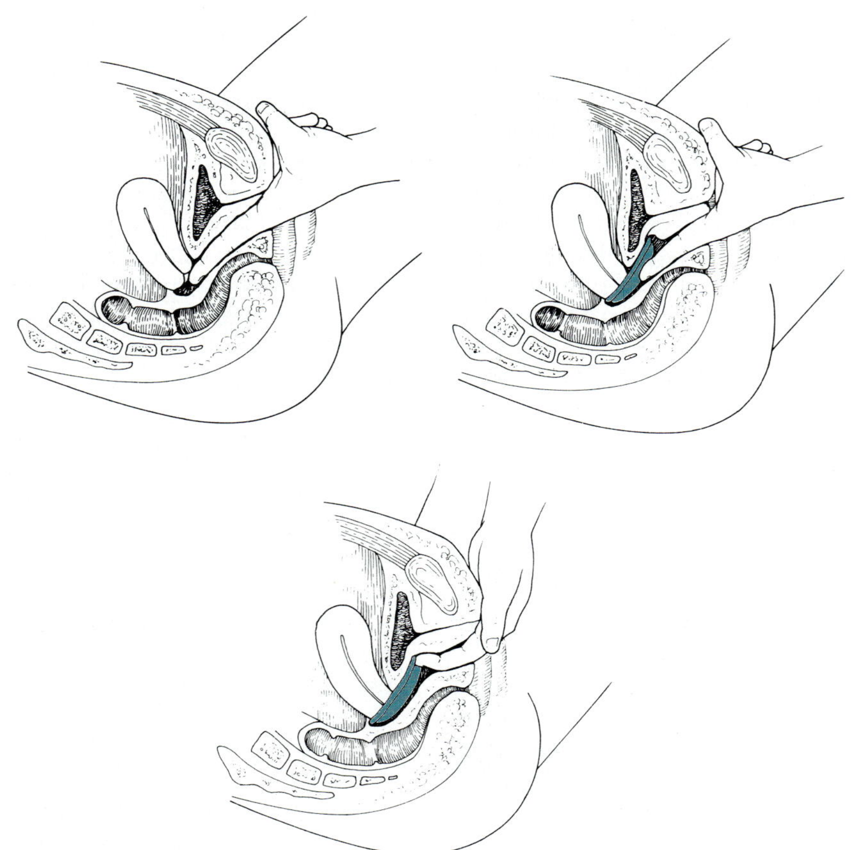

Fig. 7-3 Proper placement of diaphragm between posterior fornix and symphysis pubis. (From Fogel CI, Woods NF: *Health care of women: a nursing perspective,* St. Louis, 1981, Mosby.)

in the United States (Fig. 7-4). It is available in three sizes. The instructions state that prescriptions should be limited to women with normal Papanicolaou (Pap) tests and that users should return to their health care providers for repeat Pap tests after 3 months of intermittent use. Four percent of cap users experience abnormal changes in results of their Pap tests. If such changes occur the use of the cap is to be discontinued. The failure rate among typical users of the cervical cap is 18% for those for who have never been pregnant and 36% for those women who have given birth.

Both the diaphragm and cap hold spermicide against the cervix to immobilize and kill the sperm. Caps and diaphragms must be fitted by a physician or technician. Because of anatomical differences, not all women can be fitted satisfactorily. Both the diaphragm and cervical cap may need to be refitted after pregnancy because of subsequent changes in cervical size. The woman's ability to insert and remove these devices properly must be checked. Some women find it distasteful to insert these devices and others may be sensitive to latex.

These vaginal barriers are most effective when inserted no longer than 1 hour before intercourse, since the spermicidal application becomes less powerful with the passage of time. An additional application of spermicide should be added (without removing the device) if intercourse is repeated. The devices should remain in place for at least 8 hours after intercourse. Although the cap may remain in place for up to 48 hours, removal of both the diaphragm and cap before 24 hours is optimal. Women should not douche after intercourse, since douching washes away the spermicide.

Vaginal sponge The vaginal sponge, another type of barrier contraceptive, was approved for use in the United States in 1983. Since that time, it has achieved considerable popularity. Made of soft polyurethane the mushroom-shaped device contains 1 gm of the spermicide nonoxynol-9. This device prevents pregnancy in three ways: by slow but constant release of spermicide, by blocking the cervical opening, and by absorbing semen and destroying the sperm. It is sold over-the-counter in a single size, 2 inches (5.1 cm) in

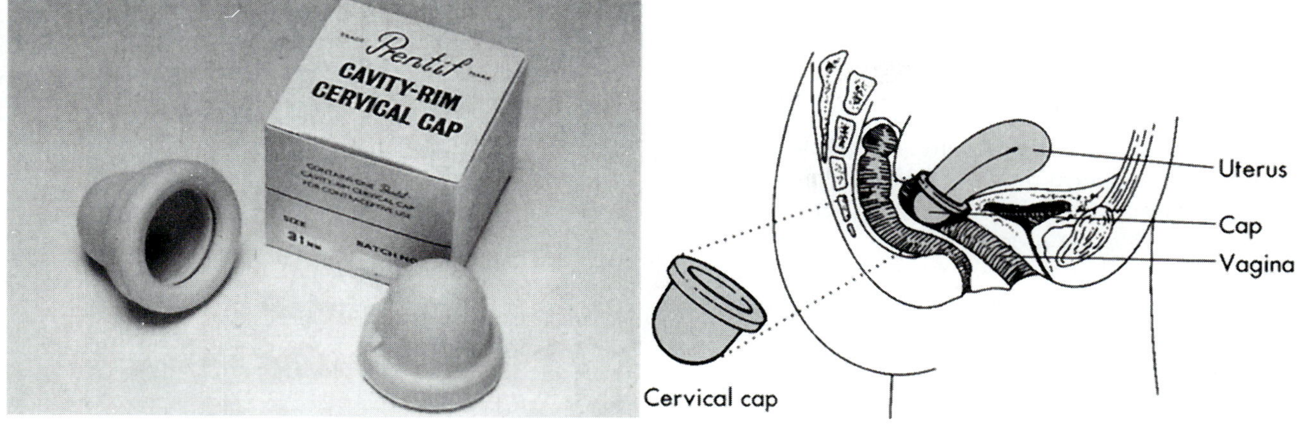

Fig. 7-4 **A,** Cervical cap; **B,** cervical cap placement. (From Dickason EJ, Silverman BL, Schult MO: *Maternal-infant nursing care,* ed 2, St. Louis, 1994, Mosby.)

SIGNS AND SYMPTOMS OF TOXIC SHOCK SYNDROME

Temperature of 101° F or more.
Diarrhea and vomiting.
Muscle and joint aches.
Weakness and faintness.
Sore throat.
Sunburn-like rash or peeling of skin on hands and feet.

diameter and ¾ inch (1.9 cm) thick. The device is relatively easy to insert over the cervix, and an attached loop aids in its removal. It must be moistened before insertion to activate the spermicide. The manufacturer's instructions should be consulted. After intercourse the sponge must be left in place for at least 6 hours. The failure rate among typical users of the vaginal sponge is the same as for the cervical cap (18% for those never pregnant, 36% for those women who have given birth).

These vaginal barrier methods of contraception should not be used during menses or when abnormal vaginal discharge is noted. The recommended 24-hour limit for cervical caps, diaphragms, and vaginal sponges is designed to reduce the complications of tissue injury, infection, and toxic shock syndrome (TSS). TSS is caused by a toxin produced by the microorganism *Staphylococcus aureus.* This disease occurs during or immediately after menstruation. Women should be informed of the symptoms of TSS, a rare but serious illness, so they can seek timely medical care (see the box above). Despite the risk of TSS, however, these vaginal barrier methods are relatively free of side effects. All vaginal barrier methods provide limited protection against STDs. If STD and HIV protection is needed, condoms should be used.

Spermicides

Other substances available in the form of creams, jellies, suppositories, foams, aerosols, and foam tablets provide both a physical barrier to sperm penetration and chemical spermicidal action. A newer type of intravaginal contraceptive recently introduced to the United States has been marketed in Europe as C-film. A small, 2-inch square of paper-thin spermicidal film (VCF) is inserted over the cervix at least 5 minutes before intercourse to allow it to dissolve. Nonoxynol-9, the spermicide used in many contraceptive products, also kills organisms that cause gonorrhea, genital herpes, trichomoniasis, syphilis, and HIV (NAACOG, 1991). Most spermicides are effective for only 1 hour and must be reapplied if intercourse is repeated. With the exception of suppositories, tablets, and cervical film, no waiting period after application is needed before the spermicide becomes effective. All substances need to remain in the vagina for 8 hours after intercourse. Be sure to read product labels carefully.

Intravaginal spermicidal/barrier agents sometimes cause local irritation or fail to melt or foam as designed. Some couples object to the foaming activity and others complain that they are messy. Spermicides are readily available and relatively inexpensive. The failure rate among typical users of this method is 21%. Spermicides are more effective and provide much better protection from STDs and HIV if used in conjunction with one of the other barrier methods. Higher pregnancy rates are thought to be attributable chiefly to inconsistent use rather than to failure of this category of contraceptive.

Douches

Vaginal irrigations are not recommended as a means of contraception. Sperm may enter the cervix 10 to 90 seconds after ejaculation. Douching may actually help to force sperm into the uterus.

Methods that Prevent Ovulation

Oral contraceptives

Oral contraceptives (OCs) are available in combinations of estrogens and progesterone-like compounds or progesterone alone. When taken orally as directed, they are designed to prevent the release of the ovum from the ovary. Other associated actions of these substances that help to prevent pregnancy in the rare instances when ovulation is not inhibited involve: the decrease in and the thickening of cervical mucus, making the uterus less hospitable to spermatozoa; and the altered maturation of the uterine endometrium, rendering it inappropriate for successful implantation. "The pill," the most widely used oral contraceptive, was first accepted for general use by prescription in the United States in 1960. It is now one of the most popular methods of contraception in the United States.

Normally the woman is given a special dispenser to help her keep a record of her medication. Two basic types of pills and programs may be prescribed. One type of tablet, the combination, includes both estrogens and progestin and is taken daily. If one pill is missed, she should take it as soon as she remembers and take the next pill at the regularly scheduled time. If two pills in a row are missed, she should take the two pills as soon as she remembers and take two pills the next day. The regular schedule should then be resumed (Hatcher, et al, 1994). If two pills are missed, a backup method of contraception must be used for 7 days. This method of contraception has a failure rate of 3% among typical users.

The second type of pill is the all-progestin "mini pill" (norethindrone), which is also taken every day. It should technically not be placed in this category, since it is less effective in inhibiting ovulation but seems to prevent sperm transport by causing cervical mucus to thicken. One of three patterns of menstrual response to the mini pill may occur: no change in menstruation may be experienced—and ovulation will still take place; irregular menstrual-type bleeding may occur associated with lack of or reduced ovulation; or the woman may become completely amenorrheic. If menstrual flow seems excessive or prolonged or if pregnancy is suspected, a physician should be consulted. A backup method of contraception must be used for 48 hours if pills are taken 3 or more hours late. This method is less effective than the combination pills (1.1% to 13.2% failure rate among typical users).

CONTRAINDICATIONS FOR THE USE OF ESTROGEN-PROGESTIN COMBINATION ORAL CONTRACEPTIVES

- Thrombophlebitis or thromboembolic disorder (or history).
- Cerebrovascular accident (CVA, stroke) (or history).
- Coronary artery or ischemic heart disease (or history).
- Known or suspected breast cancer (or history).
- Pregnancy.
- Benign or malignant liver tumor (or history).
- Known or suspected estrogen-dependent tumor (or history).
- Impaired liver function.
- Previous cholestasis (suppression of bile flow) during pregnancy.

The so-called "morning-after pill," designed to be taken after unprotected intercourse, contains diethylstilbestrol in large doses. Its effectiveness has been established. Because of diethylstilbestrol's effect on the fetus, however, abortion is advised if this method fails to prevent pregnancy. For this reason, the combination type of birth control pills are more frequently used for postcoital contraception. Ethinyl estradiol 50 µg and norgestrel 0.5 mg are taken within 12 to 24 hours of intercourse. The same dosage is repeated exactly 12 hours later. RU 486 (mifepristone) and prostaglandins may be approved in the United States for this use in the future (Baylor College of Medicine, 1993a). RU 486, a progesterone antagonist, has been used in Europe to induce abortion since 1988. Because of its use as an abortion pill, it has been controversial in the United States. Only recently was it approved for research use in the United States.

Frequently reported side effects associated with oral contraceptives include nausea, breast tenderness, weight gain or loss, mood changes, and irregular vaginal bleeding. See the box above for contraindications to the use of the combination type of oral contraceptives. The most serious complications of the combination type of OCs are heart attacks, strokes, deep vein thrombosis, and circulatory disorders, including hypertension. These complications occur because estrogen increases clot formation. Approximately 5% of women using OCs develop hypertension. For most women, this side effect is mild and returns to normal 1 to 3 months after discontinuing use. The risks for these complications is less for those using the progestin-only "mini pill."

The risk of problems occurring in women using OCs dramatically increases among women who smoke, especially those over 35 years of age. Among healthy users who do not smoke, no increased risk of heart attack seems apparent. It is still unclear whether or not there is a small increase in the risk of blood clots and stroke. OCs do not increase the risk of ovarian and endometrial cancer and appear to provide protection against these forms of cancer. The evidence is conflicting, however, for risk of breast and cervical cancer (Engel, 1990). The combination type of pills may also be used during lactation, once breast milk production is firmly established. They are not the first choice for the lactating woman's contraception, however, because they may reduce the amount of milk produced (Baylor College of Medicine, 1993b). Progestin-only OCs do not have a negative effect on lactation and can be prescribed immediately postpartum. The minimal amount of hormone that reaches the infant from either type of OC does not appear to have any negative effects on the child.

Oral contraceptives have a number of disadvantages: the patient must have the ability and motivation to take them faithfully, they are expensive, and they have a number of side-effects. Advantages of "the pill" include its high reliability and safety, the fact that its use does not interrupt the sex act, and the woman's ability to easily stop therapy when she chooses to conceive. Careful screening to determine which women are at risk for complications, the use of the lowest acceptable dose pill for each woman, and a carefully planned follow-up schedule help to prevent problems. It must be emphasized, however, that the use of OCs does not prevent STDs or HIV.

Injectable progestins

Depo-medroxyprogesterone acetate (Depo-Provera) received FDA approval for use as a contraceptive in October 1992. It has been used in Europe, however, for this purpose for many years. It contains a synthetic hormone similar to natural progesterone. Women receive intramuscular injections of the drug in the arm or buttock. Each injection protects the woman from pregnancy for 3 months. The drug's most common side effects are menstrual irregularities and weight gain. Some women also experience headache, nervousness, abdominal pain, dizziness, weakness, or fatigue. The FDA does not recommend this drug for women who have a history of acute liver disease, unexplained vaginal bleeding, breast cancer, or blood clots (*AWHONN Voice,* 1993). The failure rate of this method is 0.3%.

Implants containing progestin

Norplant, the first subdermal (under the skin) implant, received FDA approval in 1990. It consists of six Silastic, match-stick sized rods filled with powdered, synthetic progesterone. The woman is given a local anesthetic and the rods are inserted through a small incision in the skin—usually on the inside of the upper arm. The rods slowly and steadily release the progestin into the body over a 5-year period. Like the injectable form of progestin, *Norplant* helps to prevent ovulation and also thickens the cervical mucus, making it less hospitable to sperm. The most common side effects are irregular bleeding, amenorrhea, or both, although these tend to diminish over the first year. The contraindications and side effects of this method are similar to those for the injectable progestin. Drawbacks of the implant procedure include possible infection, bleeding, and the prominent appearance of the rod beneath the skin. This method has a failure rate of only 0.09%. Neither the injectable nor implant forms of progestin provide protection against STDs or HIV.

Methods that Prevent Implantation

Authorities do not agree about how intrauterine devices (IUDs) prevent pregnancy. The mechanism involved in some way interferes with the fertilization process, the readiness of a fertilized ovum to implant, or the ability of the uterine wall to receive the egg. IUDs inserted in the early 1900s often caused tissue damage and infection because of their placement or design. Their use was largely abandoned by physicians. However, in the 1960s and 1970s, with the advent of polyethylene and improved designs, they were a particularly popular method of contraception. In the 1980s, numerous lawsuits were filed against selected manufacturers related to the use of one particular IUD that is no longer on the market. Because of these legal involvements, most manufacturers have discontinued making these products and many physicians, fearful of involvement in litigation, have abandoned their use. At this writing, only two IUDs are being marketed in the United States. Long, detailed, and signed consent forms are typically required.

Currently available IUDs are either copper-bearing (good for 8 years) or hormone-releasing (good for 1 year) (Fig. 7-5). IUDs must be inserted and removed by a proficient physician or practitioner.

The use of IUDs is associated with uterine cramping,

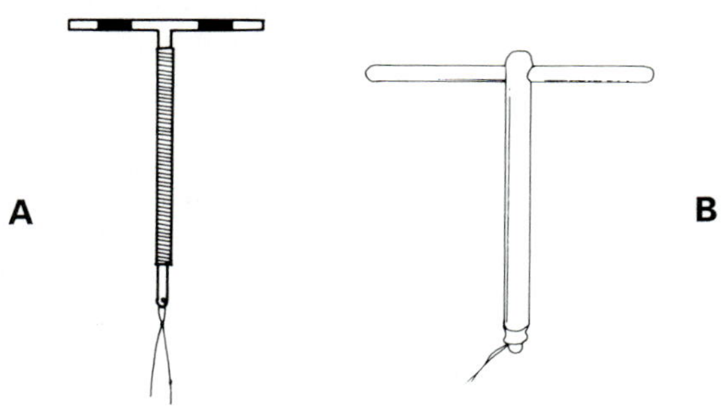

Fig. 7-5 Intrauterine devices. **A,** Copper-T 380A. **B,** Progestasert contains progesterone.

IUD WARNING SIGNS

Late menstrual period.
Missing string.
Abnormal spotting or bleeding.
Abdominal pain.
Pain with intercourse.
Abnormal vaginal discharge.
Fever, chills, and flu-like symptoms.

bleeding, and in rare instances, infection and perforation. Research indicates that the IUD should not be the contraceptive method of first choice for women who have not borne a child. In addition, use of an IUD is not advisable for women who have had pelvic infections or who are not involved in mutually monogamous relationships, increasing their risk for STDs.

IUDs may be spontaneously expelled. However, they require little care after insertion and, unless expelled, they may remain in place for months or years without untoward symptoms. The woman should be taught to check the string after every menstrual period and any time expulsion is suspected. If there is any question of expulsion, the woman should use a backup method of contraception. Ectopic pregnancies occur more frequently among wearers of IUDs than among pregnant women in general. These pregnancies are not because the device causes these abnormally placed pregnancies, but because it prevents uterine pregnancy much more efficiently than it does extrauterine gestation. If intrauterine pregnancy does occur, it is recommended that the IUD be removed as soon as possible to prevent a septic abortion. Signs of impending problems are listed in the box above right. This method does not protect the user against STDs or HIV. The failure rate of this method is 0.8% for the copper IUD and 2% for the progesterone IUD.

Clearly, no perfect method of contraception exists that is applicable to all persons and circumstances, and research continues. Equally clear is that a method must be used consistently to be effective. It is important to note that the maternal death rate associated with pregnancy and childbirth is greater than that associated with the use of any of the types of contraceptives discussed.

ABORTION

If a pregnancy occurs that for medical, psychological, economical, or social reasons is unwanted, the woman may elect to terminate the pregnancy. From the mid-1800s when abortion was outlawed until 1967 the only way that a woman could procure a legal abortion in most states was through a statement of medical agreement that continuation of the pregnancy would be a threat to her life. (A few states also considered the "health of the mother" in the wording of relevant legislation.) Laws condemning abortion were written more than 100 years ago when the operation was dangerous, even under the best auspices, and, in unskilled hands, was often catastrophic. Community concepts concerning population growth, roles of women and children, and meanings and rules surrounding sex, pregnancy, and childbirth also influenced this legislation. In the time between 1967 and 1973, several states modified their statutes to include other reasons for abortion, including the mother's physical and mental health, probable serious deformity of the baby, and cases of incest or rape. A few made abortion, with certain restrictions, a private decision between a woman and her physician.

In January 1973 the US Supreme Court decision in *Roe v. Wade* legalized abortion, noting that the decision to terminate pregnancy in the first trimester (first 12 weeks) rests only with the woman in consultation with her physician. In the second trimester, before viability of the fetus, the state recognizes a vested interest in the health of the woman and can regulate the conditions under which an abortion is performed. The state, however, cannot prohibit the procedure during this time. After "viability," which is variously considered to be after 20 or 24 weeks gestation, the state may prohibit abortion based on its interest in the life and health of the fetus. Most states do prohibit such abortions except to save the life or health of the pregnant woman.

In 1989 the US Supreme Court decided in the case of *Webster v. Reproductive Health Services* that a state may forbid the use of public money and facilities to provide abortion services. The prosecution in the case maintained what states consider to be the right of deciding not to subsidize certain medical costs. The defense in the case maintained that women who do not have financial access to private care or the ability to seek public abortion services in states that do allow the use of public funds are unduly affected. The issue of the legal availability of abortion in our society remains complicated and controversial.

The 1973 US Supreme Court decision continues to be challenged (Harrison and Naylor, 1991). Organizations such as the Right to Life Committee, the National Youth Pro-Life Coalition, and Operation Rescue actively support efforts to overturn the *Roe v. Wade* decision. They also support other antiabortion legislation, such as states' rights laws that would allow each state's legislature to determine its own abortion regulations. Meanwhile, the National Abortion Rights Action League (NARAL), Planned Parenthood, and the National Organization for Women (NOW) are groups working to maintain the 1973 court action and limit abortion restrictions by states. Legal, first-trimester abortion is safer (statistically speaking) than carrying a baby to term. The moral and political debate, however, surrounding the abortion issue is intense.

Medical and nursing personnel must be familiar with the laws regulating abortion in the area in which they practice. The question of professional participation in abortion when not done for obvious health needs of the mother is for many emotionally charged, morally disturbing, and legally complex. Most state laws have "conscience clauses" that allow physicians, nurses, and others to refuse to assist with elective abortions if it conflicts with their ethical or religious beliefs.

About half of the unintended pregnancies in the United States end in elective abortion, also referred to as induced or *therapeutic abortion* (TAB). The vast majority (91%) of women who have abortions report that they either used a contraceptive and it failed or that they recently discontinued contraceptive use (Harlap et al, 1991).

The following methods of abortion are used in hospital, clinic, or office settings for first trimester abortions:

1. *Aspiration or vacuum.* The cervix is progressively dilated enough to insert a suction catheter. The uterine contents are then dislodged by the use of the specially designed suction catheter or vacuum apparatus. The procedure is rapid (approximately 5 minutes), and blood loss is minimal. It is now the most common method used for abortions done before 13 weeks' gestation and has the fewest complications.
2. *Dilation and curettage.* The cervical canal is progressively dilated and the products of conception are gently scraped from their uterine attachments. This procedure may be done when newer aspiration equipment is not available.

NOTE: The progesterone-antagonist RU-486, is not yet available for first trimester abortions in the United States.

Methods used for second trimester abortions include the following:

1. *Dilation and evacuation.* This procedure, performed under local anesthetic between 13 and 20 weeks of pregnancy, involves a gradual dilation of the cervix and removal of the fetus by alternating suction and curettage. This is currently the most common method used in the second trimester.
2. *Prostaglandin (PG) administration.* Prostaglandin E_2 (PGE_2) or $F_2\alpha$ ($PGF_2\alpha$) will cause the uterus to contract and the cervix to soften and dilate. These actions result in the eventual expulsion of the fetus and other products of conception. PGE_2 (prostaglandin E_2) is supplied in the form of vaginal suppositories or gels applied to the cervical canal. $PGF_2\alpha$ is injected directly into the amniotic sac. Side effects include nausea, diarrhea, and fever. Lomotil or Compazine may be prescribed to help control these problems. A rare but very distressing possibility associated with prostaglandin abortions is the delivery of a live abortus.
3. *Other intraamniotic instillations.* Because of the potential for severe life-threatening maternal complications, saline intraamniotic instillations are rarely performed. However, solutions of hypertonic urea may be instilled safely into the amniotic sac (with or without $PGF_2\alpha$) after partial withdrawal of the amniotic fluid. The urea kills the fetus, and the prostaglandin helps ensure expulsion.
4. *Laminaria "tents."* Laminaria are compressed, seaweed cervical inserts that gradually swell in place causing cervical dilation with less trauma than other mechanical means. These may be used to "ripen" the cervix and be followed by PG (prostaglandin) or oxytocin administration or surgical evacuation.
5. *Abdominal hysterotomy.* A type of cesarean birth, a hysterotomy is performed in cases of failed PG or urea instillations when sterilization is desired. It usually involves a hospitalization and recovery period similar to that of a cesarean birth.

Obviously, termination of a pregnancy after the first trimester is a more difficult and hazardous procedure. Currently the majority of second trimester abortions follow determination of fetal anomalies. Of women seeking abortions, 90% do so in the first trimester.

Although complications are few, the most common complications after any abortion are excessive bleeding or infection. Women should be counseled to report excessive bleeding, cramps, or fever. Serious psychiatric problems are rare.

STERILIZATION

In some instances an individual or couple, for health, genetic, social, or personal considerations, may wish to permanently discontinue their capacity to have children. Any process that produces this result is termed *sterilization*. Many couples in the United States now complete their desired families at an early age. Rather than long-term use of contraception, couples are requesting sterilization after they have had their desired number of children. Sterilization procedures may be performed on either the man or the woman. Such procedures do not interfere with the ability to participate in sexual relations, nor do they diminish masculine or feminine characteristics. Some couples report enhanced enjoyment of sexual relations after being freed from the fear of unintended pregnancy.

Over the years, many advances have been made in the techniques of female sterilization. The following is a brief description of the three types of procedures available for tubal ligation:

1 Sterilization using a laparotomy approach, or "mini-laparotomy," involves abdominal incisions to visualize and ligate or otherwise occlude the fallopian tubes. If done during the postpartum period, this is the method most commonly chosen.
2 Sterilization using a laparoscope ("Band-Aid") surgery has been widely publicized and accepted as an inexpensive, safe, and effective method of sterilization. Under general or local anesthesia the physician observes the operative site through a laparoscope introduced into the abdominal cavity through a small incision at the base of the umbilicus. The fallopian tubes may be occluded by electrocoagulation or the placement of several types of clips or rings. This procedure may be performed in a hospital or surgi-center on an inpatient or outpatient basis.
3 Vaginal tubal sterilization may be performed by entering the peritoneal cavity through the posterior vaginal fornix (colpotomy) with or without a scope similar to the laparoscope. The basic sterilization procedure is as described for the laparoscopy technique. This technique is associated with an increased risk of infection.

Sterilization of the man by vas ligation, or vasectomy, is accomplished without entry into the abdominal cavity. It is usually done on an outpatient basis with local anesthesia. Twin surgical incisions are made in the area where the scrotum joins the body, just over the vas. The ducts are tied and separated. Portions may be excised. Follow-up sperm counts are made to confirm sterility and to determine when contraceptive techniques are unnecessary. Although vasectomy is generally a safer, simpler procedure, it is used approximately half as often as tubal sterilization.

Although sterilization procedures are intended to be permanent, occasionally a man or woman may regret his or her decision. In some cases the tubes may be rejoined and reproductive ability regained. Sterilization, however, should be viewed as a lasting intervention. To date, attempts to provide temporary sterility using various devices have been disappointing. Informed consent before undergoing a sterilization procedure is essential.

GENETIC COUNSELING

Advances in understanding genetic disorders have been rapid in the last few years. With this understanding comes an increased need and desire for genetic counseling. Genetic screening offers the possibility of reducing the suffering that results from genetic defects. Screening programs help determine whether certain people are carriers of inherited diseases such as Tay-Sachs disease and sickle cell anemia. There is no coercive action associated with the information given. What persons do with the knowledge they gain is a personal choice. Through the services of a genetic counselor the genealogy of the client or couple is investigated. Such a study is particularly helpful when a hereditary problem has been identified in a person's family but the probability of passing the defect to offspring is unknown. See Chapter 20 for a more complete discussion of genetic factors and genetic counseling.

Genetic screening services should be part of any comprehensive family planning program. Whether the subjects of screening tests are found to be carriers of genetic problems or not, psychological problems may confront them. The nurse must be aware of these possible problems. Nurses often refer clients for genetic counseling. In addition they also have many other opportunities to help couples as they go through the testing process and cope with the outcome (Williams, 1993). Genetic counseling is available in most urban areas to aid the client who has difficulty in understanding the concept of probability, psychological defense reactions, and differences in individual values. A wide range of psychological, ethical, and financial considerations are involved in genetic counseling.

INFERTILITY

The capacity to have children of one's own is desired by and meaningful to most persons. Infertility is usually defined as an inability to conceive after a year of consistent intercourse without the use of contracep-

NATIONAL HEALTH OBJECTIVE FOR THE YEAR 2000

Reduce the incidence of infertility to no more than 6.5% of married couples with wives aged 15 through 44.

tion. Infertility affects approximately 2.4 million married couples and an unknown number among unmarried couples and singles (US Department of Health and Human Services, 1992). See the box above for the related national health objective for the year 2000.

Couples who come to a fertility clinic have two outstanding needs. The first is for education about reproduction and about procedures used to evaluate fertility. The second is for counseling to help them maximize their potential for conceiving. Knowledge about reproduction provides the clients with a basis for understanding the circumstances necessary for conception and the reasons for evaluating fertility.

The first step in evaluating the infertile couple is a complete history and physical examination of both the man and the woman to rule out related endocrine problems, emotional conditions, or disease entities that may be interfering with conception.

The second step is usually an evaluation of the reproductive capacity of the man. Recent semen samples are examined microscopically to detect abnormalities in number, form, and motility of sperm. If few or no sperm are found, hormone analysis, testicular biopsy, and x-ray studies may determine whether the spermatozoa are manufactured but lack transport because of a blockage in the reproductive system. If this is the case, surgery to relieve the obstacle is sometimes possible. If sperm are not being produced or are limited in quantity, hormonal therapy may be helpful.

Evaluation of the female's capacity to conceive is more complex. The difference in the female anatomy requires a complete physical examination. This examination is followed by a determination of the ability of the woman to ovulate. Several methods may be used. These include detection of a characteristic pattern of basal body temperature readings (see Fig. 7-1); urine testing to determine a preovulatory rise in luteinizing hormone (LH) levels; microscopic examination of a biopsy of the endometrium, or lining of the uterus; and investigation of the viscosity of the cervical mucus. If ovulation is established, examination of the patency of the fallopian tubes through dye and gas studies may be performed. The uterine cavity, the vaginal canal, and the type and action of cervical and vaginal secretions may also be investigated.

If ovulation does not occur, hormonal therapy and general measures to improve health may be helpful. One example of a hormonal product that stimulates ovarian function is a follicle-stimulating hormone called menotropins (Pergonal). Another medication that has been used to promote pregnancy is clomiphene citrate (Clomid). Perganol in particular has been known to promote the maturation of more than one ovum during the menstrual cycle, causing the development of multiple births (for example, quadruplets and quintuplets). Since these infants are usually of low birth weight and very fragile, multiple births are a mixed blessing to even the most eager parents.

Surgical intervention to open blocked passageways that must be traversed by the ascending sperm or the descending egg may also be performed with varying success, depending on the area treated. Sometimes the diagnostic procedures used to detect fallopian tube obstruction also serve as therapy, causing the removal of minor blocks in the oviducts. Medical treatment of pelvic inflammatory disease may also enable conception to occur.

Alternative birth technologies

The 1978 birth of the first "test tube baby" added yet another alternative for selected clients previously unable to conceive because of oviduct defects. A *test tube baby* is a fetus that is conceived by a process known medically as *in vitro fertilization* (IVF). An egg is removed from the mother-to-be approximately 2 weeks after her last menstrual period has occurred. This is done through a process known as *laparoscopy*, or more recently, *transvaginal aspiration under sonography*. The egg is then placed in a specialized culture fluid and kept in an incubator. At an appropriate later time a specific quantity of sperm from the father-to-be is introduced into the fluid containing the egg in the incubator.

Under these circumstances, fertilization occurs. The zygote is then removed from the fertilization fluid using a microscope and placed in a fresh culture fluid for a day or two to allow time for growth and division. The microscopic multicellular embryo is then transferred into the woman's uterus.

In 1984 an important modification was developed involving transfer of egg(s) and sperm into the distal end of a patent fallopian tube directly after aspiration. This procedure is called *gamete intrafallopian transfer* (**GIFT**). In major centers where there is extensive experience with the IVF procedure the pregnancy rate is about 20%. The **GIFT** technique may increase a couple's possibility of parenthood beyond this percentage. This expensive technology is rapidly advancing and changing.

At times, persistent failure to conceive because of certain male defects can be circumvented through artificial insemination techniques using the husband's sperm. More rarely, semen from an anonymous, healthy, normal man may be used. Instances of so-called surrogate motherhood have also been reported. This is a legally precarious and controversial arrangement whereby the sperm of the husband is inseminated into another woman who carries the resulting fetus to term and then relinquishes the infant to the couple.

Nursing implications

Infertility treatment uses invasive procedures, advanced technology, surgery, and potent drugs, and is expensive. The treatment may last from 3 to 5 years and exacts a high emotional and physical toll. High-technology interventions are often not covered by conventional medical insurance. Nurses are in a pivotal position to alleviate some of the stresses that couples experience as they go through the treatment process. Health care practitioners need to engage in ongoing assessments of patients' stress and tolerance of specific treatment regimens, inquire about the impact that treatment has on other aspects of their lives, and be sensitive in their approach to clients (Blenner, 1992).

The conventional methods of formal adoption or foster parenthood, although sometimes not available to couples and often involving long waiting periods, may be a satisfying solution. Pursuing these options, however, should await the couple's resolving their feelings about their inability to conceive or carry a pregnancy to live birth (Sherrod, 1992).

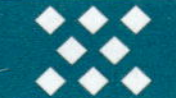

KEY CONCEPTS

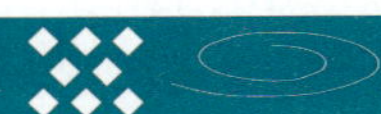

1 Fertility is the ability of the body to create and sustain new life.

2 Family planning is the effort to control fertility. Components of a comprehensive family planning program include: contraceptive education, genetic counseling, infertility counseling and methods of fertility enhancement, alternative birth technologies, and adoption.

3 Natural family planning (NFP) is characterized by avoidance of intercourse during fertile periods. The fertility awareness method (FAM) uses a barrier method of contraception during fertile intervals.

4 Contraceptive methods that prevent fertilization are abstinence, coitus interruptus, periodic abstinence, and local barrier methods. Methods that prevent ovulation include oral contraceptives and injectable and implanted progestins. Methods that prevent implantation are intrauterine devices (IUDs).

5 The most reliable methods of (temporary) contraception are those that prevent ovulation ("the pill," Norplant, Depo-Provera), condoms used with spermicidal agents, and IUDs.

6 Frequently reported side effect of oral contraceptives include nausea, breast tenderness, weight gain or loss, mood changes, and irregular vaginal bleeding.

7 The 1973 US Supreme Court decision regarding abortion *(Roe v. Wade)* specifies that the decision to have an abortion in the first trimester of pregnancy rests with the woman in consultation with her physician. In the second trimester the state can regulate conditions under which an abortion is performed but cannot prohibit the procedure before viability. The state may prohibit abortion in the third trimester except to save the life or health of the mother.

8 The 1989 US Supreme Court decision in the case of *Webster v. Reproductive Health Services* allows a state to forbid the use of public money and facilities for abortion services. This decision may impact the availability and access to abortion services for poor women.

9 Four types of surgical interventions result in sterilization. Tubal ligation or occlusion in women can be achieved via (1) a laparotomy, (2) a laparoscopy, or (3) a vaginal approach. Sterilization of the man is accomplished by vasectomy.

10 The usual definition of infertility is the inability to conceive after a year of periodic intercourse without the use of contraception. If infertility is the result of the absence of ovulation, hormonal therapy may be helpful. Surgical intervention to open blocked fallopian tubes has been performed with varying success.

CRITICAL THOUGHT QUESTIONS 

1 Develop a teaching plan for patients interested in learning more about "natural" methods of preventing conception.

2 The Lees are in their twenties, in good health, and have been married for 2 years. They want to delay having children for another 2 years. They are interested in learning about contraceptive methods that are very reliable but that do not interfere with the spontaneity of the sex act. How would you advise them? Why?

3 Elective abortion is a national issue. Some individuals maintain a pro-life stance and others maintain a pro-choice stance. Explore your own values and beliefs regarding this issue. How will they affect your ability or willingness to assist with an elective abortion?

4 Elective sterilization is possible for both males and females. If a couple chooses this option, which spouse do you think should be sterilized? Why?

5 Infertility is often a wrenching emotional issue for those affected. As a nurse, what actions would convey sensitivity to (1) a couple in their second year of intensive, unsuccessful therapy or (2) a couple experiencing their third miscarriage (spontaneous abortion) after conception achieved through infertility therapy?

REFERENCES

Association of Women's Health, Obstetric, and Neonatal Nurses: Drug approved as contraception, *AWHONN Voice* 1(1):4, 1993.

Baylor College of Medicine: RU 486: an overview of mifepristone and its potential applications, *The Contraception Report* 4(2):7-9, 1993a.

Baylor College of Medicine: Contraception during breastfeeding, *The Contraception Report* 4(5):7-11, 1993b.

Blenner J: Stress and mediators: patients' perceptions of infertility treatment, *Image* 41(2):92-97, 1992.

Engel NS: Update on cancer risk and oral contraceptives, *MCN* 15(1):37, 1990.

Harlap S, Kost K, Forrest J: *Preventing pregnancy, protecting health: a new look at birth control choices in the United States,* New York, 1991, The Alan Guttmacher Institute.

Harrison LK, Naylor KL: The laws that affect abortion in the United States and their impact on women's health, *Nurse Pract* 16(12):53, 1991.

Hatcher RA, Trussell J, Stewart GK, et al: *Contraceptive technology,* ed 16, New York, 1994, Irvington.

Institute of Medicine: *Preventing low birthweight,* Washington, DC, 1985, National Academy.

Nurses' Association of the American College of Obstetricians and Gynecologists: *Contraceptive options: OGN nursing practice resource,* Washington, DC, September 1991, The Association.

Sherrod RA: Helping infertile couples explore the option of adoption, *J Obstet Gynecol Neonatal Nurs* 21(6):465-470, 1992.

US Department of Health and Human Services: *Healthy people 2000: national health promotion and disease prevention objectives,* Boston, 1992, Jones and Bartlett.

Williams JK: New genetic discoveries increase counseling opportunities, *MCN* 18(4):218-222, 1993.

BIBLIOGRAPHY

Blenner J: Clomiphene-induced mood swings, *J Obstet Gynecol Neonatal Nurs* 20(4):321-327, 1991.

Blenner J: Health care providers' treatment approaches to culturally diverse infertile patients, *J of Transcult Nurs* 2(2):24-27, 1991.

Fehring RJ: New technology in natural family planning, *J Obstet Gynecol Neonatal Nurs* 20(3):199-205, 1991.

Frank DI: Factors related to decisions about infertility, *J Obstet Gynecol Neonatal Nurs* 19(2):162-167, 1990.

Goode CJ, Hahn SJ: Oocyte donation and in vitro fertilization: the nurse's role with ethical and legal issues, *J Obstet Gynecol Neonatal Nurs* 22(2):106-111, 1993.

Hinkle LT: Education and counseling for Norplant users, *J Obstet Gynecol Neonatal Nurs* 23(5):387-391, 1994.

Jarret M, Lethbridge D: The contraceptive needs of midlife women, *Nurse Pract* 15(2):34-39, 1990.

King J: Helping patients choose an appropriate method of birth control, *MCN* 17(2):91-95, 1990.

Lethbridge D: Coitus interruptus as a method of birth control *J Obstet Gynecol Neonatal Nurs* 20(1):80-85, 1991.

Libbus MK: Condoms as primary prevention in sexually active women, *MCN* 17(5):256-260, 1992.

Lommel L, Taylor D: Adolescent use of contraceptives, *NAACOG Clin Issues Perinat Women's Health Nurs* 3(2):199-208, 1992.

Low M: Personal values and contraceptive choices, *NAACOG Clin Issues Perinat Women's Health Nurs* 3(2):192-198, 1992.

Mueller L: Second-trimester termination of pregnancy: nursing care, *J Obstet Gynecol Neonatal Nurs* 20(4):284-289, 1991.

Prattke TW, Gass-Sternas KA: Appraisal, coping, and emotional health of infertile couples undergoing donor artificial insemination, *J Obstet Gynecol Neonatal Nurs* 22(6):516-527, 1993.

Stampfer MJ, Willett WC, Colditz GA: Past use of oral contraceptives and cardiovascular disease: a meta-analysis in the context of the Nurses' Health Study, *Am J Obstet Gynecol* 163:285-291, 1990.

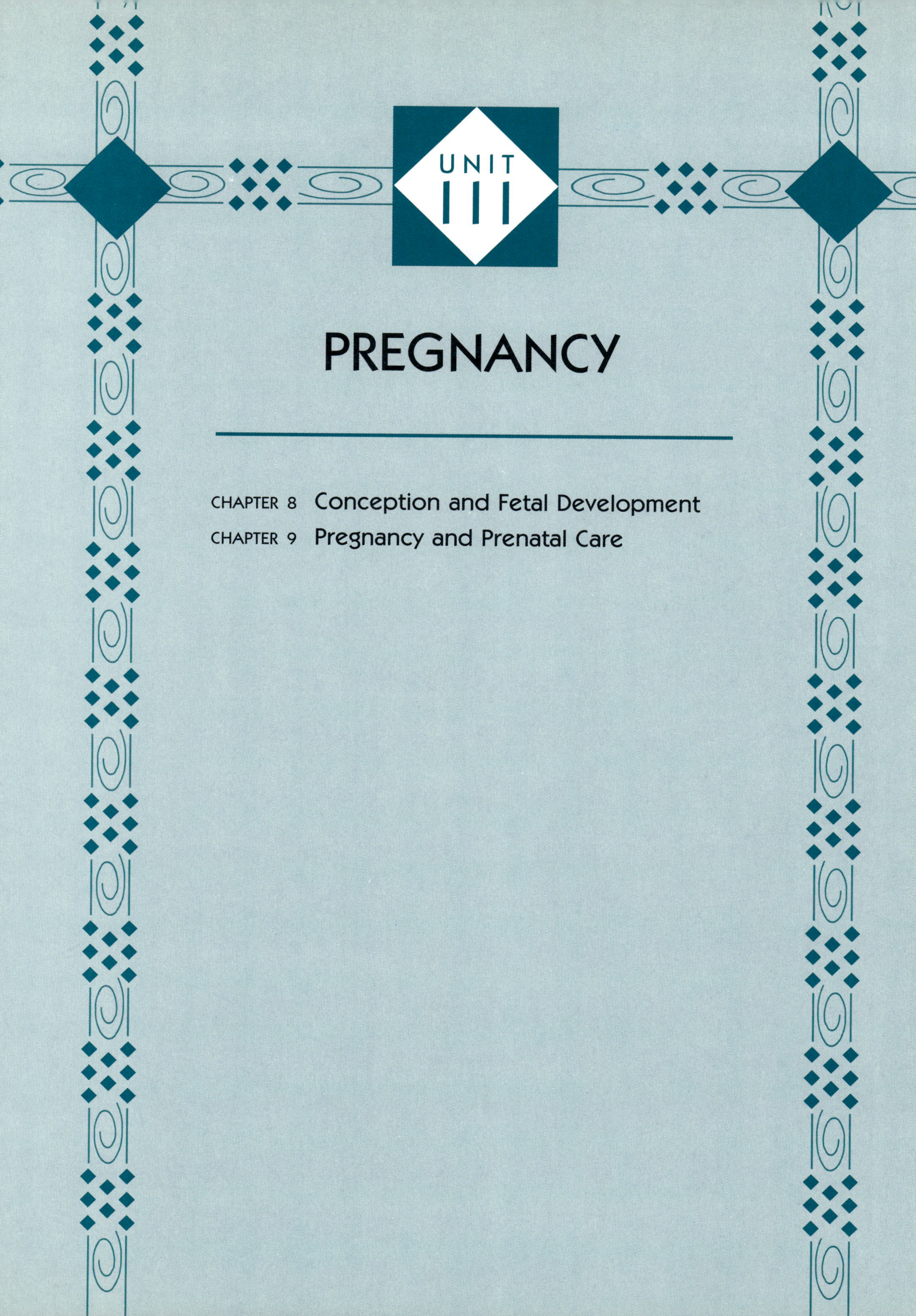

UNIT III

PREGNANCY

8

Conception and Fetal Development

CHAPTER OBJECTIVES

After studying this chapter, the student should be able to:

1. Describe the normal duration of human gestation based on menstrual history versus fertilization (conception).
2. Describe how the infant's gender is determined.
3. Define the following terms: *fertilization* or *conception, zygote, morula, implantation, decidua, embryo, fetus, placenta, chorion,* and *amnion.*
4. List the functions of the placenta and the amniotic fluid.
5. Identify the gestational week for the following stages of fetal development or progression of pregnancy:
   a. Rudimentary organ systems completely formed.
   b. Fetal heart beat heard by ultrasound fetoscope and by conventional fetoscope.
   c. Quickening felt by multiparas and primiparas.
   d. The term *fetus* can first be used to describe the growing child.
   e. Uterine fundus at or slightly above the maternal umbilicus.
   f. Lightening experienced by primiparas.
6. Explain the effect of the production of human chorionic gonadotropin (hCG) in pregnant women and hCG's influence on pregnancy tests.
7. Trace the normal fetal circulation pattern through the placenta, umbilical vein and arteries, ductus venosus, foramen ovale, and ductus arteriosus.
8. Differentiate between fraternal and identical twins.
9. Define teratogen.
10. Describe eight ways that the age, size, maturity, and well-being of the fetus may be assessed in utero.
11. List the presumptive signs of pregnancy, noting other conditions that cause similar signs or symptoms.
12. List the probable signs of pregnancy, and explain why they are only probable.
13. Indicate the positive signs of pregnancy, and explain why they are considered positive.
14. Discuss the development of parental attachment to the unborn child.

Conception, the union of the male sex cell (sperm) and the female sex cell (ovum), sets into motion a period of growth unequaled at any other time in the life of an individual. Just after fertilization, or conception, the ovum is almost as large as the period ending a sentence. Within approximately 9 calendar months, however, the ovum will increase in size approximately 200 billion times, become a highly complex structure, and attain the personality of the infant. The length of human gestation is

280 days, or 40 weeks, when calculated from the first day of the last menstrual period (menstrual or gestational age); 266 days, or 38 weeks, when calculated from conception (fertilization age)—a more difficult event to pinpoint. The time description of fetal development used in this chapter is based on development from conception.

Genetic Considerations

The nucleus of each body cell contains a certain number of threadlike strands called *chromosomes,* which are composed of strands of deoxyribonucleic acid (DNA) and protein. Genes are lengths of DNA that contain unique hereditary elements. The chromosome number is constant for each species. For example, human beings have 46 chromosomes, divided into 23 pairs, in each body tissue cell. Twenty-two pairs of chromosomes are called *autosomes* and are different in genetic content and appearance. The child inherits genetic material from both parents. The twenty-third pair contains the sex chromosomes (XX or XY). The sex cells (gametes) of the male and female, however, are unlike the rest of the cells found in the body. Through a special process called *meiosis,* the chromosome count in these cells is reduced by half. When male and female sex cells unite at fertilization the chromosome count is restored to 46 in the new developing embryo. See Chapter 20 for a more in-depth discussion of genetic influences.

Gender Determination

At fertilization, each parent donates only one sex chromosome. The mother always contributes an X chromosome; the father, however, may contribute either an X or a Y chromosome. As a result the gender of the child is determined by the type of male sex cell that penetrates the ovum or egg. When the sperm that unites with an ovum carries the Y chromosome, a boy (XY) will result; if the sperm that fertilizes the egg carries an X chromosome, a girl (XX) will result. Although research exploring possible ways to preselect the gender of one's offspring continues, such as controlling the acidity or alkalinity of the vagina or using certain techniques and timing for intercourse, the results are often unreliable. However, as knowledge of genetic potential and control expands, preselection of one's offspring is likely to become a more complex ethical issue.

EMBRYOLOGY

Conception normally takes place in the fallopian tube (Table 8-1). The fertilized cell (zygote) soon divides into two, then four, then eight cells, and so on. The fertilized egg, or zygote, assumes the bumpy appearance of a mulberry and is called a *morula* as it journeys down the fallopian tube toward the uterus.

Implantation

The journey from the ovary to the uterine cavity, where implantation occurs, takes approximately 7 days. At the end of this time the zygote, now a hollow, fluid-filled *blastocyst*, burrows into the soft uterine lining. The outer layer of the blastocyst (the trophoblast) becomes covered with fingerlike tissue projections called *chorionic villi.* These projections aid in the process of the zygote's implantation in the endometrium (known as the *decidua* during pregnancy). Implantation may cause limited bleeding, similar to menstrual spotting.

The villi also manufacture the *human chorionic gonadotropin* (hCG) that signals the corpus luteum in the ovary to continue manufacturing progesterone and estrogen, preventing menstruation and ovulation. After implantation the aggregation of the cells of the blastocyst begins to form a definite pattern. A small yolk sac forms red blood cells during the first 6 weeks of embryonic development, until the embryo's liver takes over the process. The yolk sac is then incorporated into the umbilical cord. A microscopic embryonic disk develops, marking the beginning of the child and its basic support system. Ten days after conception the zygote is developed enough to be called an embryo.

Embryonic Membranes

At the time of implantation, two fetal membranes, the chorion and the amnion, begin to form. The *chorion* is the thick, outer membrane that develops from the trophoblast. The chorionic villi on the surface of the chorion, located under the embryo, form the fetal portion of the placenta. The function of the villi is to facilitate the transfer of nutrients from maternal blood and the elimination of fetal waste. The inner layer, the *amnion*, develops from the ectoderm, a basic germ layer. The cells of the thin amnion produce amniotic fluid, in which the fetus floats. The amount of amniotic fluid is about 30 ml at 10 weeks. It ranges from 500 to 1000 ml after 20 weeks. The amniotic fluid helps control the environmental temperature of the fetus and protects it from trauma and infection. As the amnion expands with the growth of the embryo, it fuses with the chorion. Together these two form the amniotic sac, commonly known as the *bag of waters,* or the *membranes.* Normally the membranes remain intact until the time of labor and birth.

Placenta

After the implantation of a zygote the placenta, or afterbirth, develops (Fig. 8-1). The maternal portion of

◆ **TABLE 8-1**
Prenatal Calendar

General Developmental Characteristics (Schematically Pictured)		Average Weight and Size	Maternal Findings and Diagnostic Aids
Fetal growth measured from conception **Germinal stage (1 to 10 days)** **First week**			
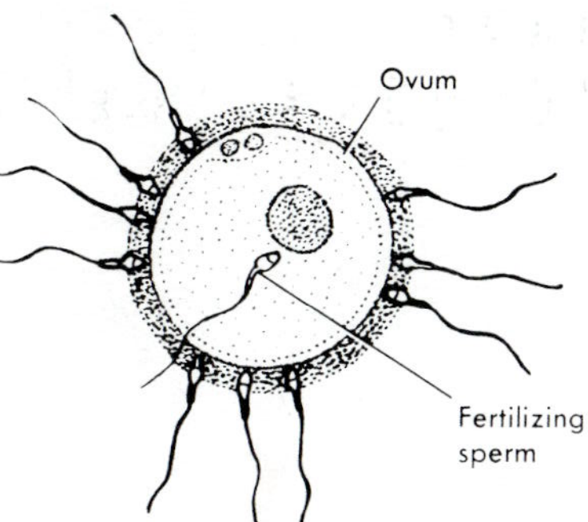	*Zygote* forms: ovum fertilized in fallopian tube undergoes cell divisions (cleavage) on way to uterus.	Just visible to eye.	Maternal changes measured using menstrual/gestational age (GA) (2 weeks added to fertilization age) or as indicated. 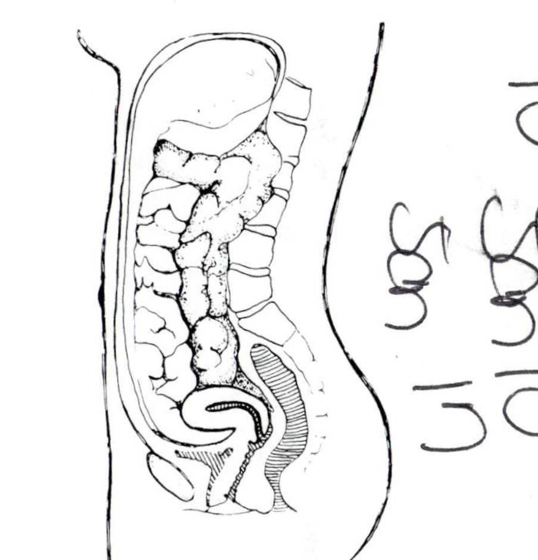 Normal female pelvis before implantation (sagittal section).
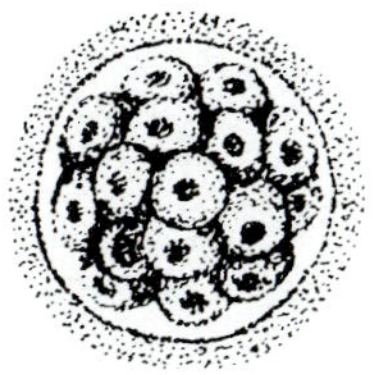	*Morula* forms: solid mass of about 16 microscopic cells resembling mulberry; enters uterus on third day.		
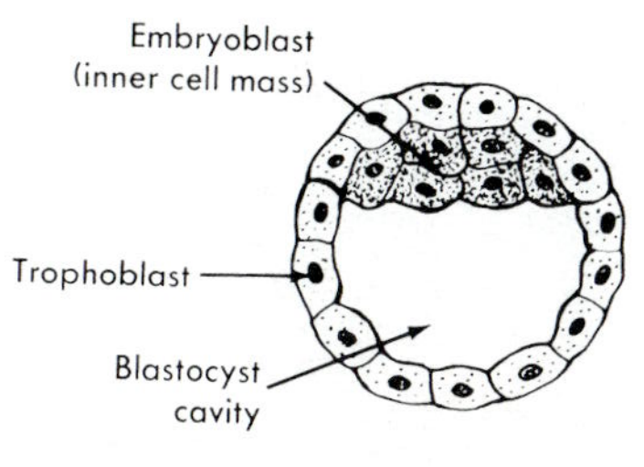	*Blastocyst:* morula develops fluid-filled cavity; *trophoblast:* outer wall of blastocyst: *embryoblast:* inner cell mass from which embryo eventually forms.		

Continued.

◆ TABLE 8-1
Prenatal Calendar—cont'd

General Developmental Characteristics (Schematically Pictured)		Average Weight and Size	Maternal Findings and Diagnostic Aids
Trophoblastic tissue; Endometrium; Inner cell mass	Beginning implantation of blastocyst in endometrium by invading trophoblastic tissue ±7 days.		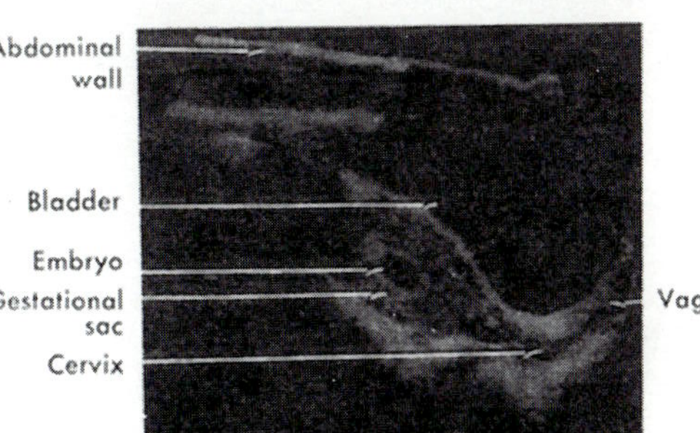 From Hertig AT, Beck J: Contr Embryol Carneg Inst, Wash 29:127, 1941.
Embryonic stage (10 days to eighth week) **Second week** 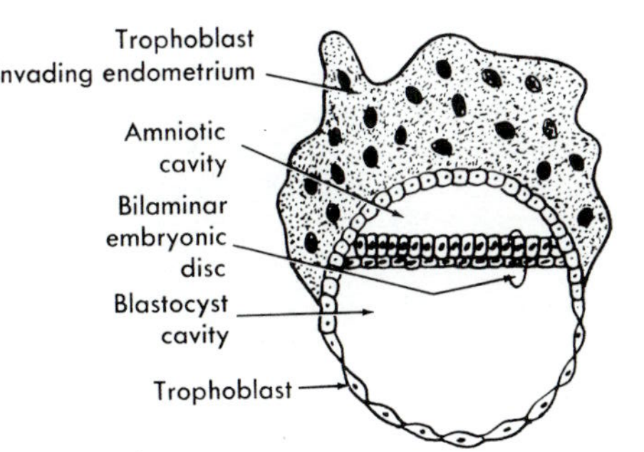	Implantation deepens and is completed; primitive uteroplacental circulation originates from enlarging trophoblast and maternal endometrial tissues. *Amniotic cavity* appears as an opening between inner cell mass and invading trophoblast; a thin lining becomes amnion. Two-layered (bilaminar) embryo called *embryonic disc* develops, formed by ectoderm and endoderm. *Yolk sac* present.		Implantation site of human embryo at about 12 days (see *arrow*). Endometrium covers blastocyst, producing elevation or wartlike bulge on uterine surface.
Third week Embryonic disc; Connecting stalk; Yolk sac Embryonic ectoderm; Intraembryonic mesoderm; Embryonic endoderm; Trilaminar embryonic disc	Thickening in midline of ectoderm gives rise to *mesoderm*, a third layer between ectoderm and endoderm forming trilaminar embryo; basic embryological beginnings of body systems and organs.	1/10 inch (2 to 3 mm)	Amenorrhea. Human chorionic gonadotropin (hCG) in urine beginning 10 days after conception; tests not always sensitive. Ultrasonogram may reveal pregnancy as early as 3 to 4 weeks postconception.

	Three basic embryonic layers: 1. *Endoderm:* forerunner of lining of gastrointestinal tract from pharynx to rectum; epithelial parts of trachea, bronchi, lungs, liver, pancreas, and urinary bladder. 2. *Ectoderm:* forerunner of mucous membrane, tooth enamel, hair, nails, mammary glands, and nervous system. 3. *Mesoderm:* forerunner of heart and blood vessels, spleen, blood and lymph cells, bones, and muscles. Neural tube, beginning of central nervous system, forms in midline of cranial portion of ectoderm.		
Fourth week	Cells group in mesoderm to form primitive blood vessels and blood cells; heart tube forms and contracts to circulate blood by end of third week; umbilical vessels pass through connecting stalk to placenta. Flat, disclike embryo folds to form typical C-shaped cylinder. Rapid development of forebrain portion of neural tube. Heart prominence seen. Arm and leg buds; forerunners of ears and eyes appear. Primitive gut formed with incorporation of dorsal yolk sac. Rudimentary lungs, kidneys.	$\frac{1}{16}$ inch (5 mm)	Nausea and vomiting. Urinary frequency. Breast tenderness, tingling, swelling. Montgomery's tubercles visible. Uterine enlargement. Increased cervical secretions.

Continued.

◆ **TABLE 8-1**
Prenatal Calendar—cont'd

General Developmental Characteristics (Schematically Pictured)		Average Weight and Size	Maternal Findings and Diagnostic Aids
Fifth through seventh weeks 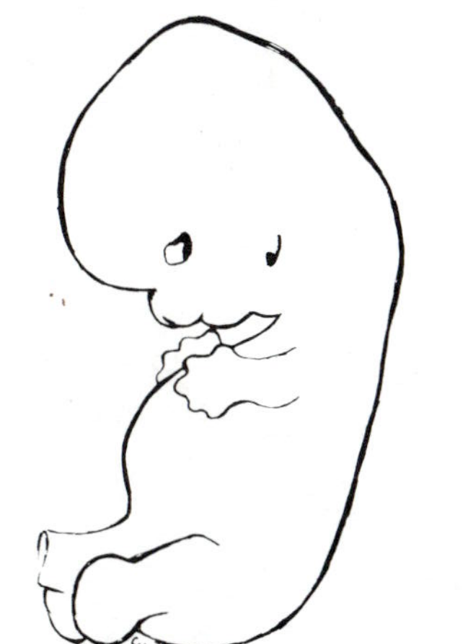 By end of seventh week all essential systems present.	Rapid brain development. Retina of eye forms. Heart becomes chambered. Fingers, toes, and eyes are becoming visible. Palate and upper lip forming. Gastrointestinal tract develops; part of intestine still in umbilical cord. Rapid formation of urogenital systems.		Softening of cervix (Goodell's sign). Softening of uterine isthmus (Hegar's sign). Violet coloration of cervix and vagina (Chadwick's sign). 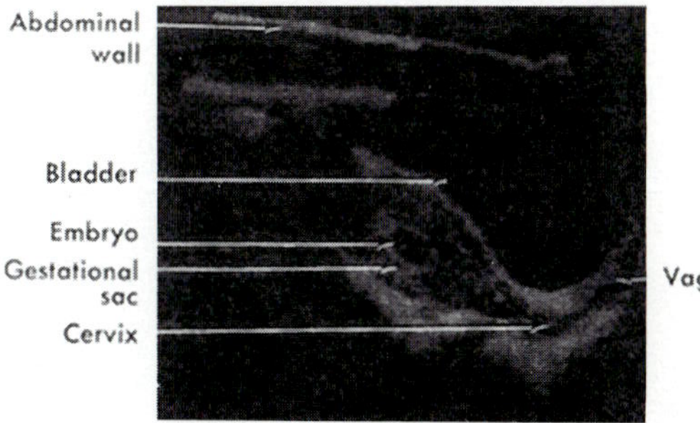 **Sonogram of 6-weeks gestational sac containing embryo.** *(Courtesy George R. Leopold, MD, University Hospital, San Diego, CA.)*
Fetal stage (eighth week to birth) **Eighth through tenth weeks**	Development mainly involves growth and maturation of structures begun in embryo; fetus less vulnerable to effects of drugs, most infections, and radiation. Head almost half fetal length at 8 weeks (see fetus within amniotic sac).	1⅛ inches (3 cm) $\frac{1}{15}$ oz (2 gm)	Chorionic villus sampling (8 to 11 weeks).

Eleventh through twelfth weeks 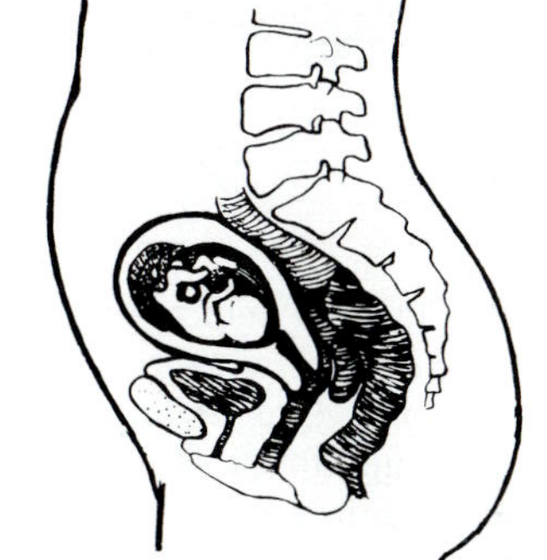 	Facial features forming. Eyelids present and fused. Intestine retracted from umbilical cord into abdomen. Palate fusion complete. External sex identification possible. Well-defined neck. Nail beds beginning. Tooth buds forming.	Crown-heel length: 4½ inches (11.5 cm) ⅔ oz (20 gm)	Frequent urination and nausea have usually disappeared. Fetal heart tone may be detected with Doppler techniques. 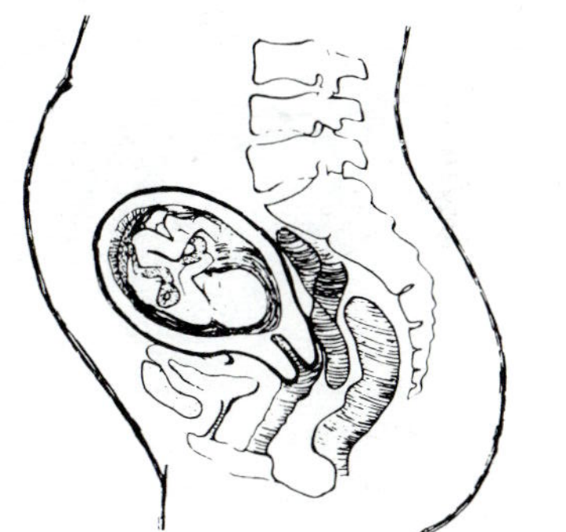 Fundus of uterus rises above pubic bone between 12 and 16 weeks.
Thirteenth through sixteenth weeks 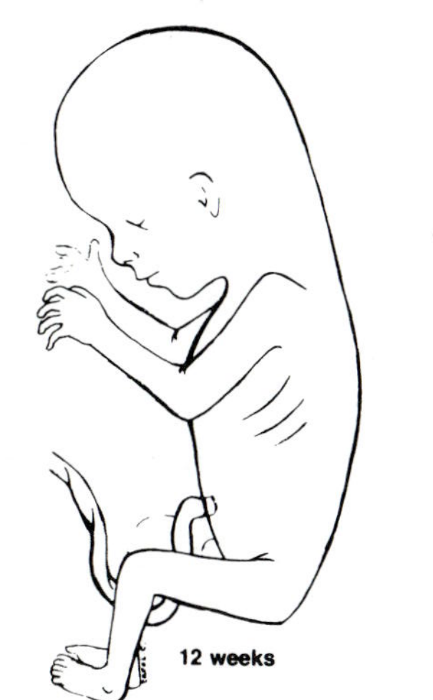	Rapid growth of limbs and trunk; head less prominent. Active fetus. Skeleton calcified on x-ray examination by sixteenth week. Increasing respiratory movement detected by sonogram. Approximately 150 to 280 ml amniotic fluid present. Placenta distinct.	7½ inches (19 cm) 3⅓ oz (100 gm)	Amniocentesis between 14 and 20 weeks. 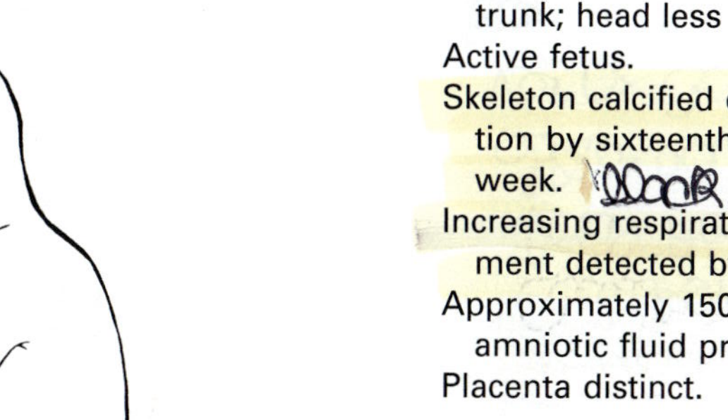 Fundus half distance between pubic and umbilicus at 16 weeks.

Continued.

◆ TABLE 8-1
Prenatal Calendar—cont'd

General Developmental Characteristics (Schematically Pictured)		Average Weight and Size	Maternal Findings and Diagnostic Aids
Seventeenth through twentieth weeks	Eyebrows, lanugo, and vernix appear. Nipples barely visible. (illustration shows placental relationship) Scalp hair visible. Fetus able to hear sounds within mother and in external world.	8¾ inches (22 cm) 10 oz (300 gm)	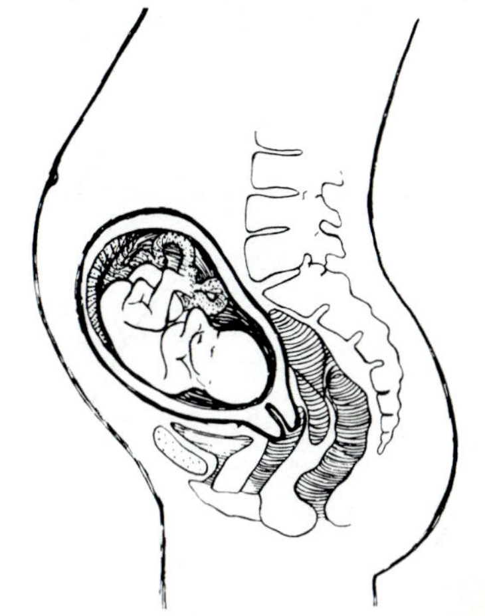 Quickening at 16 to 18 weeks. Fetal heart tone detected by standard fetoscope (18 to 20 weeks). Secondary areola prominent. Fundus at umbilicus or slightly above at 20 weeks. Chloasma (mask of pregnancy). Striae may develop.
Twenty-fourth week	External ear soft, flat, shapeless. Skin wrinkled, translucent, appears pink; blood in capillaries shows. Lanugo covers body. Alveoli begin to form.	12½ inches (32 cm) 1¼ lb (600 gm)	

Twenty-eighth week 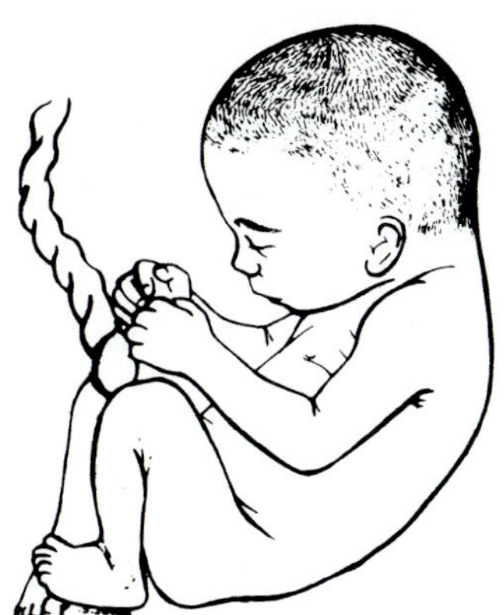	Subcutaneous fat appears, fingernails and toenails. Testes at internal inguinal ring or below. Eyes open. Scalp hair well developed.	14 inches (36 cm) 2¼ lb (1100 gm)
Thirty-second week 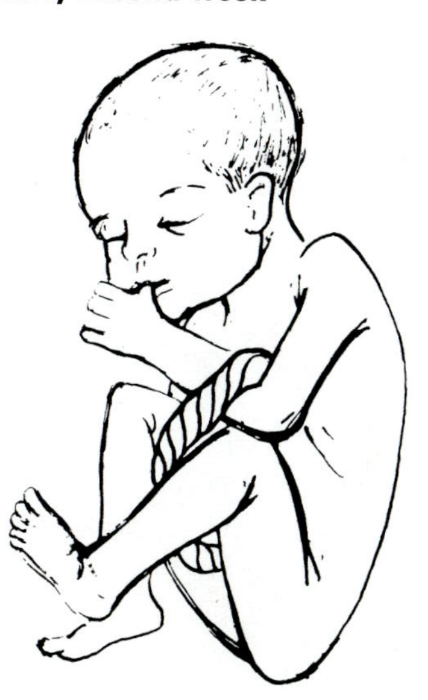	Hair fine and woolly. Nails to fingertips. Prominent clitoris; labia majora small and separated. Skin pink and smooth. One or two creases on anterior portion of soles. Breast areolae visible but flat.	16 inches (41 cm) 3¾ lb (1800 gm)

Continued.

◆ TABLE 8-1
Prenatal Calendar—cont'd

General Developmental Characteristics (Schematically Pictured)		Average Weight and Size	Maternal Findings and Diagnostic Aids
Thirty-sixth week 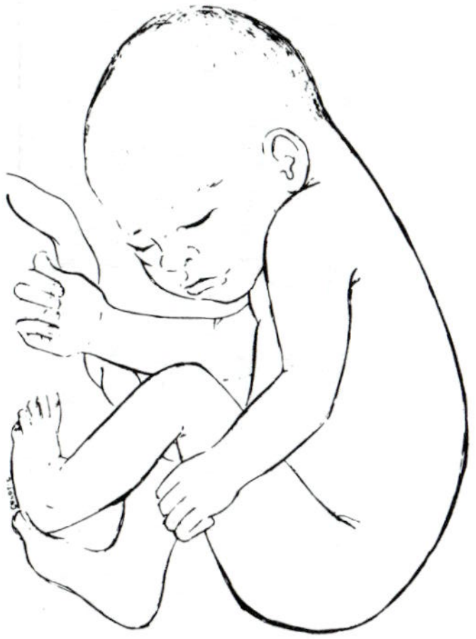	Body, limbs more rounded. Skin thicker, whiter; lanugo disappearing. Breast tissue develops under nipples. Scrotal rugae few. Testes in inguinal canal. Sole creases involve anterior two thirds of sole.	18 inches (46 cm) 4½ lb (2200 gm)	Dyspnea because of pressure on diaphragm. Lightening in primigravidas about 38 weeks. Urinary frequency returns. Increasing prominence of Braxton Hicks contractions. Colostrum may appear in breasts. In primigravida, characteristic cervical effacement may be noted by pelvic examination.
Full-term **End of thirty-eighth week (fertilization age)** 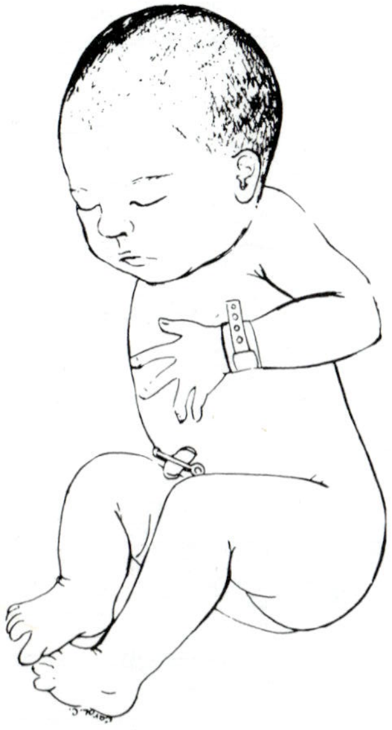	Skin whitish pink. Lanugo gone from face. Hair in single strands. Vernix decreasing. Areola 5 to 6 mm with 7 to 10 mm breast tissue. Ear well defined by outer incurving to lobe, erect from head. Testes in scrotum. Labia majora meet in midline; cover labia minora and clitoris.	20 inches (51 cm) 6.6+ lb (3200+ gm)	At term (40 weeks, GA) 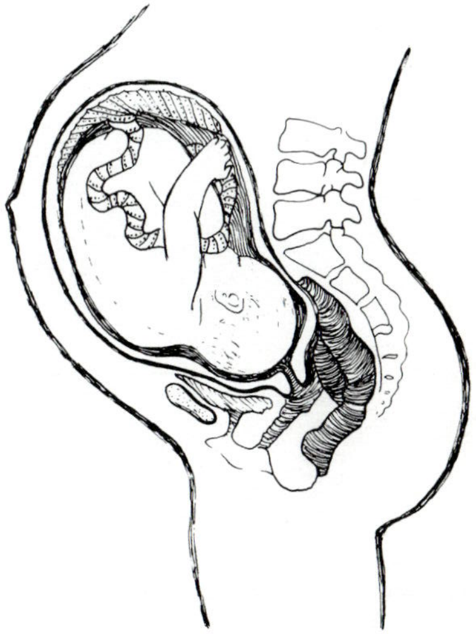

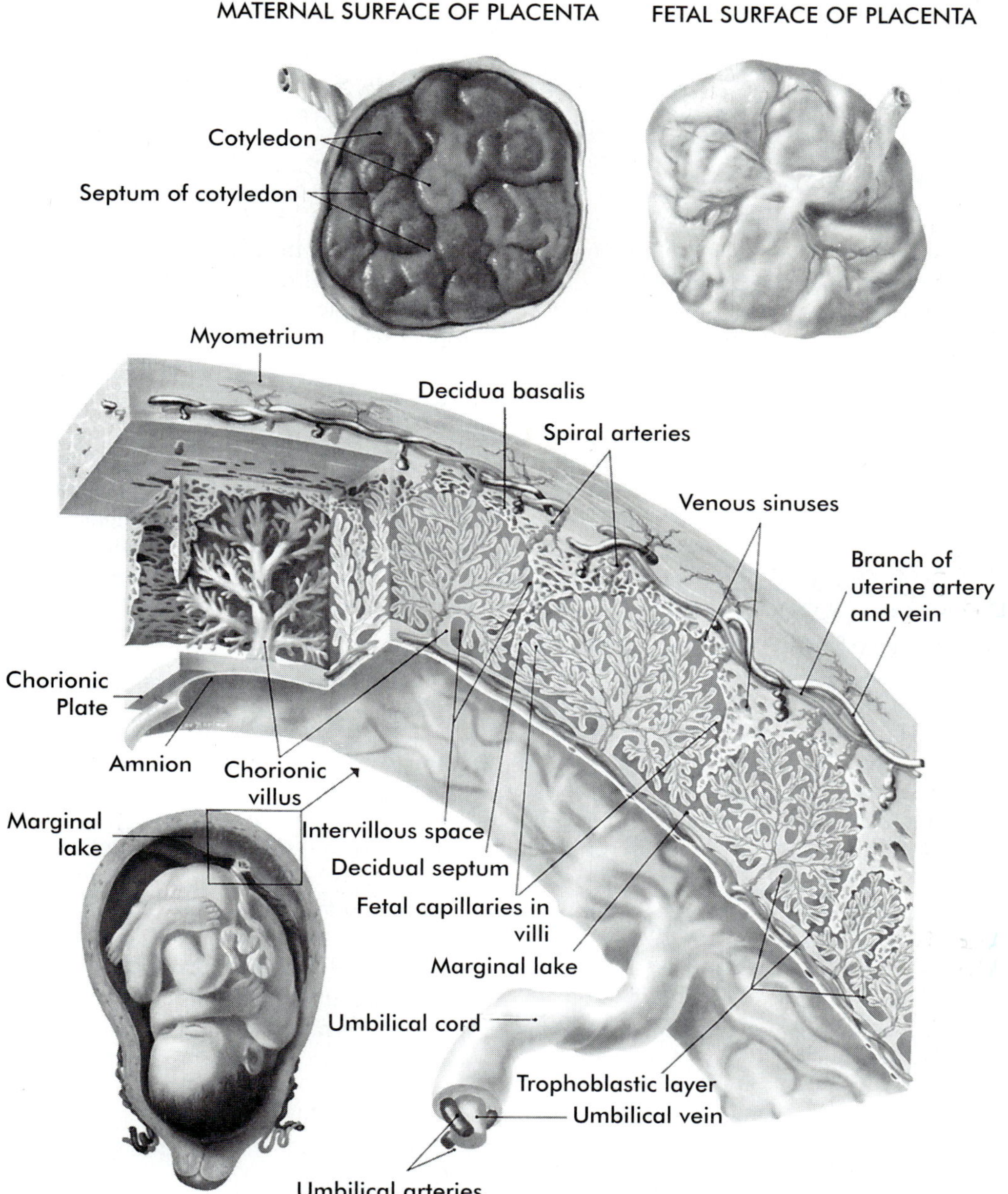

Fig. 8-1 Placental structure and circulation. (Courtesy Ross Laboratories, Columbus, OH.)

the placenta consists of the decidua and its circulation. The fetal portion consists of the chorionic villi and their circulation. Maternal and fetal blood are separated by thin layers of tissue and do not mix. Occasional breaks in this tissue, however, can allow fetal red blood cells to pass into the maternal circulation. These tissue breaks are most likely at the time of delivery. Using complex molecular processes the placenta transports nutrients and oxygen necessary for fetal growth and development from the maternal circulation to the fetal circulation. Using the same processes, carbon dioxide and other metabolic wastes are eliminated from the fetal circulation via the placenta and maternal bloodstream. The placenta provides protection from harmful substances that are not easily transported, such as drugs with high molecular weights. The placenta also functions as an endocrine organ, manufacturing estrogen, progesterone, chorionic gonadotropin, as well as other hormones and enzymes. These substances influence the growth and maintenance of the pregnancy and the maternal preparation for birth and lactation. Maternal antibodies are also thought to be transferred to the fetus during this time, providing temporary immunity to some diseases.

Umbilical Cord

The umbilical cord develops from the amnion. The cord is usually attached to the center of the placenta, although other points of insertion are possible. Oxygenated blood flows from the placenta to the fetus through the large umbilical vein in the umbilical cord. The two arteries in the umbilical cord are wound around the umbilical vein and carry fetal waste to the placenta. The number of vessels contained in the umbilical cord should be counted at delivery. If only two exist, one artery and one vein, the newborn should be evaluated for congenital malformations. Connective tissue known as *Wharton's jelly* surrounds and protects the cord vessels.

THE FETUS

From the eighth week of growth the embryo has developed enough to be called a *fetus,* meaning "young one." The fetus is less than 2 inches (about 3 cm) long and weighs a fraction of an ounce. Rudimentary body systems are formed and working. The skeleton is also becoming established (Fig. 8-2).

Fetal heart tones can be heard by electronic doppler devices between 8 and 12 weeks.

Twelve weeks

By the twelfth week the face is well formed. The gender of the fetus is clearly discernible, and the genitourinary tract is completely developed. Spontaneous fetal movements are also present.

Sixteen weeks

At 16 weeks of intrauterine development the fetus has increased in size considerably. It is approximately 7½ inches (19 cm) long and weighs about 3⅓ ounces (100 gm). The uterus is correspondingly larger, and the expectant mother may begin to wear maternity clothes. At 16 to 18 weeks' gestation pregnant women usually report feeling fetal movement, or *quickening.*

Twenty weeks

At 20 weeks of growth the fetus is about 8¾ inches (22 cm) long and weighs approximately 10 ounces (300 gm). The fetal heartbeat is heard using a standard fetoscope, and muscles are well developed. The top of the uterus (the fundus) is 20 cm from the symphysis pubis.

Twenty-four weeks

At 24 weeks the fetus is about 12½ inches (32 cm) long and weighs about 1¼ pounds (600 gm). The eye is structurally complete and will soon open. Eyelashes and eyebrows are formed. Little subcutaneous fat exists and the skin is covered with vernix caseosa. The alveoli (tiny air sacs) in the lungs are forming.

Some state laws declare that the legal threshold of viability is 24 weeks' gestation; others use 20 weeks' gestation as the lower limit. However the true length of a pregnancy may be difficult to determine. Moral-ethical dilemmas involving the rights and responsibilities of the parents and the community result, as well as

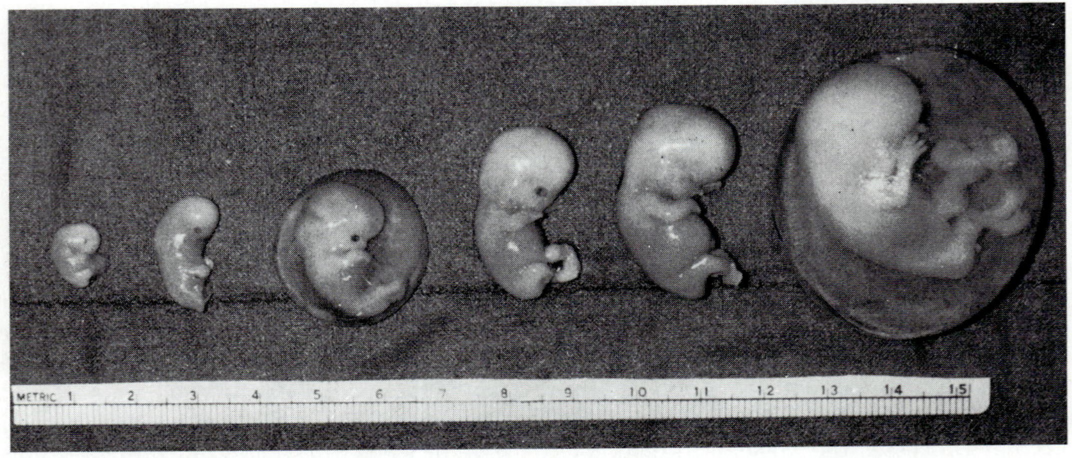

Fig. 8-2 Progressive growth of the human fetus (measured in centimeters). Two amniotic sacs are still intact. (Courtesy Jeanne I. Miller, MD, Modesto, CA.)

consideration for the life and well-being of the developing fetus. Infants of less than 24 weeks' gestation that survive delivery may make respiratory efforts. Neonatal intensive care units (NICUs) using sophisticated technology can now support and monitor body warmth, ventilation, cardiac function, and nutrition, saving fetuses of increasingly shorter gestations. Nevertheless, when all births are evaluated, such survivals are rare.

The characteristics of the premature infant and his or her grip on life depend on genetic endowment, the length in and quality of the prenatal environment, and the immediate postnatal care (see Chapters 18 and 19 for a more complete discussion of the premature newborn). Assuming the prenatal environment and fetal condition are satisfactory, each additional day the fetus is able to remain in the uterus until maturity, approximately 38 weeks' gestation, is beneficial. Each day increases the ability of the newborn to withstand the demands of extrauterine life and to adjust to the tremendous circulatory, respiratory, and digestive alterations that must take place at birth (see Chapter 16 for a discussion of these changes).

Fetal Circulation

The circulatory system of the fetus maintains blood flow to the placenta. The placenta, in turn, provides the fetus with oxygen, nutrients, and the elimination of wastes (see Fig. 16-9). The umbilical vein within the umbilical cord carries blood from the placenta to the fetus, entering the fetal body at the umbilicus. The vein travels upward, dividing to form a bypass of the liver called the *ductus venosus,* which eventually joins the inferior vena cava. The rich, oxygenated blood from the umbilical vein mixes with the oxygen-poor blood flowing from the lower extremities and abdominal cavity toward the heart. The blood enters the heart by way of the right atrium, as in postnatal circulation. Because pulmonary circulation is unnecessary for oxygenation, much of the blood entering the heart from the inferior vena cava crosses directly to the left atrium through the fetal shunt called the *foramen ovale.* This blood is then guided into the usual circulation pattern of entering the left atrium, then the left ventricle, and then flowing to the aorta.

Blood from the head and upper extremities enters the right atrium via the superior vena cava. This blood then flows primarily into the right ventricle and eventually moves into the pulmonary artery. However, the trip to the lungs is superfluous at this time. The blood is shunted from the pulmonary artery, through the ductus arteriosus, to the aorta. Relatively little blood flows to the lung fields and then back to the left heart by way of the pulmonary veins.

The blood that flows downward through the aorta is eventually channeled into the iliac arteries to the hypogastric arteries. These arteries then join with the umbilical arteries, leading to the umbilical cord and placenta.

Pulmonary circulation becomes established within a relatively short time after birth. The umbilical cord is clamped and cut, occluding the cord's blood vessels. Because of the changes in thoracic pressures initiated by postnatal expansion of the lungs the foramen ovale begins to close. The ductus arteriosus collapses and becomes a ligament within a period of days or weeks.

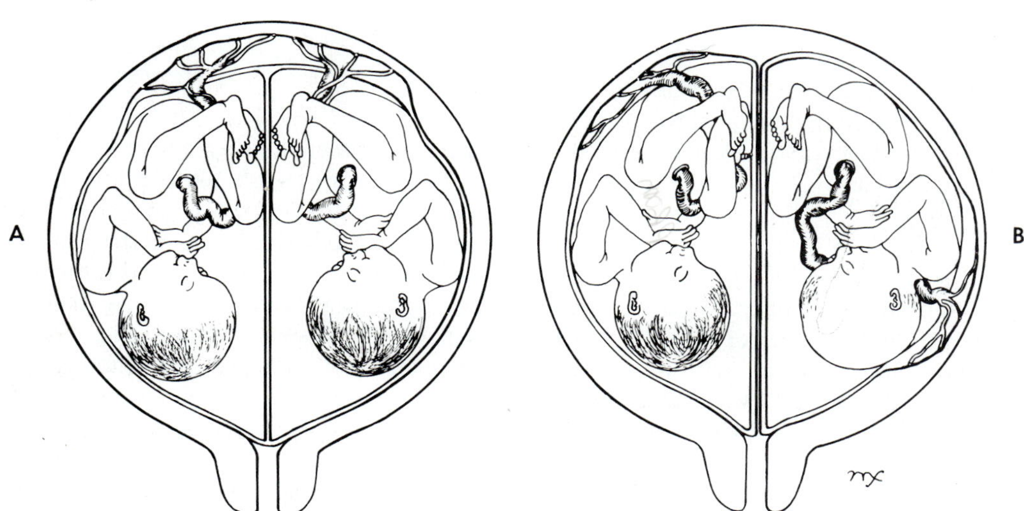

Fig. 8-3 **A,** Identical twins. **B,** Fraternal twins. Note differences in construction of amniotic sacs.

Twins

Twins occur approximately once in every 90 pregnancies. There are two types of twins, fraternal (dizygotic) and identical (monozygotic) (Fig. 8-3). Fraternal twins are the result of two simultaneous pregnancies developing from the fertilization of two separate ova by two distinct spermatozoa. They do not resemble one another any more than siblings resemble one another. They may be of the same sex or of opposite sexes. The placental circulation of each fetus is separate, although the adjoining placentas may be fused. Each fetus develops within its own amniotic sac (one chorion and one amnion each). Fraternal twins are more common than identical twins.

Identical twins result from the division of one fertilized ovum into two identical halves that develop into two individuals of the same appearance and same sex. Placental circulation is shared by the attachment of two umbilical cords. The number of amnions and chorions varies, depending on the timing of cellular division. Most commonly, each infant is encased in a separate amniotic sac but shares the chorion with his or her twin. Less often, twins will share a common amniotic sac and a common chorion. Mortality is higher in the latter instance because of the danger of cord entanglement (Creasy, Resnik, 1993).

Teratogens

A teratogen is an agent or factor that produces a major or minor deviation from normal structure or function in the developing embryo or fetus. The growing organism is most susceptible to malformation from the effects of maternal drug ingestion, radiation, or infection in the first trimester (the first 13 weeks of pregnancy), when basic organs and systems are being formed. Certain drugs may distort fetal development within 11 days of conception, before the woman realizes that she is pregnant. Many substances and infections are teratogenic (see the box at right). Others are currently under study to determine teratogenic effects.

POTENTIAL HUMAN TERATOGENIC FACTORS

SUBSTANCES
Alcohol
Amphetamines
Cocaine
Diethylstilbestrol
Heroin
Isotretinoin (Accutane)
Lithium
Marijuana
Methadone
Methotrexate
Methyl mercury
Mysoline
Phenothiazines
Phenytoin (Dilantin)
Tetracycline
Thalidomide
Tobacco smoke
Tricyclics
Trimethadione
Valium
Warfarin (Coumadin)

INFECTIONS
Coxsackie B
Cytomegalovirus (CMV)
Rubella
Syphilis
Toxoplasmosis
Varicella

OTHER
Hyperthermia
Maternal disease (such as diabetes)
Maternal malnutrition
Radiation

Drugs

Drugs, such as methotrexate and phenytoin, cause fetal structural abnormalities. Other drugs may cause hemorrhage, jaundice, neurological symptoms, and abnormal dental pigmentation. Effects of drugs taken during pregnancy may not become obvious until years later (such as vaginal malignancy in young women or sperm changes causing infertility in men whose mothers received diethylstilbestrol in early pregnancy). The pregnant woman should be cautioned not to use over-the-counter or prescription medications without first consulting her health-care provider.

Illicit drugs, such as cocaine and heroin, taken during pregnancy, may produce addiction in the newborn. Methadone, a legal drug used to treat heroin addiction, can also result in the birth of an addicted newborn. Maternal cocaine use has been associated with an increased incidence of spontaneous abortions, preterm labor, abruptio placentae (premature separation of the placenta from the uterine wall), intrauterine-growth retardation, and signs of toxicity in the neonate (Lynch, 1990). Because of conflicting evidence, more research is needed to establish whether or not a clear association between marijuana use and abnormal fetal development exists. Nurses and other health-care providers must participate in efforts to identify substance-abusing pregnant women. Health workers must educate these women about the effects of these drugs and refer them for treatment (Chasnoff, 1991).

Nicotine, alcohol, and caffeine

Smoking decreases the oxygen supply to the unborn fetus by displacing oxygen with variable quantities of carbon monoxide and by decreasing intrauterine blood flow. Utilization of calories, vitamins, and minerals, as well as the transport of amino acids, are compromised in smoking mothers. Cigarette smoking accounts for 20% to 30% of all low-birth-weight babies born in the United States (US Department of Health and Human Services, 1990). Mothers who smoke more than 10 cigarettes a day give birth to smaller infants than do nonsmoking women. Small babies of women who smoke grow faster during the 6 months after birth than do infants of nonsmokers. This growth pattern is interpreted as a response to the removal of the infant from the "inhibiting and toxic" influence of the smoking mother's uterus. Evidence also indicates that a relationship exists between mothers who smoke excessively and the incidence of pneumonia and bronchitis in their babies aged 6 to 9 months. From the perspective of general maternal and child health, smoking is an important causative factor in respiratory and circulatory diseases. Pregnant women should be encouraged to stop or decrease their habit.

Intrauterine exposure to alcohol is an important teratogen. Babies born with sufficient intrauterine exposure to alcohol often demonstrate fetal alcohol syndrome (FAS). Chronic, excessive use of alcohol has been identified as a significant cause of fetal growth retardation, impaired intellect, and congenital malformation, particularly microcephaly and facial abnormalities. Both the amount and timing of alcohol consumption by the mother, as well as her physical condition, appear to be influential. More moderate levels of alcohol consumption may result in fetal alcohol effects (FAE), characterized by the more subtle features of FAS. Moderate drinkers have a higher risk of spontaneous abortion, abruptio placentae, and low-birth-weight babies. Research has not yet determined minimum, safe amounts of alcohol intake during pregnancy (Aaronson, Macnee, 1989). Pregnant women need to be educated about the effects of alcohol consumption. Those mothers who find it difficult to stop drinking during pregnancy need referral for appropriate, rehabilitative treatment.

The use of methylxanthines by the pregnant woman, such as caffeine and theobromine found in coffee, tea, chocolate, colas, and some analgesics, has been questioned because of the teratogenic effects evidenced in animal studies. However, at normal dosages (less than 600 mg/day), teratogenic effects have not been demonstrated in humans. A cup of coffee has 75 to 155 mg of caffeine (up to 330 mg have been reported). Although data are insufficient to make specific recommendations on caffeine intake the pregnant woman should be counseled to limit consumption of foods and drinks containing methylxanthines.

TORCH infections

The **TORCH** group of infectious diseases are those that can cause serious harm to the developing embryofetus. These diseases include toxoplasmosis (TO), rubella (R), cytomegalovirus (C), and herpes simplex virus type 2 (H). (Some sources identify the "O" as other in fections.) Toxoplasmosis is a parasitic disease, transmitted to the pregnant woman by eating or handling raw meat, drinking goat's milk, and coming in contact with cat feces. As a defensive measure, an expectant mother should not handle a cat's litter box. In addition, she must wash her hands carefully after handling raw meat, cook meat well, wash fruits and vegetables before eating them, and wear gloves while gardening.

The fetus is particularly vulnerable to viral infections during the early weeks of development. Pregnant women should not knowingly expose themselves to any viral disease to which they do not have immunity, such as rubella (German measles) or cytomegalovirus (CMV). Although CMV can have teratogenic effects from placental transmission, it may also be acquired during the birth process, resulting in serious neonatal infection. Transmission of the herpes simplex virus type 2 is likely to occur only after membranes have ruptured. The herpes virus ascends from active lesions of the cervix, vagina, or vulva. For this reason, women with known active lesions at the onset of labor deliver their infants by cesarean section, preferably before the rupture of membranes. See Chapter 14 for further discussion of CMV and herpes infections.

Other factors that may cause teratogenic effects in the fetus include environmental pollutants, lead, and excessive use of vitamins A, D, and K. Although diagnostic x-ray films should not be taken unless necessary, no conclusive evidence exists confirming that the levels of exposure associated with infrequent, low-dose x-rays cause fetal injury. Lead aprons and shields should be used.

METHODS OF EVALUATING FETAL GROWTH, MATURITY, AND WELL-BEING

The maturity of a fetus at birth is important to its survival outside the uterus. Clinical assessment, com-

◆ **TABLE 8-2**
Evaluation of the Unborn Infant

Age and growth Important for medical-legal considerations (e.g., dating of prospective abortion [or elective cesarean birth]).	1. Date of first day of last normal menstrual period (Nägele's rule: count back 3 months, add 7 days to determine delivery date). 2. Fundal height (assumes normal fetal growth). 3. Appearance of fetal heart tone at 10 to 12 weeks using "Doppler" fetoscope. 4. Ultrasound measurements (transabdominal or transvaginal). a. Size of amniotic sac/uterine cavity. b. Fetal crown to rump length. c. Biparietal diameters, femur length, head-abdomen ratio (second trimester for greatest accuracy).
Maturity Various body system development may be monitored, but overall fetal maturity may be difficult to ascertain.	1. Amniotic fluid analysis (amniocentesis). a. L/S ratio usually rises to two or more when lungs have matured; other biochemical tests (e.g., amount of phospholipids) increase reliability of lung maturation evaluation in complex obstetric cases (usually mature by 35 weeks). b. Positive foam or shake test usually rules out lung immaturity. c. Fatty cell recovery percentage—low reliability. d. Creatinine levels may assist in assessment of renal maturity (normal = 2, by 37 weeks).
Well-being Indications of some specific defects and clues of general fetal well-being.	1. Fetal movement—usually reassuring if not exaggerated. 2. Ultrasound measurements. a. Evaluation of fetal presentation; multiple pregnancy. b. Detection of some structural abnormalities (e.g., central nervous system and genitourinary anomalies). c. Localization of placenta; diagnosis of placenta previa. d. Identification of excessive or diminished amniotic fluid volume: related to possible fetal abnormalities or jeopardy. e. Motion picture (real-time techniques) may confirm fetal death. 3. Amniotic fluid analysis (amniocentesis). a. Chromosomal studies may reveal the following: (1) Fetal abnormalities in chromosome number and gross structure (e.g., Down syndrome). (2) Gender of infant to help evaluate probability of sex-linked genetic disorders (e.g., Duchenne's muscular dystrophy, classic hemophilia). b. Biochemical studies may reveal the following: (1) Anencephaly-myelomeningocele, based on level of alpha fetoprotein. (2) A number of metabolic and blood diseases (e.g., thalassemia). c. Bilirubin levels to monitor severity of maternal-fetal blood incompatibility (Rh disease). 4. Chorionic villi sampling (CVS) at 9 to 11 weeks for genetic analysis and early detection of selected hereditary defects. 5. Fetal heart rate monitoring—external or internal. a. Fetal heart rate changes in response to fetal movement without uterine contractions (before labor) are consistent with fetal health and form basis of *nonstress* test. b. Positive oxytocin challenge test or nipple stimulation contraction stress test may predict fetal jeopardy in true labor. c. Helps identify episodes of hypoxia resulting from uteroplacental insufficiency or cord compression during labor (see Chapter 11). 6. Biophysical profile. 7. Maternal blood analysis helps screen alpha-fetoprotein levels for possible neural tube, abdominal wall defects, or chromosomal disorders. 8. Meconium-stained amniotic fluid; possible fetal oxygen lack (hypoxia). 9. Fetal blood sampling (microsamples drawn from presenting part, usually scalp) (in labor). a. Helps identify fetal hypoxia, retention of carbon dioxide (CO_2), and developing acidosis. b. Serial samples are more meaningful. c. pH values below 7.2 in two or more samples usually indicate need for assistance. d. Maternal acidosis may cause misleading interpretations of fetal status.

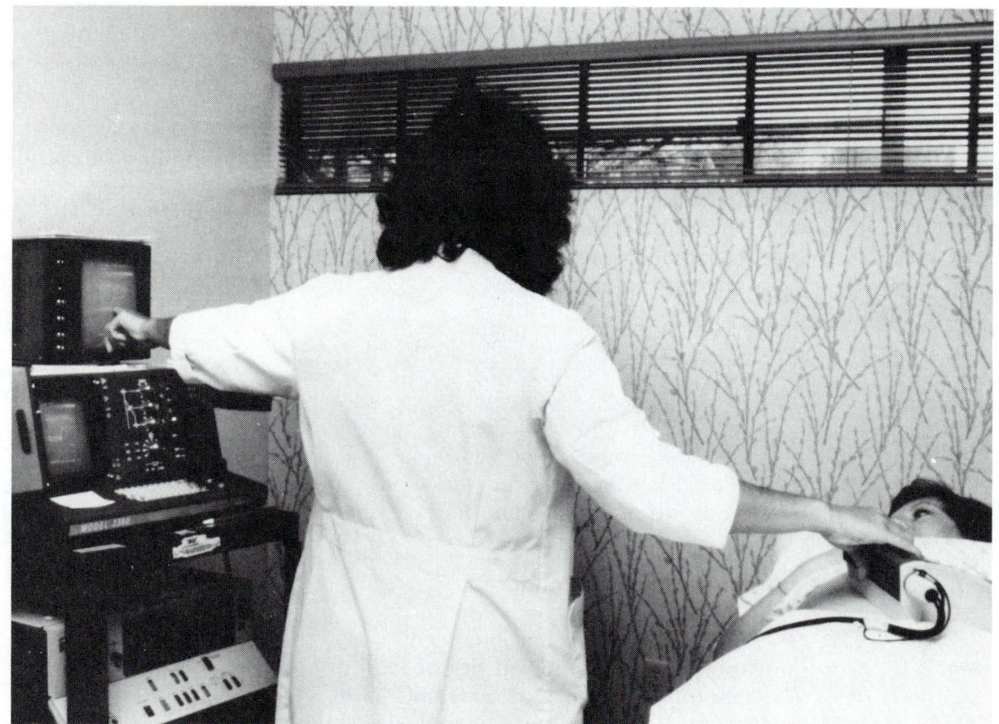

Fig. 8-4 Transabdominal ultrasound examination of fetus. A moderately full bladder lifts uterus from behind pelvis and provides the best picture. Mineral oil or a special gel is applied to the mother's abdomen. A smooth sensor (transducer) is guided over the skin, and a progressive series of ultrasonic images of uterine contents is obtained. Endosonography or transvaginal ultrasound imaging that uses a sensor introduced into the vaginal canal is also available. This technique does not require a full bladder and gives better visualization for diagnosis of certain conditions (e.g., ectopic pregnancy).

bined with technological tools, can be used to evaluate intrauterine growth and fetal well-being. The nurse must recognize that the woman is likely to be apprehensive about many of these tests. It is important to assess whether she understands the reason for the tests, and to educate her about necessary preparations and what to expect during the tests. The nurse may also need to assist with clarifying test results. Tests that assess fetal age, size, maturity, and well-being are highlighted in Table 8-2. A discussion of selected assessment technologies follows.

Ultrasound

Ultrasonography detects differences in tissue density by directing high-frequency sound waves into tissue and electrically measuring the reflected echoes from internal structures. It can be applied to the woman's abdomen or a transducer can be inserted into the vagina (Fig. 8-4). Ultrasound scanning uses static or a combination of static and real-time scanners. Real-time imaging offers the benefit of being able to visualize fetal breathing, tone, movement, urination, and cardiac activity.

Ultrasound is a valuable tool for assessing fetal age and intrauterine growth. It can also be used to visualize the placenta, confirm fetal presentation, determine amniotic fluid levels, evaluate umbilical artery blood flow, and detect congenital anomalies such as hydrocephaly. Ultrasound is a useful adjunct to other tests, such as amniocentesis and percutaneous umbilical blood sampling, providing guidance for needle placement and helping to avoid damage to the placenta or fetus.

Amniocentesis

Amniocentesis is a technique in which amniotic fluid is aspirated transabdominally or suprapubically from the amniotic sac (Fig. 8-5). The amniotic fluid contains fetal cells that are then analyzed. When done in early pregnancy (14 to 20 weeks), this procedure is usually

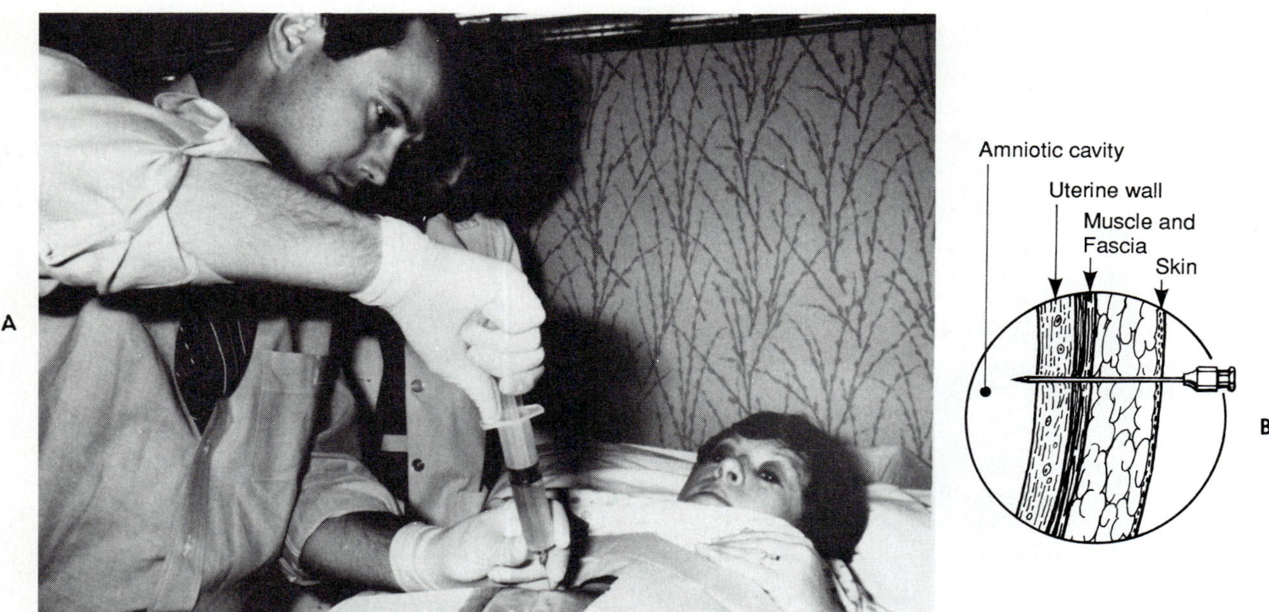

Fig. 8-5 **A,** Amniocentesis. To help lessen risk of fetal or placental trauma, ultrasound is used to locate intrauterine structures before the insertion of a needle. Amniocentesis is usually performed for genetic analysis between 14 and 16 weeks' gestation. **B,** Layers of tissue through which the needle must pass to reach amniotic fluid. (Courtesy Thomas Key, MD, Department of Obstetrics and Gynecology, University of California, San Diego.)

for the purpose of determining developmental anomalies and genetic makeup, including gender.

It can also be done in the third trimester to evaluate fetal lung maturity (the lecithin-sphingomyelin [L/S] ratio and the presence of phosphatidylglycerol [PG]). These phospholipids are components of surfactant, which lower lung surface tension, stabilizing the alveoli and preventing the lungs from collapsing. A quick, bedside test of the amniotic fluid (foam or shake test) also provides an indication of fetal lung maturity. In the foam test the amniotic fluid is mixed in a tube with ethanol and shaken. If significant bubbles remain after 15 minutes the lungs are most likely mature.

Amniotic fluid can also be tested for infection, monitored to determine the severity of Rh disease, and tested for alpha-fetoprotein (AFP) level to rule out a neural tube defect. Complications of amniocentesis are rare, but the mother must be informed of the possibility and a signed consent is usually required.

Chorionic villus sampling (CVS)

CVS is an alternative to amniocentesis for prenatal diagnosis of genetic disorders. Because CVS can be done earlier in pregnancy (8 to 11 weeks' gestation versus 14 to 20 weeks' gestation for amniocentesis) and the results are obtained more quickly (within 1 to 7 days versus 10 days to 4 weeks for amniocentesis), first-trimester abortion is possible if desired. The test is usually done using real-time imaging while the physician passes a catheter through the cervical os and aspirates chorionic villi from the placenta. A full bladder may help position the uterus for easier catheter insertion. The risk of CVS causing a natural miscarriage is slightly higher than it is for amniocentesis (Jones, 1988). Education about the procedure and a signed consent form are required.

Electronic fetal heart rate monitoring

During the third trimester, evaluation of fetal well-being is indicated for women with diabetes, pregnancy-induced hypertension, and other high-risk conditions. It is also desirable for those women who are overdue (41 or more weeks' gestation), since placental aging may compromise fetal oxygenation. The most widely accepted method of evaluating fetal status is the nonstress test (NST). The woman is placed in a semifowlers position and an electronic fetal monitor is applied to her abdomen. Fetal movement and fetal

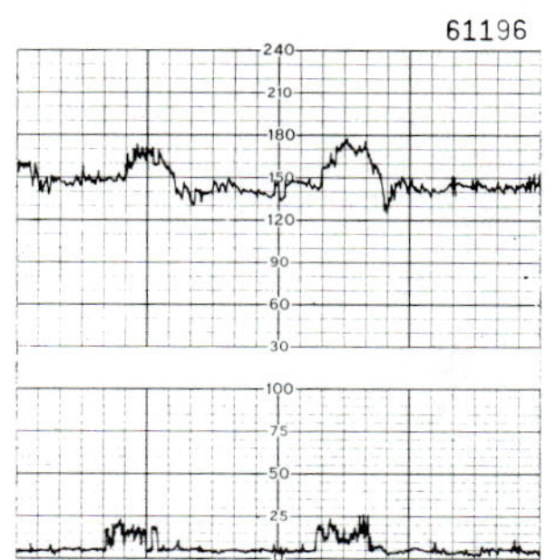

Fig. 8-6 Acceleration of FHR with fetal movement. (From Tucker SM: *Pocket guide to fetal monitoring,* St. Louis, 1992, Mosby.)

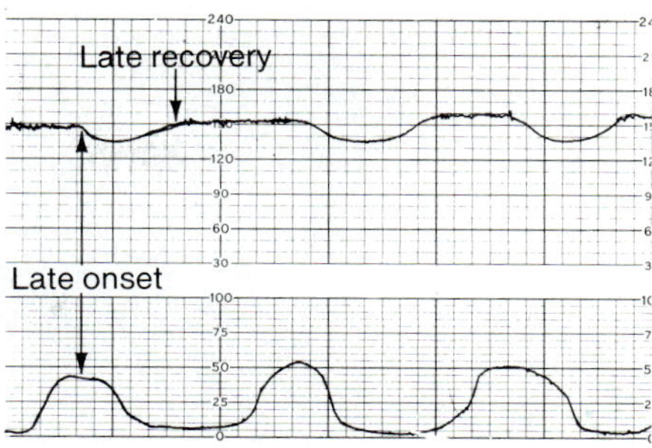

Fig. 8-7 Late decelerations of FHR, key points identified. (From Tucker SM: *Pocket guide to fetal monitoring,* St. Louis, 1992, Mosby.)

heart rate are recorded. A "reactive" NST demonstrates at least two fetal heart rate accelerations (15 second duration, 15 beats per minute increase) with fetal movements in a 20-minute period (Fig. 8-6). Accelerations of the fetal heart rate indicate an intact nervous system that is not compromised.

Increasingly, sound (acoustic) or vibration with sound (vibroacoustic) is used to stimulate the fetus during an NST. A device, such as an artificial larynx, is held to the mother's abdomen and the sound or combined sound and vibration stimulates fetal movement and fetal heart rate accelerations. This technique typically shortens the time necessary for an NST.

In the event of a nonreactive NST or other high risk condition the health-care provider may order a contraction stress test to evaluate placental functioning. Contractions are induced by nipple stimulation or an intravenous oxytocin infusion. The goal of this test is to achieve three contractions lasting 40 to 60 seconds within a 10-minute period. The fetal heart rate is observed for late decelerations, which indicate diminished fetal reserves (Fig. 8-7).

During labor the immediate status of the baby may be evaluated through simultaneous monitoring of the fetal heart rate and contraction patterns, observation of the color of the amniotic fluid, and, in certain cases, by fetal blood sampling (see Chapter 11).

Biophysical profile

The biophysical profile is a relatively new test that evaluates fetal status by measuring five fetal characteristics: fetal breathing movements, gross fetal body movements, fetal tone, and amniotic fluid volume. All of these characteristics are evaluated by real-time ultrasound. A nonstress test evaluates reactivity of the fetal heart rate. A score of two for each of the five characteristics is optimal. Some facilities also grade placental maturation.

SIGNS AND SYMPTOMS OF PREGNANCY

After conception, widespread changes take place in the woman's body, creating signs and symptoms that possess varying degrees of importance in the diagnosis of pregnancy. These signs and symptoms, usually classified according to their accuracy, form three groups: the presumptive, the probable, and the positive signs of pregnancy. No universal agreement exists, however, regarding the contents of these categories.

Presumptive Signs and Symptoms

Presumptive signs and symptoms of pregnancy are those that could easily be an indication of another condition. Presumptive signs tend to occur earlier and are more subjective than later signs and symptoms. They usually include the symptoms that follow.

Amenorrhea

Although the absence of menses may be an early sign of a developing pregnancy, it is not always a true indication. Amenorrhea may occur as a result of sudden changes in environment or occupation, emotional upset, malnutrition, fatigue, hormonal disorders, extensive exercise, and menopause.

Nausea and vomiting

Nausea and vomiting in relation to pregnancy often occur in the morning but are not limited to this time. These signs are presumably caused by changes in hormone levels in the first weeks of preghnancy. Nausea and vomiting are not confined to pregnancy, however, since they are a common occurrence during gastrointestinal tract irritation and emotional stress.

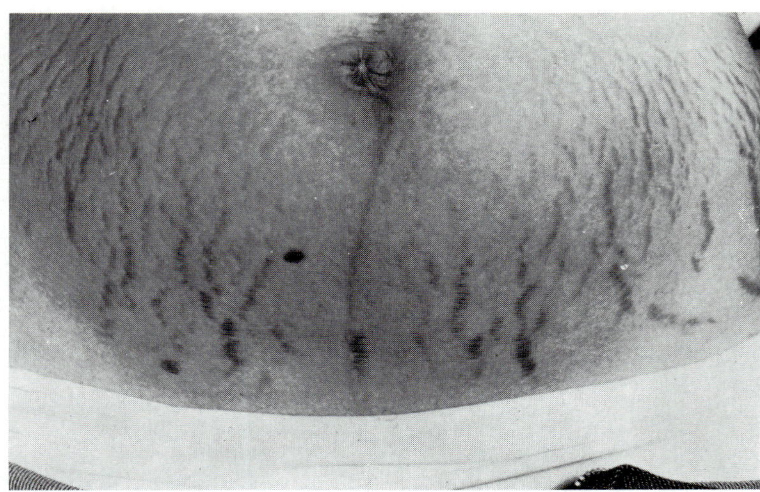

Fig. 8-8 Striae. (Courtesy Mercy Hospital and Medical Center, San Diego, CA.)

Frequent urination

Frequent urination, usually in small amounts, is ommon during the first and last weeks of pregnancy. elvic congestion and pressure of the uterus on the ladder are primary causes. Urinary frequency may also be present merely because of excitement, large fluid intake, or irritation of the urinary tract. Increased urination is also associated with diabetes mellitus.

Fatigue

Fatigue, often described as excessive, is a widespread complaint that may persist throughout the first trimester. It is thought to be due to increased hormone levels.

Probable Signs and Symptoms

The probable signs of pregnancy are more certain than presumptive signs. They are more objective. They are not, however, foolproof. The probable signs follow.

Basal body temperature elevation

Persistent basal body temperature elevation is one of the earliest diagnostic observations and is considered 97% accurate in confirming pregnancy. For this basal or waking temperature to have meaning, however, the woman must take her temperature consistently, using proper techniques both before and after ovulation to detect the relative increase in basal readings (see Chapter 7).

Breast changes

Breast tingling, swelling, and tenderness are found early in pregnancy. These symptoms may also be experienced during each menstrual cycle, just before menses. Darkening of the areola is also a common finding, influenced by hormonal changes.

Changes in the skin and mucous membranes

Commonly known as *stretch marks,* striae gravidarum is probably related more to increased production or sensitivity to adrenocortical hormones during pregnancy than to weight gain alone (Fig. 8-8). Skin changes such as these are also noted in patients with Cushing's disease and, to a lesser degree, in patients with sudden weight gains not associated with pregnancy.

Another pigmentation characteristic of pregnancy is a bronze type of facial coloration called *chloasma,* or the mask of pregnancy. Often seen on dark-haired women, development of a dark line *(linea nigra),* extending from the sternum to the pubis in the midline, is quite common. These changes in skin coloration are most likely related to hormonal alterations.

The violet coloration of the vagina, cervix, and vulva, which is apparent at approximately 6 to 10 weeks' gestation is known as *Chadwick's sign*. This condition is caused by increased circulation to the vaginal area and may be associated with any cause of pelvic congestion.

Deepened pigmentation of the areola, production of a breast secretion (colostrum), and the presence of the linea nigra may have little diagnostic value for women

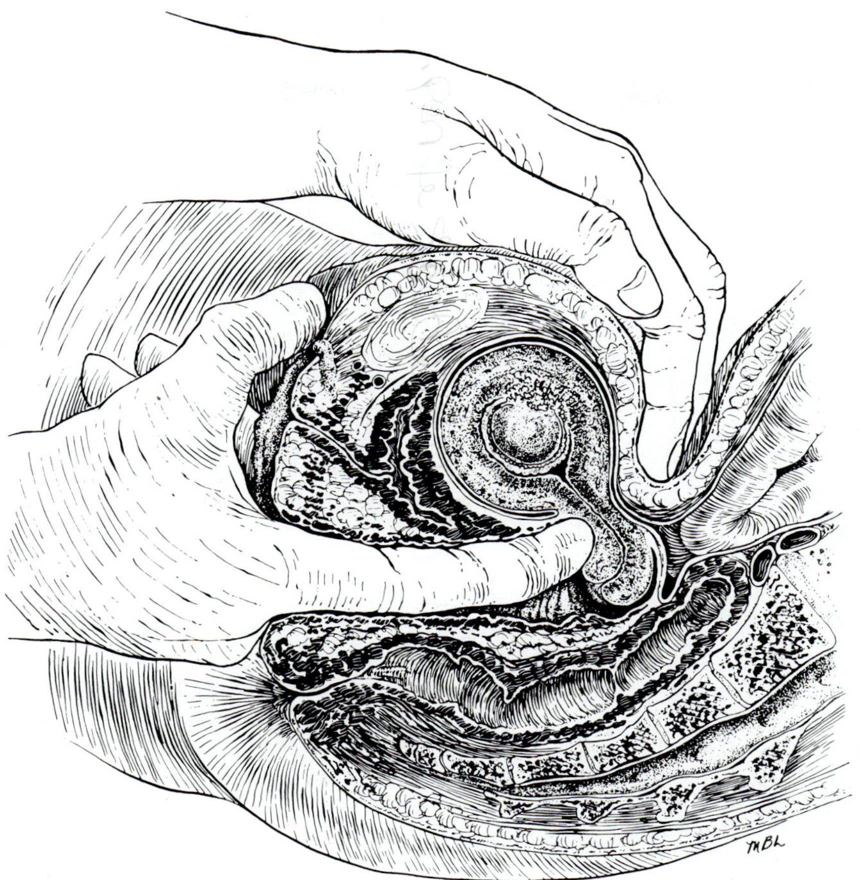

Fig. 8-9 Hegar's sign.

who have recently had children or have recently breast-fed infants.

Abdominal enlargement

Increased abdominal size is usually noted the eighth to tenth week of pregnancy. However, increased abdominal size may be due to dietary intake rather than gestation. Increased abdominal size may also be influenced by the growth of tumors or hernias.

Uterine changes

At 6 to 8 weeks' gestation a softening of the region of the uterus between the body and the cervix, called the *isthmus,* occurs. It is determined by a simultaneous abdominal and vaginal examination. This bimanual maneuver is illustrated in Fig. 8-9. The softening is termed *Hegar's sign.* Another softening of the uterus affecting the cervix is detected by the examiner's finger. In the nonpregnant state the cervix feels somewhat like the cartilage at the tip of a nose. During pregnancy the cervix changes in consistency to resemble the pliability of the ear lobe or lips *(Goodell's sign).*

Enlargement of the uterus, rather than an increase in abdominal size, is a more definitive sign of pregnancy. The fundus, or top of the uterus, is felt about halfway between the top of the pubic bone and the umbilicus at approximately 16 weeks' gestation (Fig. 8-10). The fundus is found near the umbilicus at approximately 20 weeks' gestation. After 20 weeks' gestation the examiner can determine fundal height by measuring from the symphysis pubis to the top of the uterine fundus (McDonald's method). It correlates well with the weeks of gestation between 20 and 31 (26 cm = 26 weeks' gestation). As a result, fundal height may be used as an indicator of fetal growth. When near full term the fundus is almost at the level of the tip of the sternum. A woman expecting her first baby usually experiences sudden relief from a shortness of breath approximately 2 weeks before her delivery. This is due to the fetus "dropping" and *lightening,* taking pressure off of the diaphragm and increasing pressure on the bladder.

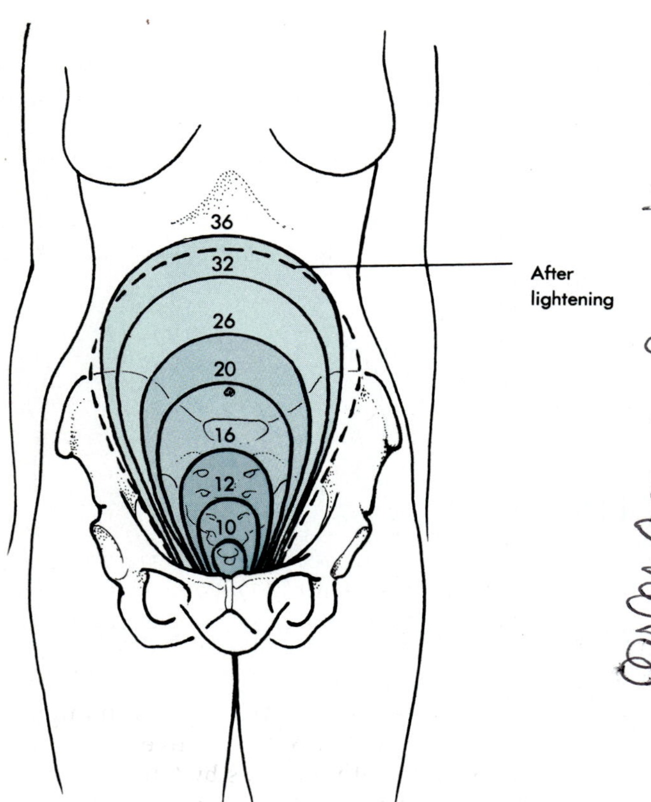

Fig. 8-10 Progressive growth of fundus during pregnancy, measured in weeks. Note that fundus is lower at term than at 36 weeks' gestation

Normally painless, irregular uterine contractions, called *Braxton Hicks contractions*, occur throughout pregnancy. After about 28 weeks' gestation these contrations can be detected by palpating the abdomen.

Ballottement

The French term *ballottement* describes "tossing up a ball in the air and catching it on its return." Near midpregnancy the small fetus is enclosed in a relatively large fluid-filled sac or bag of waters. When an examiner taps the baby's head or body, it characteristically floats away and then rebounds to nudge the examiner's fingertips. Rarely will this ball-like rebound be mimicked by the movement of a uterine tumor or polyp. It represents, therefore, only a probable sign.

Quickening

Quickening, meaning the first time fetal movement is felt by the woman, can sometimes be imitated by peristalsis or gas and be misinterpreted. By the time quickening is felt (at approximately 16 weeks' gestation by women who have already had children and 18 weeks' or more by women who are experiencing their first pregnancy), other more definite signs should be manifested.

Positive pregnancy tests

Pregnancy tests are based on the fact that the chorionic villi of an implanted ovum or of the developing placenta secrete human chorionic gonadotropic hormone (hCG). In a pregnant woman, hCG is excreted in small amounts in the urine and blood. Although the excretion of urinary hCG during pregnancy has significant individual variations, within 48 hours of implantation, hCG levels increase rapidly. The first pregnancy tests were biological, using laboratory animals. They have been replaced by immunological, radioimmunoassay, and monoclonal antibody tests that are faster and more accurate.

The most common types of immunological pregnancy tests are based on the principle that hCG in the pregnant woman's urine inhibits clumping of RBCs or latex particles. Urine tests are accurate 4 to 10 days after a missed menses. The radioreceptor assay is a 1 hour blood test that is usually accurate at the time of missed menses.

Blood tests known as *radioimmunoassays (RIAs)* may also be used to confirm pregnancy. The RIA for the β (beta) subunit of hCG is capable of diagnosing pregnancy as early as 5 days before the first missed period. These tests are the most sensitive available.

Enzyme-linked immunosorbent assay uses a specific monoclonal antibody to identify the hCG antigen in serum, plasma, or urine. These tests are popular because they are easy to use and read. They have demonstrated very accurate results as early as 1 week after implantation.

Pregnancy tests designed for home use are based on enzyme-linked, immunosorbent assay technology. Tests are usually done 3 to 9 days after the missed menstrual period and should be repeated in 2 weeks if the first results are negative. These home tests have a relatively low false-positive rate but a high (about 25%) false-negative rate. The high false-negative rate is due, in part, to the fact that many women do not carefully follow test directions.

Most pregnancy tests are only about 95% to 99% accurate. These results depend on when they are performed, the method used, and the presence of factors that may cause both false negatives and positives. For these reasons, "positive" results are usually considered probable and not positive signs of pregnancy. Although a firm diagnosis of pregnancy can often be made after the eighth week of gestation without any special chemical tests, a growing tendency exists to use the tests to help detect pregnancy as soon as possible. The earlier pregnancy can be documented, the sooner prenatal care can be initiated and an accurate estimated date of birth established. The results of pregnancy tests are especially helpful in diagnosing pregnancy outside the uterine cavity (ectopic pregnancy) or a suspected abnormal growth of the fertilized ovum (hydatidiform mole). The tests are strategic in planning surgery involving anesthesia, diagnostic or therapeutic radiation, prescription of medications potentially toxic to a developing fetus, or abortion.

Positive Signs

Positive signs are objective (can be seen, heard, or felt), and offer proof of pregnancy.

Ultrasound techniques

A gestation sac may be visible as early as 3 to 4 weeks after conception. As the pregnancy advances, fetal form and motion become progressively more apparent with real-time sonography.

Fetal heart tones

Fetal heart tones are usually heard after 18 to 20 weeks' gestation by conventional auscultation with a standard fetoscope. Fetal heart tones can be detected 10 to 12 weeks after conception using ultrasonic or Doppler-effect techniques.

Up until the twentieth week the fetal heart rate is heard best at the center of the pubic hairline.

The presence of the *funic souffle,* a rapid, repetitive, whistlelike sound not synchronous with the maternal pulse, may be evidence of the fetal heart rate. This sound, however, caused by pulsations of blood in the baby's umbilical cord, is not always heard. Another sound called the *uterine souffle,* a swishlike tone occurring at the same rate as the maternal pulse, is not diagnostic of pregnancy. This tone originates with the mother's pulsating uterine arteries and may also be detected in the presence of large vascular pelvic tumors.

Fetal movement

Fetal movement can be detected by a trained examiner after approximately 20 weeks' gestation.

PRENATAL ATTACHMENT

In maternity nursing, attachment refers to the enduring mutual affection that develops between the parents and their infant. Both parents usually begin to develop positive feelings for the child during pregnancy. After approximately 16 to 20 weeks' gestation the woman is acutely aware of the fetus through its movement. Mothers may exhibit positive feelings and attempts to interact with the fetus by talking to it and changing positions to elicit a corresponding movement. Fathers do not have the same physical awareness of the fetus but may also attempt to interact through the mother. Frequently parents call the fetus by a special nickname or by the chosen name, evidencing their attempts to personalize the unborn infant. The first fetal movements may accelerate the woman's early feelings of attachment. Research indicates that hearing the fetal heart rate and seeing the fetal outline on a sonogram have similar effects.

KEY CONCEPTS

1 The length of human gestation is 280 days (40 weeks) when calculated from the first day of the last menstrual period and 266 days (38 weeks) when calculated from the time of conception.

2 Each living thing has a certain number of threadlike strands, or chromosomes, of transmittable characteristics, or genes, within the nuclei of its tissue cells. The number of chromosomes is constant for each species.

3 Through meiosis, the number of chromosomes in the gametes (sex cells) of the male and female is reduced by half. When male and female gametes unite, fertilization takes place, and the new embryo contains the correct number of chromosomes.

4 The gender of the child is determined by the type of male sex cell that fertilizes the ovum.

5 The fertilized egg, or zygote, is called a *morula* as it moves from the fallopian tube to the uterine cavity, where implantation occurs.

6 The outer surface of the zygote becomes covered with fingerlike tissue projections called *chorionic villi.* These structures aid in the process of implantation into the endometrium and the manufacture of human chorionic gonadotropin (hCG).

7 The placenta serves as a supply and elimination system for the developing embryo or fetus. Its functions are manufacturing hormones and enzymes; transporting food, oxygen, and antibodies from the mother to the fetus; removing waste products from the fetal circulation to the maternal bloodstream; and providing limited protection from some harmful substances.

8 The fetus is surrounded by a transparent sac made up of two membranous layers called the *chorion* and the *amnion*. The amnion produces amniotic fluid, which helps to control the environmental temperature of the fetus and shield it from trauma and infection.

9 At 16 weeks' gestation the fetus is about $7\frac{1}{2}$ inches (19 cm) long and weighs about $3\frac{1}{3}$ ounces (100 gm). At 16 to 18 weeks' gestation, women usually report feeling fetal movement, or quickening.

10 At 20 weeks' gestation the fetal heartbeat can be heard using a standard fetoscope. Between 20 to 24 weeks' gestational age is considered the legal threshold of viability.

11 The umbilical vein within the umbilical cord carries oxygenated blood from the placenta to the fetus. Circulation through the fetus is relatively similar to postnatal circulation. Pulmonary circulation, however, is not completely established until after birth.

12 Fraternal twins result from the fertilization of two separate ova by two distinct spermatozoa. Each twin develops within their own amniotic sacs (one chorion and one amnion). Identical twins result from the division of one fertilized ovum. The number of amnions and chorions varies depending on the timing of cellular division.

13 The embryo or fetus is most susceptible to malformation from the effects of maternal drug ingestion, radiation, or infection during the first trimester, when organ systems are forming.

14 Technological methods of evaluating fetal status before labor include ultrasonography, amniocentesis, chorionic villus sampling, maternal blood and urine analysis, and fetal heart monitoring.

15 Presumptive signs and symptoms of pregnancy are somewhat subjective and usually include amenorrhea, nausea and vomiting, frequent urination, and fatigue.

16 Probable signs and symptoms of pregnancy usually include basal body temperature elevation, breast changes, coloration changes in skin and mucous membranes, enlargement of the abdomen and uterus, ballottement, quickening, and positive pregnancy tests.

17 Positive signs of pregnancy are objective—they can be seen, heard, and felt. Ultrasound permits visualization of the gestational sac and fetal form. Fetal heart tones can be heard after 10 to 12 weeks' gestation using an ultrasonic or Doppler technique or, after 18 to 20 weeks' gestation, with a standard fetoscope. Fetal movement can be felt by a trained examiner after about 20 weeks' gestation.

18 Feelings of parental attachment to the child begin to develop during pregnancy.

CRITICAL THOUGHT QUESTIONS

1 A pregnant woman asks you if the baby breathes in the uterus. What would you tell her?

2 Mrs. James is 20 weeks pregnant. She asks you what the baby looks like at this age. How would you respond?

3 At her first prenatal visit, the patient asks you if there are any foods or medications she should avoid during the pregnancy. How would you respond? Why?

4 A friend confides that she thought she was pregnant, but her home pregnancy test was negative. Given the negative results, she is surprised that she has not yet begun her menstrual period. What would you advise her? Why?

5 Mrs. Hanks is 37 weeks pregnant and complains to you that "It punches me to keep me awake at night." While talking to her, you discover that they have not yet discussed names for the baby or begun to prepare the home for the baby's arrival. Given these findings, what nursing diagnosis/diagnoses might be appropriate?

REFERENCES

Aaronson LS, Macnee CL: Tobacco, alcohol and caffeine use during pregnancy, *J Obstet Gynecol Neonatal Nurs* 18(4):279, 1989.

Chasnoff IJ: Drugs, alcohol, pregnancy and the neonate: pay now or pay later, *JAMA* 266:1567, 1991.

Creasy RK, Resnik R: *Maternal-fetal medicine*, ed 3, Philadelphia, 1994, WB Saunders.

Jones SL: Decision making in clinical genetics: ethical implications for perinatal nursing practice, *J Perinat and Neonatal Nurs* 1(3):11-23, 1988.

Lynch M, McKeon VA: Cocaine use during pregnancy: research findings and clinical implications, *J Obstet Gynecol Neonatal Nurs* 19(4):285, 1990.

Tucker SM: *Pocket guide to fetal monitoring*, St. Louis, 1988, Mosby.

US Department of Health and Human Services: *Healthy people 2000: national health promotion and disease prevention objectives,* Boston, 1992, Jones and Bartlett.

BIBLIOGRAPHY

Cranley M: Roots of attachment: the relationship of parents with their unborn, *Birth defects: original article series* 17(6):59-65, 1981.

Gebauer CL, Lowe NK: The biophysical profile: antepartal assessment of fetal well-being, *J Obstet Gynecol Neonatal Nurs* 22(2):115-124, 1993.

Gardner K: Twin transfusion syndrome, *J Obstet Gynecol Neonatal Nurs* 22(1):64-71, 1992.

Gegor CL, Paine LL: Antepartum fetal assessment techniques: an update for today's perinatal nurse, *J Perinat Neonatal Nurs* 5(4):1-15, 1992.

Goodwin L: Home fetal assessment, *J Perinat Neonatal Nurs* 5(4):33-45, 1992.

Mercer R, Ferketich S, May K, et al: Further exploration of maternal and paternal fetal attachment, *Res Nurs Health* 11(1):83-87, 1988.

Worthington-Roberts BS, Williams SR: *Nutrition in pregnancy and lactation*, ed 5, St Louis, 1993, Mosby.

Pregnancy and Prenatal Care

CHAPTER OBJECTIVES

After studying this chapter, the student should be able to:

1. Describe the changes in a woman's anatomy and physiology occurring during pregnancy.
2. Describe the psychological changes that a woman typically undergoes during each trimester.
3. Define the following terms: *viable, primigravida, primipara, multigravida, multipara, nullipara, antepartal*, and *prenatal.*
4. Identify the health objective related to prenatal care for the year 2000.
5. List the broad objectives and components of prenatal care.
6. Indicate the information that is obtained during a woman's first prenatal pelvic examination.
7. Determine the meaning of the five-number code often used to describe a patient's obstetric history.
8. Calculate a woman's estimated date of delivery (EDD) using Nagele's rule.
9. Identify the hemoglobin and hematocrit levels that usually signal the presence of anemia in a maternity patient.
10. Enumerate nine signs or symptoms that the pregnant woman should report to her health care provider.
11. Explain why expectant mothers are routinely weighed and checked for elevated blood pressure, albuminuria, and glucosuria.
12. List six laboratory tests that are frequently ordered to evaluate the status of an expectant mother.
13. Name four foods rich in vitamin C, three foods with significant calcium content, and two foods high in iron.
14. List weight gain recommendations for women who enter pregnancy underweight, at a normal weight, moderately overweight, and very overweight.
15. State at least two considerations that may cause a health care provider to modify weight gain recommendations for a pregnant client.
16. Describe a diet appropriate for a pregnant woman using the recommended servings from the food groups in the Daily Food Guide.
17. Discuss the reason iron supplements are prescribed during pregnancy.
18. Explain why the supine position is not recommended for rest or exercise.
19. Relate how Kegel exercises are performed and why they are beneficial.
20. Describe the guidelines for exercise during pregnancy.
21. Indicate how a woman may need to alter her clothing as her pregnancy advances.
22. Identify two concerns associated with douching, especially during pregnancy.

Continued.

CHAPTER OBJECTIVES—cont'd

23 Develop a teaching plan for the prevention or alleviation of the common discomforts of pregnancy.
24 Indicate a government agency that would be concerned with possible employment discrimination affecting pregnant workers.
25 Help plan clothing and furnishings for a first-born infant.
26 Explain the philosophy on which psychoprophylactic preparation for childbirth is based.
27 Compare cultural differences that may affect maternal-child health practices among African-Americans, Hispanics, Asians, and Native Americans.

Pregnancy causes many physical and psychological changes in a woman. The nurse who works with the pregnant woman and her family must be familiar with these changes to provide appropriate anticipatory guidance. Adequate prenatal care is the key to preventing complications and promoting a healthy pregnancy. This chapter describes the physical and psychological changes of pregnancy. It also discusses prenatal care and suggests areas for patient teaching.

The following terms are used to describe the number of times the woman has been pregnant and the number of times she has completed a pregnancy of viable age.

gravida The number of pregnancies, including this one, a woman has had, regardless of outcome.

para The number of pregnancies a woman has completed that have resulted in *viable births.* (The usual legal definitions of viable are a pregnancy of 20 or 24 weeks or more duration or the delivery of an infant weighing at least 500 gm.) The para count does not change if an infant is living or dead, if the child is born vaginally or by cesarean, or if the pregnancy produces multiple births (e.g., twins).

nulligravida A woman who has never been pregnant. (The prefix *nul* means none.)

nullipara A woman who has never delivered a viable child.

primigravida A woman who is having or has had one pregnancy. (The prefix *prim* means first.)

primipara A woman who has completed one pregnancy of a viable age. Although not technically correct, a woman who is carrying her first viable child but has not yet delivered is often referred to as a primipara, or "primip," to differentiate from a woman who has been through the birth process.

multigravida A woman who has had more than one pregnancy. (The prefix *mult* means many, or at least more than one.)

multipara A woman who has completed two or more viable pregnancies. Although not technically correct, the term is often applied to a woman who has completed one or more pregnancies, to differentiate her from a "first timer." Sometimes women who have had five or more viable births are called "grandmultips."

PHYSIOLOGY OF PREGNANCY

Reproductive System

Breasts

Estrogen and progesterone cause breast tissue to increase in size and nodularity in preparation for lactation. Superficial veins become prominent, nipples more erect, and the areola becomes darker. Colostrum, or milky secretions, may be expressed as early as 12 weeks' gestation.

Ovaries

The ovaries cease ovum production. The corpus luteum produces essential hormones that sustain the pregnancy for approximately 10 to 12 weeks, at which time the placenta assumes this role.

Uterus

The uterus grows from a small, pear-shaped organ to one large enough to accommodate a full-term infant. The growth, under the influence of estrogen, is primarily from the increase in size (hypertrophy) of existing muscle cells. The uterine walls are relatively thick during the first few months of pregnancy. The walls become thin near term, allowing easier palpation of fetal parts and position. The number and size of uterine blood vessels also increase.

Braxton Hicks contractions, described in Chapter 8, occur throughout pregnancy and aid in uterine circulation.

Cervix

The glandular tissue of the cervix increases under the influence of estrogen. This tissue secretes thick mucus, forming a mucous plug that prevents bacteria from entering the uterus. Vascularization increases, causing a bluish coloration of the cervix (Chadwick's sign), and a softening of the tissue (Goodell's sign).

Vagina

Estrogen causes the cells lining the vagina to increase in size, number, and vascularization. The latter may produce the same bluish coloration seen in the cervix. Vaginal secretions increase and are thick and white. They are also acidic, providing the mother and fetus with some protection against infection. They do, however, tend to facilitate the growth of yeast organisms, resulting in a common vaginal infection, moniliasis.

Cardiovascular System

Blood volume progressively increases throughout pregnancy, peaking at 40% to 50% above prepregnant levels, in the early part of the third trimester. Plasma volume increases more than red cell volume, resulting in hemodilution and subsequent slight reduction in hemoglobin and hematocrit levels. This phenomenon is known as physiological anemia of pregnancy and should not be confused with true anemia. Generally, hemoglobin less than 11 gm/dl and hematocrit less than 33% are diagnostic for iron deficiency anemia in pregnancy. (A more in-depth discussion of anemia can be found in the nutrition section of this chapter.)

Leukocytes (white blood cells) also increase during pregnancy. The average count is 5000 to 15,000/mm^3. Although the exact cause is uncertain, it is not unusual for this count to be significantly increased (as much as 25,000/mm^3) during labor and the immediate postpartum period. (See Appendix C to compare laboratory values for the pregnant and nonpregnant woman.)

Pulse rate increases slightly (10 to 15 beats per minute) during pregnancy. Blood pressure decreases slightly (2 to 3 mm Hg systolic, 5 to 10 mm Hg diastolic), reaching the lowest level in the second trimester, and increasing to normal levels by term. Blood pressure is highest when the woman is sitting and lowest in the left-lateral position.

Pressure of the growing uterus on the iliac veins and the inferior vena cava results in blood stasis in the lower extremities. This contributes to varicose vein formation and edema of the legs and feet.

The large uterus may also cause pressure on the vena cava when the woman lies on her back (supine), resulting in **supine hypotensive syndrome**. When this occurs, a dramatic decrease in blood pressure results and the woman experiences dizziness and lightheadedness. It can be prevented (or corrected) by having the woman lie on her side.

Respiratory System

A greater demand for oxygen is due to the increased basal metabolic rate and oxygen requirements of the pregnant woman and fetus. The diaphragm is elevated because of pressure from the enlarging uterus. To compensate the chest circumference increases by 5 to 7 cm (2 to 3 inches). The woman breathes more deeply than in the nonpregnant state. Respiratory rate is unchanged. Nasal stuffiness is frequently experienced because of edema and vascular congestion of the nasal mucosa.

Gastrointestinal System

Estrogen causes the gums to be more vascular and swollen, creating a tendency to bleed. Saliva production is not increased, but excess saliva may be associated with nausea because of decreased swallowing.

Progesterone causes smooth muscle relaxation of the gastrointestinal tract. This relaxation contributes to slowed peristalsis and constipation, as well as slowed gastric emptying and esophageal regurgitation (heartburn). Hemorrhoids may result from the pressure of the uterus, particularly if the woman is frequently constipated. The growing uterus also puts pressure on the stomach and colon.

Urinary System

Progesterone causes smooth muscle relaxation of the urinary tract. The renal pelvis and ureters dilate, causing urinary stasis and increasing the danger of pyelonephritis (inflammation of the kidney). Bladder tone is also diminished. Uterine pressure on the bladder results in reduced bladder capacity and increased urinary frequency.

Musculoskeletal System

The enlarging uterus and resulting shift in the woman's center of gravity causes compensatory changes in posture. The normal lumbosacral curve increases (lordosis) and an exaggerated forward flexion of the head results. Relaxation and increased mobility of joints also appears, resulting in the characteristic "waddle" seen in the third trimester. In some women a slight separation of the rectus muscles of the abdominal wall (diastasis recti) occurs, associated with the enlarging uterus.

PSYCHOLOGY OF PREGNANCY

Pregnancy and childbearing are developmental phases in the family life cycle, with attendant psychological changes and stresses. Many factors affect how a woman will adjust to the changes and stresses of pregnancy: her health; previous life experiences, including previous pregnancies; her characteristic way of reacting to life; her own mothering experiences and the relationship she has with her mother; social factors such as income; her culture; her relationship with her partner/father of the baby; and whether the pregnancy was planned or not. Her partner is likely to experience many of the same concerns and feelings that she does. The following is a brief summary of typical psychological changes of pregnancy by trimester.

First trimester

Whether or not the pregnancy was planned the initial response to confirmation of pregnancy is normally mixed. Feelings range from positive to negative (see the nursing care plan on p. 113). During the early weeks, these mixed feelings or ambivalence may dominate because women are anxious about the need to rework personal relationships and/or career plans, adapt to lifestyle changes, take on new parenting responsibilities, meet additional financial obligations, and cope with the pain of labor and birth. Hormonal fluctuations contribute to mood swings and increased introversion (turning in on one's self). She may be uncomfortable because of early symptoms of pregnancy such as nausea and vomiting, fatigue, breast tenderness, and other body changes. These body changes and symptoms, however, help her validate the pregnancy. She may experience decreased interest in sexual activity as a result of fatigue.

Expectant fathers experience similar ambivalence and are particularly concerned about the financial implications of impending parenthood. They are often confused by their partners' mood swings and concerned about the fatigue and diminished interest in sex.

Second trimester

During the second trimester the woman's physical discomforts usually improve and she experiences a general sense of well-being. Quickening brings a sense of excitement and is accompanied by dreams and fantasies about what the fetus will be like as a person (e.g., gender) and about herself and her partner as parents. Introversion continues. Body changes are more pronounced, providing additional confirmation of pregnancy. These changes may be a source of pride, concern, or embarrassment. The woman's interest and responsivity to sexual activity usually improves.

The expectant father, like his partner, increasingly accepts the pregnancy as a reality. Feeling fetal movements, hearing the heart beat, and seeing the fetus on sonogram may be particularly important in this acceptance. Some men find their partners' changing body appealing, whereas others do not. Expectant fathers and mothers typically sort through their own mothering and fathering experiences and choose behaviors they wish to replicate. Communication is essential as couples discuss and negotiate their new roles.

Third trimester

During the third trimester, women frequently complain of impatience with the discomforts of pregnancy and the awkwardness of their bodies. They usually have less interest in sexual activity because of the physical discomforts and fatigue. They also experience increased feelings of dependency and concerns about their own safety, the safety of the fetus, and of their partner. As labor and delivery nears, both parents experience anxiety about labor and delivery, accompanied by increased anticipation of the baby's arrival. Completing home preparations for the infant takes on a new urgency.

PRENATAL CARE

The term *antepartal* or *prenatal care* refers to the systematic examination, observation, and anticipatory guidance of a pregnant woman. "The broad objectives of prenatal care are to promote the health and well-being of the pregnant woman, the fetus, the infant, and the family up to 1 year after the infant's birth" (US Department of Health and Human Services,

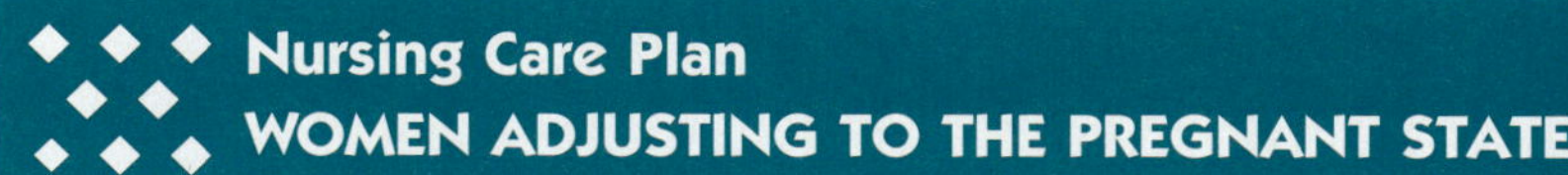

Nursing Care Plan
WOMEN ADJUSTING TO THE PREGNANT STATE

Selected Nursing Diagnoses	Expected Outcomes	Interventions
Anxiety related to emotional responses to pregnancy.	Anxiety is reduced. Woman discusses her feelings and uses positive coping mechanisms to deal with her emotional responses to pregnancy.	Provide realistic reassurance that responses are normal and encourage open discussion of concerns.
	Specific plans for selected problems are described below.	
A Early phase of maternal adaptation to pregnancy evidenced by ambivalence about being pregnant. Clinical manifestations: Expresses surprise at being pregnant. Responses to news includes mixed emotions: "Who, me? Not now!"	Woman verbalizes her concerns and exhibits positive behaviors towards pregnancy status (e.g., tells others about being pregnant, buys/wears maternity clothes).	Ask how she feels about being pregnant. Give permission to express positive or negative feeling about pregnancy (e.g., "Many women find that they do not feel quite ready when they learn that they are pregnant."). Provide appropriate place to talk. Explain near universality of ambivalence in early pregnancy.
B Alteration in self-concept: change in body image. Clinical manifestations: Feelings range from very positive to extremely negative. May worry that she is seen as fat. Feels large, heavy, and awkward as pregnancy advances.	Enlarging abdomen and other body changes are accepted as normal.	Provide information about: hormonal and uterine changes and what outcomes can be expected (e.g., most changes revert after delivery); striae don't disappear but do fade; weight can be lost and muscle tone regained with exercise. Observe for indications that the woman is not coping well with pregnancy's impact on her body (e.g., wears constrictive clothing; repeated referral to self as "fat" or "ugly," or "look what this baby is doing to me"); overly concerned with striae or pigment changes of the skin. Arrange counseling for these women to avoid inappropriate self-care and psychological stresses.

Continued.

1989). Components of optimum prenatal care are listed in the box on p. 115.

The extension of prenatal care is probably the primary factor in the improvement of maternal morbidity and mortality statistics in the United States. As indicated in Chapter 1, prenatal care is also viewed as a *key* element in achieving future reductions in infant mortality and morbidity (National Commission to Prevent Infant Mortality, 1992). (See the box on p. 115 for the national health objective for the year 2000.) As soon as a woman suspects she is pregnant, she should seek prenatal care. Women who are planning to become pregnant should seek preconceptual care in an effort to maximize their health *before* becoming pregnant.

For prenatal care to be effective, it must be available

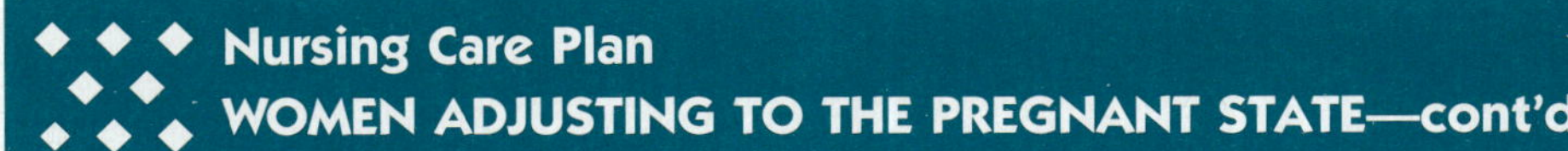

Nursing Care Plan
WOMEN ADJUSTING TO THE PREGNANT STATE—cont'd

Selected Nursing Diagnoses	Expected Outcomes	Interventions
Altered patterns of sexual expression related to physical changes of pregnancy, changes in sexual desire, or fear of injury to fetus. Clinical manifestations: Woman may ask questions about effect of pregnancy on sexuality but, more often, will not.	Woman and partner understand the reason for these changes and concerns and will maintain a mutually satisfying sexual relationship.	Explain possible causes of discomfort or lack of responsiveness in pregnancy (e.g., fatigue, nausea, and vomiting); breast tenderness in first trimester. Fatigue and enlarging abdomen in third trimester. Determine impact on sexuality of pregnancy of woman and her partner, need of couple to share concerns. Suggest alternative sexual activities and positions. Discuss issues of safety: there is no evidence that sexual intercourse during *normal* pregnancy can cause harm to fetus. Intercourse can be safely continued until membranes rupture, unless health care provider advises otherwise.

and it must be used. Currently, a need exists for health care delivery systems that encourage socioeconomically disadvantaged urban and rural clients to receive needed care and vital health instruction. Because of financial strain, transportation difficulties, child care problems, or fear and distrust of depersonalized and fragmented care systems, some expectant mothers do not obtain or use these services as often as do those who are financially and socially better prepared.

Prenatal care may be provided by a physician, a nurse practitioner, or a certified nurse midwife. In prenatal clinics and obstetrician's offices the registered nurse, and/or the licensed vocational/practical nurse (LVN/LPN), are the first to greet the patient and have a major role to play in setting the tone for the visit and in establishing a supportive environment for the woman and her family.

The First Visit

Preparation for pregnancy begins in the life of a woman before she becomes pregnant. Her basic physique is determined before her birth by her parents. Her environment leaves its physical and emotional imprint. Previous pregnancies and their spacing affect her health and her attitude toward pregnancy. Her culture, her family circle, and her close friends also influence her attitude toward pregnancy and the challenges and responsibilities of motherhood. Whether or not the pregnancy was planned the first visit to the health care provider is usually accompanied by some anxiety. Typically her first visit is the most lengthy.

Preparation for the first prenatal visit is usually made by telephone. Some prenatal programs provide, through mailings or recorded tapes, extended information regarding the upcoming appointment and helpful resources. The expectant father should be encouraged to attend the first and subsequent visits. His presence may be reassuring to the woman and his participation enables him to ask questions that may be of special concern to him. It is customary for a new patient to be asked to bring a sample of the first voided urine on the day of the appointment, if her visit will be made early in the morning.

The nurse or receptionist should talk with the client and her partner, making them feel welcome. Brief information cards for office use are usually completed. An office that emphasizes health promotion is likely to have attractive bulletin boards emphasizing nutrition and meal planning, mental health practices, good grooming, maternity wardrobe styles, and approved courses in preparation for childbirth and parenting. Up-to-date pamphlets on maternal and child care and breast-feeding literature may also be available. Not all reading material should be pregnancy-oriented, however. When waits are protracted, an offer of nutritious beverages may be appreciated. The way to the rest-

COMPONENTS OF PRENATAL CARE

1 Early and continuing risk assessment:
  - history
  - physical examination
  - laboratory tests

2 Health promotion activities:
  - counseling that promotes and supports healthful behaviors
  - education about pregnancy and parenting
  - information about the individual's proposed care and treatment

3 Medical and psychosocial interventions and follow-up

From USDHHS: *Caring for our future: the content of prenatal care,* Washington, DC, 1989, The Department.

NATIONAL HEALTH OBJECTIVE FOR THE YEAR 2000

Ninety percent of all pregnant women will obtain prenatal care within the first 3 months of pregnancy.

From USDHHS: *Healthy people 2000,* Boston, 1992, Jones and Bartlett.

room should be clearly indicated, since frequent urination is common during pregnancy and general nervousness may exaggerate this symptom.

History

Before actually seeing the health care provider the woman is usually asked to fill out a questionnaire that asks questions about previous health and health practices. She is then weighed, and height is measured. Her temperature, pulse, and respiration are checked by the nurse. In some clinics, nurses also take the blood pressures and complete the medical and obstetrical histories of new patients. Many practitioners, however, prefer to complete the blood pressures and the histories themselves. A careful history is an important screening tool in assessing reproductive risk and the need for special care. Early detection of reproductive risk is essential in preventing maternal or fetal problems. Categories of information usually gathered in a complete history are presented in the box above right. Information about the mother's current pregnancy is also gathered.

A record of previous pregnancies and their outcome

PRENATAL HISTORY: IMPORTANT CATEGORIES OF INFORMATION

MEDICAL	PSYCHOSOCIAL
Social and demographic data	Smoking
Menstrual history	Alcohol
Past obstetrical history	Drugs
Sexual history	Social support
Medical/surgical history	Stress levels
Infection history	Physical abuse
Family and genetic history	Mental illness/status
Nutrition	Pregnancy readiness
	Exposure to teratogens
	Housing, finances, etc.
	Extremes of physical work, exercise, and other activity

From USDHHS: *Caring for our future: the content of prenatal care,* Washington DC, 1989, The Department.

is important in the assessment of potential risk. One method of coding the results of previous pregnancies involves the use of five consecutive digits (the G/TPAL system). The first digit refers to the number of pregnancies (gravida) experienced, the second to the number of full-term deliveries, the third to the number of premature births, the fourth to abortions, and the fifth to children now living. For example, Mrs. Vasquez is pregnant for the fourth time, has 2 living children (1 was born full-term and 1 was born prematurely), and had 1 spontaneous abortion (miscarriage). The G/TPAL designation would be 4/1/1/1/2. The time spent in gathering historical data provides an opportunity to establish rapport, to learn about the parents' knowledge and expectations of pregnancy and the health care system, and to better evaluate the woman's health status and potential risks of pregnancy and birth.

Physical examination

The first prenatal visit usually includes a complete physical examination. The woman is asked to change into a gown that provides coverage but opens to facilitate the examination. In addition to the pelvic examination the health care provider checks the woman's blood pressure; listens to her heart and lungs; examines her mouth, eyes, nose, and throat; observes and palpates her breasts for abnormalities; and inquires about her preference for feeding the infant. The breast examination determines whether normal breast changes of pregnancy are occurring and assesses whether infection or malignancy is present. The

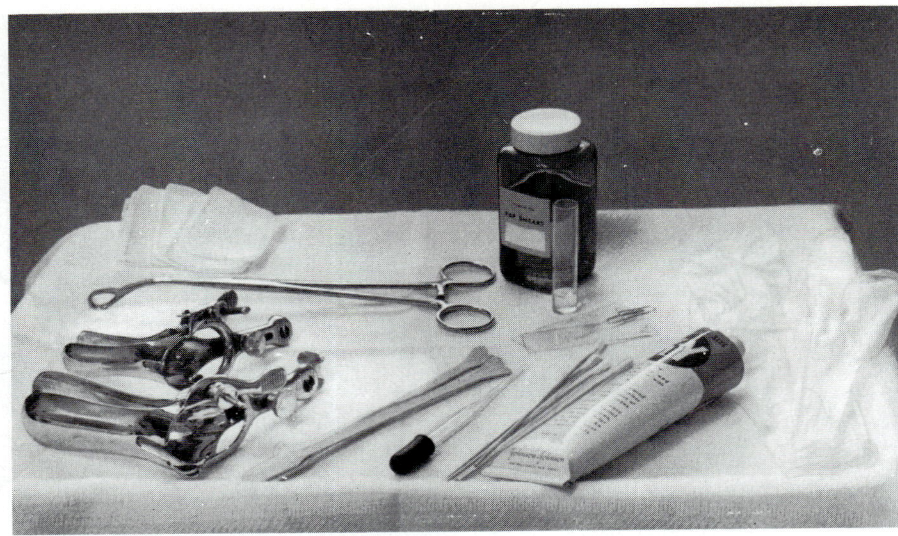

Fig. 9-1 Typical pelvic tray (sterile gloves not shown). Small test tube contains physiological saline solution for wet mount of vaginal discharge.

abdomen is palpated with the knees flexed for greater relaxation of the abdominal wall, and evaluated for changes consistent with early pregnancy. The extremities are checked for bruises, swelling, and enlarged veins.

Pelvic examination. Just before the pelvic examination the woman should have an opportunity to empty her bladder to increase her comfort and to allow more accurate assessment of pelvic organs and measurement of the height of the uterine fundus. The nurse's manner and clear explanations can help the patient relax for this examination. A drape that makes the woman feel covered, even if she is not, is usually provided. The hips should extend approximately 1 inch over the edge of the table, with the feet supported in covered stirrups. Although not always the case, a male physician may prefer to have a female nurse present during the examination. Necessary instruments should be ready (Fig. 9-1): a warmed speculum; spatula or applicator, or vaginal pipette with rubber bulb; slides and preservative for cervical cancer detection; long swabs or cotton balls; sponge sticks; both sterile and clean examination gloves; lubricant; and paper tissue wipes. A good light and a convenient stool are essential. If the woman is able to let her knees fall outward and relax, the examination will be more comfortable. Having her breathe slowly through her open mouth usually promotes relaxation.

The pelvic examination yields considerable information. First, the external genitalia are inspected. Next, if a Papanicolaou (Pap) smear for cancer detection is desired (and it is almost always part of the routine), a warmed bivalve speculum, lubricated with water, is inserted to reveal the cervix. Secretions are aspirated from the posterior fornix with the pipette or secured with the applicator or spatula from the cervix and placed thinly and evenly on one or two slides. These slides must not be allowed to dry out but should immediately be placed in a fixative (usually equal parts of 95% alcohol and ether). The mucosa will be checked for the bluish discoloration of Chadwick's sign.

The examiner will then observe the cervix and vaginal mucosa for any abnormalities or unusual discharge. Specimens of any discharge can be obtained for analysis. (Fungous infection caused by *Candida albicans* or infection initiated by microscopic organisms, or protozoa, called *Trichomonas vaginalis,* is fairly common.) Routine cultures of cervical mucus for *Neisseria gonorrhoeae,* the cause of gonorrhea, and *Chlamydia* are done to detect these so-called silent infections. Some health care providers are also routinely obtaining cervical cultures for group B streptococcus, an organism that can cause serious illness in the newborn. Cultures for herpes simplex (types 1 and 2) may be done if indicated by history or observation of lesions. Herpes lesions usually first appear as tender, painful blisters (vesicles) on the vulva, cervix, vagina, anus, or buttocks. After these vesicles break, wet ulcers form, which later crust.

After general inspection of the vulva, cervix, and vagina the speculum is gently removed and a digital examination is made with a hand protected by a lubricated glove. At this time the examiner feels the size and position of the uterus and the consistency of the cervix, and perhaps tries to elicit Hegar's sign, the softening of the uterine isthmus, through vaginoabdominal pressure. The pelvic contents are palpated to try to identify any abnormal masses or tumors. Before the examination is completed, an attempt to measure the diagonal conjugate to estimate the size of the pelvic canal, evaluate the position and bluntness of the ischial spines, and measure the distance between the tuberosities may be made (see Chapter 4 for a discussion of evaluation of the bony pelvis). At the end of the vaginal examination a rectal examination is usually done.

The time of pelvic evaluation can provide an excellent opportunity to teach the patient about her external genitalia, internal pelvic anatomy, and the normal physiological changes that take place during pregnancy. Generally, the examiner can report at the end of the pelvic examination whether the woman is pregnant, based on a number of signs and symptoms. Many examiners also include pregnancy tests as part of their initial evaluations.

Determination of delivery date

The most common method of determining the date of delivery involves a record of the menstrual cycle. The woman is asked to identify the *first* day of her last *normal* menstrual period. The caregiver then counts back 3 months and adds 7 days to calculate the estimated date of delivery or confinement (EDD or EDC). (*Confinement* is an older term used to indicate the period of labor and birth.) For example, if a woman says her last normal menstrual period occurred between May 7 and May 12, her EDD would be February 14 of the following year. This method of calculation is called Nagele's rule. Nagele's rule offers only an estimate. Approximately 4% of all babies arrive on the predetermined date using this schedule, whereas 60% appear 1 to 7 days earlier or later. Actually, infants born within 2 weeks of the EDD calculated using Nagele's rule are considered full term. Of course, if the patient cannot remember the necessary vital statistics, then the size of the uterus may be interpreted, or the time of the intercourse that preceded conception may be known. Occasionally quickening may be used as a measurable landmark, but it is not considered reliable. Ultrasound evaluation may be used if it is important to more accurately estimate the age of the fetus.

Laboratory tests

Usually at the conclusion of the physical examination, arrangements are made for the necessary laboratory tests. (See Appendix C for normal laboratory values.) A sample of venous blood is drawn. A complete blood cell count (CBC) with differential smear, a hemoglobin assessment alone, or a hematocrit may be ordered to determine the amount of hemoglobin present in the blood in relation to its volume. This test is usually repeated after 24 weeks. Any pregnant woman may be or may become anemic. Dietary deficiencies of iron are common. Prenatal testing for sickle cell anemia in previously unscreened African-American patients is recommended.

A serology test (RPR or VDRL) for the detection of syphilis is a routine screening procedure. Follow-up may utilize the fluorescent treponemal antibody absorption (FTA-ABS) test if the VDRL or RPR is reactive. Early treatment (before 18 weeks' gestation) of this disease can avoid subsequent fetal problems. In this instance, even though treatment has been instituted, the mother should be retested in the third trimester and at delivery (Stepanuk, 1994). The newborn may also be tested using serum obtained from cord blood for VDRL and FTA-ABS tests, as well as IgM-specific FTA-ABS testing.

A determination of blood group type and Rh status is made to assist in maternal care in the event of hemorrhage and to detect the possibility of blood protein incompatibility, which could threaten the life of the developing fetus or neonate. If the patient is Rh negative, Rh serum antibody levels (indirect Coombs' test) will be ordered at the initial visit and again at 26 to 28 weeks' gestation. (See Chapter 18 for more discussion of Rh disease.)

An antibody screen establishes immune status for rubella, or German measles. A history of the disease in childhood is not always reliable, since other conditions may have been incorrectly called rubella and the disease does not always manifest a rash. The presence of antibodies in a dilution greater than 1:8 or 1:10 (depending on the manufacturer) in the hemagglutination inhibition (HI or HAI) test or a value of 1000 or more as a result of the enzyme index assay (EIA) indicates immunity. Pregnant women are *not* given the available immunization against rubella. Maximum theoretic risk of fetal damage from rubella vaccination during pregnancy is approximately 2% to 5%. Women who are not immune are usually immunized during the postpartum period (see Chapter 13 for a further discussion).

Current recommendations are that all women be screened for hepatitis B (HBsAg) at the first prenatal visit. If the test is negative but the woman is at high risk for the disease, she may be immunized. If the test is positive, the baby should begin treatment within the first 12 hours of life using hepatitis B immune globulin and hepatitis B vaccine. HIV screening should also be offered to all pregnant women. The latter test is voluntary and requires a written consent.

With the rising incidence of tuberculosis, some providers are using Mantoux or tine skin testing to screen for the disease. If the skin test is positive, a full-sized, conventional chest x-ray is recommended to determine presence of active disease. Screening for tuberculosis, hepatitis, and HIV is becoming more prevalent because of increased illicit drug use and a growing immigrant population in the United States.

The urine specimen brought in the morning of the examination or secured later at the office is tested for albumin (protein) and glucose. Many health care providers also order a complete urinalysis and urine culture at the initial visit.

Health promotion activities

After all of these procedures have been completed the woman is usually tired and lengthy instructions and explanations may not be properly assimilated. One method of imparting needed information is through the use of a prenatal instruction booklet that has been approved or written by the health care provider. Some practices offer a series of teaching films that individuals or groups can check out to view at home or view while they are waiting to see the provider. Booklets and films should offer general information about physiological and emotional changes of pregnancy, sexuality, fetal growth and development, self-care for common discomforts, and referrals to early pregnancy classes dealing with some of these topics (US Department of Health and Human Services, 1989). Such guidance is absolutely necessary, but all of it need not be provided on the first visit.

Some time should be spent, however, answering questions, discussing patient expectations for the childbirth, and giving general instructions regarding dietary requirements and general health habits. In addition, the risks of self-medication, smoking, and alcohol and drug consumption should be addressed. The woman should also be given information on the timing and content of future visits, preparation for future screening and diagnostic tests, and instructed on the need to report the following **danger signs:**

1 Vaginal spotting or bleeding at any time
2 Leaking of fluid from the vagina
3 Unusual abdominal pain or cramps
4 Persistent nausea or vomiting, especially in the second or third trimester
5 Persistent headache or any blurring of vision
6 Marked swelling of the ankles and especially of the hands and face
7 Painful or burning urination
8 Foul-smelling vaginal discharge
9 Chills or fever

Subsequent Visits

During the first 28 weeks of pregnancy, most expectant mothers visit their health care provider every 4 weeks, unless special needs indicate a greater frequency. From 28 to 36 weeks' gestation, visits are scheduled every 2 weeks. In the last month, checkups are usually every week (more often if complications arise).

Subsequent visits are not as long or involved as the first. At each visit an interim history should include questions about the woman's physical symptoms and her emotional adjustment.

Physical examination

The woman is weighed by the nurse, her blood pressure is recorded, and a urine specimen is checked for albumin and glucose. The urine examination for glucose is made to detect diabetes mellitus or gestational diabetes. The weight, blood pressure, and urine protein determinations are done to screen for signs of pregnancy-induced hypertension (PIH) or preeclampsia (high blood pressure, edema, excessive weight gain, and albuminuria). (See Chapter 14 for further discussion of these complications.) The pelvic examination is usually not repeated until 38 to 40 weeks' gestation, when a manual examination may be done to ascertain whether the cervix is beginning to thin and dilate.

Fetal well-being is also evaluated at each visit. The health care provider measures the height of the uterus to see if the pregnancy is progressing at the expected rate. The Doptone may be used to evaluate the fetal heart rate. At approximately 18 to 20 weeks' gestation the fetal heart tone may be heard with a nonelectronic fetoscope. After 24 weeks' gestation the abdomen is palpated to determine the position of the fetus (Leopold maneuvers). If the woman does not have a reliable menstrual history, an ultrasound may be ordered to confirm the EDD. Intrauterine fetal death is often preceded by a period of decreased fetal movement. For this reason, most health care providers now instruct the woman to monitor fetal movement at the same time each day during the third trimester. The woman is instructed to lie on her side and count fetal movements until she feels 10 movements. Most women report feeling 10 movements within 20 minutes to 2 hours. If she does not feel 10 movements after 3 hours, she should call her health care provider.

Laboratory tests

The expectant mother should be offered a maternal serum alpha-fetoprotein (MSAFP) test between 14 and 16 weeks' gestation. This test screens for the presence of a neural tube defect such as spina bifida. If the results show an elevation, it will be followed by further evaluation of amniotic fluid levels, secured through amniocentesis.

Measurements of hemoglobin or hematocrit levels should be repeated for all pregnant women at least once after 24 weeks' gestation and perhaps again during the third trimester. Women with iron or folic acid deficiency anemias or other causes of hemoglobin reduction at the time of earlier tests may be checked more frequently to determine their response to therapy.

A blood glucose tolerance screening is usually ordered at 24 to 28 weeks' gestation, as a result of increasing fetal demands on the maternal system. It is common for pregnant women to spill some glucose in the urine during pregnancy. However, the urine glucose is not diagnostic for diabetes during pregnancy. Diagnosis of diabetes is established by blood tests.

If Rh incompatibility is a possibility, antibody titers may be indicated. Testing is done monthly during the first and second trimesters, biweekly during the third trimester, and the week before the due date. Rising titers may indicate maternal sensitization of an Rh-negative mother to an Rh positive baby and will alert the physician to developing erythroblastosis fetalis. If these titers rise the fetus is further evaluated by analysis of amniotic fluid (amniocentesis) for elevated bilirubin. Some cases of isoimmunization can be prevented by using prenatal administration of immune globulin (RhoGAM). Occasionally, tiny breaks in placental circulation result in the mixing of maternal and fetal blood. For this reason, Rh negative pregnant women are given RhoGam at approximately 28 weeks' gestation. RhoGAM is also indicated after amniocentesis, ectopic pregnancy, or abortion (spontaneous or therapeutic).

For those at risk the health care provider may decide to repeat the test for syphilis, gonorrhea, and HIV during the third trimester. Genital herpes can be transmitted to the baby as he or she passes through the birth canal. For this reason, whenever suspicious lesions are found, a test for herpes should be performed.

Other laboratory evaluations of fetal and maternal health and gestational maturity are possible but depend on the specific problems discovered.

Health promotion activities

Teaching should be based on the assessment of client needs. In general, however, continuing attention should be devoted to fetal growth and development, physiological and emotional changes, general health habits, and strategies to deal with the common discomforts of pregnancy. The following section discusses general health suggestions and gives specific recommendations to help relieve common discomforts. See the box at right for a trimester outline of patient education topics.

TOPICS FOR CLIENT TEACHING BY TRIMESTER

ALL THREE TRIMESTERS
Fetal growth and development
Physical and psychological changes
Nutrition and weight gain
Discomforts of pregnancy
Sexual activity
Sibling preparation (if applicable)

FIRST TRIMESTER
Readiness for pregnancy
Smoking, use of alcohol or drugs
Employment (if applicable)
Travel
General hygiene, bathing
Exercise and rest
Danger signs to report (e.g., spontaneous abortion)
Early pregnancy classes

SECOND TRIMESTER
Clothing
Adaptation to changing body
Fetal movement
Decisions about infant feeding
Preparation for infant (e.g., equipment)
Danger signs to report (e.g., preterm labor—see Chapter 14)

THIRD TRIMESTER
Travel
Employment
Exercise and rest
Danger signs (e.g., preterm labor)
Preparation for labor and birth (e.g., classes)
Decisions about the infant (e.g., circumcision, feeding)
Car seat and other infant safety measures
Signs of labor, when to call/come to the hospital
Preparation for hospitalization (where to go/admission, analgesia/anesthesia options, what to bring)
Postpartum physical and psychological changes
Family roles and adjustment

PATIENT EDUCATION

Because of the profound physical and psychological changes that occur during pregnancy, women are usually very motivated to learn about their bodies and about activities that will improve their chances for a healthy outcome. Although the topics women are interested in learning about will vary by parity and educational background, they are generally interested in a wide variety of information (Freda, et al., 1993). Nurses should be aware that the topics in which pregnant women are most interested may not match those the health care provider feels are of interest (Freda, et al., 1993). It is important, therefore, to assess the client's interest rather than simply teaching about areas the provider assumes are of interest or considers

◆ **TABLE 9-1**
Food and Nutrition Board, National Academy of Sciences—National Research Council Recommended Dietary Allowances,*

		Weight†		Height†			Fat-soluble Vitamins			
Category	Age (Years) or Condition	(kg)	(lb)	(cm)	(in)	Protein (gm)	Vitamin A (μg RE)‡	Vitamin D (μg)§	Vitamin E (mg α-TE)‖	Vitamin K (μg)
Females	11-14	46	101	157	62	46	800	10	8	45
	15-18	55	120	163	64	44	800	10	8	55
	19-24	58	128	164	65	46	800	10	8	60
	25-50	63	138	163	64	50	800	5	8	65
	51+	65	143	160	63	50	800	5	8	65
Pregnant						60	800	10	10	65
Lactating	1st 6 months					65	1300	10	12	65
	2nd 6 months					62	1200	10	11	65

*The allowances, expressed as average daily intakes over time, are intended to provide for individual variations among most normal people as they live in the United States under usual environmental stresses. Diets should be based on a variety of common foods in order to provide other nutrients for which human requirements have been less well defined.
†Weights and heights of Reference Adults are actual medians for the US population of the designated age, as reported by NHANES II. The use of these figures does not imply that the height-to-weight ratios are ideal.
‡Retinol equivalents. 1 retinol equivalent = 1 μg retinol or 6 μg β-carotene.
§As cholecalciferol. 10 μg cholecalciferol = 400 IU of vitamin D.
‖α-Tocopherol equivalents. 1 mg d-α tocopherol = 1 α-TE.

important. In addition to fetal development and danger signs and symptoms, presented in previous sections, the following material reviews many of the areas of interest to pregnant women. See the box on p. 119 for client teaching appropriate for each trimester.

Nutrition

Nutrition is a critical variable in determining the health of the childbearing woman, her offspring, and even that of future generations. A woman who is well-nourished before pregnancy and who augments her diet as needed during pregnancy reduces the risks of obstetrical and perinatal complications for herself and her unborn child. Maternal anemia, pregnancy-induced hypertension (PIH), preterm labor (PTL), low birth weight (LBW), intrauterine growth retardation (IUGR), and neural tube defects (NTD) are all conditions that have been linked to nutritional factors.

Nutrient requirements

The Food and Nutrition Board of the National Research Council periodically publishes a list of the nutrients needed by women of childbearing age. Table 9-1 reflects the last revision of this list, the recommended dietary allowances (RDAs). The RDAs are designed to indicate safe dietary levels of selected nutrients for a wide range of normal, healthy people. Individual differences in the dietary background or obstetrical histories of pregnant women may suggest the need for variations in these allowances. More of almost every listed nutrient is necessary during pregnancy. In 1990, the Institute of Medicine reported that pregnant women in the United States typically meet the recommended dietary allowance for protein, thiamin, riboflavin, niacin, and vitamins A, B_{12}, and C. Nutrients for which the recommended dietary allowance are least likely to be met are vitamins B_6, D, E, and folacin, as well as iron, calcium, zinc, and magnesium. The Institute concluded, however, that with the exception of iron, the RDAs for healthy pregnant women can be met with a balanced diet.

Calories. A normal, healthy, pregnant woman of any age should consume an additional 300 calories per day, particularly during her second and third trimesters. Special situations, such as depleted body reserves or changes in activity, however, may require calorie adjustments.

Protein. Protein provides the necessary amino acids for rapid fetal tissue growth and building the maternal components that support the fetus (placenta, uterus, blood volume, and breast tissue). Animal sources of protein, such as meat, fish, poultry, milk, and

Revised 1989 (Designed for the Maintenance of Good Nutrition of Practically all Healthy People in the United States)

Water-soluble Vitamins							Minerals						
Vitamin C (mg)	Thiamin (mg)	Riboflavin (mg)	Niacin (mg NE)¶	Vitamin B_6 (mg)	Folate (μg)	Vitamin B_{12} (μg)	Calcium (mg)	Phosphorus (mg)	Magnesium (mg)	Iron (mg)	Zinc (mg)	Iodine (μg)	Selenium (μg)
50	1.1	1.3	15	1.4	150	2.0	1200	1200	280	15	12	150	45
60	1.1	1.3	15	1.5	180	2.0	1200	1200	300	15	12	150	50
60	1.1	1.3	15	1.6	180	2.0	1200	1200	280	15	12	150	55
60	1.1	1.3	15	1.6	180	2.0	800	800	280	15	12	150	55
60	1.0	1.2	13	1.6	180	2.0	800	800	280	10	12	150	55
70	1.5	1.6	17	2.2	400	2.2	1200	1200	320	30	15	175	65
95	1.6	1.8	20	2.1	280	2.6	1200	1200	355	15	19	200	75
90	1.6	1.7	20	2.1	260	2.6	1200	1200	340	15	16	200	75

¶1 NE (niacin equivalent) is equal to 1 mg of niacin or 60 mg of dietary tryptophan.

eggs are complete proteins, containing the right combination of amino acids necessary for cell growth, repair, and development. They are generally good sources of vitamins B_6 and B_{12}, iron, and zinc. However, a diet including only animal sources of protein is likely to be high in saturated fat and cholesterol.

Vegetable protein is a good source of vitamin B_6, iron, zinc, folate, magnesium, and fiber. Since vegetable protein does not contain the right combination of essential amino acids, legumes (dried beans or peas), nuts, and seeds must be eaten together with other food so that all essential amino acids are consumed at the same or at the next meal. Mixing certain incomplete proteins or serving them with milk provides an adequate diet but requires careful planning. Examples of adequate protein mixes, using incomplete proteins, are combinations of cornmeal and kidney beans or whole wheat, soy beans, and sesame seeds. Pure vegetarian or "vegan" diets without any animal sources, dairy products, or eggs can, with careful planning, supply adequate protein, but other deficiencies (e.g., vitamin B_{12}) may become a problem.

Vitamin A. Vitamin A is essential for fetal growth and development, particularly of epithelial tissue such as skin and the membranes that line the gastrointestinal, urinary, and respiratory tracts. However, excessive consumption of vitamin A, particularly in the first trimester, can result in spontaneous abortion, fetal central nervous system abnormalities, fetal cardiovascular abnormalities, fetal facial abnormalities, and altered fetal growth.

Food sources rich in vitamin A include animal products such as liver, eggs, and fortified milk; fruits such as apricots, cantaloupe, and mango; and vegetables such as carrots, sweet potatoes, and dark green, leafy vegetables. These fruits and vegetables also provide fiber, which along with increased fluids can help relieve the common discomforts related to constipation.

Vitamin E. Vitamin E's primary function is to prevent the oxidation of unsaturated fatty acids. Vitamin E deficiency can lead to cell damage and eventually neurological symptoms. Rich dietary sources of vitamin E are vegetable oils and products made from them, such as margarine.

Vitamin B_6. Vitamin B_6, pyridoxine, is important for amino acid metabolism and protein synthesis. Vitamin B_6 deficiency in pregnancy has been associated with nausea, vomiting, and depression. Some evidence exists that B_6 supplementation is beneficial for those with the most severe forms of nausea and vomiting during early pregnancy (Sahakian, et al., 1991). The richest food sources of vitamin B_6 are animal and vegetable protein and whole grains. See the nursing alert on p. 122.

Nursing Alert

Long-term users of oral contraceptives may have depleted body reserves of vitamin B_6 and folate.

Folate. Folic acid is necessary for cell division and protein synthesis. One of the first signs of folate deficiency is megaloblastic anemia, characterized by abnormal cell division. Folic acid deficiency has also been associated with spontaneous abortion, preterm delivery, pregnancy-induced hypertension, low birth weight, and fetal neural tube defects.

The fetal neural tube closes 25 to 27 days after conception (Mills, et al., 1992), when many women are still unaware of the pregnancy. Growing evidence suggests that folate supplementation before pregnancy and at least through the first trimester may prevent the occurrence or recurrence of neural tube defects (Centers for Disease Control, 1992). For this reason, the Centers for Disease Control (CDC) currently recommend that *all* women of childbearing age consume 400 µg (0.4 mg) of folic acid each day. The CDC also recommends that women who have given birth to a child with brain or spinal cord defects ingest 4 mg of folic acid daily for a month before pregnancy and during the first trimester. The Food and Drug Administration has proposed that folic acid be added to enriched flour, bread, pasta, cereals, and other grain products to help ensure that women of childbearing age receive adequate amounts of this vitamin.

The pregnancy RDA for folate is 400 µg per day, an amount that can be difficult to achieve for those who consume few raw fruits and leafy vegetables—the best dietary sources. Liver, yeast, legumes, nuts, and whole grains also supply folic acid but in lesser amounts. Most prenatal vitamins now contain enough folic acid to meet the RDA.

Iron. Iron is necessary for the manufacture of hemoglobin in both maternal and fetal blood cells. The fetus needs to build an iron reserve for hemoglobin formation during the first few months of extrauterine life. An adequate amount is also necessary to compensate for maternal blood loss at delivery. Iron deficiency anemia is the most common anemia of pregnancy. This condition is associated with increased risk of low birth weight, preterm birth, and perinatal mortality. See the box above right for criteria of diagnosis of iron deficiency anemia. (See the Nursing Alert above right.)

The RDA for iron doubles during pregnancy and is difficult to achieve by dietary sources alone. The best sources of dietary iron are beef, dark turkey meat, liver, and legumes. Vitamin C-rich fruits and vegetables enhance iron absorption. Using iron cookware is another way to add iron to the diet. Excessive amounts of unleavened whole-grain products such as bran muffins and cereals, tea, and coffee decrease iron absorption. Women should be counseled to avoid consuming these foods and beverages while taking an iron supplement. Iron is best absorbed when the supplement is taken between meals or at bedtime, when the stomach is empty.

CRITERIA FOR DIAGNOSIS OF IRON DEFICIENCY ANEMIA IN PREGNANCY

	HEMOGLOBIN (GM/DL)	HEMATOCRIT (%)
1st trimester	<11.0	<33
2nd trimester	<10.5	<32
3rd trimester	<11.0	<33

Nursing Alert

Smokers and those living at high altitudes have higher hemoglobin and hematocrit levels. This compensatory phenomenon can result in the underdiagnosis of anemia for these individuals.

Because of the difficulty in meeting the RDA of iron with food sources alone, the Institute of Medicine (1990) advises supplementation of 30 mg of ferrous iron per day, beginning at approximately 12 weeks' gestation, when iron requirements begin to increase. If laboratory evidence of anemia exists at any stage of pregnancy the recommended iron supplement is 60 to 120 mg per day. Divided doses, providing 30 mg of elemental iron each, help to minimize gastrointestinal distress. Iron supplementation is often continued for 2 to 3 months after delivery to help replenish the mother's iron supply. (See the Nursing Alert below.)

Nursing Alert

Iron supplements can cause iron poisoning in small children and should therefore be kept in a child-proof container out of the reach of children.

Calcium. Additional calcium is required for the development of the fetal skeleton and teeth, with the greatest demand in the last trimester. The RDA for calcium is 1200 mg per day—400 mg higher than the nonpregnant recommendation. If the pregnant woman does not consume adequate calcium to meet fetal demands, she will give up her own calcium stores to meet fetal needs.

The best dietary sources of calcium are milk and milk products. Nonfat or lowfat products are the healthiest choices. Lesser amounts of calcium are supplied by soybeans, figs, and by dark green, leafy vegetables such as kale, cabbage, collards, and turnip greens. The woman who does not like the taste of milk can use milk flavorings, concentrate the value of what she does drink by adding nonfat dry milk solids, use milk in cooking, or select another milk product of approximate equal value. For example, 1½ slices of cheddar cheese or 2 cups of cottage cheese supply approximately the same amount of calcium as 1 cup of milk or yogurt. If a woman cannot tolerate milk or milk products, she should be encouraged to consume alternate dietary sources of calcium such as those listed in Table 9-2.

Some adults, especially African-Americans, Asians, Hispanics, and Native Americans experience a digestive intolerance to the lactose found in milk. They may develop abdominal cramping, intestinal gas, and diarrhea. However, they are often able to tolerate yogurt, low-lactose milk, or cheese. The harder or more aged varieties of cheese contain less lactose than processed types.

Because women under 25 are still adding mineral content to their bones, inadequate intake of calcium during pregnancy is of particular concern. The Institute of Medicine (1990) recommends a supplement of 600 mg per day for women who are not consuming adequate dietary calcium. Supplements are best absorbed if taken in divided doses with a meal.

Vitamin D. Vitamin D is essential for calcium balance. Regular exposure to sunlight results in synthesis of vitamin D by the skin. Many people, however, are exposed to little sunlight during certain seasons. Milk, fortified with vitamin D, is the primary dietary source of this vitamin. Pregnant women who do not drink milk and have minimal sun exposure should be counseled to increase their vitamin D-fortified milk intake or to take supplements providing 10 μg (400 IU) per day (Institute of Medicine, 1990). Excessive intake of vitamin D can result in hyperabsorption of calcium, hypercalcemia, and calcification of soft tissues.

Zinc. Zinc is necessary for cell reproduction and differentiation. The best dietary sources of zinc are protein foods and milk products (see the Daily Food Guide on p. 125). Zinc deficiency has been linked to fetal growth retardation, congenital malformations, and pregnancy induced hypertension in humans. This evidence, however, does not warrant routine supplementation (Institute of Medicine, 1990). Iron supplementation appears to diminish zinc absorption. The Institute of Medicine (1990) recommends zinc supplementation for women taking more than 30 mg of supplemental iron per day.

Magnesium. Many biochemical and physiological processes require or are influenced by magnesium. Magnesium deficiency can produce tremors and convulsions. The best dietary sources are vegetable protein, dark green, leafy vegetables, and whole grains.

◆ TABLE 9-2
Nondairy Foods Rich in Calcium

Food	Serving*
Almonds	4 oz
Beans: baked or pork and beans	2 cups
Broccoli, fresh cooked	1½ cups
Fish, canned: mackerel or salmon (with bones)	½ cup
Greens: turnip, cooked	1½ cups
Greens: bok choy, collard, dandelion, cooked	2 cups
Greens: kale, mustard, cooked	3 cups
Molasses, blackstrap	2 tbs
Oranges	5 medium
Sardines	5 medium or 2½ oz
Tofu (processed with calcium salt)	9 oz
Tortillas, corn (processed with lime or calcium carbonate)	7 medium

*Each is approximately equivalent in calcium to one serving of milk products and provides approximately 300 mg of calcium.

From California Department of Health Services, MCH/WIC: *Nutrition during pregnancy and the postpartum period*, June 1990, The Department.

Daily food guide

Nurses are frequently the primary educators of pregnant women and their families. Routine multivitamin supplementation should not be necessary if the pregnant woman consumes a varied, nutritious diet. (See the Nursing Alert below.) Because a pregnant woman cannot (as yet) go to the grocery store to purchase a package labeled "60 grams of protein" and since nutritional supplements or pills are expensive, inefficient, and unsatisfying, the expectant mother needs to be able to interpret caloric and nutrient needs

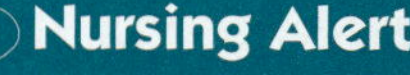

Nursing Alert

Megavitamins should be avoided during pregnancy. They can be dangerous for the developing fetus.

in terms of market commodities. The Daily Food Guide for Women (Fig. 9-2) was developed to ensure that nonpregnant, pregnant, and lactating women of average height and weight meet at least 90% of the RDAs (California Department of Health Services, 1990). The Guide provides a quick and easy means for the nurse to evaluate the adequacy of various diets. It can be used as a teaching tool to help women develop healthy eating habits for themselves and their families. A 24-hour recall of foods eaten or a few days' record of food intake can be used to compare foods eaten with those recommended by the Guide. The resulting food plan should be individualized to incorporate client preferences and be workable for her life style.

Weight gain

As indicated in the previous discussion, optimum maternal and fetal outcomes are dependent on the pregnant woman consuming sufficient nutrients to meet maternal and fetal needs. Maternal weight gain is considered an important, though imperfect, measure of adequate prenatal nutrition. Length of gestation and pregnancy weight gain are, however, the best predictors of the newborn's birth weight. Teenagers, African-American women, women who smoke, and women living in poverty are most at risk for having low-birth-weight babies. Newborns have a low birth weight either because they are delivered prematurely (before 37 weeks' gestation) or, if full-term, because their growth is retarded in utero. Inadequate pregnancy weight gain is associated with both preterm delivery and term newborns of low birth weight (under 2500 gm or 5 lb 8 oz).

Recommendations for weight gain are commonly based on prepregnancy weight for height. Table 9-3 can be used to determine if the woman is underweight, normal weight, or overweight for her height.

The following ranges provide *general* guidelines for weight gain:

Underweight	28-40 lbs
Normal weight	25-35 lbs
Moderately overweight	15-25 lbs
Very overweight	15 lbs

Short women (less than 62 inches in height) should aim for the lower end of each range. Young adolescents, African-American women, and smokers should aim for gains at the upper end of each range. Women pregnant with twins should gain 35 to 45 pounds (Institute of Medicine, 1990). Nutritional counseling should stress high quality food choices and avoidance of "empty calories"— items that contribute little or no nutrient value other than calories for energy.

Pattern of weight gain. Weight gain in early pregnancy is caused by uterine growth and expanding maternal blood volume. Toward the end of pregnancy, fetal growth accounts for the majority of weight gain. Components of weight gain in pregnancy are indicated in Table 9-4.

The usual recommended pattern of weight gain is approximately 2 to 5 pounds during the first trimester, and approximately 1 pound per week during the remainder of the pregnancy (Worthington-Roberts and Williams, 1993). A sudden increase in weight gain is usually caused by excessive fluid retention—a sign of pregnancy induced hypertension, especially if noted after 20 weeks' gestation. Weight gain charts provide visual tracking of weight gain by week of gestation. See Fig. 9-3 for an example of a grid for women with normal weight for height.

Adequate weight gain during pregnancy is important for maternal and fetal well-being. Excessive weight gain, however, can lead to health problems during and after pregnancy. Excessive weight gain during pregnancy (35% above prepregnancy weight) is associated with an increased risk for hypertension, pregnancy induced hypertension, difficult labor, and cesarean birth (Shepard, et al., 1986). After delivery the woman is likely to find it difficult to lose the remaining accumulated fat, predisposing her to long-term health problems.

Nutritional services

Low-income families may be eligible for the United States' Special Supplemental Food Program for Women, Infants, and Children, better known as WIC. This program provides food, nutrition education, and health services to pregnant and postpartum women (up to 12 months if breast-feeding and up to 6 months if not breast-feeding) and infants and children up to 5 years of age.

The registered dietitian (RD) is a valuable member of the health care team. Pregnant women with special nutritional needs or problems (e.g., diabetes, high blood pressure, PKU, or "vegan" vegetarians) should be referred for more extensive nutritional counseling.

Pica

Sometimes during pregnancy women experience special cravings for unusual foods or food combinations. Generally, these desires do not threaten good nutrition. Pica, however, refers to the compulsion to ingest non-food substances such as laundry starch or clay. Ingestion of relatively large amounts of these substances can interfere with good maternal and fetal nutrition and is associated with iron deficiency anemia. This practice is not limited to any one geographical area, race, creed, culture, or socioeconomic group.

Food Group	One Serving Equals		Recommended Minimum Servings		
			Nonpregnant		Pregnant/ Lactating
			11–24 yrs.	25+ yrs.	
PROTEIN FOODS Provide protein, iron, zinc, and B-vitamins for growth of muscles, bone, blood, and nerves. Vegetable protein provides fiber to prevent constipation.	**Animal Protein:** 1 oz. cooked chicken or turkey 1 oz. cooked lean beef, lamb, or pork 1 oz. or ¼ cup fish or other seafood 1 egg 2 fish sticks or hot dogs 2 slices luncheon meat	**Vegetable Protein:** ½ cup cooked dry beans, lentils, or split peas 3 oz. tofu 1 oz. or ¼ cup peanuts, pumpkin, or sunflower seeds 1½ oz. or ⅓ cup other nuts 2 tbsp. peanut butter	5 A half serving of vegetable protein daily	5	7 One serving of vegetable protein daily
MILK PRODUCTS Provide protein and calcium to build strong bones, teeth, healthy nerves and muscles, and to promote normal blood clotting.	8 oz. milk 8 oz. yogurt 1 cup milk shake 1½ cups cream soup (made with milk) 1½ oz. or ⅓ cup grated cheese (like cheddar, monterey, mozzarella, or swiss)	1½–2 slices presliced American cheese 4 tbsp. parmesan cheese 2 cups cottage cheese 1 cup pudding 1 cup custard or flan 1½ cups ice milk, ice cream, or frozen yogurt	3	2	3
BREADS, CEREALS, GRAINS Provide carbohydrates and B-vitamins for energy and healthy nerves. Also provide iron for healthy blood. Whole grains provide fiber to prevent constipation.	1 slice bread 1 dinner roll ½ bun or bagel ½ English muffin or pita 1 small tortilla ¾ cup dry cereal ½ cup granola ½ cup cooked cereal	½ cup rice ½ cup noodles or spaghetti ¼ cup wheat germ 1 4-inch pancake or waffle 1 small muffin 8 medium crackers 4 graham cracker squares 3 cups popcorn	7 Four servings of whole-grain products daily	6	7
VITAMIN C-RICH FRUITS AND VEGETABLES Provide vitamin C to prevent infection and to promote healing and iron absorption. Also provide fiber to prevent constipation.	6 oz. orange, grapefruit, or fruit juice enriched with vitamin C 6 oz. tomato juice or vegetable juice cocktail 1 orange, kiwi, mango ½ grapefruit, cantaloupe ½ cup papaya 2 tangerines	½ cup strawberries ½ cup cooked or 1 cup raw cabbage ½ cup broccoli, Brussels sprouts, or cauliflower ½ cup snow peas, sweet peppers, or tomato puree 2 tomatoes	1	1	1
VITAMIN A-RICH FRUITS AND VEGETABLES Provide beta-carotene and vitamin A to prevent infection and to promote wound healing and night vision. Also provide fiber to prevent constipation.	6 oz. apricot nectar or vegetable juice cocktail 3 raw or ¼ cup dried apricots ¼ cantaloupe or mango 1 small or ½ cup sliced carrots 2 tomatoes	½ cup cooked or 1 cup raw spinach ½ cup cooked greens (beet, chard, collards, dandelion, kale, mustard) ½ cup pumpkin, sweet potato, winter squash, or yams	1	1	1
OTHER FRUITS AND VEGETABLES Provide carbohydrates for energy and fiber to prevent constipation.	6 oz. fruit juice (if not listed above) 1 medium or ½ cup sliced fruit (apple, banana, peach, pear) ½ cup berries (other than strawberries) ½ cup cherries or grapes ½ cup pineapple ½ cup watermelon	¼ cup dried fruit ½ cup sliced vegetable (asparagus, beets, green beans, celery, corn, eggplant, mushrooms, onion, peas, potato, summer squash, zucchini) ½ artichoke 1 cup lettuce	3	3	3
UNSATURATED FATS Provide vitamin E to protect tissue.	⅛ med. avocado 1 tsp. margarine 1 tsp. mayonnaise 1 tsp. vegetable oil	2 tsp. salad dressing (mayonnaise-based) 1 tbsp. salad dressing (oil-based)	3	3	3

Note: The Daily Food Guide for Women may not provide all the calories you require. The best way to increase your intake is to include more than the minimum servings recommended.

Fig. 9-2 Daily Food Guide for nonpregnant, pregnant, and lactating women. Different food guides may differ in the number of animal protein servings recommended. This difference is due to a difference in calculating serving size. For example, seven *one-ounce* servings are equal to three and one half *two-ounce* servings. (From California Department of Health Services [MCH/WIC]: *Nutrition during pregnancy and the postpartum period,* June 1990, The Department.)

◆ **TABLE 9-3**
Prepregnant Weight for Height*

Height (in)	Underweight (lbs)	Normal (lbs)	Moderately Overweight (lbs)	Very Overweight (lbs)
58	94 or less	95-127	128-143	144 or more
59	97 or less	98-131	132-147	148 or more
60	100 or less	101-135	136-151	152 or more
61	102 or less	103-138	139-155	156 or more
62	106 or less	107-143	144-161	162 or more
63	109 or less	110-147	148-165	166 or more
64	112 or less	113-151	152-170	171 or more
65	116 or less	117-156	157-176	177 or more
66	119 or less	120-161	162-181	182 or more
67	123 or less	124-166	167-187	188 or more
68	126 or less	127-171	172-192	193 or more
69	131 or less	132-177	178-199	200 or more
70	134 or less	135-182	183-204	205 or more

*Height without shoes; weight without clothes.
From California Department of Health Services (MCH/WIC): *Nutrition during pregnancy and the postpartum period*, June 1990, The Department.

◆ **TABLE 9-4**
Average Weight of the Products of Pregnancy

Products	lbs		kgs
Fetus	7.5		3.4
Placenta	1.0		0.5
Amniotic fluid	2.0		0.9
Uterine weight increase	2.5		1.1
Breast tissue	3.0		1.4
Blood volume	4.0		1.8
Maternal stores	4 to 8		1.8 to 3.6
Totals	24 to 28	or	10.9 to 12.7

From Worthington-Roberts B, Williams SR: *Nutrition in pregnancy and lactation*, St. Louis, 1993, Mosby.

Women most likely to engage in the practice tend to be African-American, tend to live in rural areas, and have a childhood and family history of pica, rooted in local custom and tradition (Worthington-Roberts and Williams, 1993). Health care providers should question all women about pica behavior. Those who indicate that they engage in the practice should be counseled about the negative consequences and be monitored for anemia and poor fetal development.

Pregnancy-induced hypertension (PIH)

Historically, salt or sodium restriction was advocated in an attempt to prevent and treat the symptoms of pregnancy-induced hypertension, a serious complication characterized by edema of the face or hands, hypertension, and albuminuria, which can lead to convulsions and death (see Chapter 14 for a further discussion). Currently, considerable controversy exists regarding the cause and prevention of this disease. Although the lack of enough dietary protein is considered by some clinicians to be a major trigger in the mechanism of PIH, studies have not consistently supported this explanation as a primary cause. Other nutrients associated with incidence of PIH include thiamin, vitamins B_6 and B_{12}, calcium, magnesium, polyunsaturated fats, and zinc (Lu, et al., 1981; Newman and Fullerton, 1990). The roles of various nutritional deficiencies in the etiology of PIH require further research before definite conclusions are made. The evidence thus far suggests that women may be less at risk for this disease if they consume adequate calories, protein, calcium, magnesium, zinc, and other vitamins and minerals according to the RDAs for pregnant women (Newman and Fullerton, 1990).

General Health Habits

Rest

Pregnant women need to conserve their resources by getting adequate rest, particularly in the first and third trimester when fatigue is common. They may not be able to nap in the morning and afternoon, but should be encouraged to sit down with their feet up. With advancing pregnancy the fetus compresses the inferior vena cava and puts pressure on the diaphragm when

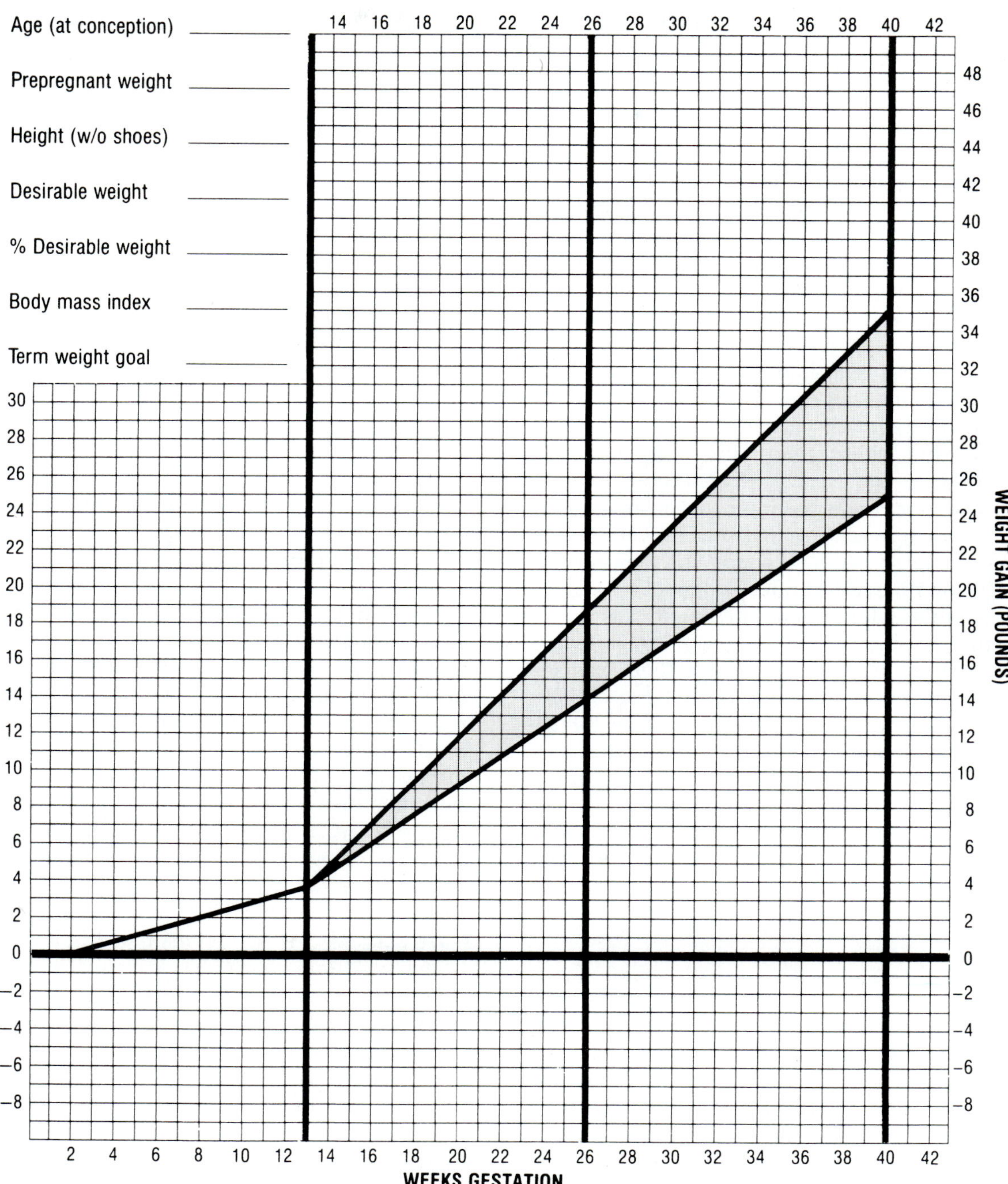

Note: Young adolescents, African American women, and smokers should strive for gains at the upper end of the recommended ranges. Short women (<62 inches) should strive for gains at the lower end of the range.

Fig. 9-3 Prenatal weight gain grid for normal weight women. To visually track weight gain: weigh the woman at each visit, look at chart, and find the total number of pounds gained. Line up the number of weeks of pregnancy with the number of pounds gained, and make a dot where the two lines meet on the chart. The goal is to keep weight gain inside the shaded area. (From California Department of Health Services [MCH/WIC]: *Nutrition during pregnancy and the postpartum period,* June 1990, The Department.)

the woman rests in a supine position. This pressure can interfere with venous blood return to the heart and placental circulation, as well as contribute to difficult maternal breathing. A side-lying position provides optimal circulation to the placenta and comfort for the woman.

Exercise

Exercise is considered safe for healthy women with uncomplicated pregnancies. It may also contribute to enhanced feelings of well-being and a quicker return to fitness after delivery (Welton, 1993). Curtailing the exercise of a previously active woman may negatively affect her physical, emotional, and mental health. Regular exercise at least three times per week is preferable to intermittent activity. Walking, golfing, bowling, dancing, and swimming, when not done to the point of fatigue, are safe activities. Horseback riding, skiing, endurance exercises, and contact sports are not recommended for pregnant women. Expectant mothers should not exercise during high heat or humidity, or when an elevated body temperature exists. After the fourth month, she should not exercise in the supine position. The American College of Obstetricians and Gynecologists (1985) suggests that women drink adequate fluids before and after each exercise session, limit their exercise periods to 30 to 45 minutes, and do not exceed 70% of their *safe* maximum attainable heart rate (SHR). SHR is usually defined as 220 minus the woman's age. For example, a 30-year-old, pregnant woman should aim for a pulse rate not higher than $(220 - 30) \times .7$, or 133 bpm. Maternal heart rate should not exceed 140 bpm unless the woman is well conditioned before pregnancy.

Kegel exercises

Frequent exercises involving the pelvic floor (particularly the pubococcygeal muscle) may facilitate childbirth, promote healing, aid in the restoration of perineal muscle tone, and help prevent stress incontinence. The mother can be taught these exercises during the prenatal period and can benefit from their daily performance for the rest of her life. The pubococcygeal muscle can be identified as the one she uses to stop a stream of urine when voiding (see Fig. 4-8 in Chapter 4). (See the Nursing Alert above right.) Ask the woman to think of her perineal muscles as an elevator on the "first floor," which she should slowly raise by contraction to the "fourth floor" and lower by slowly relaxing the muscles. A series of 10 Kegel exercises should be repeated several times each day.

Nursing Alert

Because of the tendency of urinary stasis, the pregnant woman should not practice Kegel exercises by stopping her stream of urine.

Bathing

Because women perspire more heavily and have a heavier vaginal discharge during pregnancy, daily tub baths or showers are needed. Tub baths may become a problem in late pregnancy because of the woman's awkwardness and the risk of falls. Safety mats and hand grips are helpful aids. See the Nursing Alert on page 129.

Preparation for breast-feeding

If the expectant mother is planning to breast-feed her baby, she can begin to prepare her breasts for lactation and should be given the names of community groups such as La Leche League that help breast-feeding mothers. Exposing her nipples to light and air and going without a bra for short periods can help to slightly toughen the skin. If she has inverted or flat nipples, the health care provider may recommend the use of plastic breast shields, worn for varying intervals inside the bra, to draw out the nipple and make it easier for the newborn to grasp. In the case of inverted nipples, a lactation educator may also recommend specific nipple stretching exercises. Because of the possibility of inducing premature labor, nipple manipulation should be delayed until approximately 37 weeks' gestation.

Clothing

Never before have expectant mothers had an opportunity for such an attractive, versatile wardrobe as they have today. Attractive clothing need not be expensive if the woman can sew or if she has friends who are willing to loan their maternity clothes. Clothes should be lightweight, nonconstricting, and comfortable. It is important that the pregnant woman wear a good support bra, and she will need to purchase larger sizes as the pregnancy progresses. If she plans to breast-feed her baby, nursing bras are a good investment (avoiding those with underwires).

A maternity girdle is usually not necessary. Pregnant women are advised to practice certain exercises during pregnancy (especially the "pelvic rock, or tilt") to improve posture and strengthen muscles. However, a light maternity girdle may help prevent backache for

Nursing Alert

Women should avoid hot tubs or soaking for long periods in a hot bath because of the danger of harmful fetal effects from elevated maternal core temperature.

those women with large, pendulous abdomens or for those who continue workout regimens. Specially designed garter belts are also available. Constrictive round garters should not be used because of interference in blood return from the legs.

As pregnancy progresses and the woman's center of gravity moves forward, high-heeled shoes increase the lumbar curvature and aggravate backaches. She will find lower heels less awkward and more comfortable. Shoe styles with ties or buckles may be difficult to manage towards the end of pregnancy.

Dental care

The pregnant woman should practice good dental hygiene. If she has not done so recently, she should have a dental checkup during early pregnancy so that plenty of time is available for needed repairs and instruction regarding techniques in flossing and other hygiene measures. As discussed previously, the gums may become swollen and exhibit a tendency to bleed during pregnancy. These symptoms typically recede after the eighth month.

Employment

Many pregnant women are employed. Whether they continue their employment and for how long during pregnancy depends on several factors, one of which is the type of work (e.g., heavy lifting, exposure to potential hazards of radiation or chemicals, or long hours of standing). The employment of pregnant women in certain occupations is often restricted by state law, policies of the individual employer (dependent on insurance coverage, previous experience, etc.), and the health of the employee.

Women have challenged disability benefit regulations and pregnancy leave rulings that require a working, expectant mother to resign her position because she has reached a certain month in her pregnancy. The Pregnancy Discrimination Act of 1978 prohibits discrimination on the basis of pregnancy in hiring, pay, working conditions, or other privileges of employment. Predetermined stop and start dates are illegal. Pregnancy should be treated as any other temporary disability with regard to time off and insurance. Challenges to this act have been taken as high as the Supreme Court. Complaints are directed to the Equal Employment Opportunity Commission.

Travel

Sometimes pregnant women ask whether they should restrict travel. If no complications exist and the woman is healthy, travel is usually not restricted. If a trip can be so arranged, it is best to travel during the second trimester, since the pregnant woman is normally most comfortable during that time. It is a good idea for the woman to carry a copy of her medical records with her. Car trip schedules should allow for rest stops approximately every 2 hours. The woman should walk around for a few minutes at each stop. She should always use automobile safety belts appropriately. The lap belt should be worn snug and low across the hip bones, with the shoulder belt above the pregnant uterus, resting between the breasts. Commercial airline travel is now considered as safe as other methods of transportation. Just as for car trips, she should get up and walk periodically. Travel close to term is discouraged if a history of bleeding or PIH exists, or if multiple births are expected (Barry and Bia, 1989).

Sexual relations

Couples frequently have many questions about sexual activity during pregnancy. They may be concerned about the changes in desire for sexual intercourse and may be fearful of harming the fetus. The health care provider or office nurse can allay fears, educate about the normal changes in pregnancy, and suggest alternative positions that may be more comfortable. Instructions regarding sexual intercourse during pregnancy are now much more liberal than in the past. In healthy pregnancies, no restrictions on sexual intercourse exist. Intercourse is contraindicated, however, in the case of vaginal bleeding or ruptured membranes. Those women with a history of premature labor or strong uterine contractions after orgasm should be advised of the danger of premature labor associated with orgasm after 32 weeks' gestation. Most couples find such privations stressful and may need counseling regarding alternative modes of mutual sexual gratification.

Common Discomforts of Pregnancy

Nausea and vomiting

Probably the first discomfort noted by many pregnant women is nausea and vomiting (a presumptive sign of pregnancy)—particularly in the morning, although it may occur at any time of the day. This

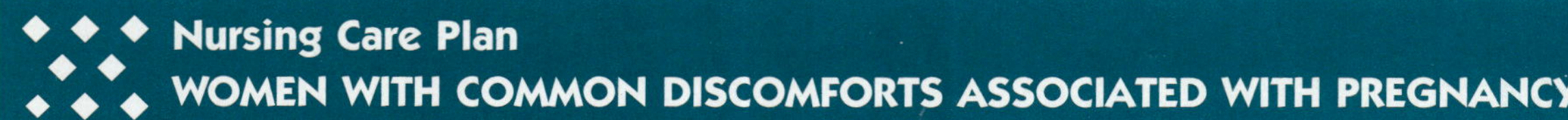

Nursing Care Plan
WOMEN WITH COMMON DISCOMFORTS ASSOCIATED WITH PREGNANCY

Selected Nursing Diagnoses	Expected Outcomes	Interventions
Knowledge deficit related to self-care strategies for coping with minor discomforts of pregnancy.	Woman verbalizes understanding of discomforts and utilizes self-care measures to lessen their impact.	Explain cause of condition and provide anticipatory guidance for self care throughout pregnancy.
		Specific plans for selected problems are described below.
A Alteration in urinary elimination pattern related to physical changes of early and late pregnancy. Clinical manifestations: Patient complains of fullness, frequent urination.	Sleep pattern is undisturbed by nocturia. Maintains adequate fluid intake. Recognizes and reports symptoms of urinary tract infection.	Collect additional information concerning urinary complaint to distinguish normal condition from possible urinary tract infection. Teach patient signs of urinary tract infection, such as burning on urination, fever, flank pain, cloudy urine, urgency. Explain importance of reporting promptly to physician if they occur. Advise patient to: Void when urge occurs—minimize urinary stasis (potential for infection). Eliminate fluid intake after 6 PM (be sure to maintain adequate intake during day). Empty bladder immediately before going to bed. Reduce intake of beverages high in caffeine (e.g., tea, coffee, cola), which acts as a urinary irritant.

Continued.

temporary condition is experienced by approximately 50% of pregnant women in the first trimester. It is associated with the hormonal changes in the body at the onset of pregnancy and psychological factors such as anxiety about pregnancy. (See the Nursing Care Plan above and on the next page.)

The most successful preventative measure seems to be eating small, frequent meals (every 2 to 3 hours) consisting of easily digested carbohydrates. Liquids are tolerated better if taken between, instead of with, meals. Eating something dry and high in carbohydrate value, like a few crackers or a piece of toast, 15 minutes before getting out of bed is usually helpful. Avoiding food odors and getting plenty of fresh air may also ease symptoms. Vitamin B_6 has helped some women. Research evidence, however, is conflicting as to the effectiveness of this treatment. Vitamin B_6 should be taken only with the advice of the health care provider (California Department of Health Services, 1990; Sahakian, et al., 1991). If the nausea persists and becomes severe, threatening the nutrition of the mother, it is considered a serious complication termed *hyperemesis gravidarum.* It may necessitate hospitalization and the administration of intravenous feedings.

Heartburn

Heartburn, or pyrosis, an uncomfortable burning sensation felt behind the sternum, often accompanied by gas and acid regurgitation into the esophagus, has nothing to do with the heart. Heartburn becomes more common as pregnancy advances. It is related to decreased peristalsis and the pressure of the growing fetus, which causes stomach acid reflux and secondary esophagitis. For this reason, lying flat

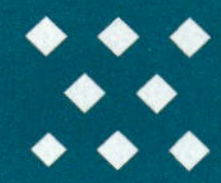

Nursing Care Plan
WOMEN WITH COMMON DISCOMFORTS ASSOCIATED WITH PREGNANCY—cont'd.

Selected Nursing Diagnoses	Expected Outcomes	Interventions
B Alteration in comfort related to varicose veins of the lower extremities, vulva or anus. Previous history or family history of varicosities. Clinical manifestations: Visible, distended, superficial veins. Discomfort varies from mild to severe; throbbing pain.	Varicose veins are prevented or their severity lessened. Discomfort from varicosities is reduced.	Explain cause of varicose veins during pregnancy: high hormone levels result in relaxed vein walls; enlarging uterus, long periods of standing or sitting, straining with bowel movements, and constrictive clothing. If varicosities common in family, patient should follow preventive measures before signs or symptoms appear. Teach patient self-care measures to prevent or treat discomfort: 1. Wear support stockings—apply in the morning before rising. 2. Rest with hips and legs elevated. 3. Avoid constricting garments. 4. Change standing or sitting positions frequently. 5. Prevent constipation by intake of increased fluid and dietary fiber. 6. Support vulvar varicosities with peripad held snugly in place by belt or maternity panty girdle.
C Alteration in comfort and potential alteration in nutrition related to nausea and/or vomiting during early pregnancy. Clinical manifestations: Transient nausea and/or vomiting: commonly called "morning sickness" but may occur at any time of the day.	Nausea and vomiting resolves after first trimester. Adequate nutritional status is maintained. Woman is able to continue with usual daily activities.	Collect additional information regarding severity and timing of nausea and vomiting. If they are continuous or severe, notify physician. Explain cause of nausea and vomiting during pregnancy: hormonal changes cause slowed gastric emptying, slowed peristalsis. Advise dietary modifications: 1. Eat high carbohydrate food before arising (e.g., soda crackers, dry popcorn). 2. Avoid greasy or spicy food. 3. Eat six small meals rather than three large meals. 4. Avoid foods or odors identified as causing problems. 5. Avoid drinking liquid with meals.

directly after eating should be avoided, as should overeating and highly seasoned, fatty, or fried foods. More frequent, smaller, leisurely meals are also recommended. With the health care provider's approval, an antacid such as Maalox (a mixture of magnesium and aluminum hydroxides) may be used, especially before bedtime. Sodium bicarbonate or other products high in sodium, often considered for such distress, should be avoided since they may upset electrolyte balance.

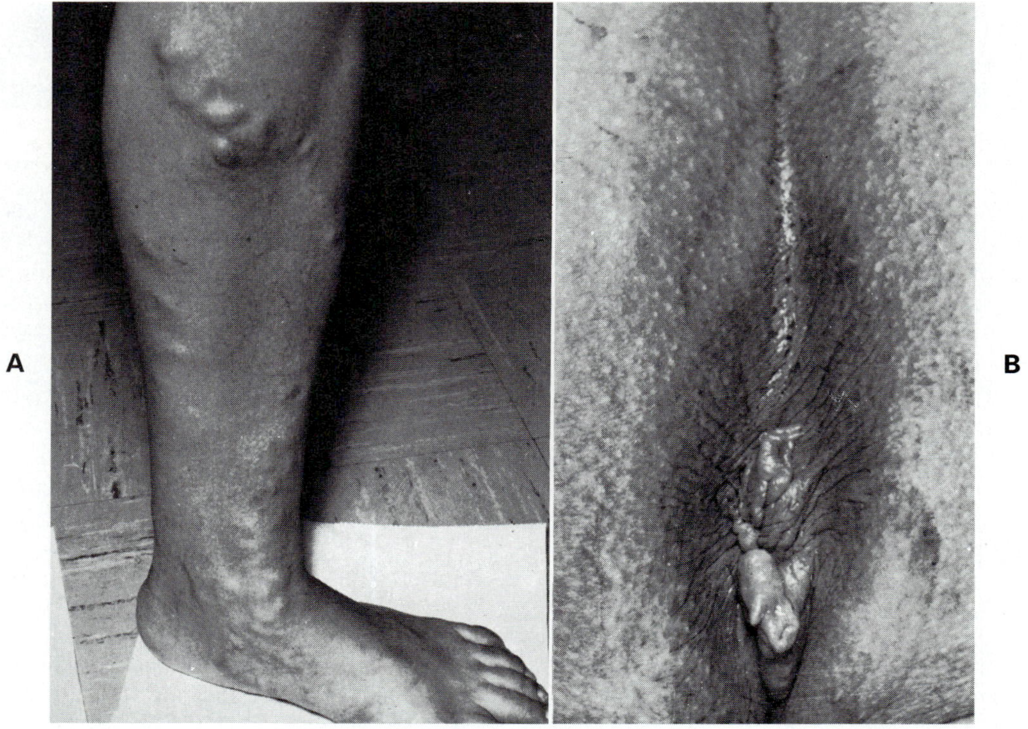

Fig. 9-4 **A,** Varicose veins of lower extremity. **B,** Varicosities of rectal area (hemorrhoids). (Courtesy Mercy Hospital and Medical Center, San Diego, CA.)

Constipation

Because of the hormonally induced, intestinal sluggishness, displacement of the intestines, and iron supplementation, constipation may also be a problem. The following four things may help: a diet that includes plenty of roughage, abundant fluids, regular exercise, and a consistent time of day set aside for unhurried evacuation. Mild laxatives may also be used. An expectant mother should, however, check with her health care provider regarding the type and frequency of such medication.

Varicosities

Many pregnant women suffer from varicosities, also called varices or varicose veins (Fig. 9-4, *A*). They most often occur in the lower extremities and rectal area but occasionally also involve the vulva and groin. These are surface veins, the walls of which are thin and greatly enlarged. Their prominence during pregnancy is common because of increased blood volume, edema, and obstruction in venous return from the lower extremities. Increased hormone levels may also cause relaxation of the smooth muscles in the walls of veins. They may appear as a swollen, purple, knotted network just under the skin. Affected lower extremities tire easily. The swollen veins may be more than a cosmetic problem, since occasionally they may be injured, may rupture and bleed, or become the point of origin for a blood clot (thrombus).

Regular exercise is recommended to promote venous return to the heart. Pregnant women should also avoid crossing their legs and standing for long periods. Lying down at intervals with her feet elevated above the level of her head will help reduce swelling and fatigue. Most women find relief by wearing support hose or applying bandages that stimulate return circulation to the heart. If elastic bandages are used, they should be applied from the foot up, with an even tension so that the bandages themselves do not become obstructions to circulation. Ideally, support hose or bandages are applied after the woman has elevated her legs for several minutes to drain the swollen veins. Round garters or knee- or calf-length elastic-topped hose should never be worn. Pooling of blood in the lower part of the body, plus dilation of the surface blood vessels, may be one cause of the fainting spells experienced by many pregnant women.

Hemorrhoids

Rectal varicosities are termed *hemorrhoids.* They may be external or internal and are produced or aggravated by the pressure of the developing fetus or constipation (Fig. 9-4, *B*). They can be painful and,

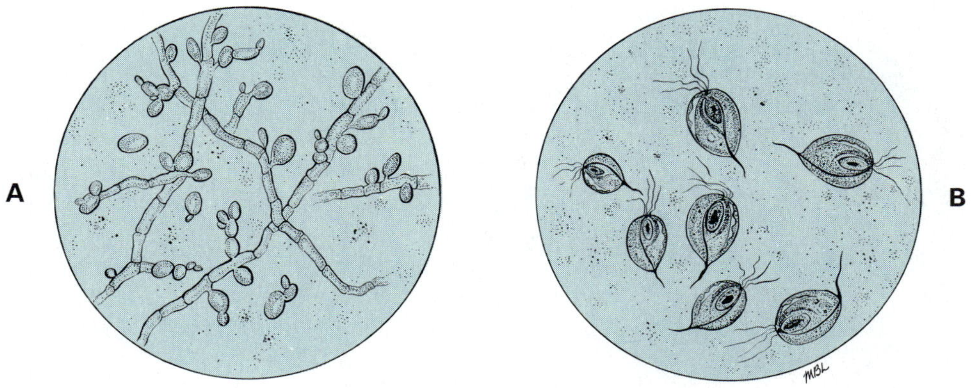

Fig. 9-5 Microscopic views. **A,** *Candida (Monilia) albicans,* a fungus. **B,** *Trichomonas vaginalis,* a protozoan.

occasionally, may become thrombosed or may bleed. In most cases, surgical treatment is not contemplated during pregnancy since the condition usually disappears or vastly improves after childbirth. Preventing constipation can help relieve or prevent hemorrhoids. Witch hazel compresses, analgesic ointments, such as dibucaine (Nupercainal), special suppositories, and sitz baths may help.

Leg cramps

Muscle cramps are often experienced during pregnancy. They usually involve the calf muscle and can be agonizing. Although the cause is unknown, it is thought that they result from a calcium and phosphorus imbalance in the body, causing a form of tetany. Magnesium deficiency may also be a contributing factor. Immediate treatment consists of straightening the leg by pushing down on the knee and pulling the ball of the foot up toward the knee. The woman should avoid excessive protein, calcium, and phosphorus by eating no more than the recommended number of servings of protein foods and milk products. She should limit the intake of processed foods and carbonated beverages, which may also be high in phosphorus. Adequate dietary magnesium can be consumed by eating at least one serving of vegetable protein, one serving of a dark green, leafy vegetable, and at least four servings of whole-grain products daily (California Department of Health Services, 1990). The patient should be advised to avoid fatigue, cold legs, and pointing her toes when stretching. She should lead with her heels when walking.

Leukorrhea

During pregnancy the hormonally stimulated cervix produces more mucus than in the nonpregnant state. This discharge, termed *leukorrhea,* may be bothersome. Women should be reassured that the discharge is normal and be advised not to douche. Even in the nonpregnant state, douching is not recommended; bacteria may be forced in a retrograde fashion through the cervix, uterus, and tubes, causing endometritis and salpingitis. Besides causing an increase in pelvic infections, douching washes away the normal vaginal flora, leading to an overgrowth of hostile organisms. The possibility of an air embolism also exists.

To prevent the development of vaginal infections the woman should keep the perineal area clean and dry by frequent bathing, wearing cotton underpants, and avoiding tight underwear and panty hose. She should report the following signs of infection: foul odor, change in color or character of the discharge, and vulvovaginal itching. Descriptions of common vaginal infections follow.

Trichomoniasis. *Trichomonas vaginalis,* a microscopic protozoan, is a common cause of leukorrhea (Fig. 9-5, *B*). This organism may inhabit the vaginal canal without causing noticeable symptoms. However, during pregnancy the increase in vaginal secretions may cause the organism to multiply rapidly and create annoying signs and symptoms. Typically, these symptoms are an irritating, profuse, thin, foamy, yellow, malodorous vaginal discharge and vulvovaginal itching or burning. The motile organism may be identified under the microscope in hanging drop slide preparations. Sometimes a simple glass slide with cover slip allows visualization of the motile parasite. *Trichomonas* is difficult to combat locally because of the structure of the vaginal folds. Metronidazole (Flagyl), administered orally or vaginally, has proved effective and is now the drug of choice in the treatment of trichomonas. Formerly, its use during the first trimester of pregnancy was not recommended. However, research involving 1020 women who were given metronidazole during the first 3 months of pregnancy has demonstrated no

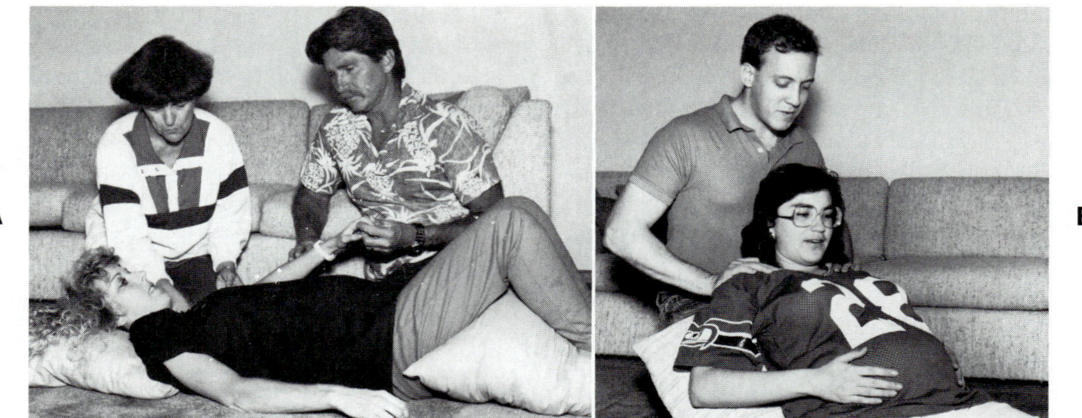

Fig. 9-6 **A,** Childbirth education instructor teaches a father to check for muscular relaxation. **B,** A young couple practices relaxation, effleurage (light massage), and breathing techniques.

increased frequency of birth defects (Rosa, et al., 1987). The expectant mother's sexual partner should be treated concurrently.

Candidiasis vulvovaginitis. Candidiasis is an infection caused by a yeast or fungus called *Candida albicans,* or *Monilia albicans.* It is easily diagnosed by direct microscopic examination of the discharge or by culture (Fig. 9-5, *A*). A *Candida* vaginal infection produces a cheesy, whitish discharge and beefy-red vulvar irritation. Like *Trichomonas, C. albicans* can inhabit the body without producing any apparent signs or symptoms. In other cases, it may spread quickly and be quite noticeable. Candidiasis is seen frequently in pregnant women, diabetics (treated and untreated), women using broad-spectrum antibiotics (e.g., penicillin, tetracycline, and erythromycin), and women living under stressful conditions. Stress is thought to affect the acid-base balance of the vaginal mucosa. Treatment includes the use of fungicidal agents applied locally in the form of vaginal suppositories and creams such as miconazole nitrate 2%, clotrimazole, or nystatin (Mycostatin). Nystatin also may be given by mouth to prevent monilial overgrowth when broad-spectrum antibiotics are prescribed or to treat an oral infection. (*C. albicans* in the oral cavity produces thrush.) Intermittent cool tap water compresses applied to the vulva may prove soothing. The woman's sexual partner should be treated concurrently.

Community Education Resources

In many communities, classes are offered to help expectant parents prepare for the changes of pregnancy and parenthood. They may be sponsored by the local Childbirth Education Association, American Red Cross, YWCA, public health departments, adult education programs, postpartum support groups, hospitals, or medical groups. Some classes concentrate on imparting an understanding of the basic anatomy and physiology of reproduction, what to expect during pregnancy, what occurs during labor and birth, how to prepare the baby's nursery and layette, how to bathe the newborn infant, techniques of breast-feeding, and how to prepare formula. Others emphasize exercises in training the body and mind for peak performance during pregnancy, labor, and childbirth, and are usually led by a physical therapist or nurse specializing in childbirth education (Fig. 9-6). Such informal group sessions with other couples facing similar experiences, expectations, hopes, and fears are especially helpful in assisting prospective fathers and mothers to gain needed instruction and self-confidence for their changing roles.

Education for childbirth

In the mid-twentieth century, few mothers in the United States remembered much of the experience of labor or delivery. Most women in the hospital setting were given types and doses of drugs designed to relieve pain, which also produced at least partial amnesia of the event. These medications were often associated with the birth of infants whose respirations were initially depressed.

Consumer demand has led to current trends in obstetrics that favor a more alert patient during labor—one who is able to participate with dignity in the experience of childbirth. To this end, greater efforts have been made to educate the woman and her designated support person for their roles, both psychologically and physically. Many different courses have been instituted to teach techniques in posture, breathing, and relaxation, as well as to impart basic information about labor and birth. Nurses should be familiar with the childbirth education programs in their community and provide program information to clients during the prenatal period.

The late, English obstetrician, Grantly Dick-Read, probably popularized the term *natural childbirth* in his book *Childbirth Without Fear* (1987). In his writings and lectures, he stressed that much of the fear pregnant women feel is caused by a lack of knowledge of what is really happening and an ensuing feeling of helplessness. He declared that fear builds tension and that tension eventually produces pain. Because of this, much of his effort was spent in educating the future mother and prescribing exercises to condition her body for labor and birth.

In 1952 the French obstetrician Fernand Lamaze became intrigued with the labor and delivery techniques based on Pavlov's theories of conditioned response that he had observed during a visit to the Soviet Union. When he returned to Paris, he introduced psychoprophylactic concepts into his practice to prepare his patients for their maternity experiences and to assist them in a conscious, rewarding participation in the birth of their children. Much of what Lamaze emphasized was also stressed by Dick-Read. However, the relaxation taught by Lamaze is based on the principle that a high level of concentrated cerebral activity can inhibit the reception of other stimuli. That is, the mind (psycho) could be induced to prevent (prophylaxis) the reception of unpleasant and painful sensations. The patient is educated (conditioned) to respond neuromuscularly to specific verbal cues. Intense preoccupation with certain muscular tension and release patterns, respiratory movements, and massage may help attain these goals. A specially prepared labor coach, sometimes called a *monitrice,* may be assigned to assist and support the patient in her efforts to utilize her training. In the United States the husband or chosen companion of the expectant mother usually fills the role of labor coach.

The absence of all forms of drug-induced analgesia or anesthesia is not a prerequisite of either the Dick-Read or Lamaze method. In fact, some women do not use any analgesic or anesthetic drugs. However, with the greater availability of epidural anesthesia in many areas of the United States, more women are using the various nonmedical techniques learned in classes during early labor and completing their labor and birth experience with epidural anesthesia. (See Chapter 12 for a discussion of epidural anesthesia.)

A third method of childbirth education was introduced by obstetrician, Robert Bradley, in 1965. The Bradley method emphasizes a quiet environment, deep body relaxation, abdominal breathing techniques, and the role of the husband-coach. The goal of this method is "true" natural childbirth—without analgesics or anesthetics.

Today many childbirth educators are emphasizing the need for increased flexibility and individualization in the labor techniques offered to their clients. This broader perspective considers the wide range of normal physiological responses found in women, their varying cultural backgrounds, and different personalities. These considerations affect their perception and tolerance of pain and the selection of coping skills. This new perspective has led to the support of more types of maternal behavior during labor. This broad teaching perspective relieves a certain rigidity (reflected especially in past teaching of respiratory patterns to coincide with contractions), which was helpful to some women, but not to all.

Those who have used psychoprophylactic techniques, or have cared for patients who were prepared, generally believe that their preparation was of value. The breathing and relaxation exercises, patterned light massage (effleurage), visual focal points or imagery, and mental and physical conditioning that these team efforts involve represent helpful tools that many mothers can profitably employ as they face the task of childbirth. If a laboring woman decides to use other alternatives (such as analgesia, tranquilizers, or anesthetics), she should not feel herself to be a failure or guilty of betraying a concept. She is not a competitor in a contest. She is a participant in an experience.

Hypnosis and acupuncture

Hypnosis, an intense altered state of receptive concentration, is greatly enhanced by high motivation. The psychoprophylactic method of childbirth preparation incorporates certain aspects of this technique. The ability to attain a trance-like state can be measured by the use of the Hypnotic Induction Profile (Spiegel, 1981). A trance may be induced by another person or self-induced. Training for this type of pain relief is typically time-consuming and expensive. The use of group sessions has made hypnosis more accessible. However, it still has not become a popular form of pain control for maternity patients.

The use of acupuncture for vaginal deliveries has received mixed reviews. Acupuncture associated with electric stimulation (electroacupuncture) in the dorsolumbar and lumbosacral areas may eliminate painful sensation during labor. It has been proposed that acupuncture releases endorphins (morphine-like compounds) from the pituitary gland and midbrain. These forms of pain relief and control are likely to be the subject of more study and research.

Transcutaneous electrical neural stimulation (TENS)

TENS is a technique in which conductive pads are placed over the appropriate nerve roots in the back. Small electrical currents stimulate the nerves in an effort to interfere with painful neurotransmission. This technique has proven unsatisfactory for labor discomfort but is still used for some postoperative pain.

Preparation for the Infant and the Hospital Visit

Infant clothing and supplies

Provided finances are not strained, preparing the layette for the new baby can be one of the most pleasurable duties of the expectant parents. Baby showers may also help in this regard. Since infants grow quickly, baby shower suggestions should include basic clothes for the 1- to 2-year-old child. If the baby is not the firstborn, infant clothes will probably be left over from the last child. A basic layette, at least enough to begin care, includes the following items:

1. Six cotton undershirts, short or long sleeves, depending on the weather (Stretch shirts cost more but can be worn longer. Some long-sleeved shirts have fold-over cuffs, enclosing the hands.)
2. Four dozen cotton gauze, bird's-eye, or flannelette diapers if a diaper service is not used; 1 dozen, if it is; or disposable diapers
3. Two or three plastic diaper covers, for use with cloth diapers (do not use if the baby has skin irritation)
4. Four long gowns with drawstring bottoms, useful in early weeks when baby's posture is very flexed
5. Four one-piece outfits with legs, opening down the front with grip fasteners
6. One hooded wrap that has leg openings—for use with a car seat
7. Three or four soft, light receiving blankets
8. One square, heavy blanket for use outdoors
9. One cap
10. Booties or heavy long socks, if the weather is cold
11. One bunting, in a climate requiring such protection (The tendency is to overdress rather than underdress infants.)
12. Two or three waterproof squares for protecting surfaces from the baby's urine
13. Three or four washcloths, just for the baby
14. Six cotton sheets and two crib blankets

Basic furniture includes a crib with closely spaced slats (2⅜ inches apart) and nontoxic paint (a bassinet, although pretty, is unnecessary), a firm and snug-fitting mattress, and cover. (Pillows should not be used because of the danger of suffocation.) Other useful items include: some type of chest of drawers for storage, a covered diaper pail, and a large plastic tub. A bath tray is a convenience, but it does not have to be expensive. Any clean tray will do. Suggested items for a tray are a jar of cotton balls; a jar of safety pins; a mild soap and soap dish; baby lotion; and a box of paper tissues. Baby powder, especially that containing talc, is not recommended. If inhaled, it can cause serious respiratory illness.

Even if the baby is to be breast-fed, equipment should be available in the home for preparing formula feedings or for storing and feeding breast milk when the mother is away. An approved infant car seat is a necessity, and a portable infant seat or baby carrier worn by the infant's caretaker can be helpful. Parents can often borrow needed items.

What to take to the hospital

The mother should have a few things ready for her trip to the hospital or birthing center. Usually, the following list suffices for today's short stays:

1. Recommended articles to assist with the Lamaze type of labor techniques (e.g., extra pillows, lip pomade, focal point)
2. One nightgown (the short type)
3. Robe and slippers
4. One brassiere (nursing type, if breast-feeding)
5. Toothbrush, dentrifice, brush, comb, cosmetics
6. Deodorant, shower cap
7. Checkbook or cash for deposit at hospital, insurance identification if applicable
8. Clothing in which to take infant home (e.g., undershirt, gown, booties, blanket or wrap)

Cross-Cultural Components Influencing Maternity Care

When caring for a pregnant woman from another culture or ethnic group the nurse must understand the variations in the mother's attitudes and behaviors that may result from cultural influences. As discussed in Chapter 3, perceptions of health and illness are culturally derived. The care given should fit the prospective mother's cultural life-style when possible and take into account her customs and beliefs. For example, nutritional guidance must consider food practices and the symbolic significance of food. In some cultures, certain foods are not to be eaten (taboo) during pregnancy (Andrews, 1989). Certain groups do not assign an active role to the father in prenatal care or labor and delivery. In some cultures, grandmothers may have a primary support role during labor and, later, in child-rearing. Likewise, the nurse teaching infant health care should identify who the principal care provider is as she works with different families and groups.

Although individuals must not be stereotyped, it is helpful for the nurse to briefly review some of the childbearing beliefs and practices of a few ethnic groups. Of course, practices and views associated with childbearing also vary with individuals, their personal values, and their economic resources. Discussing cultural influences with the parents will help the nurse to better plan for cultural preferences and needs.

African-American practices

The cultural patterns of African Americans in different socioeconomic groups largely resemble the patterns of the majority of members of these groups. Extended family members typically help provide support to childbearing families.

Black Muslim women often follow meat-restricted diets. Their prenatal nutrition, as well as that of the breast-feeding mother, should be explored. They characteristically wear long, modest garments and cover their hair. Nurses should recognize the importance of protecting the modesty of these women.

Native American practices

The traditional Native-American woman often finds fulfillment through her role in pregnancy, childbirth, and rearing healthy children. Support is received from her family and community. Female family members are especially involved in these concerns.

In caring for these families, it is important to be acquainted with the tribe's cultural beliefs and taboos. Many of these can be accommodated safely. For instance, for some tribes it is important not to palpate the infant's anterior fontanel in the presence of the family. As with other cultures, taboos against certain foods exist during pregnancy. Native-American women generally believe contraception should not be implemented until after the first child.

Hispanic practices

Hispanics are the largest ethnic group in the United States. They have come from many different Spanish-speaking regions of the world. Some of these families have adopted the middle-American culture, whereas others have retained the concepts and lifestyles of their Hispanic heritages. Again, large extended families are common and important. The advice given by a family member may be accepted by the mother in preference to that given by a member of the health team. The "hot-cold theory" of disease and health can influence the mother's prenatal diet and her compliance with dietary recommendations. Certain foods are considered hot or cold, though these concepts may have no relationship to their actual temperatures. The mother may seek a balance between these foods. Since pregnancy is viewed as normal, going to the physician may be delayed. This group is characterized by male-dominant relationships. Large families are often desired.

Asian practices

Asian families in the United States currently represent particularly diverse cultures and socioeconomic levels. The extended family is dominant. Although some taboos govern food and activity during pregnancy, pregnancy is seen as a normal, healthy process in which family members should have the major role. When caring for patients from the Asian culture, nurses should particularly protect the modesty of the patient. Male participation in the direct care of the mother is usually minimal but does not represent a noncaring attitude. Politeness and propriety characterize Southeast Asian people. Direct confrontation is avoided. Harmony with nature and dualist concepts of disease are part of the health beliefs and practices. The concepts of yin and yang (in some ways similar to the "hot-cold theory" of disease and health) and the need to balance these contrary forces in an individual's life can affect diet, hygiene, and activity, particularly in the postpartum period. Culturally sensitive explanations to the client and her family members are essential to nursing care.

Arab practices

Arab families feel strong family unity among extended family members and rely on this bonded-family for help before going outside the family. The experience of pregnancy and birth is usually seen as an exclusively female affair. Having children, especially sons, is an important function of women. Arab women feel a special need for modesty. Often families from the Arab culture are oriented to the present; planning ahead for the care of the coming child is not part of the culture. This should not be viewed as showing less concern for the infant. It is an aspect of the culture, perhaps prompted by ancient high infant mortality rates. This emphasis on the present rather than the future should also be remembered if contraception is to be taught. Including other adult family members in health teaching is helpful. Having both husband and wife together during such discussions may increase compliance.

KEY CONCEPTS

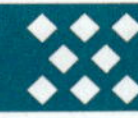

1. Significant physiological and psychological changes occur during pregnancy.
2. The broad objectives of prenatal care are to promote the health and well-being of the pregnant woman, the fetus, the infant, and the family.
3. The basic components of prenatal care include early and continuing risk assessment, health promotion activities, and medical and psychosocial interventions with followup.
4. Signs and symptoms that a pregnant woman should be instructed to report to her health care provider are vaginal spotting or bleeding; leaking of fluid from the vagina; unusual abdominal pain or cramps; persistent nausea or vomiting; persistent headache or blurring of vision; marked swelling of the ankles, hands, and face; painful or burning urination; foul-smelling vaginal discharge; and chills or fever.
5. After the first prenatal visit, health care visits are scheduled every 4 weeks for the first 28 weeks' gestation; every 2 weeks from 28 to 36 weeks' gestation; and every 1 week from 36 weeks' gestation until delivery. Routine assessments during these visits include taking vital signs, urine examination for protein and glucose, measurement of the height of the uterus, and assessment of fetal heart rate.
6. Good nutrition during pregnancy reduces the risk of obstetrical and perinatal complications. The National Research Council's Recommended Dietary Allowance (RDA) suggests dietary adjustments for pregnancy.
7. Physiological anemia of pregnancy should not be confused with true anemia.
8. Although routine multivitamin supplementation is normally unnecessary, supplemental iron is recommended. Folic acid may also be prescribed. Megavitamin supplements may be dangerous and are not recommended.
9. The Daily Food Guide provides easy-to-follow guidelines for proper nutrition. It is also a helpful tool for assessing the adequacy of the pregnant woman's dietary intake.
10. The suggested total weight gain during pregnancy ranges from 25 to 35 pounds for the woman who enters pregnancy at normal weight for her height. Prepregnancy weight, height, age, race, smoking, and multiple pregnancy all influence what is considered a healthy weight gain during pregnancy.
11. In later pregnancy, resting or exercising in a flat, supine position may interfere with venous blood return to the heart and placental circulation. It may also contribute to difficult respirations. A side-lying position provides optimal circulation to the placenta and comfort for the mother.
12. Some exercise is encouraged during a normal pregnancy. The type and frequency depend on the woman's health, exercise habits, and obstetrical history.
13. Kegel exercises facilitate childbirth, promote healing, aid in the restoration of perineal muscle tone, and help prevent stress incontinence.
14. Maternity clothes should be lightweight, nonconstrictive, and comfortable. As the pregnancy progresses the woman may require a larger brassiere size and will find that low-heeled shoes without ties or buckles are more comfortable and easier to put on and remove.
15. Douching is not generally recommended because of the possibility of predisposing the woman to vaginal infections and an air embolus.
16. Whether a pregnant woman should continue her employment and for how long depends on several factors, including the type of work. Discrimination on the basis of pregnancy in hiring, pay, conditions, or other privileges of employment can be reported to the Equal Employment Opportunity Commission.
17. Participation in community education classes is recommended to help parents prepare for labor and birth and to care for their newborn.
18. Psychoprophylactic preparation for childbirth is based on the principle that a high level of concentrated cerebral activity can inhibit reception of unpleasant and painful sensations. Knowledge of the birth process reduces stress and anxiety. Conditioning exercises during pregnancy and breathing and relaxation techniques during labor can reduce physical discomfort.
19. Basic necessities for the newborn include the following: undershirts, diapers, gowns, blankets, cap, booties or long socks, waterproof squares, washcloths, bed linens, crib, chest of drawers, diaper pail, bath tray, equipment for preparing formula or storing breast milk, and an infant car seat.
20. The concepts of transcultural nursing need to be applied to maternity care. Cultural differences regarding childbearing influence factors such as food practices, the father's role, and the need for modesty.

CRITICAL THOUGHT QUESTIONS

1 The cost of medical care often is a reason given for delayed or inadequate prenatal care. If you agree that prenatal care is essential, what do you think should be done to guarantee that all women receive adequate care during pregnancy? How can nursing help accomplish the prenatal care goal for the year 2000?

2 Pregnancy is a normal physiological condition. It may require, however, a woman to change some of her activities and in some way alter her normal lifestyle. Your friend, Jane, enjoys her daily aerobics classes. Now that she is pregnant, she is concerned that she will gain too much weight if she stops taking the classes. What would you suggest to her? Why?

3 Identify the most common assessments performed during pregnancy. Your patient states "you keep doing these tests each time I come to the doctor." How would you explain these repeated assessments and their significance?

4 Culture plays an important part in maternal-child health practices. Select a culture other than your own that is common in your locale. Discuss the practices that are in keeping with good basic prenatal care and also those that may be harmful during pregnancy. What could you do if harmful practices are discovered?

REFERENCES

American College of Obstetricians and Gynecologists: *Home exercise programs: exercise during pregnancy and the postnatal period,* Washington, DC, 1985, ACOG.

Andrews MM: Culture and nutrition. In Boyle JS, Andrews MM: *Transcultural concepts in nursing care,* pp. 333-355, Glenview, IL, 1989, Scott Foresman.

Barry M, Bia F: Pregnancy and travel, *JAMA* 261:728, 1989.

California Department of Health Services (MCH/WIC): *Nutrition during pregnancy and the postpartum period,* June 1990, The Department.

Centers for Disease Control: Recommendations for the use of folic acid to reduce the number of cases of spina bifida and other neural tube defects, *MMWR* 41(RR-14):1, 1992.

Dick-Read G: *Childbirth without fear,* ed 5, New York, 1987, Harper & Row.

Food and Nutrition Board, National Research Council: *Recommended dietary allowances,* ed 10, Washington, DC, 1989, National Academy.

Freda MC, Andersen HF, Damus K, Merkatz IR: What pregnant women want to know: a comparison of client and provider perceptions, *J Obstet Gynecol Neonatal Nurs* 22(3):237-244, 1993.

Institute of Medicine, National Academy of Sciences: *Nutrition during pregnancy: part I weight gain, part II nutrient supplements,* Washington, DC, 1990, National Academy.

Lu JY, Cook DL, Javia JB, et al: Intakes of vitamins and minerals by pregnant women with selected clinical symptoms, *J Am Diet Assoc* 78(5):477-482, 1981.

Mills JL, et al: Maternal vitamin levels during pregnancies producing infants with neural tube defects, *J Pediatr* 120(6):863-871, 1992.

National Commission to Prevent Infant Mortality: *Troubling trends persist: Shortchanging America's next generation,* Washington, DC, 1992, The Commission.

Newman V, Fullerton JT: Role of nutrition in the prevention of preeclampsia: review of the literature, *J Nurse-Midwifery* 35(5):282, 1990.

Rosa FW, Baum C, Shaw M: Pregnancy outcomes after first trimester vaginitis drug therapy, *Obstet Gynecol* 69(5):751, 1987.

Sahakian V, Rouse D, Sipes S, et al: Vitamin B_6 is effective therapy for nausea and vomiting of pregnancy: a randomized double-blind placebo- controlled study, *Obstet Gynecol* 78(1):33-36, 1991.

Shephard MJ, Hellenbrand KG, Braken MB: Proportional weight gain and complications of pregnancy, labor and delivery in healthy women of normal prepregnancy weight, *Am J Obstet Gynecol* 155(5):947-954, 1986.

Spiegel H: Obstetrics, pain and hypnosis. In Cosmi E, editor: *Obstetric anesthesia and perinatalogy,* New York, 1981, Appleton-Century-Crofts.

Stepanuk K: Congenital syphilis: Are we missing infected newborns? *MCN* 19(5):272-274, 1994.

US Department of Health and Human Services: *Caring for our future: the content of prenatal care,* Washington, DC, 1989.

US Department of Health and Human Services: *Healthy people 2000: national health promotion and disease prevention objectives,* Boston, 1992, Jones and Bartlett.

Welton A: Is exercise safe during pregnancy? *AWHONN Voice* 1(10):8, 1993.

Worthington-Roberts BS, Williams SR: *Nutrition in pregnancy and lactation,* ed 5, St Louis, 1993, Mosby.

BIBLIOGRAPHY

Artal R, Subak-Sharpe GJ: *Pregnancy and exercise,* New York, 1992, Delacorte.

Association of Women's Health, Obstetric, and Neonatal Nurses: *Competencies and program guidelines for nurse providers of perinatal education,* Washington, DC, 1993, The Association.

Beal MW: Acupuncture and related treatment modalities: II.

applications to antepartal and intrapartal care, *J Nurse Midwife* 37(4):260, 1990.

Belizan JM, Villar J, Gonzalez L, et al: Calcium supplementation to prevent hypertensive disorders of pregnancy, *N Engl J Med* 325(20):1399-1405, 1991.

Bradley R: *Husband-coached childbirth*, ed 3, New York, 1981, Harper & Row.

Centers for Disease Control: Use of folic acid for prevention of spina bifida and other neural tube defects—1983-1991, *MMWR* 40:513, 1991.

Giotta MP: Nutrition during pregnancy: reducing obstetric risk. *J Perinat Neonatal Nurs* 6(4):1-12, 1993.

Heaney RP, Smith KT, Recker RR, Hinders SM: Meal effects on calcium absorption, *Am J Clin Nutr* 49:372-376, 1989.

Hoffman JA: Iron deficiency anemia: an update, *J Perinat and Neonatal Nurs* 6(4):13-20, 1993.

Jimenez SLM: *The pregnant woman's comfort guide: safe, quick, and easy relief from the discomforts of pregnancy and postpartum*, Wayne, NJ, 1992, Avery.

Karmel M: *Thank you, Dr. Lamaze*, New York, 1983, Harper & Row.

Spadt SK, Martin KR, Thomas AM: Experiential classes for siblings-to-be, *MCN* 15(3):184-186, 1990.

Middlemark RA, Wiswell RA, Drinkwater BL, Repovich WE: Exercise guidelines for pregnancy. In Mittlemark RA, Wiswell RA, Drinkwater BL, editors: *Exercise in pregnancy*, pp. 299-311, Baltimore, 1991, Williams & Wilkins.

Newman V, Lee D: Developing a daily food guide for women, *J of Nutr Educ* 23(2):76-82, 1991

O'Brien B, Naber S: Nausea and vomiting during pregnancy: effects on the quality of women's lives, *Birth* 19(3):138-143, 1992.

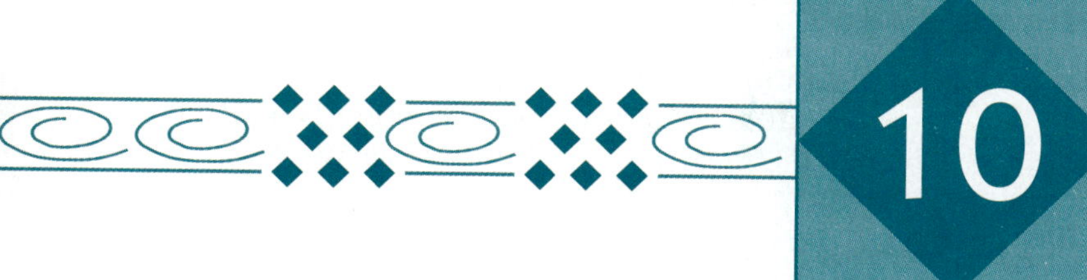
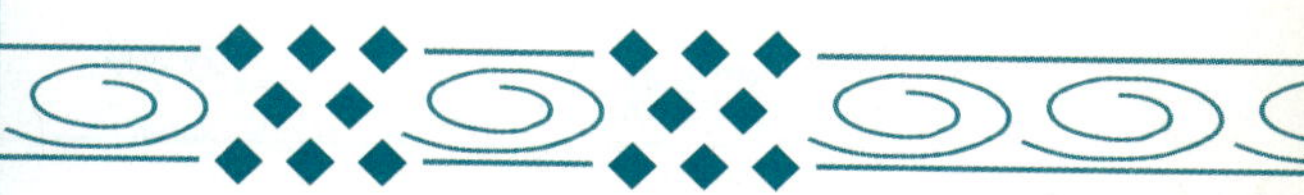

10

Mechanics of Labor and Birth

CHAPTER OBJECTIVES

After studying this chapter, the student should be able to:

1. Indicate four major factors that determine the progress of labor.
2. Define the following terms: *fetal lie, presentation, position, attitude,* and *station; cervical effacement* and *dilation.*
3. Use a pelvic model and fetal mannequin to depict the following fetal positions: LOA, ROP, ROT, LSA, RMP; and identify the most common position.
4. Describe three types of breech presentations.
5. Describe the cardinal movements in the mechanism of labor and birth, using an LOA fetal position as an example.
6. Explain the differences between true and false labor.
7. Explain the origin and significance of bloody show.
8. Describe the effects of maternal fear and anxiety and position on the progress of labor.
9. Define the four stages of labor and indicate the approximate duration of each for primiparas and multiparas.
10. Identify the two labor measurements that graph a patient's progress on the Friedman labor curve.
11. Indicate four options that a health care provider has when labor is not progressing normally.
12. Explain the difference between a precipitous delivery and a precipitous labor and the dangers of both.
13. List four signs of the separation of the placenta from the uterine wall during the third stage of labor.
14. Identify a potential complication of the third and fourth stages of labor.

The progress of labor and birth depends on several factors: the size of the *passage,* or bony pelvis; the size and position of the fetus, or *passenger;* the rhythm and strength of the uterine contractions, or *powers;* and the mental preparedness, or *psyche,* of the woman. The nurse must have a basic understanding of how these factors interact to accurately assess the woman's progress in labor and to effectively support her efforts.

PASSAGE

The maternal bony pelvis and the muscles of the pelvic floor and perineum make up the passageway that the fetus must travel during labor and birth. The diameters of the pelvic inlet, midpelvis, and outlet must be adequate for the size and position of the fetus if the infant is to deliver vaginally. See Chapter 4 for a review of the muscular and bony anatomy of the pelvis, classification of pelvic types, and methods of assessing pelvic adequacy.

PASSENGER

Fetal head

The fetal head is the largest part of the fetus. It is composed of several bones: the two frontal bones, two temporal bones, two parietal bones, and the occipital bone (Fig. 10-1, *A*). These bones are not fused, but are separated by membranous spaces called *sutures.* The suture lines meet at the anterior and posterior fontanels (Fig. 10-1, *B*). The sutures allow the fetal head to mold slightly as it passes through the bony pelvic canal. The examiner can determine the position of the fetal head by palpating the sutures and fontanels during a vaginal exam. The diameters of the fetal head (biparietal, occipitomental, occipitofrontal, and suboccipitobregmatic) may vary slightly as the head molds during its passage through the bony pelvic canal (Fig. 10-1, *A* and *B*).

Lie

The lie refers to the relationship of the long axis of the fetus to the long axis of the mother. If the cephalocaudal length of the fetus is parallel with the woman's spine the lie is longitudinal. However, if the fetal spine is perpendicular to the maternal spine, the lie is transverse.

Attitude

Fetal attitude refers to the degree of flexion of the body, head, and extremities (Fig. 10-2). The normal attitude is complete flexion.

Presentation

The term *presentation* is often used synonymously with the phrase presenting part—the part of the infant that is coming through the pelvic canal first. Headfirst placement is referred to as a *cephalic presentation.* When the feet or buttocks come first the presentation is called *breech.* Approximately 96% of all births are cephalic; approximately 3.5% are breech. Shoulder or transverse presentations are rare (0.5%) and account for the remaining births. Presentation is usually assessed by abdominal palpation and vaginal or ultrasonic examinations.

Four types of cephalic presentations exist. Vertex presentation, when the head is completely flexed on the chest, is the most common (Figs. 10-2 and 10-3). A well-flexed head presents the smallest longitudinal cephalic diameter (suboccipitobregmatic) and, therefore, fewer mechanical problems in descent and delivery. The military (median) presentation occurs when the head is neither flexed nor extended, presenting the occipitofrontal diameter (see Fig. 10-2). The brow presentation occurs when the head is partially extended, presenting the occipitomental diameter (see Fig. 10-2). The face presentation occurs when the head is hyperextended and the longest diameter, the submentobregmatic, presents to the maternal pelvis (Fig. 10-4). Brow presentations are associated with longer, more difficult labors, and a higher incidence of cesarean birth. Face presentations are rarely delivered vaginally because of a significant risk of injury to the infant's cervical spine.

Three types of breech presentations exist (see Fig. 10-4). A complete, or full breech, involves the flexion of the fetus's legs, usually tailor fashion so that the buttocks and feet appear at the vaginal opening. A frank, or single, breech is the most common type and occurs when the thighs are flexed on the abdomen with the extended legs against the trunk and the feet against the face (foot-in-mouth posture). The term *incomplete breech* indicates the initial appearance of either the feet or knees. The presentation of one or both feet is labeled a single or double footling, respectively.

Vaginal births are seldom attempted for breech presentations, since they carry greater risks for the infant (see Chapter 11 for a discussion of the implications of breech presentation). If the fetus is breech the woman is likely to be scheduled for a cesarean birth or the obstetrician may attempt to turn the breech presentation into cephalic. This is done by external manipulation, called *version.* The simultaneous availability of electronic FHR monitoring, continuous real-time sonograms, and medications (tocolytics) that help relax the uterus have substantially increased the safety and success of versions and offer another alternative to cesarean delivery. (See the nursing alert below.) A version, however, may be contraindicated for a number of reasons (e.g., if another condition also exists that calls for a cesarean birth [an abnormally positioned placenta], if more than one infant occupies the uterus, or if the fetus is exceptionally large).

Nursing Alert

If the infant is in a breech position the physician may offer to attempt to convert to cephalic presentation by a version. The woman should be fully informed of all risks and has the right to decline the procedure.

Position

The position of the fetus is the relationship of a certain point of reference on the presenting part of the

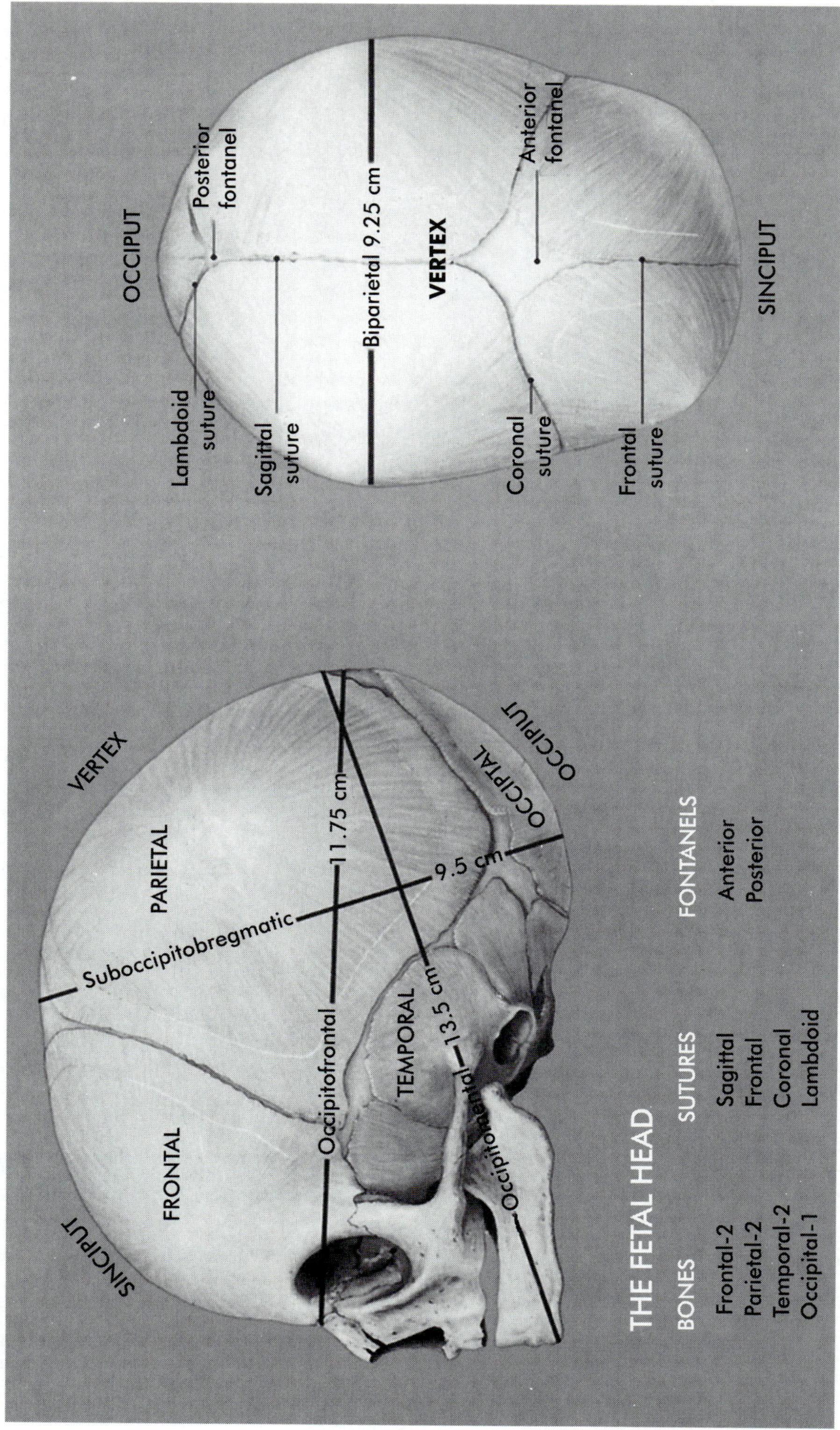

Fig. 10-1 The fetal head. **A,** Side view showing bones and longitudinal diameters; **B,** top view showing sutures and transverse diameter. (From *Clinical teaching aid no. 13.* Columbus, OH, 1970, Ross Laboratories.)

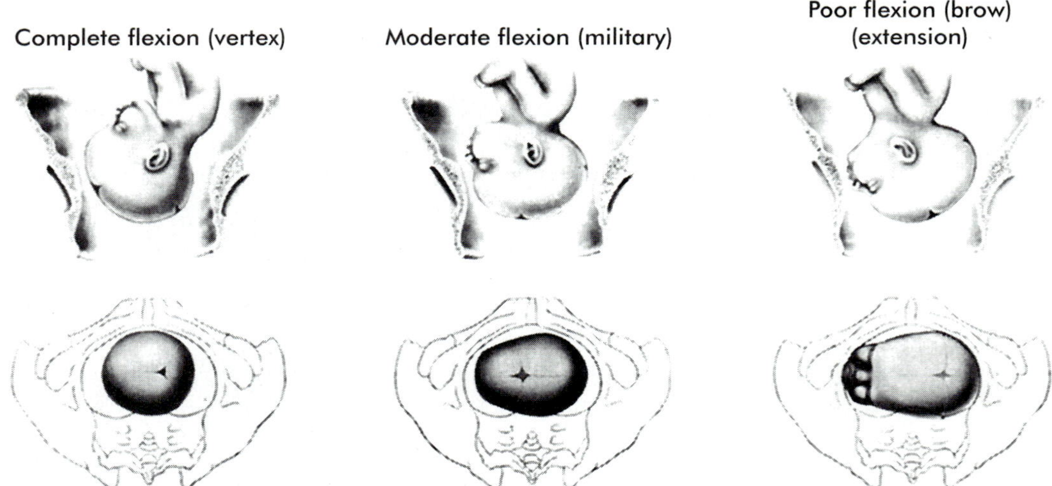

Fig. 10-2 Cephalic presentations showing head diameters in varying degrees of flexion. (From *Phenomena of normal labor,* Columbus, OH, 1964, Ross Laboratories.)

fetus to the pelvic quadrants of the mother (see Figs. 10-3 and 10-4). The position gives more detailed information about fetal progress, since the presenting part adapts to the shape and size of the various parts of the birth canal. The maternal pelvic quadrants are identified as right and left posterior, and right and left anterior (Fig. 10-5). The pelvic quadrants never change location. The point of reference, of course, varies according to the presenting part discussed and the amount of flexion present. In the event of a well-flexed cephalic or vertex presentation the point of reference is the occipital bone, or occiput, which can be palpated during a vaginal examination. After sufficient cervical dilation has occurred, it is fairly easy to follow the suture lines of the fetal skull with a gloved finger and determine the placement of the occiput. The sutures trace as a "Y." The occiput is found between the top shafts of the "Y," behind the triangular posterior fontanel (see Fig. 10-1, *B*).

References to the various positions begin with either right or left (of the mother's pelvis), followed by the fetal point of reference, and the adjectives anterior, posterior, or transverse (referring again to the part of the mother's pelvis toward which a particular point on the fetus is directed). The most common position in a vertex presentation is left occiput anterior (LOA). Each presenting part has the possibility of eight positions following the same pattern. Only the middle initial or code letters representing the point of reference need to be changed (see Figs. 10-3 and 10-4). For example, the following are the possible positions for a vertex presentation:

1 Right occiput* anterior ROA
2 Left occiput anterior LOA
3 Right occiput posterior ROP
4 Left occiput posterior LOP
5 Right occiput transverse ROT
6 Left occiput transverse LOT
7 Occiput at sacrum (occiput posterior) OP
8 Occiput at the pubis (occiput anterior) OA

In the rare case of cephalic presentations demonstrating less flexion, other points of reference are used, since the occiput is no longer available or meaningful to the examiner. In a brow presentation the letter "F" for fronto is used, referring to the frontal bones. In a face presentation the letter "M" for mentum, or chin, is used. Breech presentations use the sacrum or coccyx as a point of reference and the code letter "S" (see Fig. 10-4).

Note that a transverse position is *not* the same thing as a transverse lie. In a transverse lie the shoulder is usually the presenting part. A shoulder presentation, involving the scapula or its upper tip and the acromion as the reference point, "Sc" or "A" is the code. The fetus lying crosswise in the uterus may be positioned with his or her back toward the front or back of the mother. The fetal scapula, posteriorly located, indicates the position of his or her back. Sometimes the terms *dorsoanterior* or *dorsoposterior* may be used to clarify this fetal position. A fetus whose shoulder and head occupy the right side of the mother's pelvis and whose back is toward her front is in the right acromiodorsoanterior position (RADA) (see Fig. 10-4). The fetus in a transverse lie cannot be delivered vaginally.

Station

Another measurement related to the location of the fetus in the passageway is station. Station is the

* Sometimes the term *occipito* is used instead of *occiput.*

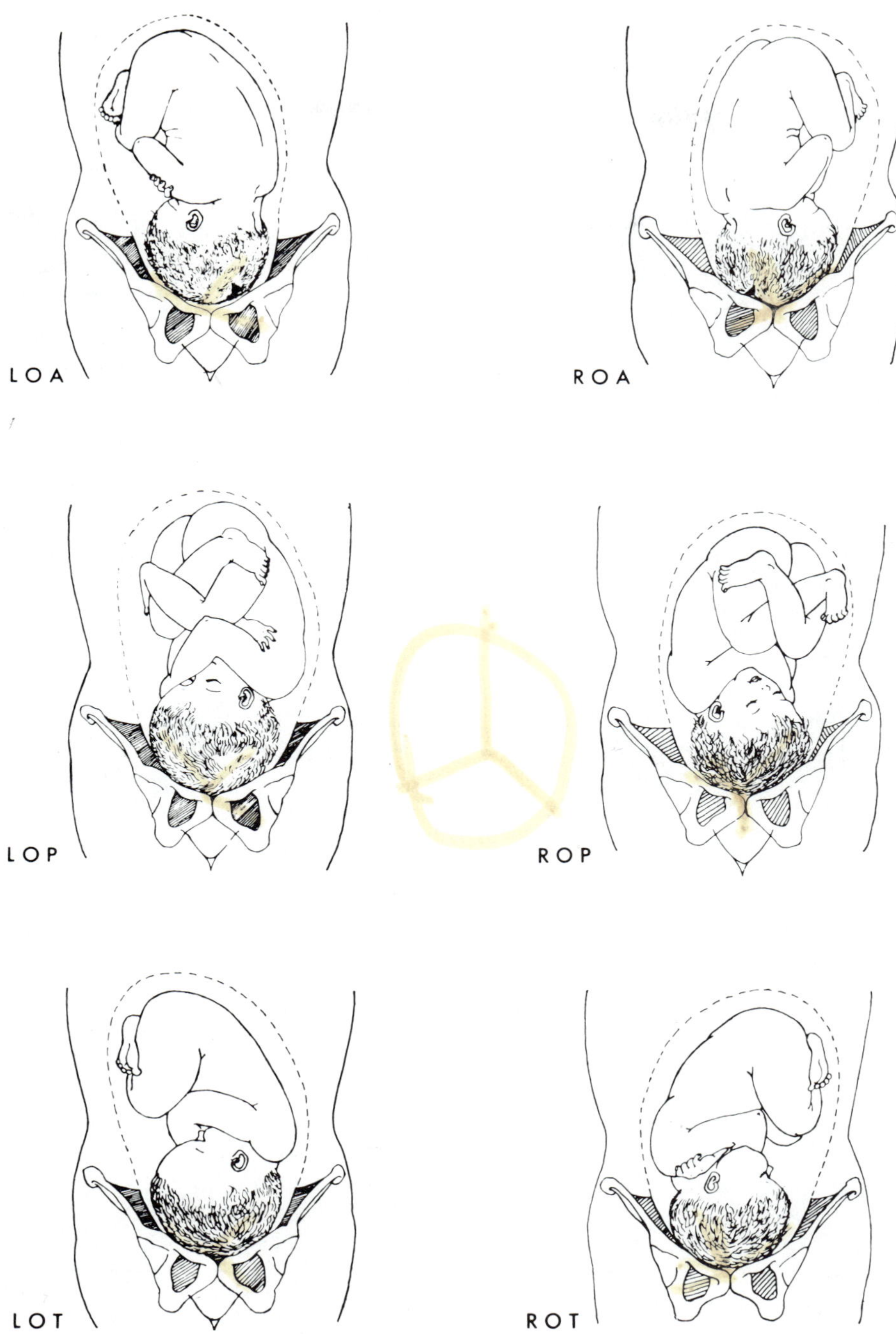

Fig. 10-3 Cephalic presentations (vertex) in varying positions.

relationship of the fetal presenting part to the ischial spines of the mother's mid-pelvis. When the largest diameter of the presenting part is at the level of the ischial spines, it is considered *engaged*, and the station is 0. If the presentation is above the ischial spines, the station is –1 or –2, etc., labeling an estimate of its location in centimeters above the ischial spines. If the presenting part is below the ischial spines, the station is coded as +1 or +2, etc., again making an estimate in centimeters (Fig. 10-6). The station can be assessed through vaginal examination.

Mechanism of labor

The cardinal movements in the mechanism of labor describe the series of passive position adjustments the fetus makes as it accommodates to the space in the passageway. In the vertex presentation, these move-

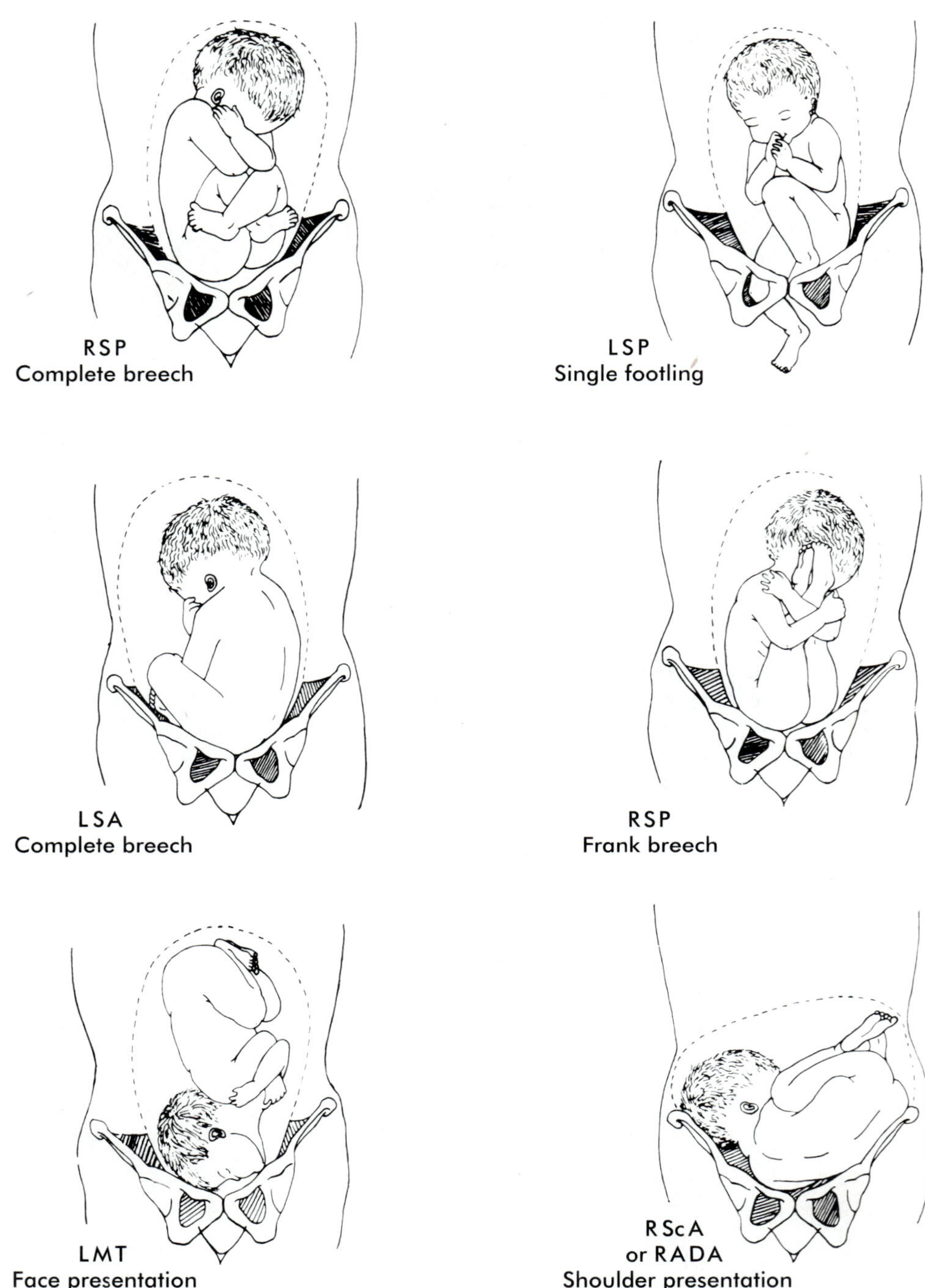

Fig. 10-4 Breech presentations in varying positions; face presentation and transverse (shoulder) presentation with positions indicated.

ments include the following: descent, flexion, engagement, internal rotation, extension, external rotation, and expulsion (Fig. 10-7). The first four movements are not necessarily in order, since flexion may be present before descent and may increase thereafter. Descent and internal rotation also continue after engagement. These mechanisms can occur concurrently and defy a consecutive order.

Descent, flexion, and engagement. Flexion of the fetal head is the normal attitude of the fetus. In a primigravida, descent of the fetus into the true pelvis usually occurs approximately 2 weeks before the actual birth of the child. This descent is referred to as lightening and results in engagement of the presenting part. The pregnant woman may refer to this change in fetal location with the phrase "the baby dropped." In

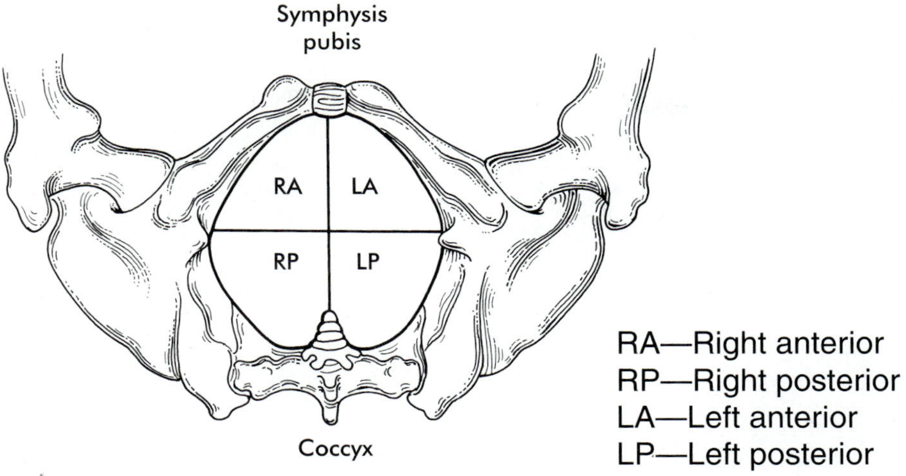

Fig. 10-5 Quadrants of the maternal pelvis, viewed from pelvic outlet.

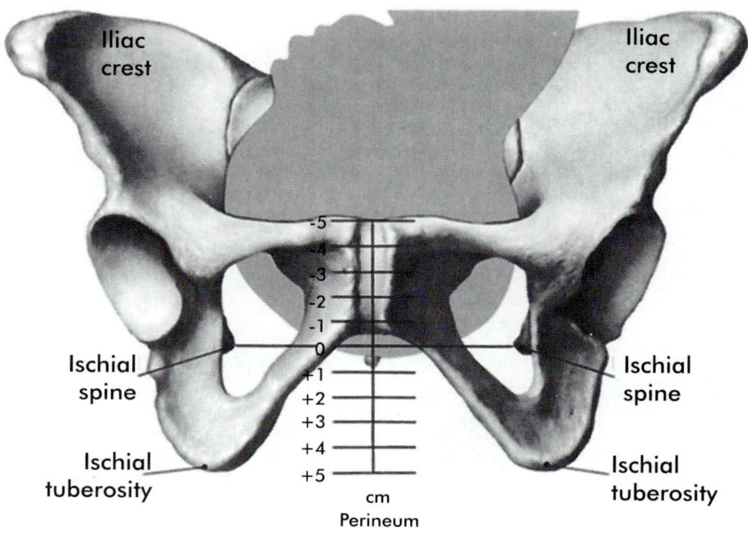

Fig. 10-6 Stations of presenting part or degree of engagement. Stations are expressed in centimeters above *(minus)* and below *(plus)* the level of the ischial spines *(zero).* The head is considered engaged when it reaches the level of the ischial spines. (From *Clinical teaching aid no. 13,* Columbus, OH, 1970, Ross Laboratories.)

a multipara, descent and engagement may not occur until dilation of the cervix begins.

Internal rotation. The amount of internal rotation will depend on the position of the fetus and the way the head rotates to accommodate itself to the changing diameters of the pelvis. The most common rotation is that which involves the turning of the head to the occiput anterior position. If the fetus begins its descent in the LOA or LOT position, this rotation represents only a short distance of 45 to 90 degrees. However, if the internal rotation involves moving from a posterior position, it may mean a turn of 135 degrees. For this reason, posterior positions usually entail a longer labor and more lower back discomfort for the mother. Occasionally, instead of rotating to an anterior position, the occiput turns to the sacrum. The child is then born in the OP position—a delivery that is usually slower and causes more trauma to the maternal tissues. Often the occiput will complete the longer rotation from the posterior position to the pubis. Sometimes the occiput lingers unduly in the posterior position, which is called *persistent posterior,* or stops its rotation in transverse, referred to as *transverse arrest.* These positions can occur at almost any station or depth in the pelvic canal and may necessitate manual rotation or the use of

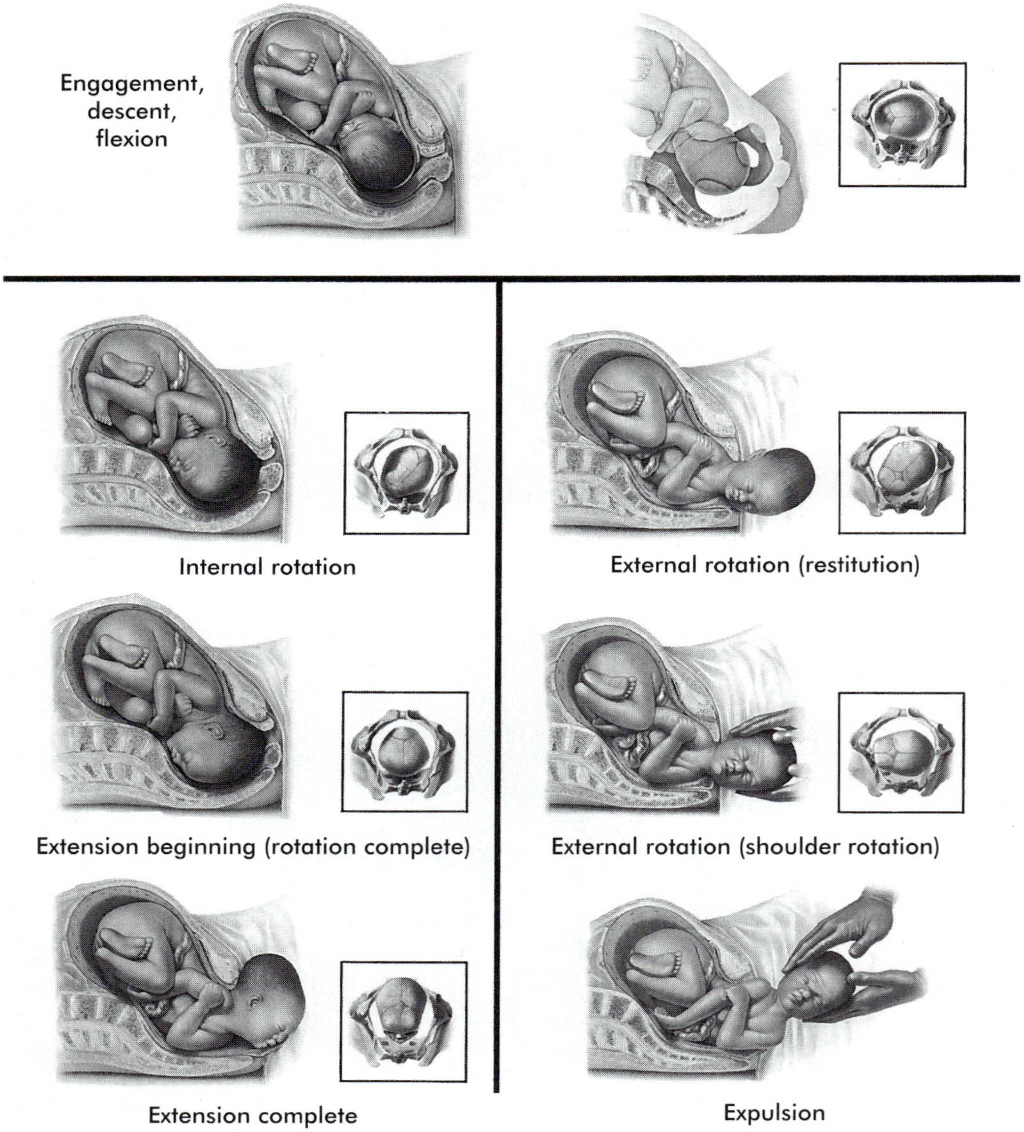

Engagement, descent, flexion

Internal rotation

External rotation (restitution)

Extension beginning (rotation complete)

External rotation (shoulder rotation)

Extension complete

Expulsion

Fig. 10-7 Mechanism of normal labor, LOA position showing head rotation in square inserts. (From *Clinical teaching aid no. 13,* Columbus, OH, 1970, Ross Laboratories.)

rotation forceps by an obstetrician. (See the nursing alert below.)

> **Nursing Alert**
>
> When the fetus is in an occiput posterior (OP) position, having the mother move to a hands-and-knees position may facilitate fetal rotation to a more anterior position.

Extension. In a vertex presentation the head is delivered by extension. During descent the head is normally forced into a flexed attitude by the pressure of the cervix, pelvic walls, and floor. Once the occiput has rotated to the anterior position and moved under the pubic arch, the head cannot make any further progress unless extension occurs. Because of this extension and the natural curve of the lower pelvis the infant's head is born pushing upward out of the vaginal canal. The rate of extension is controlled, in part, by the health care provider. If the bag of waters (membranes) has not broken during labor, it must be broken at this point to prevent the infant from aspirating amniotic fluid. If an episiotomy, a surgical incision extending the soft tissue vaginal opening, is necessary to avoid tearing of the perineum, it is performed just before the birth of the head (see Chapter 11 for a more thorough discussion of an episiotomy).

External rotation. When the perineum slides over the chin of the baby and the neck is at the outlet, more room is available for head movement. Usually, without the coaxing of the birth attendant, the back of the infant's head turns to line up with his or her back. This movement is called *restitution.* The turning movement of the head generally continues and influences the location of the back, helping to line up the unborn shoulders in anteroposterior position just beneath the pubis. This process of alignment is called *shoulder rotation.*

Expulsion. Usually the top of the anterior shoulder is just under the pubis—generally aided by the health care provider, who may exert gentle but firm downward traction on the head. The head is then gently raised to clear the posterior shoulder, and the entire body follows without difficulty. Expulsion of the infant is completed.

POWERS

The uterine contractions are the primary powers of labor. The factors contributing to the onset of labor contractions are not well defined. A number of theories exist. It appears that hormones of both maternal and fetal origin play a role, as does the stretching of the uterus and the pressure of the presenting part on the lower uterine segment. Contractions begin in the uterine fundus and rapidly radiate downward over the body of the uterus.

Each contraction has a rhythmic pattern: a gradual increase in strength until reaching peak intensity, and a gradual decrease in strength until the uterus resumes its resting state. Assessing the *frequency* (the time from the onset of one contraction to the onset of the next), the *duration* (from the beginning to the end of a single contraction), and the *intensity* (degree of peak tightness or hardness) of contractions is part of the nurse's responsibility and gives valuable information concerning the progress of labor. Contractions may be monitored by palpation with the nurse's hands, by electronic means, or by a combination of both. (See Chapter 11 for a more thorough description of evaluating uterine contractions.) At the beginning of labor the contractions are usually mild, short, and relatively infrequent.

More frequent and progressively longer and stronger uterine contractions create the effacement (shortening and thinning) and *dilation* of the cervix to an opening approximately 10 cm (approximately 4 inches) in diameter. Early effacement and dilation (1 to 3 cm) may occur "silently," as the result of unobtrusive Braxton Hicks contractions before the onset of more definitive, vigorous labor. The disappearance, or effacement, of the cervical canal, as its walls move upward to become part of the lower uterine segment, is expressed in percentages. The cervix of a primipara (nullipara) usually effaces completely (100%) before dilating (Fig. 10-8). The cervix of a multipara, on the other hand, typically effaces and dilates simultaneously (Fig. 10-8). After complete cervical dilation, uterine muscles continue to contract and the mother adds the power of her voluntary pushing efforts to move the fetus through the pelvic canal.

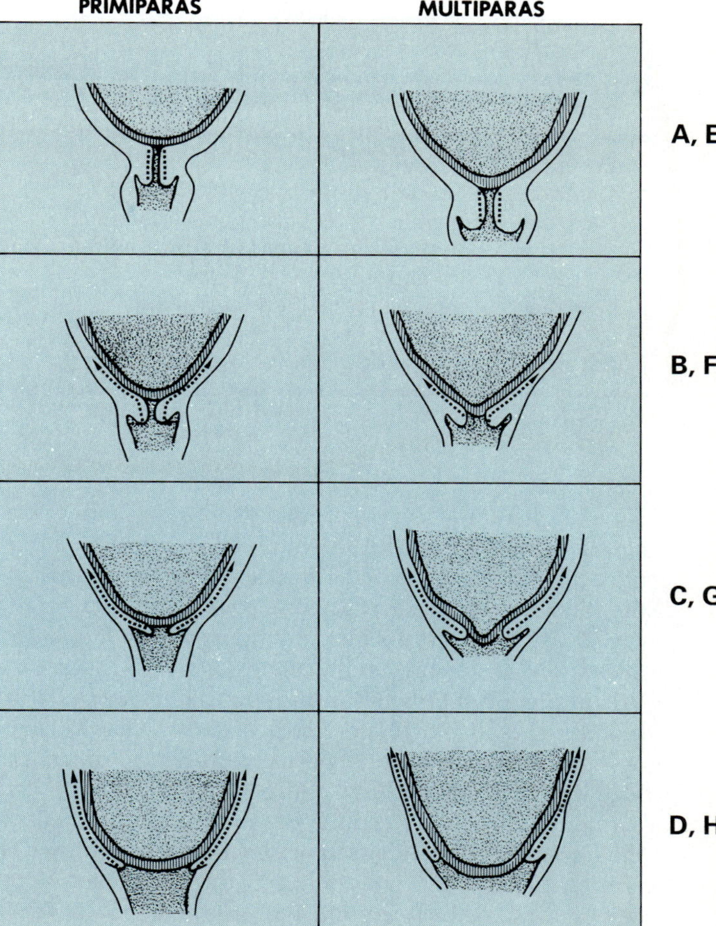

Fig. 10-8 The columns above compare the typical progress of cervical effacement and dilation demonstrated by women in labor with their first child compared with that of women in labor with their second or subsequent child. **A** and **E,** Long cervix. Multiparas usually have a relaxed cervical canal. **B** and **F,** Effacement or shortening of cervix begins. **C** and **G,** Cervix thins in primiparas but little dilation occurs. Effacement and dilation are simultaneous in multiparas. **D** and **H,** Effacement and dilation are complete.

◆ TABLE 10-1
Differences Between True and False Labor

True Labor	False Labor
Contractions are regular.	Contractions are irregular.
Contractions become more frequent.	Frequency is usually unchanged.
Contractions increase in duration and intensity.	Duration and intensity unchanged.
Discomfort begins in the lower back and radiates around to the abdomen.	Discomfort is primarily in the abdomen.
Contractions usually intensified by walking.	Walking does not effect, or may lessen, the frequency and intensity.
Cervical effacement and dilation are progressive.	Little or no cervical change.

Dilation of the cervix is usually accompanied by *bloody show.* When the cervix begins to dilate, the cervical mucus plug that has protected the uterus is discharged. As the cervix continues to dilate, small capillaries in the cervix break, staining the mucus with blood. The faster the cervix dilates and the closer it is to complete dilation the more abundant and red the bloody show. However, bloody show should not assume the proportions or characteristics of frank bleeding or contain clots.

In summary, to determine the progress of the fetus, the nurse and the physician or certified nurse midwife is interested in the presentation, the body part that comes first; the position, the relationship of the presenting part to the pelvic quadrants; and the station, the depth of the presenting part in the pelvic canal. If these elements are known, in addition to the relative size and shape of the pelvis and fetus, the effacement and dilation of the cervix, and the frequency, duration, and intensity of the uterine contractions, the health care provider has a good basis to evaluate the progress of the labor and the mechanisms involved.

PSYCHE

The woman's preparation for labor, her usual patterns of coping with pain and stressful situations, her culture, and her attitude and expectations about labor and birth will determine how she reacts to her labor. If a woman is highly anxious, that anxiety can alter not only her perception of the labor but also the progress of the labor itself. Research indicates that high levels of anxiety prompt the secretion of catecholamines, hormones that may, in turn, decrease the frequency, duration, and intensity of uterine contractions (Lederman, et al., 1978; Lederman, et al., 1985).

Those who attend childbirth education classes enter labor equipped with factual information, less anxiety, and more confidence in their ability to positively deal with the labor and birth (Nichols and Humenick, 1988). The presence of supportive friends or family, and the care of an experienced nurse can also reduce anxiety and promote comfort and feelings of confidence in her ability to have a satisfying labor and birth experience.

Differences Between True and False Labor

The uterus contracts and relaxes intermittently all during pregnancy. Its contractions, however, are usually mild and not uncomfortable for the woman. However, in the last few weeks of pregnancy, these uterine contractions may become uncomfortable, even painful. If they do not serve to progressively dilate the cervix, they are called false labor, or Braxton Hicks contractions, after the British obstetrician who described them. It is often difficult for the pregnant woman to distinguish false labor from the real thing. It is particularly discouraging for a woman to go to the hospital or birth center, only to be sent home. See Table 10-1 for the major differences between true and false labor.

STAGES OF LABOR

Labor has traditionally been divided into three stages. Some clinicians also describe a fourth stage.

Stage 1—from the onset of regular labor contractions, beginning with effacement and dilation of the cervix to complete dilation at 10 cm. Stage one is further divided into three phases:
- (a) the latent phase—from the start of true labor to cervical dilation of 3 cm to 4 cm
- (b) the active phase—from cervical dilation of 4 cm to 7 to 8 cm
- (c) the transition phase—from 8 cm to 10 cm.

Stage 2—from complete dilation to the birth of the infant.

Stage 3—from birth of the infant to the expulsion of the placenta and membranes.

Stage 4—a 1-hour to 4-hour period of transition, stabilization, and initial recovery from childbirth.

See Chapter 11 for further discussion of the stages of labor.

Friedman Labor Curve

As indicated earlier, the progress of labor depends on a number of factors. Emmanuel Friedman studied thousands of labors and births to determine patterns of normal labor. The guidelines he developed for judging whether the progress of labor is within normal limits were translated into the well-known Friedman curve. Friedman noted that two measurements, when serially repeated and graphed, reveal whether or not the journey through the pelvic passageway is proceeding satisfactorily. These two measurements are cervical dilation and station. In most facilities the labor is not actually graphed, but the following norms serve as mental guidelines for the nurse, certified nurse midwife, and physician. The nurse should be aware that these guidelines must be used in concert with assessment of other clinical signs of labor, and of maternal and fetal well-being.

Changes in cervical dilation

Friedman identified two similar S-shaped curves, based on the speed of cervical dilation of multiparas and primiparas (nulliparas). When the rate of an individual woman's cervical dilation is plotted against the appropriate curve, disturbances in labor progress are more readily apparent. Both curves are divided into sections describing different phases of the labor process (Fig. 10-9). The vertical side of the graph indicates the cervical dilation of 0 to 10 centimeters and the horizontal side indicates the number of hours in labor. The mean, or average, length of labor is much shorter for multiparas, accounting for the variance in the curves.

Two main phases are described for the first stage of labor: the relatively slow-moving, flat first section called the *latent phase,* involving cervical softening, effacement, and early dilation (tracing the period extending from onset of labor until more rapid dilation manifests itself at approximately 2 cm to 3 cm); and a second section, the active phase (4 cm to 10 cm), which is indicated by the sudden upswing and steep ascent of the tracing, ending with a brief rounding at the apex. This active phase of dilation has, in turn, been divided into three phases: (1) the acceleration phase (4 cm to 5 cm) is the curve upward from the latent phase that first indicates more rapid cervical dilation; (2) the phase of maximum slope (5 cm to 9 cm) is the steepest part of the tracing; and (3) the deceleration phase (9 cm to 10 cm) is the rounding of the apex, which represents a slowing of the dilation just before the cervix is completely dilated. Existence of the deceleration phase is disputed and has often been characterized as short or absent in multiparas. (The transition phase is not defined as a separate phase in the Friedman model of labor.)

It is sometimes difficult to determine when the latent phase begins, since effacement and early cervical dilation are "silent," or false labor may confuse the issue. The patient's labor graph is usually begun when a nullipara's (primipara's) contractions are regular at 3- to 5-minute intervals or when a multipara attains regular contractions at 5- to 10-minute intervals.

Although the condition of the mother and the fetus is considered more important than the passage of time, comparing the cervical dilation of a maternity patient to the appropriate Friedman curve may be helpful in identifying problems affecting labor. Using this standard, a labor is considered prolonged if:

1 The latent phase lasts
   - a 14 hours or more for multiparas
   - b 20 hours or more for nulliparas
2 The rate of maximum slope is
   - a 1.5 cm/hr or less for multiparas
   - b 1.2 cm/hr or less for nulliparas
3 The maximum slope shows no progress in dilation for 2 hours or more (secondary arrest—the most damaging dilation pattern)
4 The deceleration phase lasts
   - a More than 1 hour for multiparas
   - b More than 3 hours for nulliparas

These abnormalities are shown in Fig. 10-10. When these conditions exist the health care provider will evaluate the probable cause and, depending on the cause, may decide to:

1 Intensify maternal and infant assessment
2 Use sedation for the mother
3 Stimulate uterine contractions with oxytocic medication
4 Prepare for cesarean birth

(See Chapter 14 for a more thorough discussion of management of labor problems.)

Changes in station or descent

Friedman's study of descent rate of the fetus through the pelvic canal produces a curve that is divided in almost the same way as the dilation curve. The descent curve is sometimes superimposed on the dilation graph to show that the phase of maximum slope for cervical dilation normally corresponds to the phase of acceleration for descent (Fig. 10-11).

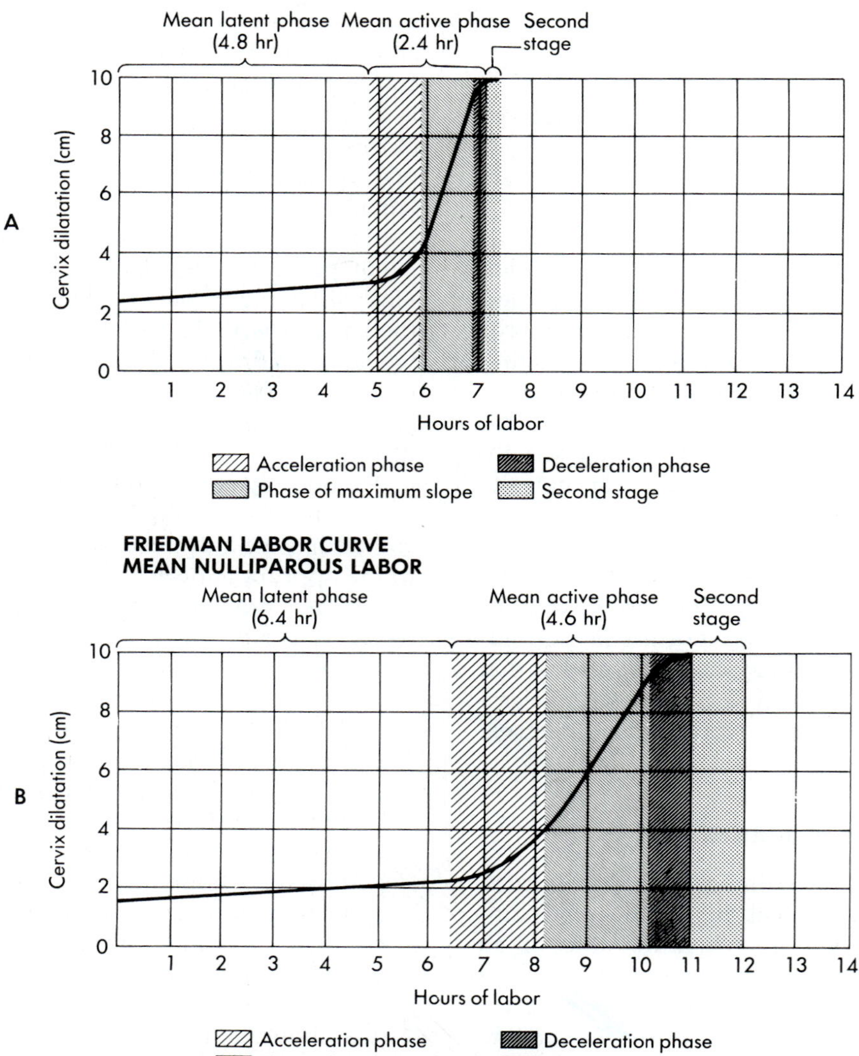

Fig. 10-9 The Friedman labor curve formed by plotting the rate of cervical dilation of the mean multiparous labor **(A)** and mean nulliparous (primiparous) labor **(B)** (*mean* indicates average). (Based on revised mean labor statistics in Friedman EA: *Labor: clinical evaluation and management,* ed 2, New York, 1979, Appleton-Century-Crofts; and personal correspondence.)

Descent abnormalities occur alone or in conjunction with problems in dilation. Descent is considered to be abnormally slow or arrested if:

1. During the maximum slope the rate is
   a. 2 cm/hr or less for multiparas
   b. 1 cm/hr or less for nulliparas
2. During descent labor progress is stopped for 1 hour or more

If problems in descent occur, the physician or certified nurse midwife reevaluates fetal presentation and position and the adequacy of the maternal pelvis. Changes in the woman's posture or activity of the mother are usually helpful. For example, walking is likely to improve the quality of the contractions during the first stage of labor, and sitting (more than 30 degrees) or squatting improves the angle for pushing during the second stage of labor (Biancuzzo, 1993). If more conservative methods fail, oxytocics may be ordered or a cesarean birth scheduled.

NOTE: Too rapid of a descent or precipitous labor (not to be confused with precipitous delivery, which means a birth without adequate preparation) can also be a

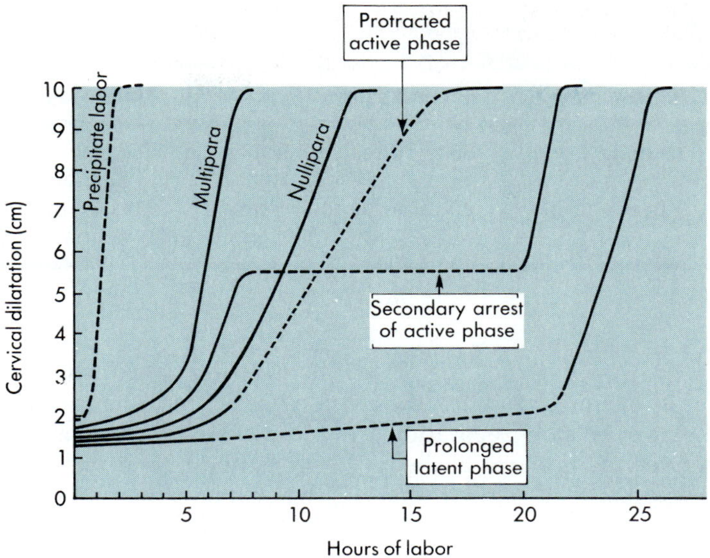

Fig. 10-10 Deviations in rate of cervical dilation (as described by Friedman). The prolonged deceleration phase is not pictured.

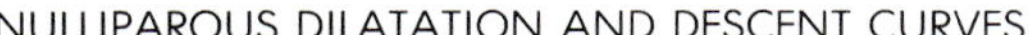

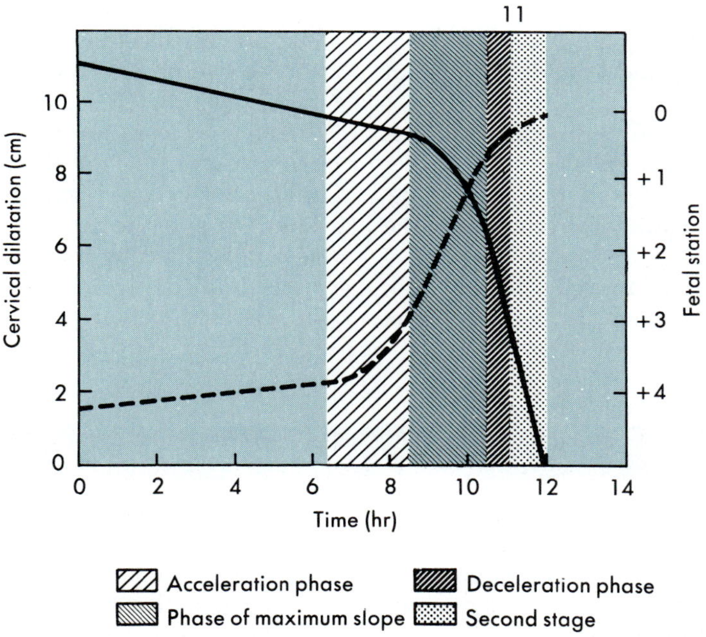

Fig. 10-11 Shows approximate relationship of cervical dilation rate to fetal descent rate in average nulliparous (primiparous) labor. (Adapted from Friedman EA: *Labor: clinical evaluation and management,* ed 2, New York, 1978, Appleton-Century-Crofts.)

problem. A precipitous labor is defined as a labor of less than 3 hours, which may be accompanied by uterine and perineal lacerations, lowered fetal oxygenation, and infant birth injury (especially cerebral hemorrhage).

Experienced nurses, midwives, and physicians are reluctant to make specific predictions regarding the length of the stages of labor. However, Table 10-2 may be useful in estimating typical time intervals.

◆ TABLE 10-2
Usual Duration of the Stages of Labor

	First Stage	Second Stage	Third Stage
Primiparas (nulliparas)	10 to 12 hours	30 minutes to 2 hours	5 to 20 minutes (often aided by oxytocics or manual pressure)
Multiparas	6 to 8 hours	20 minutes to 1½ hours	5 to 20 minutes (often aided by oxytocics or manual pressure)

Third Stage of Labor

The third stage of labor is characterized by the separation of the placenta and its expulsion. Separation of the placenta from the uterine wall is accomplished by the contraction of the uterus. The site of the placental attachment suddenly becomes reduced, but the placenta itself remains the same size, causing a separation of the two structures. The placenta slides down into the lower portion of the uterus and vagina. The signs of placental separation, include the following:

1 The rise of the uterus to the umbilicus or above—pushed up by the bulky placenta in the vagina
2 The increased firmness and rounded shape of the fundus
3 The lengthening of the umbilical cord from the vagina as the placenta descends
4 The sudden appearance of moderate, temporary vaginal bleeding, originating from the site of the placental separation

After the placenta is separated from the uterine wall, it is pushed out by the mother during a uterine contraction when she is instructed again to "bear down." Often, she is assisted by the health care provider, who—*after* separation of the placenta—carefully exerts abdominal pressure with one hand just above the pubic bone, momentarily pushing the uterus higher to help the placenta slip further down the birth canal. The provider gently pulls on the umbilical cord with the other hand (the Brandt-Andrews maneuver), causing the placenta's expulsion. At times the health care provider may elect to help deliver the placenta through cautious intravaginal, intrauterine, or abdominal maneuvers. Manual extraction may be necessary in cases of abnormally retained placenta or excessive uterine bleeding. The cervix is visually inspected for lacerations and the placenta is checked for abnormality, completeness, and number of cord vessels.

The third and fourth stages of labor are probably the most dangerous for the mother, since hemorrhages most often occur during this time. To prevent excessive blood loss, oxytocics, medications that help contract the uterus, are frequently added to existing intravenous fluids or given intramuscularly after the placenta is delivered.

KEY CONCEPTS

1 The progress of labor depends on the size of the passage (bony pelvis), the size and position of the passenger (fetus), the rhythm and strength of the powers (uterine contractions), and the woman's psyche (mental preparedness).
2 The lie refers to the relationship of the long axis of the fetus to the long axis of the mother.
3 Presentation, or presenting part, refers to the part of the baby entering the pelvic canal first. Most births are headfirst, or cephalic (96%); approximately 3.5% of births are breech; the remainder are shoulder or transverse (0.5%).
4 Three types of breech presentations may occur. With a complete or full breech the fetus' legs are flexed so that the buttocks and feet appear at the vaginal opening almost simultaneously. A frank or single breech occurs when the thighs of the fetus are flexed on the abdomen, with the extended legs against the trunk and the feet against the face. Incomplete breech may indicate that either the feet or the knees are presenting.
5 Attitude refers to the degree of flexion of the body, head, and extremities. The normal attitude is complete flexion.
6 The position is the relationship of a certain point of reference on the presenting part of the fetus to the pelvic quadrants of the mother.
7 The phrase describing fetal position comprises three terms: (1) right or left (of the mother's pelvis), (2) the fetal point of reference, and (3) the adjective

anterior, posterior, or transverse (referring to the part of the mother's pelvis toward which a particular point on the fetus is directed). The most common vertex position is left occiput anterior (LOA).

8 Station refers to the relationship of the presenting part of the fetus to the ischial spines of the mother's pelvis.

9 Uterine contractions cause cervical effacement (shortening and thinning) and dilation (widening to an opening approximately 10 cm [4 in] in diameter).

10 As the cervix dilates the mucus plug is discharged and becomes blood-tinged as a result of the breakage of small capillaries in the cervix. This discharge is referred to as *bloody show.* The faster the cervix dilates and the closer it is to complete dilation, the more abundant and red the bloody show.

11 The cardinal movements in the mechanism of labor describe the series of passive position adjustments the fetus makes as it accommodates to the space in the passage way.

12 Descent is when the fetus moves into the true pelvis. Descent results in engagement, or the passage of the largest diameter of the presenting part into the true pelvis.

13 The amount of internal rotation depends on the position of the fetus and the way the head rotates to accommodate to the changing diameters of the pelvis.

14 In a vertex delivery the head is delivered by extension, with the head pushing upward out of the vaginal canal.

15 After the head has been delivered, it usually turns, helping to line up the unborn shoulders. This movement is called *external rotation* and allows for delivery of the rest of the infant, or expulsion.

16 Labor is divided into four stages. Stage 1 begins with the onset of regular labor contractions and ends with complete cervical dilation. Stage 2 begins with complete dilation and ends with the birth of the infant. Stage 3 begins with the birth of the infant and ends with the expulsion of the placenta and membranes. Stage 4 is the period of transition, stabilization, and initial recovery from childbirth.

17 The Friedman labor curve employs two measurements—cervical dilation and station—to graph a woman's progress during the first two stages of labor. The curve can be used, along with other assessment data, to determine if the progress of a woman's labor falls within normal, healthy limits.

18 Two main phases of cervical dilation are described in a patient's labor graph: the latent phase and the active phase. The active phase is divided further into three phases: acceleration phase, phase of maximum slope, and deceleration phase.

19 Using the Friedman labor curve, the following dilations indicate prolonged labor: latent phase lasts longer than 14 hours in multiparas or 20 hours in nulliparas; rate of maximum slope is 1.5 cm/hour or less for multiparas, or 1.2 cm/hr or less for nulliparas; or the maximum slope shows no progress in dilation for 2 hours or more.

20 When labor is not progressing normally the health care provider may decide to intensify maternal and infant assessment, use sedation for the mother, stimulate uterine contractions with oxytocic medications, or prepare for cesarean birth.

21 Fetal descent is considered to be abnormally slow or arrested if either of the following occurs: the rate during maximum slope is 2 cm/hr or less for multiparas or 1 cm/hr or less for nulliparas, or labor progress is stopped for 1 hour or more during descent.

22 Both precipitous labor, which is too rapid of a descent, and precipitous delivery, which is birth without adequate preparation, can present problems for mother and fetus.

23 Usual duration of the first three stages of labor are as follows: the first stage lasts approximately 10 to 12 hours in primiparas and 6 to 8 hours in multiparas; the second stage lasts approximately 30 minutes to 2 hours in primiparas and 20 minutes to 1½ hours in multiparas; and the third stage lasts approximately 5 to 20 minutes in all women.

24 Signs of placental separation include the following: the rise of the uterus to the umbilicus or above, increased firmness and rounded shape of the fundus, lengthening of the umbilical cord from the vagina, and the sudden appearance of moderate and temporary vaginal bleeding.

CRITICAL THOUGHT QUESTIONS

1 The physician has just examined your labor patient and determined that the fetus is in the LOP position. Your patient asks you to explain what the physician meant by LOP position and the significance of this finding for her labor. How would you explain the LOP position and its significance so that she understands?

2 Abnormal presentations are most commonly found

in multiple pregnancies, in cases of pelvic deformity, and in situations in which the placenta is abnormally located. Why do you think these conditions are significant to fetal presentation?

3 If your patient's fetus is LOA, what is the presentation, lie, and attitude? How are all of these related?

4 Mrs. Janes comes to the birth center, sure that she is in true labor with her second child. She is *very* disappointed when the examiner tells her that her cervix is dilated to 1 cm, 50% effaced (no change from the midwife's examination 2 days ago), and decides to send her home to await the "real thing." As the nurse, how could you help this woman deal with her disappointment and feel confident about her ability to judge true labor?

5 Mrs. Ho is admitted to the birth center in early labor with her second child. She tells you that she had a long difficult labor with her first child and is fearful that this labor will be just as long and difficult. She asks your opinion. What would you tell her? Why?

REFERENCES

Biancuzzo M: Six myths of maternal posture during labor, *MCN* 18(5):264-269, 1993.

Friedman EA: *Labor: clinical evaluation and management,* ed 2, New York, 1979, Appleton-Century-Crofts.

Lederman R, Lederman E, Work B, McCann D: Anxiety and epinephrine in multiparous women in labor: relationship to duration of labor and fetal heart rate pattern, *Am J Obstet Gynecol* 153(8):870-877, 1985.

Lederman R, Lederman E, Work B, McCann D: The relationship of maternal anxiety, plasma catecholamines, and plasma cortisol to progress in labor, *Am J Obstet Gynecol* 132(5):495-500, 1978.

Nichols FH, Humenick SS: *Childbirth education: practice, research, and theory.* Philadelphia, 1988, WB Saunders.

BIBLIOGRAPHY

Biancuzzo M: The patient observer: does the hands-and-knees posture during labor help to rotate the occiput posterior fetus? *Birth* 18:40-47, 1991.

Creasy RK, Resnik R: *Maternal-fetal medicine,* ed 3, Philadelphia, 1994, WB Saunders.

Lowe N: Maternal confidence in coping with labor, *J Obstet Gynecol Neonatal Nurs* 20(6):457, 1991.

Oxhorn H: *Human labor and birth,* ed 5, New York, 1986, Appleton-Century-Crofts.

Labor and Birth

CHAPTER OBJECTIVES

After studying this chapter, the student should be able to:

1. Discuss the advantages and disadvantages of various childbirth settings.
2. List the signs and symptoms of impending labor.
3. Discuss the factors that influence when a woman in labor should go to the hospital or center where she plans to give birth.
4. Indicate the admission data that the nurse must gather to adequately assess the status of the labor and maternal and fetal well-being.
5. Describe how the uterus is evaluated for contraction frequency, duration, and intensity, and uterine-resting tone.
6. Use diagrams to differentiate the three classic, fetal-heart-rate (FHR) patterns called early, late, and variable FHR decelerations.
7. Discuss the significance and recommended nursing interventions for early, late, and variable FHR decelerations.
8. Discuss the possible causes and significance of diminished baseline FHR variability.
9. List six signs of possible fetal distress during the labor process.
10. Define the following terms associated with psychoprophylactic labor techniques and prenatal exercises: *cleansing breaths, focal point, effleurage, sacral support*, and *pelvic rock.*
11. Define the four stages of labor and discuss how stage length may differ for women having their first babies and for those who have given birth before.
12. Discuss the nursing care appropriate for each stage of labor.
13. Describe appropriate nursing interventions if there is a question of ruptured membranes.
14. Explain how the nurse can assist the patient and the health care provider with a vaginal examination and artificial rupture of the membranes.
15. List four possible indications of the onset of the second stage of labor.
16. Describe at least two ways the nurse can intervene to enhance parent–infant attachment in the perinatal period.
17. Differentiate among first, second, third, and fourth degree perineal lacerations.
18. Explain the Apgar evaluation of the newborn, listing the five features assessed.
19. Describe major considerations involved in precipitous delivery and how the nurse can best help the mother and newborn.
20. Enumerate indications for induction of labor.
21. Discuss the emergency preparation of a labor patient for cesarean birth, including procedures and psychological support.
22. State three complications associated with breech birth.
23. Indicate how preparations for a twin birth may differ from those for a single child.

CHILDBIRTH SETTINGS

As indicated in Chapter 1, a trend toward making maternity services more family-centered is underway. This trend evolved in response to consumer demand for more natural childbirth and more family participation and control over their birth experiences. Families frequently "shop" for services that meet their needs and desires. These services may include a relaxed, personal atmosphere and more flexibility in the types of care offered; policies that permit the presence of other family members and friends (including, in some instances, sibling presence at the birth); less medical intervention (e.g., choices about fetal monitoring, administration of drugs, artificial rupture of the bag of waters, routine transfer from the labor area to a delivery room, episiotomy, and forceps application); having the newborn room-in; and lower costs.

Alternatives to Traditional Birth Settings

Home birth

Alternatives to "traditional" hospital birth vary in availability and safety. Some parents decide to give birth at home. The birth attendant may be a physician, certified nurse midwife, lay midwife, friend, or father of the baby. The legality and proficiency of the attendant differ, depending on locale and circumstances. Although a minority of physicians and nurse midwives will attend home births for selected low-risk women, most will not. They contend that, although other developed countries, such as Great Britain and the Netherlands, offer home birth to certain women, the health care system in the United States is not organized to safely render such care. In support of their argument, they cite the small but important percentage (5% to 10%) of mothers and infants who, although not considered high risk, develop problems during the labor–birth period. These health care workers are concerned about professional backup in the event that they cannot attend the birth and about the threat of malpractice judgments. They are also influenced by the accessibility of hospital facilities and perinatal centers in the event that complications arise.

Alternative birth center (or room)

An alternative to a home birth or a traditional hospital birth is the alternative birthing room or alternative birth center (ABC). These alternative facilities are part of or near a hospital or clinic where emergency equipment and staff are available if needed. They are typically designed to care for uncomplicated births in a home-like setting. These rooms serve for labor, birth, and early postpartum care. Such centers have liberal visitation policies and usually discharge the mother and baby several hours after birth. Often, follow-up nursing visits are made to the home. Many of these centers use nurse midwives, as well as physicians, to monitor the labor and assist at the birth.

Single Room Maternity Care

The traditional hospital labor and delivery unit is based on the surgical transfer model. In this model the mother is moved from room to room, often during the most critical biological or psychological moments of the birth experience. In contrast, Single Room Maternity Care provides for the labor, birth, recovery, and initial postpartum care in one location (Machol, 1989) (Fig. 11-1). Mother, baby, and her support person stay in one or, at the most, two rooms during the entire hospital stay. Unlike other alternative birth options, this system is not limited to uncomplicated or low-risk clients. Since the mother and her baby are in a hospital setting, with life-sustaining equipment and health personnel available, all women who are having vaginal deliveries can be taken care of in the Single Room Maternity Care system. This concept combines the science and safety of modern medicine, the knowledge of skilled caregivers, and the needs of the family into one package. Hundreds of hospitals across the United States have initiated one of the two types of Single Room Maternity Care options described in the following text.

LDR (labor, delivery, recovery). In the LDR setting the mother is admitted to a birthing suite and remains there for her labor, delivery, and recovery. The rooms are decorated much like hotel rooms, but with all of the necessary medical equipment readily available. Following recovery the mother and her infant are moved to a Mother–Baby Unit, where the goal is to enable one nurse to care for the mother and baby together.

LDRP (labor, delivery, recovery, postpartum). The LDRP setting is similar to the LDR, but the mother and infant are not transferred to another unit after the recovery period. After the family is admitted to the LDRP, labor, delivery, recovery, and postpartum care take place in one room.

There are many advantages to single room maternity care (LDR or LDRP). This system encourages both parents to get to know their baby and begin functioning as a family unit under the guidance of skilled maternity personnel. Nursing care is less fragmented in these settings. Assessments, treatments, and teaching are more easily coordinated when one nurse knows the status of both the mother and child. By minimizing the number of people receiving a report on each patient

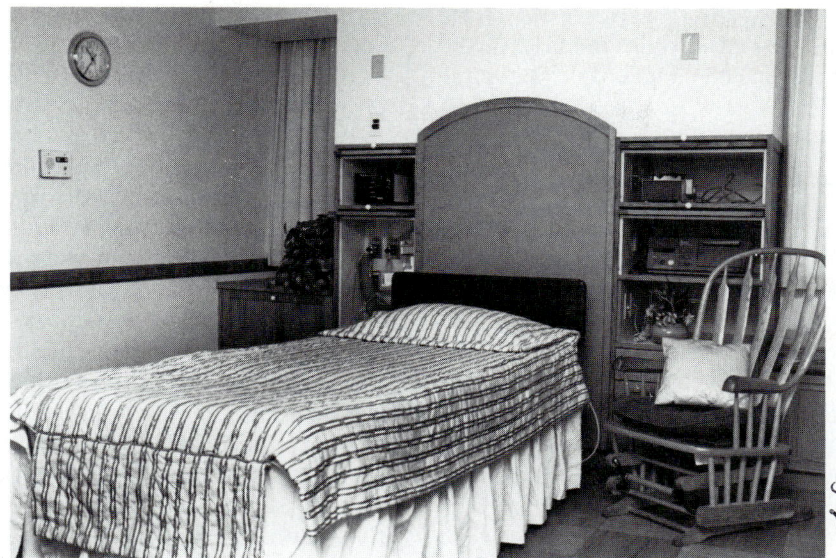

Fig. 11-1 This LDRP room has the equipment needed for a normal delivery. (Courtesy Grossmont Hospital, La Mesa, CA.)

the chances for error are reduced. The risk of infection is also lessened when mother and baby remain together. The following discussion of nursing care for the laboring woman assumes, except where indicated, a single room maternity care setting (LDR or LDRP).

SIGNS OF IMPENDING LABOR

As the time of labor and birth approaches the pregnant woman should be alerted to the signs of imminent labor. She should be instructed when to call the health care provider and when to come to the hospital or birth center. Several signs and symptoms usually precede the onset of true labor. These early signs are generally welcome. At the end of a full-term pregnancy the mother is often impatient to end her increasingly uncomfortable pregnancy and greet the newborn. She has feelings of anxiety, however, as she contemplates the actual period of labor and birth. Signs and symptoms that should alert the woman that true labor is near follow.

Lightening

A woman bearing her first infant will feel a relative change in fetal location, occurring approximately 2 weeks before birth. The fetus "drops" into the true pelvis and the presenting part becomes engaged. After lightening she finds herself able to breathe more freely. Pressure of the presenting part, however, causes more frequent urination, backache and leg pain, and edema of the legs and feet. Primigravidas are expected to experience lightening and engagement before true labor begins. If this does not occur the possibility of too small of a pelvic inlet or too large of a presenting part (fetal-pelvic disproportion) is a concern. Multigravidas may not undergo lightening until just before or during true labor.

Braxton Hicks contractions

Toward the end of pregnancy, Braxton Hicks contractions may become more uncomfortable, resulting in "false labor." Walking usually lessens the discomfort. These contractions, together with hormonal changes, result in early cervical changes or "ripening". The cervix moves from a posterior to a more anterior position, becomes softer, thins (50% or so), and dilates somewhat (1 to 2 cm).

Gastrointestinal upsets

Women frequently experience diarrhea, indigestion, or nausea and vomiting in the few days before the onset of labor. These upsets may be accompanied by a 2- to 3-lb weight loss.

Burst of energy

Many women experience a phenomenal "burst of energy" 24 to 48 hours before going into labor. They engage in house cleaning and last minute preparations for the baby (nesting behavior).

Bloody show

As the cervix "ripens" the early dilation and effacement result in bloody show. This is usually a late sign of imminent labor.

Ruptured membranes or bag of waters

Occasionally the amniotic membranes will rupture before the onset of labor. Once membranes have ruptured, most women will go into spontaneous labor within 24 hours. If membranes rupture and labor does not begin within this time frame the health care provider may decide to induce labor to avoid the risk of infection. The latter course of action is taken only when the pregnancy is full term. See Chapter 14 for a discussion of ruptured membranes in a less than full-term pregnancy.

HOSPITAL ADMISSION

The time at which the woman should go to the hospital or birth center depends on her reported labor progress, the distance she must travel, how many babies she has had, and the history of her previous labors. Usually health care providers instruct the woman to come to the health facility if the amniotic membranes (bag of waters) is leaking or ruptures, vaginal bleeding or bloody show is experienced, and if uterine contractions are regular and frequent (from 5- to 10-minute intervals or less for at least 1 hour in primigravidas and 10- to 15-minute intervals for 1 hour in multigravidas). (See Chapter 10 for a list of the differences between true and false labor).

The woman may take advantage of the waiting period before coming to the hospital to relax in a shower, confirm arrangements for transportation and/or child care, and recheck her packed bag. She should rest as much as possible and limit her intake to clear liquids until she is evaluated. Limiting solid food is advised because of the slowing of the digestive process that occurs during labor. Such precautions may also help prevent aspiration if general anesthesia is required in an obstetrical emergency.

Many hospitals suggest that the pregnant woman preregister before labor. This policy makes the later admission process much shorter and eliminates the need for a labor partner to complete admission procedures when he or she could be providing needed support to the laboring woman. The health care provider should tell the woman what the admission procedures involve so that she is prepared. Usually only one consent signature is needed—that of the woman herself—for permission to perform the routine procedures necessary during labor and birth. Routine procedures do not include a cesarean birth, for which separate permission is required.

All women harbor anxiety about their labor experience. Some women are very nervous and fearful. The nursing staff should do everything in its power to alleviate this anxiety and make the woman and her partner or family feel welcome and secure. A calm, pleasant greeting instills confidence and makes a lasting impression. Unfortunately, so does a rude, thoughtless, or disorganized admission experience. Some facilities assess the status of the mother and fetus in a triage area, whereas other facilities perform the assessment in the room in which she will labor, if she is admitted. If she desires, her chosen companion should be allowed to remain with her during the initial assessment and admission procedure. Other family members or friends are usually shown a place where they can comfortably wait until the completion of the admission assessment and procedures.

Admission Assessment

The nurse usually helps the patient remove her clothes and put on a hospital gown. Valuables, such as watches and eyeglasses, are noted. If the woman phoned before coming to the facility the nurse may have already reviewed her prenatal record. If she did not call first the nurse should ask the name of the health care provider and secure the patient's prenatal record. The record should be reviewed for (1) the obstetrical history—the number of viable births she has had, previous difficulties, the rapidity of former labors, and Rh status; (2) the record of the current pregnancy—the expected date of birth, laboratory results, present physical or psychosocial problems, and any known allergies; (3) plans for the labor and birth—type of anesthesia, if desired, and whether she has attended childbirth education classes; (4) accommodations preferred, method selected for feeding the infant, and the name of the physician or nurse practitioner who will care for the baby; and (5) marital status.

The nurse's first priority is to assess the labor status. The status of labor contractions, in particular, determines whether or not the rest of the admission process can proceed in a more leisurely fashion or must be abbreviated. Relevant information includes:

1 Time of onset of the contractions (obtained through patient interview).
2 Current frequency, duration, and intensity of the contractions (obtained through the nurse's palpation of uterine contractions).
3 Whether or not the amniotic membranes are ruptured (obtained through patient interview and tests performed on pooled vaginal fluid).
4 Presence of bloody show or vaginal bleeding

(obtained through patient interview and nurse's observation of vaginal fluid). NOTE: Vaginal examinations should be delayed if the woman indicates vaginal bleeding other than normal bloody show (see Chapter 14 for information on the significance of third trimester bleeding).

5 Cervical dilation, effacement, and fetal station, position and presentation (obtained through the nurse's vaginal examination; real-time ultrasound if there is a question about presentation, number of fetuses, or placental placement).

6 Woman's perception of pain and her coping behaviors.

If the question of ruptured membranes exists, vaginal fluid is obtained for testing. The nitrazine test for pH uses a pH-sensitive test strip to differentiate amniotic fluid, which is slightly alkaline, from urine or vaginal secretions, which are slightly acidic. Wearing a sterile glove, lubricated only with water, the nurse holds the test paper at the cervical os or uses a sterile, cotton-tipped applicator to obtain fluid from the vagina. Amniotic fluid will cause the test strip to turn a deep blue color. In the ferning test a drop of amniotic fluid is placed on a glass slide and allowed to dry. The slide is then examined under a microscope for the appearance of a fern pattern, characteristic of amniotic fluid.

If membranes have ruptured the nurse should inquire about and observe the color of the fluid. It is normally clear and without odor. Greenish amniotic fluid indicates passage of meconium (fetal stool), which is often associated with fetal distress. See the nursing alert at right. A foul odor may indicate infection. If the membranes are ruptured and the fetus' presenting part is not engaged the woman is usually asked to remain in bed. This precaution helps avoid the risk of a prolapse of the umbilical cord into the vagina—an obstetrical emergency.

The nurse must monitor maternal *and* fetal status throughout the labor. On admission the mother's temperature, pulse, respirations, and blood pressure are taken and the fetal heart rate is assessed (more information on fetal heart rate monitoring is presented later in this chapter). The nurse should determine whether the patient has recently eaten. In most maternity services, a voided urine specimen is obtained for urinalysis at the time of admission. The nurse should also check the urine for protein, ketones, and glucose using a dipstick. Proteinuria (a 2+ reading or more) in the presence of edema and/or elevated blood pressure may be a sign of pregnancy-induced hypertension, providing that the specimen is not contaminated with amniotic fluid or blood. High proteinuria levels should be reported to the physician. Some providers also order a blood specimen to check

Nursing Alert

Meconium staining with a breech presentation is usually not considered significant, since the pressure exerted on a breech during its passage through the pelvic canal may cause the discharge of meconium.

hemoglobin (Hgb) and hematocrit (Hct) levels, and a complete blood count (CBC).

As soon as possible the patient is properly identified, usually with a wrist band. The woman and her partner should be oriented to the treatment room and to the usual procedures for ongoing care (e.g., when to expect vaginal and vital sign examinations). During the admission process the nurse should reaffirm the woman's childbirth education and expectations for labor and birth. Some health care providers and childbirth education classes provide a checklist of options for the birth experience (Fig. 11-2). If the woman has completed such a checklist the nurse should review it with her.

The nurse reviews the individual orders for the health care provider regarding the types of analgesia and anesthesia and the expected delivery setup. The nurse also relays information regarding the arrival of the patient at the maternity service, unusual vital signs, and pertinent information gained from the pelvic examination and other assessments of the mother and fetus.

Vaginal prep and enema

Some health care providers leave standing orders for a mini prep. Preparation consists of shaving the perineal hair surrounding the vaginal orifice and the anus. The purpose of these preps is to prevent infection by cleansing the perineal area and to facilitate the cutting and repair of an episiotomy. The use of preps is increasingly controversial, since hair in this area is usually minimal and shaving may nick the skin, contributing to increased risk of infection. Furthermore, no increase in infection is present when the patient has not been shaved. Most health care providers no longer order these preps and rely on careful perineal cleansing just before the birth. If a mini prep is done the nurse should explain the procedure and provide privacy and support. See the box on p. 163 for details regarding the mini prep procedure.

Routine administration of an enema is also controversial. The purposes of the enema are to empty the lower bowel to make descent of the fetal head easier, to avoid the mother's embarrassment at expelling bowel contents during pushing, and to prevent contamination of the sterile field during birth. The enema may

	WOULD LIKE	NO STRONG VIEWS	WISH TO AVOID	STRONGLY OPPOSE	DOCTOR'S COMMENTS
DURING LABOR					
Presence of more than one friend or family member.	______	______	______	______	______
Choice of walking, sitting, or other position for labor.	______	______	______	______	______
Continuous monitoring of baby's heart rate.	______	______	______	______	______
Pain medications.	______	______	______	______	______
Epidural anesthesia.	______	______	______	______	______
FOR DELIVERY					
Presence of more than one friend or family member. (you may wish to specify who they will be). ______	______	______	______	______	______
Episiotomy	______	______	______	______	______
Photography or videotaping by my coach or friend.	______	______	______	______	______
AFTER DELIVERY					
Cord cut by father or support person.	______	______	______	______	______
Baby placed on mom's abdomen.	______	______	______	______	______
Dimmed room lights.	______	______	______	______	______

OTHER: Please feel free to mention any additional ideas or preferences that you have about your labor and delivery. ______

______

______

______

______

______

Do you have a strong preference for either a Doctor or a Certified Nurse Midwife to attend your birth? _____ Yes _____ No

If you have had any formal childbirth preparation course, please indicate which one: ______

Fig. 11-2 Birth plan checklist. (Courtesy Kaiser Permanente Hospital, San Diego, CA.)

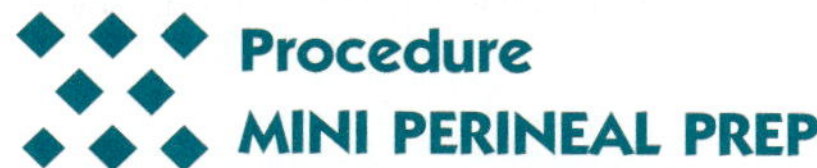

Procedure
MINI PERINEAL PREP

EQUIPMENT/SUPPLIES
- Adequate lighting (overhead spotlight or gooseneck lamp)
- Waterproof pad
- Bath blanket or small pillow
- Small basin of clean, warm water
- Sudsing, antiseptic solution
- Disposable, safety razor
- Two or three clean, dry cotton balls or gauze squares
- Soft paper or cloth towels
- Several paper towels or a plastic bag for waste disposal
- Clean, disposable, sized gloves

STEPS
1 Explain the procedure to the patient.
2 Adjust lighting to avoid shadows (e.g., opposite side of the bed from where you will stand).
3 Place the waterproof pad under her hips.
4 Place a small pillow or rolled bath blanket at her back so that she is not lying completely flat.
5 Draw a privacy curtain to screen the patient from the door. Drape the patient for maximum privacy. A sheet may be over the lower legs and feet; the patient's gown is turned up to just above the perineal hairline.
6 Put on gloves.
7 Have the patient bend her knees and drop her legs sideways—heels toward one another.
8 Question the patient about the presence of perineal moles or warts (and observe for them during the procedure).
9 Lather the perineal hair. Create tension on the skin with a dry gauze square with one hand and shave the area with the other. Place the razor at a 30-degree angle to the skin. Use short strokes rinsing the razor frequently. Cleanse away any collection of smegma (cellular debris found in the labial folds). Avoid getting any solution into the vagina.
10 Wipe off the prepped area with a soft towel dampened with water to remove the solution, which may be irritating. Use a different surface for each stroke and dry with the second soft towel, using the same technique. Never return to the vulva after passing over the rectal area.
11 Turn the patient on her side to finish the perianal region. Repeat the procedure for the area between the vagina and anus, the *true perineum* (the area cut if an episiotomy is performed).

also stimulate uterine contractions. Others question whether the enema accomplishes any of these goals. Most health care providers no longer order an enema unless the patient complains of constipation and asks for one (see the box on p. 164 for details regarding the enema procedure). Enemas are contraindicated in the event of rapidly progressing labor, vaginal bleeding, or a high presenting part (unengaged), especially if membranes are ruptured. Some providers prefer that no enemas be given when membranes are ruptured, even after engagement, because of the increased danger of infection.

The nurse should ascertain the woman's wishes regarding the prep and enema procedures and function as a client advocate in conveying that information to the health care provider. After the woman is admitted and settled into the labor room the nurse's primary responsibilities include assessing the labor progress and monitoring for maternal or fetal complications. It is also the nurse's responsibility to provide comfort measures and assist the family and support person(s) in their efforts.

EVALUATION OF LABOR PROGRESS

The primary means of evaluating the labor progress is to assess the frequency, duration, and intensity of labor contractions. Evaluating contractions serves other purposes as well. Contraction evaluation helps detect abnormalities such as a lack of uterine relaxation, which may lead to maternal and fetal complications; detect fetal distress by simultaneous observation of contraction and fetal heart rate patterns when internal or external electronic monitors are used; reassure the patient and her family by the nurse's presence and interest; and provide an opportunity to support her labor efforts with comfort measures, teaching, encouragement, and assisting the coach to meet her labor needs.

The nurse evaluates uterine contractions by palpating with her hands and also with the aid of external or internal electronic monitors. The woman should be informed about the purpose and technique of each method.

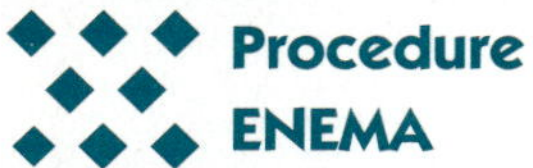

Procedure ENEMA

EQUIPMENT/SUPPLIES
- Small, prepackaged enema
- Waterproof pad
- Clean, sized gloves

STEPS
1 Explain the procedure to the patient.
2 Place the waterproof pad under her hips.
3 Position her on her left side.
4 Follow package directions for administering the enema.
5 Assist the woman to the bathroom to expel the enema.
6 Show her how to operate the emergency bathroom call light.
7 Assist the woman back into bed.
8 Assess the FHR and uterine contraction pattern.

Palpation of contractions

When palpating the uterus for contractions the nurse's hands should be clean and warm. In a full-term pregnancy the strongest muscular contraction can be felt at the fundus. The nurse's hand should rest in this area to best evaluate the frequency, duration, and intensity of the uterine contractions. As the uterus contracts and the uterine muscle fibers shorten the nurse may see or feel the fundus rise in the abdominal cavity and become quite firm at the peak of the contraction. The degree of firmness or hardness at the peak is called the *intensity* of a contraction. Contraction intensity is usually described as mild, moderate, or strong, depending on the indentability of the uterus at peak intensity. The nurse will not be able to indent the uterine fundus with her fingertips if the contraction is strong.

The *duration* of the contraction is the period from the beginning to the end of the contraction, when the uterus is discernibly firm or tight. The interval or *frequency* of contractions is from the beginning of one contraction to the beginning of the following contraction. The time between contractions is called the *relaxation time,* a period equally as important as the frequency or duration. During the relaxation period the nurse should assess the *resting tone* of the uterus by depressing the uterine wall with her fingertips. The wall should be easy to indent at this time. If the relaxation time is very short or nonexistent the fetus may suffer from a lack of oxygen, since the placenta is not adequately perfused with blood. A continuously contracted, hard uterus may be a symptom of abruptio placentae, a condition in which the placenta separates prematurely from the uterine wall (see Chapter 14). The contraction and relaxation periods and the interval between them are diagrammed in Fig. 11-3. Contractions may be more difficult to palpate if the woman is obese.

Electronic monitoring of contractions

Both external and internal monitors are available for the continuous monitoring of uterine contractions. When the external (indirect) method is used, a tocodynamometer ("toco") is attached to a belt, which holds it in place over the uterine fundus. The toco is a disk that is sensitive to uterine tightening and transmits this information to a monitor, which records the contraction wave on graph paper. When the indirect method of monitoring uterine frequency and duration is used, neither the intensity of the contraction nor the resting tone between contractions is measured. The advantage of this method is that it can be used before the rupture of membranes. The disadvantages are that the belt may be uncomfortable and it does not assess the contraction intensity or uterine resting tone.

The internal (direct) method of monitoring uses a small polyethylene catheter inserted directly into the uterine cavity (some require filling with sterile water and others do not). The increased pressure of the uterine contraction is translated to the monitor, which records the contraction wave on graph paper. The advantage of internal monitoring is that it measures the contraction intensity and uterine resting tone (in mm of mercury). It also measures the frequency and duration of the contractions. The disadvantage of internal monitoring is that membranes must be ruptured before the internal catheter is inserted. Internal monitoring is preferred for women who are at risk for hyperstimulation of the uterus because of oxytoxic (Pitocin) induction or augmentation of labor. It may also be indicated if the labor is prolonged and more accurate information is needed as to the quality of the contractions.

Electronic monitoring must not be used in place of nursing assessment. No machine works perfectly at all times. The nurse must also periodically palpate the uterus and compare the findings with those recorded on the monitor strip.

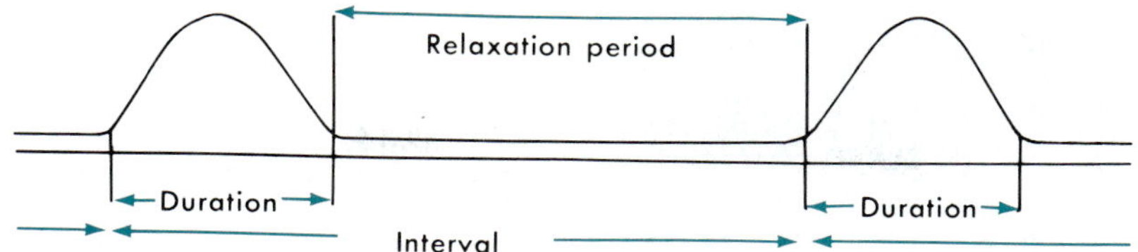

Fig. 11-3 Diagram of uterine contraction and relaxation.

◆ **TABLE 11-1**
Typical Uterine Contraction and Dilation Relationships and Danger Signals

Cervical Dilation (cm)	Contraction Duration (sec)	Contraction Interval (min)
Fingertip to 2	20 to 30	6 to 8
2 to 4	30 to 35	5 to 6
4 to 6	40 to 50	4 to 5
6 to 8	45 to 60	3 to 4
8 to 10 (Most difficult period, including fatigue, nausea, vomiting, irregular or intensive contractions, and "transition")	50 to 90	2 to 3 (Tends to be irregular)

Danger signals to report:

Contraction duration more than 2 minutes or intensity greater than 90 mm Hg, measured by internal monitor.
Relaxation period less than 30 seconds.
Poor relaxation quality (intrauterine resting tone greater than 20 mm Hg).

Whether contractions are assessed by palpation or electronically monitored, a relationship between the duration and frequency of uterine contractions and the dilation of the cervix typically exists. It follows the approximate pattern shown in Table 11-1. Documentation of uterine contractions should include the frequency or interval, duration, and intensity and the mother's reaction to them. For example, "Mild contractions q 5-6 minutes lasting 35 seconds. Patient relaxing well between contractions and using slow-breathing techniques effectively."

Other signs of labor progress

The amount of bloody show and the laboring woman's perception and expression of increasing discomfort and pain will also assist the experienced nurse in evaluating labor progress. Since the risk of infection is increased with vaginal examinations, they are not routinely done to determine cervical dilation, effacement, and fetal descent. They are indicated, however, when the nurse or health care provider anticipates that significant progress has been made or to confirm a suspected lack of progress and need for medical intervention. The nurse can also evaluate labor progress by plotting cervical dilation on the Friedman curve (see Chapter 10 for a review of this process).

EVALUATION OF FETAL WELL-BEING

The primary method of evaluating the fetus during labor is the assessment of the fetal heart rate (FHR). The FHR may be assessed using varied equipment, ranging from fairly simple hand-held fetoscopes to electronic devices capable of continuous visual and printed records. Research indicates that intermittent FHR monitoring is comparable to continuous monitoring in detecting problems, provided that the nurse is adequately educated in the use of the technique and an appropriate nurse-to-patient ratio exists (1:1 ratio for at-risk, laboring women) (American Academy of Pediatrics and American College of Obstetricians and Gynecologists, 1992). Recommendations for the frequency of intermittent auscultation of the FHR and the proper documentation of findings are indicated in Table 11-2.

◆ TABLE 11-2
Frequency of Intermittent FHR Assessment and Documentation

Low-Risk Clients	High-Risk Clients
First stage of labor: Latent phase: every hour Active phase: every 30 minutes	**First stage of labor:** Latent phase: every 30 minutes Active phase: every 15 minutes
Second stage of labor: every 15 minutes	**Second stage of labor:** every 5 minutes

Labor Events

Assess FHR *before*:
- initiation of labor-enhancing procedures (e.g., artificial rupture of membranes)
- periods of ambulation
- administration of medications
- administration or initiation of analgesia or anesthesia

Assess FHR *after*:
- rupture of membranes
- recognition of abnormal, uterine-activity patterns
- evaluation of oxytocin (maintenance, increase, or decrease of dosage)
- administration of medications (at time of peak action)
- expulsion of enema
- urinary catheterization
- vaginal examination
- periods of ambulation
- evaluation of analgesia or anesthesia (maintenance, increase, or decrease of dosage)

From NAACOG: *Fetal Heart Rate Auscultation, OGN nursing practice resource*, Washington, DC, March 1990, The Association. Reprinted with permission of AWHONN.

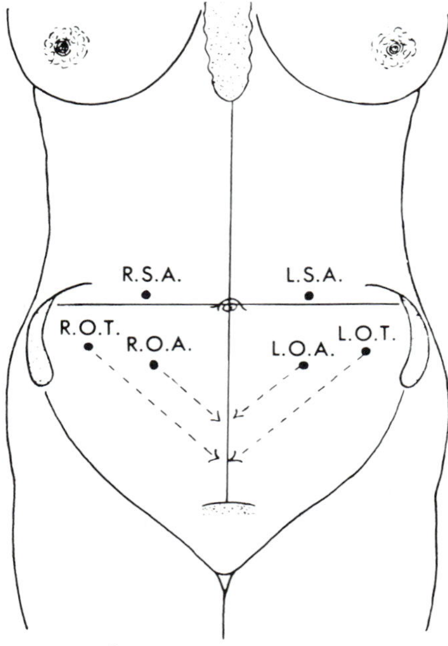

Fig. 11-4 Fetal heart tone locations on abdominal wall, indicating corresponding fetal positions and effects of internal rotation of the fetus.

FHR location on the abdominal wall

The abdominal area, where the FHR may be heard best, is over the fetal back and is related to the following (Fig. 11-4):

a. **Presentation.** In headfirst (cephalic) presentations the FHR is found in the mother's lower-abdominal quadrants, below the umbilicus. In breech presentations the FHR is usually found at the level of the mother's umbilicus or above.
b. **Position.** If the back of the infant is toward the mother's left side (LOA or LOP position), the FHR will probably be heard best on the mother's left. If the infant's back points to the mother's right side, the FHR will most frequently be heard best on her right. Just because an FHR can be heard in more than one place does not necessarily mean that more than one baby is involved. The nurse, however, may want to check the possibility of a multiple birth by having another nurse listen simultaneously, using a finger-wagging technique to be sure that the pattern heard in both areas is the same. Suspicious findings can be confirmed with a sonogram.
c. **Station.** As internal rotation and descent occur, the location of the FHR changes, swinging gradually from the right or left quadrants to the midline and dropping until immediately before birth. The FHR is then found just above the pubic bone.

The following section discusses the use of hand-held fetoscopes, as well as basic principles of simultaneous, electronic fetal heart and contraction monitoring.

Intermittent auscultation of FHR

The following hand-held fetoscopes may be used to intermittently auscultate (listen to) the FHR:

1 Leffscope—a stethoscope with a large, heavily weighted bell (Fig. 11-5, *A*)

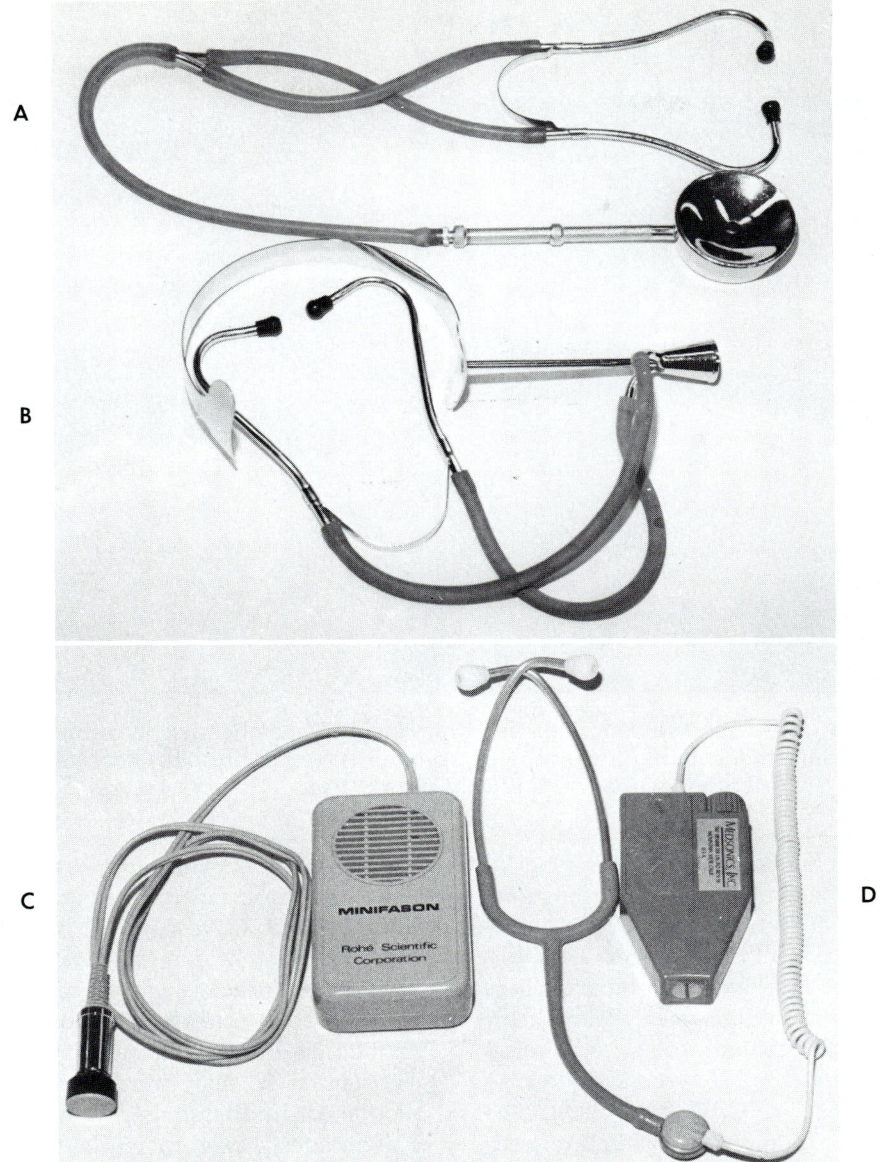

Fig. 11-5 **A,** Leffscope; **B,** DeLee-Hollis head scope; **C,** electronic ultrasound fetoscope amplifies FHR so that it is heard by all in area; **D,** electronic ultrasound fetoscope transmits FHR by means of ear pieces. (Courtesy Grossmont Hospital, La Mesa, CA.)

2 DeLee-Hollis head scope (Figs. 11-5, *B* and 11-6)—uses bone conduction to amplify the FHR sounds
3 Various ultrasonic fetoscopes, which amplify the FHR (Fig. 11-5, *C* and *D*)—the end is lubricated with a water-soluble gel to improve the signal

NOTE: The fetoscopes described and pictured in Fig. 11-5, *A* and *B* and 11-6 are not used often in present health care settings but are included since the nurse may occasionally encounter them.

The nurse should explain to the family that the purpose of listening to the FHR is to check the fetus' general condition and tolerance of labor contractions. The nurse should listen to the FHR immediately after a contraction and occasionally listen during, as well as immediately after the contraction to detect decelerations. The pressure exerted on the abdominal wall during a contraction by the Leffscope or the DeLee-Hollis fetoscope, however, may be uncomfortable and not easily tolerated by many laboring women. The electronic, hand-held fetoscope (Fig. 11-5, *C* and *D*) is better tolerated because it requires less pressure to detect the FHR during a contraction (NAACOG, 1990).

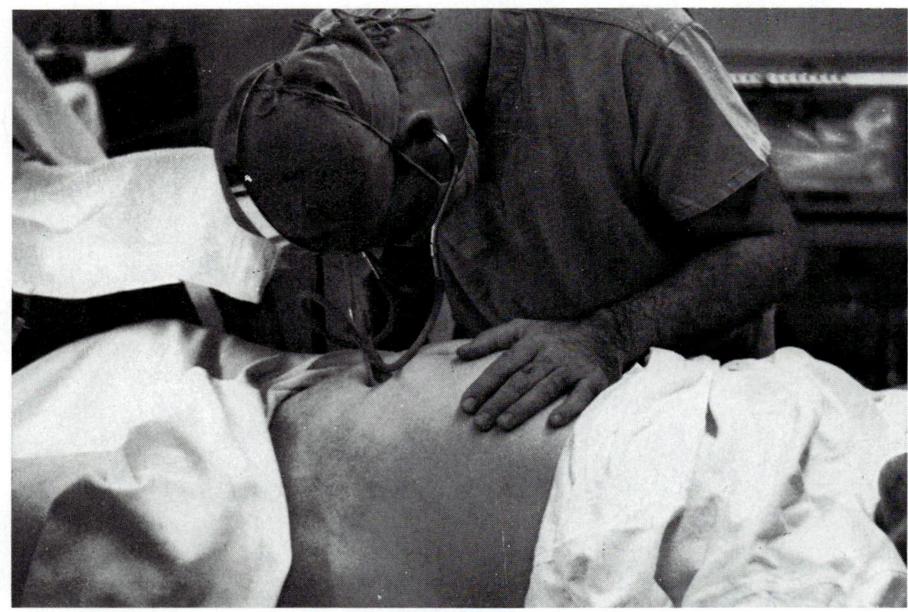

Fig. 11-6 Physician listens to fetal heart rate (using DeLee head scope) shortly before birth. Note location of the scope on abdominal wall. (Courtesy Grossmont Hospital and Martin M. Greenberg, MD, La Mesa, CA.)

The nurse may also choose to use the ultrasonic or Doppler attachment of the continuous, electronic fetal monitor for intermittent FHR assessment.

Regardless of the instrument used the nurse should listen for 30 to 60 seconds between contractions and multiply as necessary to obtain the baseline heart rate for 1 minute. The FHR should also be counted during a contraction and for 30 seconds after to determine fetal response (NAACOG, 1990). The FHR sounds are much softer when using the Leff-scope or the DeLee-Hollis fetoscope, and require considerable concentration to hear them until one is accustomed to using these instruments. Friction noises distort the sound and can be avoided by keeping fingers off of the bell and pressing firmly on the abdominal wall.

Other sounds heard in the mother's abdomen may be mistaken for the FHR. The pulsation of the uterine arteries produces a "sh" sound, with the same rhythm as the maternal pulse. A rapid, maternal heart rate may be mistaken for the FHR. The nurse should place a finger on the mother's radial pulse to differentiate it from the FHR.

Continuous electronic monitoring of FHR

Like electronic monitoring of contractions, electronic monitoring of the FHR may be external (indirect) or internal (direct). The most common external method uses an ultrasound transducer (Doppler), which produces sound waves and is placed on the woman's abdomen and held in place with a belt (Fig. 11-7). A water-soluble gel is placed on the underside of the transducer to improve the conduction of fetal heart sounds. The sound waves bounce off of the fetal heart. The signal is then translated by the monitor and displayed simultaneously on a screen and graph paper. Advantages of external FHR monitoring are that it may be used before the membranes rupture and, therefore, is less invasive. External FHR monitoring also provides a continuous record of fetal condition. The disadvantages are similar to those for external monitoring of uterine contractions. If the fetus is very active, the woman is obese, or more amniotic fluid than normal is present, the tracing may be of poor quality. The Doppler may frequently have to be readjusted as the woman changes position, the labor progresses, and the fetus descends.

Internal fetal electrocardiography requires the rupture of maternal membranes, 1 to 2 cm of cervical dilation, and a presenting part no higher than –2 station. A physician or specially trained nurse attaches the spiral electrode to the presenting part (scalp or buttock), penetrating the infant's epidermis by a tiny metal spiral or clip, during a vaginal examination (Fig. 11-8). Infection and soft tissue injury are possibilities

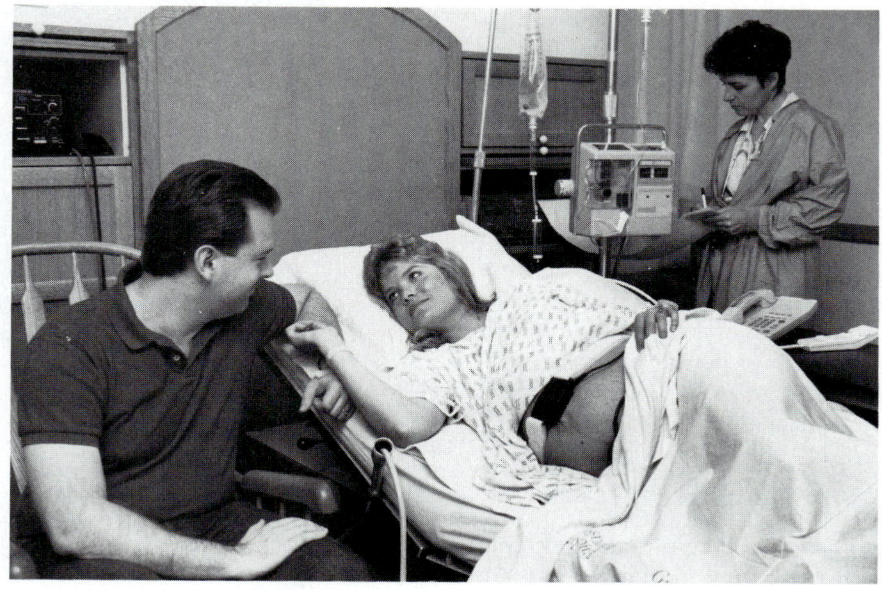

Fig. 11-7 The beginning of a labor induction with oxytocin (Pitocin). Double IV set up in place. External contraction monitor (toco) positioned over fundus. External fetal heart rate monitor (doppler) in place but not completely visible under sheet. (Courtesy Grossmont Hospital, La Mesa, CA.)

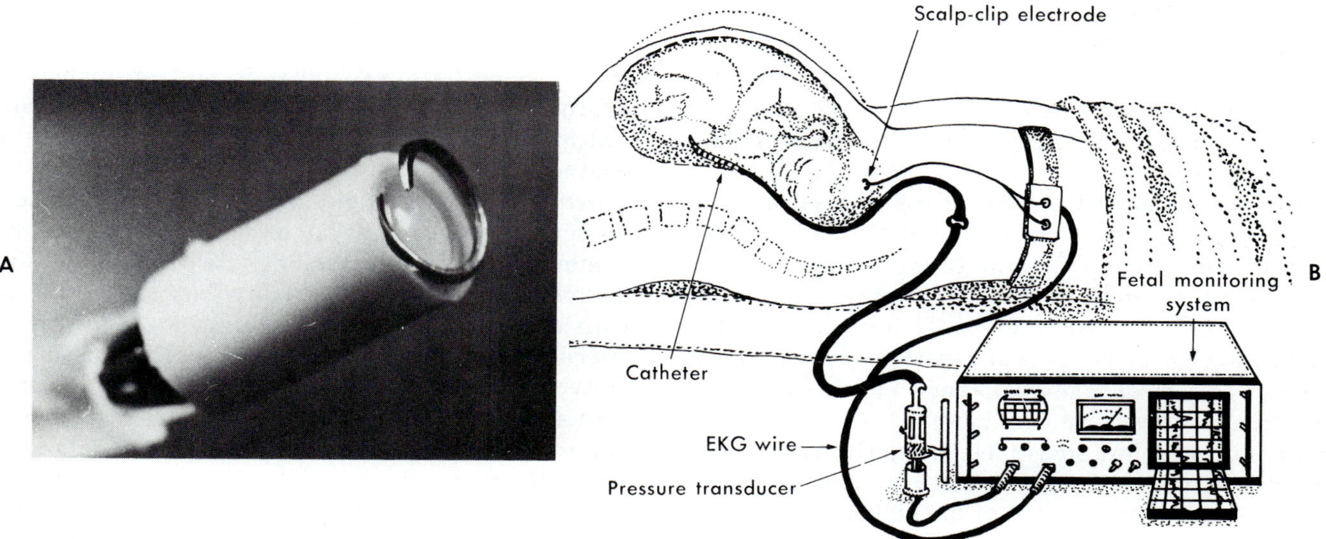

Fig. 11-8 **A,** Spiral electrode used to attach FHR monitor to fetal presenting part; **B,** diagram of internal fetal heart and contraction monitoring. Internal monitoring indicates fetal ECG and intensity, as well as frequency of uterine contractions. (**A,** Courtesy Corometrics Medical Systems, Inc, Wallingford, CT.)

but have not been significant problems. This method provides continuous recording of the FHR and a clearer recording than that of an external Doppler.

Telemetry is a portable method of electronic FHR and uterine contraction monitoring that allows the woman to be ambulatory, yet provides continuous monitoring. With this system the FHR can be monitored directly or indirectly, and the contractions can be monitored indirectly.

During labor, both the FHR and uterine contraction patterns should be evaluated. As indicated earlier the FHR is an indicator of the fetus' general condition and also reflects how well the fetus is tolerating the stress of labor contractions. With electronic monitoring, uterine contraction patterns interpreted by either an external toco transducer or an internal pressure catheter can be recorded concurrently with the FHR, making this evaluation easier (Fig. 11-9).

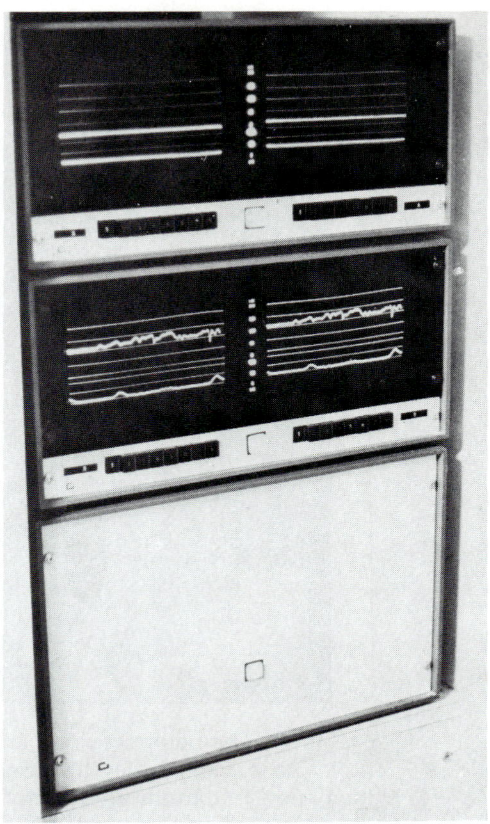

Fig. 11-9 A central monitor at the nurses' station, capable of displaying FHR and contraction patterns of four different labor patients. Two different patients' patterns are shown here. (Courtesy Corometrics Medical Systems, Inc., Wallingford, CT.)

Electronic monitor strip FHR patterns

The FHR is evaluated by assessing both the baseline rate and the changes that occur periodically, usually in response to uterine contractions or fetal activity. The following section gives basic definitions related to this procedure and explains concepts that facilitate interpretation of electronic fetal monitor strip patterns.*

Baseline FHR. The baseline FHR is the FHR range determined either before labor begins or between uterine contractions, over a 10-minute period of monitoring. The baseline rate does not include the FHR during decelerations or accelerations (periodical changes). The normal baseline rate is usually 120 to 160 beats per minute. The following baseline changes that persist for 10 minutes or more may indicate fetal distress and should be evaluated by the health care provider: tachycardia is a baseline rate of 160 bpm or greater, and bradycardia is a baseline rate less than 120 bpm.

Baseline variability. FHR variability is one of the most important parameters of fetal well-being. A certain amount of irregularity in the baseline FHR is considered an indication of a healthy, autonomic nervous system. Long-term variability refers to the fluctuations of the FHR that occur from 2 to 6 times per minute and have a normal range of 6 to 10 beats per minute. Long-term variability of less than 5 beats per minute may be a sign of fetal jeopardy, particularly when lack of variability is found in conjunction with periods of late deceleration of the FHR.

Short-term variability refers to the rate differences from beat-to-beat and usually vary by 2 to 3 beats per minute. This variability is classified as either present or absent. Short-term variability is best evaluated by internal fetal scalp electrode. Loss of short-term variability is particularly ominous when accompanied by fetal tachycardia.

Reduced long-term and short-term variability may be signs of fetal distress but are also produced by the administration of certain analgesic or sedative drugs to the mother. Long-term variability (but not short-term variability) may be decreased during 20- to 30-minute intervals of "fetal sleep" or inactivity (Fig. 11-10 and 11-11).

Fetal heart rate accelerations. An FHR acceleration is an increase of 15 beats per minute that lasts at least 15 seconds. Periodical accelerations are usually considered benign and indicative of fetal well-being. Accelerations typically occur in response to fetal movement, uterine contractions, or maternal abdominal contractions. Recall that this type of acceleration is the basis of the nonstress test (see Chapter 8, Fig. 8-6).

* For a more detailed discussion of the evaluation of FHR patterns, students should be referred to Tucker SM: *Pocket guide to fetal monitoring*, St. Louis, 1992, Mosby.

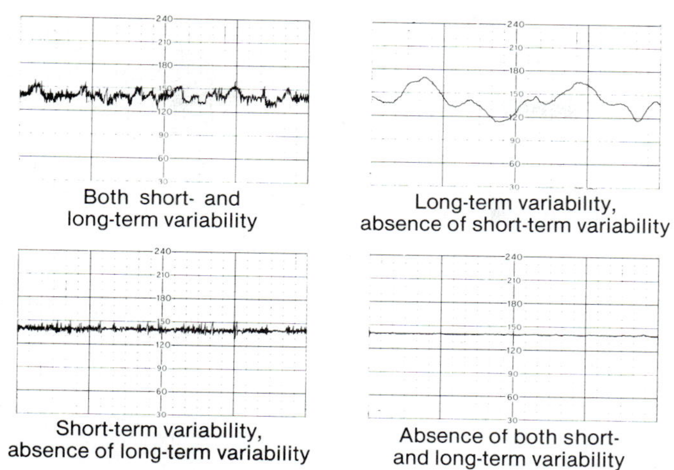

Fig. 11-10 Variations in short– and long–term FHR variability. (From Tucker SM: *Pocket guide to fetal monitoring,* ed 2, St. Louis, 1992, Mosby.)

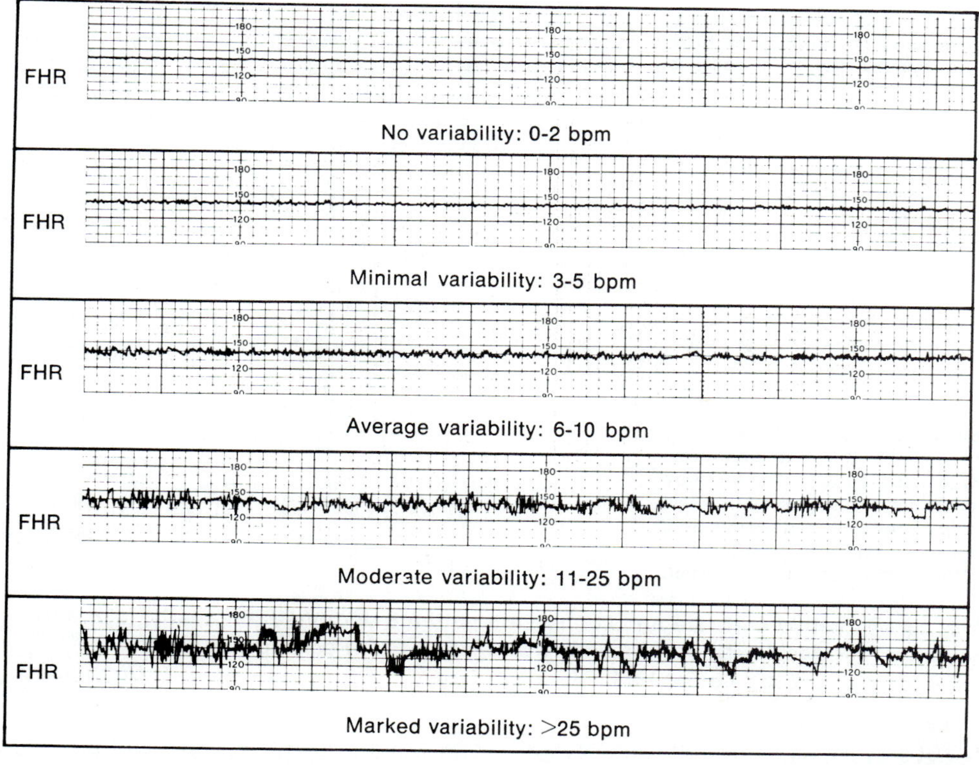

Fig. 11-11 Degrees of FHR variability. Short– and long–term variability tend to increase and decrease together. (From Tucker SM: *Pocket guide to fetal monitoring,* ed 2, St. Louis, 1992, Mosby.)

CLASSIC FETAL HEART RATE AND CONTRACTION PATTERNS

Early decelerations (benign)
"Mirror" coincidental contractions; lowest point in FHR corresponds to peak of contraction curve. More common between 4 and 7 cm dilation and second-stage labor.

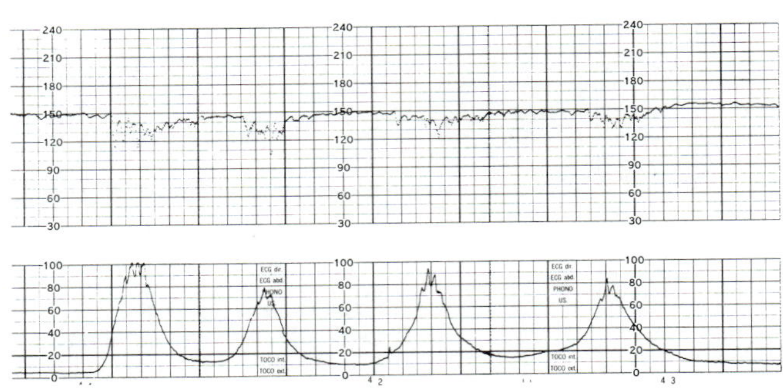

Late decelerations (ominous)
Mimic somewhat shape of associated contractions, but onset and lowest point in FHR occur after peak of contractions. Return to FHR baseline often exceeds 20 seconds after end of contractions. Tachycardia, bradycardia and/or depressed baseline variability poor signs.

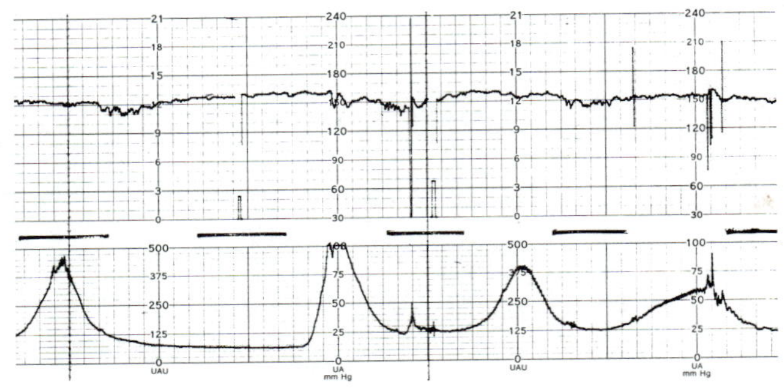

Variable decelerations (varying significance)
Usually V- or U-shaped with abrupt fall and recovery of FHR. Severe if below 70 bpm, last for more than 30 seconds or if recovery sloped or slow. No consistent relationship to contraction pattern noted. Tachycardia, bradycardia, depressed baseline variability poor signs. More common in advanced labor.

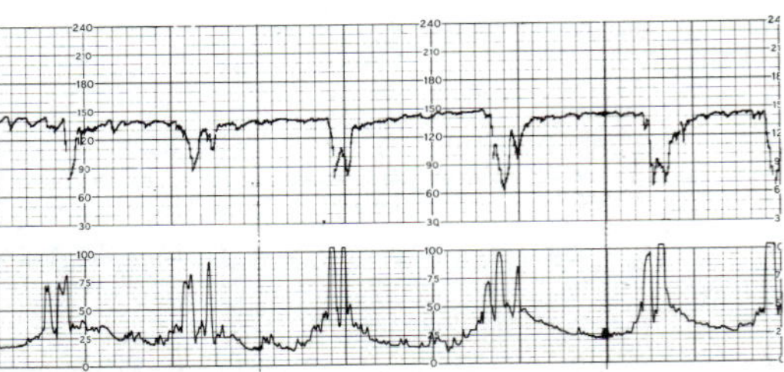

Fig. 11-12 Fetal heart rate and contraction patterns demonstrating early, late, and variable FHR decelerations. (Tracings from Tucker SM: *Pocket guide to fetal monitoring,* ed 2, St. Louis, 1992, Mosby.) *Continued.*

Fetal-heart-rate decelerations. Periodical FHR decelerations are categorized as early, late, and variable, according to their relationships to uterine contractions and their shapes. These decelerations may be detected through continuous monitoring devices. (See Fig. 11-12 for tracings, explanations, and nursing interventions.)

Early decelerations start at the onset of a contraction and end when the contraction ends. They have a uniform, smooth shape and are usually within the normal FHR range of 120 to 160 beats per minute. This

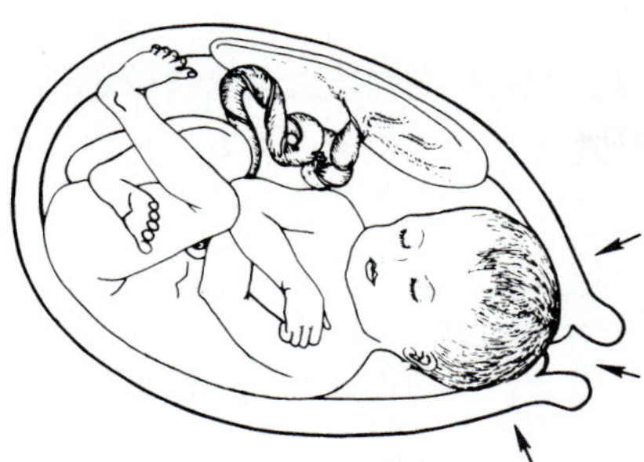
Head compression

Intervention

No intervention indicated

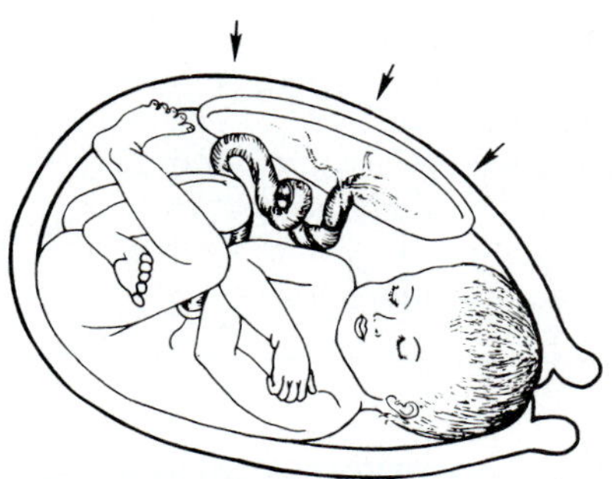
Uteroplacental insufficiency

Notify health-care provider
Turn patient to either side (left preferred)
Oxygen 8 to10 liters/min
Stop oxytocin infusion
Elevate legs (if hypotensive), increase IV rate
Possible fetal blood PH
Possible vaginal examination for scalp stimulation to increase FHR

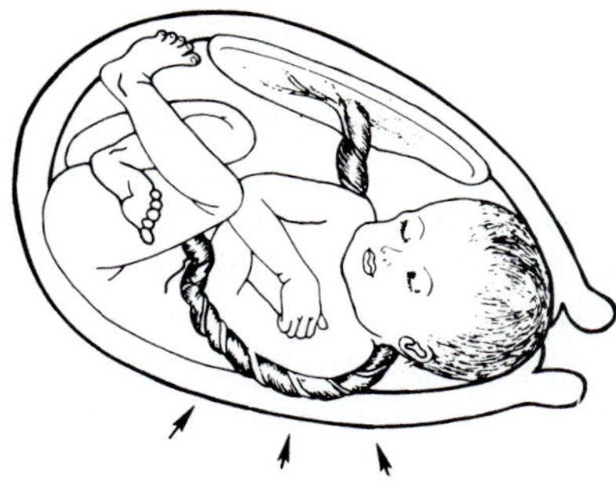
Umbilical cord compression

Notify health-care provider
Reposition patient
Possible vaginal examination to check for and protect prolapsed cord.
Possible fetal blood pH, scalp stimulation
Oxygen 8 to 10 liters/min
If moderate, possible amnioinfusion

Fig. 11-12—cont'd.

pattern is due to fetal head compression as the fetus travels down the birth canal. This deceleration is generally benign, resulting from increased intracranial pressure. This deceleration is seen most frequently at the end of labor, when the fetal head is at the perineum. It does not call for an intervention on the part of the obstetrical team. The nurse, however, must carefully observe to differentiate it from a late deceleration (Fig. 11-12).

Late decelerations are characterized by a slowing of the fetal heart after the peak, or acme, of the uterine contraction and by a delayed return to baseline after the contraction ends. Like early decelerations, late decelerations have a smooth, uniform shape and are within the normal FHR range of 120 to 160 beats per minute. As fetal distress increases the range and frequency of the FHR deceleration increase. This pattern is due to uteroplacental insufficiency and is always considered an ominous sign. These decelerations are frequently associated with uterine hyperactivity caused by oxytocin administration, maternal hypotension, or other high-risk conditions that affect placental function. Nursing interventions to decrease or eliminate fetal distress are indicated in Fig. 11-12. The nurse should promptly notify the health care provider when these decelerations are noted.

Variable decelerations are characterized by a periodical, unpredictable slowing of the FHR that shows neither a consistent, sequential relationship to the uterine contractions, nor a regular, repetitive range or duration. The shape of this deceleration typically traces a steep-sided "V" or "U." This type of pattern is the result of umbilical cord compression. These decelerations usually fall below the normal range of 120 beats per minute and may be mild, moderate, or severe. Repetitive, variable decelerations that worsen as labor progresses are cause for concern. Nursing interventions are indicated in Fig. 11-12. The nurse should notify the health care provider if these decelerations are moderate or are not lessened by these interventions. In cases of severe variable decelerations, an amnioinfusion may alleviate the pattern. In this procedure, sterile, normal saline is infused into the uterine cavity via an intrauterine-pressure catheter in an effort to protect the umbilical cord from compression (Haubrich, 1990). See the nursing alert below.

Documentation on monitor strip

If continuous, electronic monitoring is used the monitor strip must be evaluated frequently and initialed by the nurse evaluating the strip. The frequency of this evaluation, like that for FHR auscultation, varies according to anticipated risk. The American Academy of Pediatrics and the American College of Obstetricians and Gynecologists (1992) recommend that the strip be evaluated using the same schedule as that for auscultation (see Table 11-2). The monitor strip is a legal part of the birth record and a convenient flow sheet for recording labor events (Chez and Verklan, 1987). See the box above right for information that the nurse should document on the monitor strip. See the nursing alert at right.

Other signs of fetal distress

As indicated earlier, fetal distress may also manifest itself by the passage of meconium-stained amniotic fluid. This sign, however, is not consistently reliable. Sudden, exaggerated fetal movement has also been

> **Nursing Alert**
>
> Amnioinfusion is contraindicated in cases of severe fetal distress.

> **MONITORING STRIP DOCUMENTATION**
>
> **THE FOLLOWING SHOULD BE DOCUMENTED ON THE MONITOR STRIP:**
>
> 1. Maternal position change
> 2. Maternal vital signs
> 3. Spontaneous or artificial rupture of membranes and characteristics of the amniotic fluid
> 4. Vaginal examinations (dilation, effacement, station, and position)
> 5. Adjustments of the toco transducer and/or Doppler device
> 6. Switch to internal monitoring (application of internal-spiral electrode and/or internal-pressure uterine catheter)
> 7. Medications, oxygen, IV fluids, analgesia, and anesthesia
> 8. Maternal events (e.g., vomiting, pushing)
> 9. Voiding or catheterization
> 10. Time of birth, type of birth (e.g., vaginal, cesarean), Apgar scores

> **Nursing Alert**
>
> When ominous FHR patterns (e.g., late decelerations, lack of variability) exist the nurse must document the interventions and subsequent return to normal.

considered a sign of fetal difficulty. In the presence of the FHR and contraction patterns that denote fetal distress, fetal-scalp stimulation is replacing fetal-scalp vein sampling as a faster, simpler way to confirm (or disconfirm) fetal jeopardy. The examiner, using a gloved hand, locates the fetal scalp and applies firm pressure to the head. FHR accelerations in response to scalp stimulation are reassuring. The absence of accelerations in response to this stimulation indicates a compromised fetus (Harvey, 1987). Fetal scalp sampling is a more complicated procedure, requiring that the examiner obtain a blood sample from a scalp vein. The presence of an acid-base imbalance, evident by pH values below 7.20, in two or more samples usually indicates fetal acidosis requiring prompt delivery by low forceps or cesarean section.

EVALUATION OF MATERNAL WELL-BEING

After admission is completed, unless birth is imminent, a prolonged period of waiting and observation

◆ TABLE 11-3
Assessments of Maternal Physical Well-Being During the First and Second Stages of Labor

First stage:	
Latent Phase	Temperature taken every 4 hours. If elevated or membranes are ruptured, assess temperature every hour. Blood pressure, pulse, and respirations every hour if in normal range. Assess mucous membranes (should be moist) every hour. Monitor bladder for distention every hour. Evaluate uterine contractions every 30 minutes.
Active Phase	Temperature taken every 4 hours. If elevated or membranes are ruptured, assess every hour. Blood pressure, pulse, and respirations every hour if in normal range. Assess mucous membranes for moisture every 30 minutes. Monitor bladder for distention every hour. Evaluate uterine contractions every 30 minutes.
Transition	Blood pressure, pulse, and respirations every hour if in normal range. Assess mucous membranes for moisture every 30 minutes. Monitor bladder for distention every hour. Evaluate uterine contractions every 15 to 30 minutes.
Second stage:	Blood pressure, pulse, and respirations every 15 minutes. Monitor bladder for distention every 30 minutes to 1 hour. Evaluate uterine contractions continuously.

ensues, during which the physical and emotional support of the woman and preparation for the birth are paramount. During this time the nurse must monitor the physical well-being of the mother, as well as the fetus. Table 11-3 outlines maternal, physical assessments during the first and second stages of labor.

Elevated maternal temperature may be indicative of dehydration or infection. Hypertension may be related to increasing pain or, more likely, the onset of pregnancy-induced hypertension. Hypotension may be the result of maternal supine position or regional anesthesia. Dry mucous membranes indicate normal dryness from mouth-breathing techniques or may be a sign of dehydration. Bladder distension is common secondary to pain or regional anesthesia. Each of these conditions suggests the need for nursing interventions and should be reported to the health care provider.

NURSING CARE

Psychoprophylactical Techniques

The presence of the woman's mother, husband, or chosen companion at the bedside can be a source of support. Often the husband or companion may have attended classes in preparation to be the woman's labor coach and, as such, is extremely important in sustaining the morale and comfort of the parturient. If visitors are not supportive or if they appear to antagonize or upset the patient the nurse should privately confirm this observation with the patient. The nurse should then be creative in arranging for the visitor(s) to have a "rest." Several techniques make use of breathing patterns and relaxation as a method to help women cope with the discomfort of labor. Couples who have practiced these techniques in preparation for labor usually need only occasional reminders and positive reinforcement for their efforts. Those who have no preparation benefit from the nurse's instruction and coaching.

Currently, the emphasis is on doing what feels natural versus using rigidly programmed breathing patterns. No one technique is superior to another. Use of any technique is better than not using a technique. During the first-stage of labor, use of a psychoprophylactical technique (see Chapter 9) promotes relaxation of abdominal and perineal muscles. During the second stage of labor, breathing patterns may be used to increase the effectiveness of pushing efforts. A summary of some techniques is presented in Table 11-4. The following text is an explanation of the terms included:

cleansing breath Deep breaths taken in through the nose and out through the mouth; used at the beginning and end of contractions to ready the body for special breathing, to help with relaxation, and to restore normal breathing and gas exchange.

◆ **TABLE 11-4**
Summary of Suggested Breathing and Relaxation Techniques

Labor Phase	Breathing-Relaxation Techniques, Instructions to Patient	Suggestions and Diagrams
Stage I		
Early 0 to 4 cm	Practice distraction When contractions cannot be ignored, use deep chest or abdominal breathing 1. Cleansing breath 2. Focal point 3. 6 to 9 slow breaths/min (in nose, out pursed lips) 4. Possible effleurage 5. Cleansing breath Pelvic rocking, sacral support Relaxation checks	If possible (membranes intact), stay up—walk, play games, plan a vacation, make out the grocery list, etc. 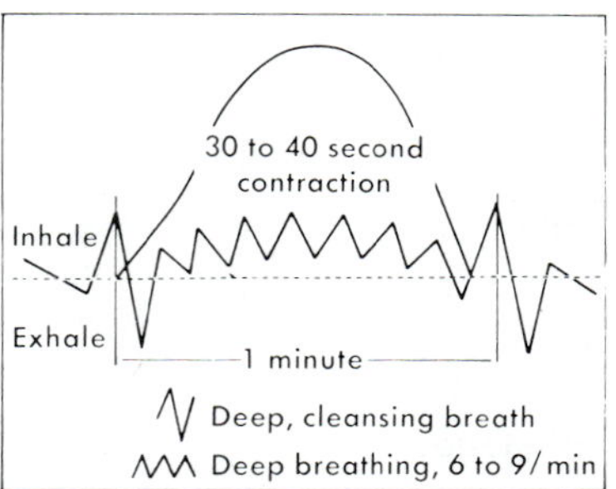
Midlabor 4 to 8 cm	Begin when needed: Accelerated-decelerated shallow panting 1. Cleansing breath 2. Focal point 3. Rhythmic slow acceleration-deceleration with contraction 4. Effleurage 5. Cleansing breath Sacral support Relaxation checks Increasing coach support	Mouth care Cool cloth 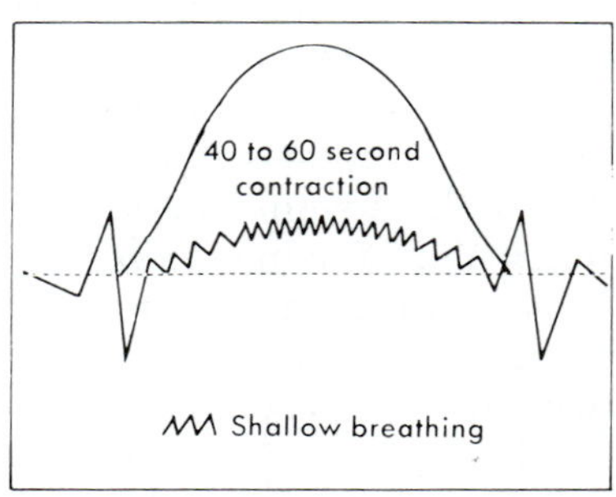
Transition 8 to 10 cm	Begin when needed: Pant-blow breathing 1. Cleansing breath 2. Focal point 3. 4 to 6 shallow breaths, then short blow during length of contraction 4. Cleansing breath Intensified coach support	Mouth care Cool cloth 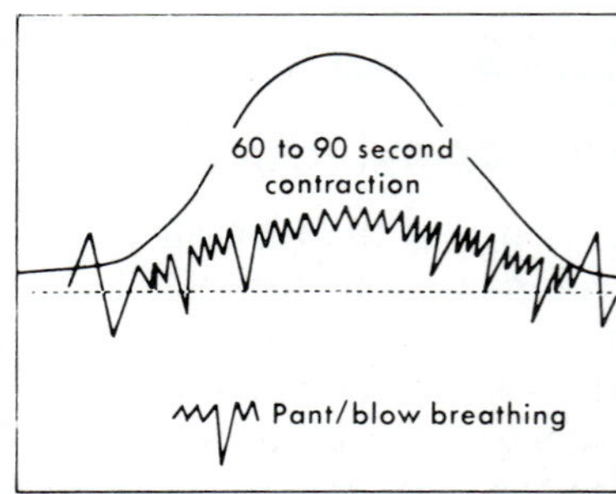

Continued.

◆ **TABLE 11-4**
Summary of Suggested Breathing and Relaxation Techniques—cont'd.

Labor Phase	Breathing-Relaxation Techniques, Instructions to Patient	Suggestions and Diagrams

Stage II

From complete dilation to birth of baby

Breathing techniques that enhance bearing down efforts

Natural

Begin when urge to bear down is present
Use any position preferred
1. Push only when urge to push is felt
2. Push only during expiration with glottis open
3. Push no longer than 5 to 6 seconds
4. Do a series of short pushes with each contraction

Recommended to avoid fetal hypoxia and maternal fatigue
Indicated when fetus is at risk (compromised)

Vigorous

Begin when completely dilated
1. Cleansing breath
2. Elevate head and back; second deep breath
3. Hold no longer than 5 to 10 seconds, trapping air in chest; bend and drop knees to side; pull on thighs, knees, or bed rails while pushing down; keep hips motionless on bed
4. Take another breath
5. Repeat 3 and 4 until contraction is over
6. Cleansing breath

Rest; doze between contractions
Recommended to shorten second stage when necessary and when regional block is used

focal point Point or object somewhere in the room used as center of visual concentration; may be the coach's face, a picture, furniture, etc; serves to maintain cerebral input; concentration is usually enhanced if the woman does not close her eyes during contractions.

effleurage Light, patterned abdominal massage; usually done with the tips of fingers.

sacral support Counterpressure exerted to lift the sacrum slightly off of the bed if the patient is supine, or firm lower back pressure; may use objects such as hands, towels, or rolling pins to relieve lower back discomfort.

pelvic rock An exercise in which the woman alternately increases and then flattens the lumbar sacral curve of the back to relieve lower back discomfort.

Occasionally, symptoms of hyperventilation may be associated with some of the rapid-breathing techniques. The woman may complain of tingling hands and feet, which cause annoyance or loss of concentration and may, in fact, decrease fetal oxygenation. Slowing respirations and temporarily breathing into cupped hands or a paper bag helps relieve these problems. Symptoms related to hyperventilation are not frequent because rapid-breathing patterns have been modified to include slower acceleration and deceleration periods and shallower respirations.

Regardless of the method of childbirth education the coach and the labor staff should work as a team for the realization of a constructive, dignified, and satisfying parturition. The attending nurses should be knowledgeable about the aims of the techniques employed. The methods used may differ, but it is helpful if nurses acquaint themselves with the different types of programs available in their communities and the ways in which expectant parents are taught.

Women trained for labor need support and encouragement from nurses who will enhance their efforts, help evaluate and aid relaxation, render sacral pressure as directed, share information regarding progress in labor, and be sincerely supportive of the idealism and efforts manifested by laboring women and their partners. In addition, the nurse should render the careful physical assessment and comfort care that all laboring women require.

Nursing interventions that provide emotional and physical support for the laboring woman are organized according to the various phases and stages of labor. Table 11-5 shows the relationships between stages of labor, patient behavior and coping techniques, and suggested nursing interventions.

◆ TABLE 11-5
The Typical Woman in Normal Labor

Stages of Labor	Physical and Psychological Characteristics, Contraction Patterns	Suggested Activity, Including Relaxation and Breathing Techniques	Recommended Nursing Care, Common Physician Orders
Stage I cervical effacement and dilation to 10 cm			
Time range Primipara—10 to 12 hours Multipara—6 to 8 hours Early labor 0 to 4 cm	Cervical dilation begins; minimal bloody show; contractions variable, approximately 20 to 35 seconds at 5- to 8-minute intervals; possible backache; intensity of contractions increasingly strong but tolerable Alert, talkative, nervous; may welcome diversion, conversation; coach at bedside	If membranes not ruptured: may prefer to be up and about labor room or unit; when contractions cannot be ignored, slow, deep chest or abdominal breathing, and other relaxation techniques If membranes ruptured: if presenting part not engaged—confined to bed; relaxation techniques as above; if possible, turn to side, elevate head slightly; should not remain flat on back	*Admission procedures:* Welcome, orientation, individual patient assessment Review of prenatal records—TPR, BP, FHR; presentation, cervical dilation, membranes, station, contractions, bloody show Opportunity to void—urine specimen, enema, perineal preparation, electronic monitor application as ordered *Follow-up nursing responsibilities:* TPR at least every 4 hours; BP hourly FHR, contraction pattern, bloody show, amniotic fluid, labor tolerance every 15 to 30 minutes or less; teach breathing, relaxation Check on need to void every 2 hours or less
Midlabor 4 to 8 cm	Contractions approximately 40 to 60 seconds at 3- to 5-minute intervals; intensity increasing but may still be manageable Becoming less outgoing, more introverted, concentrating on breathing patterns Increased reliance on nurse and coach	May be confined to bed; more concentration needed; increased emphasis on breathing and relaxation techniques; accelerated shallow panting, effleurage; continued need for encouragement	*Follow-up nursing responsibilities:* As above, evaluation of efficacy of breathing, relaxation, teach simple techniques prn; encourage and praise husband/coach and patient; assess need for medication IV if ordered

Continued.

First Stage of Labor

Early labor (latent phase)

The woman in early labor (usually defined as up to 4-cm cervical dilation) is characteristically alert, talkative, and nervous. She is generally most eager to cooperate with the health care provider and nurses. Her contractions, although perhaps uncomfortable, are tolerable. If her membranes are not ruptured, her contractions are not very frequent or intense, and bloody show is not remarkable, she will probably be more comfortable being mobile (after baseline FHR determination). She should not automatically be con-

◆ **TABLE 11-5**
The Typical Woman in Normal Labor—cont'd.

Stages of Labor	Physical and Psychological Characteristics, Contraction Patterns	Suggested Activity, Including Relaxation and Breathing Techniques	Recommended Nursing Care, Common Physician Orders
			Other possible nursing responsibilities: Mouth care, cool cloth, back support, massage, encouragement, aid in maintaining concentration; vaginal examinations as indicated; prepare room for delivery; maintain electronic monitoring, if used
Transition 8 to 10 cm	Most difficult period during labor Fatigued, perhaps nauseated; fears loss of control; contractions may be irregular, very forceful, as frequent as every 2 to 3 minutes, lasting 80 seconds or more; bloody show increases; needs much encouragement	Switching to more intensive breathing patterns—high chest, pant-blow transition techniques	*Scheduled nursing responsibilities:* As above plus increased emotional support, observation for onset of stage II, descent of baby, increased bloody show, complaints of rectal pressure, desire to push, bulging perineum and caput Finalize delivery room preparations
Stage II from complete dilation (10 cm) to birth of baby			
Time range Primipara—30 minutes to 2 hours Multipara—20 minutes to 1½ hours	Cervix completely dilated; patient desires to push; perineum bulging, anus dilated, contractions long but less frequent; bloody show at maximum of normal Encouraged by progress made; using all resources for pushing; perhaps dozing between contractions or intensely aware and alert regarding progress of labor	Pushing patterns Rest, doze between contractions—head elevated if supine	Scheduled nursing duties Check perineum frequently during contractions for signs of progress, FHR every 5 to 10 minutes; stay with patient; sterile perineal prep; assist physician/nurse-midwife Possible anesthesia offered; subarachnoid, epidural, pudendal block, local

Continued.

fined to her bed just because she has been admitted to the hospital. A warm shower or jacuzzi bath may increase comfort. When in bed she should lie on her side to enhance maternal and fetal circulation, urinary function, and uterine efficiency. A number of nursing assessments and procedures (manual FHR determination and checking the cervical dilation or perineum) are more easily carried out if the patient intermittently

◆ **TABLE 11-5**
The Typical Woman in Normal Labor—cont'd.

Stages of Labor	Physical and Psychological Characteristics, Contraction Patterns	Suggested Activity, Including Relaxation and Breathing Techniques	Recommended Nursing Care, Common Physician Orders
Stage III from birth of baby to delivery of placenta			
Time range Primipara—5 to 20 minutes Multipara—5 to 20 minutes (time depends on techniques employed)	Excited, extremely anxious and curious about infant; reactions vary according to individual and type of birth preparation and anesthesia received Unaware of contractions Separation and delivery of placenta	Inspection and touching of newborn, possible breast-feeding; may recommence pushing to deliver placenta when separation occurs Resting, visiting with husband or companion and baby	Oxytocics as ordered; care for infant, allowing parents to observe; check for abnormality, warmth, identification, cord, Apgar evaluation; assist physician in obtaining cord blood, preparing to suture lacerations or episiotomy as needed; observe mother for relaxed fundus, hemorrhage, problems in delivery of placenta, and interaction with infant
Stage IV from delivery of placenta to postpartum "stabilization"			
Time range 2 to 4 hours	Fundus firm, at or below umbilicus Lochial flow moderate Relieved that labor has ended Animated or exhausted; great individual differences seen	Quiet, recovery period Visit with husband or companion and baby, if possible Refreshing bath Light meal or snack	Temperature check Provide period for more interaction with infant if desirable BP, P, R, lochial flow and fundus check every 15 minutes for at least 1 hour; ice pack to perineum? Observe for voiding problems Observe response to type of analgesia, anesthesia

turns to the supine position. If the patient is going to be supine for an appreciable length of time, the head of the bed should be elevated at least 30 degrees to prevent circulatory and respiratory difficulty.

This early labor period is an excellent time to assess the family's preparation for labor, to teach breathing and relaxation techniques, and prepare them for the procedures to come. The mother's anxiety will be lessened if the nurse and other care givers explain all procedures, the results of examinations, and so forth. Maternal and fetal assessments should be carried out according to the schedules indicated in Tables 11-2 and 11-3 or more often if individual history or indications warrant. The mother should conserve her energy for the more demanding period of labor to come. Backrubs and frequent change of position contribute to her general comfort. Clear fluids or ice chips are usually allowed to maintain hydration and prevent dry mucous membranes from mouth breathing. An intravenous infusion (IV) may be delayed until the onset of more active labor. The woman should be encouraged to void approximately every 2 hours to prevent bladder distension and its associated discomfort. The amount and character of any bloody show or amniotic drainage should be noted. If a question of ruptured membranes exists, the amniotic fluid tests indicated in the hospital admission section of this chapter should be done.

Rupture of the membranes (spontaneous). If the bag of waters breaks at any time while the patient is in the labor area, she should be instructed not to get out of bed or sit completely upright until evaluated. The nurse inspects the perineum for signs of a prolapsed cord or, in the case of advanced labor, evaluates signs of the advance of the presenting part (e.g., bulging perineum, appearance of the fetal scalp) and the amount and color of the amniotic fluid.

Normal amniotic fluid is very light yellow in color. If any meconium is in the fluid, staining it a brownish-green, it should be reported immediately to the health care provider. As indicated earlier, meconium-stained amniotic fluid in cephalic presentations is considered a sign of fetal distress—the response of the fetus to lack of oxygen. The appearance of red-tinged amniotic drainage, old, dark blood, bright red, frank bleeding, or blood clots at any time during labor should also be reported. Fetal heart tones should be checked immediately after the rupture of the membranes to try to detect possible cord prolapse and compression.

The fact that the bag of waters appears to have ruptured should be documented and reported. If meconium or blood is present in the fluid the health care provider may elect to use the internal mode of FHR monitoring. Since rupture of membranes may stimulate labor, contractions should be evaluated for increased frequency, duration, and intensity. The perineum should be cleaned and dry linens provided to prevent infection and increase comfort for the laboring woman. Since fluid continues to be produced it is likely to continue to leak throughout the labor. Attention should be paid to perineal hygiene. If the presenting part of the baby is tight against the cervix and the health care provider so orders, the laboring mother may ambulate.

Rupture of the membranes (artificial). At times, in an effort to induce or hasten labor or to apply an internal monitor lead, the health care provider artificially ruptures the membranes during a vaginal examination. This is done, however, only under certain conditions. The cervix should be effaced, and some dilation must be present. The head should be engaged to prevent a cord prolapse.

The actual rupture of the bag of waters causes no pain since no nerves are located in the membranes. The pressure exerted to perform the vaginal examination and to position the instrument, however, may cause some discomfort. The woman may need some encouragement during the procedure. If rupture of the membranes is anticipated at the time of a vaginal examination the patient should be placed on several bed-protecting pads to catch the drainage. The physician or nurse midwife ordinarily uses a sterile instrument with a small, hook-like end. The membranes are ruptured between contractions. The fluid flow is controlled to avoid the cord being swept out of place by a sudden gush of "water." Care after the procedure is the same as that for a spontaneous rupture of membranes.

If severe bradycardia and prolonged variable FHR deceleration is present after spontaneous or artificial rupture the woman should be checked vaginally for presence of a prolapsed cord. In the event of a prolapse the nurse may attempt to lift the fetal head off of the cord with her gloved fingers until the health care provider arrives. Oxygen should be administered to the mother and she can be placed in a Trendelenburg or knee-chest position to utilize the forces of gravity while she is being transported to the operating room. An immediate cesarean section is usually indicated.

Vaginal examinations. As previously indicated, vaginal examinations are kept to a minimum, since they are uncomfortable and may introduce infection. Student nurses are not routinely taught these techniques because they are unable to practice the technique frequently enough to be able to correctly interpret the findings. In addition, the patient should not have the discomfort of duplicate examinations.

When a vaginal examination is indicated the nurse or health care provider positions the woman supine with her head slightly elevated. The nurse may encourage the woman to use breathing techniques to help her relax. The examiner washes his or her hands before putting on a sterile examining glove. The glove is lubricated with a sterile, water-soluble lubricant. The vulva should be cleansed, and disinfectant is poured over the gloved fingers and vulva. Care should be taken not to touch anything but the vaginal canal so that organisms from anal or other areas are not introduced into the canal. Cervical dilation and effacement, and fetal station, presentation and position are usually evaluated. After the examination the patient's perineal area should be cleansed and dried. The woman should be told the results of the examination, encouraged, and reassured.

Active labor

As labor progresses, contractions are more frequent and intense. Increasingly the woman's attention is focused on meeting the demands of these contractions. She is anxious about whether she has the physical and psychological resources to continue to deal with them. The nurse can help by providing comfort measures, encouraging her, and listening to her concerns. Her labor support coach is likely to need increasing support as well. A quiet, calm environment will help the patient to relax and concentrate on her efforts. If she has had no previous training in breathing and relaxation techniques, she may still benefit from some simple instruction. These techniques may ease her discomfort and help her relax. If the woman is unfamiliar with breathing methods the nurse should observe for signs of hyperventilation, likely with the rapid breathing patterns, and help her correct the pattern. She should be encouraged to void every 1 to 2 hours. The nurse should give her positive reinforcement for her efforts, and frequently share signs of her labor progress with her and her family members.

Probably the most difficult period of labor is called *transition,* lasting approximately from 8 to 10 cm dilation. The laboring patient is now fatigued and usually discouraged. She wonders if she is ever going to have her baby and worries about her performance when she does. Her contractions may be irregular, at times seeming to come one right after another. Nausea and vomiting are common. She may suddenly become very irritable and may not want to be touched, yet fear being left alone. She is usually most grateful for the presence of the nurse or labor coach. Although she may not tolerate touching she is likely to appreciate cool, fresh pillowcases, cool gauze sponges or an ice chip to ease the dry mouth, and a cool cloth on the forehead. The husband or the chosen companion can often help with these simple methods of relieving distress. The nurse should continue to be alert for bladder distention. If the woman cannot void, she may need to be catheterized before the pushing involved in the second stage of labor. Distention may delay fetal descent or traumatize the bladder, causing edema of the trigone area and inability to void in the postpartal period.

Second Stage of Labor

During transition the patient needs to be assessed frequently for signs of the onset of the second stage of labor, the period of expulsion. The health care provider and other nursing staff should be informed of the patient's progress. The second stage will ordinarily be heralded by an increase in bloody show, an involuntary urge to push or bear down with each contraction as the cervix completely dilates and the presenting part descends, fetal heart tones heard just above the pubic bone in cephalic presentations, and late signs (e.g., the bulging of the perineum, the dilation of the anus, the appearance of caput or the fetal scalp) (Fig. 11-13). The experienced nurse knows that when the actively laboring woman says "The baby's coming!" she is normally correct.

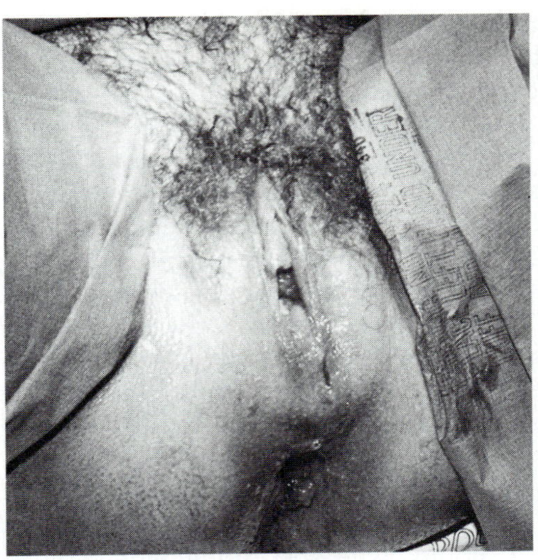

Fig. 11-13 Bulging of perineum and appearance of fetal head (caput) in second stage of labor. (Courtesy Grossmont Hospital and Martin M. Greenberg, MD, La Mesa, CA.)

Although she may wish to do so, a woman should be urged not to bear down or push before complete dilation of the cervix is determined. To do so could cause greater fatigue for the mother, greater strain on the fetus, and swelling and injury to the cervix. After complete dilation and preparations for the birth are made the woman is instructed to push. Most women are relieved by pushing and cooperate well in following instructions, if they are not confused by too many instructors. (See Table 11-4.) The woman should be positioned comfortably in a relatively upright position (or squatting in some cases) to allow gravity to assist her. When vigorous pushing is required, the woman should not hold her breath longer than 5 to 10 seconds. When her breath is held for longer periods than this, the exchange of gases across the placenta is significantly reduced. The labor coach should be encouraged to help the mother in her efforts and watch the progress of the birth with her in an overhead mirror. Not all men want to see their children being born. For those who do, it is usually a memorable, positive experience. In some cultures the woman's mother or other female support people fulfill this important, supportive role.

To avoid a last minute rush the delivery table should be set up when the multipara is approximately 6 to 7 cm dilated. If the woman is a primigravida the nurse can wait to set up the table until she is pushing, since the period between complete dilation and the birth of the infant may be relatively protracted. If the woman is delivering in a traditional hospital setting, she

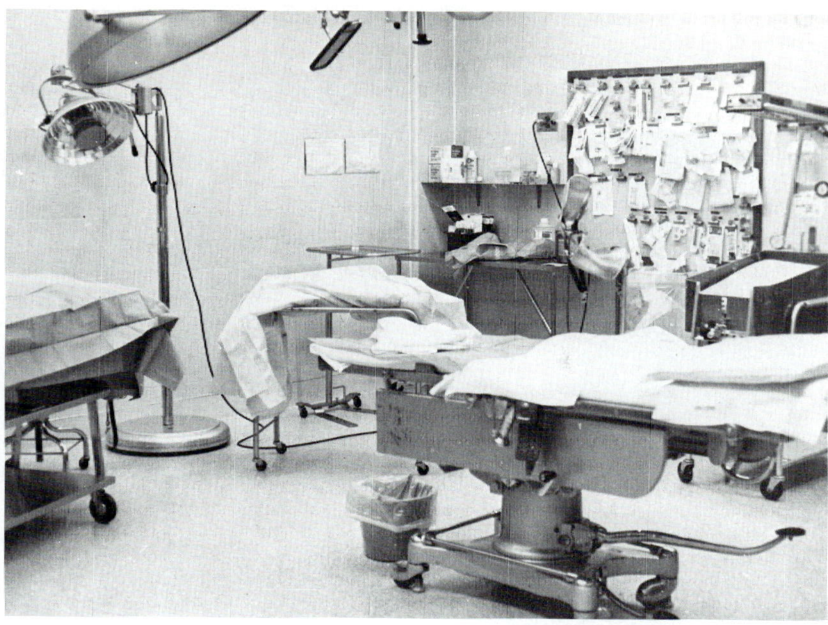

Fig. 11-14 View of so-called traditional delivery room. The patient labors elsewhere and is transferred to the delivery room shortly before the birth. After giving birth she is transferred again for recovery and postpartum care. Not seen are anesthesia machine and maternal and fetal monitors.

should be transferred to the delivery room at the same time given for table set-up.

Preparation of the delivery room

The responsibility of preparing the delivery room may be that of the registered nurse or a licensed vocational nurse (Fig. 11-14). The nurse must have a clear concept of the principles of sterile technique, know where supplies are kept, and know the patient's special needs and the attending physician or nurse midwife's desires. The nurse should have some idea of when the delivery is likely so that this work can be planned. Regardless of the setting, similar preparations for delivery and the same principles of asepsis apply to setting up the delivery table.

The room should be set up to accomplish the following goals:

1. To provide an aseptic field for the anticipated birth, and subsequent newborn and maternal care.
2. To ensure the convenient placement and operation of all necessary articles to promote safety, speed, and staff confidence on behalf of the physical and emotional care of the mother and child.
3. To aid in the necessary legal and statistical recording of the event.

Capsule review of principles and practice of aseptic technique. The practice of asepsis is not difficult if the appropriate equipment and supplies are available and if conscientious, knowledgeable people are involved in their use and care. It is, however, a serious responsibility that involves evaluation of the environment, including the nurses' dress and personal health problems that may threaten the safety of the patient. Four simple rules sum up aseptic technique:

1. Know what is sterile.
2. Know what is not sterile.
3. Keep the two apart.
4. Remedy contamination immediately.

Review the methods of unwrapping and placing supplies (Figs. 11-15 and 11-16). When approaching a sterile field to add sterile supplies, take care to avoid accidentally brushing or touching the area. When passing a sterile field, keep a safe distance away and, if possible, face the field. Never turn your back on a sterile area. Avoid turning your back toward an associate who is gowned in a sterile manner.

If contamination of a sterile area does occur the event must be reported immediately. It is not a terrible sin to contaminate. It is dangerous and irresponsible to contaminate a sterile field, to know it, and to do nothing about it. No one at the time may see the lapse of asepsis. Ultimately, however, the patient may suffer from its results. The medical-nursing team should be

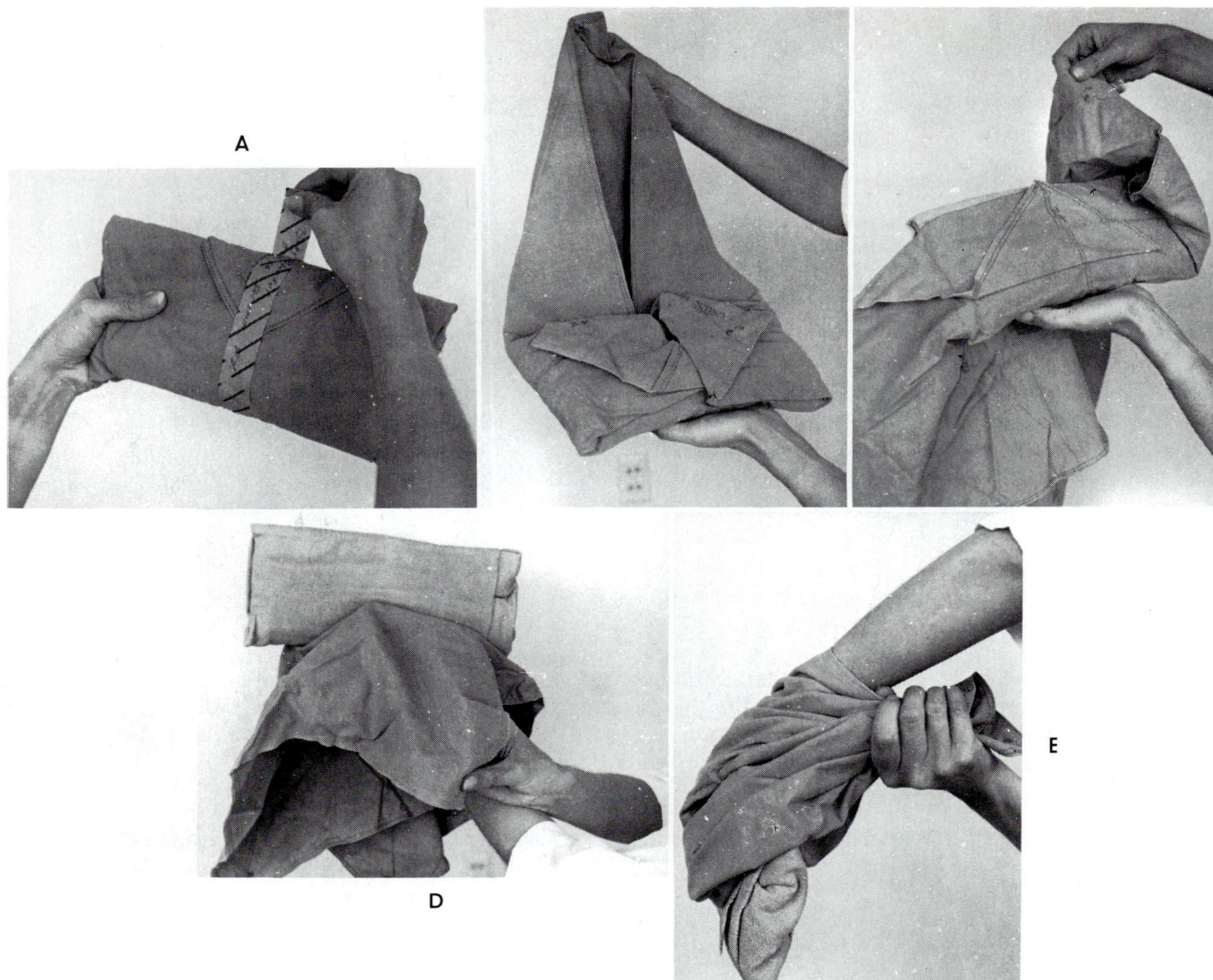

Fig. 11-15 Opening sterile packages. **A,** Remove heat-sensitive tape closing package, checking tape for color change, label, and date. Start unwrapping package with point of the wrapper facing you. In this way the part of package next to you will remain covered and protected for longest period possible. **B,** Pull back the point and let it drop down after assuring yourself that the outside of dangling wrapper will not contaminate any nearby sterile surface. **C,** Pull back two side folds by little turnbacks designed for your use. Uncover the end on side of supporting hand first, then the side next to active hand. If you are preparing inner package for drop onto sterile surface, stabilize pack by bringing your thumb over top of wrapper before completely exposing inner pack. **D,** Pull back the last fold covering inner wrap to expose sterile surface. The inner pack can now be picked up by gloved associate or it can be "scooted" onto sterile table while the ends of outer wrapper are held back to prevent contamination. **E,** If hand-thumb grip is used, the pack can be dropped in manner pictured. Care must be taken not to get too close to sterile table or field while adding supplies. (Courtesy Grossmont Hospital, La Mesa, CA.)

glad to have breaks in technique or inadvertent contamination called to their attention so that they may correct the situation. See the box on p. 186 for the procedure to set up the delivery room.

Transfer and immediate predelivery care

If the woman is transferred to a separate delivery room for delivery, the move should be done as smoothly and safely as possible. Her privacy and modesty should be protected by covering her lower body with a sheet during the transfer. If the patient has a strong desire to push and it is not considered appropriate at the time, she should be instructed and assisted to pant through her open mouth. The transfer from a bed or cart to the delivery table should be done between contractions. The woman can usually help considerably in the move to the delivery table if she has

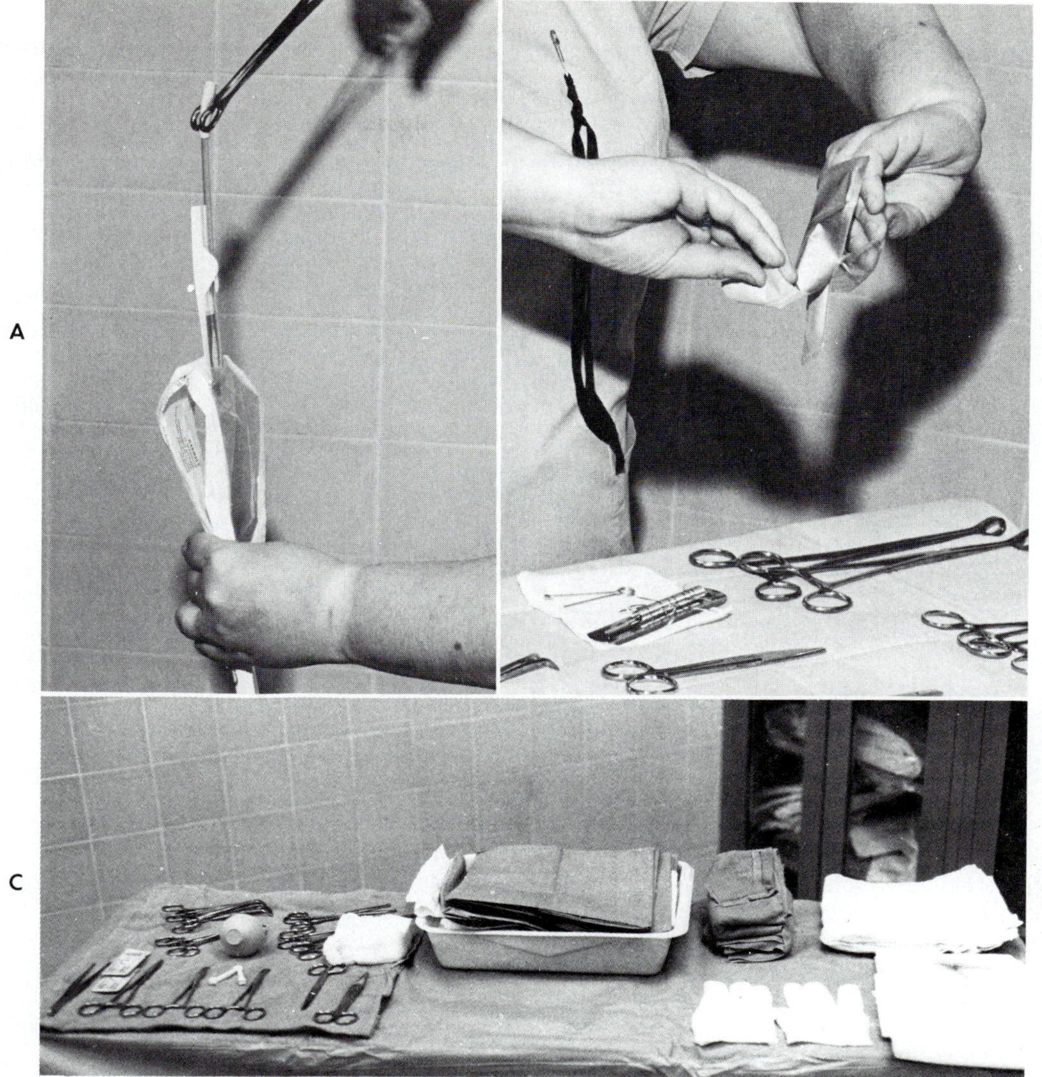

Fig. 11-16 **A,** Extracting sterile catheter from commercially prepared peel-back package; **B,** dropping sterile suture from commercially prepared peel-back package; **C,** one way to set up basic delivery room table. (Courtesy Grossmont Hospital, La Mesa, CA.)

not had a regional anesthesia or if the level of that anesthesia allows adequate lower body movement. The bed or cart should be locked and the patient securely supported during the transfer. Once on the table, a specially designed wedge is placed under one side of the patient's back to prevent her from being in a completely supine position. Assessment and recording of maternal pulse and blood pressure, as well as FHR patterns, should continue in a consistent manner (at least every 15 minutes) after the patient has been transferred to the delivery room.

While the patient is being prepared for delivery the physician or nurse midwife is usually dressing and scrubbing for the delivery. The physician or anesthesiologist may administer a spinal anesthesia for the delivery itself. The nurse uncovers the sterile table and basin set and turns on the necessary lights. The physician or nurse midwife generally advises the staff when the patient should be positioned for delivery.

Positioning. Ideally, two nurses assist in lithotomy positioning, although it can be accomplished by one. If crutch or stirrup leg supports are used, both of the patient's legs should be raised or lowered at the same time to prevent strain on her back. Coaching her to bend her knees as her legs are raised helps. The supports must be fitted to the patient, not the patient fitted to the supports. Most delivery tables have some method of dividing in half, temporarily eliminating the foot portion of the table to allow the buttocks to hang over the end of the upper part of the table and the provider to stand directly in front of the perineum. As soon as the patient's legs are adequately secured in the

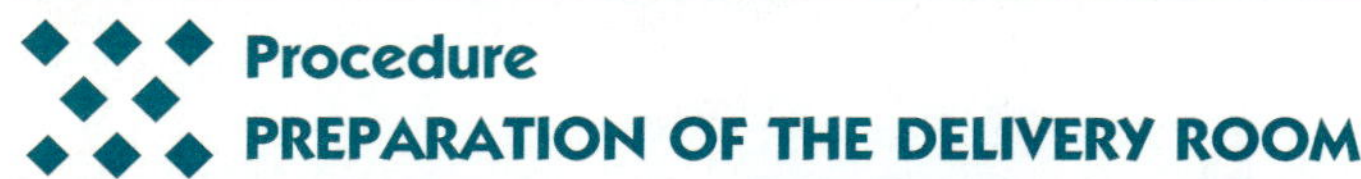

Procedure
PREPARATION OF THE DELIVERY ROOM

EQUIPMENT/SUPPLIES

Delivery table:
- Sterile delivery pack (drapes, towels, gown that is impervious to fluids or has a plastic splash apron)
- Sterile gloves (appropriate size for physician or nurse midwife)
- Instruments
- Basins (2) (one for the placenta and one for lubricating obstetrical forceps, rinsing gloved hands, or cleansing the patient)
- Sterile, warm water for the basin
- Perineal preparation tray (cleansing solution, sterile gauze sponges, sterile gloves)
- Anesthesia supplies (if appropriate)
- Bulb syringe
- Cord clamp

Other supplies:
- Obstetrical forceps (if indicated)
- Sutures
- Disposable mask with eye shield or goggles for those in the "splash zone"
- Disposable hat and shoe covers for the health care provider
- Hat, mask, and sterile gloves sized for the nurse setting up the delivery table
- Pitocin and syringe for adding to IV or giving IM after the placenta is delivered, and a medication label
- Syringe, needle, and specimen tubes for collection of cord blood (if necessary)

Supplies for the newborn:
- Radiant warmer (prewarmed)
- Warmed blankets and hat
- Thermometer for assessing the newborn's temperature
- Scale (weight not always measured in the delivery room)
- Oxygen
- Suction equipment and catheters
- Emergency equipment (laryngoscope with a working light and blades; endotracheal tubes; bag set-up for resuscitation)

STEPS

1. Put on the mask. Be sure all hair is covered by a hat.
2. Wash hands carefully.
3. Open necessary sterile packs for the delivery table. Check outside tapes on packs for proof of sterilization (if this type of tape is used). Check dates on packs to avoid outdated materials.
4. Put on sterile gloves.
5. Arrange the equipment on the table.
6. Add additional sterile equipment to the table as needed (e.g., bulb syringe, cord clamp, anesthesia supplies).
7. Cover the table with a sterile drape.
8. Remove the hat, mask, and gloves and prepare the rest of the room.
9. Place forceps and suture material so they are readily available.
10. Check that equipment is in working order (e.g., bed, lights, mirror, oxygen, suction, newborn emergency equipment).
11. Prepare infant identification materials so they are ready for last minute additions.
12. Prepare delivery paper work so that it is ready for delivery entries.
13. Turn on radiant warmer and get warm newborn blankets and a scale shortly before the birth.
14. Add warmed, sterile water to the basin shortly before the birth.
15. Draw up Pitocin and prepare medication label (if added to IV).

supports, the table is so adjusted. This is called "dropping" or "breaking" the table.

Giving birth in the lithotomy position is not an anatomical necessity. It is, however, the position that is associated with the use of spinal anesthesia and forceps and is the most familiar to many health care providers in the United States. In Great Britain, a modified side position is often used. In some cultures the mother gives birth in a squatting position. In parts of Europe a modified Fowler's position is typically used, with flexion and abduction of the lower extremities. These last two postures allow gravity to aid the mother in her efforts to push the fetus to the outside world. The newer, adjustable combination labor-delivery beds or chairs that are commonly available in LDRs and LDRPs assist the mother to maintain a more advantageous physiological birth position (Fig. 11-17).

Perineal preparation. As soon as the table or delivery bed is "dropped" the nurse cleanses the thighs, lower abdomen, and complete perineal area of the mother with a soap or antiseptic solution. This prep is carried out in slightly different ways in different institutions. It involves sterile gloving and the use of sterile gauze pads or sponge sticks. The principles are

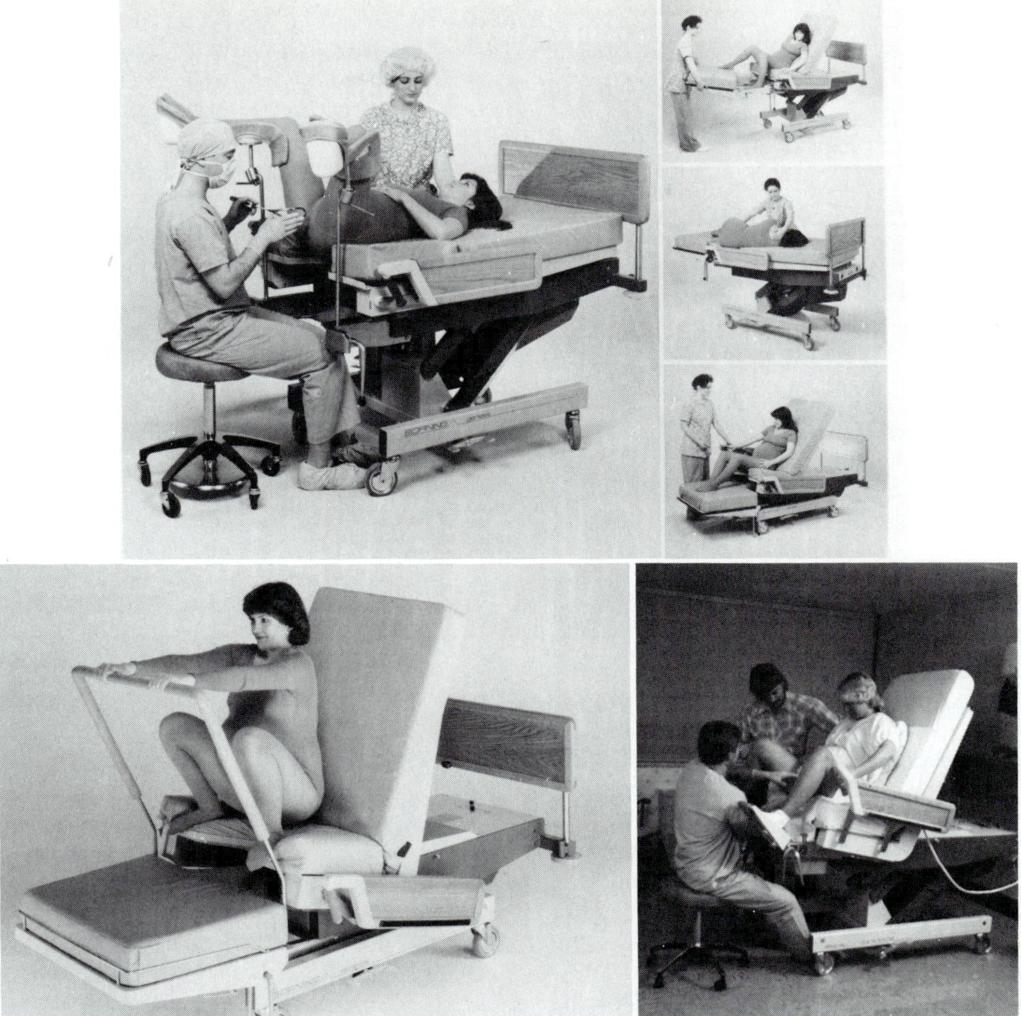

Fig. 11-17 The versatility of the maternity bed called *Genesis* is demonstrated here. Some maternity services remove the head board permanently to allow easy access to the patient's head by an anesthesiologist. (Courtesy Borning Corporation, Spokane, WA.)

the same: to help prevent infection and to increase the visibility of the area involved. To prevent contamination of the birth canal, care should be taken to ensure that no sponge is used in the anal-rectal area and then returned to the vulvar region. Usually the first sponge is used to cleanse side to side from the pubic bone to the lower abdomen (Fig. 11-18). It is then discarded. The second and third sponges are used in cleansing the thighs with an up-and-down motion from the labia majora to the midthigh. Each is discarded directly after use. The fourth and fifth sponges are used to clean the labia on the right and left of the vagina, avoiding the rectum, and then discarded. The last cleansing sponge passes directly over the vagina and anus.

The perineum may be rinsed and dried and perhaps sprayed or painted with an additional antiseptic. The purpose of this preparation should be kept in mind. The object is not to go through so many prescribed motions but to clean the skin. On the other hand, it must be performed rather swiftly, or the infant may arrive before one is finished. The gowned health care provider is usually ready to drape for delivery as soon as the nurse is finished.

All personnel attending the delivery should adhere to *universal precautions* (OSHA, 1991): those in the "splash zone" are those close enough to be splashed with blood or amniotic fluid and should wear a gown impervious to fluid or a plastic apron, a face mask with eye shield or goggles, and gloves. Those likely to be exposed to body fluids or to handle the newborn

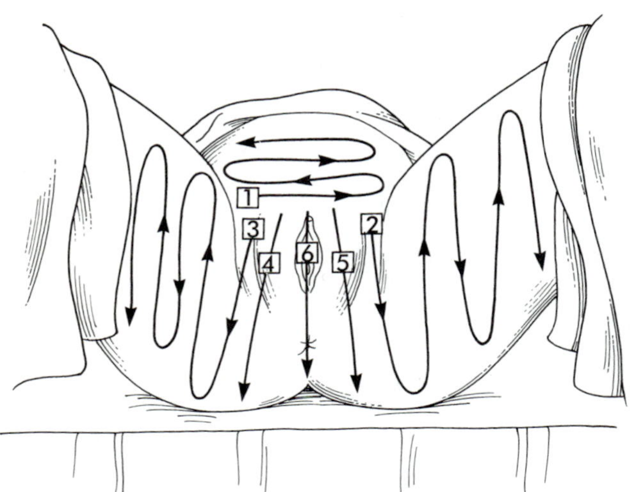

Fig. 11-18 Cleansing the perineum in preparation for birth. The numbered diagram shows the order and direction of each stroke. A new sponge should be used for each area. This perineal scrub can be done with the woman in any delivering position.

should also wear gloves. Shoe covers are not required for universal precautions, but they will protect the shoes from becoming soiled.

Draping. During the draping procedure the nurse provides a stool for the physician or nurse midwife, pushes the sterile supply table and basin rack into position, adjusts the light and mirror, unwraps the forceps if they are desired, secures any needed additional supplies, and begins the written record of the delivery (Fig. 11-19). The nurse also supports the woman's pushing efforts during this time and encourages the woman's labor coach. After the woman is draped, no part of the exposed side of the sterile linen (or paper) covering the patient should be touched by anyone not properly gloved or gowned. If the nurse needs to palpate contractions or apply fundal or suprapubic pressure she must reach under the sterile drape, avoiding the exposed perineum. After the infant is born, if she is placed on her mother's abdomen, the nurse may reach under the covering drape and, using the drape as a hand guard, hold on to an arm or leg to help give support while the newborn's airway is aspirated or the cord is clamped.

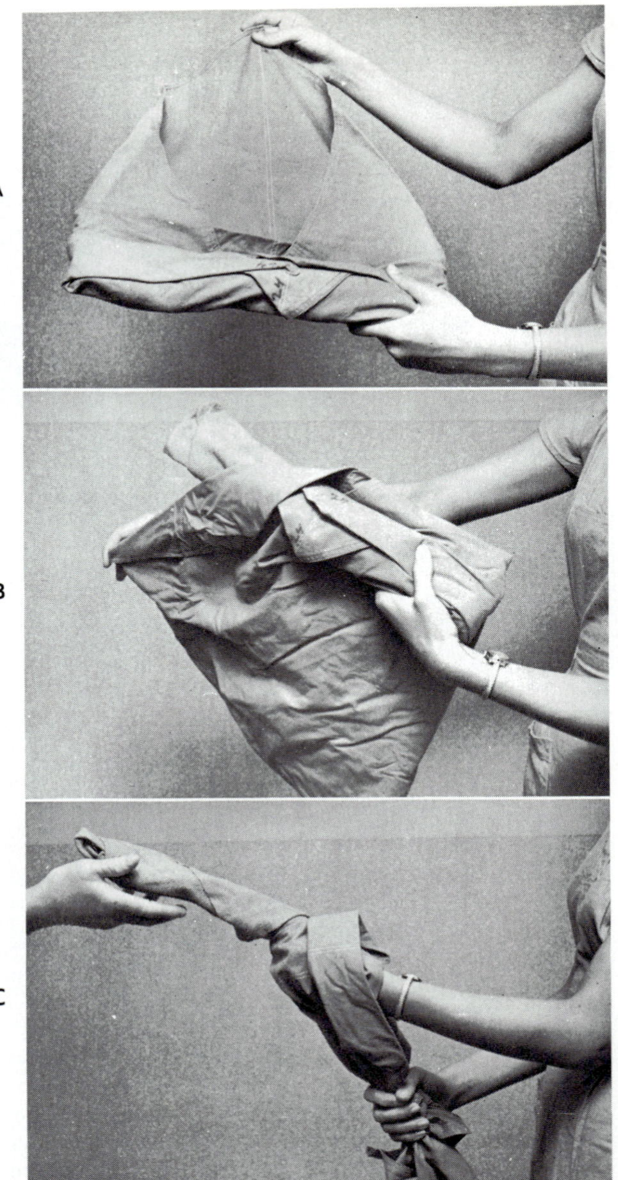

Fig. 11-19 Steps in unwrapping sterile forceps to hand to physician. **A,** Grasp one end of package, remove outer tape, and unwind outer wrapper. **B,** Pull back inner turnback at top of package and continue to uncover inner wrap. **C,** Grasp carefully all dangling ends of outer wrap and pull them out of the way toward your wrist. Do not touch inner wrap. (Courtesy Grossmont Hospital, La Mesa, CA.)

Delivery forceps, vacuum extraction, and episiotomies

After the sterile preparation and draping are complete, if the mother's bladder needs to be emptied or a urine specimen is necessary, the provider will perform a catheterization before the birth of the baby.

At times, especially if the mother is bearing her first child, the physician may use outlet forceps to lift out the infant's head (Fig. 11-20 *A, B, C, E*). Judicious application of these forceps may shorten the second stage of labor considerably if the mother is finding it difficult to push effectively or if the fetus or mother's condition makes more rapid delivery advisable.

Vacuum extraction may be preferred over forceps to shorten the second stage of labor. However, the use of

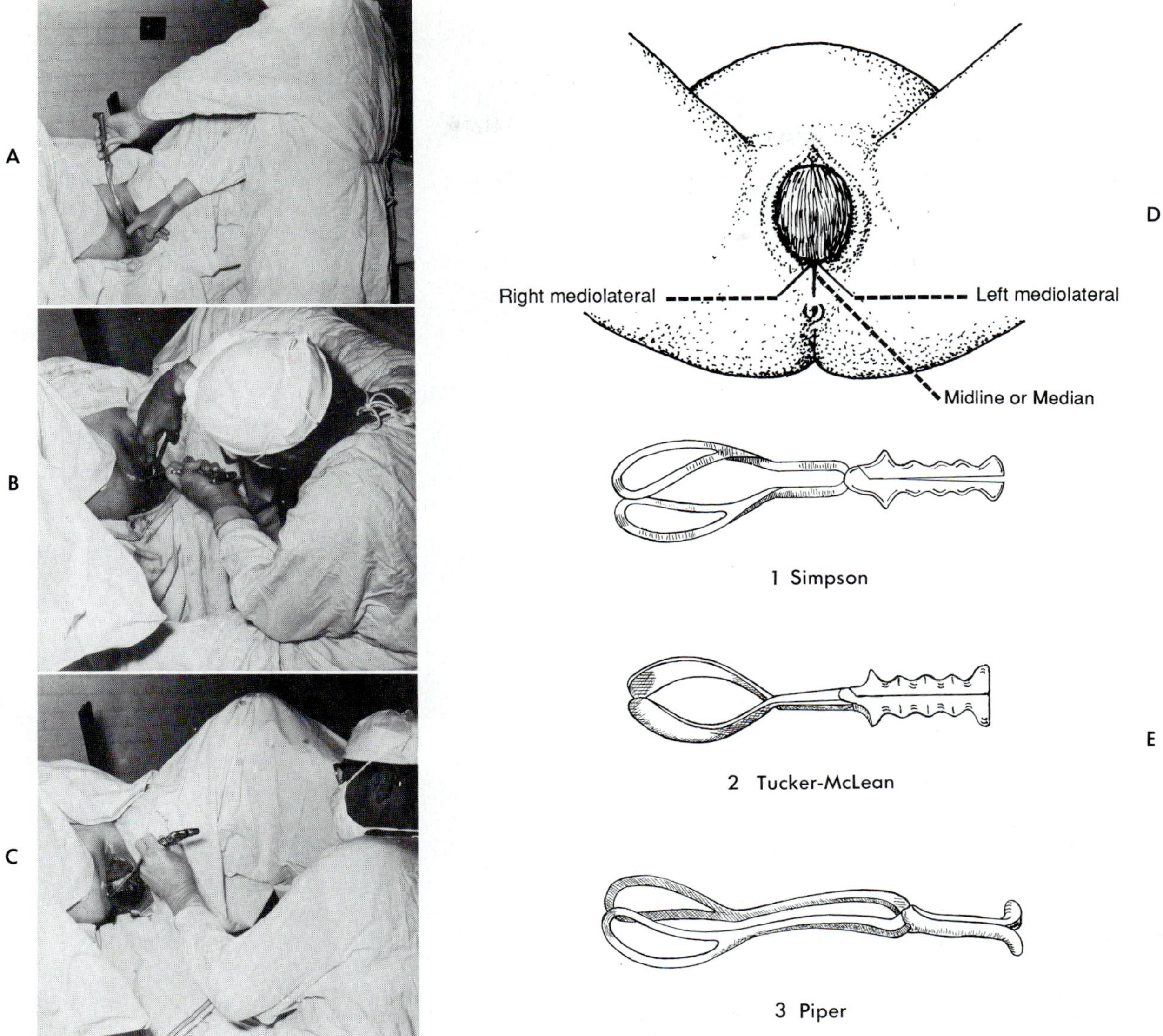

Fig. 11-20 **A,** Insertion of one forceps blade; **B,** cutting midline episiotomy (one blade of the forceps has been inserted); **C,** use of outlet forceps; **D,** various types of episiotomies; **E,** three kinds of obstetrical forceps: 1, Simpson; 2, Tucker-McLean; 3, Piper (sometimes used to deliver after-coming head in breech presentation). (**A** to **C,** Courtesy Wayne B. Henderson, MD, San Diego, CA.)

outlet forceps or vacuum extraction just to save time is unwarranted. The vacuum extractor consists of a soft suction cup attached by tubing to a suction pump. The cup is placed over the occiput of the fetal head and suction is applied with a contraction. The vacuum extractor is contraindicated in face and breech presentations.

Forceps are usually applied in conjunction with a planned incision of the perineum to enlarge the vaginal opening, called an *episiotomy.* An episiotomy may be performed with or without the use of forceps. It is done to prevent lacerations or damage to the perineum, to avoid possible prolonged pressure on the infant's head, and to hasten delivery. If the woman does not have an epidural or spinal anesthesia in place, the provider will use local infiltration or a pudendal block to provide pain relief for the episiotomy procedure. Two main types of episiotomies include: (1) the midline or median, which features an incision from the vaginal opening straight down toward but not extending into the anus, and (2) the mediolateral, which begins at the midline above the anus but angles to the left or right. (Fig. 11-20, *D*). The midline type is easier to repair and more comfortable for the mother but occasionally it may extend during the birth, tearing the anal sphincter. The mediolateral type of episiotomy is designed to prevent this complication but is considered more difficult to repair and is usually more painful during the postpartum period. It is rarely used in the United States. The *routine* use of outlet forceps and/or episiotomy is controversial and has stirred considerable debate (Simpson, 1988). The birth of many infants does not involve the use of either forceps or episiotomy.

Delivery mechanisms

If forceps are not used for the complete delivery of the head, the child is delivered manually between contractions by slow gentle extension (Fig. 11-21). The woman may be asked to pant to avoid too rapid expulsion of the fetal head, which can result in perineal lacerations. In some cases, she may be asked to gently bear down between contractions to facilitate the passage of the head from the vaginal canal. The provider manually supports the perineum during the birth of the head. After the head is delivered the physician checks to see whether the umbilical cord is wound around the infant's neck. If it is, it must be slipped over the infant's head or clamped and cut to avoid strangulation or excessive pulling. Before the entire body of the infant is delivered the mouth is aspirated to clear the airway for the first breath. Restitution and external rotation occur after the delivery of the head. The provider may assist by gently turning the infant's head to the side so that the occiput lines up with his back. The physician or nurse midwife then gently but firmly pulls down to deliver the top (anterior) shoulder and then gently pulls up to deliver the bottom (posterior) shoulder. Once the shoulders are delivered the rest of the infant follows easily. Further aspiration of the newborn's airway may be necessary. The infant usually cries very soon after birth. The umbilical cord is clamped in two places and cut between the clamps. A plastic cord clamp can then be applied about ½ to 1 inch from the newborn's umbilicus and the metal clamp closest to the newborn removed. The newborn is placed on the mother's abdomen or handed to the nurse for further care under a radiant warmer (Fig. 11-22).

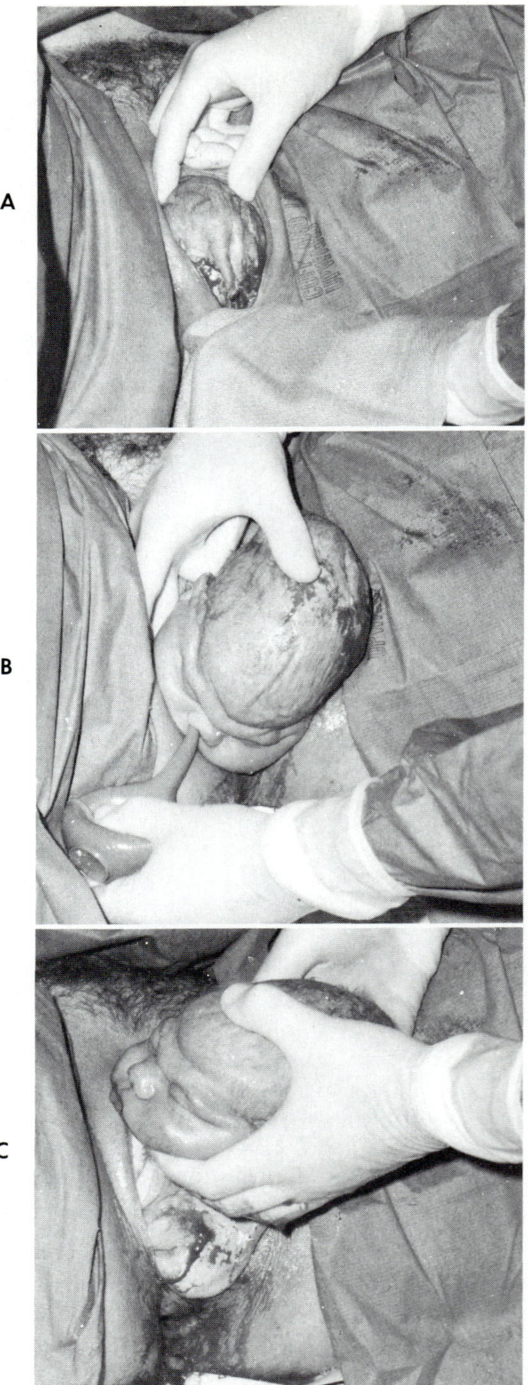

Fig. 11-21 Delivery sequence (LOA) **A,** Crowning; **B,** delivery of head and clearing airway (delivery of anterior shoulder not pictured); **C,** delivery of posterior shoulder. (Courtesy Grossmont Hospital and Mark A. Treger, MD, La Mesa, CA.)

Immediate Care of the Newborn

Immediate priorities for newborn care are to establish respiration and to provide and maintain body warmth. In most cases, this immediate care can be accomplished while the newborn is held by the parents or under the radiant warmer (placed so parents can see the infant). The first task is to clear the airway. No amount of oxygen, mouth-to-mouth resuscitation, or intermittent positive pressure will stimulate a newborn infant to breathe if its airway is not open. Conversely, if the airway is not clear but filled with amniotic fluid, meconium particles, or blood, and the infant does try to take a breath and inhale, the respiratory tract may become plugged,

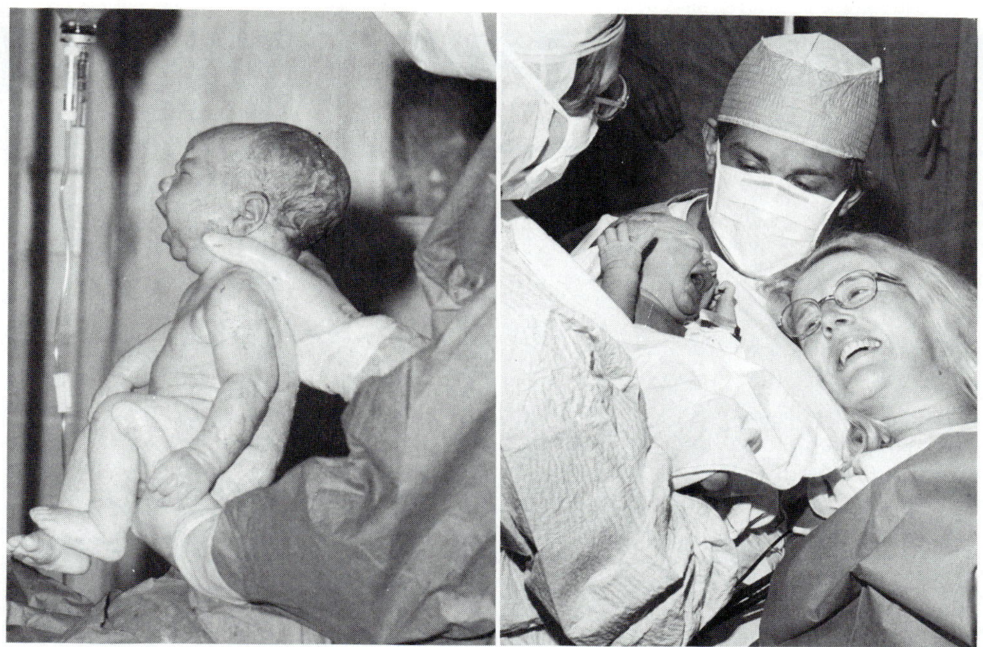

Fig. 11-22 The long-awaited parent-newborn introduction. (Courtesy Grossmont Hospital, Mark A. Treger, MD, and Martin M. Greenberg, MD, La Mesa, CA.)

irritated, or contaminated. The airway may be cleared by using the following methods:

1. Wiping off the infant's nose and mouth at the time of the birth of the head, usually performed by the physician or nurse midwife.
2. Gently suctioning first the mouth and then the nose with a bulb aspirator or a soft catheter attached to a trap and low-wall suction before birth is complete (see Fig. 17-1).
3. Holding the child's head down to drain immediately after birth while gently compressing the throat toward the mouth to milk out secretions.
4. Visualizing the larynx with a laryngoscope and suctioning the trachea, done by trained personnel for unresponsive infants or when meconium stained amniotic fluid is present.

Establish and maintain respiration

If respiration does not occur spontaneously after the airway is clear the newborn should be stimulated to cry. Many infants respond to gentle rubbing of the back or gentle suctioning of the nose with a soft catheter. If breathing is not initiated soon after stimulation, methods of breathing for the infant must be employed. Usually this means the use of intermittent positive pressure using an orotracheal tube or mask and bag. Sometimes the operator will blow directly through a patent endotracheal tube. No matter what method is used, it should be emphasized that an airway must be maintained through proper head positioning and/or the use of a small oropharyngeal airway to keep the infant's tongue from falling back and obstructing the pharynx. (For cardiopulmonary resuscitation of the newborn infant, see Chapter 28.)

When a child is being resuscitated, is breathing poorly on his or her own, has generalized cyanosis, or has a heart rate under 100 beats per minute, supplementary oxygen should be administered.

Provide and maintain warmth

The newborn should be dried immediately after birth with a warm towel or blanket. The stimulation from this activity may initiate or help maintain respiration. Once dried, the infant can then be placed skin-to-skin on the mother's abdomen or chest and covered with prewarmed blankets and a cotton hat or placed on a dry, warm blanket under the radiant heat unit. These two steps, which should be done for all infants after delivery, require only a few seconds to accomplish and can prevent the infant from becoming cold-stressed as a result of evaporative, convective, and radiant heat losses. Even healthy, term infants are limited in their ability to produce heat when exposed to a cold environment, especially during the first 12 hours of life (see Chapter 17 for a more thorough discussion of thermoregulation of the newborn).

Warming units are open, provide easy access for care, and use overhead radiant heat panels to provide heat. While under a radiant warmer the infant should not be covered. Covering prevents the radiant heat

◆ TABLE 11-6
Modified Apgar Scoring Chart to Evaluate Newborn Status 1 and 5 Minutes After Birth

New Name	Traditional Sign	0	1	2
A Appearance	Color	Blue, pale	Body pink Extremities blue	Completely pink
P Pulse	Heart rate	Absent	Slow (below 100)	Over 100
G Grimace	Reflex response (e.g., to catheter in nostril)	No response	Grimace	Cry, cough, or sneeze
A Activity	Muscle tone	Flaccid	Some flexion of extremities	Actual motion
R Respiratory effort	Respiratory effort	Absent	Slow, irregular	Good, crying

Total score: 1 min ______________________

5 min ______________________

Severely depressed	0 to 3
Moderately depressed	4 to 6
Vigorous	7 to 10

This Apgar scoring chart incorporates a concept first introduced at the University of Kentucky Medical Center, Lexington, Kentucky, by Robert Beargie, MD. Modified from Campbell SJ: New use for the APGAR name, *Point of View/Ethicon* 17:6, 1980.

waves from reaching the skin. Mother-infant skin-to-skin contact is believed to promote attachment and is effective in maintaining the infant's body temperature. A study by Phillips (1974) compared heat loss in heated cribs with heat loss in the mother's arms, confirming that the mother is a reliable source of heat for the normal, dry, wrapped infant placed on her chest. Given these findings, the healthy infant should be given to the mother or father to hold soon after birth.

Apgar assessment

The Apgar method of evaluating the newborn infant was designed in 1952 by Virginia Apgar. Its purpose is to ascertain the physical condition of the newborn and the need for resuscitation. The newborn is evaluated at 1 and 5 minutes after birth using the following criteria: heart rate, respiratory effort, muscle tone, reflex irritability, and color (see Table 11-6). The heart rate is the most important criteria and color the least important. This scoring may be done by the physician, anesthesiologist, or nurse. The nurse, however, is thought to be the more impartial and available observer, especially for the 5 minutes' evaluation. Infants receiving a score of 7 to 10 are considered vigorous. Scores of 4 to 6 denote mild- to moderate-depression, whereas 0 to 3 indicates severe depression. Apgar believed that few newborn infants deserve a 1 minute rating totaling 10 because she believed that few babies are completely pink at 1 minute after birth.

Continuing care

The newborn's body must make many adjustments to adapt to extrauterine life (see Chapter 16). The nurse should frequently assess the child's ability to adapt during the immediate period after birth. Vital signs are usually taken every half hour for the first hour, then hourly until stable. A brief physical assessment should be done to observe for anomalies (e.g., cleft palate). The nurse must also attach the appropriate identification (usually arm and wrist bands) approved by the hospital. Some facilities may also require the mother's fingerprints and the newborn's footprints. Eye medication to prevent infection and vitamin K injection, once done immediately after delivery, are usually delayed to enhance the parent-infant attachment process and early breast-feeding (see Chapter 17 for these procedures).

The Leboyer method of birth and immediate newborn care

The French obstetrician Frederick Leboyer (1976) critiqued the traditional birth experience and immediate treatment of the newborn in his book and film, *Birth Without Violence.* He called for more consideration of the sensory needs of the newborn at birth. For normal births, he advocates the following: a quiet and dimmed atmosphere, gentle handling and support for the infant's spine, maternal-child skin-to-skin contact, delayed clamping of the umbilical cord until pulsation has ceased, newborn body massage, and a gentle body temperature water bath followed by warm wrapping and breast-feeding. Objections most often voiced regarding his recommended techniques involve the dimmed environment, which may inhibit an adequate ability to observe; the difficulty of maintaining the water bath at the right temperature; and the additional time and space needed to carry out his recommendations in busy maternity services. The method was more popular in the late 1970s and early 1980s. Some couples, however, currently seek out health care providers sympathetic to Leboyer's principles. Most labor-delivery units will use this technique if parents request it.

Third Stage of Labor

The third stage of labor is from the birth of the infant until the expulsion of the placenta (Fig. 11-23). The signs of placental separation from the uterine wall are reviewed in Chapter 10. As indicated in Chapter 10, once the placenta has separated from the uterine wall the placenta may be delivered through the bearing-down efforts of the mother or it may be expressed by the health care provider. If an inspection of the placenta reveals that it is not complete, the health care provider will usually internally palpate for retained fragments. Retained placental fragments can interfere with the ability of the uterus to contract effectively, resulting in maternal hemorrhage. After the delivery of the placenta the nurse usually adds ordered oxytocin (Pitocin) to an existing IV or gives it IM to promote uterine contraction.

Fourth Stage of Labor

The fourth stage of labor is the initial 1 to 4 hour period of immediate stabilization and recuperation after the delivery of the placenta.

Perineal repair

During the first part of this period any necessary perineal (or cervical) repair is done (Fig. 11-24). Generally, if an anesthetic was used for a delivery, the same one can be employed for the repair. Sometimes, however, a local anesthetic is administered. If a local is used the provider will need a syringe, some infiltration needles, the local anesthetic of choice, and the sutures and other materials involved in a perineal repair. A seat and good light are essential.

In spite of precautions, lacerations or episiotomy extensions occasionally occur. Some maternal tissues tear more easily than others. Very large infants or unusual fetal positions are a special threat to the perineum. Lacerations of the perineum are described as first, second, third, and fourth degree. First-degree lacerations, involving a tear in the mucous membrane and skin only, are fairly common and usually of no permanent consequence. Second-degree lacerations include a tear into the muscles of the perineal body but exclude the rectal sphincter. Adequately repaired, they usually heal well with little problem. Third-degree lacerations, however, which by definition involve the circular anal sphincter muscle, are more difficult to repair and may result in permanent damage to the perineum and sphincter (review the anatomy of the pelvic floor in Chapter 4). Fourth-degree lacerations also involve the rectovaginal wall. To avoid third- and fourth-degree lacerations or episiotomy extensions that are uncontrolled and more difficult to repair, some providers purposely cut the rectal sphincter, performing an episioproctotomy (also known as a proctoepisiotomy) when the perineum is endangered.

Lacerations may involve areas other than the true perineum. Tears of the labia, interior vaginal wall, and cervix are not uncommon. All of these areas should be inspected for such tears after a birth. An adequate, early repair of obstetrical injuries to the birth canal or its supports is important to continuing good health. Inadequate repair can lead to early hemorrhage, hematoma, infection, and later in life, to urinary and bowel problems.

Hygiene and comfort

With the termination of any repair and the cleansing of the perineum the nurse realigns the head and foot of the delivery table and removes the patient's legs from the stirrups or supports. If an episiotomy or laceration occurred, an ice pack may be ordered and applied to the patient's perineum to help prevent swelling and discomfort. The perineal pads are then attached. The nurse replaces the hospital gown with a clean one and places clean absorbent pads beneath her hips. She is covered by a warm blanket for comfort and to minimize the normal shaking that may occur.

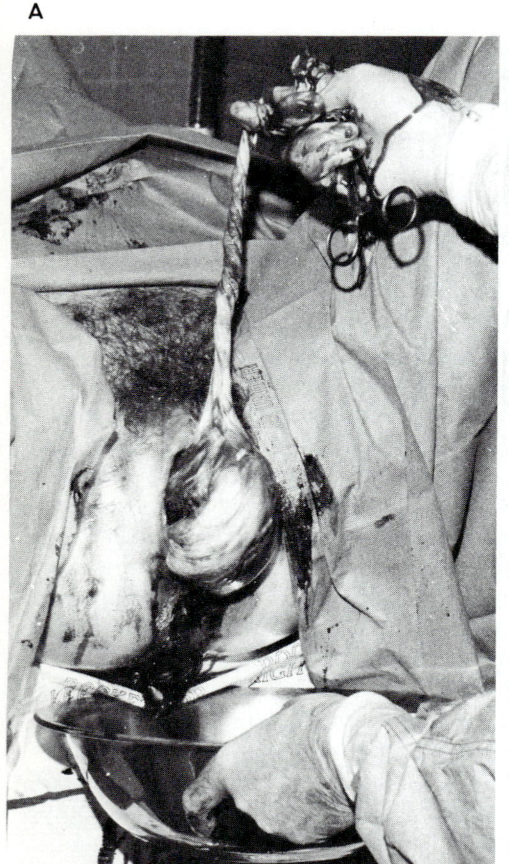

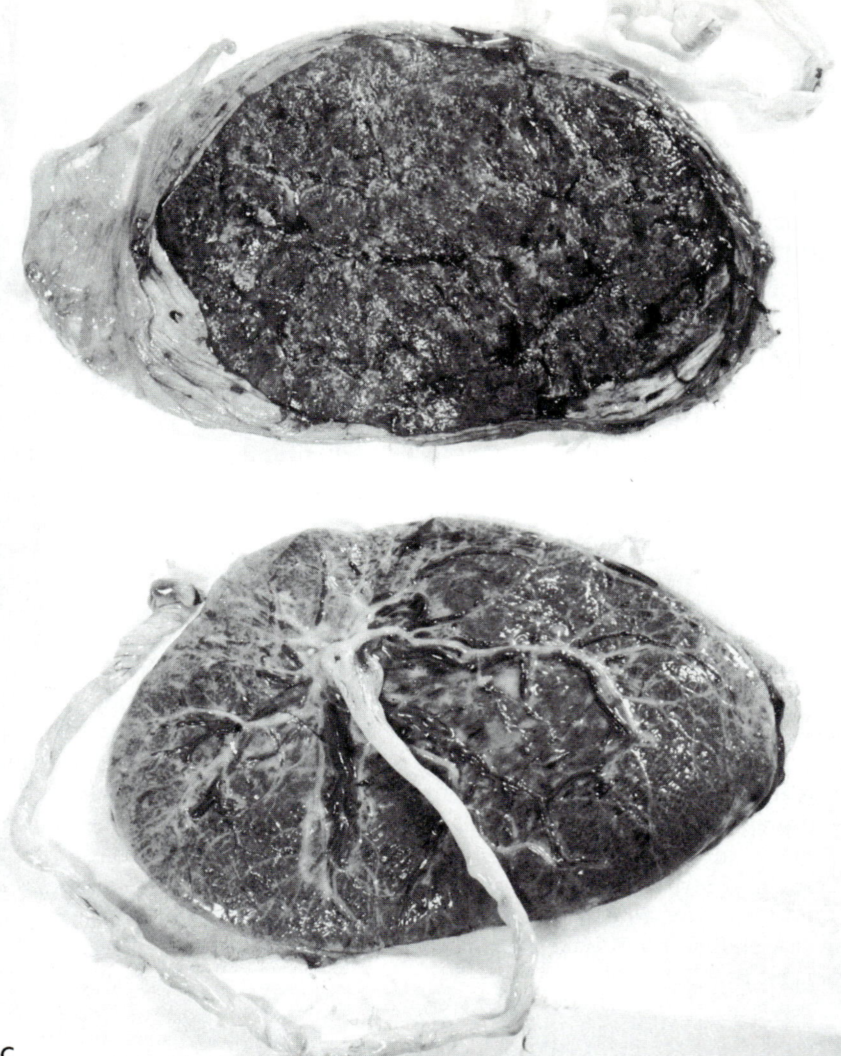

A B C

Fig. 11-23 **A,** Delivery of placenta (afterbirth); **B,** maternal side showing cotyledons and membranes pulled to one side. The cord attaches on opposite side. If this side appears first at outlet, placenta has separated by Duncan's mechanism; **C,** fetal side showing insertion of cord. If this side appears first at outlet, placental separation is by Schultz's mechanism. (Courtesy Grossmont Hospital and Martin M. Greenberg, MD, La Mesa, CA.)

Women who deliver in an LDR or LDRP will receive early recovery care in those rooms. Women who deliver in a traditional delivery room usually receive early recovery care in a special recovery room in the labor and delivery area. In the latter case, care must be exercised during the transfer from the delivery table to the recovery bed. Several hands may be needed if the patient has an IV infusion and is temporarily unable to use her legs properly because of the lingering effects of spinal or epidural anesthesia. The IV should be handled carefully to ensure that the needle is not dislodged during the transfer.

Nursing assessment

Throughout this early recovery period the patient is assessed for excessive bleeding and signs of shock. Maternal blood pressure, pulse, and respirations are frequently assessed. The uterine fundus is palpated frequently to assess for relaxation of the muscles, a condition that can result in subsequent heavy blood loss. If an IV infusion is in place, it is carefully monitored for rate of administration and possible infiltration. Many of these infusions contain an oxytocic (Pitocin) and should not be given rapidly. The box on p. 196 presents an outline of important nursing care

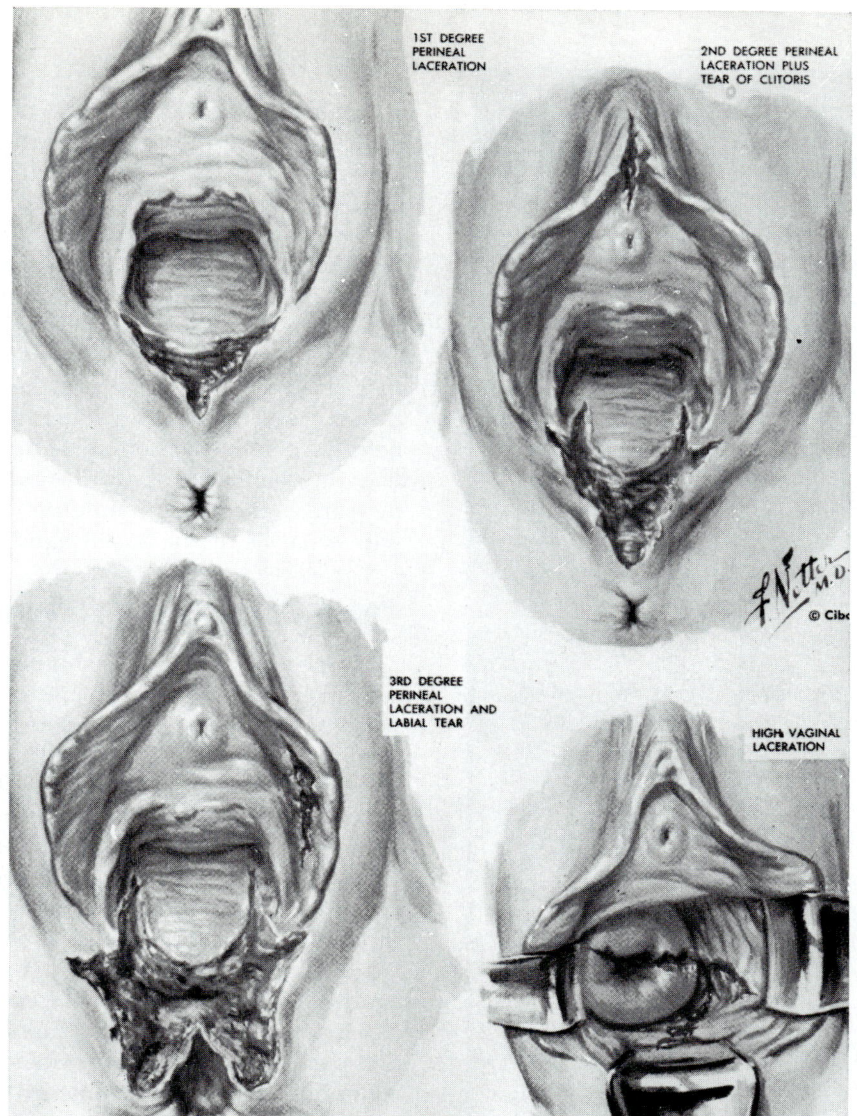

Fig. 11-24 Obstetrical lacerations—vagina, perineum, and vulva. (From the CIBA collection of medical illustrations, by Frank H. Netter, MD, Copyright CIBA.)

during the fourth stage of labor. See Chapter 13 for a more detailed description of nursing care during this early postpartum period.

Parent-Infant Attachment

The birth of an infant is a special occasion. Although the neonate needs to be protected against infection and over-handling, the way the newborn is introduced to the parents and siblings is important. If possible, both the father and the mother should have an opportunity to see and handle the infant without hurry directly after birth.

The importance of this early postpartum period to the formation of positive mother-child and mother-father-child relationships has been studied over the past 30 years. The newborn is often more alert during the first hour after birth than in subsequent hours. If the mother is also alert, willing, and the circumstances of the labor and birth are conducive, this early period is an opportune time to begin the patient-infant acquaintance process and breast-feeding. Breast-feeding directly after delivery of the placenta also has physiological benefits, since stimulation of the breasts causes the uterus to contract and helps prevent blood loss. The nurse is in an excellent position to assist with breast-feeding and to assess and facilitate the early attachment process.

Numerous investigators have described the typical, initial exploratory behavior of human mothers and

NURSING ASSESSMENT FOR THE FOURTH STAGE OF LABOR

The following maternal assessments are customary for the first hour after vaginal birth or until the woman is stable.

1 Pulse, respirations, and blood pressure measurements taken every 15 min during the first hour and thereafter until her condition is stable.
2 Temperature taken once.
3 Consistency and location of the fundus checked every 15 min.
4 Type and amount of vaginal discharge (lochia) and the appearance of the perineum every 15 min.
5 Signs and symptoms of distention of the urinary bladder every 15 min (intake and output should be recorded carefully during this period).
6 Rate of flow and condition of any IV infusion present, and amount and type of any medication.
7 General condition of the patient: color, feel of her skin (warm or cold, dry or clammy), level of consciousness (drowsy, apprehensive, unresponsive), and presence of nausea or vomiting.
8 Emotional status: depression or joy (quality of interactions with infant, family, and friends).
9 Pain (requests for pain medication or nonverbal signs of pain).
10 Recovery from anesthesia, if any (return of motion, sensation, or consciousness).
11 Nutritional and fluid status.

fathers. Gentle fingertip touching of the hands and feet progresses to massage-like motions of the palm on the infant's trunk. Eye-to-eye contact is remarkable, and a characteristic "en face" position is often demonstrated (the mother's face poised directly in front of and in line with that of her infant). This eye-to-eye observation helps establish the newborn's identity as a person and provides rewarding feedback to the parent. Dimming the room lights and delaying the eye prophylaxis are two methods of facilitating this early eye contact. If for some reason such early interaction is not possible, one should remember that human beings are very adaptable. Parents are able to forge strong relationships without the benefit of this early contact.

SPECIAL SITUATIONS

We now consider some special situations that occasionally arise in the labor-delivery setting.

Precipitous Delivery

A precipitous delivery is a birth that occurs with such speed that the usual preparation for and medical supervision of the event are lacking. A multipara with a relaxed perineal floor may have an extremely short period of expulsion. Two or three powerful contractions may cause the infant to appear. In this instance, the nurse may be the only one at the bedside or delivery table to assist the patient. In no instance should the nurse leave the woman alone but should turn on the call light or use the intercom to call for assistance. If it is obvious that the infant will be born before the delivery room is set up (e.g., the patient has had three children [para 3] and the head is almost delivered), the nurse should do the best he or she can with what he or she has at hand.

Birth of the baby in a vertex presentation

If time allows the nurse should wash, put on gloves, and place a sterile drape under the woman's hips. However, this basic preparation is not always possible. The mother is likely to be frightened and a calm manner and clear instructions from the nurse will reassure her. The infant's head should not be forcibly held back, since this may cause fetal distress and aspiration. It is important, however, to maintain flexion of the fetal head to avoid trauma to maternal periurethral and perineal tissue. This restraint can usually be achieved by allowing the infant to emerge slowly against a guiding hand placed on the top of the advancing head. The nurse should support the woman's perineum with the other hand. If the bag of waters is not broken, it must be pinched or torn to release the fluid and protect the infant from aspiration. The actual delivery of the head should be accomplished between contractions, with the mother panting or lightly bearing down. As soon as the head is born the nurse should wipe off the newborn's face and, if possible, suction the mouth and nose. The nurse should also check to determine whether the cord is around the neck. If it is, it should be slipped over the head or shoulders to prevent choking. Rarely it may be too tight to slip over with the fingers. If this happens, it must be clamped and cut (by this time, assistance in the form of personnel and the emergency delivery pack containing scissors and clamps should have arrived). The mother should be firmly instructed to pant through her open mouth and not push during this interval.

After the head is delivered, the infant's face wiped, suction employed, and the location of the cord determined, the rest of the baby's body usually emerges without further assistance. The body should be supported during delivery. However, if there seems to be no further progress and external rotation has not occurred, the nurse can gently assist by turning the head in the direction of least resistance to line up with the child's back. There is no need to hurry. The head should then gently but firmly be directed downward to deliver the anterior shoulder. After the anterior shoulder is expelled, the infant is lifted up toward the pubic bone to release the posterior shoulder. The rest of the child can then be delivered without any particular problem. Before the birth of the infant, it is helpful if the mother's hips can be elevated (or the foot portion of the table lowered a few inches) by another person to give more room for perineal support, facilitate the gentle up-and-down maneuvers described above, and to help keep the infant's face free of vaginal and anal drainage.

Immediate care of the newborn and placental delivery. As soon as possible, the infant's airway should be cleared. If a suction bulb is available, it is usually quite effective. The newborn's body should be supported on the nurse's hand and arm at the level of the mother's uterus and tilted to allow mucous and amniotic fluid to drain (without placing tension on the umbilical cord). The nurse must be careful to have a good grip since the wet newborn will be very slippery. After the airway is clear the infant should be quickly dried with a towel or blanket and placed on his or her side—the head slightly lower than the body—on the mother's abdomen. Most of these babies cry immediately, but the drying process provides stimulation to breathe and promotes warmth.

No haste is needed to cut the cord or, for that matter, to deliver the placenta. The cord can wait until sterile equipment is available. The nurse should wait for delivery of the placenta unless professional aid is very long in arriving or excessive bleeding occurs. However, if no professional help is forthcoming, if the signs of separation of the placenta have occurred, and if the uterus is firm, the nurse should ask the mother to bear down to deliver the placenta. It should be supported as it is expelled so that the membranes are not torn. The cord can be clamped and cut at this time if sterile equipment is available. The nurse should inspect the placenta for completeness, and save it for later evaluation by the physician or nurse midwife. The nurse then checks the firmness of the uterus. It can be gently massaged to increase uterine contractions and the newborn can be encouraged to breast-feed for the same reason. Usually the physician or nurse midwife arrives in time to complete the delivery of the placenta and repair any lacerations.

Birth of the infant in a breech presentation

As discussed in Chapter 10, the incidence of breech presentations is low (3.5%). A vaginal birth of an infant in breech presentation involves more risk to the infant than a cephalic birth. The mother is likely to have a longer, more tiring labor, and a larger episiotomy. As a rule, greater possibility of prolapse of the umbilical cord exists during breech labor. During the delivery of the infant, it may be compressed against the pelvic outlet. The infant may try to take a breath before the head is born and aspirate tenacious vaginal secretions. The primary concern, however, is that the largest part of the body (the head) presents last and may become trapped in the cervix. A special type of forceps called *Piper's forceps,* applied to the aftercoming head, may be used for a breech birth. Because of these risks, physicians usually elect to deliver babies in breech presentations by cesarean section.

Occasionally, however, a mother may arrive at the birth center in very active labor and the breech birth will be precipitous. In this instance, the nurse should call for assistance and proceed calmly as described for delivery of a baby in a vertex presentation. The buttocks usually present and, after they are born, the nurse should support the breech with both hands. The body can be lifted slightly upward to facilitate the delivery of the posterior shoulder and arm, then lowered to allow delivery of the anterior shoulder and arm. Before these body manipulations the nurse may need to pull down a loop of the cord to prevent tension on the point of insertion.

While supporting the infant's body with one arm and hand, the nurse should apply suprapubic pressure with the other hand to keep the infant's head flexed until it is born. The head is often delivered so that the infant almost seems to do a guided, half somersault over the mother's abdomen. Care of the newborn and delivery of the placenta are the same as those described for a precipitous delivery of an infant in vertex presentation.

Usually no harm results from a precipitous delivery. Every effort should be made, however, to prevent its occurrence. In such births the advantages of antisepsis and asepsis are largely lost. There is greater risk of injury to the maternal tissues and of aspiration and injury to the infant. All patients should be evaluated frequently for progress during labor. Signs of the approach of the second stage of labor should not be ignored.

Induction of Labor

Occasionally, medical indications for artificially stimulating uterine contractions before the onset of spontaneous labor may arise. Indications for an induction of labor may include: (1) pre-existing maternal disease (e.g., diabetes mellitus, pregnancy induced hypertension, heart disease), (2) premature rupture of the membranes after 37 weeks' gestation without spontaneous onset of contractions, (3) chorioamnionitis, (4) postmaturity (pregnancy of 42 weeks' gestation or more), (5) suspected fetal jeopardy (e.g., intrauterine growth retardation, nonreassuring fetal testing, fetal hemolytic disease), or (6) fetal death without labor onset. Occasionally the risk of rapid labor or difficulty getting to the birthing center may also be indications for induction. Induction planned for the convenience of the patient or the physician is not considered valid (American College of Obstetricians and Gynecologists, 1991).

Methods and nursing care

Labor can be induced by artificial rupture of membranes or, more often, by IV administration of the synthetic pituitary hormone oxytocin (Pitocin). If the cervix is favorable (soft, effaced 50%, dilated 2 cm or more, anterior position), and the vertex is engaged, the likelihood of success is high (NAACOG, 1988). If the cervix is not favorable the physician may elect to prepare or "ripen" it so that it will be more likely to respond to oxytocin. The application of prostaglandin E_2 gel (PGE_2) within the cervical canal or intravaginally, as close to the cervix as possible, is usually effective in ripening the cervix (Miller and Lorkovic, 1993). At times, the application of PGE_2 alone may initiate labor. See the nursing alert at right.

If the membranes are artificially ruptured and labor does not begin within 24 hours, increased possibility of infection exists and the physician or nurse midwife may elect to stimulate the labor with IV oxytocin. Whether or not the membranes are ruptured, the procedure for induction of labor with oxytocin is the same. A primary IV infusion is established. The oxytocic Pitocin (usually 10 units per 1000 ml of Ringer's Solution) is given per infusion pump by a secondary line. This piggyback set-up allows the nurse to discontinue the uterine stimulation if necessary, while still maintaining access to the vein. The current recommended starting dose of Pitocin is 0.5 to 1 mU per minute. The nurse gradually increases the dose in increments of 1 to 2 mU per minute at 30- to 60-minute intervals until an optimal labor pattern is reached (contractions every 2 to 3 minutes, duration of 40 to 90 seconds, an intensity of 40 to 90 mm Hg intrauterine pressure, and resting uterine tone of less than 20 mm Hg) (Brodsky and Pelzar, 1991). Once the woman's cervix is 5 to 6 cm dilated and the labor pattern is good, the rate of the oxytocin infusion may gradually be decreased. Before the introduction of oxytocin, a baseline FHR strip should be obtained. Once the oxytocin infusion has begun, the labor should be electronically monitored and the FHR, frequency, duration, and intensity of contractions, and uterine resting tone evaluated and documented (usually every 15 minutes). Maternal blood pressure should also be evaluated at 30- to 60-minute intervals—whenever the dosage is evaluated.

> **Nursing Alert**
>
> The Food and Drug Administration has approved the use of intracervical application, but not yet intravaginal application, of PGE_2. Informed consent is necessary for this procedure.

The greatest risk from oxytocin administration is the possibility of uterine hyperstimulation. The nurse monitoring the labor must be familiar with the effects of oxytocin and able to identify both maternal and fetal complications. Uterine contractions lasting more than 90 seconds or occurring more frequently than every 2 minutes, exaggerated contraction intensity and resting uterine tone, and/or non-reassuring FHR patterns call for the oxytocin infusion to be stopped immediately (NAACOG, 1988). The health care provider should be notified and the woman reevaluated. In the case of non-reassuring FHR patterns the nurse should also place the woman in a lateral semirecumbent position and administer oxygen at 8 to 10 liters per minute. Unit protocols regarding use of oxytocin for induction need to be determined and followed. The physician should be readily available in the event of problems.

Cesarean Birth

With the decreasing risk involved in the performance of cesarean birth (removal of the child through incisions in the abdominal and uterine walls), the operation is used more frequently in modern obstetrics. Cesarean rates vary considerably from hospital to hospital, but the current rate is approximately 20% of births (Tighe and Sweezy, 1990). The rise in cesarean births has been attributed to (1) a more aggressive approach to poor progress in labor, (2) an increased tendency to use cesarean for all breech births, (3) a rise in repeat cesarean births, and (4) the medical malpractice climate. Electronic fetal monitoring may also be a factor (Afriat, 1990). High cesarean rates have come under scrutiny from consumers and the insurance industry.

The most common reason for cesarean birth in the United States has been a previous cesarean birth. Currently more physicians are less reluctant to consider a trial of labor and vaginal birth if the reasons for the former cesarean birth do not persist, if the mother so wishes, and if the previous uterine incision was not vertical. If these conditions exist, research indicates that vaginal birth after cesarean (VBAC) is a safe alternative to a repeat cesarean section (Afriat, 1990). The mother may choose, however, to have a repeat cesarean.

Needless to say, a mother entering the hospital for a repeat cesarean is usually not enduring the stress of an unexpected surgery hastily arranged because of an obstetrical complication. However, an emergency cesarean is sometimes indicated because of conditions such as abruptio placentae, placenta previa, fetal-pelvic disproportion, abnormal presentations, a prolapsed umbilical cord, uterine inertia (failure of the uterus to contract sufficiently to continue progress in labor), or signs of fetal distress. Conditions that indicate acute fetal distress or maternal jeopardy demand the prompt and rapid preparation of the patient once the condition has been discovered and the course of action determined. A patient who has an emergency cesarean delivery is subjected to many procedures in the space of a few minutes. Everything should be done as calmly and quickly as possible. Patient teaching and support must be done at the same time the nurse is preparing the patient for the operating room. The patient and her family will probably be frightened.

As much as is possible the woman and her partner should be informed about the usual sequence of events, sensations she will experience, and how the health care team will assist them to cope with the stressors and to participate in the birth (Tighe and Sweezy, 1990). The nurse should not lose sight of the fact that a cesarean birth is a birth. Women wish to have family present and hold the infant as soon as possible. Many women feel disappointed or that they have failed when a cesarean birth is necessary (Fawcett, Pollio, and Tully, 1992). The sensitive nurse, however, can do much to enable the parents to have a positive birth experience.

Preparation for cesarean birth

The following procedures are routinely carried out in preparation of the surgery. Some may be done in the labor room, whereas others take place in the operating room.

1. Signing of the operative permit by the patient or responsible party
2. Blood type, crossmatch, and hemoglobin determination
3. Removal of any hairpins or hard objects from the hair; application of a surgical cap; removal of cosmetics, and any jewelry, glasses, contact lenses, etc, to be given to the family; taping of wedding and engagement rings to the fingers without impeding circulation
4. Removal and safekeeping of any dentures
5. Preoperative medications as ordered
6. Preoperative assessment by anesthesiologist
7. IV infusion if one is not already in place
8. NPO status
9. An abdominal-perineal prep, which starts at the nipple line and includes the entire abdomen from side to side as well as the perineal area visible when the legs are parallel—sometimes done in the operating room
10. Insertion of an indwelling catheter—sometimes done in the operating room after anesthesia

Removal of nail polish so that nailbeds may be checked for cyanosis is infrequently done because of the increasing availability of the oximeter, the vogue of artificial nails, and the recognition that nail cyanosis is a relatively late sign of poor oxygenation. Patients may be transferred to an operating room suite for surgery, or a delivery room may be prepared for the procedure. During all of the busy preparations, family members should not be forgotten. Provisions should be made for them to wait in as much mental and physical comfort as possible. Many hospitals permit the father or designated support person to stay with the mother during the birth, providing general anesthesia is not used. In many areas, classes are now available to parents anticipating or interested in cesarean birth.

Twins or Multiple Births

Multiple pregnancies have a much higher perinatal mortality rate than do singleton pregnancies. The high rates of prematurity and intrauterine-growth retardation in multiple gestation are also associated with significant neonatal morbidity (Creasy and Resnik, 1994). Approximately 54% of twins are premature, and the risk of intracranial hemorrhage, developmental respiratory distress syndrome, and other neonatal difficulties is relatively high. Mortality for a second-born twin is approximately three times higher than it is for the first-born sibling, probably because of a greater incidence of malpresentations. Thus the nursery should be alerted when a twin birth is anticipated. With the increased use of prenatal ultrasound, multiple birth "surprises" are less likely than they used to be.

Maternal complications are also greater in multiple pregnancy. Mothers of twins are more likely to suffer from hyperemesis gravidarum (excessive nausea and vomiting), pregnancy induced hypertension, anemia, polyhydramnios (excessive amniotic fluid), and placenta previa. Greater distention of the uterus makes these women more often victims of preterm labor and postpartum hemorrhage.

Preparation for multiple birth. Depending on the presentations of the fetuses, the gestational age, and the presence of maternal complications, multiple births may be vaginal or cesarean. In almost one half of all twin births, both infants are cephalic presentations. Any combination of presentations and positions, however, may exist. When twins are expected, two sets of identification should be ready with double newborn record sheets. Two sterile, infant receiving blankets, two cord clamps, two aspirator bulbs, and two sets of emergency resuscitation equipment should be available. Physicians and nurses experienced in treating small or premature infants should be present for the delivery.

KEY CONCEPTS

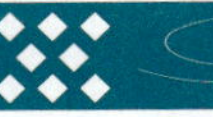

1 Couples seek alternatives to traditional hospital births for various reasons, including the following: a desire for a more relaxed atmosphere and flexible policies that allow family participation, a wish for a birth with less medical intervention, a desire to have the newborn near at hand, and the high cost of hospitalization.

2 Alternatives to traditional hospital birth include the following: home birth, birthing rooms or alternative birth centers (ABCs), and single room maternity care (LDR or LDRP).

3 Impending labor is signaled by lightening, Braxton Hicks contractions, gastrointestinal upsets, a burst of energy, bloody show, and/or a ruptured bag of waters.

4 The woman in labor should be instructed to go to the hospital if the bag of waters ruptures, vaginal bleeding or bloody show exists, and/or uterine contractions are regular and frequent. Other factors to consider are the distance she must travel, how many children she has had, and the history of her previous labors.

5 On admission the nurse must assess the status of the labor contractions, determine if membranes are ruptured, and evaluate the presence of bloody show, cervical dilation, effacement, fetal station, position, and presentation, as well as the woman's perception of her pain and her coping abilities.

6 Uterine contractions are timed to help determine the progress of labor, to detect abnormalities, to help detect fetal distress, and to reassure the patient and family.

7 Normal baseline fetal heart rate (FHR) is 120 to 160 beats per minute.

8 Baseline FHR variability is an important parameter of fetal well-being. Diminished long-term and short-term variability may be an indicator of fetal distress or drug administration to the mother. Diminished long-term (but not short-term) variability is also associated with short periods of fetal sleep.

9 Three types of FHR decelerations may be detected by continuous monitoring devices. Early decelerations have a smooth shape, start at the onset of a contraction, and end when the contraction ends. They indicate fetal head compression and are benign. Late deceleration patterns are characterized by a smooth shape, slowing of the FHR after the peak of the contraction, and by a delayed return to baseline. They suggest uteroplacental insufficiency and are ominous. Variable deceleration patterns are characterized by a periodical, unpredictable slowing of the FHR that shows neither a consistent sequential relationship to the contractions nor a regular repetitive range or duration. They indicate umbilical cord compression and may be mild or severe.

10 The monitor strip is a legal part of the patient record and should be frequently evaluated. Care should be documented directly on the strip.

11 Signs of possible fetal distress during labor include the passage of meconium-stained amniotic fluid when the infant is in the cephalic position, sudden exaggerated fetal movement, diminished long- and short-term baseline FHR variability, FHR tachycardia or bradycardia, and late or variable deceleration patterns. A combination of any of these factors indicates greater distress than any one singly.

12 Several techniques make use of breathing patterns and relaxation as a method to help women cope with the discomfort of labor.

13 The first stage of labor is characterized by three classic periods: early labor (0 to 4 cm cervical dilation), mid or active labor (4 to 8 cm dilation), and transition (8 to 10 cm dilation).

14 When the membranes rupture the nurse should do the following: check the FHR; inspect the perineum for signs of a prolapsed cord, the advance of the presenting part, and the amount and color of the amniotic fluid; give perineal care; and report that the membranes have ruptured.

15 During a vaginal examination the nurse prepares and assists the patient and helps her to relax.

16 Indications of the onset of the second stage of labor include the following: an increase in bloody show; an involuntary urge to push with each contraction; the fetal heart tone is heard just above the pubic

bone in cephalic presentations; and late signs that include bulging of the perineum, dilation of the anus, and appearance of the fetal scalp.

17 To properly prepare the delivery room for birth the nurse must understand the principles of aseptic technique, know where supplies are located, and be aware of the patient's special needs and the health care provider's specific requirements.

18 In preparation for delivery the nurse assists with transferring the woman to the delivery room (in traditional settings), positioning her, and cleansing the perineal area.

19 Forceps, which are sometimes used to lift out the infant's head, are usually applied in conjunction with an episiotomy, although an episiotomy may be performed when forceps are not used. Vacuum extraction may be preferred over forceps.

20 Immediately after birth the nurse must assist in establishing and maintaining newborn respirations, provide warmth for the infant, perform a brief physical assessment, and identify the infant per hospital policy.

21 Using the Apgar score, the newborn's heart rate, respiratory effort, muscle tone, reflex irritability, and color are recorded 1 and 5 minutes after birth. Infants receiving a score of 7 to 10 are considered vigorous; scores of 4 to 6 denote mild-to-moderate depression; and a score of 3 or less indicates severe depression.

22 Lacerations of the perineum are described as first, second, third, and fourth degree. First-degree lacerations involve a tear in only the mucous membrane and skin, and are usually of no permanent consequence. Second-degree lacerations include a tear into the muscles of the perineal body, and usually heal well if adequately repaired. Third-degree lacerations involve the circular anal sphincter muscle and may result in permanent damage. Fourth-degree lacerations also involve the rectovaginal wall.

23 Parent-infant attachment may be promoted by maternal-infant skin-to-skin contact immediately after birth, delaying eye prophylaxis and dimming the room lights to help the parents relate to a more responsive newborn, and facilitating breastfeeding shortly after birth.

24 If precipitous delivery is imminent the nurse should remain calm, reassuring, and do the following: turn on the call light, guide the emerging head, break the bag of waters (if not already ruptured), make sure the cord is not around the infant's neck, clear the infant's airway, help deliver the body, and dry off and wrap the infant in a towel or blanket.

25 Indications for induction of labor include the following: preexisting maternal disease, premature rupture of the membranes after 37 weeks' gestation without spontaneous onset of contractions, chorioamnionitis, postmaturity, suspected fetal jeopardy, and fetal death without onset of labor.

26 Preparation for emergency, cesarean birth should include the following: signing of the operative permit; abdominal-perineal prep; insertion of an indwelling catheter; blood type, crossmatch, and hemoglobin determination; removal of hairpins, cosmetics, jewelry, glasses, dentures, and the like; application of a surgical cap; preoperative medications; and as much patient teaching as possible.

27 Complications that may be associated with breech birth include the following: longer labor, prolapse of the umbilical cord, aspiration of vaginal secretions, difficulty in extracting the arms or head, and entrapment of the fetal head.

28 In preparation for the delivery of twins, two of each of the following should be readied: identification sets, record sheets, receiving blankets, cord clamps, aspiration bulbs, and emergency resuscitation equipment.

29 Mothers of twins (or other multiples) are more likely to suffer from hyperemesis gravidarum, pregnancy induced hypertension, polyhydramnios, placenta previa, preterm labor, and postpartum hemorrhage.

30 Twins (and other multiples) have a higher mortality and morbidity rate than do single infants.

CRITICAL THOUGHT QUESTIONS

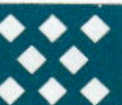

1 You are working in a prenatal clinic. Ellen Jackson is 38 weeks pregnant with her second child and has had an uncomplicated pregnancy. Her first labor was approximately 8 hours in length. She lives 30 minutes from the birth center. What signs of impending labor would you discuss with her? How will you explain the difference between true and false labor? At what point in her labor would you suggest she leave for the birth center?

2 Modern obstetrical care has changed dramatically in the past few years. Locate individuals who gave birth within the past few months, 5 years ago, 10

years ago, and 20 years ago (or more). What are the differences apparent in preparation for childbirth, physical care in labor (such as enemas, perineal preps, and so on), delivery/birthing rooms, presence of significant others, length of hospital stay and any other areas that you feel are significant?

3 Janet Etcheson is in very active labor. Her boyfriend is with her and has been actively coaching her. She suddenly tells him, in a very irritable tone, not to touch her. He seems bewildered by her behavior and retreats to a chair in the corner. What is the likely reason for this change in her behavior? As the nurse what would you do to assist him in his role as labor coach?

4 You are monitoring a patient in labor and everything appears to be progressing normally. Suddenly the FHR begins to decrease. What action would you take first? Next? Explain your reasons.

5 Your neighbor is pregnant with her third child. On your day off she calls you and excitedly tells you that her bag of waters has just broken and her contractions are one on top of the other. Her husband has taken the other children to their grandmother's and she is alone. When you arrive, you ascertain that she is in the second stage of labor, frightened, and trying to resist the urge to push. How would you proceed? Give your reasons for your actions.

REFERENCES

Afriat C: Vaginal birth after cesarean section: a review of the literature, *J Perinat Neonatal Nurs* 3(3):1-13, 1990.

American College of Obstetricians and Gynecologists: *Induction and augmentation of labor,* Technical Bulletin No. 157, Washington, DC, 1991, The College.

American Academy of Pediatrics and American College of Obstetricians and Gynecologists: *Guidelines for Perinatal Care,* ed 3, Washington, DC, 1992, The Academy and The College.

Campbell SJ: New use for the APGAR name, *Point of view/Ethicon* 17:6, 1980.

Chez BF, Verklan MT: Documentation and electronic fetal monitoring: how, where, and what? *J Perinat Neonatal Nurs* 1(1):11-28, 1987.

Creasy RK, Resnik R: *Maternal-fetal medicine,* ed 3, Philadelphia, 1994, WB Saunders.

Fawcett J, Pollio N, Tully A: Women's perceptions of cesarean and vaginal delivery: another look, *Research in Nursing & Health* 15(6):439-446.

Freeman R: Intrapartum fetal monitoring—a disappointing story, *New Engl J Med* 322(9):625, 1990.

Harvey CJ: Fetal scalp stimulation: enhancing the interpretation of fetal monitor tracings, *J Perinat Neonatal Nurs* 1(1):13-21, 1987.

Haubrich KL: Amnioinfusion: A technique for the relief of variable deceleration, *J Obstet Gynecol Neonatal Nurs* 19(4):299-303, 1990.

Leboyer F: *Birth without violence,* New York, 1976, Knopf.

Machol L: Single-room maternity care gains converts, *Contemp OB/GYN* 34(5)62, 1989.

Miller AM, Lorkovic M: Prostaglandin E_2 for cervical ripening, *MCN* Special Supplement, Sept/Oct:23-30, 1993.

Nurses Association of the American College of Obstetricians and Gynecologists: *The nurse's role in the induction/augmentation of labor: OGN nursing practice resource,* Washington, DC, 1988, The Association.

Nurses Association of the American College of Obstetricians and Gynecologists: *Fetal heart rate auscultation: OGN nursing practice resource,* Washington, DC, 1990, The Association.

Occupational Safety and Health Administration (OSHA): Bloodborne pathogens standard—29–CFR-1910. 1030. *The federal register,* December 6, 1991.

Phillips CRN: Neonatal heat loss in heated cribs vs mother's arms, *J Obstet Gynecol Neonatal Nurs* 3:11, 1974.

Simpson D: Examining the episiotomy argument, *Midwife Health Visit Commun Nurse* 24(1):6, 1988.

Tighe D, Sweezy SR: The perioperative experience of cesarean birth: preparation, considerations, and complications, *J Perinat Neonatal Nurs* 3(3):14-30, 1990.

Tucker SM: *Pocket guide to fetal monitoring,* St. Louis, 1992, Mosby.

Wuitchik M, Hesson K, Bakal DA: Perinatal predictors of pain and distress during labor, *Birth* 17(4):186-191, 1990.

BIBLIOGRAPHY

Chapman LL: Expectant fathers' roles during labor and birth, *J Obstet Gynecol Neonatal Nurs* 21(2):114-120, 1992.

Griese ME, Prickett SA: Nursing management of umbilical cord prolapse, *J Obstet Gynecol Neonatal Nurs* 22(4):311-315, 1992.

McKay S, Barrows T: Holding back: maternal readiness to give birth, *MCN* 16(5):251-254, 1991.

Penny DS, Perlis DS: Shoulder dystocia: when to use suprapubic or fundal pressure, *MCN* 17(1):34-36, 1992.

Reichert JA, Baron M, Fawcett J: Changes in attitudes toward cesarean birth, *J Obstet Gynecol Neonatal Nurs* 22(2):159-167, 1993.

Snydal SH: Responses of laboring women to fetal heart rate monitoring, *J Nurse-Midwifery* 33(5):208-216, 1988.

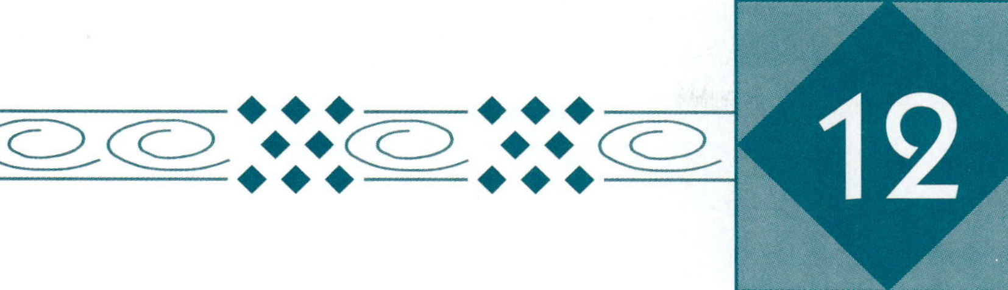

Pharmacological Pain Management

CHAPTER OBJECTIVES

After studying this chapter, the student should be able to:

1. Define the following terms: *analgesic, tranquilizer, hypnotic, agonist, amnesic,* and *anesthetic.*
2. Indicate at least three factors that influence the timing and dosage of analgesia given during labor.
3. Name an analgesic commonly given during labor and indicate why it is often given with tranquilizers.
4. Differentiate between subarachnoid (spinal or saddle) and epidural regional anesthesias in timing of administration, effect on the patient, possible complications, and nursing care.
5. Describe indications for the use of local anesthesia and pudendal block for the alleviation of pain. Explain their safety and effectiveness.

METHODS OF PAIN RELIEF

The subject of modern childbirth would be incomplete without a discussion of the pharmacological methods most commonly used to make the experience of labor and birth easier and more comfortable for the mother. Nonpharmacological methods are discussed in Chapters 9 and 11.

The following definitions will be useful in the discussion of pain-relieving drugs and procedures:

agonist A drug that stimulates a cell receptor site and produces a physiological activity.

antagonist A drug that stimulates a cell receptor site and prevents or reverses a specific physiological activity.

amnesic A technique or medication that causes memory loss of varying degrees.

analgesic A technique or medication that reduces or eliminates pain.

anesthetic A technique or medication that partially or completely eliminates sensation or feeling. It may be a nerve-blocking type (local or regional anesthesia) or a sleep-producing type (general anesthesia).

hypnotic A technique or medication that causes sleep.

tranquilizer A technique or medication that relieves anxiety and quiets the patient.

Labor Discomfort

The nurse should have a basic understanding of the physiological origin of discomfort in labor. Labor discomfort results partly from intermittent muscular contractions of the uterine fundus and the stretching of muscle fibers of the cervix, lower uterine segment, and vagina. Pain during the first stage of labor is carried by the T10 through L1 spinal segments. Pain during the

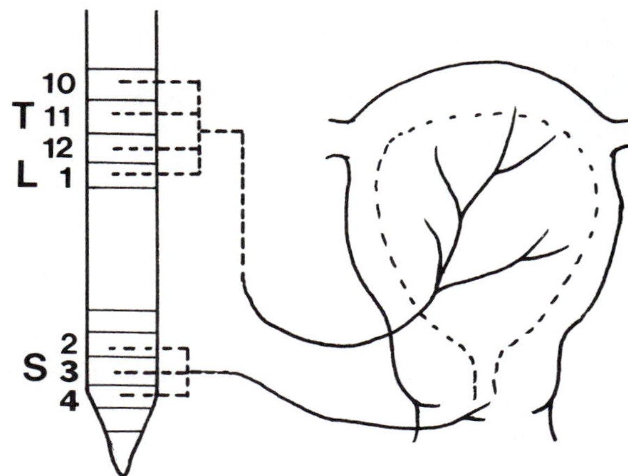

Fig. 12-1 Pain pathways for the first and second stages of labor. (From Datta S: *The obstetric anesthesia handbook,* St. Louis, 1992, Mosby.)

second stage of labor is carried by the S2, S3, and S4 spinal segments (Fig. 12-1). The amount of painful stimuli produced is also influenced by the individual woman's pelvic anatomy; the size and flexion of the fetal head; the strength, duration, and frequency of uterine contractions; and the presence or absence of obstetrical deviations or complications.

A person's pain threshold may also be significantly altered by the level of available endorphins, morphine-like hormonal substances in the body. These special proteins appear to interfere with the transmission of pain-producing impulses to the brain or the brain's sensitivity to those impulses. The endorphin level falls in the presence of anxiety, tension, fatigue, or extended negative stimuli. This phenomenon may offer a physiological basis for the woman's perception of pain. Her resulting behavior is greatly influenced by her interpretation of what is occurring, the childbirth education she has received, her cultural background, and the emotional support she gains from those around her.

Therefore methods of pain relief during labor and birth involve more than the administration of drugs. Pain relief also includes ways of helping the laboring woman understand the process of childbirth and to consciously cooperate with what her body is trying to accomplish. A clean, calm, attractive environment, techniques of relaxation, application of counterpressure to the mother's lower back, position changes, close supervision and encouragement from a concerned nursing staff and health care provider, and the companionship of those she loves will help decrease the need for administration of analgesic and anesthetic medications.

The pharmacological method of pain relief used depends on the woman's special needs and wishes, the preference of the health care provider, and the availability of someone with the expertise and willingness to use the selected method. Consideration of risks versus benefits and financial constraints should be incorporated in the selection process. The health care provider should review pain relief options with the family before labor. During labor the health care provider or anesthesiologist must obtain informed consent before ordering or administering an analgesic or anesthetic agent. The nurse can assist the family in making an informed decision by clarifying and describing the medications or procedures under consideration. The box above outlines the types of analgesia and anesthesia used in the first and second stages of labor.

PHARMACOLOGICAL METHODS BY STAGE OF LABOR AND TYPE OF BIRTH

FIRST STAGE
Systemic Analgesia
- Narcotics
- Agonist-antagonists
- Tranquilizers (potentiators)

Regional Analgesia/Anesthesia
- Lumbar epidural block
- Paracervical (rare)
- Inhalation (self-administered) (rare)

SECOND STAGE (VAGINAL BIRTH)
Regional Analgesia/Anesthesia
- Local infiltration
- Pudendal block
- Subarachnoid (spinal) block
- Lumbar epidural block
- Epidural and spinal narcotics
- Inhalation (self-administered)

SECOND STAGE (CESAREAN BIRTH)
Regional Anesthesia
- Subarachnoid (spinal) block
- Epidural block
- Epidural and spinal narcotics

General Anesthesia

Obstetrical Analgesia (First and Second Stages of Labor)

The prescription and administration of analgesic drugs during the first stage of labor must be carefully considered and performed, since the health care provider is caring for two patients. Systemic analgesics cross the maternal blood-brain barrier and the placental barrier, resulting in a hypnotic effect not only on the mother but also on her fetus. The choice of drug, dosage, and timing must be considered so that the baby will not be too sleepy to breathe on its own at the time of birth. Before birth, sleepiness of the fetus is not crucial, since the fetus does not have to breathe; the fetus receives oxygen from the mother. After birth, however, the maternal oxygen supply is no longer available. Failure of the newborn to breathe adequately is called *asphyxia neonatorum.* It can be treated by artificial ventilation or a narcotic-reversal drug called *naloxone.*

Fetal maturity must also be considered when selecting pharmaceutical methods of pain relief. If a premature birth is expected the mother is encouraged to continue her labor with a minimum amount of systemic analgesia. The premature infant does not detoxify drugs well and may exhibit respiratory depression at birth. Even a full-term newborn may have difficulty detoxifying large amounts of systemic analgesics. See the Nursing Alert at right.

Another consideration in the administration of systemic, inhalation, or regional analgesic or anesthetic drugs during the first stage of labor is the possible effect of the medication on the progress of labor. Given too soon during the latent phase, many analgesics and anesthetics may unnecessarily slow down or even stop contractions. This problem makes most health care providers reluctant to give any drug before the contractions are strong, frequent, and regular; the cervix is thinning; the fetal head is descending; or the woman is receiving oxytocin (Pitocin) for augmentation or induction of her labor.

Systemic analgesics

Two groups of systemic analgesic drugs exist that are given to women in labor. One is the narcotic agonist group, including meperidine and fentanyl. The other is the agonist-antagonist group, including butorphanol and nalbuphine.

Merperidine (Demerol) is one narcotic that is commonly used in labor. It can be given either intravenously (dosage 25 to 50 mg; onset in less than 1 minute, peak effect within 5 to 20 minutes) or intramuscularly (dosage 50 to 100 mg; onset within 1 to 5 minutes, peak effect within 30 to 50 minutes). For either method of administration the effect duration is 2 to 4 hours. Meperidine produces respiratory depressing active metabolites (breakdown products which have activity of their own) that may be difficult for the newborn to metabolize. Regardless of the mode of administration, less neonatal respiratory depression results if the birth occurs less than 1 hour or more than 4 hours after administration of meperidine.

> **Nursing Alert**
>
> Labor nurses should inform nursery and postpartum nurses of the type, level, and timing of analgesia and anesthesia used in labor and delivery.

Fentanyl (Sublimaze) is a newer, shorter-acting narcotic that is beginning to be used in labor. It is usually given intravenously (dosage 50 to 100 μ; onset in less than 30 seconds; peak effect within 5 to 15 minutes; duration of 30 to 60 minutes). Although no active metabolites from fentanyl exist the best time for delivery is less than 10 minutes or more than 30 minutes after fentanyl administration. Fentanyl can also be used in a "patient-controlled analgesia" infusion device, where the woman controls the amount of analgesia she needs within preset limits.

Agonist-antagonist systemic drugs, such as butorphanol and nalbuphine, prevent or reverse the analgesic and the unwanted side effects of narcotics. They have some limited analgesic effects of their own and limited respiratory depressant effects on the newborn.

Butorphanol (Stadol) is usually given intravenously (dosage ½ to 2 mg; onset within 1 to 5 minutes; peak effect within 5 to 10 minutes; duration of 2 to 4 hours). Butorphanol frequently causes sedation and may cause euphoria (a sense of well-being), dysphoria (a sense of malaise), or hallucinations. It may also interfere with the analgesic effects of subsequent spinal or epidural narcotics.

Nalbuphine (Nubain) is usually given intravenously (dosage 5 to 10 mg; onset within 2 to 3 minutes; peak effect within 5 to 10 minutes; duration of 3 to 6 hours). It causes less sedation and dysphoria than butorphanol. Like butorphanol it may interfere with the analgesic effects of subsequent spinal or epidural narcotics. It is frequently used as an intravenous infusion to counteract undesirable side effects of spinal or epidural narcotics.

Systemic analgesics are frequently given in combination with a tranquilizer such as promethazine (Phenergan) or hydroxyzine (Vistaril). These combinations are more effective because they increase the analgesic effect of other drugs and counteract the nausea and itching often associated with the narcotic. Promethazine may be given intramuscularly (dosage of 25 to 50 mg; onset within 15 to 30 minutes) or intravenously (dosage of 12½ to 50 mg; onset within 2 to 5 minutes). Hydroxyzine is only given intramuscularly (dosage of 25 to 50 mg; onset within 15 to 30 minutes). The peak effect for both of these drugs when given intramuscularly is less than 2 hours and the duration is 2 to 6 hours.

Many systemic drugs, such as analgesics or tranquilizers, will decrease the beat-to-beat variability of the fetal heart rate for a period of time, during which the usefulness of this method of fetal monitoring is reduced.

Narcotic antagonists

Antagonistic medications such as naloxone hydrochloride (Narcan) are available to counteract the depressive action of narcotic agonists or narcotic agonist/antagonists on the mother and the newborn infant. Naloxone may be given to the mother intravenously or intramuscularly to counteract her respiratory depression or the anticipated respiratory depression in the newborn (titration dose 0.1 to 2 mg every 2 minutes up to 0.4 to 10 mg; onset intravenously is 1 to 2 minutes, intramuscularly is 2 to 5 minutes; peak within 5 to 15 minutes; duration of 1 to 4 hours). Since the drug reverses the effect of the narcotic the mother will experience a return of her discomfort. It can also be given to the newborn through the umbilical vein or intramuscularly in the thigh (dosage of 0.1 mg/kg). It has no known detrimental action in newborns except when used to treat addicted newborns. In this case, it may precipitate acute withdrawal symptoms. A narcotic-dependent mother may also experience withdrawal symptoms if she receives a narcotic antagonist during labor. See the Nursing Alert at the right.

Inhalation analgesia

Intermittent, inhalation analgesia used in the latter portion of the first and during most of the second stages of labor, although rarely used in the United States, has had considerable popularity in certain areas of the world. The woman breathes anesthetic gases through a mask or a mouthpiece. When these gases are properly administered in low concentrations the woman does not become unconscious but experiences a reduction in discomfort. Nitrous oxide (laughing gas) may be self-administered by the patient using a specially designed dispenser. It may also be administered by an anesthesiologist or nurse-anesthetist using an anesthesia machine. It is important that such analgesia does not become anesthetic in depth, since regurgitation and aspiration (the inhalation of gastric contents into the lungs) can become a deadly complication. If self-administered the nurse should remain with the patient but never administer the gas for her. Instructions for the use of various types of gases and equipment must be carefully followed. When used in the second stage of labor, inhalation analgesia relieves the mother's pain but still allows her to bear down with her contractions. Inhalation analgesia usually does not provide sufficient relief for the entire second stage of labor. Often its analgesic effects are augmented by a pudendal block or infiltration of the perineum with a local anesthetic.

> **Nursing Alert**
>
> The nurse must carefully monitor the laboring woman and her fetus for the depressant effects of systemic analgesics. If narcotic agonists or agonist-antagonists are used during labor, a narcotic antagonist should be readily available for administration to the mother or newborn infant.

Obstetrical Anesthesia (First, Second, and Third Stages of Labor)

Anesthesia is the province of a trained physician, anesthesiologist, or nurse-anesthetist. Nurses should not attempt to function in this area without advanced training.

General anesthesia

General anesthesia is seldom used for uncomplicated births. Regional anesthetics are safer and allow parental participation in the birth process. However, when the condition of the fetus requires emergency cesarean birth or when rapid uterine relaxation is needed for obstetrical maneuvers, general anesthesia may be favored. It does not cause the maternal hypotension that sometimes accompanies regional conductive anesthetics and may be administered rapidly with good results.

Special considerations. When a general anesthetic is planned, it is important to know when the labor started and how recently the woman has eaten, because of the danger of aspiration, obstruction of the airway (asphyxiation), and pneumonia. The nurse should give the woman nothing by mouth unless it is ordered, since digestion slows during labor and recent meals may remain in the stomach. Even if a woman in labor has not eaten recently, her highly acidic, gastric secretions may still pose the threat of acid aspiration pneumonitis (Mendelson's syndrome). To counteract this possibility, some health care providers order oral administration of 15 to 30 ml of an antacid, such as sodium citrate (Bicitra), before receiving general anesthesia. Chilling the liquid antacid may increase its palatability. The nurse should be sure that contact lenses, chewing gum, and dentures are removed before administration of the anesthetic. A wedge should be placed under the woman's right hip to displace the uterus to the left, thereby preventing compression of the aorta and vena cava by the pregnant uterus. The compression of these vessels interferes with the circulation of the mother's blood and eventually reduces placental perfusion, depriving the fetus of oxygen. The resulting maternal hypotension, dizziness, pallor, and clamminess have been called the *aortocaval* or *supine hypotensive syndrome.*

During the period when a patient is being anesthetized (the period of induction), the delivery room should be as quiet as possible to make the induction smooth and without patient distraction. Undue confusion and noise should also be avoided at the time of emergence.

Thiopental (Pentothal) produces a rapid induction by intravenous injection. If thiopental is given for only brief periods the brain of the fetus is bypassed and little neonatal depression is seen.

Propofol (Diprivan) is a newer, shorter-acting induction agent that has almost supplanted thiopental in the last few years. It works better in controlling the increase in blood pressure frequently associated with light, general anesthesia under thiopental. There is also no resulting neonatal depression with propofol.

Nitrous oxide is usually used in moderate concentrations before the delivery, and then in approximately 70% concentrations after delivery. It may have some depressant effects on the newborn, but the nitrous oxide is quickly eliminated through the lungs.

Halothan (Fluothane) and isoflurane (Forane) are anesthetic gases that are useful in producing rapid uterine relaxation when used in higher concentrations. In low concentrations, these gases can be used to decrease awareness during operative deliveries if a light general anesthetic is desired. Oxygen must always be mixed with gas anesthetics to supply the bodily needs of the mother and her unborn child (Fig. 12-2).

Ketamine hydrochloride (Ketaject), given by intravenous injection, produces rapid anesthesia and is used primarily for emergencies. It is useful when maternal blood pressure tends to be low. It should not be used with hypertensive patients. Ketamine hydrochloride may be associated with dreamlike episodes and hallucinations during emergence. Reduced stimulation during emergence is essential. It is usually given with a relaxant drug, such as diazepam (Valium) or midazolam (Versed), which decreases the unpleasant side effects of ketamine.

Since all anesthetics cross the placenta and, if given in sufficient concentration, produce symptoms in the infant, they should not be started soon before the expected birth. Usually general anesthesia is induced by an intravenous injection of a sleep dose of propofol (Diprivan) or thiopental (Pentothal) and a paralyzing dose of succinylcholine (Anectine). This procedure is followed by rapid placement of a cuffed endotracheal tube into the mother's trachea. The nurse may be asked to help at this time by pushing on the cricoid cartilage of the larynx (just below the "Adam's apple"). This helps close off the esophagus (Fig. 12-3). Both cricoid pressure and endotracheal intubation help prevent aspiration. The anesthesia is then maintained with nitrous oxide, oxygen, a muscle relaxant, and perhaps halothane. Once the baby is delivered, a narcotic and a tranquilizer are given intravenously to complete the anesthetic, oxytocin (Pitocin) is given to make the uterus contract, and an antibiotic is given to prevent infection. In case of vomiting the woman's head should be turned to the side and the emesis suctioned.

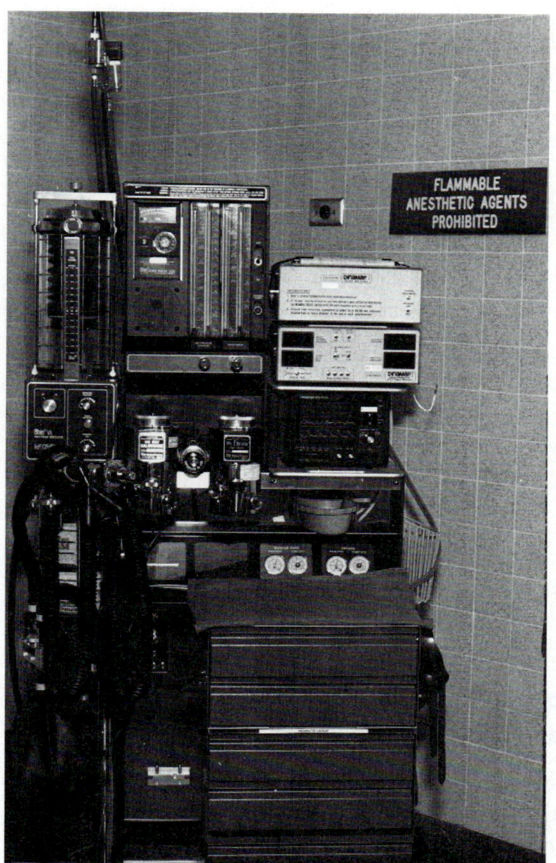

Fig. 12-2 General anesthesia machine capable of providing a number of gas anesthetics. Most hospitals no longer use flammable gases. (Courtesy Alex Pue, MD, Donald N. Sharp Memorial Community Hospital, San Diego, CA.)

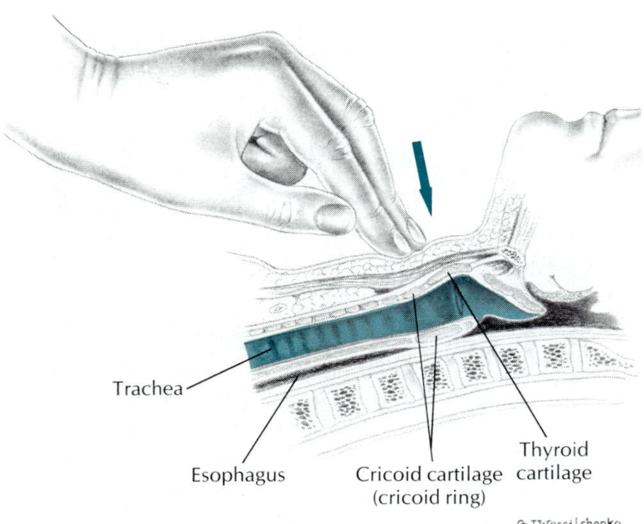

Fig. 12-3 Technique of applying pressure on cricoid cartilage. (From Bobak IM, Jensen MD: *Maternity and gynecologic care,* ed 5, St. Louis, 1992, Mosby.)

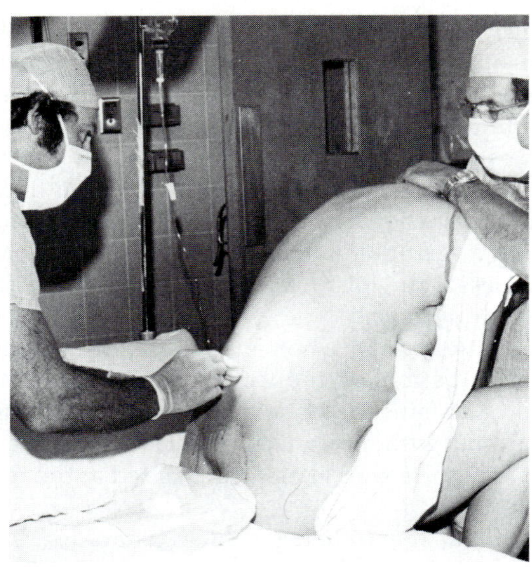

Fig. 12-4 Administration of subarachnoid (spinal or saddle) anesthetic. (Courtesy Grossmont Hospital, Martin M. Greenberg, MD, La Mesa, CA.)

Regional (conductive) analgesia/anesthesia

Regional or conductive anesthetics for labor and birth have become popular in recent years. They provide good pain relief and do not affect the central nervous system, thus the woman can be an active participant in the birth process. Neonatal effects result primarily from maternal hypotension that reduces placental perfusion, and rarely from maternal sensitivity to local anesthetics or narcotics used in regional anesthesia.

Subarachnoid block. The use of a subarachnoid block, commonly called a *spinal* or *saddle,* is often the choice for delivery, but not labor. The woman is hydrated with intravenous fluids before the injection of the anesthetic to decrease the potential for hypotension. The mother is supported in a sitting position on the edge of the delivery table or lies on her side with her curved back facing the administrator (Fig. 12-4). Next, a thin, sterile spinal needle (with or without a larger introducing needle) is inserted between the vertebrae at about the level of the iliac crests, below the level of the spinal cord. Its tip is placed in the subarachnoid space, which is identified by the appearance of cerebrospinal fluid dripping from the needle's hub (Fig. 12-5). Between contractions, an anesthetic that is heavier than the cerebrospinal fluid, such as lidocaine (Xylocaine), is injected into the subarachnoid space. The patient is then positioned on her back with a wedge under her right hip to displace the uterus to her left side. Her head and shoulders are elevated and her legs are positioned for delivery. After injection, maternal blood pressure, pulse, respirations, and fetal heart rate must be checked every 5 to 10 minutes.

Classically a saddle block is supposed to affect only those areas of the body that would be touched by a saddle if a person were riding a horse. In practice the anesthesia is usually more extensive. Low spinal anesthesia commonly numbs the abdominal and pelvic areas below the umbilicus, affecting the abdomen, perineum, legs, and feet. It takes effect immediately and gains maximum potency in 3 to 5 minutes. How long low spinal anesthesia lasts (1 to 3 hours) depends on the medication used. For cesarean birth a subarachnoid block that is designed to go higher (up to the nipples) is frequently used. Vertebral abnormalities or past back surgery can make some women bad candidates for spinal anesthetics. Sometimes a lack of time or qualified medical personnel precludes the use of this type of anesthetic.

The so-called spinal headache is a complication often feared by women. The actual incidence of spinal headache has been estimated as less than 5%, and is decreasing. The use of an intravenous infusion to promote better hydration of the patient and the use of the new thin, pencil-tipped spinal needles have significantly reduced the incidence and severity of spinal headaches. The conservative treatment of spinal headaches includes bedrest and increasing the woman's fluid and salt intake. The latter helps replenish spinal fluid volume. Occasionally, intravenous caffeine and abdominal binders are also used. The definitive treatment of the spinal headache is the epidural blood

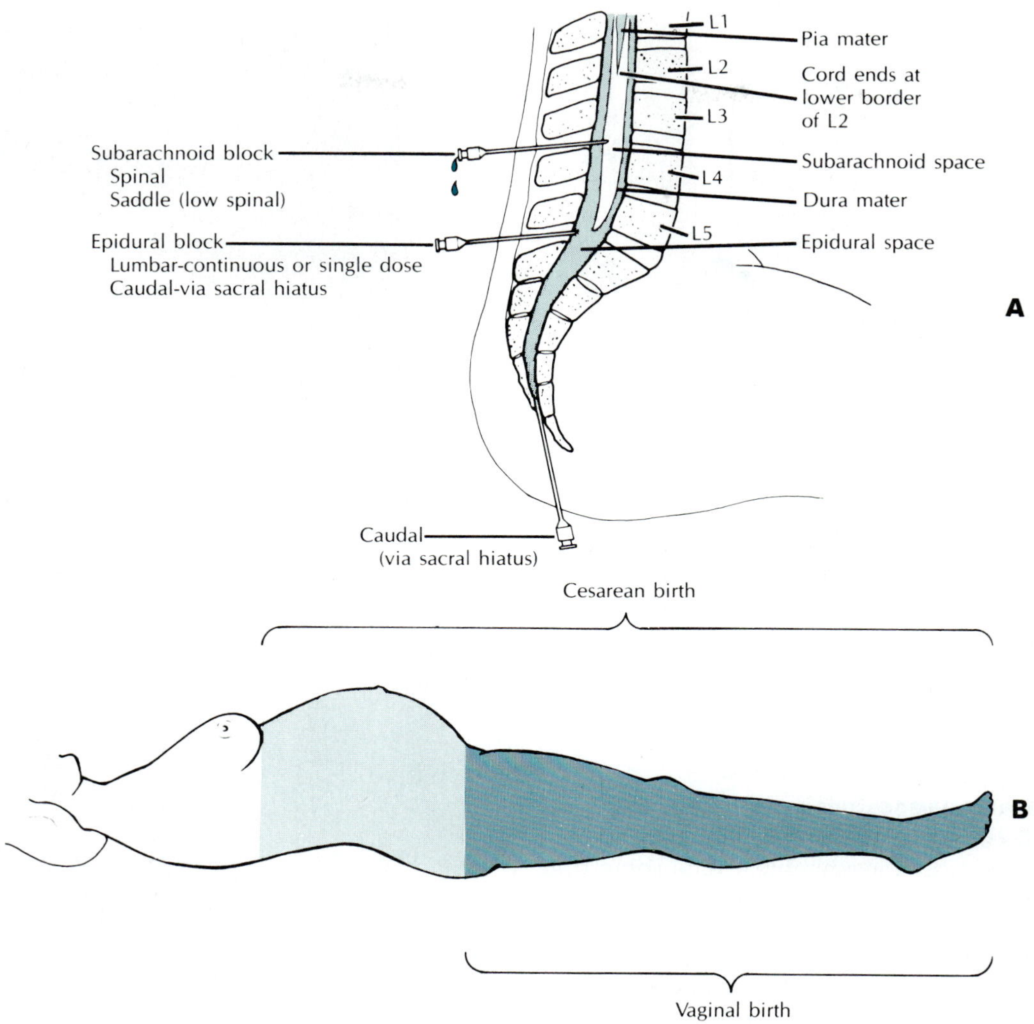

Fig. 12-5 A, Regional block analgesia and anesthesia in obstetrics. B, Level of anesthesia necessary for cesarean birth and for vaginal birth. (Courtesy Ross Laboratories, Columbus, OH.)

patch. In this procedure, 10 to 20 ml of sterile blood from the mother is placed in the epidural space at the site of the spinal, forming a clot to prevent further fluid loss (Fig. 12-6). This is an invasive procedure, however, and has the theoretical risk of infection and nerve damage. It is only used if conservative treatments do not work, or if little time exists for conservative treatments.

Subarachnoid block anesthesia does entail certain other inconveniences as well. During the procedure the mother must sit or lie curled up, with her back pushed out, and must not move. This is difficult to do during the second stage of labor, even with the support of an understanding nurse. Subarachnoid block anesthesia does not stop contractions, but the woman does not feel them and must be instructed when to bear down. She may find it difficult to push properly. Usually, outlet forceps or a vacuum extractor are used. On the other hand, a saddle block is frequently used to provide adequate anesthesia when a forceps or vacuum delivery is necessary. Occasionally, a woman's blood pressure may drop, possibly affecting the baby's oxygen supply, or the woman may have trouble breathing because of a high level of anesthesia. In the immediate postpartum period the woman may find it more difficult to void spontaneously. (See Chapter 13.)

Many practitioners believe that the positive aspects of subarachnoid anesthesia outweigh the negative aspects. The baby is not in danger of being put to sleep and of having a difficult time breathing at birth as a result of the anesthetic. The mother is awake for the birth of her baby. Regional anesthetics are safer than

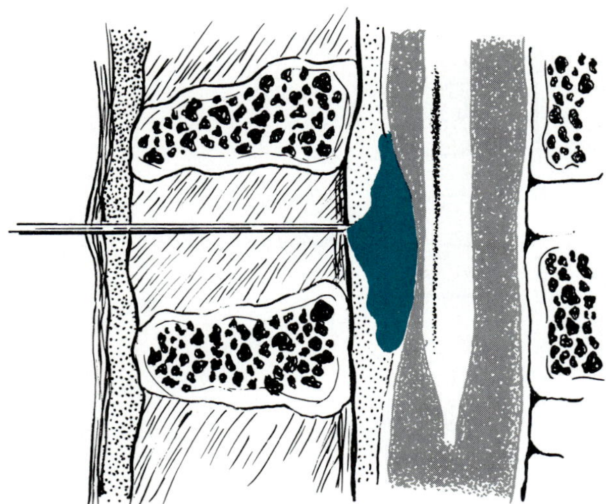

Fig. 12-6 Blood patch therapy for postspinal headache. (From Bobak IM, Jensen MD: *Maternity and gynecologic care,* ed 5, St. Louis, 1993, Mosby.)

gas anesthetics for obstetrical patients. Nausea and vomiting during and after use of regional anesthetics are minimal. The patient is awake and less likely to choke or aspirate, even if she does vomit.

Epidural analgesia/anesthesia. Other types of regional anesthetics are available for relief of both labor and delivery pain. In considerable vogue some time ago was continuous caudal anesthesia, or one-shot caudal (Fig. 12-5). This technique introduced local anesthetic agents into the epidural space of the sacral canal, where nerves travel outside the meninges or spinal cord coverings. This procedure is rarely used today.

Another kind of regional anesthesia, less difficult to administer than a caudal, is called a *lumbar epidural block.* As with a subarachnoid block the woman is hydrated with 500 to 1000 ml of IV fluids before the injection of anesthetic to reduce the risk of hypotension. The drug is then injected into the epidural space, usually between the second and third or the third and fourth lumbar vertebrae, while the mother lies on her side or is supported in a sitting position (Fig. 12-5). After careful identification of the desired location, a nylon or plastic catheter is threaded through the needle at the insertion site and the needle is removed. The catheter is carefully secured in position with tape (Fig. 12-7). After a small test dose, cautious instillation of the anesthetic is begun. Most commonly, a short acting narcotic such as fentanyl or sufentanyl is added to a more dilute solution of bupivacaine to achieve appropriate pain relief without excessive motor block during labor.

During the first stage of labor the dosages are adjusted to limit the block to the T10 and upper lumbar segments and to avoid interfering with the internal rotation of the fetal head. During the second stage of labor the block can be extended to the sacral area to allow perineal relaxation and episiotomy repair.

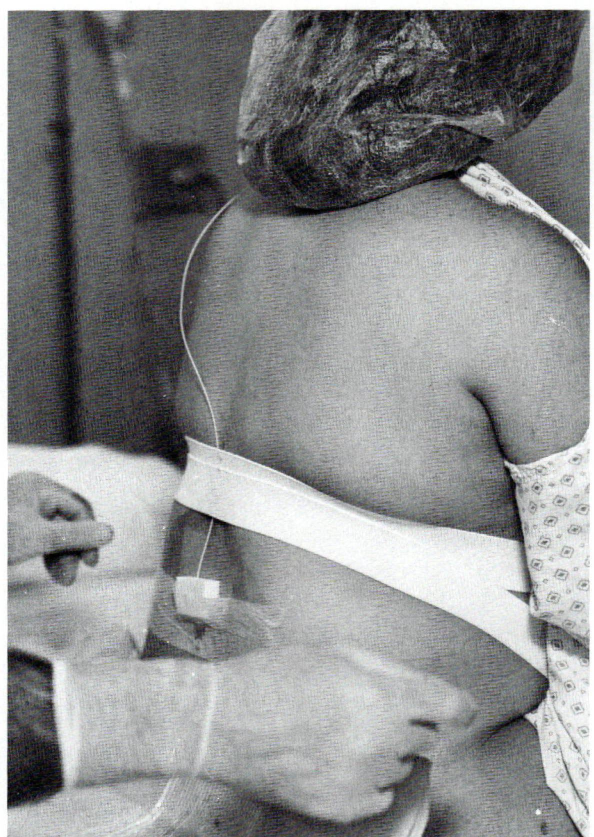

Fig. 12-7 The epidural catheter has just been inserted and is taped securely in place. The white belts help support the external fetal heart and contraction monitors. (Courtesy Alex Pue, MD, Donald N. Sharp Memorial Community Hospital, San Diego, CA.)

The woman should be informed about what she may experience during the initiation of the epidural. She may detect a burning or stinging sensation at the site of the injection of the local anesthesia before the insertion of the needle and cannula, local pressure during insertion, and a "crazy bone" feeling in her leg, hip, or back if the flexible catheter touches a nerve as it advances into the epidural space.

An expected, although not frequent, immediate side effect of an epidural is a drop in maternal blood pressure. This hypotension is caused by the epidural blocking sympathetic nerve fibers as they pass through the epidural space and go to the blood vessels in the lower body. For this reason the mother's blood pressure must be taken frequently for 10 to 30 minutes after each bolus of local anesthetic. See the Nursing Alert on p. 211.

Nursing Alert

To prevent supine hypotensive syndrome, laboring women should never be positioned flat on their backs. It is particularly important to avoid supine positioning when the woman receives epidural or spinal anesthesia, since these methods are also likely to cause hypotension. Maternal hypotension reduces placental perfusion and, thus, fetal oxygenation.

A rare complication of an epidural is the injection of the epidural medicine into the subarachnoid space, caused by unintentional penetration of the spinal sack (duramater). The larger amounts of anesthetic routinely used during epidural techniques could rapidly cause hypotension and dangerously high anesthesia levels, compromising respirations and maternal and fetal oxygen supplies. For this reason the mother should be watched for rapid pain reduction and loss of leg mobility in the first 5 minutes after each test dose. A dural puncture could also predispose the mother to spinal headache. (See the preceding discussion of subarachnoid block.)

Another rare complication associated with an epidural is the unintentional injection of the anesthetic into a blood vessel. The woman may indicate ringing in the ears, light-headedness, circumoral tingling or numbness, and the sudden recognition of a metallic taste. Convulsions may follow, at which time the woman is placed in a side-lying position, the airway is preserved, and oxygen is given. Diazepam (Valium), midazolam (Versed), propofol (Diprivan), or thiopental sodium (Pentothal) may be administered to stop the convulsions.

After the epidural anesthetic has been administered the woman may remain on her side with her head slightly raised for labor. If she is close to delivery, she may be assisted to a sitting position. These postures are assumed to help control the level of anesthesia and to prevent the weight of the uterus from compressing the maternal aorta and vena cava, causing hypotension and reduced placental perfusion. The nurse must always be alert for developing maternal hypotension. The anesthetic may be infused through the catheter in small continuous amounts using an infusion pump or given intermittently, whenever analgesic action lessens. Blood pressure and pulse are taken every 2 minutes for 10 to 15 minutes after the administration of each intermittent dose, then every 10 to 15 minutes until stable. In some situations, a patient-controlled epidural anesthetic may be used. In this case the woman pushes a special button and receives a small dose of epidural drug. The patient on a continuous infusion should have blood pressure and the ability to raise her leg checked every 30 minutes for the duration of the anesthetic. Usually pain relief begins within 10 minutes of injection. Full effect is obtained within 15 to 20 minutes. Many women will confirm sensations of abdominal or perineal pressure and note weakness or numbness in their legs (Taylor, 1993).

Contraindications to using an epidural anesthesia include patient or health care provider refusal, current anticoagulant therapy, the presence of hemorrhage or shock, septicemia or local infection in the area of the proposed injection, and various spinal problems.

Epidural techniques can be used to good advantage in the latter part of the first stage of labor and continued into the second and third stages. For a cesarean birth the effects of an epidural block may be extended by injecting more local anesthetic until the level of numbness is felt up to the nipple line (T4 level). The woman with epidural anesthetic is typically alert and comfortable. Little effect on the fetus results, unless the woman experiences prolonged hypotension or sensitivity to the anesthetic agent (very rare). Women wishing medication during their labors are usually enthusiastic regarding the method. Use of epidurals is growing in most areas of the United States.

However, epidural anesthesia requires the supervision of an anesthesiologist, a special apparatus, and continuous maternal-fetal monitoring and support by the nurse. The nurse must detect signs of maternal hypotension and evaluate the duration and quality of uterine contractions, progress in labor, and fetal-heart-rate response. The loss of normal pelvic sensation, together with routine intravenous hydration, causes many women to experience urinary distention. They should be asked to empty their bladders before the epidural is begun and should be watched carefully for bladder distention. Catheterization may be necessary. The mother's urge and ability to push may be impaired. Forceps deliveries are more common than in those women who have received no anesthesia before delivery. Usually, ambulation should be delayed until complete sensation and control of the legs returns. However, some very light, narcotic-only techniques may allow the mother to ambulate (the walking epidural). (See the following discussion.)

Epidural and subarachnoid narcotics

Injecting narcotics, along with local anesthetics, into the subarachnoid (spinal) or epidural spaces to manage pain during both vaginal and cesarean births and to provide postoperative pain control is fairly common. One technique uses long-lasting morphine (Duramorph) or other, shorter-acting narcotics such as

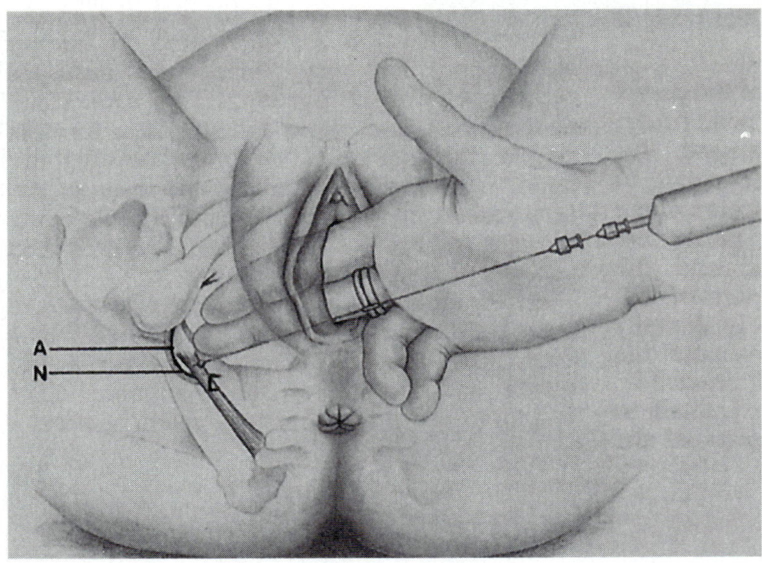

Fig. 12-8 Pudendal block. (From Al-Azzawi F: *Atlas of childbirth and obstetric techniques,* St. Louis, 1990, Mosby.)

fentanyl (Sublimaze) or sufentanyl (Sufental). It can provide very effective analgesia. Side effects, however, such as itching, nausea, and vomiting, occur frequently when narcotics are used in this way. Occasionally, urinary retention may also result. The major concern is a rare but potentially fatal complication—delayed respiratory depression (Nicholson, 1990). The possibility of this problem, when narcotics are injected into the subarachnoid or epidural spaces, increases the need for respiratory patterns of the patient to be carefully monitored over an extended period. Protocols for special observation and care should be in place.

Local anesthesia and nerve blocks

Local anesthesia by direct infiltration of the perineal tissues or infiltration of those nerves that serve to relay sensation initiated in the perineal area to the brain is probably the safest anesthesia for both mother and baby available today. Local anesthetics have no effect on maternal vital signs or fetal heart rate.

Local anesthesia. Local anesthesia of the perineal area can be achieved through injection of the anesthetic agent directly into the tissues of the perineum. It is generally used for episiotomy repair.

Pudendal block. Pudendal block stops sensory impulses from the pudendal nerve through bilateral infiltration of a local anesthetic with a long needle into the area just below the pudendal plexus (Fig. 12-8). Although a pudendal block does not relieve contraction pain, it does provide analgesia of the perineum. With its use, an episiotomy may be performed. The urge to bear down may be somewhat diminished, but the woman is able to do so with coaching.

Paracervical block. Another type of analgesic technique is called a *paracervical block.* It features injections of local anesthetic into the lateral fornices of the vagina at the junction of the vaginal wall and the partially dilated cervix. Although it may relieve discomfort from contractions, the technique in most instances is not sufficient to meet the total needs of most laboring women. Even more important, the paracervical block has been associated with episodes of fetal bradycardia and a few fetal deaths. For all these reasons, this type of block is infrequently undertaken.

KEY CONCEPTS

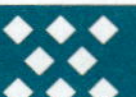

1 Dosage and time of administration of analgesics during labor are affected by the following factors: the need to ensure that the baby will be alert enough to breathe at birth, the maturity of the infant, and the possible effects on the progress of labor.

2 The narcotic meperidine (Demerol) is frequently given in combination with a tranquilizer, since the combination increases the analgesic effect and counteracts the nausea often associated with the narcotic.

3 Drugs used for general anesthesia include thiopental (Pentothal), profol (Diprivan), nitrous oxide (laughing gas), halothane (Fluothane), isoflurane (Forane), and ketamine hydrochloride (Ketaject).
4 A subarachnoid (saddle) block is administered during the second stage of labor and commonly numbs the mother's abdominal and pelvic areas below the umbilicus, affecting the abdomen, perineum, legs, and feet. Possible complications include hypotension, difficulty in pushing, spinal headache, respiratory difficulty, and problems with spontaneous voiding in the postpartum period.
5 Epidural anesthesia can be administered during the latter part of the first stage of labor and continued into the second and third stages. Normal pelvic sensation may be lost, but many women still confirm sensations of abdominal or perineal pressure and note weakness or numbness in their legs. Possible complications include bladder distention, hypotension, and a decreased urge and ability to push.
6 A pudendal block stops sensory impulses from the pudendal nerve by infiltration of a local anesthetic. It does not provide relief from uterine contractions but does provide perineal analgesia. The mother's urge to push may be diminished.
7 Paracervical block involves injections of local anesthetic. This technique is rarely sufficient to meet the total needs of most patients during labor and has been associated with a few fetal deaths. It is infrequently used.

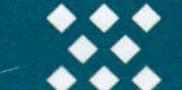

CRITICAL THOUGHT QUESTIONS

1 Compare and contrast the different types of analgesia and anesthesia commonly used during labor and birth. Given the advantages and disadvantages of each, which would you choose for yourself and why?
2 Maria Hernandez is in early labor and has been admitted to the labor and delivery unit. She has not received education regarding types of pharmacological pain relief measures. As she becomes more uncomfortable, she asks you if she can be "put to sleep" like she was last time. How would you respond?
3 The nurse midwife explains the various pain relief options to Anna Garcia, but quickly realizes that there is a communication problem because of the patient's limited English. What is the midwife's legal responsibility to this patient? How can the labor nurse assist?
4 Hanna Jackson has just received a lumbar epidural for relief of her labor pain. She is resting comfortably in a supine position. The nurse notices a sharp drop in her blood pressure. What nursing intervention should be done *first.* Why?

REFERENCES

Datta S: *The obstetric anesthesia handbook,* St. Louis, 1992, Mosby.

Taylor T: Epidural anesthesia in the maternity patient, *MCN* 18(2):86-93, 1993.

Nicholson C: Nursing considerations for the parturient who has received epidural narcotics during labor or delivery, *J Perinat Neonat Nurs* 4(1):14-26, 1990.

BIBLIOGRAPHY

Henrikson ML, Wild LR: A nursing process approach to epidural analgesia, *J Obstet Gynecol Neonatal Nurs* 17(5):316-320, 1988.

Kirby-McDonnel A: *Epidural anesthesia for labor & delivery, NAACOG Update Series #6,* Washington, DC, 1989, The Association.

The Organization for Obstetric, Gynecologic, and Neonatal Nurses: *Position statement on the role of the registered nurse in the management of analgesia by catheter technique (epidural, intrathecal, intrapleura, or peripheral nerve catheters),* Washington, DC, 1990, The Association.

Powell AH, Bova MB: How do you give continuous epidural fentanyl? *Am J Nurs* 89(9):1197-1200, 1989.

Stampone D: The history of obstetric anesthesia, *J Perinat Neonat Nurs* 4(1):1-13, 1990.

Wild L, Coyne C: The basics and beyond: epidural analgesia, *Am J Nurs* 92(4):26-34, 1992.

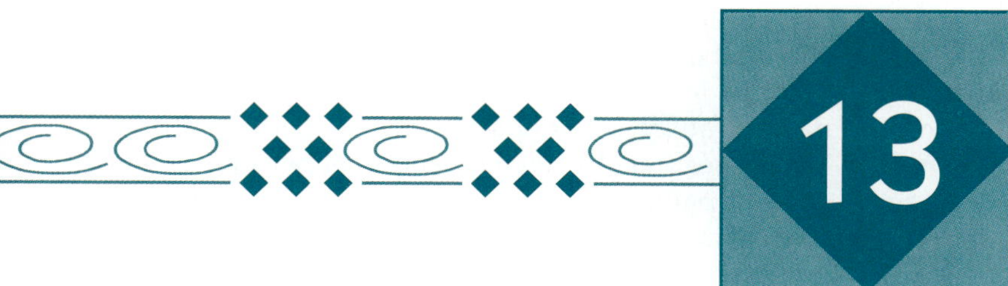

13

Postpartum

CHAPTER OBJECTIVES

After studying this chapter, the student should be able to:

1. Define the following terms: *postpartum, puerperium, involution, lochia, fundus, engorgement,* and *let-down reflex.*
2. Describe nursing assessments and their rationale for the early postpartum period (fourth stage of labor).
3. Discuss four factors that may influence the position of the uterus.
4. Describe four interventions to promote uterine contractility and, thus, minimize excessive bleeding.
5. Explain how to correctly massage a relaxed uterine fundus.
6. Demonstrate how to record the postpartum position and consistency of a patient's uterus.
7. List the principles of postpartum, perineal cleansing.
8. Describe the care for perineal lacerations.
9. Describe methods that breast-feeding and nonbreast-feeding mothers may use to lessen the discomfort of breast engorgement.
10. Indicate methods of preventing or treating constipation in the postpartum period.
11. Indicate the advantages of early postpartum ambulation.
12. List four support groups or agencies that help parents assume their new roles.
13. Prepare a discharge teaching plan that can be adapted to meet the educational needs of postpartum families.
14. Explain how the nursing care of a mother who has given birth by cesarean section differs from that of a woman who gave birth vaginally.
15. Describe behaviors that may indicate that a mother is developing postpartum psychosis.
16. Describe ways that the nurse can support grieving parenpts.

The postpartum period, or *puerperium,* is the interval from the birth of the baby until 6 weeks after. These days are numerated, starting with the first day after birth. This 6-week interval is characterized by the development of lactation and the return of the reproductive organs to their approximate, prepregnant positions. Of course, some mothers, not wishing to or unable to breast-feed their babies, do not experience the full development of lactation. The return of the reproductive organs to the nonpregnant state is called the process of *involution.*

This period is also a time when parents become acquainted with and further their attachment to their newborn. Today the average patient's postpartum in-hospital stay is very short, posing challenges and opportunities for nurses who must assure that the woman's physical and psychological recovery is progressing normally, the parents' educational needs are met, and the family is adjusting to the infant.

This chapter discusses early postpartum care (the fourth stage of labor), continuing in-hospital care, discharge teaching, and special situations.

EARLY POSTPARTUM CARE

As indicated in Chapter 11 the early postpartum period is sometimes referred to as the fourth stage of labor. It is the initial 1- to 4-hour period after delivery of the placenta, during which the woman's body stabilizes. Nursing assessment during this period focuses on the mother's physiological status. If the newborn is present the assessment also includes the early mother-infant acquaintance process. The following tasks are performed frequently during the first hour after birth or until the woman is stable (see Chapter 11). If the newborn remains with the mother the nurse will also monitor the child's adaptation to extrauterine life (see Chapters 16 and 17 for a further discussion).

Vital signs

Blood pressure should return to its prelabor level. Occasionally the blood pressure is elevated shortly after delivery. This condition may be the result of a variety of factors including the excitement of the birth and seeing the baby, the type of oxytocic the patient received or is still receiving intravenously, pain, urinary retention, or pregnancy-induced hypertension. It is important to know the patient's vital signs before labor and birth so that a baseline for comparison exists. Increased blood pressure, especially when accompanied by headache, may suggest pregnancy-induced hypertension. Blood pressures over 130 mm Hg systolic or 90 mm Hg diastolic should be reported to the health care provider.

If the mother's blood pressure is lower than her prelabor baseline, it may be a sign of excessive blood loss during birth or current bleeding. Any pressure of 100 mm Hg systolic or below should be reported. Normal pressures that begin to fall should also be reported for evaluation. Falling blood pressures are accompanied by an initially rising pulse. However, if the patient continues into shock, the pulse will gradually slow, weaken, and have a thready quality. Abnormally dilated pupils; pale, cyanotic, or clammy skin; apprehension; and unconsciousness are also signs of shock.

The normal pulse rate is slightly lower than during labor but is of good quality and is not associated with other signs of shock. This lower pulse rate (normal range is 40 to 80 beats per minute) is related to decreased cardiac strain and is not significant. As previously mentioned, a rising pulse rate accompanied by a falling blood pressure is a sign of blood loss. Tachycardia alone may be related to a long, difficult labor or may indicate infection.

The respiratory rate should be at prelabor levels. Respirations should be regular and breath sounds should be clear. Bradypnea (respiratory rate of less than 14 to 16 per minute) may occur secondary to narcotic analgesic or epidural narcotic administration. Tachypnea (respiratory rate above 24 per minute) may suggest pain, infection, excessive blood loss or shock, or respiratory compromise because of pulmonary emboli or pulmonary edema.

The temperature is taken shortly after birth, before the woman has anything hot or cold to drink. If it is not elevated, it is usually not repeated until the next routine shift assessment. An initial temperature of 100.4°F (38°C) is likely the result of the exertion and dehydration from labor. Rest and fluids will usually restore the normal body temperature. After the first 24 hours a maternal temperature of 100.4°F (38°C) suggests infection.

Uterine contractility

After the completion of the third stage of a normal, full-term labor the fundus should be firmly contracted and located at or below the umbilicus. A firm uterus prevents excessive bleeding by compressing the large vessels that brought blood to and from the placental sinuses before the placenta separated and delivered. A high, soft fundus suggests uterine bleeding. A high, firm fundus often indicates urinary retention. Since the uterine ligaments are still stretched, a distended bladder, located just below the uterus, causes the fundus to rise (usually to one side and often to the right). It is an important cause of postpartum hemorrhage and should be prevented. If the woman cannot void the nurse may have to catheterize.

If a fundus is large, soft, or boggy (seems to contain excess blood), it should be massaged gently with one hand until it is firm, whereas the other hand is positioned at the symphysis pubis for support (Fig. 13-1). If clots are suspected, once the fundus is firm it is gently grasped and, still supporting the lower uterus, pressure is then exerted in the direction of the pelvic canal to push out the clots that were emptied from the uterus into the lower uterine segment and vagina. Supporting the uterus with the lower hand during fundal massage and expulsion of clots helps prevent the uterus from inverting or prolapsing into the vagina. The nurse should avoid over-stimulating the uterus with continuous massaging. See the Nursing Alert on p. 217.

In the event of excessive vaginal bleeding, uterine massage is the first measure used to control hemorrhage. If intravenous oxytocin (Pitocin) is infusing the rate may be increased until bleeding is stable. Putting the infant to breast will also stimulate the uterine muscles to contract. The bladder should be emptied.

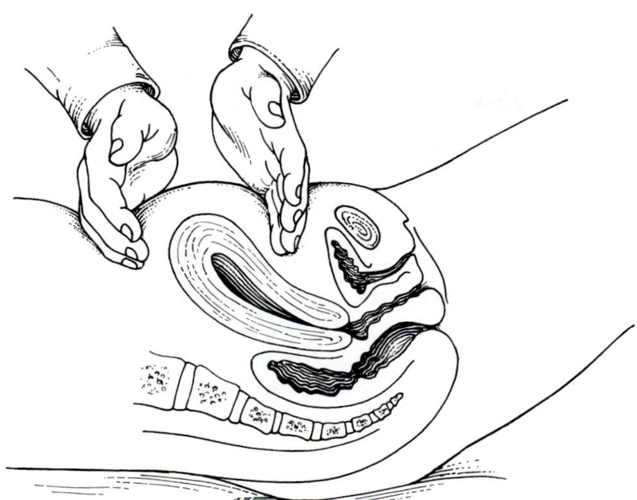

Fig. 13-1 Massaging the uterine fundus. One hand anchors the lower uterine segment just above the symphysis. The other gently massages the fundus.

See Chapter 14 for additional information on the causes and treatment of postpartum hemorrhage.

Lochia

The nurse should wear gloves when assessing the amount and character of vaginal drainage, or lochia. The nurse examines the patient's drainage by checking the perineal pad and observing the pad under the patient's hips. Much of the drainage may not be on the perineal pad but may soak into the pad underneath the hips. The perineal area should be observed for bleeding and clots whenever the uterus is massaged or attempts are made to express clots. Shortly after delivery the drainage should be dark red with a fleshy, but not foul, odor. The presence and size of clots should be documented and reported to the health care provider. Accurate visual assessment of the amount of lochial flow is often difficult. Estimating the amount by measurement of the stain on the peripad may be complicated by the different types of pads used and how often they are changed. Saturation of one perineal pad (peripad) within 1 hour, however, is usually considered heavy drainage. The patient usually wears two peripads that are changed once or twice during her first 2 hours postpartum. These should always be removed and applied from front to back to avoid contamination of the perineum.

Perineum

When assessing the lochia the nurse should also assess the perineum for swelling and bruising. If an episiotomy or laceration exists, check for approximation of the suture line. An ice pack, if ordered to decrease edema, should be reapplied as necessary. The ice pack should be wrapped with clean, waterproof material and a fairly thin, absorbent outer layer and intermittently applied directly to the perineum. It may be held in place by its own attachments or by an encircling sanitary pad. Commercial perineal ice packs are available. They need to be fairly comfortable, durable, and able to provide cold temperatures for reasonable periods. If no such pads are available the nurse can fill a rubber glove with cracked ice and water, close it tightly, and wrap it in a light, clean plastic covering and a clean towel. Ice packs must be changed often.

If the woman complains of extreme pain in the perineal area the nurse should examine the perineum for the development of a hematoma (localized collection of blood, usually clotted, in the tissue) (see Chapter 14, for more information regarding postpartum hemorrhage).

> **Nursing Alert**
>
> Continuous massaging of the uterus can lead to over-stimulation, resulting in uterine relaxation and hemorrhage.

Bladder distention

The most common cause of a high fundus is a full bladder. A distended bladder may interfere with the normal contraction of the uterus and predispose the patient to hemorrhage. Even if a woman is catheterized just before birth, she may have a full bladder soon afterward, especially if she is receiving or has had intravenous infusions. Signs of urinary distention are a puffy area just above the pubic bone, complaints by the patient that she feels she should void but cannot, or the voiding of amounts less than 200 ml. The latter is called *dribbling* and usually indicates a full bladder that can contract only partially to release limited amounts of urine. The nurse should measure any voiding and assess the height of the fundus after voiding to evaluate, by a change in the position, the efficiency of the emptying process.

If a patient appears to have a full bladder, every effort should be made to help her void without resorting to catheterization. Catheterization, especially repeated catheterizations, may cause inflammation even in the best of circumstances. The following techniques may help the woman to void.

If the patient cannot get up to go to the bathroom because of her general condition or because she has had spinal anesthesia and does not as yet have an ambulation order, the problem of initiating natural voiding is particularly difficult. Sometimes, if the health care provider knows that a choice must be made between catheterization and probable success in voiding, she or he orders earlier ambulation. Patients who have had saddle block or epidural anesthesia also experience more problems voiding because they have lost normal feeling in the bladder area.

If a metal bedpan must be used, it should be warmed. Patients who have had a subarachnoid block are raised just enough so that their hips are not higher than their heads while positioned on the pan. Privacy should be maintained, and, if possible, water should be left running into a washbowl to provide psychological stimulation. Giving an ordered analgesic such as oxycodone (Percodan) or acetaminophen (Tylenol) with codeine approximately 20 minutes before the bedpan is offered often solves the problem. Having the patient blow bubbles through a straw into a glass of water or pretend to blow up a balloon while she is on the bedpan sometimes relaxes the sphincter muscle, as does pouring a measured amount of warm water over the perineum.

For the woman who can ambulate the previously mentioned techniques, a sitz bath, or taking a shower may help the patient void. If not, these efforts help clean the area before catheterization. Encouraging the patient to drink amounts of fluid exceeding normal requirements before she voids usually adds to rather than relieves the problem and is not recommended.

If none of the preceeding methods bring about the desired result, and the bladder is distended, catheterization must be performed. Before catheterization the nurse should check the orders to see if a specimen should be saved for laboratory analysis. Individual differences of opinion still exist regarding how much urine should be removed from the bladder during the catheterization of a postpartum patient. The most common practice is to empty the bladder completely but slowly. Although a mild sympathetic response of slightly lowered blood pressure may occur when more than 1000 ml is removed, this has not been found to be significant in postpartum patients (Sands, 1972). If urine remains in the bladder the problems that result outweigh any mild, sympathetic response. See the box on p. 219 for the catheterization procedure. If the woman must be catheterized more than once the provider may order a Foley catheter for 12 to 24 hours to avoid additional catheterizations.

Anesthesia recovery

The patient who received spinal or epidural anesthesia should be observed for return of sensation to her legs and buttocks. Only after she has a return of complete sensation and movement should she ambulate. The nurse should assist her when she walks for the first time.

Pain

Although most patients are able to describe discomfort, it is important to make a systematic assessment of the presence, cause, type, and location of pain. Asking the patient to rate her pain on a scale of 1 to 10 is one way for her to convey the extent of her discomfort. Elevations in the patient's blood pressure and pulse may also indicate the existence of pain. Nursing measures such as positioning, warm blankets, a sponge bath, and emptying the bladder may ease discomfort. Applications of cold or heat, as ordered, may also be helpful. And, of course, ordered analgesics should be given when needed. The success of measures to relieve pain must be evaluated and documented.

Hydration and nutrition

Most women will have an intravenous line with Pitocin infusing during the early postpartum period. If the woman is stable the health care provider will usually order the intravenous line discontinued within a few hours. The nurse should monitor the rate while it is infusing and check for signs of infiltration. Oral fluids and sometimes a light snack are offered if the woman is not bleeding excessively. The nurse should assess the woman's preference for hot or cold beverages and food after delivery. In many cultures (e.g., Asian American and Hispanic American) hot is preferred to restore the body's balance between hot and cold.

Psychological status

The labor experience is often a most demanding period for a woman. Sometimes women are disappointed in their ability to cope with the discomfort. The nurse should offer opportunities for her to talk about and integrate the experience. She may need reassurance that she behaved appropriately. If the newborn remains with the mother the nurse should continue to facilitate and assess the early attachment behaviors of the parents (see Chapter 11 for a further discussion). The mother may need to rest during this period and the nurse can provide the opportunity for her to do so. Research indicates that new mothers get relatively little uninterrupted sleep during their time in the hospital (Lentz and Killien, 1991). The postpartum woman must have her own psychological and physical needs met so that she may meet those of her baby.

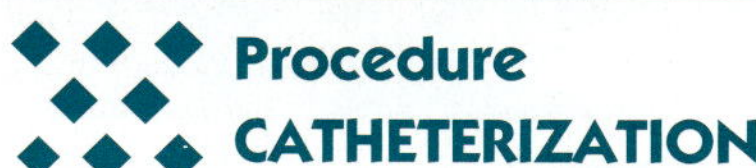

Procedure CATHETERIZATION

EQUIPMENT/SUPPLIES
- Sterile catheterization set
- Good light

STEPS
1. Check the health care provider's order regarding catheterization.
2. Explain to the patient, in simple terms the purpose of the procedure, what you will be doing, and what she is likely to feel. Assure her that she will be more comfortable afterwards.
3. Provide privacy with curtains and draping.
4. Adjust the lighting.
5. Wash your hands.
6. Open the catheterization set, being careful not to contaminate the inside.
7. Place the sterile drape under the patient's buttocks.
8. Put on the sterile gloves.
9. Prepare the rest of the catheterization materials (e.g., put antiseptic agent on cotton balls, lubricate the catheter).
10. Using one hand (considered contaminated once it has touched the skin), separate the labia so that you can adequately see the urinary meatus. Be gentle, since some patients have little feeling because of residual anesthesia, others are very sensitive, and still others have stitches in the vagina and true perineum.
11. Holding the labia back with a cotton ball under one supporting finger may help maintain the position. Technically, if the labia closes after the area has been washed with antiseptic, the area must be rewashed, since it has been contaminated by the enfolding tissue. It is, therefore, important to maintain the labia in the drawn back position.
12. With the other hand, using the forceps provided in the set, cleanse the area from the outside to the inside. Use one cotton ball for each downward stroke, then discard. The last cotton ball or two should be reserved for cleansing directly over the meatus.
13. Insert the lubricated catheter. It should be inserted no more than 4 inches to avoid puncturing the bladder. If obstruction is encountered, the catheter should never be forced. An abnormality of the canal may exist (e.g., presence of a tumor or stricture), or the meatus may not be properly identified.
14. A slight downward incline of the catheter may aid insertion, since the urethral canal slopes downward when the patient is in the dorsal recumbent position.
15. Allow the urine to slowly drain into the basin.
16. When the urine stops, withdraw the catheter and remove the materials.
17. Reposition perineal pads, ice pack, etc. and make the patient comfortable.
18. Measure the amount of urine obtained. Send any requested specimen to the laboratory.
19. Note the height of the uterine fundus and document it, along with the amount and color of the urine obtained.

CONTINUING CARE

The basic care of the postpartum patient is an extension of the care given during the first few hours after birth. If the woman will be transferred from the delivery area to a mother-baby unit for the remainder of her stay, it is important for the labor nurse to report the type of delivery (vaginal or abdominal) experienced; the kind of anesthesia used, if any; the status of her recovery; the status of the infant; and any other pertinent information to the postpartum nurse. The patient's personal effects are carefully transferred so that nothing is lost in the move.

After the initial period of recovery and stabilization, nursing assessments for the woman who has delivered vaginally are usually completed every 8 to 12 hours. If the woman delivered by Cesarean section, these assessments may be ordered every 4 hours. See Table 13-1, for a list of the factors assessed, usual findings, and deviations from normal.

Physiological Adaptation and Nursing Care

As the nurse assesses the mother's condition and intervenes to promote comfort and prevent complications, many opportunities arise to teach the woman about her recovering body and self-care activities.

Ambulation

Ambulation of the postpartum patient is determined by the orders of the attending physician or nurse midwife. It also depends on the type of anesthetic given during delivery and the general condition of the

◆ **TABLE 13-1**
Postpartum Nursing Assessment

Assessment	Usual Findings	Deviations
Vital Signs		
Blood pressure	90/60 to 140/90 (check prenatal values)	Hypotension or hypertension
Temperature	36.8 to 37.8° C (98.2 to 100° F)	>37.8° C (100° F)
Pulse	60 to 100 beats/minute (bpm)	<60 or >100 bpm
Respirations	14 to 24 breaths/minute	<14 or >24
Neurological		
Level of consciousness	Alert, oriented (may be drowsy)	Stuporous, coma, disoriented
Pain level	Mild to moderate discomfort	Severe pain, complaint of continuous headache
Vision	Clear	Visual disturbances (blurring, spots)
Deep tendon reflexes	2+, no clonus	0 or 4+, clonus
Respiratory		
Breath sounds	Clear and equal sounds	Crackles, wheezes, snoring type of sounds
Cardiovascular		
Skin	Warm and dry	Cool, pale
Peripheral pulses (radial, pedal)	Regular, strong pulse	Irregular pulse; weak, thready pulse; bounding pulse
Homan's sign	Negative	Homan's positive; localized redness or tenderness in legs
Edema	Absent	Present (2+ to generalized)
Incision (cesarean)	Intact, edges approximated; dressing dry (if one is used)	Edges not approximated; redness, pus; dressing stained with blood, drainage
Gastrointestinal		
Bowel sounds	Present	Absent
Pain	No tenderness	Epigastric pain
Reproductive		
Breasts	Soft; or slightly firm if after 48 hours	Hard, engorged
Nipples	Soft, supple, intact; everted, flat, inverted	Dry, cracked, bleeding
Uterus	Firm fundus, position midline	Boggy fundus, displaced to right or left
Uterine involution	Should decrease in size with subsequent examinations	Not decreasing in size
Perineum	Intact episiotomy, slight edema and redness; nonbleeding hemorrhoids	Gaps in suture line, edges not approximated; swollen; extremely painful; continuous bleeding.
Lochia	Rubra, scant to moderate amount	Foul smelling, large amount with increasing clots or tissue
Urinary		
Bladder	Nondistended, voiding adequate amounts	Distended; voiding amounts <200 cc
Foley catheter	Clear, adequate amounts of amber urine	Hematuria, oliguria, discolored

Continued.

◆ TABLE 13-1
Postpartum Nursing Assessment—cont'd.

Assessment	Usual Findings	Deviations
Extremities		
Intravenous lines	Nonreddened site, intact	Infiltration
Range of motion	Adequate at all points	Immobility
Psychosocial		
Emotions	Talkative, cheerful; tearful at times, especially at 48 to 72 hours postpartum	Constant sobbing, does not interact with infant, family, or nurse; anxious, withdrawn; refuses care
Support network	Visitors; patient mentions support, assistance from family, friends. Partner (father of baby) involved in patient and infant care.	No support persons visible or mentioned
Attachment	Participates in infant care, attentive to infant needs, holds child close, en face position; positive comments about infant.	Refuses to care for infant; handles roughly, does not promptly attend to infant needs; negative comments about infant.
Infant caregiving	Performs infant care correctly; verbalizes signs and symptoms to report to pediatrician or nurse practitioner	Care performed incorrectly; unable to recount signs and symptoms of complications that should be reported

patient. Patients who have received subarachnoid spinal (saddle block) anesthesia may be confined to bed, flat or with only one pillow, for 8 to 12 hours after the birth. The restriction of ambulation and posture is chiefly to prevent the leakage of spinal fluid through the puncture site in the dura, causing a decrease of fluid and pressure related to the onset of spinal headache. With better anesthesia technology, these ambulation and posture restrictions are encountered less often than in the past.

New mothers who have had epidural anesthesia may usually ambulate with assistance when the anesthetic has worn off and they have full return of sensation to their legs. Those who have had local or no anesthetic may ambulate as soon as they wish.

The pendulum has swung a long way from 40 years ago, when 5 to 10 days passed before the new mother stirred from her bed. Early ambulation of postpartum patients lessens the incidence of respiratory, circulatory, and urinary problems, prevents constipation, and promotes the rapid return of strength. When the patient first ambulates, *the nurse should not leave her alone.* These patients may experience a sudden drop in blood pressure when they stand erect (orthostatic hypotension) and, as a result, become dizzy and faint. The nurse can prevent falls resulting from orthostatic hypotension by evaluating the woman's blood pressure and pulse in the supine position, then raising the bed to a high Fowler's position and, after 2 to 3 minutes, retaking the blood pressure and pulse. A significant fall in blood pressure (15 to 20 mm Hg) and rise in pulse (20 bpm) with this position change indicates the likelihood of orthostatic hypotension. If her pressure and pulse remain stable after a few minutes of sitting with her legs dangling, she can usually safely ambulate. If the patient does become faint, she should be eased onto a chair, her bed, or even gently to the floor. Spirits of ammonia may be useful to revive her—the nurse should have one handy. She should never be left alone. If she is on a chair the nurse can support her while she lowers her head to her knees. Until she feels stronger the patient should be instructed to rise slowly and sit on the side of the bed for a few minutes before ambulating. No matter how many days postpartum the nurse should always evaluate the new mother's ability to ambulate safely. See the nursing alert below.

The first time the postpartum patient gets out of bed, she may experience a sudden, temporary gush of vaginal discharge. If it is dark red, it is probably not significant. It reflects the patient's change in posture after being recumbent for several hours when the uterine drainage was not as efficient. However, the

Nursing Alert

Injuries from falls are the most common cause of malpractice litigation in the United States.

patient should be evaluated for excessive bleeding and signs of shock.

Early ambulation has significantly reduced the incidence of thrombophlebitis (inflammation of a vein often associated with a clot). The new mother has higher levels of clotting factors, however, and is therefore at increased risk for clot formation. As a result the nurse should assess her for signs of thrombophlebitis by inspecting the legs (a common site) for red, warm, tender areas and by testing for *Homan's sign.* Homan's sign is positive if the patient reports calf pain when her foot is firmly dorsiflexed while the leg is supported in an extended position with the knee slightly bent. A positive Homan's sign should be reported to the health care provider. (See Chapter 14 for further discussion of thrombophlebitis.)

Hygiene

Cleanliness, comfort, and observation for infection are prime considerations for the new mother. The postpartum patient is likely to perspire heavily. It is one way in which the body rids itself of excess fluids acquired during pregnancy. A sponge bath or shower should be offered in a timely manner. If a sponge bath is done, special attention should be given to the two areas that are easily infected—the breasts and the perineum. If the patient delivered by cesarean the incision line constitutes a third area susceptible to infection. The mother should be instructed to bathe daily, paying particular attention to these areas of the body.

Breast care

Whether the mother showers or has a sponge bath, she should be instructed in the care of her breasts. Usually only clear water is used in washing the breasts. Soap may have a drying effect and cause cracked nipples. If the woman is breast-feeding the nurse should carefully assess the nipples for signs of trauma—bruising, cracks, fissures—which can predispose her to a breast infection (see Chapter 14 for a further discussion). Nipple trauma is usually the result of incorrect breast-feeding techniques and can be prevented with good teaching and support. See Chapter 17 for additional breast care suggestions for the breast-feeding mother. Whether breast-feeding or not, postpartum patients should begin wearing a well-fitting support bra soon after delivery. Absorbent breast pads may help keep the breasts dry once the milk is in but should be changed frequently to prevent bacterial growth and subsequent breast infection. The woman should be taught to promptly report cracked and bleeding nipples and signs of breast infection (e.g., redness, hardness, and elevated temperature [38.4°C, 101°F]).

Anatomy of the breasts. A brief description of the anatomy of the breast permits a greater understanding of the basics of breast care, the technique of nursing an infant, and the principles involved in pumping the breasts. The breasts, or mammary glands, are divided into segments, or lobes, which in turn are divided into lobules (smaller lobes). These contain the actual milk-producing glands known as *acini,* or alveoli (Fig. 13-2). *Prolactin* is the hormone primarily responsible for milk production. Infant suckling at the breast provides the stimulus for the anterior pituitary gland to release prolactin. The breasts are richly supplied with blood vessels, lymphatics, and nerves.

Each segment of the breast radiates from the central darkly pigmented portion, known as the *areola,* which rings the sensitive erectile tissue known as the *nipple.* Milk ducts from the acini travel toward the areola and open out onto the surface of the nipples. Each nipple usually has 15 to 20 such openings. As each major milk duct approaches the areola, it widens temporarily, forming a small reservoir, or *sinus.*

When the baby begins sucking, *oxytocin* from the posterior pituitary is released (Fig. 13-3). Its action stimulates the contraction of muscles around the milk ducts, allowing the milk to flow into the sinus to be readily available to the baby. This physiological response is called the *letdown reflex.* It may be accompanied by a tingling or shivering sensation. It occurs in both breasts, even though the baby is only nursing at one. The oxytocin also stimulates the uterine muscles to contract, thus lessening the possibility of hemorrhage and increasing the rapidity of involution. When a mother pumps her breasts manually, she obtains the best flow if she first presses the breast tissue back with her thumb and fingers and then squeezes the breast. Properly holding the breast with one hand during breast-feeding not only allows the baby to breathe more comfortably but also encourages secretion of milk. For more information about breast-feeding, see Chapter 17.

Breast engorgement. Breast engorgement may occur at the third day postpartum and is often attributed to the milk "coming in." The tenderness and swelling, however, do not result entirely from the presence of more milk. Engorgement results, for the most part, from the increased venous and lymphatic congestion in the breast tissue. With engorgement the breasts feel hard and nodular. Engorgement usually resolves within 48 hours. In the meantime the following strategies can help the woman to manage the associated discomfort.

The woman who is breast-feeding can ease discomfort by wearing a good support bra and feeding frequently. The breasts can be softened before feeding by applying a warm, wet washcloth, taking a hot shower, or manually expressing a small amount of

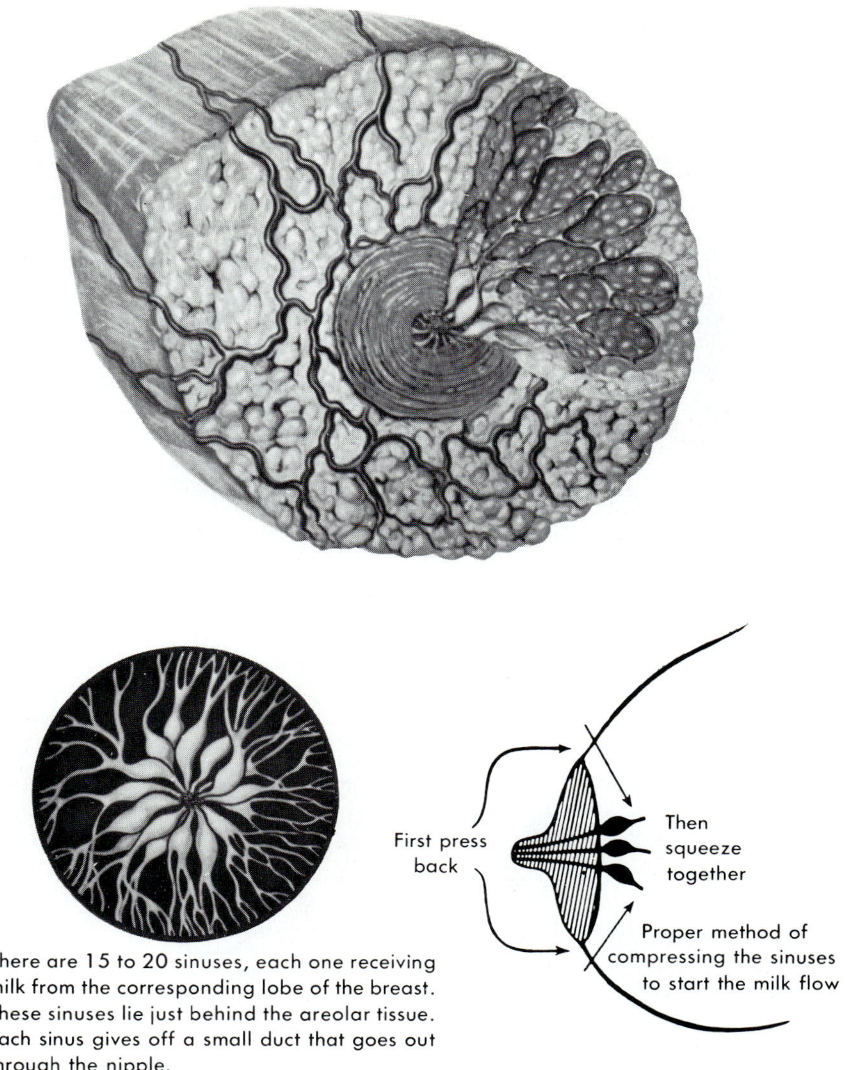

Fig. 13-2 Lactating breast. (Courtesy Carnation Company, Los Angeles, CA.)

milk. The best strategy for alleviating engorgement is frequent (every 2 to 3 hours) feedings of the newborn. An oxcytocin nasal spray may enhance the let-down reflex. Pumping the breasts is not advised to relieve engorgement in nursing or nonnursing mothers, since emptying the breasts stimulates more milk production.

Analgesic drugs may also be prescribed to relieve pain. Many medications can pass through the milk to the nursing infant with varying effects. A breast-feeding mother should always check with her health care provider before taking any kind of medication.

Mothers who are not breast-feeding can alleviate engorgement discomfort by wearing support bras, appling ice packs to the breasts, and taking analgesics. Avoiding breast and nipple stimulation, such as heat, massage, or pumping the breasts, will help suppress lactation.

The prescription of oral estrogenic compounds, such as chlorotrianisene (TACE), or intramuscular injection of androgenic compounds (Deladumone OB) to suppress lactation is infrequent and not recommended. The incidence of painful engorgement experienced by nonnursing mothers who did not receive such medications is low. Other means of treating the discomfort are preferable. Research indicates that a causal relationship may exist between a reported increased occurrence of thromboemboli after the use of estrogens, especially after cesarean birth, and also between the later development of endometrial cancer and the use of estrogens. Informed patient consent is required by the Federal Drug Administration before estrogens are given.

A nonhormonal drug, bromocriptine mesylate (Parlodel), which suppresses lactation by preventing the secretion of prolactin, is sometimes prescribed. However, it has been associated with sudden episodes of hypotension, nausea, vomiting, and other side effects.

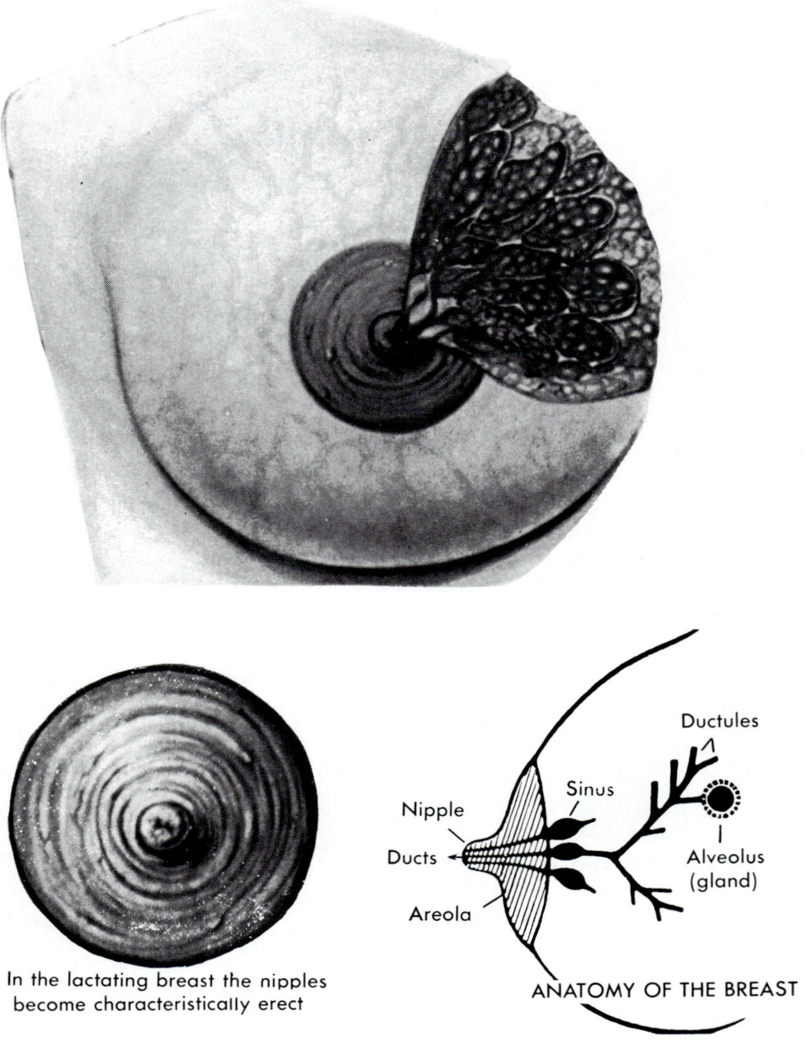

Fig. 13-2—cont'd.

Most health care providers believe that the best therapies available to relieve the discomfort of the nonbreast-feeding mother are the mechanical aids previously described, in addition to the "tincture of time."

Pumping the breasts. If the newborn cannot breast-feed because of illness or prematurity the mother may be encouraged to pump her breasts to maintain or encourage her milk supply. A mother may express milk manually or use a hand or electric pump as shown in Fig. 13-4. Whatever method is used, she should be supported comfortably in a sitting or side position with her hands and breasts freshly washed. Any equipment that touches her breasts should be sterilized before use. If the milk is saved for the baby, it should be collected in a sterile container, using aseptic technique. See Chapter 17 for more information about breast milk storage. The mother should be instructed on how to empty her breasts using the preferred pumping method. If an electric breast pump is used the nurse must make sure that the suction is not too great. It should be increased gradually. A record of the amount of milk obtained should be kept with the patient's chart. Mothers are sometimes surprised by the color of their milk. They should be assured that, although human breast milk looks thinner and more bluish than cow's milk, it is perfectly suited for the baby. Colostrum, the first secretion from the breast, is more creamy or orange in appearance.

Uterine involution

On the first postpartal day the fundus is usually felt at the umbilicus or slightly below. The fundus then

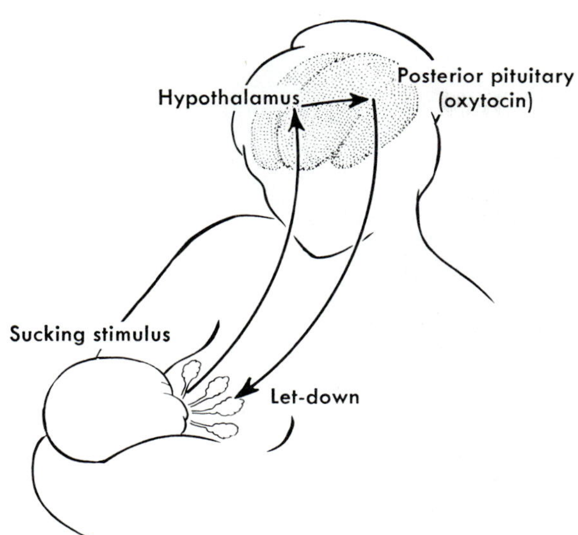

Fig. 13-3 The letdown reflex. The sucking stimulus arrives at hypothalamus, which promotes release of oxytocin from posterior pituitary. Oxytocin stimulates contraction of myoepithelial cells around milk ducts, allowing milk to flow into the lactiferous sinuses, where it is available to the nursing infant. (From Worthington-Roberts BS, Williams SR: *Nutrition in pregnancy and lactation,* ed 5, St. Louis, 1993, Mosby.)

becomes smaller and descends approximately one finger width further into the pelvis on each successive day. At the end of 10 days, it is down behind the pubic bone again and not palpable (Fig. 13-5). The position of the fundus is usually coded by counting finger widths above or below the umbilicus in the following manner. If the fundus (which feels somewhat like a large cantaloupe through the abdominal wall) is two finger widths above the level of the umbilicus, it is recorded as "+2." If it is located one finger width below the level of the umbilicus, it is recorded as "–1." If the fundus is found at the level of the umbilicus, it is recorded as "@ umbilicus." A typical record of the condition of the fundus would be "Fundus: firm –2 midline."

The location of the fundus may be influenced by the size of the patient's infant, the condition of her uterine muscle, the content of the urinary bladder, and abnormal conditions such as retained placental fragments and the development of uterine infection. Barring complications the uterus returns to its nonpregnant size by 4 to 6 weeks after birth.

Multiparas often complain of *afterpains,* or cramping caused by the contraction of the uterus in the process of involution. These mothers are more often bothered by cramping than are primiparas, who possess better muscle tone. Breast-feeding mothers may experience more afterpains because of the stimulation of the uterus during the process of nursing. These cramps usually diminish within 48 to 72 hours. Keeping the bladder empty and taking mild analgesics help relieve the discomfort.

Lochia

The dark red *lochia rubra* persists for the first 2 or 3 days postpartum. A few small clots, the size of a nickel or less, are normal during this period. Large clots, however, are not normal. The lochia becomes pinkish-brownish from approximately the third to the tenth day postpartum and is called *lochia serosa.* For another week or two the lochia becomes lighter in color—a creamy yellow—and is known as *lochia alba.* The nurse should educate the patient about these normal changes. Reappearance of bright red blood after lochia rubra has stopped indicates subinvolution or possibly a delayed postpartum hemorrhage. Any foul smell to the lochia indicates infection. Both conditions should be promptly reported to the woman's health care provider. When the cervix returns to its closed position the lochia stops and the woman is less vulnerable to uterine infection.

Douching is not necessary and should never be done before 6 weeks postpartum. The menstrual cycle will return in approximately 4 weeks to 3 months if the woman is not breast-feeding. For the breast-feeding mother, menses will return from 6 weeks to 10 months but may be delayed until the infant is completely weaned (Lawrence, 1994). This does not mean, however, that she cannot become pregnant during this period. Mothers who breast-feed *exclusively* and *frequently* during the first 6 months postpartum are less likely to ovulate, but should not rely on this method to prevent conception. (See Chapter 7 for further discussion of contraceptive methods that do not interfere with breast-feeding.)

Perineal care

At least once each shift the nurse should assess the perineum of the patient who gave birth vaginally for signs of infection (redness, edema, or unusual discharge), for signs of trauma, for approximation of any suture line, and for hemorrhoids. A hematoma in the area may develop slowly. The patient should lie in the Sims' position and the nurse should lift the upper buttock to expose the perineum and anus. Sufficient light is necessary to see the area clearly—a penlight is helpful.

The principles involved in perineal care should be the same whether they are done by the nurse or the patient herself. Perineal cleansing is performed to prevent infection, eliminate odor, observe the area and

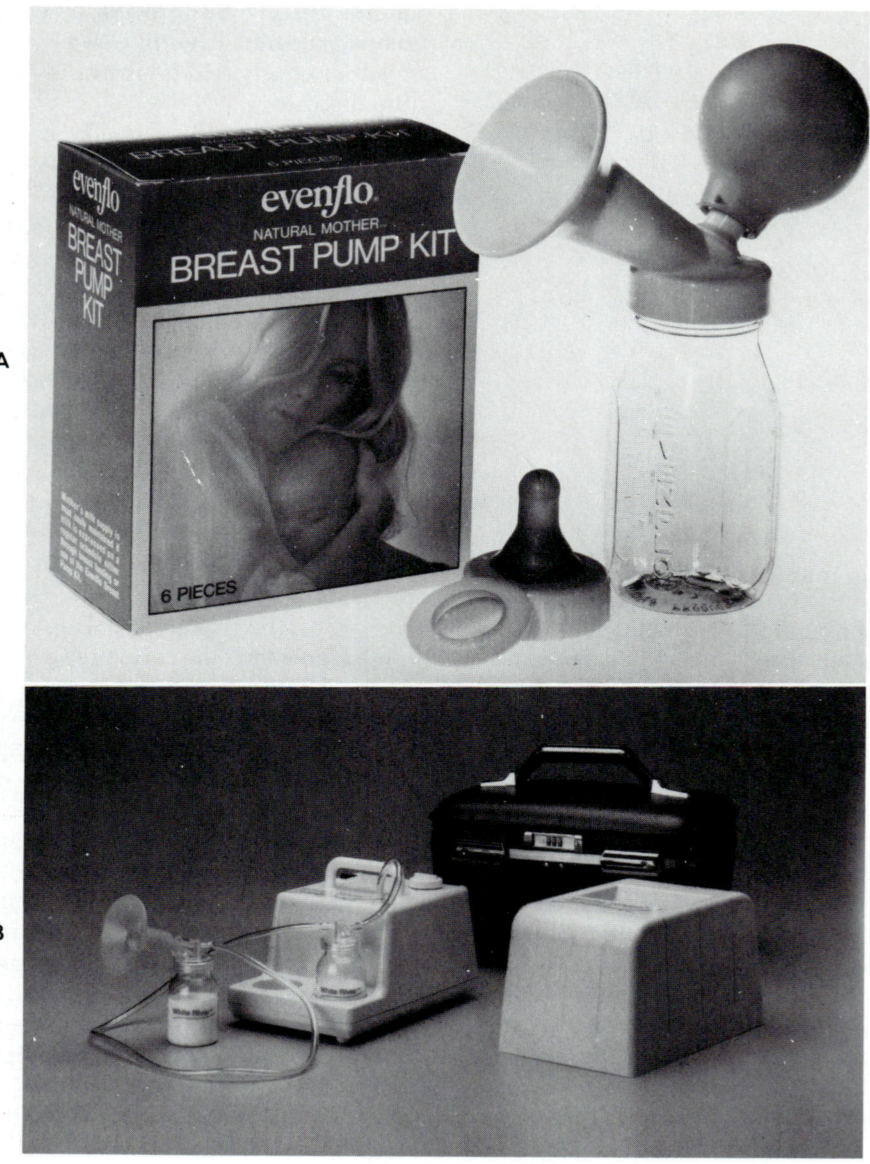

Fig. 13-4 **A,** Manual breast pump-bottle combination. **B,** The White River Breast Pump Kit features a flexible cup and a pumping action, which simulates a nursing neonate. It weighs under 10 lbs. (**A,** Courtesy Evenflo Products Company, Ravenna, OH. **B,** Courtesy Elena Grant, Natural Technologies, Laguna Hills, CA.)

lochial flow, and ease the patient's discomfort. Any equipment used by one patient should be absolutely clean and should not be used by another. Reusable equipment, rare today, should be sterilized between patients. In most instances the mother is taught perineal cleansing on her first trip to the bathroom. She should be taught to continue this routine cleansing until the lochia stops.

Hands of the patient and/or nurse should be washed before and after care. Nurses should use gloves. The patient should be taught to cleanse the perineal area after each voiding or bowel movement. Some maternity services issue plastic squeeze bottles for antiseptic solution or warm tap water, plus cellulose wipes. Water temperature should be tested on the thigh or wrist to ensure comfort and prevent burns. Other health care services provide wall-mounted surgigators with soap cartridges. Still others provide individually wrapped, moist towelettes impregnated with rapid-drying antiseptic. If a bed rest regimen is necessary the patient may be placed on a bedpan and warm water poured over her perineum, taking care to

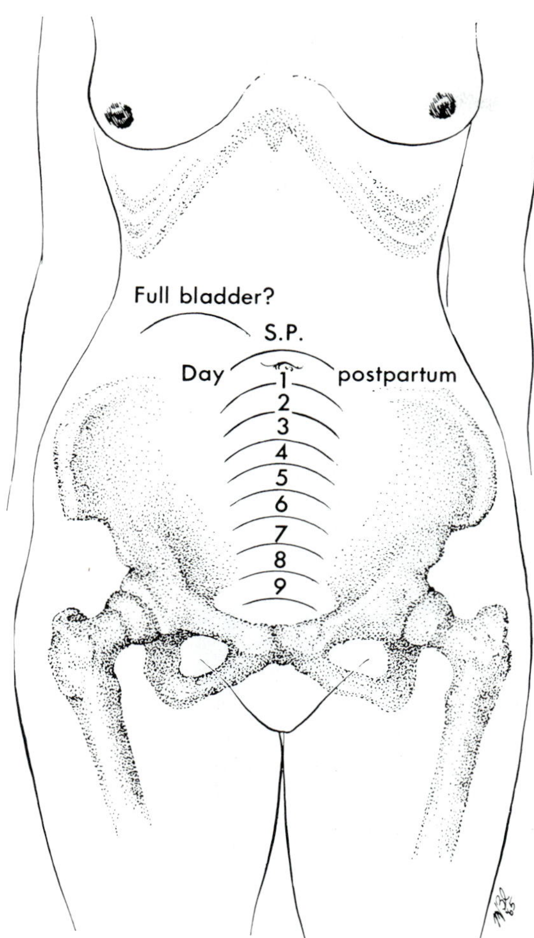

Fig. 13-5 Involution of uterus, showing positions of fundus on various postpartum days. S.P., Level just after separation of placenta from uterine wall, before its delivery.

avoid filling the birth canal with water. The patient may then be patted dry from the front to the back with a clean wash cloth or tissue. After cleansing the perineal pad should be changed (tampons should not be used for the first 6 weeks). Care should be taken in cleansing the perineum and in removing and applying perineal pads so that bacteria are not introduced to the vulva. This means, for both nurse and patient, wiping from front to back once only with each cleansing surface. The nurse or patient should remove and apply perineal pads from front to back and not touch the surface that is next to the perineum.

Episiotomies and lacerations. For patients who have undergone episiotomies or laceration repairs, perineal care usually involves more than just cleansing. Many hospitals provide an antiseptic and analgesic benzocaine perineal spray such as Dermoplast or Americaine. Other local analgesics such as dibucaine

> **Nursing Alert**
>
> Topical anesthetics (sprays or ointments) should be applied *after* heat lamp treatments or burns may result.

(Nupercainal) ointment may also be ordered. Witchhazel pads (Tucks) help reduce the swelling and discomfort associated with episiotomies, lacerations, and hemorrhoids. The health care provider may order sitz baths and/or a perineal lamp ("peri light") to increase circulation and ease perineal discomfort (Fig. 13-6). Each can be used several times a day for 15- to 20-minute intervals to improve circulation, promote healing, and ease discomfort. Lamps and sitz baths are usually not offered until 12 hours after birth. If given too early, they may stimulate additional bleeding. This consideration may mean that many mothers will be discharged before such treatments are received. However, the woman can be taught to use the sitz bath at home. The nurse should caution her to test the water temperature for comfort. Recent research indicates that a cool sitz bath may be just as effective as a warm one in promoting comfort (LaFoy and Geden, 1989).

When perineal lamps are used, care must be taken that they are no closer than 18 inches (41 cm) from the perineum. A 25- to 40-watt lamp should be used. To protect the skin the thighs should always be draped before the lamp is used. See the nursing alert above.

Mothers with third- and fourth-degree perineal lacerations (extending into the rectal sphincter and the anterior rectal wall, respectively) are likely to experience more discomfort than those with lesser lacerations. Great caution must be exercised in giving these patients any type of ordered enema, suppository, or cathartic.

Patients with episiotomies and lacerations usually respond well to the combination of cleansing, heat lamp or sitz bath, analgesic spray, and witchhazel pads. Oral analgesics may also be helpful. At first, sitting may be quite uncomfortable. Advising the mother to tense her buttocks and tuck in her pelvis before sitting down often lessens the pull and discomfort of the perineum. She should be taught to inspect her episiotomy/laceration site daily for signs of infection—easily seen with the use of a hand mirror.

Elimination

Urinary output increases during the first 12 to 24 hours postpartum as the kidneys eliminate approximately 2000 to 3000 ml of extracellular fluid characteristic of a normal pregnancy. Voidings of postpartum patients are usually measured until two or three

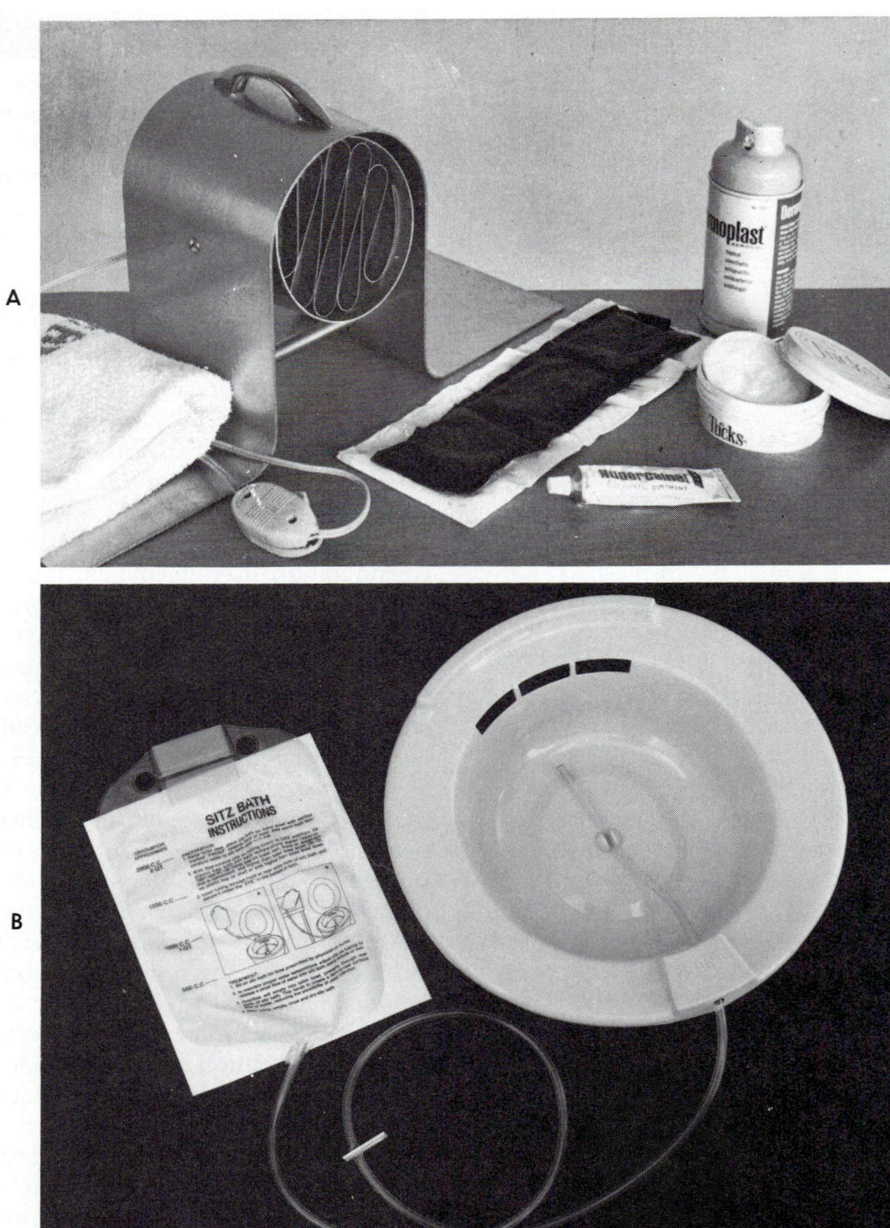

Fig. 13-6 **A,** Aids in relieving perineal discomfort through local application: perineal lamp (hood is draped with towel when used), perineal ice pack (unwrapped for better view), Nupercainal anesthetic ointment, Dermoplast antiseptic-anesthetic spray, and Tucks (lightweight witchhazel-impregnated compresses). **B,** Sitz bath easily portable for use in hospital or home. (Courtesy Grossmont Hospital, La Mesa, CA.)

voidings of over 300 ml are recorded and a fundus check after the voidings indicates that the patient is emptying her bladder well. See the nursing alert on p. 229. During the second day postpartum the patient may experience diuresis with a urinary output as high as 3000 ml. The woman should be encouraged to void every 3 to 4 hours, to drink adequate fluids (2 to 3 quarts per day), and to report any associated pain, burning, or difficulty which may indicate an infection.

Constipation, caused by diminished intestinal and abdominal muscle tone, may be a problem to the postpartum patient. Health care providers often order a stool softener the evening after delivery or the first postpartum day to prevent the discomfort of a hard

Nursing Alert

The urine of a woman who has had a long labor and associated dehydration or who is diabetic may test positive for acetone. A urine specimen contaminated with lochia may test positive for protein.

stool. Early ambulation, adequate fluids (2 to 3 quarts per day), and a diet containing raw fruits and vegetables and other foods high in fiber will help prevent constipation. If stools are difficult to pass, a stool softener may be recommended for use at home.

Immunizations

If the mother is Rh negative and her newborn infant is Rh positive (determined by testing cord blood) the nurse will give her *Rh immune globulin* specific for D antigen (RhoGAM), within 72 hours of birth. This immunization prevents the mother's sensitization to the Rh factor and prevents hemolytic disease of the newborn in subsequent pregnancies. This drug is a one vial dose, given intramuscularly.

If the mother's prenatal test for immunity to rubella indicates that she is not immune the most opportune time to immunize her is during the postpartum period. *Rubella* virus vaccine is a live vaccine that comes in a single-dose vial and is given subcutaneously. The nurse should ascertain if the woman is sensitive to neomycin since the vaccine contains neomycin. See the nursing alert above right. Because of the danger of fetal teratogenic effects from live vaccines the woman should also be counseled to avoid becoming pregnant for the three months following vaccination.

Nursing Alert

Rubella vaccine (a live vaccine) should not be given to a woman who is immunosuppressed or has received a blood transfusion within the last 3 months. If given to a woman who is also receiving Rh immune globulin (RhoGAM), antibodies to rubella may be suppressed.

Cesarean Birth

The physical care of the post-cesarean-birth patient is similar to that of any patient who has had a vaginal delivery. However, she has also had abdominal surgery and the nurse must attend to those special needs.

The immediate care of the post-cesarean-birth patient is usually given in a Post-Anesthesia Care Unit (PACU). If possible the family should be able to stay together and the parents given time to interact with the newborn. Blood pressure, pulse, and respiration rate are taken at least every 15 minutes for a minimum of 2 hours and until stable. The temperature is also monitored. The dressing should be observed for drainage and any staining should be reported. The lochia must be observed and evaluated. As a rule, cesarean-birth patients have less lochial flow. After the placenta is extracted during surgery the uterus is inspected and gently sponged, emptying the cavity of some of the drainage that would otherwise be expelled vaginally. The fundus may be gently palpated after surgery to determine its position, but it should not be routinely massaged. In some centers, electrocardiograms (ECGs) and pulse oximetry are also done.

If the woman has received regional anesthesia the nurse should assess the level of anesthesia every 15 minutes and assist the patient with safe positioning. The mother who has had a general anesthetic must be monitored for level of consciousness and assisted to turn, cough, and deep breathe. Elevating the head of the bed slightly may assist her in breathing more deeply. Splinting the incision with pillows lessens the pain of coughing. As soon as she is awake, she should be able to see her family and the newborn. After the woman is stable, she is transferred to the mother-baby unit.

The patient usually receives intravenous fluids during the first 24 to 48 hours. The first ordered fluids may contain an oxytocic to cause the uterus to contract. The intravenous infusion should be frequently observed for rate of flow and signs of infiltration. An indwelling Foley catheter is usually maintained for 12 to 24 hours or until the intravenous fluids are discontinued. The catheter should be checked for rate of flow and urine characteristics. Blood-tinged urine indicates trauma to the bladder and should be reported to the health care provider. The catheter tubing must be stabilized, without dependent loops. As long as the intravenous fluids or Foley catheter are in place the nurse should maintain accurate intake and output records. The nurse should assess the patient's ability to ambulate before removing a Foley catheter. Once the Foley catheter is removed the nurse measures the first three voidings, as for the vaginally delivered patient.

Pain control

Traditional nursing comfort measures, such as positioning and bathing, help make the recent cesarean-birth patient more comfortable. However, timely analgesia is also important. The nurse must carefully assess the patient's needs for pain medication and its effectiveness. A variety of medications and methods of administration are used. Intramuscular injections or, more commonly, intravenous infusions of narcotics are traditional. Increasingly, patient-controlled analgesia (PCA) by intravenous route or epidural narcotic administration just before the removal of the indwelling epidural catheter after surgery are alternatives. (See Chapter 12.) Once the patient is tolerating oral fluids she is usually switched to oral analgesics.

Psychological support

Although the initial physical care of the new cesarean-birth mother is the primary priority, emotional and maternal needs of the patient must not be forgotten. As indicated in Chapter 11 the woman who did not anticipate a cesarean birth may experience disappointment and a sense of failure (Fawcett, Pollio, and Tully, 1992). The nurse should allow her to talk over her experience and express her feelings. She should be praised for her labor efforts and reassured that she did the best she could given the circumstances. According to her strength and desires, she should be given the opportunity to see, handle, and breast-feed her infant. As she regains strength and mobility, she can assume infant care for longer periods.

Dietary considerations

Although orders may vary considerably the new cesarean-birth patient is initially given nothing by mouth. She is then gradually given a progressive diet based on her toleration of oral feedings, return of bowel sounds, and ability to pass flatus. This means progressing from sips of water to a clear liquid, to a soft diet, and then to a regular diet, over a period of approximately 2 to 3 days. Because of their reputations as gas-formers, milk, ice water, and citrus juices are often omitted from the maternal diet, along with other foodstuffs such as green peppers, cauliflower, and brussels sprouts. Some observers believe that drinking through straws may also increase flatus.

Ambulation

Although orders to ambulate may not be written until the day after cesarean birth, planned movement in bed should be carried out. The patient is periodically encouraged to breathe deeply and cough as soon as she is put to bed after surgery. She is assisted to turn at least every 2 hours and perform leg exercises. How long she remains flat depends on the anesthetic used, her general condition, and her physician's orders. When she is first allowed out of bed, she should briefly dangle her feet, then stand and march in place. Only then should she walk a short distance with the nurse's support. Walking the patient to a chair two steps away for a 15-minute period of sitting is not considered the best interpretation of "ambulate." The sitting position does not aid the circulation in the lower extremities. It is important to follow orders for progressive ambulation. Just because a patient is hesitant does not mean that ambulation should not be attempted. The nurse does not need to list off all of the complications the health care provider seeks to avoid through early ambulation. Usually if the nurse simply states that the activity will help the patient feel stronger faster and prevent or relieve gas pain, the needed motivation is provided.

Abdominal distention

Abdominal distention caused by trapped flatus can be distressing to any patient who has undergone abdominal surgery. Frequently, it is the chief complaint of the cesarean-birth patient. Medications, such as morphine or meperidine hydrochloride (Demerol), used for incisional pain and sometimes for the relief of pain from trapped flatus, can actually contribute to the problem by slowing bowel motility. The nurse should assess the condition of the abdomen. Evaluate whether the area just above the dressing is hard, bloated, and tender, or soft and relatively flat. Establish the presence of bowel sounds. A variety of methods are used to prevent or relieve distention: ambulation, a diet of low-gas-forming foods, small enemas, the Harris flush technique, antiflatulent medication (simethicone), and suppositories. Research indicates that mothers who rocked in a rocking chair (and also ambulated earlier) in combination with either diet modification or antiflatulent medication had less difficulty with gas pain (Thomas et al, 1990).

Incision

The cesarean patient should cleanse the perineum just as the vaginal-birth patient does. Sprays, sitz baths, or heat lamps, however, are not necessary since no suturing or trauma occurred in the perineum. The abdominal dressing is usually removed the first day after surgery. Once it is removed the nurse should periodically assess the incision line for approximation and for signs of infection. Many providers are allowing cesarean section patients to shower relatively soon after delivery, with a plastic protector over their abdominal dressing. Abdominal staples are removed at approximately the third postoperative day and are replaced with adhesive Steri-strips. The latter will eventually fall off. If they do not the mother may remove them at approximately 10 days postpartum. She should inspect the incision daily, after her shower, with a hand mirror and report any redness, swelling, or drainage to her health care provider. It is normal for the incision and abdomen above it to feel numb for several months.

Complications

Cesarean births result in a low rate of maternal mortality. Neonatal mortality, however, is higher. The results depend on the condition of the mother and the fetus, the equipment available, and the skill of the operator and nursing staff. Related maternal problems reported include sepsis, hemorrhage, thrombus formation, embolism, and complications of anesthesia. Occasionally, afibrinogenemia, causing bleeding problems, complicates the recovery.

Psychological Adaptation

All postpartum patients, regardless of their different individual backgrounds and specific strengths and problems, must respond successfully to challenges related to changes in body image, roles, and responsibilities before they can develop a satisfactory sense of progress, wellness, and fulfillment. Ramona Mercer (1981) speaks of the mother's need to review and integrate her childbirth experience into her total self-concept. Mothers must also put aside the fantasies that they may have entertained regarding their unseen infant by identifying, claiming, and learning to care for their real infant. Mercer indicates that as the mother adapts to the reality of her changing body and her new role as both mother and mate, she is performing a type of necessary "grief work." The nurse can be an important force in helping the mother cope with these changing perceptions and her developing maternal identity.

Fathers must also adjust psychologically to the birth experience and get acquainted with their newborn infants. One father's perspective, written a few days after the birth of his second child, is included in the box at right.

A FATHER'S PERSPECTIVE

The whole birthing process continuously challenged me to "stay involved and bond with the mother and child." I was moved around the room like a floor lamp until the baby was born. I thought my name was "Stand Here!" until the nurse handed me the baby and congratulated me by name. Seriously, it was very moving to see the woman I love deliver a child that we created together. All of the months of careful dieting, purposeful activity, and positive thinking by Ellen culminated in the appearance of a beautiful child.

As a parent and witness to the birth, it is difficult not to have first impressions. The doctor did not stimulate the baby immediately, in order to clean out the mouth and throat. As a result little Jennifer did not immediately announce her presence. After some brief tears I was charmed to see her react to our verbal attempts to soothe her. She became quiet and calmly looked in the direction of our voices. She appeared content and focused on what we were saying to her. What a valuable quality! I will remind her of this ability many times as she is growing up. I am sure that many of you will remark or reflect on the changes that are possible when people decide to have a family. After a few nights without sleep, I had to admit that we are no longer a couple with a kid. We are a *family.* This was a very sobering thought to me. I realized that like the TV show suggested, I will probably never buy underwear in a tube again. My politics will be exaggerated. I will have to learn to like "fast food." I will have to learn some tolerance for new clothing and grooming ideas. Worst of all, *I* will have to monitor what my kids see on television. All of this sounds like issues better addressed by Oliver North and Hillary Clinton!

Despite the numerous challenges, we are actually looking forward to the road of parenthood. Little Jennifer has moved us to another point as a family. As I held her tonight in a lamp-lit room, I was conscious of her trust and contentment as she opened her eyes for a moment and then went back to sleep. It was an opportunity to enjoy her company in a long list of opportunities to come.

(Used with permission.)

Postpartum "blues"

As the mother's hormonal levels change and the responsibilities of an enlarging family and infant care suddenly make themselves felt, many new mothers experience some degree of transitory depression, commonly called *postpartum blues.* This condition usually occurs around the third to tenth day postpartum—often after the patient is discharged. These feelings are in stark contrast to the excitement and euphoria experienced in the first few days after the birth (Mead-Bennett, 1990). Symptoms may include tearfulness that she cannot explain, sadness, irritability, and disturbances in appetite and sleep. The new mother is often surprised by these feelings. The nurse can help prepare her for their normal occurrence. With understanding and support the postpartum blues usually resolve spontaneously. Symptoms that last longer than 2 weeks may be a sign of major depression or postpartum psychosis and should be addressed by a health care worker (Beck, 1992; Unterman et al, 1990).

Postpartum depression and psychosis

Labor and birth often comprise a physically and emotionally exhausting period even for the normal, healthy woman. For a small but seemingly growing minority of women the weeks after delivery represent a special period of unresolved stress that can result in progressive symptoms of a mental disorder. For some the intensity of their distress may eventually bear the label of "postpartum psychosis." These mothers become withdrawn and uninterested or belligerent and suspicious. They are often victims of unreasonable fears. In severe cases, they may become dangerous to themselves and others.

Because of increasingly early discharge practices the nurse in the hospital setting rarely sees the anxiety and developing delusions. The causes of these disturbances are probably long-standing and multiple, including genetic, physiological, and psychosocial factors. The crises of parenthood may serve as only the triggering mechanism for the maladaptive patterns of behavior observed. Often these patients have had histories of previous emotional instability or illness. Depression has a more gradual onset. Psychosis, on the other hand, often has an abrupt onset, most often occurring between 3 and 14 days postpartum. Much more needs to be learned about these conditions and their origins.

Discharge Teaching

Discharge from the birth center on or before the second postpartum day is routine in many parts of the United States, and short stays of 24 hours or less are common for the vaginally delivered patient. The cesarean birth patient may be discharged as early as the third day postpartum. Parent education for early discharge is likely to be more effective if it is based on thorough assessment of learning needs, individualized teaching, and follow-up home visits or telephone calls (Harrison, 1990). If the new mother does not have adequate support or help at home, a home health or social service referral may also be indicated.

The new mother must learn self-care measures, as well as the basics of infant care. At her arrival in the mother-baby unit the nurse should begin to assess the mother's learning needs. It is important to focus on the individual mother's needs, since the time available is often short (McGregor, 1994). The nurse should include interested family members in teaching (Fig. 13-7). The box on p. 233 offers areas for suggested teaching topics. After teaching, it is important to gain feedback from the mother to evaluate what she has learned. Listening to the mother describe what she has learned in her own words or observing her as she performs a skill are two ways of evaluating her learning.

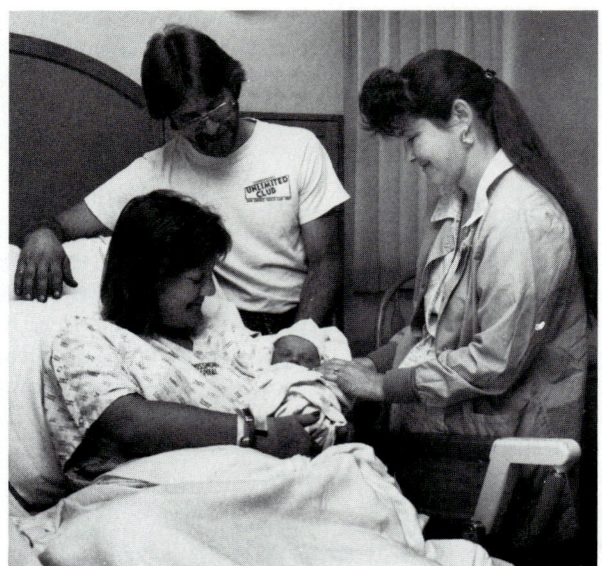

Fig. 13-7 Nurses can do a great deal to educate new parents. (Courtesy Grossmont Hospital, La Mesa, CA.)

Maternal self-care

Six areas of self-care not discussed elsewhere in this text are included in the following sections: weight loss, nutrition, physical activity, exercise, resumption of sexual activity, and signs of illness to report to the health care provider.

Weight loss. One of the first things the mother wishes to investigate after she has seen her infant and recovered some of her strength is her own weight loss. She is usually dissatisfied with her loss the first time she steps on the scale. Most of the initial weight loss (10 to 12 lbs) is the result of the delivery of the infant, the placenta, and amniotic fluid. Pueriperal diuresis will result in the loss of approximately another 5 lbs during the early puerperium. She needs to be reassured that, under normal conditions, she will approximate her prepregnant weight in approximately 6 to 8 weeks if she has not gained more than the average 25 to 30 lbs. If she has gained excessive weight, a referral to a dietitian may help her establish realistic weight loss goals (usually 1 to 2 lbs per week) and strategies.

Nutrition. Nutritional needs of new mothers differ based on whether or not they are breast-feeding. Nutritional requirements for the breast-feeding mother are discussed in Chapter 17. See also the Daily Food

PATIENT EDUCATION—MATERNAL SELF-CARE TOPICS

PHYSICAL CHANGES (PROCESS OF INVOLUTION)
- Breast
- Uterine
- Lochia

SELF-CARE
- Breast (breast-feeding and nonbreast-feeding)
- Perineal
- Incisional (episiotomy, laceration, cesarean)
- Hemorrhoids
- Bowel and bladder

ACTIVITY

EXERCISES

WEIGHT LOSS

NUTRITION (BREAST-FEEDING AND NONBREAST-FEEDING)

RESUMPTION OF SEXUAL ACTIVITY

CONTRACEPTION

SIGNS OF ILLNESS TO REPORT

PSYCHOLOGICAL ADAPTATION

Guide for Women in Chapter 9 to review the recommended number of food group servings for the lactating woman. Nutritional needs for the woman who is not breast-feeding return to prepregnancy levels. Once she has recovered from the birth, it is customary to advise her to reduce her calorie intake by approximately 300 kcal and to follow the Daily Food Guide for Women's recommendations for the nonpregnant woman (see Daily Food Guide for Women in Chapter 9). Adequate fluids, raw vegetables and fruit, and other foods high in fiber will minimize problems with constipation.

Part of the nurse's nutritional assessment should include a review of the patient's *hemoglobin* and *hematocrit* values after birth. Regardless of whether the woman is breast-feeding or formula feeding, hemoglobin values should return to prepregnant levels within 2 to 6 weeks of birth. Hematocrit levels will gradually rise because of the hemoconcentration that occurs secondary to puerperal diuresis. Nonnursing mothers should be advised to continue their prenatal vitamins and iron supplements for the first 2 months to replenish stores depleted during pregnancy and birth; breast-feeding mothers should continue them until the baby is weaned. The hematocrit may be checked again at the 6-week postpartum visit to detect anemia.

Physical activity. New mothers should be advised to increase their activities gradually and to avoid fatigue, lifting heavy objects and older children (over 15 lbs), frequently climbing stairs, and strenuous activity. Cesarean birth mothers are usually also advised not to drive for the first 3 weeks postpartum. Mothers should be encouraged to have midmorning and midafternoon naps—sleeping when the baby does can accomplish this goal. Ideally, they will have extra help at home to take care of household chores. New mothers have a tendency to try to do too much and become overly fatigued. Most women are physically able to resume all previous activities by 4 to 6 weeks postpartum, and usually delay returning to work until after the 6-week postpartum examination.

Exercise. Return to prepregnant weight does not necessarily coincide with the return of the prepregnant shape. Because of the stretching of the abdominal muscles, time and effort are required to regain abdominal muscle tone. Occasionally, a hernia develops because of the separation of the rectus abdominis muscles, which are supposed to support the abdominal contents. This condition adds to the "pregnant look." The mother should be encouraged to begin simple exercises to restore muscle tone and to improve circulation, promote involution, and regain general strength. These exercises are graded according to difficulty, ranging from deep breathing and gentle range of motion to pelvic tilts, leg lifts, and modified sit-ups. Kegel exercises help to restore the tone of the pelvic floor musculature and can begin immediately after birth (see Chapter 9 for a discussion of Kegel exercises). The progression of exercises should be directed by the health care provider because some may be too strenuous or even dangerous if done too early. (The knee-chest position done in early puerperium has been associated with a few cases of air embolism.) Exercise routines differ for those who have had a cesarean birth.

Resumption of sexual activity. Currently couples are advised to wait until lochial discharge has stopped and the episiotomy has healed (approximately the end of the third week postpartum) before resuming sexual intercourse. Because the vagina is still relatively dry, they should be counseled that some form of water soluble lubricant, such as K-Y jelly, may be necessary. The female superior or side-by-side positions allow the woman to control the depth of penile penetration and may initially be more comfortable. Breast milk can spout from the nipples during orgasm because of the release of oxytocin. If the couple finds the release of milk disturbing, it can be reduced by breast-feeding the baby before sexual activity or the mother may choose to wear a bra.

Fatigue, poor body image, lingering discomfort, changes in sexual response because of hormone fluctuations, and the distractions of the infant may interfere with the woman's sexual desire. Couples should be forewarned about these changes and encouraged to discuss their needs and concerns openly. They should be encouraged to express their affection in other ways (holding, kissing) and to make time for each other.

Methods of contraception are usually discussed at the 6-week examination. Since many couples do not wait very long to resume sexual activity, the nurse should also assess the need for contraceptive information, particularly those methods recommended during the first 6 weeks. Condoms with spermicide offer good protection with the added benefit of vaginal lubrication during this period. See Chapter 7 for additional information on contraceptive methods.

Signs of illness to report. Indications of infection, subinvolution, and other problems have been emphasized throughout this chapter but are summarized here. The mother should be instructed to report the following: severe fever (temperature over 101°F) and chills; increased swelling, redness or tenderness in breasts, legs, or sutures; green or foamy vaginal drainage; foul smelling vaginal drainage; frequent and burning urination; episodes of fainting; excessive or prolonged vaginal bleeding (two or more pads saturated within an hour); persistent pain that does not go away; extended periods of postpartum blues or depression.

Infant care

The average primipara and her partner have had less opportunity than their predecessors of past generations to learn the art of child care in their own family circles. Often their first sustained contact with a newborn infant arrives with the birth of their own child. Family-centered care, unlike the rooming-in concept, is a flexible concept of individualized care, which permits the parents to share the childbearing experience and to have access to their infant during the postpartum period to the extent they desire. This setting does not preclude the infant from being taken to a nursery when the parents so wish. Family-centered postpartum care makes it possible for both parents to get to know their child and to begin functioning as a family unit under the guidance of skilled maternity nursing personnel. Because the infant is cared for at the mother's bedside, she has an opportunity to observe and ask questions of the nurse. Visiting regulations vary in different hospital settings; however, siblings and other family members are often encouraged to visit and hold the new family member. Good hand washing should be done by anyone touching the infant. Cover gowns may or may not be used, as dictated by hospital policy. Multiple studies have shown no increased infection rate when gowns are not used (Renaud, 1983). See Chapter 17 for discharge teaching related to newborn care.

Educational resources

All postpartum staff members should be engaged in patient education and be aware of the importance of their teaching roles. In addition to teaching done by individual staff, many hospitals have a discharge class that covers aspects of mother and infant care. Unfortunately not all parents choose to or are able to attend. Some maternity departments also have closed-circuit television classes, which are available throughout the day. Printed instruction booklets outlining mother and infant care are also increasingly common and are valuable references once parents are home. Follow-up telephone contacts or home visits after discharge are sometimes included in routine postpartum care but are often reserved for women with complications. A great need exists for such educational follow-up (Evans, 1991).

Community resources can be valuable adjuncts to in-hospital teaching. Introducing parent-craft courses into the regular school curriculum may help prepare young adults for parenthood. Prenatal and postnatal courses offered by such community agencies as adult school programs, childbirth education associations, the YWCA, the American Red Cross, and public health departments provide many opportunities for learning about parenting, sibling preparation, and infant and childhood growth and development. Nurses should be aware of these resources in their communities and educate families about them.

Discharge

The discharge of the mother and child from the maternity service is an exciting time for the family. Before the patient leaves the physician's or nurse-midwife's discharge order for the mother (and one for the infant) should be verified and discharge teaching completed. The nurse's final assessment of the mother is documented and any laboratory tests or immunizations completed. Great care should be taken that all of her belongings leave with her.

The infant is identified again and dressed for the short trip outdoors to the car. The mother is usually discharged in a wheelchair. For maximum safety the infant should ride home in an approved infant seat, not in her mother's arms.

SPECIAL SITUATIONS

Grief and Loss

Not all parents leave the health-care facility with healthy infants. Some leave without a child because the infant did not survive birth or died in the early hours of life. Some leave without their child because their infant is premature or has some abnormality. It is especially sad when new parents who have waited for their child with anticipation find that, for all of the waiting and care, they have either no child, a child with a major anomaly, or fear that the child they have will not survive. If the infant must remain in the intensive care nursery because of prematurity or other problems, frequent communication with the nursery is essential. Her partner should be encouraged to visit the baby in the nursery. She should also be given a picture of the newborn and taken to the nursery by wheel chair as soon as possible. Often this patient feels very isolated and fearful regarding her offspring (see Chapter 19).

Parents need each other at this time. If nurses are to give parents the support they need in these crises, they must acknowledge their own difficulties with loss. Supportive nurses who are available, who listen, who recognize the stages of mourning, and who respond to the patient's cues, by touch or voice, are in a position to give a great deal of help and support to parents during infant sickness or death. Most parents have an overwhelming need to talk about the experience and should be allowed to do so with whomever they choose. Listening is probably the most important part of emotional support; platitudes are not helpful. A simple, "I'm sorry about your baby's death" acknowledges their grief. Some of the things a nurse can do to facilitate the parents' acceptance of a child's illness, deformity, or death are showing concern, allowing the parents to cry, relaxing visiting hour regulations, supporting the parents in their need to see, touch, and hold the infant, providing adequate and appropriate information, and allowing expressions of anger (recognizing these to be part of the grief process). Many of these parents have only a brief time to meet and then let go of their child. The nurse can help to provide positive memories by offering momentos such as photos of the infant, a lock of hair, and footprints.

One parent—often the father—feels compelled to suspend his own grief to comfort his partner (Page-Lieberman and Hughes, 1990). The nurse needs to be aware of this phenomena and encourage each parent to acknowledge their loss and talk openly about it. Parents may also need counsel in how to explain an illness, deformity, or death to the newborn's sibling(s). Explanations should be simple and honest. The age of the sibling will determine his or her beliefs and fears. Younger children may feel guilty or responsible, especially if they had ever wished the infant dead. Parents need to encourage the child to talk openly about feelings, allow expression of those feelings, and help the child deal with his or her feelings and emotions.

Groups of bereaved parents (Empty Cradle, Compassionate Friends) are available in many localities. These groups are designed to allow parents to share feelings and benefit from the support and counsel of those who have experienced similar losses. Parents should be given the names of these resources.

Relinquishing

Some mothers leave the maternity area without babies because they are not keeping their infants. These mothers also experience grief and loss. If a mother is planning to give up her child for adoption the nursing staff should be alert to her wishes for spending time with and caring for her infant. An emotionally healthy mother with support of friends and family may work through the crisis better when given an opportunity to perform caretaking activities for her infant (Lauderdale and Boyle, 1994).

KEY CONCEPTS

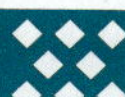

1 The postpartum period, or *puerperium,* is usually considered the interval extending from birth until 6 weeks after birth. During this period the reproductive organs return to the nonpregnant state. This process is called *involution.*

2 During the recovery period the nurse should monitor the patient for the following: vital signs, consistency and location of the uterine fundus, type and amount of vaginal discharge, appearance of the perineum, signs and symptoms of urinary bladder distention, recovery from any anesthesia, pain, hydration and nutritional status, and psychological status.

3 Vaginal drainage after delivery is called *lochia.* Immediately after birth, lochia should be moderate in quantity and dark or bright red. The presence of clots should be reported.

4 After the completion of the third stage of a normal, full-term labor the fundus should be below or at the umbilicus. The location of the fundus may be influenced by the size of the infant, the condition of the uterine muscle, the content of the urinary

bladder, and abnormal conditions such as retained placental fragments and the development of uterine infection.

5 The position of the fundus is usually recorded by counting finger widths above or below the umbilicus. The consistency of the fundus is usually described as soft, firm, or boggy.

6 If the fundus is large, soft, or boggy, it should be gently massaged with a circular motion until firm while one hand is held against the top of the pubic bone to prevent uterine inversion or prolapse. Other measures to promote uterine contractility include: administration of oxytocin, emptying the urinary bladder, and breast-feeding the newborn.

7 A variety of perineal cleansing techniques are available. The acceptance of a particular technique for perineal cleansing should be based on its safety, adequacy, simplicity, expense, and aesthetic satisfaction.

8 Patients with episiotomies and lacerations usually respond well to a combination of cleansing, heat lamp use or a sitz bath, and analgesic spray. Mothers with third-degree (those extending into the rectal sphincter) or fourth-degree (those extending into the anterior rectal wall) lacerations experience greater discomfort. Caution must be exercised in giving these patients any type of enema, suppository, or cathartic. Oral and topical analgesics may be ordered.

9 Breast engorgement results, for the most part, from increased venous and lymphatic congestion in the breast tissue. Nursing mothers experiencing breast engorgement may find that the following measures provide relief: manual expression of a small amount of milk to soften the breast before feeding; frequent nursing; good breast support worn continuously; warm, moist compresses; a warm shower; and the use of an oxytocin nasal spray to enhance the letdown reflex. Nonnursing mothers may be made more comfortable by supportive brassieres, the application of ice "caps" to the breasts, and analgesics. They should avoid any breast stimulation until engorgement resolves.

10 Constipation may be a problem for the postpartum patient. Early ambulation, increased fluids, and a diet containing raw vegetables and fruit and other high fiber foods may prevent constipation. Stool softeners may be used to prevent the discomfort of a hard stool.

11 Early judicious ambulation of postpartum patients decreases the incidence of respiratory, circulatory, and urinary problems; prevents constipation; and promotes the rapid return of strength.

12 Postpartum parent education needs to include the following topics: physical changes of involution; breast and perineal care; incisional care; fluid needs, nutrition, and weight loss; rest and activity; exercise; resumption of sexual activity and contraception; signs of illness to report; psychological adaptation; and infant care and feeding.

13 The physical care of the post-cesarean-birth patient is similar to that of the patient who has had a vaginal delivery. However, special needs exist related to her abdominal surgery. She usually receives intravenous fluids during the first 24 to 48 hours postpartum and has an indwelling Foley catheter for 12 to 24 hours. She is gradually given a progressive diet based on her tolerance of oral feedings, bowel sounds, and ability to pass flatus. Abdominal distention is frequently the chief complaint of these patients. Staples are removed approximately the third postoperative day and replaced with Steri-strips.

14 Postpartum blues is a normal, transient condition resulting from shifting hormonal levels and the increased responsibilities of parenthood. It usually resolves spontaneously. Postpartum depression and psychosis are more serious, characterized by withdrawal and disinterest and sometimes delusions and suicidal thoughts. They require prompt medical attention.

15 The nurse may effectively support grieving parents by empathetic listening, clear explanations, recognizing stages of mourning, and responding to patient cues.

CRITICAL THOUGHT QUESTIONS

1 When performing early postpartum checks, you discover that the uterus is "boggy," 2 cms above the umbilicus, and displaced to the side. What nursing measure would you institute first? Next? After that? Give rationales for your choices.

2 Compare and contrast recommended treatment of breast engorgement for nonbreast-feeding mothers and breast-feeding mothers.

3 With early discharge becoming increasingly common, postpartum observation by a nurse may last only 1 or 2 days. Identify the signs and symptoms that might indicate maternal complications. Discuss

how and when you could best communicate these danger signs to a new mother.

4 Changes in body image, fatigue, and emotional swings are common in the postpartum patient. How could you help a new mother cope with these?

5 A primigravida has prepared for childbirth by attending a series of natural childbirth classes. Because of cephalopelvic disproportion, she delivers by cesarean. She appears somewhat depressed and verbalizes significant disappointment about her birth experience. What feelings may she be having regarding the birth experience? How could you help her deal with her feelings?

REFERENCES

Beck C, Reynolds M, Rutkowski P: Maternity blues and postpartum depression, *J Obstet Gynecol Neonatal Nurs* 21(4):287-293, 1992.

Evans CJ: Description of a home follow-up program for childbearing families, *J Obstet Gynecol Neonatal Nurs* 20(2):113-118, 1991.

Fawcett J, Pollio N, Tully A: Women's perceptions of cesarean and vaginal delivery: another look, *Research in Nursing and Health* 15(6):439-446, 1992.

Harrison LL: Patient education in early postpartum discharge programs, *MCN* 15:39, 1990.

LaFoy J, Geden EA: Postepisiotomy pain: warm versus cold sitz bath, *J Obstet Gynecol Neonatal Nurs* 18(5):399-403, 1989.

Lauderdale JL, Boyle JS: Infant relinquishment through adoption, *Image* 26(3):213-217, 1994.

Lawrence RA: *Breastfeeding: a guide for the medical profession,* ed 4, St. Louis, 1994, Mosby.

Lentz MJ, Killien MG: Are you sleeping?: sleep patterns during postpartum hospitalization, *J Perinat Neonatal Nurs* 4(4): 30-38, 1991.

Mead-Bennett B: The relationship of primigravid sleep experience and select moods on the first postpartum day, *J Perinat Neonatal Nurs* 19(2):146-145, 1990.

McGregor LA: Short, shorter, shortest: improving the hospital stay for mothers and newborns, *MCN* 19(2):91-96, 1994.

Page-Lieberman J, Hughes CB: How fathers perceive perinatal death, *MCN* 15(5):320-323, 1990.

Renaud M: Effects of discontinuing cover gowns on a postpartal ward upon cord colonization of the newborn, *J Obstet Gynecol Neonatal Nurs* 12(6):399, 1983.

Sands JP: Bladder pressure and its effect on mean arterial blood pressure, *Invest Urol* 10:14-18, 1972.

Thomas L, Ptak H, Giddings L, et al: The effects of rocking, diet modifications, and antiflatulent medication of post-cesarean section gas pain, *J Perinat Neonatal Nurs* 4(3):12, 1990.

Unterman R, Posner N, Williams K: Postpartum depressive disorders: changing trends, *Birth* 17(3):131, 1990.

BIBLIOGRAPHY

Auerback K: The effect of nipple shields on maternal milk volume, *J Obstet Gynecol Neonatal Nurs* 19(5):419-427, 1990.

Damrosch SP, Perry LA: Self-reported adjustment, chronic sorrow, and coping of parents of children with Down Syndrome, *Nursing Research* 38(1):25-30, 1989.

Lawson LV: Culturally sensitive support for grieving parents, *MCN* 15:76-79, 1990.

Maguire DP, Skoolicas SJ: Developing a bereavement follow-up program, *J Perinat Neonatal Nurs* 2(2):67-77, 1988.

Martell LK: Postpartum depression as a family problem, *MCN* 15(2):90-93, 1990.

Miovech SM, Knapp H, Borucki L, et al: Major concerns of women after cesarean delivery, *J Obstet Gynecol Neonatal Nurs* 23(1):53-59, 1994.

Ryan PF, Côté-Arsenault D, Sugarman LL: Facilitating care after perinatal loss: a comprehensive checklist, *J Obstet Gynecol Neonatal Nurs* 20(5):385-389, 1991.

Spadt SK, Martin KR, Thomas AM: Experiential classes for siblings-to-be, *MCN* 15(3):184-186, 1990.

Williams LR, Cooper MK: Nurse-managed postpartum home care, *J Obstet Gynecol Neonatal Nurs* 22(1):25-31, 1993.

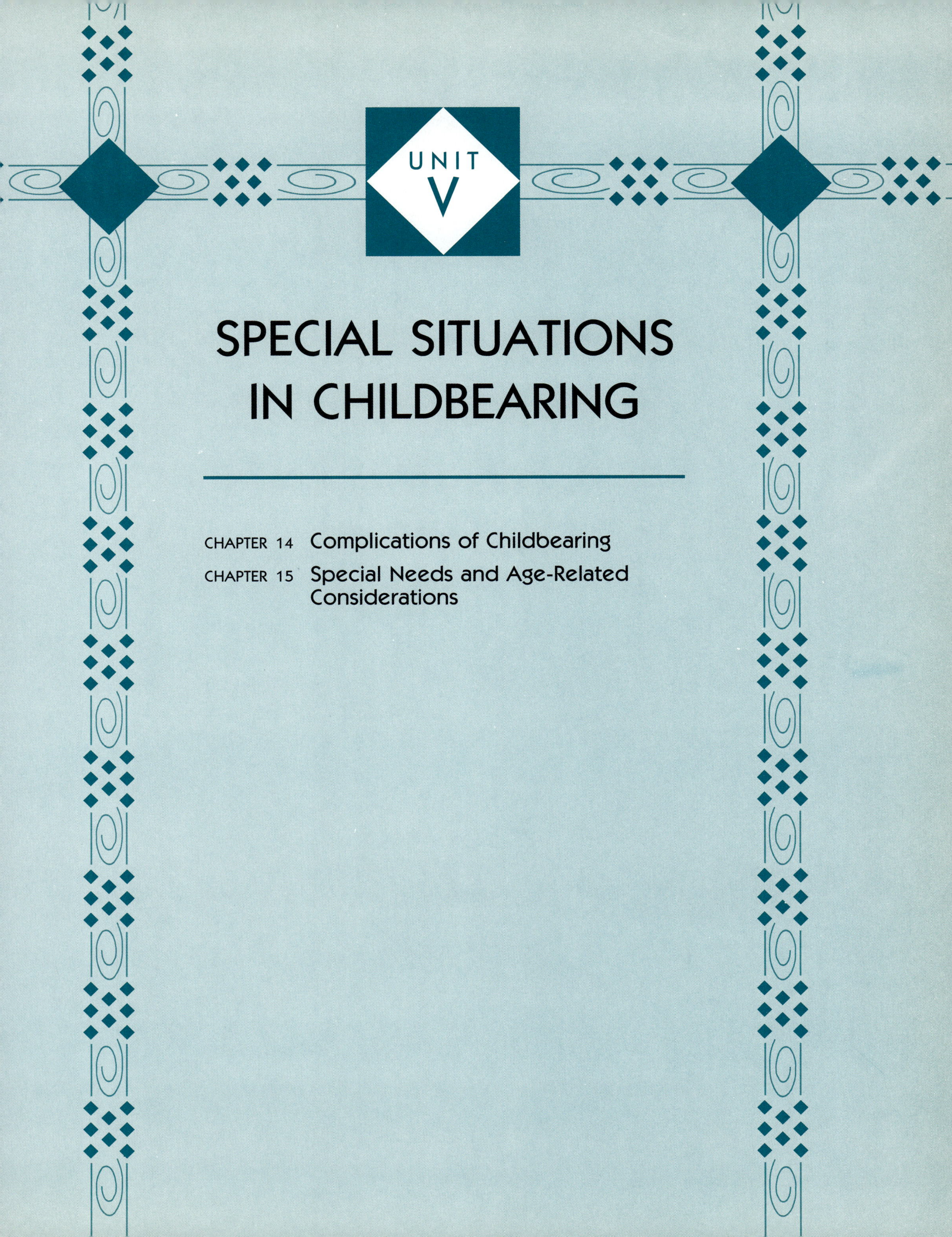

UNIT V

SPECIAL SITUATIONS IN CHILDBEARING

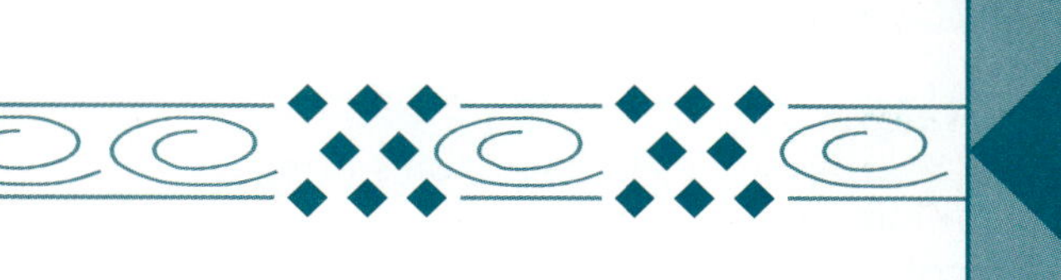

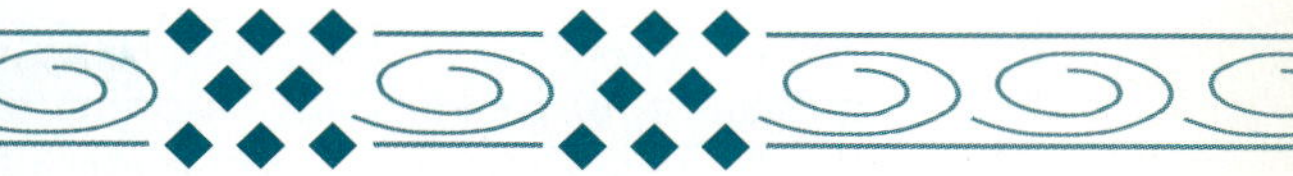

14 Complications of Childbearing

CHAPTER OBJECTIVES

After studying this chapter, the student should be able to:

1 Identify three psychosocial factors, three medical factors, and three obstetrical factors that place the pregnant woman and her fetus at increased risk for complications of pregnancy, birth, and postpartum.
2 Outline the needs of the pregnant woman with diabetes regarding insulin dosage, urine testing for ketones, blood glucose monitoring, diet, and exercise.
3 Indicate four analyses or procedures used to help evaluate the status of a diabetic mother's unborn child.
4 Indicate the point in pregnancy that a pregnant woman with heart disease is most likely to exhibit signs of cardiac decompensation.
5 Differentiate between bladder and kidney infections with regard to signs, symptoms, and treatment.
6 Explain efforts to protect the mother and unborn child from syphilis, indicating methods of transmission, disease identification, and treatment.
7 Identify three dangers of gonorrheal infection and why it affects reproductive capacity.
8 Identify the potential dangers of chlamydia trachomatis for the newborn.
9 Discuss dangers posed by the herpes simplex virus to the fetus and to the newborn.
10 Describe the risks of cytomegalovirus (CMV) for the fetus.
11 Describe the women most at risk for human immunodeficiency virus (HIV) infection.
12 Describe the recommended treatment for infants born to hepatitis B-infected mothers.
13 Define the various types of abortion: *spontaneous, induced, threatened, inevitable, complete, incomplete, recurrent,* and *missed.*
14 Describe the major threat to the mother's life during the rupture of a tubal type of ectopic pregnancy and note the signs and symptoms of such a situation.
15 Contrast in three ways placenta previa and abruptio placentae, the two obstetrical abnormalities associated with the attachment of the placenta to the uterine wall.
16 List at least five nursing considerations that must be remembered when caring for a maternity patient experiencing abnormal bleeding.
17 Cite the three major signs of preeclampsia, or pregnancy-induced hypertension (PIH), and state four indications of worsening patient status.
18 Indicate four categories of expectant mothers who are most likely to develop preeclampsia-eclampsia.
19 Explain why a maternal side-lying position is advantageous to the fetus.
20 Note the action and uses of magnesium sulfate in the treatment of PIH, as well as its side effects and the recommended antidote.
21 Describe the three primary causes of dysfunctional labor.
22 Indicate the primary risks of preterm, premature rupture of membranes to the mother and fetus.

Continued.

CHAPTER OBJECTIVES—cont'd

23 Indicate four reasons why a premature birth should be avoided and two methods that may be employed to halt labor.
24 Indicate the major causes of postpartum hemorrhage.
25 Describe the signs and symptoms of puerperal infection.
26 Describe the signs and symptoms of thrombophlebitis.

The goal of perinatal medical and nursing care is to ensure that healthy mothers give birth to healthy infants. This goal is met in most cases. Occasionally, however, complications arise during pregnancy, birth, or the postpartum period that result in poor outcomes for either mother, infant, or both. Many of these complications can be prevented or minimized with prompt recognition and treatment.

Nurses have a significant role to play in identifying those at risk for developing complications, in assessing developing signs of complications, in educating the patient and family, in carrying out the treatment plan, and in evaluating maternal and fetal responses. Nurses can also help families cope with the additional challenges posed by childbearing complications. Referral to the newly formed national support network for high-risk pregnancy patients, Sidelines, may be appropriate (AWHONN, 1993). This chapter discusses the most frequently encountered prenatal, labor and birth, and postpartum complications.

RISK ASSESSMENT

Risk assessment involves identifying those characteristics or conditions of the prospective mother or her child that place them at risk for complications. Some of these factors can be detected at the onset or shortly after the beginning of gestation. The amount of risk is determined by considering the number of and relationships among medical risk factors (e.g., chronic disease), obstetrical risk factors (e.g., poor reproductive history), and psychosocial risk factors (e.g., young age and low level of education). The box on p. 243 highlights factors that can place the woman and her fetus at increased risk.

Patients designated at increased risk may be referred to regional perinatal centers where specialists and sophisticated equipment are available. These centers are commonly associated with neonatal intensive care units, capable of caring for the premature or ill newborn. Maternal, fetal, and infant mortalities have decreased with prompt identification of risk factors, referral when necessary, and appropriate treatment.

PREGNANCY COMPLICATIONS

Diabetes Mellitus

Nearly 1 in 300 pregnancies is complicated by diabetes mellitus, an endocrine disorder characterized by high levels of blood glucose owing to insufficient insulin production by the pancreas or inability to use insulin to metabolize glucose. Three major types of diabetes exist (Table 14-1). The age at which the diabetes was diagnosed and the degree of vascular change resulting from the disease are important considerations during pregnancy.

Before to the implementation of insulin therapy, few diabetic women conceived. Many of those who did conceive did not survive pregnancy. Insulin improved fertility and decreased maternal mortality, but perinatal mortality remained high (approximately 40%). In recent years, technological advances have dramatically altered the management of diabetic pregnancies. Today, mothers receiving optimal care, who demonstrate diabetes before their pregnancy, experience a perinatal mortality of approximately 5%. Those who develop signs of diabetes during pregnancy (gestational diabetes) have no greater perinatal mortality than those without this condition. These improved outcomes are only possible with careful management (Gabbe, 1990).

Diagnosis of diabetes

Normal pregnancy is often referred to as a diabetogenic state. The hormonal changes of normal pregnancy cause resistance to insulin use, which increases blood sugar. High blood levels of glucose cause increased insulin production, which increases the rate of fat breakdown and protein synthesis. In this manner, additional amounts of glucose and amino acids are made available for fetal consumption, and an alternative source of fuel—free fatty acids—is provided for maternal energy requirements. Women with marginally productive pancreatic cells may not be able to meet the additional needs for insulin and develop gestational diabetes that resolves after delivery. Other

SOME CONDITIONS OR CHARACTERISTICS THAT CONSTITUTE INCREASED RISK FOR A MOTHER AND HER UNBORN CHILD

1 Low socioeconomic, educational status (influencing especially nutrition, prenatal care supervision, and compliance)
2 Little or no prenatal care
3 Maternal age less than 18 or more than 35 years of age
4 More than four pregnancies (especially if more than 35 years of age)
5 Conception within 2 months of last delivery
6 Living at high altitude
7 The presence of coincidental maternal disease or significant health problems involving
  - **a.** Cardiovascular disease
  - **b.** Renal disease
  - **c.** Diabetes mellitus
  - **d.** Tuberculosis or other pulmonary disease
  - **e.** Herpes simplex, syphilis, viral infections
  - **f.** Hereditary anomaly or possible carrier state (e.g., sickle-cell anemia, myelomeningocele, cystic fibrosis, osteogenesis imperfecta)
  - **g.** Use of drugs: alcohol, nicotine, and street drugs
  - **h.** Ingestion of fetotoxic medication, exposure to radiation or toxic chemicals
  - **i.** Obesity (more than 20% greater than standard weight for height)

8 Previous obstetrical complications that may recur, such as
  - **a.** Preeclampsia-eclampsia (pregnancy-induced hypertension)
  - **b.** Severe anemia, clotting problems, intrapartum or postpartum hemorrhage
  - **c.** Cephalopelvic disproportion

9 Previous poor fetal outcome (repetitive fetal loss, stillbirth)
10 Deviations in the current pregnancy such as
  - **a.** Twinning or other multiple pregnancies
  - **b.** Premature or small-for-date fetus
  - **c.** Postmature fetus (more than 42 weeks)
  - **d.** Breech presentation
  - **e.** Polyhydramnios or oligohydramnios
  - **f.** Preterm or prolonged rupture of membranes
  - **g.** Any of the complications noted in number 8 above
  - **h.** Obstetrical complications (e.g., placenta previa, abruptio placentae, abnormal presentation, Rh or blood group sensitization)

◆ TABLE 14-1
National Institutes of Health Classification of Diabetes

Classification	Definition	Treatment in Pregnancy
Type I: IDDM	Insulin-dependent diabetes (usually juvenile onset) Insulin deficient (prone to ketosis)	Diet control and insulin
Type II: NIDDM	Non-insulin-dependent diabetes (usually adult onset) Pancreatic cells unable to meet demand for insulin over time or with stress (resistant to ketosis and to insulin)	Diet control and insulin
Type III: GDM	Gestational diabetes—develops during pregnancy (carbohydrate intolerance)	Diet control alone or Diet control and insulin

Modified from Heppard M, Garite T: *Acute obstetrics: a practical guide*, St. Louis, 1991, Mosby; Creasy RK, Resnik R: *Maternal-fetal medicine,* ed 3, Philadelphia, 1994, WB Saunders.

women may not be aware that they have preexisting diabetes.

Ideally, screening for hyperglycemia begins before conception with a fasting blood sugar or 50-gm, 1-hour glucose screen (see the nursing alert on p. 244). If the woman is not screened before pregnancy, screening begins with the first antenatal visit and continues throughout pregnancy. Screening includes risk assessment, urinalysis to detect glycosuria (each prenatal visit includes a urinalysis for glucose), and a 50-gm, 1-hour glucose screen between 24 to 28 weeks' gestation. A blood sugar level of 140 mg/dl or more on the 1-hour screen should be followed with a 100-gm, 3-hour glucose tolerance test (see the nursing alert

NORMAL BLOOD GLUCOSE VALUES DURING PREGNANCY

TEST	VALUE
Fasting blood sugar	< 90 mg/dl
50 gm glucose, 1-hour	< 140
3-hour glucose tolerance	
Fasting	< 105
1 hour	< 190
2 hour	< 165
3 hour	< 145
Glycosylated hemoglobin	<7%

Nursing Alert

Some brands of oral contraceptives impair carbohydrate metabolism.

at right). Gestational diabetes is confirmed if two or more of the blood glucose levels are elevated (see the box above for normal blood glucose levels). Risk factors associated with the development of gestational diabetes are included in the box at right (Creasy and Resnik, 1994; Gilbert and Harmon, 1993; Howard, 1992).

Glycosylated hemoglobin is a blood test that determines the percent of hemoglobin A that has become glucose-coated during its 120-day life span, reflecting adequacy of glucose control for a 4- to 6-week period. It is used to screen women with preexisting diabetes before conception or at the initial prenatal visit (Gilbert and Harmon, 1993). Some perinatologists (specialists in high-risk pregnancy conditions) also use this test to monitor long-term glucose control during pregnancy (Creasy and Resnik, 1994).

Effect of pregnancy on the diabetic state. In women with preexisting diabetes, pregnancy does not worsen the diabetic state, unless the diabetes is poorly controlled. It does, however, significantly affect insulin control of the disorder. The diabetic woman's need for increased amounts of injected (exogenous) insulin varies during pregnancy. Until approximately 18 weeks' gestation, insulin needs are reduced because of the large amounts of glucose and amino acids that are transported to the fetus. The pregnant diabetic is most at risk for *hypoglycemia* during this period. After that time the developing placenta produces increasing amounts of hormones that cause resistance to insulin use so that from 20 weeks' gestation until term insulin needs both fluctuate and increase. *Ketoacidosis,* characterized by hyperglycemia, ketonemia, and acidosis, is

RISK FACTORS ASSOCIATED WITH GESTATIONAL DIABETES

Maternal age > 25 years
Previous macrosomic infant (larger than 9 lbs)
Previous infant with anomalies
Previous unexplained stillbirth
Previous pregnancy with GDM
Family history of diabetes mellitus
Recurrent monilial vaginitis
Obesity
Hypertension
Glucosuria on two successive prenatal visits
Fasting glucose > 140 mg/dl or random glucose > 200 mg/dl

Nursing Alert

The woman should have nothing by mouth except water after midnight prior to the 3-hour glucose tolerance test. She should avoid caffeine-containing beverages, which increase blood glucose, not smoke for 12 hours before the test, and rest for 30 minutes prior to the test.

more common in the second half of pregnancy in women with Type I diabetes (Harvey 1992). Immediately after the expulsion of the placenta, insulin needs drop abruptly and remain low for a period of time. Less insulin is required by the breast-feeding mother.

Effect of diabetes on fetus, neonate, and mother. The risk of complications is directly related to glucose control during pregnancy. Chronic hyperglycemia has vascular effects. These vascular changes also affect the placenta. The result is placental insufficiency of varying degrees. Hyperglycemia *early in pregnancy* may cause spontaneous abortion or adversely affect embryonic development. Congenital anomalies are five to six times more common in infants of diabetic mothers. Congenital anomalies are less likely if the diabetes is well controlled in the 3 month period *prior* to conception and during the first 2 months of pregnancy (Gilbert and Harmon, 1993). Hyperglycemia *late in pregnancy* is associated with intrauterine death (especially after 36 weeks' gestation); delayed fetal lung maturity (often not mature until 38 to 39 weeks' gestation); large infants (above 9 lbs); and neonatal hypoglycemia, hypocalcemia, hyperbilirubinemia and polycythemia. See Chapter 19 for discussion of the nursing care of the infant of a diabetic mother. Fetal exposure to hyperglycemia may also result in children with lower intelligence, motor impairment, and a tendency to develop childhood obesity and Type II diabetes later in life (Cousins et al, 1991).

Diabetes (hyperglycemia) increases the woman's risk of infection, especially pyelonephritis and monilial vaginitis. The probability is higher that she will experience pregnancy-induced hypertension or polyhydramnios, with their attendant risks of placental detachment, amniotic fluid embolism, and disseminated intravascular coagulation (DIC). The pregnant diabetic woman is also more likely to have a cesarean birth because of pregnancy complications, fetal distress, fetal macrosomia, and induction failures before 40 weeks' gestation (Gilbert and Harmon, 1993).

Medical management and nursing care

The goal of treatment of diabetes during pregnancy is to achieve and maintain normal maternal glucose levels (60 to 120 mg/dl during a 24-hour period) to prevent maternal and fetal complications. Management is a team effort. The patient's commitment is essential. Both a perinatologist and an endocrinologist usually monitor the diabetic woman's pregnancy. Other members of the team typically include a dietitian to manage nutrition, diet compliance, and weight gain, and a nurse who has a critical role in patient education. A social worker may be helpful in locating community resources. Effective education and control of the disease during pregnancy promotes optimal outcome and may enhance the woman's ability to control the disease for the rest of her life (Leff, Gagne, and Jefferis, 1991). Home control and management include the following five aspects: urine testing for ketones, blood glucose monitoring, insulin administration, diet control, and exercise modified to gain glucose control.

Urine testing. The woman should test the first voided specimen of the day for ketones, at least two to four times a week (Gilbert and Harmon, 1993). If ketones are present in two consecutive specimens the physician should be notified. Ketonuria may reflect insufficient dietary intake or ketoacidosis.

Urine sugar is not a reliable indicator of complications during pregnancy. Blood sugar should be monitored directly.

Blood glucose determination. At home blood glucose determination is done two to ten times per day depending on difficulty of control. This can be done by either of two methods: color-stable strips or the use of Glucostix and a reflectance meter. The latter method is associated with fewer hospitalizations for blood sugar stabilization.

Insulin management. Insulin is secreted by the islets of Langerhans in the pancreas. Failure of these cells to produce insulin results in hyperglycemia because insulin is required to carry glucose across the peripheral cell membranes. Two types of medication are used to correct hyperglycemia. One is the administration of exogenous insulin. The other is an oral hypoglycemic medication that lowers blood sugar by stimulating the pancreatic cells to produce more insulin. However, oral hypoglycemics are discontinued during pregnancy since this class of medication may be teratogenic and produce neonatal hypoglycemia. Rapid- and intermediate-acting insulin are both used during pregnancy. Insulin administration may be by multiple, subcutaneous injections or continuously through the use of an insulin pump.

Dietary management. The woman's adherence to dietary recommendations is essential in maintaining adequate glucose control. Dietary recommendations are based on prepregnancy weight, general health status, dietary habits, activity level, and insulin therapy (Gilbert and Harmon, 1993).

During pregnancy calories should be increased by approximately 300 per day (see Chapter 9 for pregnancy RDAs). The ratio of nutrients (e.g., carbohydrates, proteins, and fats) is important in diabetes. Current recommendations are 40% carbohydrates, 20% protein, and 40% fat (Worthington-Roberts and Williams, 1993). Complex carbohydrates are preferred, since they provide more sustained glucose release than do simple sugars. Saturated fats should be limited. To avoid hypoglycemia and ketoacidosis, a consistent pattern of meals and snacks should be distributed throughout the day. Each should contain complex carbohydrates and protein to even out the subsequent release of glucose (Worthington-Roberts and Williams, 1993).

Exercise. Exercise assists in establishing and maintaining glucose control. In Type II and gestational diabetes, exercise improves sensitivity to insulin (Winn and Reece, 1989). Type I diabetics may be limited to only mild activity because of the danger of placental ischemia during exercise.

Fetal surveillance

Fetal surveillance intensifies after 26 weeks' gestation and is essential for judging the most favorable time for delivery. Ultrasound examinations estimate fetal size, fetal growth rates, and the volume of amniotic fluid. Daily fetal movement counts done by the mother indicate fetal well-being. Nonstress tests, contraction stress tests, and biophysical profiles evaluate fetal well-being and placental sufficiency. If delivery is contemplated before term, amniocentesis may be used to obtain an amniotic fluid specimen to determine pulmonary maturation (L/S ratio).

Among the factors that influence perinatal survival are the severity of the diabetes, blood glucose control during pregnancy, placental function, the occurrence of other obstetrical complications or congenital abnormalities, and prematurity.

Labor and postpartum management

When labor occurs, insulin is infused continuously with an infusion pump. Hourly blood sugar assessment is used to compute insulin dosage, and the fetus is monitored electronically. After delivery, blood sugar levels continue to be the basis for determining insulin dosage. Breast-feeding mothers require more calories and less insulin. Breast-feeding women can avoid periods of hypoglycemia after feedings by drinking a glass of milk or the equivalent before feeding. The increased demands of parenthood can lead to poorly controlled glucose levels once the patient is home. The diabetes pregnancy team should arrange close follow up after discharge (Creasy and Resnik, 1994).

Cardiac Disease

The incidence of heart disease in obstetrical patients varies from 0.5% to 2.0%. Individuals with heart disease are classified according to the amount of activity that causes disability or distress (see the box at right). During pregnancy, cardiac output is increased by more than one third, reaching a peak by approximately 20 weeks' gestation. The maternal heart rate accelerates by 10 beats per minute (bpm), and blood volume is expanded by more than one third, reaching a peak between 28 to 30 weeks' gestation (Creasy and Resnik, 1994). After birth, readjustment in vascular volume occurs. The periods of maximum cardiovascular stress and the times that some measure of decompensation most likely will occur are near 28 weeks' gestation, during labor, and in the hours immediately after birth.

CLASSIFICATIONS OF CARDIAC DISEASE

CLASS I
Asymtomatic with all activity
Uncompromised

CLASS II
Asymptomatic at rest; symptomatic with heavy physical activity
Slightly compromised

CLASS III
Asymptomatic at rest; symptomatic with ordinary activity
Markedly compromised

CLASS IV
Symptomatic with all activity; symptomatic at rest
Severely compromised

Modified from Criteria Committee of the New York Heart Association: *Nomenclature and criteria for diagnosis of diseases of the heart and great vessels,* ed 8, New York, 1979, The Association.

Medical management and nursing care

The goal of medical management in pregnancy is to reduce the cardiac workload. The woman should be followed carefully by both the obstetrician and a cardiologist. Cardiac medications may need to be changed to avoid untoward fetal effects. For example, heparin is the only anticoagulant drug that is safe for the fetus. A dietitian may also be involved to monitor adequate nutrient intake and weight gain. The latter should be sufficient to meet the needs of the pregnant woman and fetus without being excessive. Activity restrictions are usually based on the degree of symptomatology. Bed rest may be necessary for women with Class III or IV cardiac disease. The nurse can play a critical role in educating the patient about her medications, activity restrictions, and the signs of cardiac decompensation.

Signs and symptoms of cardiac decompensation are a heart rate greater than 100 bpm and respirations greater than 28 per minute, often associated with dyspnea severe enough to limit activity and inspire coughing, rales at the base of the lungs, chest pain, edema, palpitations, and pallor or cyanosis. Decompensation must be treated to avoid overt heart failure. The nurse, in collaboration wih the physician, should carefully assess the patient for signs of cardiac decompensation at each visit.

Labor management. As in pregnancy, the goal of medical management and nursing care during labor is to reduce cardiac work load. The woman is usually positioned on her left side, and regional anesthesia is the analgesic/anesthetic of choice. The fetus is electronically monitored. Forceps may be used to shorten the work of the second stage of labor.

When cardiac disability is minimal, maternal and perinatal mortality are only slightly increased. With marked degrees of cardiac disease, maternal mortality ranges from 5% to 50% (Creasy and Resnik, 1994). Fetal and neonatal outcomes are directly related to the severity of the mother's cardiac disease and the resulting intrauterine oxygenation.

Urinary Problems

Urinary problems in pregnancy typically result from infections and/or preexisting renal disease.

Urinary tract infection

Asymptomatic bacteriuira occurs in 2% to 10% of pregnant women. If left untreated, these women are likely to develop symptoms of acute urinary tract infection (UTI). Symptomatic bacteriuria occurs in another 1% to 1.5% of pregnant women. Urinary tract infections can be of the lower urinary tract (the bladder—cystitis) or of the upper urinary tract (the kidneys—pyelonephritis) (Creasy and Resnik, 1994).

Pregnancy puts a strain on the urinary system. The developing uterus may pinch or kink the dilated ureters (particularly on the right because the growing uterus rotates to the right during pregnancy). Stoppage or slowing of normal urinary flow predisposes the system to infection. If the kidneys are already damaged by a previous pathological condition the added strain imposed by the excretion of fetal waste may be significant. Infection is most often caused by *Escherichia coli,* bacteria from the colon that contaminate the urethra when perineal hygiene is done incorrectly. It can, however, also be caused by other organisms.

Infection of the urinary tract may manifest itself in several ways. A bladder infection is usually accompanied by urinary frequency, pain on voiding (dysuria), urgency of urination, and lower abdominal pain. A kidney infection is characterized by chills and fever, nausea, vomiting, and flank pain, which may occur with or without urinary frequency, dysuria, and urgency.

Medical management and nursing care. Symptomatic or asymptomatic bacteriuria is diagnosed by obtaining a clean-catch urine specimen for culture. Infection is indicated by the presence of numerous white blood cells and bacteria (100,000+ colonies per ml) (Creasy and Resnik, 1994). Infection of the bladder and kidney usually responds well to measures such as bed rest, fluids, urinary sedatives or analgesics, and antibiotic therapy based on sensitivity studies. A repeat urine culture is done after the course of antibiotics. If hospitalized, these patients are routinely on intake and output measurement and undergo frequent blood pressure and daily weight determinations. Recurrent infection may necessitate urological tests to rule out urinary tract obstruction or other nonpregnancy-related causes. Untreated infection may prompt premature labor and delivery.

Nurses can play a significant role in educating women to prevent urinary tract infections. Pregnant women should be taught correct perineal hygiene and the signs and symptoms of infection to report. If infection occurs, they will also need to learn about medications and the regimen of treatment.

Preexisting renal disease

Renal disease may be inflammatory or degenerative. Any chronic condition that interferes with the blood supply to the kidneys will present symptoms in time. Conversely, any significant damage to the kidney will reflect itself in a change in the body's circulatory system, particularly an elevation of the blood pressure, as more and more pressure is exerted in an attempt to maintain adequate filtration. The onset of significant hypertension is related to a worsening prognosis for both fetus and mother.

Medical management and nursing care. Patients whose renal disease is not caused by a current infection (e.g., glomerulonephritis) receive much the same nursing care as those with a diagnosed bacterial invasion. Antibiotics are often given prophylactically. They are also treated with antihypertensives and diuretics when necessary. Chronic or advanced renal disease should be frequently evaluated by renal function tests. It may pose a real threat to both the mother and her unborn child. The fetus is frequently evaluated by nonstress tests, contraction stress tests, and daily fetal movement records.

Nurses can help pregnant women minimize the complications of chronic renal disease. Educating women about the effects of pregnancy on their disease, ways to avoid urinary tract infection, and the importance of following the medical regimen will optimize pregnancy outcomes.

Tuberculosis

Tuberculosis (TB) is still an important health problem throughout the world. In 1990 the United States reported the largest annual increase (9.4%) in reported cases since 1953 (Summers, 1992). Tuberculosis is frequently associated with poverty, overcrowding, and poor nutrition. Its resurgence in the United States is attributed to homelessness, drug abuse, poverty, and human immunodeficiency virus (HIV). Of particular concern has been the relatively high rates of disease affecting African-Americans, Hispanic-Americans, and recent immigrants to the United States.

Tuberculosis is spread through air-borne TB germs from the coughs or sneezes of a person with infectious tuberculosis. A susceptible person who shares the same air with an infected person for a prolonged period of time may eventually breathe in TB germs and become infected. Only 5% of *newly* infected people progress to active disease within 1 to 2 years after infection. The other 95% control the infection and are *not* infectious but remain at risk of progressing to active disease for the rest of their life. From this group, another 5% progresses to active disease if they do not complete a full course of preventive therapy.

Persons with a positive tuberculin skin test (Mantoux) should receive a chest x ray and be evaluated for preventive therapy with isoniazid (INH). INH is taken for 6 to 12 months to prevent the progression of infection to active disease. Preventive therapy for pregnant women is usually postponed until after delivery.

General symptoms of TB are fever, weight loss, fatigue, and night sweats. Symptoms of pulmonary disease include these same general symptoms with the addition of cough, sputum production, hemoptysis, and chest pain. Treatment for active disease must include a minimum of two to three antituberculosis drugs. A pregnant woman with active disease needs effective drug treatment to protect herself and her fetus. Length of treatment varies depending on the regimen to which the patient is assigned, drug susceptibility results, and patient response to treatment. Regimens vary from a 4-drug/6-month protocol to a 2-drug protocol lasting 18 months or more. Current recommendations from the Centers for Disease Control and American Thoracic Society are available at the local Health Department Tuberculosis Control Program.

Breast-feeding is not discouraged, but antituberculosis drugs in breast milk are not considered effective treatment for disease or as preventive treatment for the infant (Summers, 1992). The infant is usually treated with prophylactic isoniazid for 3 months (Creasy and Resnik, 1994).

Sexually Transmitted Diseases

The incidence of sexually transmitted diseases (STDs) has increased in recent years for the following reasons: improvement in laboratory diagnostic techniques, increase in the size of the population most at risk—15 to 24 year olds, sexual activity beginning at younger ages, and more varied means of sexual expression (Killion, 1994). More than one infection may co-exist. STDs are more prevalent among adolescents, young adults, and those of low socioeconomic status (Tillman, 1992). Many city and county health departments provide free, confidential STD diagnosis and treatment for minors without parental consent, relying on their right under law to care for persons of all ages suffering from communicable diseases. However, not all states have laws that permit private and hospital physicians to treat minors for STDs without parental consent.

The rising incidence of STDs has placed pregnant women and their fetuses at risk. Because of physiological changes in cervical and vaginal cells that occur during pregnancy, pregnant women are more vulnerable to contracting STDs if exposed and to worsening of symptoms if already infected (Killion, 1994). Unfortunately, these infections may be asymptomatic and lesions go unnoticed because of the internal nature of the female reproductive tract. The extent to which the fetus is affected depends on the gestational age. Infection in the first trimester can cause fetal malformation or spontaneous abortion; infection in later pregnancy may result in preterm labor, premature rupture of membranes, or possibly stillbirth. Some neonatal infections may be acquired during exposure to maternal serum and secretions at birth with symptoms developing later (Killion, 1994).

The goals of treatment during pregnancy focus on eradicating the infection(s) and preserving the future fertility of the woman, *without* harming the fetus (Killion, 1994). The nurse's strict adherence to universal precautions and principles of asepsis is essential in preventing the spread of STDs. The nurse must also educate the woman in strategies known to prevent the spread of STDs—condom use, careful partner selection, limiting the number of partners, and the avoidance of risky sexual practices (e.g., anal sex) (Nolte, Sohn, and Koons, 1993). The following sections discuss the STDs that can have a significant negative effect on the outcome of pregnancy.

Syphilis

The incidence of syphilis peaked during World War II. In the 1950s, it was believed that the problem of syphilis had been largely solved because of routine prenatal screening and the successful introduction of antibiotics in its treatment (see Chapter 9 for a further discussion of screening methods). As a result, education of the public and the related necessary casework were not continued with the same diligence. Because of this reduced effort and the previously noted reasons for the increase in STDs the number of reported syphilis cases almost doubled from 1986 to 1990 (Centers for Disease Control, 1991).

Transmission. The infectious agent, a corkscrew-like organism, or spirochete, called *Treponema pallidum,* invades the mucous membranes, skin, or both. The spirochete cannot live for more than a few hours in an environment deprived of moisture and is destroyed by drying. It is also killed by many chemicals, including soap. Though primarily a sexually transmitted disease, syphilis may be acquired through accidental inoculation by contaminated needles or exposure to infectious skin lesions by professional personnel or others.

Transplacental syphilis infection of the fetus may occur at any time during pregnancy.

Stages. The disease is divided into three different stages of development, or progression. The first stage, the period of *incubation,* usually varies from 10 to 90 days after exposure. The average length of this stage is 3 weeks (Creasy and Resnik, 1994).

The *primary stage* occurs when the characteristic lesion or *chancre,* a relatively hard, raised, painless area crowned by a craterlike depression, develops at the site of entry. This lesion is not always visible, however. It may be hidden from view in the folds of the vaginal or urethral canals. Although rare, the chancre may develop on the lips or breast. It is highly infectious. The chancre (or sometimes multiple chancres) disappears after 2 to 6 weeks. The spirochete may be identified in its secretions in dark-field microscopic studies. However, at this time the findings of the serology test are usually negative. If the chancre is not treated the organisms will multiply and spread throughout the body via the blood stream.

The *second stage* of syphilis occurs 2 to 12 weeks after the first exposure. It is characterized by a bronze- or rose-colored flat or raised scaly rash that may be quite faint, appearing on different body areas, but most significantly on the palms of the hands and soles of the feet. This eruption is often accompanied by enlargement of the lymph nodes. Flattened, moist, wartlike lesions called *mucous patches,* or *condylomata lata,* may also appear on the skin and mucous membranes. These contain the spirochete and are highly infectious. The person does not feel well and may have a headache, sore throat, and aching joints and muscles. Spotty loss of hair may occur. These signs and symptoms may fade away after several weeks, never to return in the same way, or they may reappear at irregular intervals for a period of up to 4 years. During the second stage of syphilis the serology test is routinely positive.

When the secondary stage subsides the disease enters a period where it produces no visible symptoms and is considered latent. The serology test will be positive. If untreated, approximately one third of these cases will develop *third stage* or *tertiary* syphilis, which may occur anywhere from 2 to 40 years after the initial contact with the spirochete. Approximately 30% of those patients in the tertiary stage develop widespread serious disorders of the heart, brain, central nervous system, and occasionally the liver, bones, and skin (Gilbert and Harmon, 1993). They are usually not infectious at this stage. The serology test is positive.

Adequate treatment with penicillin in the first or second stages of syphilis brings an optimistic prognosis. Third stage syphilis is also treated with penicillin, but the outcome is less favorable.

Congenital syphilis. Approximately 50% of infants will be born with syphilis if the mother has untreated primary or secondary syphilis. The incidence is 40% in latent syphilis and 10% in tertiary cases (Tillman, 1994). Although initial, prenatal maternal serology examination can be successful in identifying most potential cases the incidence of congenital syphilis continues to rise, reflecting the increased incidence of maternal disease. The problem has increased because of a growing number of women who, for various reasons, are not receiving prenatal care or who are not receiving adequate serological testing, treatment, or response to treatment. Current CDC guidelines recommend screening all pregnant women early in pregnancy and retesting at-risk women in the third trimester and again at delivery. Previous maternal infection and treatment do not produce immunity or protection of the fetus. Screening umbilical-cord blood to identify newborns with possible infection is not as effective as screening maternal blood at delivery (Stepanuk, 1994).

The untreated syphilitic mother is more likely to have a spontaneous abortion, stillbirth, or premature birth. If born alive the affected child may suffer from various problems. The most common characteristic of the syphilitic infant is the presence of a thick, almost continuous, sometimes blood-tinged nasal discharge associated with a sniffing sound on respiration. For this reason the manifestation is called *snuffles.* The skin, especially over the palms of the hands and soles of the feet, may be blistered and peeling. Sore fissures around the lips and anus may present. The joints are sometimes very tender. The liver and spleen are usually enlarged and the infant jaundiced. The causative organism has been found in lesions of the skin and mucous membranes. All syphilitic infants should be isolated until at least 24 hours after adequate treatment is begun. Secretion and universal precautions should be in place. More permanent but later-appearing signs indicating the prior presence of congenital syphilis are notched teeth (Hutchinson's teeth) and a so-called "saddle nose." Penicillin is again the drug of choice in the treatment of congenital syphilis. (See Chapter 19 for a further discussion.)

Gonorrhea (GC)

In many communities, gonorrhea has now reached epidemic proportions, particularly among the teenage and young adult population. The incidence of the disease in pregnancy ranges from 0.5% to 7% (Creasy and Resnik, 1994).

Gonorrhea is caused by a coffee bean-shaped diplococcus, *Neisseria gonorrhoeae.* Transmission is almost entirely by sexual contact. In females, it may produce an irritating, purulent, infectious vaginal discharge, and, since it often infects the Skene glands, may initiate burning on urination. The disease may spread into the reproductive tract and cause inflammatory changes. It may produce abnormal narrowing of the fallopian tubes and may be responsible finally for ectopic pregnancy (a pregnancy that develops outside the normal uterine placement) or sterility. In males, it generally produces a urethral irritation or discharge. However, asymptomatic carriers of either gender are possible. Gonorrhea may also become a more generalized infection, spreading through the bloodstream and lymphatic system. It is not innocuous, occasionally causing serious complications, spreading abscesses, arthritis, and other inflammations in both genders.

In pregnancy, untreated gonorrhea can result in *amniotic infection syndrome,* characterized by premature rupture of membranes, premature delivery, and a high rate of infant morbidity. The newborn may acquire gonorrhea during passage through an infected cervical canal, resulting in *ophthalmia neonatorum.* If the newborn's eyes are not treated shortly after birth, corneal ulceration and scarring occur, resulting in blindness (Creasy and Resnik, 1994). See Chapter 17 for a discussion of routine eye care for the newborn.

Pregnant women should be screened on the first prenatal visit (see Chapter 9 for a further discussion). Women considered at high risk should be screened again in the third trimester. Previous disease confers no immunity in the event of additional exposures. The incubation period extends from 1 to 14 days. Resistant strains of the gonoccoccus do not respond to the previously effective regimens of penicillin or tetracycline. The Centers for Disease Control (1989) recommend treatment with ceftriaxone, with reculturing in 2 to 3 months to identify reinfection (Creasy and Resnik, 1994). Alternatives to ceftriaxone include cefuroxime axetil, spectinomycin, ceftizoxime, and cefotaxime (see the Nursing Alert below). When the latter drugs are used, follow-up cultures from infected sites are recommended within 3 to 7 days of treatment (Creasy and Resnik, 1994).

Chlamydia

Today the bacterial microorganism *Chlamydia trachomatis* (CT) is the cause of the most common sexually transmitted disease in the United States—over 4 million new cases are estimated to occur each year. It easily surpasses gonorrhea in the number of persons affected, although it shares some of its characteristics and outcomes.

> **Nursing Alert**
>
> Doxycycline and quinolones such as ciprofloxocin and norfloxacin, drugs sometimes used in the treatment of gonorrhea, are contraindicated during pregnacy.

Like gonorrhea, CT is often present without creating noticeable signs or symptoms, but is also capable of producing much pain and anguish. In men, it may be associated with urethritis, epididymitis, and possible sterility. In women, CT may initiate pelvic inflammatory disease (PID), leading to ectopic pregnancies and infertility. Women under 20 years of age who have recently become sexually active and who have multiple sex partners are especially at risk for acquiring CT disease. Almost 50% of women diagnosed as infected with CT also have gonorrhea. It is recommended that patients with either disease receive treatment for both (Creasy and Resnik, 1994).

Controversy exists over the effects of CT on pregnancy outcomes. Some evidence suggests an association between CT and premature rupture of membranes, preterm labor and delivery, low birth weight, increased perinatal mortality, and late-onset endometritis (Creasy and Resnik, 1994). Pregnant women should be screened for the disease (see Chapter 9 for a further discussion). Extended erythromycin therapy is advocated for chlamydia infections during pregnancy. The organism is transmitted to the infant during passage through the infected birth canal, often resulting in conjunctivitis and/or pneumonia (see Chapter 19 for a further discussion).

Herpes genitalis

Herpes simplex virus type 2 (HSV-2) characteristically infects the lower genital tract. The lesions are similar to those of the related common fever blister caused by herpes simplex type 1 (HSV-1). Type 1 may also cause genital lesions but not as commonly as HSV-2, although rates worldwide appear to differ considerably. Regardless of the agent's type, the lesions, which typically involve the vulva, perineum, and cervix, are painful blisters that rupture to reveal shallow ulcerations that later crust. Healing of primary lesions is usually complete in 2 to 4 weeks.

The first episode of infection (*primary infection*) typically is accompanied by fever, dysuria, lymphadenopathy, and flu-like symptoms. *Recurrent* lesions are not as painful and last approximately 10 days. Often these infections are asymptomatic. Infected persons shed the virus irregularly and indefinitely. The virus is identified by tissue culture of scrapings from the base of a lesion or by detection of typical giant cells in a Papanicolaou smear.

During early pregnancy, a primary attack of herpes genitalis may be responsible for an increased incidence of spontaneous abortion (see Chapter 8). Later in pregnancy a first infection increases the risk of premature birth. Acyclovir (Zovirax) is usually considered the most effective drug in hastening the healing of primary lesions. Its use during pregnancy has not been adequately studied and is not recommended for mild cases. Some evidence exists that it may be used in severe cases without increased risk of birth defects (Andrews, Yankaskas, and Cordero, 1992). Sitz baths and/or heat lamps may provide comfort. HSV-2 is associated with later cervical dysplasia and may be linked with the development of cervical cancer. Follow-up observation is essential.

The infant may acquire the infection during vaginal birth. The infant born vaginally to a mother suffering from *primary* genital herpes has about a 50% chance of neonatal infection. However, the risk of neonatal infection in the case of *recurrent* maternal disease is much lower—4% to 5%. When neonatal infection occurs the probability that an infant will die is over 50%. An infant who survives may exhibit significant neurological damage.

Because of the severity of neonatal infections and the lack of satisfactory therapy, current recommendations are for rapid cesarean delivery for women who have *active* lesions near or at term and who are in labor or have ruptured membranes (American College of Obstetricians and Gynecologists, 1988).

After delivery, depending on the patient's labor and delivery history and on hospital policies the infected mother and infant may be cared for in a private room. The mother is taught the principles and procedures of drainage and secretion precautions to protect her baby and others from the infection. She may safely breastfeed.

Cytomegalovirus (CMV)

Cytomegalic inclusion disease (CID) is caused by cytomegalovirus (CMV), one of the herpesvirus group. CID is the most prevalent infection of the **TORCH** group (see Chapter 8 for a further discussion). An individual may shed the virus for several years. CMV infection is common in adults and children and is usually asymptomatic. It causes serious illness only in fetuses and those who are immunosuppressed (Creasy and Resnik, 1994). The virus is found in urine, saliva, cervical mucus, semen, and breast milk. It is transmitted by close bodily contact such as kissing, sexual intercourse, and breast-feeding.

CMV is present in 2% to 18% of pregnant women. It may be transmitted by asymptomatic women across the placenta to the fetus, causing serious fetal damage, retardation, and even death. Primary infection is more dangerous to the fetus than recurrent CMV. The infant may also acquire the virus by exposure to infected cervical mucus during vaginal birth. Infants may be asymptomatic or symptomatic at birth. The prognosis for symptomatic infants is poor (Creasy and Resnik, 1994).

Because the disease is typically asymptomatic, pregnant women are seldom diagnosed with CID. There is not satisfactory treatment for maternal or neonatal CMV.

Human immunodeficiency virus disease (HIV)

Human immunodeficiency virus (HIV), which causes acquired immunodeficiency syndrome (AIDS), is a growing problem among pregnant women. Estimates of births to HIV-infected women range from 2 per 10,000 to 66 per 10,000 (Ellerbrock and Rogers, 1990). Over 80% of children infected with HIV acquire the disease in utero (Butler, 1991).

Transmission. HIV is transmitted from person to person through exchange of body fluids—primarily blood, blood products, semen, vaginal fluid, and urine. In the United States, HIV in women typically results from intravenous drug use or sexual exposure secondary to a partner's high-risk behaviors (Nolte, Sohn, and Koons, 1993). See the box below for HIV risk factors for women (Acosta et al, 1992; Nolte et al, 1992). HIV affects certain T cells, thereby lowering the individual's immunity and making the person susceptible to secondary or "opportunistic" infections, which may cause death.

Transmission to the fetus or neonate can occur transplacentally and, less often, by exposure to blood and vaginal secretions at delivery, and/or exposure to maternal secretions such as breast milk (Bastin et al, 1992). Cesarean section does not appear to prevent the transmission of the virus (Creasy and Resnik, 1994).

HIV RISK FACTORS FOR WOMEN

1. Sexual activity with: intravenous drug user, known HIV-positive male, bisexual male, hemophiliac, person born in country with high rate of heterosexual transmission (African or Caribbean country)
2. Intravenous drug use (past or present)
3. Blood or blood products received from 1977 to 1985 (before strict screening)
4. Born in country with high rate of heterosexual transmission (African or Caribbean country)
5. Sexually transmitted disease (STD) history or at risk for STDs by exposure to multiple sexual partners

Not all babies born to HIV-positive mothers will be infected. However, at birth the infant of any HIV-positive mother will have maternal antibodies against the virus and will not completely shed them for 12 to 15 months (Ross and Dickason, 1992). Infected infants are usually asymptomatic at birth but are likely to develop symptoms and AIDS by 2 years of age (Bastin et al, 1992).

Medical management and nursing care. The Centers for Disease Control and the American College of Obstetricians and Gynecologists recommend that all pregnant women who are at increased risk for the virus be screened as early in pregnancy as possible. Currently, controversy exists regarding the wisdom of offering the testing to all pregnant women. See the Nursing Alert at right. Women who are seropositive need to be counseled about the likelihood of transmission to the fetus and the prognosis for an infected newborn so that they may make an informed decision about terminating or continuing the pregnancy.

Pregnant, HIV-infected women should receive pneumovax, influenza, and hepatitis vaccines and should be screened for sexually transmitted diseases. They should also be monitored for immune status each trimester. If immune status falls the physician may elect to prescribe azidothymidine (AZT) to delay the onset of illness (Creasy and Resnik, 1994). The nurse should teach these women risk-reduction strategies, such as condom use to avoid repeated exposure to the virus. Additional exposure during pregnancy increases the risk of transmitting the disease to their newborns. Seropositive women should be encouraged to maintain optimal nutrition and a healthy lifestyle and may also need information about recommended drug therapy. Infants born to HIV-positive women are followed and tested periodically for at least 2 years to determine whether they have contracted the disease (Ross and Dickason, 1992).

Little evidence exists that pregnancy accelerates the mother's disease. The best indicator of pregnancy outcome is the stage of the disease at the time of pregnancy. Women who are more immunodeficient are more likely to have problems such as prematurity, low birth weight, stillbirth, and fetal demise (Tinkle, Amaya, and Tamayo, 1992).

Hepatitis B (HBV)

Hepatitis B is increasingly recognized as a threat to the fetus and neonate. In the United States, acute infection occurs in 1 to 2 pregnancies in 1000 and chronic infection in another 5 to 15 pregnancies in 1000. Most infections are asymptomatic or symptoms are relatively mild with low-grade fever, joint pains, and liver and spleen enlargement.

> **Nursing Alert**
>
> HIV testing is voluntary and must be accompanied by informed consent procedures and pretest counseling. Results are strictly confidential.

In the United States, transmission of HBV is through contact with blood and feces and during sexual intercourse (Ross and Dickason, 1992). The course of the disease is not altered by pregnancy. The primary concern in pregnancy is the transmission of HBV to the neonate through exposure to maternal blood and/or feces during delivery. Even if the neonate does not acquire the disease during delivery, 30% to 60% will become infected during the first 5 years of life if the mother is not treated and the infant is not vaccinated (Crawford and Pruss, 1993).

All pregnant women should be tested for the presence of hepatitis B surface antigen (HBsAg) (see Chapter 9 for a further discussion). No specific treatment exists for hepatitis other than rest and a high-protein, low-fat diet (Creasy and Resnik, 1994). If the woman tests negative but has been exposed or is not immune to hepatitis B, she should be given a course of HBV vaccine.

Infants born to women who have hepatitis B during pregnancy and who are HBsAg positive should be given hepatitis B immune globulin (HBIG), which provides temporary protection. In addition, hepatitis B vaccine should be given to the infant within 12 hours of birth and repeated at 1 and 6 months of age. Routine hepatitis B vaccination is also recommended for all neonates born to HBsAg-negative women (Centers for Disease Control, 1991).

Bleeding Disorders

During pregnancy, vaginal bleeding is always considered a potential threat to the well-being of both the fetus and the mother. Bleeding in the first half of pregnancy may be caused by abortion, ectopic pregnancy or hydatidiform mole. In the latter half of pregnancy particularly in the third trimester, bleeding is most often related to placenta previa or abruptio placentae.

Abortion

Spotting or bleeding during the early months of pregnancy is often related to abortion, defined as loss of the fetus before 20 weeks' gestation. Abortions may be *spontaneous*, occurring naturally (called *miscarriages* by the public), or *induced*, (also referred to as

◆ TABLE 14-2
Clinical Classification of Spontaneous Abortions

Classification	Definition	Manifestations
Threatened	Condition in which continuation of pregnancy is in doubt	Vaginal bleeding or spotting, which may be associated with mild cramps of back and lower abdomen Closed cervix Uterus that is soft, nontender, and enlarged appropriate to gestational age
Inevitable	Condition in which termination of pregnancy is in progress	Cervical dilation Membranes may be ruptured Vaginal bleeding Mild to painful uterine contractions
Complete	Condition in which products of conception are totally expelled from uterus	
Incomplete	Condition in which fragments of products of conception are expelled and part is retained in uterus	Profuse bleeding because retained tissue parts interfere with myometrial contractions
Missed	Condition in which embryo or fetus dies during first 20 weeks of gestation but is retained in uterus for 4 weeks or more afterward	Amenorrhea or intermittent vaginal bleeding, spotting, or brownish discharge No uterine growth No fetal movement felt Regression of breast changes
Septic	Condition in which products of conception become infected during abortion process	Elevated temperature of 100.4° F (38° C) or greater Foul-smelling vaginal discharge
Recurrent	Condition in which two or more successive pregnancies have ended in spontaneous abortion	

From Gilbert ES, Harmon JS: *High risk pregnancy and delivery,* St. Louis, 1993, Mosby.

therapeutic) indicating artificial interruption. See Chapter 7 for a discussion of induced abortion.

Spontaneous abortions are further classified by the following types: threatened, inevitable, complete, incomplete, missed, septic, and recurrent. (Table 14-2). Approximately 50% of all threatened abortions terminate as abortions. Approximately 50% to 60% of such fetal loss is associated with some defect in the developing child. Spontaneous abortion seems to be one way that nature tries to rectify a basic error. Approximately 10% to 15% of all pregnancies end in spontaneous abortions with no known causes. General improvement of maternal physical and mental health, prior immunization against infectious diseases, avoiding teratogenic substances, and proper prenatal care may increase the chances that a woman will not experience a spontaneous abortion. If loss after the first trimester is caused by premature dilation of the cervix (incompetent cervix) the cervix may be closed by various suturing techniques and released only when the fetus is ready for birth (e.g., Shirodkar and Würm and Lash procedures).

Medical management and nursing care. In a spontaneous abortion the patient usually presents with vaginal bleeding that may be dark or bright red. Pain may come and go or be persistent, and may be experienced as a low backache, pelvic pressure, or tenderness over the uterus (Gilbert and Harmon, 1993). The first task for the health care provider is to determine whether the bleeding is the result of a threatened abortion or another cause. Patients with inevitable abortion are admitted to the gynecological service. However, if the viability of the fetus is debatable, the patient may be referred to the obstetrical service.

The nursing care of a woman who is *threatening* spontaneous abortion includes bed rest; avoidance of stress; observation for uterine cramping and loss of amniotic fluid; temperature, pulse, and blood pressure records; careful determination of the presence and

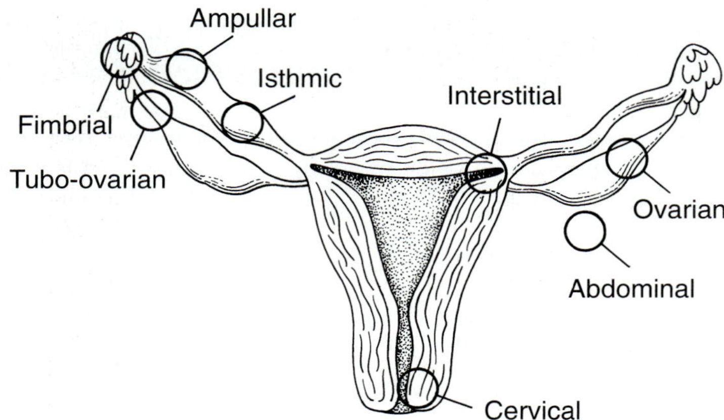

Fig. 14-1 Sites of implantation of ectopic pregnancies.

amount of vaginal bleeding (the health care provider may wish all pads and soiled linen to be saved to evaluate extent of blood loss or frequent hematocrit and hemoglobin checks); and watchfulness to secure any passed tissue for diagnosis. Periodical checks for fetal heart tone with a doppler device may be ordered if the pregnancy is beyond 10 weeks' gestation. Sedatives may be ordered.

Inevitable abortion may be speeded by use of oxytocic drugs to stimulate the uterus to contract or by surgical intervention, especially in the presence of hemorrhage. From the time an abortion becomes inevitable until it is complete (naturally or by surgical intervention) the woman is at risk for hemorrhage and/or infection. Vigilance for an elevated temperature is essential. Iron medication or blood transfusions may be indicated. Intravenous fluids may be ordered to replace fluid loss. Sedatives and antibiotics may also be used.

If the abortion is *incomplete* the remainder of the products of conception must be promptly removed from the uterus. Failure to do so increases the chance of hemorrhage and infection. See Chapter 7 for a description of methods used to induce abortion. In the event of a missed abortion beyond 12 weeks' gestation, labor may be induced with prostaglandins and intravenous oxytocin to deliver the dead fetus.

Rh-negative women who are not sensitized should receive immune globulin (RhoGam) within 72 hours of a spontaneous or induced abortion. A patient who aborts must continue to be closely observed for bleeding and infection for several hours or days, depending on her general condition and the circumstances of her loss. She should be taught the signs and symptoms of infection and excessive bleeding and report them promptly. The nurse should be aware that a woman frequently experiences significant grief and loss with spontaneous abortion, regardless of gestational age. Family members and friends may not understand the depth of these feelings, making it more difficult for her to express them and to grieve. The nurse should acknowledge the possibility that she is grieving, encourage her to express her feelings, and reassure her that they are normal.

Ectopic pregnancy

The term *ectopic pregnancy* refers to any pregnancy that does not occupy the uterine cavity. In the majority of pregnancies the migrating egg is fertilized by the sperm in the fallopian tube and usually nests or implants in the lining of the uterine wall. However, if the tubes are abnormally narrowed, stenosed from inflammation, tumor, or congenital origin, then the tube may allow the sperm to ascend but be too narrow to allow the passage of the fertilized egg into the uterus. The majority of ectopic pregnancies (approximately 95%) are located in the fallopian tube. The egg develops in the tube and soon causes rupture. Rarely, the embryo may continue growing as an abdominal pregnancy, which in unusual cases produces a full-term child who may survive if delivered through an abdominal incision. See Figure 14-1 for possible ectopic pregnancy sites.

The incidence of ectopic pregnancy in the United States is 2% and increasing every year (Trustem, 1991). It terminates almost invariably with fetal loss and is the leading cause of maternal mortality in the first trimester in the United States (Stock, 1990). The incidence is higher in women with tubal damage from pelvic infection or tubal surgery, endometriosis, altered hormones that impede ovum transport in the tube, contraceptive failure from an intrauterine contraceptive device (IUD), and those who smoke.

Medical management and nursing care. If tubal rupture or abortion occurs the patient, who may or may not be aware that she is pregnant, characteristically suffers severe knife-like pain in either lower abdominal quadrant. This may or may not be followed by spotting or bleeding. Shoulder pain from blood irritating the diaphragm or the urge to defecate are classic symptoms. The physician may be able to palpate a mass in the cul de sac or aspirate bloody fluid from the sac. Abdominal ultrasound may aid diagnosis by ruling out an intrauterine pregnancy. Transvaginal ultrasound is increasingly used to locate the misplaced gestational sac *before* rupture. Hemoglobin and hematocrit levels may drop and leukocyte levels may increase. Human chorionic gonadotropin (hCG) titers are lower than in an intrauterine pregnancy.

The danger of hemorrhage in ectopic pregnancy is extremely serious. The amount of vaginal bleeding observed does not always reveal the true condition of the patient, since much blood loss can be hidden within the abdominal cavity. As a result, the signs of shock that develop are out of proportion to the amount of visible blood loss. If the patient has profuse internal hemorrhage she will rapidly develop the classic signs of circulatory shock that include: pallor; cold, clammy skin; rapid, weak pulse, which will slow if shock deepens; falling blood pressure (a systolic reading of 90 mm Hg or under is usually considered shock, depending on previous readings obtained); apprehension; loss of consciousness; and dilated pupils. If the bleeding is slow the abdomen will become rigid and tender and signs of shock develop more gradually. Rapid surgical treatment and blood-loss replacement are usually indicated once diagnosis is confirmed.

The nurse must monitor the amount of vaginal bleeding, vital signs, and the woman's general condition for signs of overt hemorrhage and hypovolemic shock. Preparations for surgery are the same as those for any abdominal procedure. Rh-negative women who are not sensitized should receive immune globulin (RhoGam) within 72 hours. The woman with an ectopic pregnancy may experience feelings of grief and loss much like those experienced with spontaneous abortion.

Hydatidiform mole

Another complication that may produce hemorrhage is called *hydatidiform mole* (usually shortened to hydatid mole). It is fairly rare in the United States, but much more common in parts of Asia. In this condition, for some unknown reason, the developing embryo and placenta deteriorate and usually lose their identity. Instead, a mass of abnormal, rapidly growing, trophoblastic tissue develops. It is theorized that formation of the mole is preceded by the death of the embryo and the disappearance of fetal circulation, whereas maternal circulation continues to sustain residual trophoblastic tissue. However, a mole can exist with a normal pregnancy.

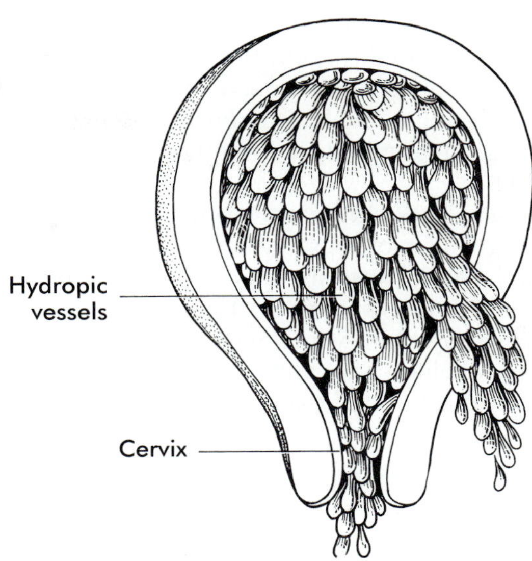

Fig. 14-2 Hydatidiform mole. In this figure some of the hydropic vesicles are being passed.

Medical management and nursing care. At times this tissue may resemble a cluster of small grapes or vesicles, or it may be of tapioca consistency (Fig. 14-2). Its presence may be suspected when the growth of a pregnancy seems abnormally rapid (a 3-month pregnancy may equal the size of a 5-month gestation), when no fetal heart tone or movement is detected, when nausea and vomiting are excessive or persistent, and when pregnancy-induced hypertension develops before 24 weeks' gestation. Vaginal bleeding may be continuous or intermittent and is usually brownish but may be bright red. Quantitative human chorionic gonadotropin (hCG) levels in the urine are greatly elevated. Diagnosis is made with ultrasound studies that identify the characteristic vesicles. The fetal skeleton is absent. If part of the abnormal tissue is expelled from the uterus, pathological examination is indicated. Rarely this growth erodes the uterus and causes rupture. The treatment is to evacuate the uterus by suction and sharp curettage.

Aside from the loss of the pregnancy the significance of a molar pregnancy for the woman is the possibility of developing a malignant tumor from the trophoblastic tissue (choriocarcinoma), which may spread to the lungs and other body parts. After the mole's removal, hCG levels are carefully monitored for a year to see whether any trophoblastic tissue is still active in the body and producing hormones. Regular chest x rays are done to detect metastasis, and the patient is advised to avoid pregnancy for at least a year. If the woman has completed her desired childbearing the physician may advise removal of the uterus (hysterectomy) because of the risk of choriocarcinoma. Fortunately, spreading choriocarcinoma is often curable with the use of anticancer chemicals such as methotrexate and actinomycin D.

The nurse in the antepartum setting should be aware of the signs of molar pregnancy. When the woman is hospitalized the nurse should monitor the amount and type of bleeding and vital signs. The woman may experience grief for the pregnancy loss and fear for her own well-being. She and her family will require information and emotional support.

Placenta previa

Two main types of obstetrical hemorrhage are associated with the location of the placenta and its attachment. In the condition known as *placenta previa* the placenta implants low on the interior of the uterine wall. A total placenta previa covers the cervical opening; a partial or incomplete placenta previa impinges on but does not cover the cervix; and a marginal placenta previa is low-lying, close to the dilating cervix (Fig. 14-3). Placenta previa occurs once in approximately 200 births. The cause is unknown but is more common in multiparous women.

In the latter part of pregnancy the uterine contractions, which are always taking place to some degree though not always felt by the mother, may loosen the attachment of this abnormally positioned placenta and cause bright red, painless bleeding. The presence of placenta previa in other cases may not be detected until the onset of true labor and the dilation of the cervical canal.

Medical management and nursing care. The health care provider must first identify the cause of bleeding. A placenta previa is most commonly diagnosed by ultrasound. When the cause of vaginal bleeding is uncertain, a vaginal examination should never be done because it can further exacerbate bleeding. If ultrasound is not available, the fetus is term, and bleeding is heavy the provider may elect to do a vaginal examination using a *double set-up* procedure. The delivery room is prepared for a vaginal examination and for cesarean birth in case the examination precipitates profuse bleeding.

If the woman is diagnosed with a placenta previa, bleeding is minimal, and she is less than 37 weeks' gestation, birth should be delayed until the fetus is term. She will be placed on bed rest, and the nurse will carefully monitor vital signs, fetal heart rate, and vaginal bleeding. If the placenta is not implanted too low, if bleeding is minimal, and if the fetus is well but premature, some obstetricians may adopt a "wait-and-see" attitude and eventually deliver the patient vaginally. It is possible that as the uterus enlarges during the pregnancy the placenta may move up. However, if profuse bleeding occurs or if signs of fetal distress exist, a cesarean birth will be performed. Cesarean birth is always necessary in the case of a total placenta previa. Infection and emboli are other possible complications of placenta previa that should be considered.

As in other cases of bleeding during pregnancy the nurse should monitor the amount and type of vaginal bleeding, vital signs, and fetal heart rate. Important nursing functions are to provide emotional support and information about the condition and treatment regimen for the woman and her family.

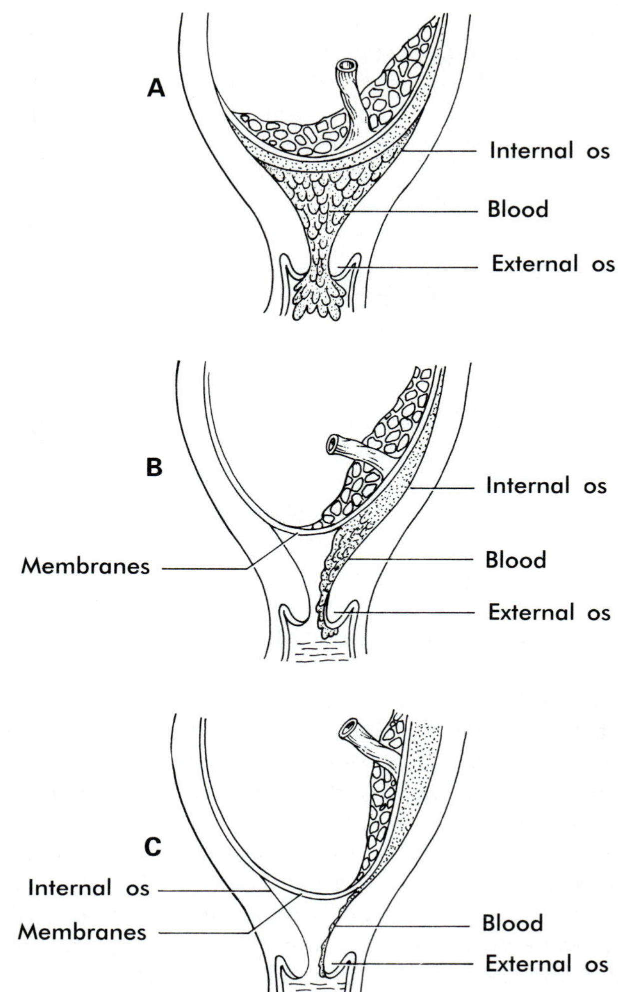

Fig. 14-3 Types of placenta previa after onset of labor. **A,** Complete, or total; **B,** incomplete, or partial; **C,** marginal, or low-lying.

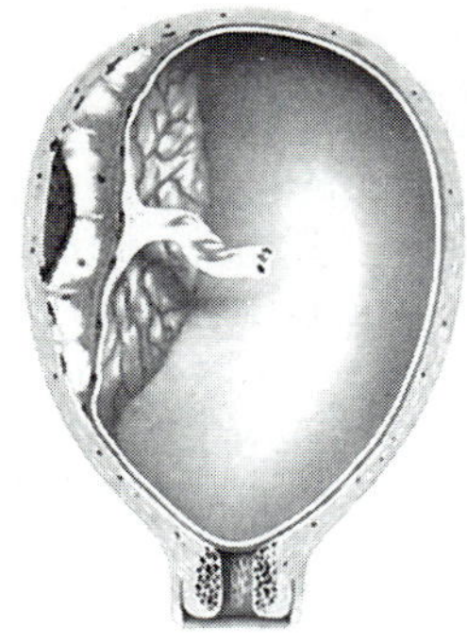

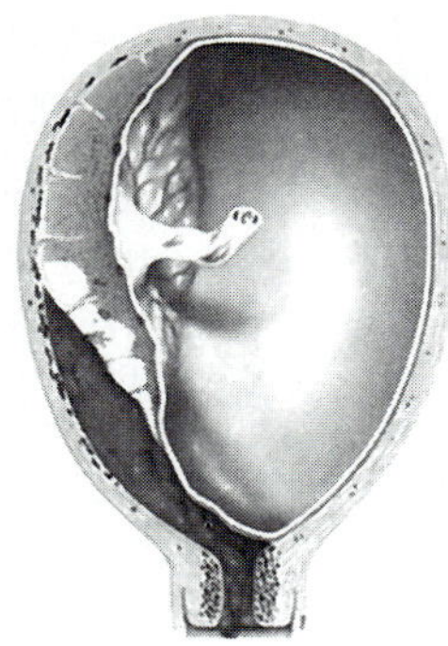

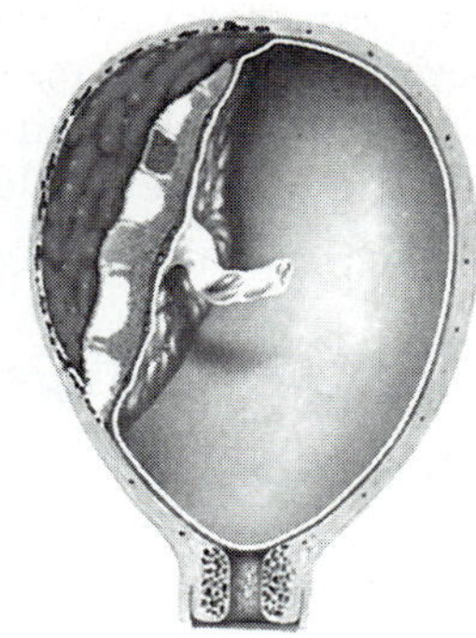

Fig. 14-4 Abruptio placentae. Premature separation of normally implanted placenta. (Courtesy Ross Laboratories, Columbus, OH.)

Abruptio placentae

The other type of hemorrhage related to placental attachment results from *abruptio placentae,* also called *ablatio placentae* or *premature separation of the placenta.* In this condition the placenta is implanted in the correct place but for some reason (e.g., chronic high blood pressure, pregnancy-induced hypertension, glomerulonephritis, dietary deficiency, local injury, rapid changes in intrauterine pressure, fetal pressure on the maternal vena cava) it becomes detached (Fig. 14-4). Although its name implies that the detachment occurs suddenly, this is not always the case. Separation of the placenta from the uterine wall may occur over a period of time. Detachment may occur first at the center of the placenta, resulting in hidden hemorrhage at first, or it may begin at the rim or outer portion, causing vaginal bleeding of varying amounts. Old blood, which has been trapped behind the separating placenta, appears dark when it finally escapes from the vaginal canal. Fresh bleeding usually is bright red (amniotic fluid may become portwine colored). Bleeding from a premature separation of a normally implanted placenta may be severe enough to cause rapid maternal circulatory shock, death, or brain damage to the infant because of lack of oxygen, and even danger of maternal mortality. The incidence of abruptio placentae is approximately 1 in 90 to 200 pregnancies (Lowe and Cunningham, 1990).

Medical management and nursing care. The first sign of abruptio placentae during labor may be an alteration in the contraction pattern. The contractions become very strong and almost constant. Little relaxation period, if any, may be detected. The uterus becomes tender and boardlike if enlarged with retained hemorrhage. There may or may not be external bleeding from the vagina. The symptoms of shock may be greater than the amount of visible bleeding would indicate. The fetal heart rate is either greatly accelerated or slowing. Late decelerations on the fetal monitor indicate diminishing placental function. The fetus, in its struggle to obtain more oxygen, may be very restless and active. If the amniotic sac, or bag of waters, is ruptured, meconium may be seen in the amniotic fluid—another sign of fetal distress. As shock from blood loss develops the blood pressure falls, and the pulse increases and weakens. Abruptio placentae in its more severe forms is an obstetrical emergency. The treatment often, although not inevitably, includes delivery by cesarean birth and blood replacement.

A serious complication of abruptio placentae that has been encountered often enough to warrant mention is *hypofibrinogenemia,* an abnormally low fibrinogen level in the blood that makes normal blood clotting impossible. Treatment may include fibrogen replacement or use of cryoprecipitate (containing both fibrinogen and clotting factor VIII). A rare but serious associated complication, possible in other obstetrical and medical situations as well, is *disseminated intravascular coagulation* (DIC). This problem begins with the excessive triggering of coagulation mechanisms, most commonly encountered in abruptio placentae, pregnancy-induced hypertension, retained intrauterine fetal demise, saline abortion, and amniotic fluid embolism (Sisson, 1992). This overstimulation of the coagulation system leads to rapid formation of massive numbers of clots. As a result the clotting factors are used up and generalized hemorrhage occurs. These multisite hemorrhages can result in maternal shock and even death. Expert medical management and intensive nursing care are needed in these precarious circumstances.

Care of the bleeding patient

Before leaving the topic of blood loss during pregnancy and labor, a review of the care of patients who are bleeding would be helpful. Presented below are some important "dos" and "don'ts" that all nurses should know.

1. Never examine a bleeding patient vaginally. The physician should perform any needed pelvic examination. Never give a bleeding patient an enema as part of the routine admission. Unnecessary manipulation of the area may increase the bleeding (especially in patients with placenta previa). Institute a regimen of bed rest and give the patient no food or fluids until ordered otherwise.
2. Observe the patient carefully and frequently:
   a. Take pulse and blood pressure determinations. Compare the results obtained with the patient's blood pressure reading on her prenatal record. Check for falling blood pressure and rising pulse.
   b. Check for type and amount of vaginal bleeding or amniotic drainage. If it is possible, save the evidences of bleeding for evaluation by the physician.
   c. Apply the electronic fetal heart monitor routinely in any situation in which fetal stress or distress is a potential problem.
   d. Monitor the character of any contraction and relaxation period by frequent palpation. Check for any special uterine tenderness or rigidity and for poor or absent uterine relaxation.
3. Keep the charge nurse and physician informed of changes in the patient's condition.
4. Expect possible orders for intravenous fluids, blood analyses, and cross match for blood transfusion. Record intake and output. Know if any religious scruples preclude transfusion (e.g., if the patient is a Jehovah's Witness).
5. Maintain a calm, supportive manner.
6. Recognize the patient's fear for her own and the fetus' well-being and her grief for the potential or actual loss of the pregnancy or newborn.
7. Provide accurate information regarding the condition and the ordered treatment.

See the accompanying nursing care plan on p. 259 for acute bleeding in the third trimester.

Pregnancy-Induced Hypertension (PIH)

Hypertensive disorders of pregnancy can significantly compromise maternal and fetal well-being. Gestational hypertensive disorders are categorized in the box on p. 260. Hypertension alone is usually benign (Working Group on High Blood Pressure in Pregnancy, 1990). Chronic hypertension increases the risk of placental insufficiency, abruptio placentae, and superimposed preeclampsia-eclampsia (Gilbert and Harmon, 1993). Of all of the gestational hypertensive disorders, preeclampsia and eclampsia carry the greatest risk of negative outcomes for both mother and fetus. The discussion here focuses on preeclampsia and eclampsia.

Preeclampsia affects approximately 7% of the entire maternity population in the United States, although in some areas, particularly the Southeast, and in some other parts of the world, the incidence is considerably higher. Preeclampsia occurs most frequently in the nulliparous woman. Approximately 5% of those demonstrating preeclampsia develop eclampsia. Approximately 8% of those mothers who become eclamptic succumb to the disease or its complications. Preeclampsia-eclampsia, or the older term *toxemia of pregnancy*, has long been listed among the first three causes of maternal mortality. Chief causes of maternal death associated with preeclampsia-eclampsia are aspiration (pneumonia), cerebral hemorrhage, cardiac failure with pulmonary edema, hepatic rupture, or obstetrical hemorrhage associated with abruptio placentae. A surviving infant may suffer from intrauterine growth retardation. Perinatal mortality usually results from placental insufficiency and abruptio placentae.

Etiology

Many theories exist regarding the causes and the mechanisms of preeclampsia-eclampsia. A limited list includes explanations involving lack of normal blood supply to uterine and placental tissues (ischemia); the presence of superabundant chorionic villi or the first exposure to such tissue; malnutrition; hormonal changes; autoimmune mechanisms; and genetic considerations. The consensus of opinion is that the disease is probably caused by a combination of factors. Risk factors for the disease are included in the box on p. 260. Patients considered at risk for the disease are currently advised to take low-dose aspirin (60 to 80 mg/day) to prevent the development of hypertension and proteinuria (Creasy and Resnik, 1994).

Signs and symptoms. Different types of pathological conditions, especially cardiovascular and renal disorders, may mimic certain aspects of preeclampsia.

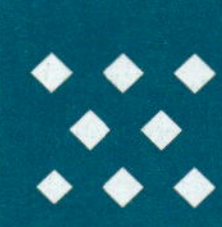

Nursing Care Plan
ADMISSION OF PREGNANT PATIENT WITH ACUTE THIRD TRIMESTER BLEEDING—AN OBSTETRICAL EMERGENCY

Selected Nursing Diagnoses	Expected Outcomes	Interventions
A Potential fluid volume deficit related to hemorrhage.	Harmful effect on mother and infant will be minimized.	*No routine enema, vaginal or rectal examination on admission*—such manipulation can worsen bleeding.
B Potential altered fetal tissue perfusion—oxygen deficit. Clinical manifestations: diagnosis? *If abruptio placentae:* Vaginal bleeding (dark red) may or may not be present. Possible portwine-colored amniotic fluid. Abdominal pain—mild to severe. Uterus firmly contracted and tender to palpation. Vital sign changes—increased pulse and decreased blood pressure. (Changes may be greater than amount of visible bleeding would indicate.) Fetal heart rate and pattern changes. Increased fetal activity. *If placenta previa:* Vaginal bleeding (bright red), varies in amount. No abdominal pain or tenderness, uterus soft between contractions if in labor. Vital sign changes—increased pulse and decreased blood pressure depending on amount of bleeding. Fetal heart rate and pattern changes.	Delivery of infant with Apgar of 7 or above. Maternal vital signs, hematocrit within normal limits.	Notify physician promptly of admission and initial assessments. Review obstetrical history—course of present pregnancy. Keep patient NPO and on bedrest. Frequent observation of: Level of consciousness; behavior. Vital signs. Skin color and temperature. Urinary output (possible Foley catheter). Fetal heart rate and (if present) contraction patterns electronically monitored. Vaginal bleeding—note color-presence of clots; count or weigh blood-stained pads. Other abnormal bleeding—petechiae, purpura, epistaxis, bleeding gums (possible signs of DIC). Localized abdominal pain. Uterine contractions? Evaluation for need of analgesia. Patient response to administration of IV fluids and acceptance and preparation for blood products as ordered. Expect follow-up blood and coagulation studies. Assist physician with ultrasound and other medical, diagnostic and therapeutic interventions. Alert pediatrician and nursery staff of impending delivery, possible cesarean delivery. Review preparation, secure permits as needed.
C Anxiety related to potential life-threatening situation. (See Nursing Care Plan for psychosocial nursing care of the high-risk patient during labor and delivery.)		Provide emotional support to woman and family.

HYPERTENSIVE DISORDERS OF PREGNANCY

PREGNANCY INDUCED HYPERTENSION (PIH)

Hypertension	Development of hypertension after 20 weeks' gestation without proteinuria
Preeclampsia	Development of hypertension accompanied by proteinuria, edema, or both after 20 weeks' gestation or during the early postpartum period; may occur before 20 weeks' gestation in molar pregnancy
Eclampsia	Development of convulsions or coma, without coincidental neurological disease, in preeclamptic patient

CHRONIC HYPERTENSION

Hypertension and/or proteinuria before pregnancy, before the twentieth week of pregnancy in the absence of a molar pregnancy, or that persists for more than 42 days postpartum

CHRONIC HYPERTENSION WITH SUPERIMPOSED PREECLAMPSIA-ECLAMPSIA

Development of preeclampsia or eclampsia in patient with chronic hypertension

Compiled from Working Group on High Blood Pressure in Pregnancy, 1990.

RISK FACTORS FOR PREECLAMPSIA-ECLAMPSIA

Nulliparity
Low socioeconomic status
Older age
Family history
Diabetes
Multiple gestation (e.g., twins)
Chronic hypertension
Hydatidiform mole
Rh incompatibility

When any of the three classic signs of preeclampsia (hypertension, proteinuria, or edema) occur *singly,* it is not sufficient to warrant a diagnosis of preeclampsia. Two of the three classic signs must be present to justify the diagnosis.

Hypertension that predates the twentieth week (except in multiple coexistent or molar pregnancies) is usually not considered indicative of true preeclampsia either—although later the trio of signs may be superimposed on a preexisting chronic hypertension, causing a particularly dangerous variety of the disorder. The signs and symptoms of pregnancy-induced hypertension may, of course, extend beyond the classic three manifestations. Table 14-3 compares the findings that help determine the relative seriousness (mild or severe) of the disorder and therefore influence the types of treatment. It should be pointed out that a number of clinicians do not consider the usual criteria of hypertension (a blood pressure at or above 140 systolic or 90 diastolic) to be appropriate during pregnancy because blood pressure levels normally are reduced—especially during the second trimester. A 30 mm Hg systolic elevation or a 15 mm Hg diastolic rise, obtained two different times at least 6 hours apart after a period of rest, as indicated in Table 14-3, is a better indication of mild preeclampsia.

One is struck by the total body involvement that this potentially lethal progressive disorder demonstrates. The kidneys, heart, lungs, liver, and brain may become prominent direct and indirect targets of the disease process, which is characterized by erratic narrowing of the microscopic arteries. This pervasive vasospasm of the arterioles probably accounts for many of the abnormalities found. However, its onset may be very subtle, with no remarkable initial signals that a patient may notice. Pregnant patients should be asked to report any swelling of the hands (tight rings), puffiness of the face, headache, or visual problems, such as blurred vision or "spots before eyes." However, these signs usually appear late in the disease process.

Regular and frequent prenatal supervision is needed for verification or interpretation of hypertension, proteinuria, and weight gain. Sudden weight gain often signals edema. Edema is associated with a rising hematocrit as more fluid from the blood transfers to the tissue spaces. As fluid leaves the bloodstream, less blood is processed by the kidneys, and a fall in urine production occurs. Proteninuria, often the last sign of the three classic clinical findings to be noted, is thought to appear as a blood vessel spasm and hypertension affects the kidneys. Abnormal neurological signs and symptoms are probably related to lowered blood-oxygen levels to the brain, minimal to massive cerebral hemorrhages, and edema. Abdominal pain is associated with swelling and vascular involvement of the liver. Thus pain, nausea, vomiting, and pulmonary edema are often noted before the onset of seizure or coma. The appearance of fever indicates a general worsening of the patient's status.

The **HELLP** syndrome refers to a severe form of PIH in patients who develop multiple organ damage (Harvey and Burke, 1992). **HELLP** is an acronym for Hemolysis, Elevated Liver enzymes, and Low Platelet

◆ TABLE 14-3
Comparison of Signs and Symptoms of Mild and Severe Preeclampsia-Eclampsia (PIH)*

Characteristics	Mild Preeclampsia	Severe Preeclampsia
Blood pressure	Greater than 140/90 but less than 160/110 mm Hg 30 mm Hg systolic rise; or 15 mm Hg diastolic rise over baseline readings of early pregnancy (Above readings obtained after rest in a sitting position two times at least 6 hours apart.)	Blood pressure greater than 160/110 mm Hg
Proteinuria (albuminuria)	300 mg/L/24 hours or two separate random daytime specimens 6 hours apart (true clean catch) of 1+, 2+	5 gm or more per 24 hours, 3+, 4+ in true clean-catch or catheterized specimen
Edema	Weight gain of more than 3 lbs (1.4 kg) per week or 6 lbs (2.72 kgs) per month—any sudden weight gain is suspicious Minimal or marked edema 1+, 2+ of lower extremities	Weight gain advances at accelerated rate Edema more pronounced, especially of hands, face 3+, 4+ (as condition worsens, edema of lungs, brain, and other organs)
Urine output	Not below 500 ml/24 hours	Oliguria less than 500 ml/24 hours
Neurological signs and symptoms	Absent or only occasional headaches, blurred vision, or spots before eyes Normal peripheral reflexes	More persistent headaches, blurred vision, and spots before eyes—retinal arteriole spasms on ophthalmic examination Hyperactive knee jerk and other tendon reflexes +3, +4 with clonus Irritability, tinnitus
Other organ involvement		Liver involvement causing epigastric or right upper quadrant abdominal pain, nausea, vomiting (often said to precede convulsion/coma or onset of eclampsia) Pulmonary edema manifested by respiratory distress, rales, cyanosis

*These criteria are not uniformly accepted by experts in the field.

count. The condition is confirmed by laboratory studies. The hematocrit, normally elevated in PIH because of the decrease in circulating plasma volume, drops as red blood cells are destroyed in the spasmed blood vessels. Platelets are used up as they try to repair the widespread vascular damage. Elevated liver enzymes signal increased liver impairment.

Medical management and nursing care. Treatment of preeclampsia depends on the severity of the symptoms encountered, the philosophy of the physician, and the understanding and compliance of the patient. She and her family deserve careful teaching regarding her problem, its observation, and its treatment. Regular, adequate prenatal care is the best insurance for control of the complication.

In *mild* forms of preeclampsia, if a patient is conscientious in carrying out her physician's instructions, treatment may be possible on an out-patient basis, but many physicians prefer to hospitalize these patients until symptoms are controlled. Treatment is directed toward relieving the edema and hypertension and restoring normal kidney function. Bed rest in a side-lying position to increase renal and placental blood flow is usually helpful in decreasing high blood pressure. Bed rest is often very difficult for a mother to maintain at home, especially if she has small children. Attention must be paid to her sources of help and support, or this important ingredient in her care will be lost. Improvement of her diet, emphasizing high-quality protein, vitamin, and mineral intake, and avoidance of empty calories, is to be encouraged. Salt intake should not exceed normal dietary levels (4 to 6 gms/24 hours). Salt restriction below 2 gms/24 hours, however, is not recommended (Newman and Fuller-

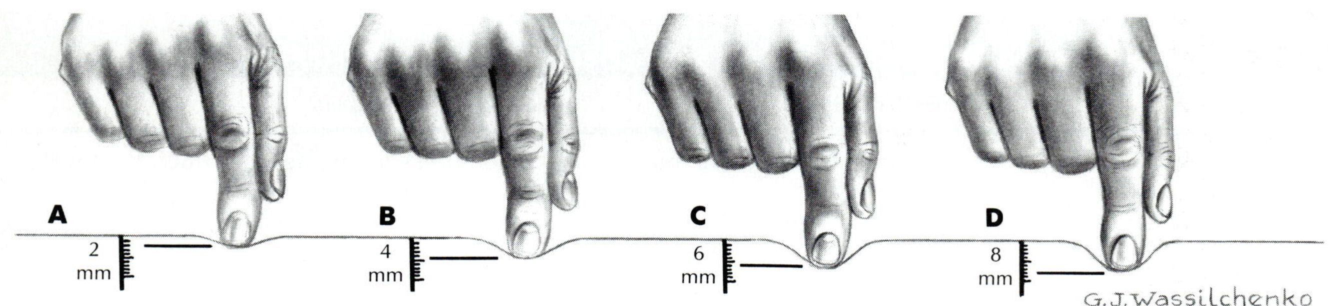

Fig. 14-5 Assessment of pitting edema. (From Bobak IM, Jensen MD: *Maternity and gynecologic care,* ed 5, St. Louis, 1993, Mosby.)

ton, 1990). Diuretics, except in select cases, are considered to be of little value and may cause harm to the patient and the fetus.

When preeclampsia patients are hospitalized, a bed rest regimen in a quiet room is usually advised. Bed rest patients should be observed particularly for sacral edema (see Fig. 14-5 for assessment of pitting edema). Blood pressure and fetal heart rate are taken at least every 4 hours. Blood pressure should be taken with the patient in the *sitting position* with her arm resting on a table at heart level. The lungs should be listened to with a stethoscope to identify crackling sounds—evidence of pulmonary edema. A daily weight determination and urinalysis to check for proteinuria are common. Deep tendon reflexes (DTRs) should be monitored for evidence of hyperreflexia (Fig. 14-6). Table 14-4 reviews grading of DTRs. Twenty-four-hour urinary protein levels, creatinine clearance tests, and uric acid levels that measure renal function are usually ordered. Intake and output records should be maintained. The patient should be assessed for the appearance of symptoms, such as dyspnea, headache, blurred vision, abdominal pain, or nausea that indicate a worsening of the condition. Intermittent tests of fetal maturity and well-being may provide information needed to direct the care of the unborn infant and the mother.

The only cure for preeclampsia is termination of the pregnancy. Although for many physicians the treatment for this disease currently remains almost as controversial as its proposed causes, all agree that the birth of a viable child as soon as possible is the best therapy. The rationale of treatment is to improve the condition of the mother to allow a vaginal or abdominal delivery at term. However, if her condition continues to deteriorate, induction of labor or a cesarean birth may be necessary.

For a patient with *severe preeclampsia* the room should be quiet and dimmed. An emergency tray should be close at hand, containing the following equipment: airway, percussion hammer (to test reflexes), and a padded tongue blade. (A tongue blade or "bite block" is still standard equipment in most hospitals, but unless it can be inserted without force, its use is to be avoided. The tongue heals—teeth do not.) The tray should also include the following medications: emergency anticonvulsants, sedatives, antihypertensives, and heparin-containing drugs, with appropriate equipment for their administration. An oxygen mask or cannula, a suction apparatus, and possibly emergency delivery equipment should be nearby. The drug of choice to prevent seizures is magnesium sulfate. Rules regarding its use and that of its antidote, calcium gluconate, are highlighted in the box on p. 265. Hydralazine (Apresoline) is the antihypertensive drug of choice and may be given if the diastolic pressure exceeds 110 mm Hg.

To measure urinary output and character more accurately, an indwelling catheter is inserted and attached to a urinometer. The blood pressure cuff is left in place. Frequent blood pressure, pulse, and respiration checks are made. Typically the patient is heavily sedated. An intravenous infusion is instituted and fluid restriction is ordered. Electronic fetal monitoring should be ongoing. A severely preeclamptic or eclamptic patient should never be left alone. Certain patients may convulse in response to loud noises, jarring of the bed, or bright lights. Conversation should be minimal. Routine bed baths, unnecessary procedures, or patient stimulation should be avoided.

Fortunately the occurrence of seizure is rare today. Increase in blood pressure, severe headache, abdominal pain, apprehension, twitchings, and hyperirritability of the muscles often precede seizures. If a seizure does occur the patient's entire body or head should be turned to the side. Suctioning is rarely necessary, but aspiration is a danger. During the periods of rigidity and muscle contraction (tonic and clonic phases) the patient should be restrained only enough to keep her from hurting herself or rolling off the bed. The sides of

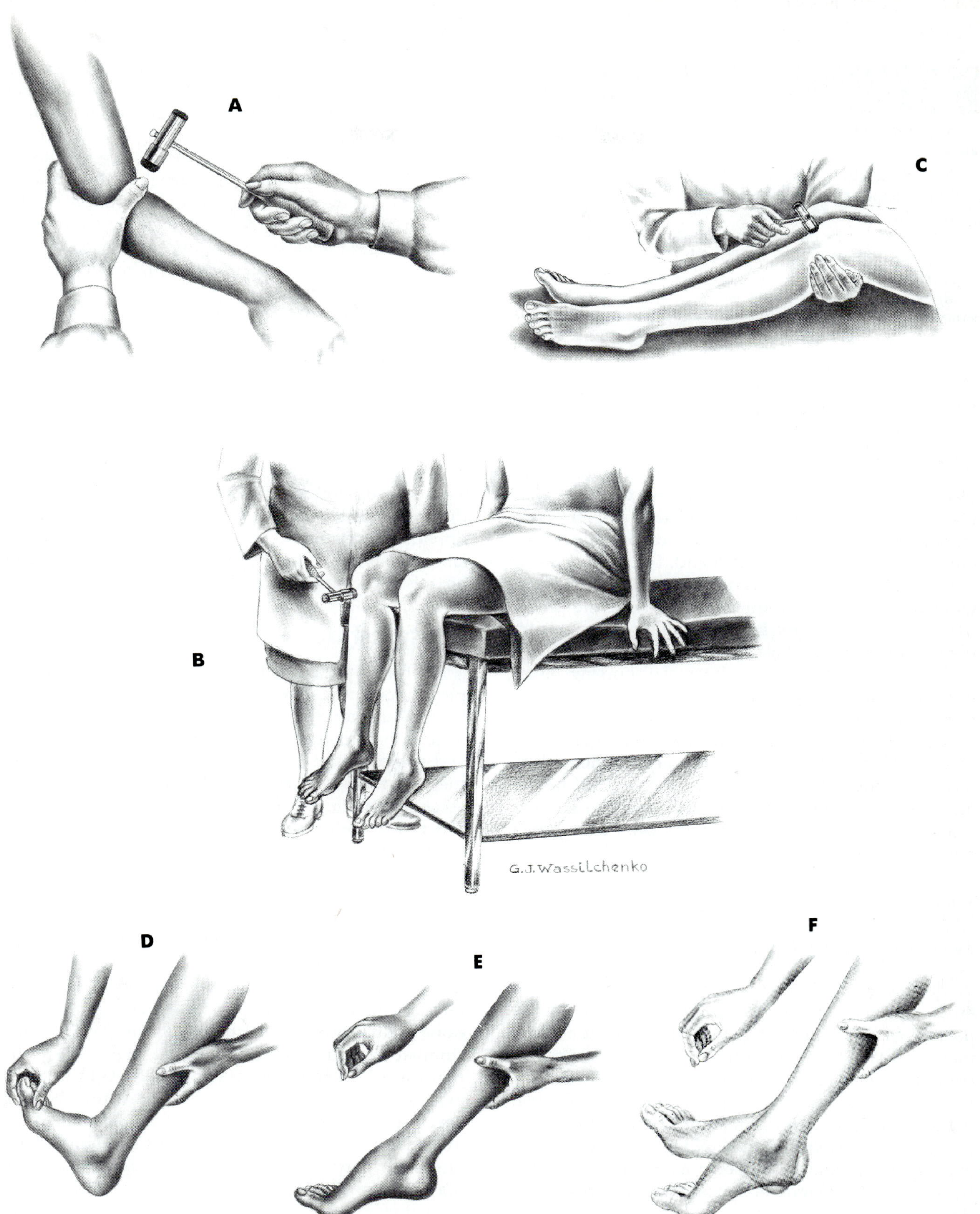

Fig. 14-6 **A,** Biceps reflex. **B,** Patellar reflex with client's legs hanging freely over end of examining table. **C,** With client in supine position. **D,** Hyperactive reflexes (clonus) at ankle joint. **E,** Normal (negative clonus) response. **F,** Abnormal (positive clonus) response. (From Bobak IM, Jensen MD: *Maternity and gynecologic care,* ed 5, St. Louis, 1993, Mosby.)

◆ TABLE 14-4
Deep Tendon Reflex (DTR) Grading

Physical Finding	Grading
No response	0
Slow response, sluggish or dull	1+
Normal, active response	2+
More than normal, brisk response	3+
Hyperactive response, brisk with transient clonus	4+
Brisk with sustained clonus	5+

the bed should be padded with pillows. Be aware that labor may progress rapidly and that infants have been born suddenly during a convulsive episode.

As soon as the patient's convulsions are controlled the condition of the fetus (if the seizures occur before birth) is ascertained, and plans for the birth are considered. The patient may labor and deliver spontaneously or the labor may need to be induced or augmented with oxytocin (Pitocin). If the progress of labor is sufficient and the conditions of the mother and fetus are satisfactory, vaginal birth may be the procedure of choice. After birth the possibility of convulsion diminishes with the passage of time. Convulsion 72 hours after birth is rare. Intensive nursing must continue during the early postpartal period, but improvement is usually rapid.

The nurse needs to be aware that these patients are often quite fearful about the outcomes for themselves and the fetus. See the nursing care plan on p. 266 for the admission of a primipara with PIH, and the nursing care plan on p. 267 for the psychosocial care of the high-risk patient during labor and delivery.

LABOR COMPLICATIONS

Dysfunctional Labor

Dysfunctional labor, also known as *dystocia,* refers to an abnormal or difficult labor. Dysfunctional labor is usually related to ineffective uterine contractions, fetal malpresentations or positions, or small pelvic size relative to the size of the fetus. The primary maternal risk from a lengthy labor is exhaustion and infection. A higher incidence of cesarean birth for women with dysfunctional labors is also noted. The fetus may experience hypoxia or birth trauma. See Chapter 10 to review normal length of labor and pattern of fetal descent information.

Ineffective uterine contractions. *Hypotonic* contractions are those that are insufficiently strong to effect cervical effacement and dilatation. Augmentation with oxytocin (Pitocin) may improve the pattern and enable the woman to give birth vaginally. *Hypertonic* contractions are frequent, strong, painful, but uncoordinated contractions that are ineffective in accomplishing cervical effacement and dilatation. Resting the uterus by sedating the mother may resolve the pattern. Occasionally the use of oxytocin will improve the coordination and alter the pattern. Adequate hydration, changing maternal position, and encouraging ambulation may also be effective in improving the quality of contractions.

Fetal malpresentation or position. The fetal malpresentations or positions that result in the greatest problems are occiput posterior position; and face, brow, shoulder, and breech presentations. See Chapter 10 for a review of the methods of dealing with these problems.

Small pelvis. Occasionally the pelvic diameters will be too small for the size of the fetus. See Chapter 4 for a review of normal diameters. Because it is often difficult to anticipate this problem, especially in primigravidas, the woman will usually be given a trial of labor before the difficulty is confirmed and a cesarean birth is determined necessary.

Ruptured Uterus

Rupture of the gravid uterus may occur during late pregnancy but is most often reported during labor and birth. The nurse should know under what circumstances this emergency is most likely to occur, the signs and symptoms most often seen, and the usual treatment pursued. Uterine rupture is most frequently associated with previous uterine surgery (e.g., cesarean births with classic uterine incisions, myomectomies), injudicious use of obstetrical forceps or oxytocin, a tempestuous or prolonged labor (e.g., fetal-pelvic disproportion), or grand-multiparity.

Typically the patient experiences a period of strong, almost unremitting contractions that, in spite of their force, produce little progress in the descent of the fetus in the birth canal. The uterus becomes extremely tender, and a weakening of its lower segment may cause a distention above the pubic bone, which may simulate the appearance of a full bladder. At the moment of rupture the patient may exclaim that she experienced a sharp pain and "felt something giving way." If rupture is complete—that is, the wall of the uterus is torn through—contractions suddenly cease. However, partial ruptures are more common. These may not be detected until postpartum intrauterine palpation.

Classically the patient, after experiencing momentary relief from pain, develops signs of profound circulatory shock resulting from intraabdominal hem-

USE OF MAGNESIUM SULFATE (EPSOM SALTS, $MGSO_4$) IN TREATMENT OF PREECLAMPSIA-ECLAMPSIA (PIH)	
Action and uses	Reduces transmission of nerve impulses from brain to muscles. Used primarily to prevent or treat convulsions. Some vasodilation and smooth muscle relaxation observed but not used chiefly for these effects.
Intent	To administer enough to prevent convulsions but avoid dangerous *nervous system* and *respiratory depression* caused by excessive magnesium serum levels in the body—either respiratory or cardiac arrest could occur.
Administration	May be ordered by intramuscularly (now rare) or intravenously, intermittent or continuous drip. Introductory (bolus) and maintenance dosages prescribed based on clinical observations and serum levels. *Extreme care* must be used to be sure the concentration and volume of solutions to be given are understood. Intramuscular dosages should be given with long (3-inch) needles using Z-track technique. With physician approval, lidocaine may be injected with $MgSO_4$ to relieve pain.
Antidote	10% solution calcium gluconate 10 to 20 ml, given intravenously, injected slowly (over 3 minutes to prevent ventricular fibrillation).
Monitoring side effects and patient response	Blood pressure, pulse, respiration every 15 to 30 minutes while on continuous intravenous infusion; before and after on varying schedules for intermittent intravenous or intramuscular therapy; an initial decrease in blood pressure may be noted because of vasodilation. Patient may complain of generalized warmth, exhibit diaphoresis. Level of consciousness: anxiety may become disorientation, drowsiness, slurring of speech, coma. Frequency and intensity of uterine contractions may diminish. Repeat doses should not be given and physician should be notified if any of the below exist: 1 Patellar knee-jerk absent 2 Respirations below 14/minute 3 Urine output for previous 4 hours less than 100 ml 4 Signs of fetal distress 5 Elevated magnesium serum levels—above 10 mg/dl (therapeutic levels 4 to 10 mg/dl)

see" policy. The orrhage. Some of this blood loss may be visible vaginally. Signs and symptoms of rupture depend on the extent and depth of the tear, the location of the fetus, and the stage of labor in which the complication occurs. Occasionally, the onset of symptoms will be delayed. Almost all the unborn babies and one third of their affected mothers die when a classic rupture occurs.

Treatment of severe cases usually consist of immediate laparotomy, possible hysterectomy, antibiotics, and massive blood transfusions.

Amniotic Fluid Embolism

A complication that few women survive involves the spontaneous, accidental infusion of amniotic fluid into the endocervical or uterine veins after the bag of water has ruptured. This may occur anytime during the labor-delivery or immediate postpartum period but has been most often reported near the end of the first stage of labor. Amniotic fluid containing particles of meconium, vernix, and lanugo may enter the large blood sinuses in the placenta through defects in the placental attachment. These emboli gain access to the mother's general circulation and lodge in the lungs. Although the entire disastrous mechanism is not clear, it appears that this foreign matter also produces profound shock and disseminated intravascular coagulation (DIC), leading to lowered fibrinogen levels in the blood and subsequent hemorrhage. This complication is more frequently associated with tumultuous uterine contractions and has been described in a disproportionate number of cases in which oxytocin has been administered to initiate or stimulate labor.

Symptoms manifest themselves suddenly. The patient may complain of chest pain or dyspnea and become extremely restless and cyanotic, occasionally expectorating frothy, blood-tinged mucus. Profound circulatory shock from hemorrhage may occur rapidly. Fetal death may result, and maternal death is almost always the outcome. Fortunately this complication is rare—occurring only once in several thousand births.

Emergency care includes intravenous administration of fibrinogen, blood, and other substances that

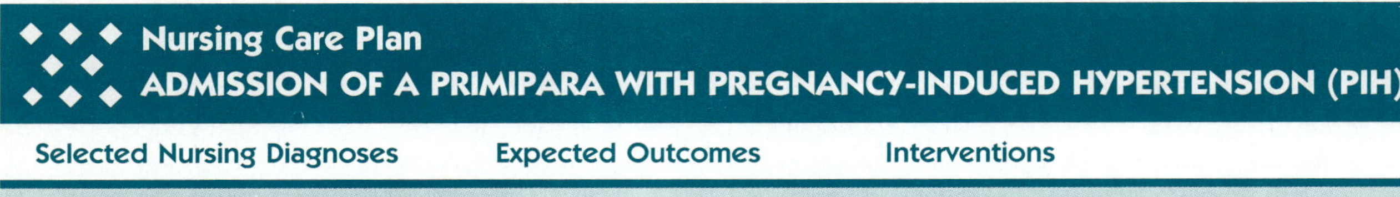

Nursing Care Plan
ADMISSION OF A PRIMIPARA WITH PREGNANCY-INDUCED HYPERTENSION (PIH)

Selected Nursing Diagnoses	Expected Outcomes	Interventions
Potential for injury:		
A Maternal, related to organ dysfunction as a result of generalized vasospasm.	Decreased maternal blood pressure, proteinuria, and edema.	Maintain patient on bed rest in left- or right-lateral position to increase blood flow to fetus and kidneys.
B Fetal, related to impaired maternal placental perfusion. Clinical manifestations: Rising blood pressure. Increasing proteinuria. Hyperactive reflexes. Complaints of headache, visual disturbances, epigastric pain. Decreased urinary output. FHR changes indicating distress.	Absence of convulsions or coma. Safe delivery of viable infant.	Monitor progress: Blood pressure frequency depends on severity of condition/orders Record hourly urine output, via catheter; report if <30 ml/hr Test for urine protein every hour or as ordered. Weigh daily and assess edema, especially in sacral area. Record intake and monitor intravenous fluids and infusion site. Assess response to magnesium sulfate therapy. Monitor fetal well-being: Continuous FHR monitoring. Assist with assessment of fetal welfare and maturity (NST, ultrasound, amniocentesis). Maintain seizure precautions, quiet, darkened room, emergency tray with airway, oxygen, and suction immediately available, padded side rails. Observe for spontaneous onset of labor—need emergency delivery pack.

will help restore normal clotting mechanisms, which paradoxically in DIC may include heparin, epsilon-aminocaproic acid (EACA), and oxygen therapy. If the infant is not yet born, he or she is delivered as soon as possible.

Umbilical Cord Prolapse

When the umbilical cord precedes the presenting part of the fetus during labor the blood circulating within the vessels of the cord may be clamped off against the pelvis by the continued descent of the fetus creating an obstetrical emergency. This condition, termed *prolapse of the cord*, occurs in approximately 0.4% of labors. See Chapter 11 for a discussion of appropriate nursing interventions in this situation.

Preterm Premature Rupture of Membranes (PPROM)

Premature rupture of membranes (PROM) is defined as rupture of the amniotic sac before the onset of labor. In most cases, patients with PROM who are full term will go into labor within 24 hours. The cause of premature rupture of membranes is often unknown. The risk of an intraamniotic infection is the major maternal risk. In the event that this occurs, it must be promptly treated to avoid septicemia and death (Gilbert and Harmon, 1993).

Approximately 20% of PROM cases occur before 36 weeks' gestation (Allen, 1991). If the fetus is not mature, there are no signs of infection, and no fetal distress the physician is likely to adopt a "wait-and-see"

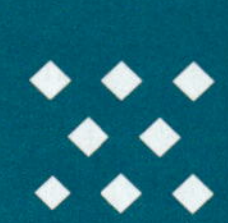

Nursing Care Plan
PSYCHOSOCIAL NURSING CARE OF THE HIGH-RISK PATIENT DURING LABOR AND DELIVERY

Selected Nursing Diagnoses	Expected Outcomes	Interventions
Fear and anxiety related to specific high-risk condition and uncertainty of outcome for mother and infant. Clinical manifestations: Expresses concern for condition of infant and self. Increased verbalization and questions or withdrawn and uncommunicative. Crying, restless, irritable, trembling. Difficulty in concentrating when directions given. Unable to relax and control breathing without continual reminders.	Patient will use effective coping mechanisms: Able to cooperate during procedures. Verbalizes understanding of risks to infant and self and rationale for plan of care.	Stay with woman. Indicate concern with eye contact, touch, as well as verbal communication according to patient's cultural background. Speak slowly and clearly. Provide simple, accurate explanations of procedures to woman and family. Allow her to express feelings in her own way: talking, crying, moaning. Help her to focus on relaxation breathing. Praise her for positive efforts. Offer information on condition and progress: emphasize hopeful findings (e.g., FHR within normal limits) but avoid false reassurance. Recognize needs of support person/family: demonstrate support techniques, provide respite if needed. Need for food, sleep, shower? Explore possible family desires for added spiritual support, involvement of clergy, prayer.

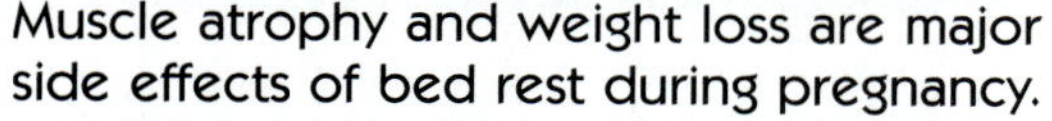

Nursing Alert

Muscle atrophy and weight loss are major side effects of bed rest during pregnancy.

policy. The medical treatment is bed rest with bathroom privileges and careful monitoring for signs of maternal infection and fetal compromise (see Nursing Alert above). Some physicians will order antibiotic prophylaxis. The nurse must educate the woman in careful perineal hygiene, and the signs and symptoms of infection and preterm labor to report. Fetal surveillance is likely to include periodic fetal heart rate monitoring, fetal movement monitoring, nonstress tests, biophysical profiles, and amniotic fluid determinations.

The goal is to lengthen the pregnancy in hopes of increasing fetal lung maturity before birth is necessary. Even with this conservative treatment, approximately half of patients with preterm PROM will go into labor and deliver within 1 week. The risk of preterm PROM for the fetus is the likelihood of premature birth with increased morbidity and mortality associated with respiratory distress syndrome.

Premature Labor and Birth

An infant born before the end of the thirty-eighth week of gestation is considered premature or preterm. Approximately 10% of all infants are born prematurely. In about half the cases the cause of preterm labor cannot be identified (Gilbert and Harmon, 1993). The multiple factors that predispose a patient to premature birth are listed in the box on p. 268.

Premature birth represents a special threat to the life or future health of the infant, special physical, psychologic, and economic stress on the family, and a challenge to community resources. Premature infants are more likely to suffer trauma during birth, to be victims of respiratory distress syndrome, intraventricular hemorrhage, necrotizing enterocolitis, and other problems, and to require longer supportive hospital care (see Chapter 19 for care of the premature infant).

PREDISPOSING FACTORS OF PRETERM LABOR

HISTORY
Previous preterm labor (single most important factor)

DEMOGRAPHIC AND LIFE-STYLE PRACTICES
Low socioeconomic status
Age (less than 19 or more than 40)
Nonwhite
Nutrition that leads to low maternal weight gain
Smoking
Illicit drug use (especially cocaine)

STRESS
Emotional stress
Long, tiring commutes
Two or more children at home
Heavy work

UTERINE FACTORS
Decreased blood flow
- Abruptio placentae
- Placenta previa
- Diabetes
- Renal disease
- Cardiovascular disease
- Preeclampsia

Overdistention of the uterus
- Multiple gestation
- Polyhydramnios

Abdominal trauma
Abdominal surgery
Premature rupture of membranes
Diethylstilbestrol (DES) exposure in utero resulting in uterine abnormalities
Incompetent cervix
Uterine anomalies

INFECTIONS
Urinary tract
Vagina/uterus/fetus
Febrile illness

Modified from Gilbert ES, Harmon JS: *High risk pregnancy and delivery,* St. Louis, 1993, Mosby.

Medical management and nursing care. For these reasons, in most cases attempts are made to prevent or halt a premature labor, unless continuing the pregnancy would jeopardize the mother or fetus or the labor is considered to be inevitable. If evidence exists of intrauterine infection, hemorrhage, or cervical dilatation beyond 3 or 4 cm, these efforts would not be appropriate. Bed rest and hydration may inhibit progression in many cases. If the bag of waters is ruptured, the use of tocolytic drugs is controversial.

Tocolytic drugs most commonly used to quiet uterine contractions are beta-adrenergic agents, terbutaline sulfate (Brethine) and ritodrine (Yutopar); and magnesium sulfate ($MgSO_4$). Two other drugs are also used, particularly if the previously mentioned tocolytics are not effective or contraindicated because of preexisting disease (e.g., beta-adrenergics are not used in diabetes because of their effect on glucose metabolism). Indomethacin, a prostaglandin inhibitor, may be useful as a tocolytic drug in women less than 34 weeks' gestation. After 34 weeks the drug may cause narrowing of the ductus arteriosus resulting in fetal compromise. Nifedipine, a calcium-channel blocker is also effective. All the drugs mentioned for suppression of labor have important side effects. Patients receiving them should be carefully observed. A maternal cardiac monitor may be appropriate. See accompanying nursing care plan for the patient with preterm labor.

Once stabilized the patient may be discharged home on oral tocolytics or tocolytics administered continuously by a portable parenteral infusion pump (Cowan, 1993). She must be thoroughly instructed in self-palpating for uterine contractions and the early signs of preterm labor and must follow the bed rest and hydration recommendations. Some health care providers also recommend home electronic uterine contraction monitoring when it is available.

The administration of a glucocorticoid, betamethasone (Celestone), to the mother will hasten maturity of fetal lungs by promoting earlier formation of lung surfactant. This therapy may diminish the probability of serious neonatal respiratory distress syndrome. If labor cannot be terminated, little analgesic medication is given because the premature infant's body cannot detoxify drugs well, and respirations at birth must not be depressed. A type of spinal anesthesia may be given at delivery. A deep episiotomy may be performed to minimize head compression at expulsion. The nursery must be notified of an impending premature birth. Ideally a pediatrician particularly skilled in the immediate care of immature newborns (neonatologist) is present at the birth. Transport to a neonatal intensive care nursery is usually indicated.

Special attention to the psychological needs of the mother is essential. Her labor is all the more demanding and difficult because her body is not prepared for the event, the outlook is precarious, and analgesic aids are minimal.

POSTPARTUM COMPLICATIONS

Postpartum Hemorrhage

Uterine atony (relaxation) or inertia is the most common cause of early postpartum hemorrhage. Pa-

Nursing Care Plan
ADMISSION OF A MULTIPARA IN EARLY PRETERM LABOR

Selected Nursing Diagnoses	Expected Outcomes	Interventions
A Knowledge deficit related to potential for premature labor and delivery. Clinical manifestations: Gestation of more than 20 but less than 38 weeks. Contractions every 10 minutes or less, lasting more than 30 seconds for more than 1 hour. Cervical dilatation less than 4 cm (greater dilatation indicates imminent delivery). Rupture of membranes? *Absence* of maternal medical condition (i.e., PIH). Absence of maternal fever or foul vaginal drainage (signs of intrauterine infection). Patient frightened and asking questions about her condition.	Labor is arrested. Pregnancy is maintained as long as possible with maternal and fetal benefit. Patient demonstrates understanding of situation and management plan.	Help patient maintain bedrest. Patient should try to remain on side on flat bed, with only small pillow to enhance blood flow to the fetus and decrease pressure on the cervix. Adjust external monitor for FHR and uterine contractions. Explain treatment plan (patient should be given written instructions for hospital and home.) Administer fluid orally or intravenously as ordered. I & O maintained. Adequate hydration needed but avoid overhydration. Assist with diagnostic examinations, cultures to r/o cervical or urinary tract infection which may cause uterine irritability. Test clear vaginal drainage, if alkaline may be amniotic fluid, membranes ruptured—greater possibility of infection and early delivery. Monitor maternal temperature-intrauterine infection precludes tocolysis. Monitor following unit protocol response to tocolytic medication used. Notify physician if signs and symptoms below are noted. Magnesium sulfate: Respirations less than 14 Urinary output less than 30 ml/hr Reflexes absent Hypotension develops Ritodrine (Cardiac monitor may be applied). Maternal tachycardia, over 100; irregular pulse. Severe anxiety, tremors, palpitations. Respiratory distress, chest pain. Nausea, diarrhea, epigastric distress. Terbutaline sulfate: Maternal tachycardia Nervousness, hypertension, palpitations, muscle cramps, weakness, continuous nausea/vomiting. If unable to stop labor, assist with preparation for delivery. If labor stops, prepare patient for discharge (see B and C).

Continued.

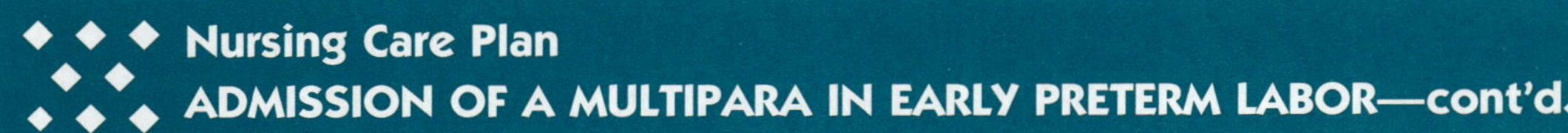

	Selected Nursing Diagnoses	Expected Outcomes	Interventions
B	Potential noncomplicance with treatment regimen related to lack of support at home.	Patient verbalizes understanding of risk recurrence and treatment plan.	Nurse should explain risks of recurrence and treatment plan—expect anger, guilt, anticipatory grief. Avoid false reassurance.
C	Potential alteration in family processes related to decrease maternal activity and concern for fetal well-being. **Home Plan** Patient to be discharged at risk for recurrence of preterm labor. Medical orders include restriction of activity, medication, monitoring for uterine conditions, adequate hydration.	Patient follows recommendations to identify and treat premature labor. Family and significant others will share feelings and provide mutual support to minimize stress.	Teach patient self-care: 1. Recognition and prompt reporting of warning signs of labor.* Palpate uterus for contractions Menstrual-like cramps Low dull back ache (constant or intermittent) Increase pelvic pressure Increase or change in vaginal discharge Abdominal cramping with or without diarrhea Patient should report any of the above if present for more than 1 hour. Early intervention may prevent the birth of "premie" needing care in an intensive care unit. 2. Maintain adequate hydration and elimination. Dehydration and/or full bladder may stimulate uterine contractions. Patient should drink 2-3 quarts of water or juice each day and void every 2 hours. 3. Limit activity as ordered, possible bed rest with only BRP or rest periods 2-3 times/day. 4. Avoid sexual stimulation (stimulation of breasts or genitalia may cause uterine contractions). Discuss needs with partner. 5. Take oral tocolytic medication as ordered, monitor for side effects. 6. Identify support system—she may need help (child care or household assistance). 7. Consider appointment with social worker to learn of community resources or deal with other family problems.

*Some services are evaluating the home use of external contraction monitors.

tients who have a history of uterine atony, more than four children, closely spaced pregnancies, multiple pregnancy, large babies, long or induced labors, precipitous labor and delivery, uterine dystocia, pregnancy induced hypertension with magnesium sulfate infusion, or general anesthesia are especially at risk for uterine inertia and should be carefully observed. Retained placental fragments also interfere with uterine contractions, resulting in atony.

If bleeding continues to be excessive and the uterus remains firm, a cause other than uterine atony must be sought to explain the blood loss. Excessive bleeding may develop because of a previously undetected cervical or vaginal laceration or a defective suture or repair. An abnormally bleeding patient may be returned to the delivery room for inspection of the uterus and vaginal canal. Repair of any lacerations, and in some cases a dilatation and curettage of the uterus to remove retained tissue may be necessary.

If no lacerations or retained tissue are evident, treatment is usually confined to the administration of additional oxytocics, such as intravenous oxytocin (Pitocin) or intramuscular methylergonovine (Methergine) or prostaglandin (Prostin). These drugs combat the lethargy of the uterine muscles. See Chapter 13 for discussion of the role of uterine massage, bladder emptying, and breast-feeding in controlling postpartum hemorrhage.

Hematomas

Perineal hematomas may follow damage to a blood vessel during birth and result in collections of 250 to 500 ml of blood, sometimes accompanied by signs of shock. The affected area will feel firm and be very painful to the touch. Large hematomas may have to be evacuated surgically. Women who are anesthetized may not complain of pain, so visualization of the perineum is especially important in these women. Suspicion of a developing hematoma should be promptly reported.

Postpartum hemorrhage, whatever the cause, can prolong the mother's recovery and predispose her to infection.

Puerperal Infection

The term *puerperal infection* may be used to describe any infection of the reproductive tract during the puerperium. In the past, a patient was considered to have a puerperal infection if she had a temperature of 100.4° F (38° C) or more on 2 successive days during the first 10 days postpartum, excluding the first 24 hours—unless another source of the temperature was determined. Now with early discharge and frequent use of antibiotics, some authorities define a puerperal infection differently using various criteria (such as temperature elevations of more than 101° F after the second day, signs and symptoms of infection, or a positive culture). The appearance of a puerperal infection is always a serious development. It may involve the perineum proper, the uterine lining (endometritis), or the pelvic area outside the uterus (parametritis). It may extend by means of blood vessels and lymphatics to areas relatively far removed, as in the case of septic thrombophlebitis of the leg. It is most often localized, but it can become a generalized peritonitis or septicemia.

Although the classic causative organisms implicated are the *streptococci* and *staphylococcus aureus*, puerperal infections may be caused by multiple organisms. Many times the bacteria that invade the uterine wound at the former site of the placenta and produce infection are those also commonly found in the intestines or colonized on the cervix, vagina, and perineum of the patient without causing any local tissue invasion or damage.

The incidence of puerperal infection is thought to be influenced by numerous factors, including the length of time the bag of waters has been ruptured before delivery, the number of vaginal examinations performed, the types and number of incisions and lacerations, the amount of blood loss, and the general health of the mother. Delivery by cesarean section has been associated with higher rates of infection than vaginal birth. The use of prophylactic antibiotics before and/or after surgery has decreased infection rates markedly. Careful handwashing and aseptic techniques continue to be an important priority. The mother must be educated in careful perineal (and incisional) hygiene and the signs and symptoms of worsening infection.

Accompanying signs and symptoms. Along with the appearance of fever, pelvic infection is often accompanied by abdominal tenderness or pain, foul-smelling lochial drainage, an abnormally large uterus, and the presence of chills. The patient may complain of general malaise and lack of appetite and display a rise in pulse rate. Such signs and symptoms should be reported immediately. Detection of a puerperal infection should initiate isolation procedure and perhaps even the removal of the patient from the maternity service proper. Such a diagnosis may also affect the nursing procedures in the care of the infant. Treatment of a case of puerperal infection depends on the extent of involvement. Antibiotics to which the causative organisms are sensitive are ordered. In cases of pelvic infection the patient most often is placed in Fowler's position to encourage drainage of the affected area. Observation for signs of the extension of the infection or generalized peritonitis should be constant. Such indications are increased abdominal tenderness and distention, and nausea and vomiting, as well as those previously listed.

Breast infections

Most breast infections are introduced at the nipple area, which may be fissured or cracked because of poor breastfeeding techniques or exceptionally fragile breast tissue. Pronounced breast engorgement results in stasis of blood and lymph and may put the woman more at risk for infection if there is a break in nipple tissue.

Breast infections are most often caused by the organism *Staphylococcus aureus.*

Because of early discharge practices, breast infection is usually not found while the patient is in the hospital or birthing center. An infection can manifest itself in inflammation of localized areas or an abcess. Fortunately, most cases of mastitis do not progress as far as abscess formation. The nurse should emphasize prevention—correct breast-feeding techniques, breast hygiene and care, and relief of engorgement. The patient should be taught to promptly report signs of inflammation or cracked and bleeding nipples. The application of cold or heat to the breast may be ordered. The treatment prescribed depends on the stage of the infection and the organism cultured. Systemic antibiotics are commonly given. Breastfeeding is usually continued.

Thrombophlebitis

Not all cases of thrombophlebitis involve the presence of infection but many do. Clots may form anywhere in the body where a slowdown in circulation, a repair of damaged tissue, or a plugging of bleeding vessels occurs. During the postpartum period, clots or thrombi may form in the pelvis or the lower extremities. They may localize and interfere with local circulation, set up areas of inflammation, or actually become foci of infection. Rarely, they may break away from the original site of formation and travel about in the circulation. Then they are called *emboli.* These clots are particularly dangerous because they may enter some small but vital vessel and cause grave damage or sudden death. This most often occurs in the case of an embolus or emboli to the lung field or brain. Pulmonary embolism is the leading cause of maternal mortality in the United States. Classic signs of pulmonary embolism include tachypnea, dyspnea, pleuritic chest pain, apprehension and cough (Witry, 1992). These signs and symptoms should be promptly investigated.

Fairly common sites of deep vein thrombophlebitis are the calf or the thigh. The patient may experience calf pain when her foot is firmly dorsiflexed while her leg is supported in an extended position (positive Homans' sign). Sometimes circulation is so impeded that the leg swells considerably, is extremely painful, and may demonstrate red streaks or locally inflamed areas. The skin may be so tense that it appears lighter in color. Signs and symptoms may vary considerably. Treatment of thrombophlebitis usually involves bed rest with elevation of the affected leg, analgesics, and the possible application of heat with a heat cradle. Antibiotics may be indicated. Some physicians may prescribe anticoagulants to cut down on the formation of further thrombi. The nurse must recognize that use of anticoagulants for a postpartum patient significantly increases the possibility of postpartum hemorrhage. Observations of any abnormal bleeding must be quickly reported. Blood pressure should be taken periodically. Laboratory prothrombin determinations are routine.

After the acute phase when ambulation is approved, an order for support stockings is common. Applied correctly, they help speed the venous circulation back to the heart and discourage the formation of clots. No massage of the legs is permitted for fear of dislodging previously formed clots. Ambulation is ordered only after assessment of the day-by-day progress of the patient, revealed by the presence or absence of fever and her general condition. Thrombophlebitis may occur in all degrees of severity. As a preventive measure, some health care providers automatically order that elastic stockings be applied to the legs of their patients who have had difficulties with varicosities.

KEY CONCEPTS

1 The degree of risk for developing childbearing complications is determined by considering the number of and relationships among medical, obstetrical, and psychosocial risk factors.
2 The diabetic woman's need for injected insulin varies during pregnancy. Until about 18 weeks of gestation, insulin needs are reduced; from 20 weeks until term, insulin needs both fluctuate and increase.
3 Ketosis in the pregnant diabetic is monitored by testing the urine for the presence of ketones. Blood glucose determination can be done at home with color-stable strips or with a Glucostix and a reflectance meter.
4 Ultrasound examinations, amniocentesis, fetal movement monitoring, stress, and nonstress tests are helpful in evaluating fetal status in the diabetic pregnant woman.
5 The pregnant woman with cardiac disease is most at risk for cardiac decompensation near 28 weeks, during labor, and in the hours immediately after birth.
6 Normal physiological changes of pregnancy predispose the woman to develop urinary problems.

7 Syphilis may be acquired through sexual contact or by accidental inoculation by contaminated needles. Transplacental syphilis infection of the fetus may occur at any time during pregnancy. Presence of the disease can be determined by a serological test. Adequate treatment with penicillin in the first or second stage of the disease is usually effective. Results of treatment in the third stage are less successful.

8 Gonorrheal infection may produce abnormal narrowing of the fallopian tubes in females and may be responsible for ectopic pregnancy or sterility.

9 Chlamydia infection may produce conjunctivitis and/or pneumonia in the newborn.

10 A first attack of herpes genitalis during early pregnancy may result in spontaneous abortion. Later in pregnancy such a primary infection increases the risk of premature birth. The infant born vaginally of a mother with primary genital herpes has about a 50% chance of neonatal infection. More than 50% of infected newborns die.

11 Cytomegalovirus (CMV) seldom causes symptoms in adults but can cause retardation and death in the fetus.

12 Human immunodeficiency virus disease (HIV) is most likely to affect women who are intravenous drug users or who have sexual intercourse with partners who engage in high-risk behaviors.

13 Infants of mothers infected with hepatitis B should be given hepatitis B immune globulin (HBIG) and started on a course of hepatitis B vaccine.

14 Abortions may be spontaneous or induced. A threatened abortion may possibly be halted; loss of the fetus cannot be prevented in an inevitable abortion. An incomplete abortion refers to the retention of some of the products of conception, whereas a complete abortion involves elimination of all products of pregnancy. Women who have experienced more than three abortions at about the same stage of development are said to be victims of habitual or recurrent abortion. A missed abortion occurs when a very young fetus dies in utero and remains there 2 months or longer before being expelled.

15 The danger of hemorrhage in ectopic pregnancy is extremely serious. If tubal rupture occurs, the woman characteristically experiences severe knifelike pain in the lower abdomen, which may or may not be followed by spotting or bleeding. Shoulder pain and the urge to defecate are classic symptoms.

16 In placenta previa the placenta implants low on the interior of the uterine wall. Bright red, painless bleeding may occur late in pregnancy, or the condition may not be discovered until the onset of true labor. Cesarean delivery may be the treatment of choice.

17 With abruptio placentae the placenta is properly placed but becomes detached. The first sign of this occurrence during labor may be strong, almost continuous contractions with or without external vaginal bleeding. Treatment often includes cesarean delivery and blood replacement.

18 When caring for a maternity patient experiencing abnormal bleeding, the nurse must remember the following: never administer a routine enema; never examine the patient vaginally; observe the patient carefully and frequently; keep the charge nurse and physician informed of changes; expect possible orders for intravenous fluids, blood analysis, and cross match for blood transfusion; record intake and output; maintain a calm, supportive manner, and provide accurate information and emotional support.

19 The three classic signs of preeclampsia, or pregnancy-induced hypertension (PIH), are hypertension, proteinuria, and edema.

20 The following women are more likely to develop preeclampsia-eclampsia: those of lower socioeconomic status, older nulliparas, those with multiple pregnancy, chronic hypertension, diabetes, a family history of PIH, hydatidiform mole, and those with Rh incompatibility.

21 Mild forms of preeclampsia may be treated on an out-patient basis. Bed rest in a side-lying position to increase placental blood flow usually helps to decrease blood pressure.

22 Magnesium sulfate reduces transmission of nerve impulses from brain to muscles and is used primarily to prevent or treat convulsions in PIH. The antidote for magnesium sulfate is calcium gluconate.

23 Premature babies are more likely to suffer trauma during birth, to be victims of respiratory distress syndrome, and to require longer supportive hospital care. The birth of such an infant places psychologic and economic stress on the family and presents a challenge to community resources.

24 Bed rest may inhibit progression of premature labor. Certain tocolytic drugs are also used in an attempt to quiet uterine contractions.

25 Postpartum hemorrhage may be the result of uterine atony, retained placental fragments, cervical or vaginal lacerations, or hematomas.

26 Puerperal infection may be demonstrated by temperature elevations of more than 101° F after the second day, signs and symptoms of infection, or a positive culture. Signs and symptoms may include abdominal tenderness or pain, foul-smelling lochia, an abnormally large uterus,

chills, general malaise, lack of appetite, and elevated pulse rate.

27 Possible signs and symptoms of thrombophlebitis include calf pain, swelling, red streaks, locally inflamed areas, and tense skin that appears lighter in color. Treatment usually involves bed rest with elevation of the affected leg, analgesics, and application of heat. Antibiotics and anticoagulants may also be prescribed.

CRITICAL THOUGHT QUESTIONS

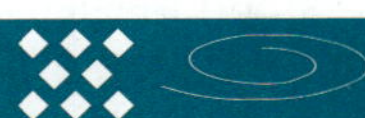

1 What questions should the nurse ask a woman, 12 weeks pregnant, who calls to report a small amount of vaginal bleeding? Give your rationale. What instructions should the nurse give her?

2 Mrs. Jones is admitted at 36 weeks with possible abruptio placentae secondary to cocaine use. You are the nurse admitting her. How would you approach her? Would your feelings and opinions interfere with your ability to carry out your professional responsibilities?

3 Ann Foley is a single 24-year-old woman, pregnant with her first child. She confides in you that her boyfriend uses intravenous heroin but that she does not. The physician advises all her patients to be tested for HIV infection. Ann asks you for your opinion. How would you advise her and why?

4 Loss of a pregnancy places physical and psychologic stress on a woman. Identify the various types of abortions. How would you deal with the psychological needs of these individuals?

5 The placenta supplies oxygen and nutrients to the fetus. If there is an abnormal placement of the placenta or premature separation of the placenta from the uterine wall problems may occur. How would you recognize these conditions? Compare and contrast the signs and symptoms of placenta previa and abruptio placentae.

REFERENCES

Acosta YM, Goodwin C, Amaya MA, et al: HIV disease and pregnancy: part 2, antepartum and intrapartum care, *J Obstet Gynecol Neonatal Nurs* 21(2):97-103, 1992.

Allen S: Epidemiology of premature rupture of the fetal membranes, *Clin Obstet Gynecol* 34(4):685-693, 1991.

American College Obstetricians and Gynecologists: *Perinatal herpes simplex infections, Tech Bull 122.* Washington, DC, 1988, The College.

Andrews EB, Yankaskas BC, Cordero J: Fetal acyclovir in pregnancy registry: six years' experience, *Obstet Gynecol* 79:7, 1992.

Association of Women's Health, Obstetric, and Neonatal Nurses: program targets high-risk pregnancy, *AWHONN Voice* 1(9):2, 1993.

Bastin N, Tamayo OW, Tinkle MB, et al: HIV disease and pregnancy: part 3, postpartum care of the HIV positive woman and her newborn, *J Obstet Gynecol Neonatal Nurs* 21(2):105-111, 1992.

Bobak IM, Jensen MD: *Maternity and gynecologic care,* ed 5, St. Louis, 1993, Mosby.

Butler K: Transmission, diagnosis and treatment of HIV infection in children, *J Intravenous Nurs* 14(3):13-24, 1991.

Centers for Disease Control: Hepatitis B virus: a comprehensive strategy for eliminating transmission in the United States through universal childhood vaccination, *Morbidity and Mortality Weekly Report* 40:1-24, 1991.

Centers for Disease Control: *Morbidity and Mortality Weekly Report* 39 (January 4):952, 1991.

Centers for Disease Control: 1989 Sexually transmitted diseases treatment guidelines, *Morbidity and Mortality Weekly Report* 38 (Suppl 81), September 1, 1989.

Cousins L, Baxi L, Chez R, et al: Screening recommendations for gestational diabetes, *Am J Obstet Gynecol* 165:493-496, 1991.

Cowan M: Home care of the pregnant woman using terbutaline, *MCN* 18(2):99-105, 1993.

Crawford NG, Pruss AM: Preventing neonatal hepatitis B infection during the perinatal period, *J Obstet Gynecol Neonatal Nurs* 22(6):491-497, 1993.

Creasy RK, Resnik R: *Maternal-fetal medicine,* ed 3, Philadelphia, 1994, WB Saunders.

Ellerbrock TV, Rogers MF: Epidemiology of human immunodeficiency virus infection in women in the United States, *Obstet Gynecol Clin North Amer* 17:523-543, 1990.

Gabbe SG: Diabetes mellitus: ways of individualizing care, *Contemp OB/GYN* 36(1):68, 1990.

Gilbert ES, Harmon JS: *High risk pregnancy and delivery,* St. Louis, 1993, Mosby.

Harvey MG: Diabetic ketoacidosis during pregnancy, *J Perinat Neonatal Nurs* 6(1):1-13, 1992.

Harvey CJ, Burke ME: Hypertensive disorders in pregnancy. In Mandeville LK, Troiano NH (eds): *High-risk intrapartum nursing,* Philadelphia, 1992, JB Lippincott.

Heppard M, Garite T: *Acute obstetrics: a practical guide,* St. Louis, 1991, Mosby.

Howard ED: Gestational diabetes mellitus screening tests: a

review of current recommendations, *J Perinat Neonatal Nurs* 6(1):37-42, 1992.

Killion C: Pregnancy: a critical time to target STDs, *MCN* 19(3):156-161, 1994.

Leff EW, Gagne MP, Jefferis SC: Type I diabetes and pregnancy, *MCN* 16(2):83-87, 1991.

Lowe T, Cunningham G: Placental abruption, *Clin Obstet Gynecol* 33(3):406-413, 1990.

Newman V, Fullerton J: Role of nutrition in the prevention of preeclampsia: review of the literature, *J Nurse Midwifery* 35(5):282-291, 1990.

Nolte S, Sohn MA, Koons B: Prevention of HIV infection in women, *J Obstet Gynecol Neonatal Nurs* 22(2):128-134, 1992.

Ross T, Dickason EJ: Vertical transmission of HIV and HBV, *MCN* 17(4):193-195, 1992.

Sisson M: Disseminated intravascular coagulation. In Mandeville LK, Troiano NH (eds): *High-risk intrapartum nursing*, Philadelphia, 1992, JB Lippincott.

Stepanuk KM: Congenital syphilis: are we missing infected newborns? *MCN* 19(5):272-274, 1994.

Stock R: Ectopic pregnancy: a look at changing concepts and problems, *Clin Obstet Gynecol* 33(3):448-453, 1990.

Summers L: Understanding tuberculosis: implications for pregnancy, *J Perinat Neonatal Nurs* 6(2):12-24, 1992.

Tillman J: Syphilis: an old disease, a contemporary problem, *J Obstet Gynecol Neonatal Nurs* 21(3):209-213, 1992.

Tinkle MB, Amaya MA, Tamayo OW: HIV disease and pregnancy: part 1, epidemiology, pathogenesis, and natural history, *J Obstet Gynecol Neonatal Nurs* 21(2):86-92, 1992.

Trustem A: When to suspect ectopic pregnancy, *RN* 54(8):22-25, 1991.

Winn H, Reece E: Integrating management of diabetic pregnancies, *Contemp OB/GYN* 33(1):91-102, 1989.

Witry SW: Pulmonary embolus in pregnancy, *J Perinat Neonatal Nurs* 6(2):1-11, 1992.

Working Group on High Blood Pressure in Pregnancy: National high blood pressure education program working group report on high blood pressure in pregnancy, *Am J Obstet Gynecol* 163:1689-1712, 1990.

Worthington-Roberts B, Williams S: *Nutrition in pregnancy and lactation*, ed 5, St. Louis, 1993, Mosby.

BIBLIOGRAPHY

Davies K: Genital herpes: an overview, *J Obstet Gynecol Neonatal Nurs* 19(5):401-406, 1990.

Harvey M: Critical care for the maternity patient, *MCN* 17(6):296-309, 1992.

Hodgman DE: Management of urinary tract infections in pregnancy, *J Perinat Neonatal Nurs* 8(1):1-11, 1994.

Keohane NS, Lacey LA: Preparing the woman with gestational diabetes for self-care, *J Obstet Gynecol Neonatal Nurs* 20(3):189-193, 1991.

Libbus MK: Condoms as primary prevention in sexually active women, *MCN* 17(5):256-260, 1992.

Maloni JA: Bed rest during pregnancy: implications for nursing, *J Obstet Gynecol Neonatal Nurs* 22(5):422-426, 1993.

Plattner MS: Pyelonephritis in pregnancy, *J Perinat Neonatal Nurs* 8(1):20-27, 1994.

Stainton MC: Supporting family functioning during a high-risk pregnancy, *MCN* 19(1):24-28, 1994.

Vomund SL, Witter SE: Advanced techniques for the treatment of severe isoimmunization, *MCN* 19(1):18-23, 1994.

Zenker PN, Berman SM: Congenital syphilis: trends and recommendations for evaluation and management. *Pediatr Infect Dis J* 10:516-522, 1991.

Special Needs and Age-Related Considerations

CHAPTER OBJECTIVES

After studying this chapter, the student should be able to:

1. Outline the normal characteristics of adolescent physical and psychosocial development.
2. Discuss the factors that contribute to the high rate of adolescent pregnancy in the United States.
3. Cite the national health objectives, related to teenage pregnancy and sexual activity, for the year 2000.
4. Identify the physical and psychosocial risks associated with childbearing in adolescents.
5. Describe how prenatal care for the pregnant adolescent may differ from that of an adult pregnant woman.
6. Identify nursing interventions that may promote the adolescent's positive parenting skills.
7. Discuss the factors that contribute to delayed childbearing.
8. Identify the physical and psychosocial risks associated with childbearing in the women over 35 years of age.
9. Describe how prenatal care for the older pregnant woman may differ from that of younger adult pregnant women.
10. Identify nursing interventions that may promote the older parent's positive parenting skills.

When pregnancy occurs in young women under 19 years of age or in women over the age of 35, the expectant mother and her fetus are at risk for age-related complications (Smith, 1993). This chapter focuses on the incidence of pregnancy, contributing factors, and special needs and risks associated with pregnancy at these two extremes of the childbearing years. Many of these risks can be minimized with adequate prenatal care and current technology. The nurse has a special role to play in educating these women to promote healthy outcomes for mother, baby, and family.

ADOLESCENT CHILDBEARING AND PARENTING

Adolescent sexual activity and pregnancy have become major health concerns in the United States. Adolescents make up approximately 18% of all sexually active women. One out of 10 American females ages 15 through 19 becomes pregnant each year (more than 1 million annually). There is also a high rate of repeat pregnancy within 2 years of the first birth. Women under 20 account for 26% of all abortions, 15% of all births, and about 46% of all out-of-wedlock births

RISK FACTORS FOR UNWED TEEN PREGNANCY

Developmental level—focused on present, feels invulnerable
Gap between sexual maturity and time of marriage
Pervasive sexual messages in the popular media
Lack of knowledge regarding reproductive function, risk of pregnancy
Social and economic deprivation (perceives few life options)
Perception of pregnancy and parenthood as way to achieve adult status
Family and/or school conflict
Drug and alcohol abuse

in the United States (Henshaw and Van Vort, 1989). Most single teenage mothers (90% to 96%) keep their babies, whether or not they have family assistance (Castiglia, 1990). Only a small number opt for adoption (4% to 10%) (Farber, 1991).

Contributing factors

Many factors are related to the incidence of early marriage or out-of-wedlock births (see accompanying box). Improved nutrition and less disease has led to early physical development and age of menarche—averaging 12½ years (see Chapter 5). Young people are also deferring marriage to complete education and career goals. The combination of earlier menarche and later marriage results in a 5- to 10-year gap between sexual maturity and sexual activity within marriage. Society's changing attitudes toward sexual topics has led to pervasive sexual images in the popular media—music, videos, television, and movies. Sexual activity outside of marriage is often portrayed as the norm, with little attention to sexual responsibility. Many young people are not waiting for marriage to initiate sexual activity. The average age of first sexual intercourse is 15 years, and is frequently attributed to peer pressure. See Nursing Alert above right.

Although improving, the use of contraception among adolescents is typically erratic or absent (Biro, 1992). Teenagers often know where to get contraceptive counseling and devices but frequently have misconceptions about reproductive function and pregnancy risk. In addition, adolescents value spontaneity and tend to feel invulnerable to risk. This view of being somehow unique and invulnerable to the possibility of becoming pregnant extends to the risk of contracting sexually transmitted diseases (STDs). The highest rates of STDs are seen among sexually active adolescents

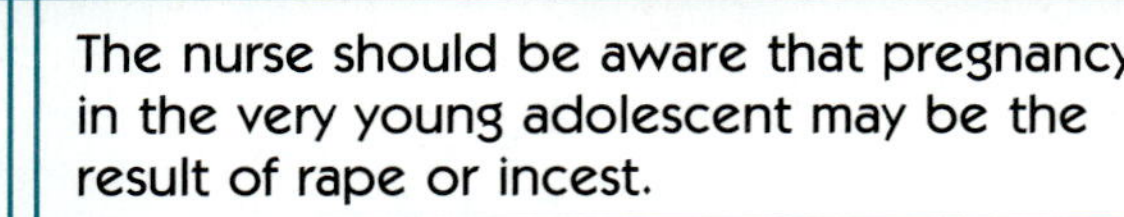

Nursing Alert

The nurse should be aware that pregnancy in the very young adolescent may be the result of rape or incest.

aged 15 to 19 years (Futterman and Hein, 1990). Teenagers who abuse alcohol and drugs are more sexually active than teenagers who do not abuse, thus increasing their exposure to STDs and pregnancy.

Not all teenage pregnancies are unplanned. There is a higher incidence of pregnancy among adolescents of lower socioeconomic status. Teenagers who perceive fewer social and economic life options may view early parenthood more positively than those who have more resources. Others are influenced by cultural values that equate pregnancy and birth with adult status. Still others are rebelling from troubled family relationships and problems in school.

Adolescent development

Maturation is a three-fold process: physical, emotional, and intellectual. Unfortunately physical maturity does not always coincide with emotional and intellectual maturity. Adolescent progress toward adulthood is often divided into three phases; each characterized by advancing physical, emotional, and cognitive maturation. Successful progress through these phases enables the adolescent to complete his or her psychological developmental tasks: establishing a secure sense of identity; developing meaningful relationships with others; and achieving emotional independence of parents and other adults (see Chapter 3).

Early adolescence (12 to 15 years). Rapid growth and development of secondary sex characteristics often occur during this period, creating a need for the girl to incorporate these changes into her self-image. Thinking tends to be focused on the present and on herself. Her primary reference group is her peers and she makes initial attempts at being independent from her family.

Middle adolescence (15 to 17 years). Physical changes are often completed during this period. She remains self-centered but is able to problem solve and begins to think about the future. At the same time, she is testing the limits of parental control in her personal behavior. Pregnancy and parenthood before age 16 is more likely to be unplanned and to deter the social, emotional, and educational development of the young woman.

Late adolescence (17 to 20 years). The older adolescent is future oriented and has a more mature view of the consequences of her own behavior. She usually has a well-developed sexual identity and a better idea of her role in society. There is ordinarily less conflict with family members and stable relationships with peers. The adolescent who becomes pregnant during this period frequently has a close relationship with the father of the baby and greater potential for growth and maturation with pregnancy. She is also more likely to complete her high school education than is the younger adolescent.

Risks and consequences of adolescent pregnancy

In general, the younger the adolescent at the time of pregnancy and childbirth, the more serious the physical health risks and the more profound the psychosocial consequences. Poverty will further compound these risks and consequences.

Physical health risks. Pregnant adolescents are more at risk for anemia because of poor nutrition. Poor dietary practices are characteristic of teenagers who are often influenced by societal preferences for being "thin" and the teenager's normal preoccupation with body image. Adolescents require additional calories to nurture the pregnancy and meet their own continuing growth needs (see Chapter 11 for weight gain and dietary recommendations for the pregnant adolescent). Poor nutrition likewise places the adolescent at increased risk for having a premature and/or low–birth-weight baby. It may also contribute to the increased incidence of pregnancy-induced hypertension noted among pregnant adolescents (Nance, 1990).

The very young teenager (under 15) is thought to be more susceptible to labor and delivery complications secondary to an underdeveloped pelvis. The cesarean birth rate is higher in this age group (Greydanus and Shearin, 1990).

The *key* to preventing physical complications in adolescents (as in adults) is adequate prenatal care, begun in the first trimester. Unfortunately teenagers often delay seeking care until late in pregnancy. Denial of the pregnancy, difficulty in planning for the future, and difficulty in accessing prenatal care may all contribute to late care (March of Dimes, 1990). Poorer adolescents and those engaging in substance abuse are especially likely to receive late or no prenatal care.

Psychosocial consequences. Although less common than in the past, teenagers sometimes marry after pregnancy or birth has occurred. The divorce rate for these unions is very high. This is not meant to imply that no successful marriages begin in the teenage years. It does, however, indicate that the chances for a satisfactory, continuing family relationship are slim. Once separated or divorced, these young mothers are less likely to receive child support payments from fathers and to return to school than are older mothers (Patch, 1990). Single-parent adolescent families frequently live in poverty, and even those who marry are more at risk for economic problems.

Pregnancy and parenting is likely to disrupt, delay, or end the education of adolescent females. Although education may be interrupted, many do eventually go on to complete their education. The cost of this delay in economic terms, is significant, and they may never "catch-up" to their peers who avoided pregnancy. Those who receive support from their own families and remain at home fare better educationally and financially than those who do not have such support.

There is less social stigma associated with adolescent pregnancy than in the past. As a result, communities are more aware of the needs of the young parent, married or not. A number of programs are available that make it possible for the pregnant adolescent to continue her formal education. These programs may also supervise prenatal care; prepare these young women for their experiences during pregnancy, labor, and birth; provide education in mothering skills; and assist them with needed personal, educational and vocational planning. The goal of such programs is to foster healthy pregnancy, infant, and family outcomes and prevent repeat adolescent pregnancies (Moore, 1989).

The adolescent father must complete the same developmental tasks as his female counterpart. He is often equally unprepared to be a parent and uneducated about reproductive risk. Like his partner, he is less likely to achieve educationally and occupationally at the same level as his peers who do not become fathers. Many adolescent fathers care about their partners and want to assume their parental responsibility but need support in doing so.

In addition to the physical and psychosocial costs to adolescents, the economic cost of adolescent pregnancy and parenting to society is great. The United States spends billions each year in Aid For Dependent Children (AFDC), Medicaid, food stamps, payments to health care providers, housing, foster care, and day care (Capitulo, 1992).

Given these risks and consequences of adolescent sexual activity and pregnancy, two national health care objectives have been set for the year 2000 (see box on p. 280).

Implications for nurses

The nurse must have an understanding of the normal adolescent maturational process; knowledge of that process should guide interactions. Listening attentively to her concerns and maintaining a nonjudgmental approach are essential to establishing a trusting relationship with the adolescent. Treating her with

NATIONAL HEALTH OBJECTIVES FOR THE YEAR 2000:

- Reduce pregnancies among girls aged 17 and younger by 30%.
- Reduce the proportion of adolescents who have engaged in sexual intercourse to no more than 15% by age 15 and no more than 40% by age 17.

respect and facilitating her problem-solving and decision-making efforts can help promote self-esteem and taking responsibility for self-care. Explanations of examinations, tests, and the expected plan of care should be geared to her level of understanding and need for information. Teenagers are often curious about their own bodies and the first visit and pelvic examination are excellent opportunities for teaching about reproductive anatomy and early signs of pregnancy. Later they can be encouraged to listen to the fetal heart rate and palpate the abdomen for fetal parts. Because of the teenager's tendency to be self-centered, teaching about important pregnancy health habits may be more effective if benefits to the adolescent are stressed, rather than benefits to the fetus. Helping her identify ways to adapt pregnancy health instructions to her life-style is likely to increase her willingness to follow them. One-to-one teaching sessions may be more effective for the younger teenager and group sessions with peers more appropriate for the older adolescent.

Prenatal. Although prenatal care for adolescents is similar to that for adults, the nurse must be alert for the special risks associated with adolescent pregnancy. For example, it is important to assess nutritional habits and status, including hemoglobin and hematocrit levels; be alert for signs and symptoms of pregnancy-induced hypertension (edema, elevated blood pressure, proteinuria); and monitor indicators of appropriate fetal growth (weight gain, fundal height, results of sonogram examinations). It is also important to assess the adolescent's risk for sexually transmitted disease, provide appropriate education, and encourage safe behavior. Substance abuse should be discussed and the teenager educated about the effects of drugs and alcohol on the fetus.

The nurse must also assess the teenager's support system. If parents, other family members or sympathetic adults, and/or boyfriend are important resource persons she may wish to have them included in her care. Parental involvement may be especially important for the very young adolescent. The nurse can be instrumental in helping mother and daughter communicate effectively. Referral to social service agencies may be necessary.

Labor and birth. The laboring adolescent may have difficulty coping with pain and be fearful of procedures such as catheterization and intravenous fluids. Explanations that are appropriate to her developmental level, encouraging the presence of her support person, and providing adequate pain relief may help her to adapt to this stressful period.

Postpartum. After birth, the adolescent mother may recuperate quickly but be disappointed in her

CHECKLIST FOR ASSESSING ADOLESCENT MOTHERING BEHAVIORS

EXPRESSING POSITIVE FEELINGS WITH THE CHILD

Does she display positive nonverbal behavior?

Does she express pleasure with the infant's activities and developing abilities?

Are expressions of negative feelings balanced with expressions of positive feelings?

RECOGNIZING AND INTERPRETING DEVELOPMENTAL NEEDS AND BEHAVIORS

Does she volunteer developmental information (to nurse, others)?

Does she interpret the meaning of her child's behavior (to nurse, others)?

RESPONDING APPROPRIATELY TO THE CHILD'S CUES

Does she bring appropriate supplies (to an office visit, etc.)?

Does she console her child during uncomfortable procedures?

Does she respond appropriately to negative child behaviors (not punitively)?

Does she respond appropriately to positive child behaviors (need to explore, etc.)?

ABILITY AND WILLINGNESS TO CONSIDER CHILD'S NEEDS BEFORE HER OWN

Does she adjust her daily routine to the child's sleep/wake/feed pattern?

Does she assist with painful procedures (immunizations, etc.)?

Does she risk social disapproval by being assertive with others about what is right for the child?

Adapted from Fleming BW, Munton MT, Clarke BA, Strauss SS: Assessing and promoting positive parenting in adolescent mothers, *MCN* 18(1):32-37, 1993.

weight loss and body shape. She needs careful discharge teaching about the normal process of involution, self-care, and newborn care (see Chapters 13 and 17). Home follow-up is helpful in preventing physical and parenting problems. The box on p. 280 presents a checklist to aid the nurse in assessing the adolescent's mothering behaviors.

Parenting. Teenage parents do have strengths that nurses should foster. They report higher gratification in the mothering role than older mothers during the first 8 months, and pleasure and astonishment at their infants' rapid growth and development (Mercer, 1986). The nurse can encourage this natural interest in their infants by demonstrating infants' abilities and reflexes. For example, if the nurse uses a rattle to demonstrate the way a newborn will turn towards the sound, the mother will realize that the infant can hear. Teaching about different infant sleep and awake states can educate the young mother that the infant will feed best and attend best to his environment when in the quiet, alert state (see Chapter 16). Adolescent mothers need to know that all parents become frustrated with lack of sleep and infant crying. They should be encouraged to call a friend, take a break (when possible), or seek assistance when frustrated. They need to know that infants do not understand physical punishment and cannot be spoiled by quickly attending to their needs or picking them up. When fathers are involved, they should be included in this teaching.

It is essential that the teenager be given positive reinforcement for appropriate parenting behaviors. The nurse should also minimize "dos and don'ts" and reinforce that parenting is a gradual learning process (Fleming et al, 1993). Referral to a teenage parent support group, if available, may help adolescents adjust to the demands of parenting. With appropriate support and guidance the adolescent mother can successfully mother her child as she continues her own psychosocial growth.

CHILDBEARING AND PARENTING AFTER AGE 35

Recent technological advances have made it possible for some women in their early fifties to bear children. In the twenty-first century the question of where birth will take place will be easier to answer than the question of *when* (in the woman's life cycle) it should occur (Freda, 1994). Although the majority of first births are to women in their twenties, the number of first births to women over 30 increased by 50% during the 1980s (Chen and Morgan, 1991). In addition, many women who have already borne a child have additional children after age 35.

Contributing factors

A number of factors are responsible for the increased number of women who choose to delay childbearing until their mid-thirties.

- Effective birth control methods.
- Increased numbers of women pursuing advanced educational goals and careers. Many of these women wait to begin their families until after they are established professionally.
- Cost of living. Many couples wait until they are more financially secure to begin their families.
- Later age for both first marriages and second marriages.
- An increased number of women in this age group.

Women who voluntarily delay childbearing tend to be white, middle class, and college educated. They are often established in their careers, in a stable marriage, and financially secure (Ventura, 1989). In most cases, they have given considerable thought to the consequences of having a child at this time of their lives and the pregnancy is planned.

Fertility declines with advancing age and women who undergo lengthy treatment for infertility may also find themselves older when they finally become pregnant. See Chapter 7 for information regarding fertility treatment. Obviously this delay is not by choice. In contrast to first pregnancies after age 35, repeat pregnancies are often unplanned, particularly for those who lack contraceptive knowledge and are poor (Jones and Forrest, 1989).

Risks and consequences of pregnancy after age 35

Generally speaking, the older the woman when she begins childbearing, the more likely she is to experience physical complications. Preexisting chronic disease compounds the risk for physical problems. Psychosocial consequences vary depending on a number of factors.

Physical health risks. As a woman ages the risk of spontaneous abortion increases significantly. There is also an increased risk for conceiving a child with Down syndrome (trisomy 21) and other chromosomal anomalies. Most health care providers will suggest that the woman over 35 receive genetic counseling and will offer amniocentesis or chorionic villous sampling for prenatal diagnosis of anomalies (see Chapter 8 for a discussion of these techniques). Multiple gestation is also more likely after age 35, particularly for those undergoing treatment for infertility.

Preexisting chronic diseases, such as diabetes and hypertension, are more significant than maternal age in determining the outcome of pregnancy. There is however, an increased incidence of gestational diabetes and pregnancy-induced hypertension (PIH) in older pregnant women (Fonteyn and Isada, 1988; Haines, Rogers, and Leung, 1991). Although medical advances have increased the ability to manage both gestational diabetes and PIH more effectively, both carry maternal and fetal risks (see Chapter 14). Older women are more at risk for preterm labor because of chronic maternal disease such as diabetes and renal disease. Fibroid tumors are more prevalent in older women and also contribute to the risk of preterm labor. These benign tumors within the uterus may enlarge during pregnancy and lead to malpresentation, difficult labor, and early postpartum hemorrhage (Creasy and Resnik, 1994).

As women age there are changes in uterine musculature and vascularization. As a result older women have more problems with dysfunctional labor and placental problems such as placenta previa and placentae abruptio. There is also an increased rate of cesarean birth for older women (Ventura 1992). These and other complications may slow postpartum recovery.

In spite of these increased risks, medical and technological advances have significantly improved the chances of older women having healthy babies. Healthy older women who do not have chronic disease or obstetrical complications have maternal and neonatal outcomes similar to their younger counterparts.

Psychosocial consequences. Older couples tend to have more concerns about health risks for mother and fetus. If there were problems conceiving or a previous spontaneous abortion, the couple may avoid emotional investment in the pregnancy until they are convinced that the danger of abortion is past or test results confirm a normal fetus. If the pregnancy was planned they usually feel psychologically ready to have a child and make dietary and life-style adjustments to ensure the health of the fetus. If the pregnancy was unplanned they may face additional financial burdens, have concerns about their ability to parent as they get older, and awkward with friends who have older children. If there are other children in the family they may be concerned about their reactions to the pregnancy.

Many older first-time parents have little experience with newborns and wonder about their ability to parent. They may be surprised at the extent that the newborn disrupts their well-established routine, and have concerns about the potential changes in their couple relationship (Broom, 1984; Mercer, 1986). First-time mothers tend to be better prepared for parenthood, yet report less gratification with the mothering role than their younger counterparts and a less positive self-concept over the first 8 months (Mercer, 1986). Older multiparous women, on the other hand, report feeling more competent in the mothering role (Pridham and Chang, 1992).

Implications for nurses

Nurses need a basic understanding of the reasons for delayed childbearing. It is important to identify whether or not a pregnancy was planned, and assess the family's readiness for having the first or subsequent child. Nurses should keep in mind that older parents are often acutely aware that there are additional risks for mother and fetus. Women who have experienced difficulty conceiving, have had prior unsuccessful pregnancies, or who have preexisting chronic disease may be particularly concerned about health risks.

Prenatal. Genetic counseling and testing is encouraged for older pregnant women. The nurse should recognize that the decision to have counseling and testing is related to personal beliefs about abortion, and respect the woman's decision (Smith, 1993). If the woman elects to have testing, the nurse will need to educate her about the procedure and support her as she awaits the results.

Prenatal care for the older woman is similar to that for younger adults, but the older woman will usually be followed more closely to detect developing problems, and fetal growth and well-being, will be monitored more frequently. If the woman is healthy, the nurse should treat the pregnancy as normal unless complications arise. It is important to educate the woman about health practices that reduce pregnancy risks (e.g., nutrition, exercise, prenatal care) and reassure her that there is much she can do to enhance chances for a healthy outcome.

The nurse should be alert for indications of gestational diabetes and PIH, both more prevalent in older mothers. If the woman has preexisting chronic disease she should be monitored for signs of developing complications and fetal well-being. The nurse should educate her about the effects of pregnancy on the disease process, the effects of the disease on the pregnancy, and ways to minimize complications (see Chapter 14 for a discussion of specific complications). The nurse should also be alert for signs of third trimester bleeding and preterm labor. The mother should be taught the signs and symptoms of complications to promptly report (see Chapter 9 for a list of danger signals to report).

The nurse should also assess the woman's ability to balance the conflicting demands of career and/or other children, and evaluate her support system. The woman who is used to being self-sufficient may have difficulty asking for assistance with child care or household chores. She may also find the emotional swings of pregnancy unnerving. Incorporating other family members in her care and teaching may increase the probability that she will get the physical and emotional support she needs.

Labor and birth. Encouraging women to attend

childbirth education classes will help them feel more prepared for and in control of this event. The nurse must recognize the potential for dysfunctional labor and placental problems in older women and work collaboratively with the health care provider to minimize complications. The woman may need creative comfort care during a long difficult labor; the coach will also need support. Delaying confinement to bed as long as possible may improve the chances of a shorter labor.

Postpartum. If the woman experiences complications or has a cesarean birth, her recovery will be slower. Because she is older she may experience more fatigue and take longer to "bounce back" than a younger woman. She may need reassurance that she is progressing normally toward full physical recovery. Adequate discharge teaching in self-care and newborn care is as essential for these women as for all others. The older mother, particularly the multiparous woman, may need assistance in identifying ways to conserve her energy for the increased demands of a newborn. She should be encouraged to get help with household chores, if finances permit; share care of the newborn (and older children) with her partner; sleep when the infant sleeps; and eat nutritious meals. Referral to community services may be necessary if the woman has limited resources or is a single parent.

Parenting. Because older first-time parents may have little experience with newborns and high expectations of themselves, they will need appropriate teaching and reassurance of their capabilities. The nurse can emphasize that although they may initially feel insecure about their caretaking skills, parenting is a learned behavior, and their maturity a strength. Helping new parents learn about their newborn's behavioral states and learn to read infant cues will promote feelings of increased competence in the parenting role. Because they may be the only couple with an infant in their circle of friends, referral to parenting classes may help them locate other new parents who are experiencing some of the same frustrations and joys. Many older women will experience conflicting feelings as they prepare to return work. They may need information about child care, continuing breast-feeding while employed, and reassurance that their feelings are normal.

Medical and technological advances have reduced the physical risks of pregnancy after age 35. These older parents bring many strengths to the parental role. With appropriate care and anticipatory guidance they can successfully balance personal and family goals.

KEY CONCEPTS

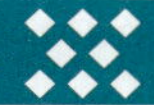

1 Adolescence is a period of significant physical, emotional, and cognitive maturation. Successful maturation enables the adolescent to complete the psychological developmental tasks specific to this period: establishing a secure sense of identity, developing meaningful relationships with others, and achieving emotional independence of parents and other adults.

2 Factors contributing to teenage pregnancy include the widening time period between menarche and marriage, lack of appreciation regarding the role and responsibilities of sexuality in the media and in society, lack of knowledge about reproductive function, family and school conflicts, social and economic deprivation, and drug and alcohol abuse.

3 Adolescent pregnancy is associated with a higher incidence of anemia, pregnancy-induced hypertension, and premature or low–birth-weight infants, The key to preventing physical complications is adequate prenatal care. These pregnancies often result in failure to complete educational goals, family instability, and dependency on government welfare.

4 Prenatal care for the adolescent includes careful monitoring for anemia, pregnancy-induced hypertension, and adequate fetal growth, and assessing for risk of sexually transmitted disease and substance abuse. The nurse must carefully evaluate the adolescent's support system. Teaching should be geared to the adolescent's developmental level.

5 Positive parenting may be facilitated by educating adolescent parents about their infant's normal growth and development, reinforcing that parenting is a gradual learning process, minimizing the "dos and don'ts", and giving positive reinforcement for appropriate parenting behaviors.

6 Delayed childbearing is the result of a variety of factors: effective birth control methods, desire to complete education and career goals, desire to be financially secure, later age for both first and second marriages, increased numbers of women in the 35 and older age group, infertility. Repeat pregnancy after age 35 is often due to lack of contraceptive knowledge and socioeconomic factors.

7 Older pregnant women are more at risk for having a child with chromosomal anomalies, multiple gestation, spontaneous abortion, gestational diabe-

tes, pregnancy-induced hypertension, preterm labor, third trimester bleeding, and dysfunctional labor. These risk factors are increased in women who have preexisting chronic disease. Psychosocial consequences will vary depending on whether or not the pregnancy was planned, the woman's previous childbearing history, number of other children, the extent of career investment, and the amount of previous experience with infants and children.

8 Prenatal care for the older pregnant woman includes genetic counseling and testing, frequent monitoring for complications of pregnancy and for fetal growth and well-being, emphasis on appropriate health habits and the importance of prenatal care. Older mothers are often very aware that they are at increased risk during pregnancy and childbirth. They need reassurance when the course is normal, and education about ways to minimize risks.

9 Older adults' parenting can be facilitated by teaching them about the infant's behavioral states and cues, positive reinforcement of appropriate parenting behaviors, and acknowledging the strengths they bring to parenting. Referral to parenting classes may be appropriate. Women may need information to ease the transition back to work.

CRITICAL THOUGHT QUESTIONS

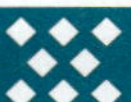

1 Ann Taylor is a 16 year old who is 12 weeks pregnant and lives with her parents who are supportive. She remains at her prepregnant weight and her hemoglobin is low. How would you work with her to improve her nutritional status?

2 Jesus and Maria are both 16, married, and the parents of a 5-week-old infant. At a home visit you notice that the infant spends most of his time in an infant seat; there are no toys nearby; and the parents are slow to respond to the infant's distress signals, stating that they don't want to spoil him. How would you handle this situation?

3 JoAnn and Brian Bilbray are expecting their first child. JoAnn is 37 years old and has a well-established law practice. This was a very carefully planned pregnancy. The physician has recommended genetic counseling and amniocentesis to rule out chromosomal anomalies. They are having difficulty making a decision whether or not to follow the physician's recommendation. As the nurse, how would you advise them? What is your rationale?

4 Mary Center is 38 years old, single, and a successful business woman. She was artificially inseminated and is now 12 weeks pregnant. What are your assumptions about this woman and your opinions about her course of action?

REFERENCES

Biro FM: Adolescents and sexually transmitted diseases, *Maternal and Child Health Technical Information Bulletin,* National Center for Education in Maternal and Child Health, August 1992, US Department of Health and Human Services.

Broom BL: Consensus about the marriage relationship during transition to parenthood, *Nursing Research* 33(4): 223-228, 1984.

Capitulo KL: *Adolescent pregnancy, module 2,* White Plains, NY, 1992, March of Dimes Birth Defects Foundation.

Castiglia PT: Adolescent mothers, *J Pediatric Health Care* 4(5):262-264, 1990.

Chin R, Morgan S: Recent trends in the timing of first births in the United States, *Demography* 28(4):513.

Creasy RK, Resnik R: *Maternal-fetal medicine,* ed 3, Philadelphia, 1994, WB Saunders.

Farber NB: The process of pregnancy resolution among adolescent mothers, *Adolescence* 26(103):697-716, 1991.

Fleming BW, Munton MT, Clarke BA, Strauss SS: Assessing and promoting positive parenting in adolescent mothers, *MCN* 18(1):32-37, 1993.

Freda MC: Childbearing, reproductive control, aging women, and health care: the projected ethical debates, *J Obstet Gynecol Neonatal Nurs* 23(2):144-152, 1994.

Futterman D, Hein K: Medical management of adolescents. In Pizzo P, Wilfret C (eds): *Pediatric Aids,* Baltimore, 1990, Williams and Wilkins.

Greydanus D, Shearin R: *Adolescent sexuality and gynecology,* Philadelphia, 1990, Lea and Febinger.

Henshaw SK, Van Vort J: Teenage abortion, birth and pregnancy statistics: an update, *Fam Planning Perspect* 21(2):85, 1989.

Jones E, Forrest J: Contraceptive failure in the United States, *Fam Planning Perspect* 21(3):103, 1989.

March of Dimes Birth Defects Foundation: *Facts you should know about teenage pregnancy,* White Plains, New York, 1990, Author.

Mercer RT: *First-time motherhood: experiences from teens to forties,* New York, 1986, Springer.

Moore ML: Recurrent teen pregnancy: making it less desirable, *MCN* 14(2):104-108, 1989.

Nance NW: Caring for the woman at risk for preterm labor or with premature rupture of the membranes. In Martin EJ (ed): *Intrapartum management modules: a perinatal education program.* Baltimore, 1990, Williams and Wilkins.

Pridham K, Chang A: Transition to being the mother of a new infant in the first 3 months: maternal problem solving and self-appraisals, *J Advanced Nurs* 17:204, 1992.

Patch L: Adolescent pregnancy, psychosocial issues, *Indiana Medicine* 83(1):30-33, 1990.

Smith JE: Age-related concerns. In Mattson S, Smith JE (eds): *Core curriculum for maternal-newborn nursing,* Philadelphia, 1993, WB Saunders.

Ventura W: First births to older mothers: 1970-1986, *Am J Public Health* 79(12):1675-1677, 1989.

Ventura S: *Advance report of new data from the 1989 birth certificate: Monthly Vital Statistics Report 40(S),* Washington, DC, 1992, US Department of Health and Human Services.

BIBLIOGRAPHY

Arnold L, Brecht M: Legislative issues affecting parenting: an overview of current policies, *J Perinat Neonatal Nurs* 4(2):24, 1990.

Barnes L: Pregnancy over 35: special needs, *MCN* 16(5):272, 1991.

Killien M: Working during pregnancy: psychological stressor or asset? *NAACOG Clinical Issues in Perinat and Woman's Health Issues* 1(1):6-13, 1990.

Mercer R: *Parents at risk,* New York, 1990, Springer.

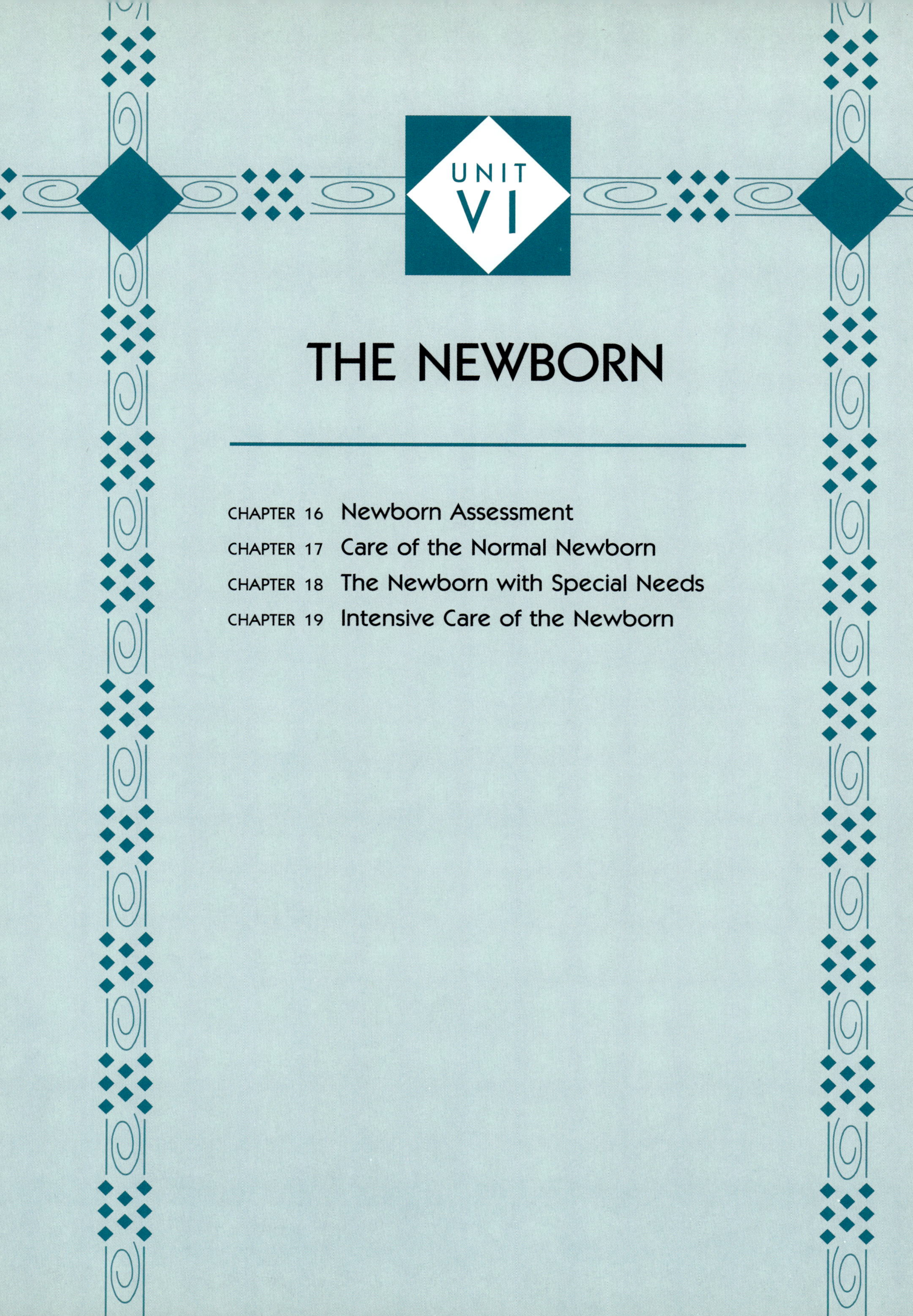

UNIT VI

THE NEWBORN

Newborn Assessment

CHAPTER OBJECTIVES

After studying this chapter, the student should be able to:

1 Describe the major respiratory and circulatory changes that must occur in order for the fetus to adapt to extrauterine life.
2 State average birth weight and length of male and female newborns.
3 Describe the following features involving the infant's head: molding, overriding sutures, fontanels, caput succedaneum, cephalhematoma, and seborrheic dermatitis (cradle cap).
4 Indicate the normal range of the head and chest circumferences of a newborn.
5 Describe common newborn skin manifestations, such as vernix caseosa, lanugo, erythema toxicum, Mongolian spots, petechiae, milia, and acrocyanosis.
6 Contrast physiological and pathological jaundice in the newborn according to the usual time of onset and the maximum acceptable level of serum bilirubin.
7 Note the normal axillary temperature range for the newborn expressed in centigrade and Fahrenheit, the normal apical pulse range, the normal respiratory range (regardless of activity), and the normal blood pressure range.
8 Describe respiratory retractions and explain their significance.
9 Compare and contrast the normal stools of breast-fed and formula-fed newborns.
10 Recall two neonatal conditions that are responses to the passage of maternal hormones across the placenta to the infant.
11 Describe five inborn or primitive reflexes.
12 Critique physical examination findings for departures from the norm.
13 Discuss the sensory capabilities of the newborn with regard to touch, sight, taste, smell, and hearing.
14 Perform a gestational age assessment and compare findings with the infant's gestational age based on mother's menstrual history.
15 Distinguish the six (sleep and awake) states.
16 Describe normal newborn behavioral patterns.

PHYSICAL ASSESSMENT OF THE NEWBORN

At birth the newborn must undergo rapid, profound physiological changes in order to adapt to extrauterine life. Understanding these physiological changes is important for the nurse who must assess whether or not the newborn is making a successful transition. Nurses at all levels are increasingly performing comprehensive newborn physical and behavioral assessments. The first assessment of the newborn is done immediately after birth to ascertain the neonate's immediate adaptation to extrauterine life and determine the need for resuscitation (see Chapter 11 for discussion of this initial assessment). A second more thorough exam is done within the first hour or so after birth, usually as part of the admission process. The admission assessment includes a physical examination and gestational assessment. A third assessment is done by the physician or nurse practitioner before discharge. In addition to these major assessments, most facilities require brief newborn assessments each shift. The nurse can foster the parents' acquaintance process with their newborn by sharing and explaining assessment findings (NAACOG, 1991).

This chapter reviews techniques and normal findings for physical and gestational assessment and discusses normal neonatal behavior. The physiological changes that occur during transition to extrauterine life are discussed under the appropriate body systems.

NEWBORN VITAL SIGNS

TEMPERATURE
Axillary: 36.5-37 C (97.7-98.6 F)
Rectal: 36.6-37.2 C (97.8-99 F)

PULSE
120-160 beats per minute (Count apical pulse for one full minute.)
If crying, as high as 180; if sleeping, as low as 100.

RESPIRATION
30-60 per minute (Count for 1 full minute.)

BLOOD PRESSURE
80-60/45-40 mm Hg at birth

Health History

Before beginning the admission assessment of the newborn, the nurse should collect pertinent information about the mother's pregnancy, labor, and delivery. The labor room nurse should provide a description of the type of labor and delivery, as well as information about complications such as nuchal cord or meconium-stained amniotic fluid, Apgar scores, and resuscitative measures.

Vital Signs

Temperature

Before birth the temperature of the fetus is about 1° F higher than that of the mother. With exposure to the outside world the newborn infant's body temperature immediately drops. Prompt drying and warming is necessary to prevent the temperature from dropping to a subnormal range (see Chapter 11 for immediate care of the newborn). The internal organs of the neonate are poorly insulated, and the skin is relatively thin. The newborn's heat-regulating center and circulatory system have not yet matured, and his or her body temperature rapidly reflects that of the environment. See Chapter 17 for discussion of the dangers of cold stress and methods of preventing heat loss.

When the neonate is dried and placed in a radiant warmer or wrapped in warm blankets, body temperature usually stabilizes within 8 to 12 hours. Rectal temperatures are sometimes done on admission as a check for imperforate anus. Rectal temperatures, however, are not advocated as a means of monitoring core temperature in newborns because of the danger of intestinal perforation if inserted more than 3 cm (1.5 inches). The axillary route is recommended as a safe and practical method for routine monitoring of deep body temperature (NAACOG, 1990). If a glass thermometer is used, it must be held firmly in place for 3 to 5 minutes to ensure an accurate axillary temperature. See accompanying box for normal temperature ranges. The infant's temperature should be taken shortly after delivery, during the admission process, and at least every 4 hours until the infant is stable, and then every 8 hours until discharge (NAACOG, 1990).

A newborn infant's feet and hands are bluish (acrocyanotic) for about 6 to 12 hours after birth because circulation is particularly poor in the extremities. For this reason one should not attempt to judge an infant's temperature by feeling the feet or hands. Evaluating the warmth of the trunk is more accurate.

Pulse

Apical pulse readings are routinely taken with a stethoscope over the heart (precordium) region. Newborn infants' pulse rates vary with the rate of respirations and with activity. The rate should be determined by listening for a full minute, preferably when the infant is sleeping or quiet. See the box above for normal pulse rates.

Respirations

A newborn infant's respirations are irregular and usually abdominal or diaphragmatic in character, typically ranging from 30 to 60 breaths per minute. Because of the irregularity, respirations should be counted for a full minute. Transient tachypnea (respiratory rate of 60 or more) for the first hour or so after birth is relatively common, as excess lung fluid is absorbed. Nasal flaring, costal or sternal retractions (sucking in of the chest wall in the rib or sternal area on inspiration), and/or grunting on expiration are abnormal and an indication of respiratory distress (see Chapter 19 for discussion of respiratory distress syndrome).

Blood pressure

In many hospitals the blood pressure of the newborn is routinely measured with a Doppler device after birth. The usual blood pressure at birth is 80-60/45-40 mm Hg. If blood pressure is abnormal, the physician or nurse practitioner should be notified. As a person grows older, pulse and respiratory rates decrease, whereas blood pressure readings rise.

General Appearance

There is a wide range of variability in the general appearance of the normal newborn infant. Approximately 106 male infants are born for every 100 female infants. However, male newborns have a higher mortality rate than females. The average male newborn infant weighs about 7½ pounds (3.40 kg) at birth, whereas the average female weighs about ½ pound less, or 3.18 kg. The average length of the male is 20 inches (50.8 cm), ½ inch longer than the female newborn. These figures are just averages, and much depends on the heredity of the child. African-Americans and Asians usually have smaller babies, whereas Caucasians and Hispanics tend to have larger newborns.

When parents first see their newborn infant, certain reactions are fairly common: "He seems to be all head." "Where is her chin?" The head is large in proportion to the rest of the body, the facial bones are underdeveloped, the chin is almost nonexistent, and the neck is short and creased. The torso of the normal newborn infant displays a relatively small thorax and a soft, rather protuberant abdomen. The genitalia are small but may be swollen. The extremities are short in relation to body length. The feet are always flat because of the presence of a fatty pad that normally disappears by the time a child has been walking for 6 to 12 months. See figure 16-1.

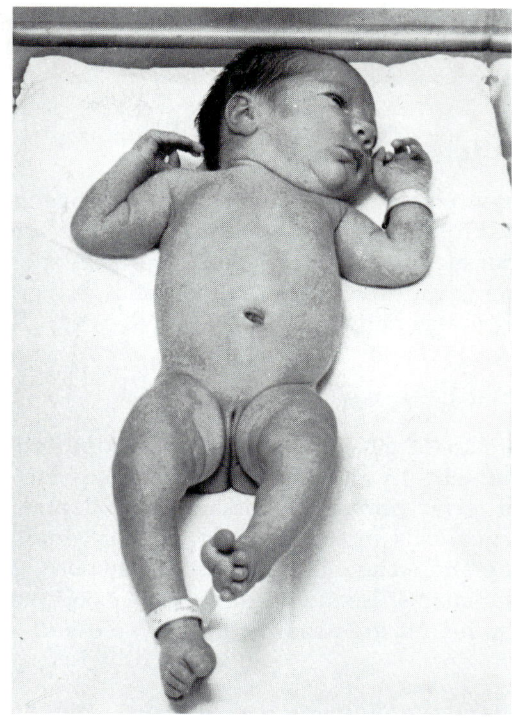

Fig. 16-1 Representative newborn infant, 3 days old. (Courtesy Grossmont Hospital, La Mesa, CA.)

Skin

The full term newborn's skin is relatively thin but few veins are visible because of the layer of subcutaneous fat. In contrast, the skin of preterm infants appears thin and transparent, with many veins visible over the abdominal area. Peeling, especially over the hands and feet, is indicative of post-maturity. The more immature the baby is, the less developed the layer of subcutaneous fat. For this reason babies who are a few hours old, when oxygenation is optimal, tend to be pink or ruddy in color. The smaller the baby, the redder she tends to be—especially when upset and crying. Nurses should be aware that African-American babies are lighter in color at birth and darken gradually. The skin of the neonate will be *mottled* (lacy pattern of dilated blood vessels under the skin) in appearance if the environment is cool. *Acrocyanosis* (blueness of the hands and feet) is not unusual in the first 12 hours of life because of poor peripheral circulation.

Jaundice

After the first 24 hours, the full-term neonate's skin may develop a yellow cast. This icterus, or jaundice, is not usually considered pathological but is thought to be associated with normal breakdown of red blood cells. This *physiological jaundice* occurs in 50% of full-term and 80% of preterm newborns and is characterized by a rise in the serum bilirubin to a maximum level of 12 mg/100 ml. (Jaundice is usually not evident unless bilirubin is above 5 mg/100 ml.) The condition usually resolves within 7 to 10 days (Korones, 1986). If jaundice is present before 24 hours of age, it is considered pathological, and the possibility of Rh factor, blood group incompatibility (ABO), or hepatitis should be recognized and determined. No matter what the age of the baby, the fact that the baby is jaundiced should be reported and evaluated.

Jaundice is usually first noticed in the head and then progresses to the trunk. The skin should be inspected in good light. It can be further evaluated by blanching the tip of the nose, the forehead, or the sternum. If jaundice is present, the area will appear yellowish as pressure is released.

Skin turgor

Turgor refers to the elasticity of the skin. It should be assessed to determine hydration status. The skin over the abdomen is lightly pinched. The skin should be elastic and quickly return to its original shape. "Tenting" indicates dehydration.

Vernix caseosa

The skin of the fetus is protected from its watery environment by a whitish cheese-like sub-stance named *vernix caseosa.* This is an accumulation of old cutaneous cells mixed with an early secretion from the oil glands. The more mature the newborn, the less vernix remains, frequently only in the body creases. Preterm infants are usually thick covered with vernix at birth.

Milia

Plugged sebaceous glands called *milia* appear as tiny raised white spots over the nose, and less frequently, other facial areas. Parents should be cautioned not to squeeze them. They will gradually disappear.

Lanugo

A relatively long, soft growth of fine hair called *lanugo* is often observed on the shoulders, back, forehead, and cheeks of the newborn infant. The more premature the infant, the more conspicuous this extra growth of hair. This hair disappears early in postnatal life.

Erythema Toxicum

Another skin manifestation that can be puzzling but is considered harmless is a condition known as newborn rash, or *erythema toxicum.* The cause is unknown. The lesions consist of red blotches that may become hive-like elevations and may later develop tiny blisters containing clear fluid in the center. These lesions may appear on the day of birth and persist for hours or days. They are most often seen on the trunk but may appear elsewhere. They are not contagious and are most frequently seen on vigorous, healthy babies. The adjective *toxic* is misleading as smears and cultures reveal eosinophils but no bacteria. No treatment is needed.

Mongolian spots

About 90% of infants of African, Indian, Asian, or Mediterranean ancestry and 10% of Caucasian infants exhibit blue-black colorations on their lower backs, buttocks, anterior trunks, and, rarely, fingers or feet. These spots are not bruises or signs of abuse, nor are they associated with mental retardation. These so-called mongolian or Asian spots usually fade in early childhood, but may persist indefinitely.

Petechiae

Petechiae are small blue-red dots caused by the breakage of minute capillaries during a difficult or rapid birth. If present, they are usually seen on the face. If petechiae are accompanied by jaundice or begin to increase measurably after birth, they may be a sign of hematological disease or infection. True petechiae do not blanch on pressure.

Birthmarks

Small reddened areas are sometimes present on the eyelids, mid-forehead, and nape of the neck. They are probably the result of a local dilation of skin capillaries and thinness of the skin. Because of the frequent involvement of the nape of the neck, they are sometimes called *stork bites* (Fig. 16-2). Other terms used to describe this phenomenon are *salmon patch* and *telangiectasia.* In contrast to port-wine stain or nevus flammeus (Fig. 16-2), stork bites are lighter in color, blanch on pressure, and often fade during early childhood. Some are noticeable only when the person blushes, is extremely warm, or becomes excited.

Another common birthmark is the so-called strawberry mark, which may not be present at birth but may develop days or weeks late (Fig. 16-2). It is characterized by a dark or bright red, raised, rough surface. Since it is formed by a collection of capillaries at the skin's surface, it may be classified as a blood vessel tumor, or *hemangioma.* The first signs of a strawberry mark may be a grouping of red dots that eventually coalesce, forming the clear-cut raised lesion. Most often this mark disappears spontaneously in early childhood without treatment. Rapid growth resulting in pressure on a vital structure or obstruction of a body orifice may warrant surgical excision or laser therapy to reduce or remove the strawberry mark. A "wait-and-see" attitude is advocated because most lesions regress spontaneously and all methods of removal cause scarring.

Additional birthmarks that may sometimes cause concern are various flat or raised, frequently pigmented irregularities of the skin that are generally termed *moles,* or *nevi* (singular, nevus). These lesions are often benign. Change in color, rapid growth, size

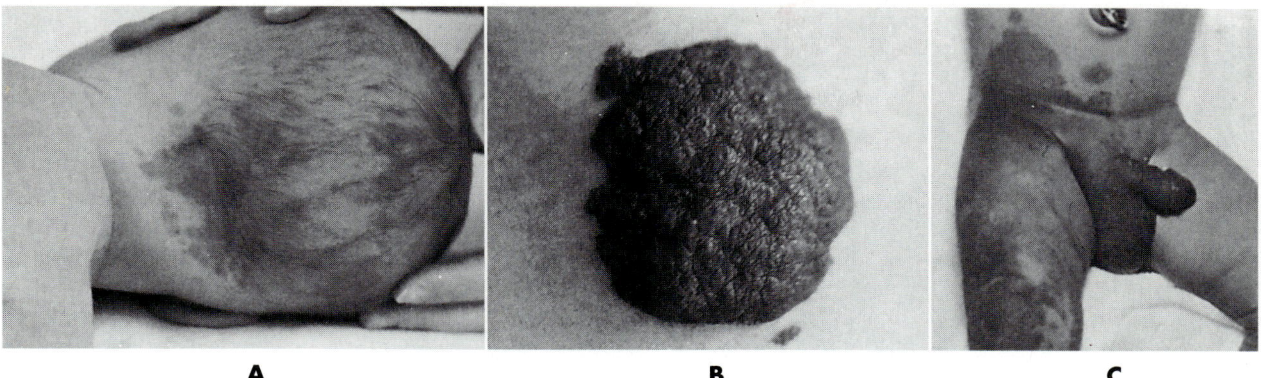

Fig. 16-2 **A,** Telangiectatic nevus (stork bite); **B,** strawberry mark, or nevus vasculosus; **C,** port-wine stain, or nevus flammeus. (Courtesy Mead Johnson & Co., Evansville, IN.)

exceeding 3 mm, or increased irregularity of the border of the nevus, however, warrants a dermatology referral. There is one type of blue-black mole that is considered precancerous, and any such lesion must be evaluated by the physician.

Head

The head of a newborn infant represents one fourth of its total length (Fig. 16-1), but in adulthood the head equals only one eighth of the individual's total height. The newborn infant's occipital-frontal head circumference (OFC) normally ranges from 13 to 14 inches (33 to 35.5 cm). It usually exceeds that of the chest by 1-2 cm. once molding has resolved (see Fig. 16-3). The head's rate of growth averages 1 cm each month during the first year.

The shape of the baby's head can also cause parents' needless concern. Cesarean-born and breech newborns usually have rounded heads. However, infants who are born vaginally in cephalic presentations, particularly those who are firstborn, usually undergo considerable head *molding*. This molding is caused by the compression of the head in the birth canal during labor (Fig. 16-4). The infant skull, because of the soft membranous seams (sutures) separating the skull bones, becomes shaped as it passes through the canal. In response to the pressure of the cervix and bony pelvis, the head usually elongates, and the skull bones may overlap in places (Fig. 16-5). This phenomenon is called *overriding sutures.* The sutures should be palpated to determine the extent of overlapping. The molding gradually resolves during the first week of life.

Two *fontanels,* or soft spots, where sutures cross or meet, can be felt and identified: the anterior diamond-shaped fontanel, through which a pulse is sometimes visible (fontanel means "little fountain"), and the smaller posterior fontanel just above the occiput. The larger anterior fontanel ranges in size from 3 to 4 cm long by 2 to 3 cm wide and closes at 9 to 18 months of age. Occasionally it is the site of seborrheic dermatitis (cradle cap). This occurs when the parent or nurse is fearful of cleaning this soft area, and secretions from the oil glands and cellular debris build up. Actually the cartilage covering the fontanels is tough. The parent should be assured that no harm will come from shampooing the area well. The small triangle-shaped posterior fontanel averages 1 cm and closes by 6 weeks of age. The anterior fontanel may swell when the newborn cries or may pulsate with the heartbeat—both normal findings. A bulging fontanel when the infant is at rest may indicate increased intracranial pressure, and a depressed or sunken fontanel indicates dehydration.

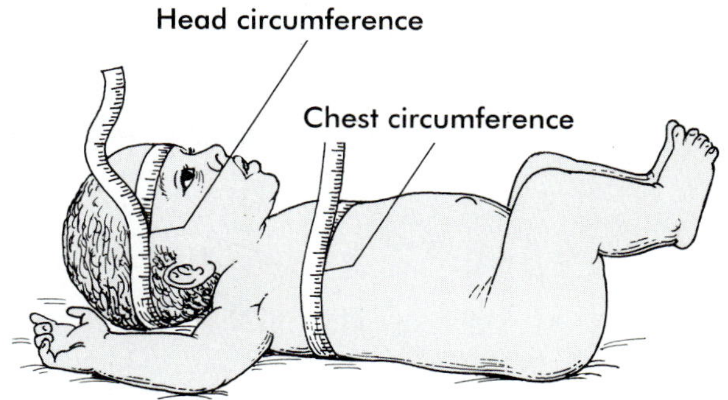

Fig. 16-3 Measuring head and chest circumference.

Two other temporary conditions involving the head may manifest themselves and cause parental anxiety. These are usually caused by the continued pressure of the undelivered head against the partially dilated cervix. The first and less important is called *caput succedaneum* or *caput.* Caput is an abnormal collection of fluid under the scalp that may or may

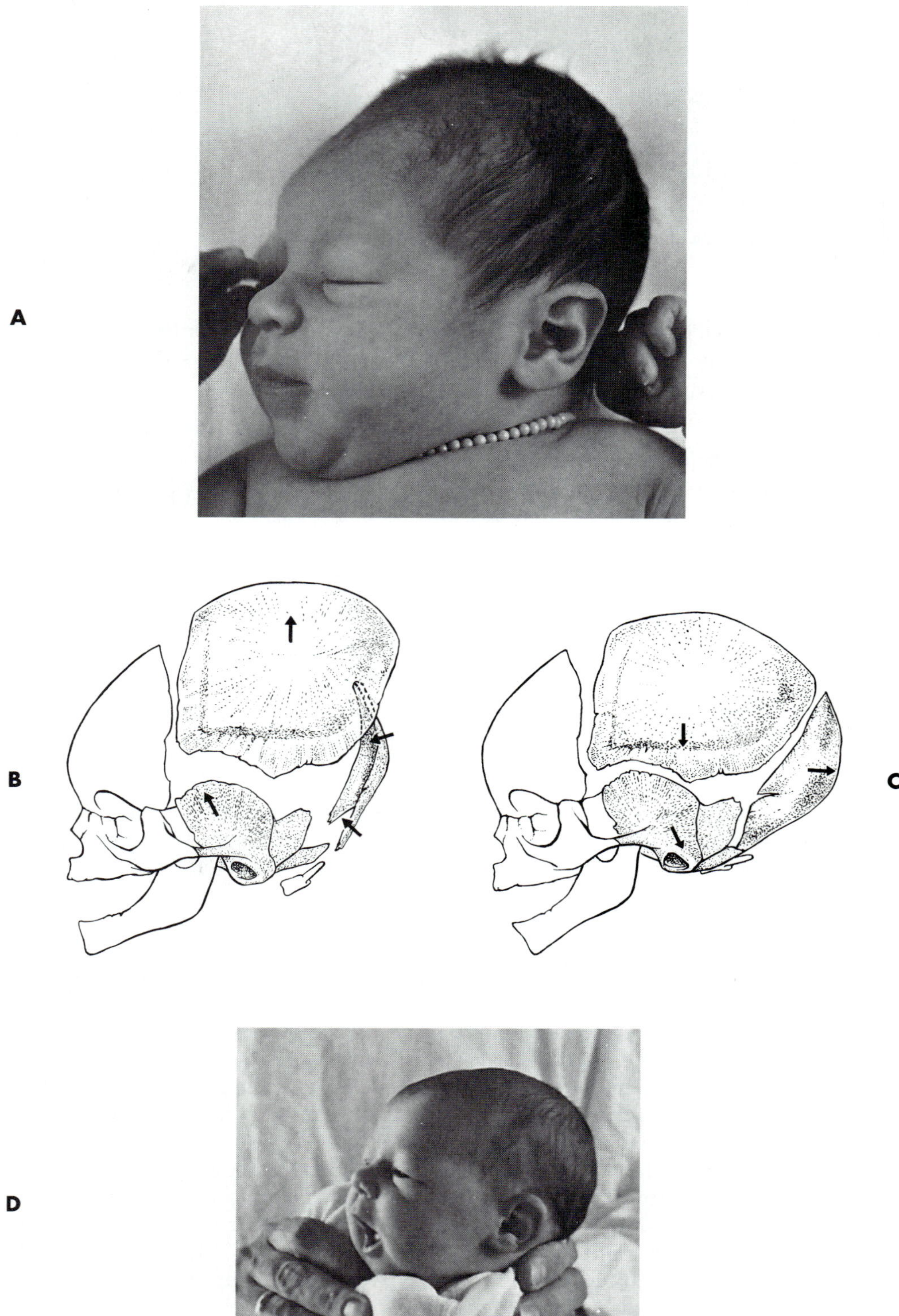

Fig. 16-4 **A,** Molding after vaginal birth; **B,** movement of cranial bones during molding; **C,** return of cranial bones to alignment; **D,** absence of molding. (Courtesy Mead Johnson, Evansville, IN.)

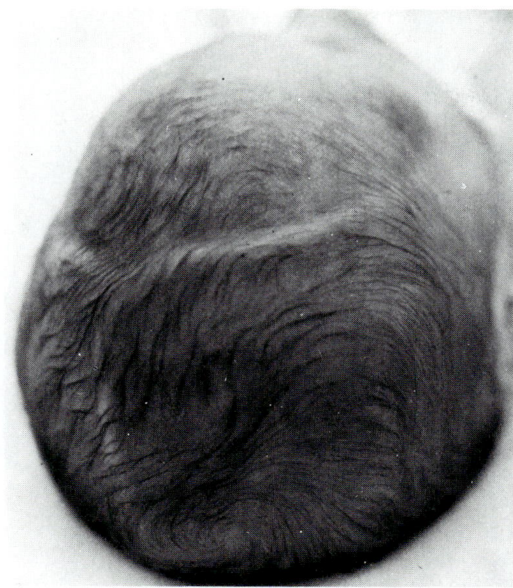

Fig. 16-5 Overlapped cranial bones producing visible ridge in a small premature infant. Easily visible overlapping does not often occur in term infants. (From Korones SB: *High-risk newborn infants: the basis for intensive nursing care,* ed 4, St. Louis, 1986, Mosby.)

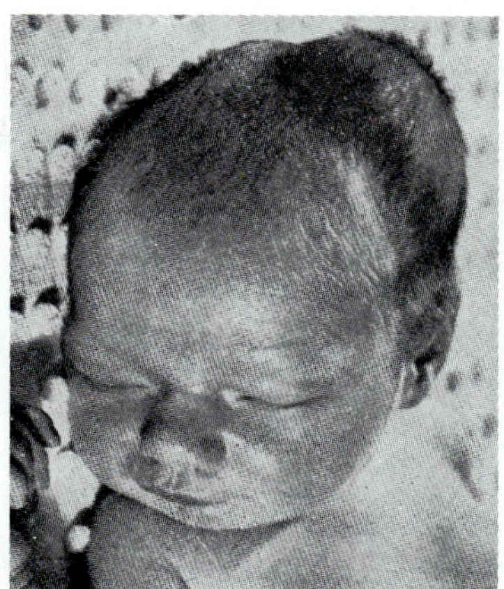

Fig. 16-6 Cephalhematoma over parietal bone. (From Davis ME, Rubin R: *DeLee's obstetrics for nurses,* ed 17, Philadelphia, 1962, WB Saunders.)

not cross suture lines, depending on its size. The accumulation is usually absorbed over a period of days and requires no treatment. The second condition is *cephalhematoma* (Fig. 16-6), caused by a collection of bloody fluid between a flat cranial bone and the periosteal membrane. It is normally restricted to one bone. If it crosses a suture line, a skull fracture may be suspected. It usually develops when labor is particularly prolonged and the pelvis and neonatal head circumference are disproportionate. As a result of the trauma, small blood vessels under the periosteum may break. A cephalhematoma may not be apparent at the time of birth because of the presence of a more inclusive caput. Like caput, cephalhematoma, although temporarily disfiguring, is not harmful and requires no treatment. Cephalhematoma takes longer to resolve than caput, usually disappearing slowly within 3 weeks to a few months. It is important to note the infant's blood values, since excess bleeding into the cephalhematoma may cause some lowering of hemoglobin and hematocrit levels. The bilirubin should be monitored and the neonate should be observed for jaundice.

Face

The newborn's face should be assessed for symmetry when the newborn is at rest and when crying. Eyes should be at the same level, nostrils equal size, cheeks full, and chin receding. The cheeks of the newborn infant have a chubby appearance because of the development of fatty sucking pads that persist until use of the cup is well established. Movements should be symmetrical. Facial paralysis becomes apparent when the newborn cries; the affected side is immobile. Paralysis may result from forceps delivery or pressure on the facial nerve during a vaginal delivery. It usually disappears within a few days to 3 weeks.

Eyes

The eyes may not track properly and may cross (strabismus) or twitch (nystagmus). These symptoms are usually not considered significant unless they persist beyond the first 4 months of life. The irises of neonates are slate blue, grey, or dark brown. True eye color is seldom established until 3 to 6 months of age. Light shined into the eyes should cause the pupils to constrict equally and the eyelids to blink. Blinking is an inborn protective reflex. The nurse should also observe the neonate's pupils for whiteness and visualize the red reflex. Red reflex is a red-orange flash of color observed when the opthalmascope light reflects off the vascular retina. A white pupil and absence of the red reflex may indicate congenital cataracts. The lacrimal glands function only minimally at birth, and the newborn infant's cries are characteristically tearless until about 2 months of age.

Occasionally, an eye discharge is apparent, caused by eye irritation from the prophylactic against *ophthalmia neonatorum* (a condition that results from a gonorrheal infection in the mother). The prophylactic, which is required in most states is an ophthalmic ointment containing erythromycin, 0.5%. Edema of the eyelids can result from birth trauma or irritation

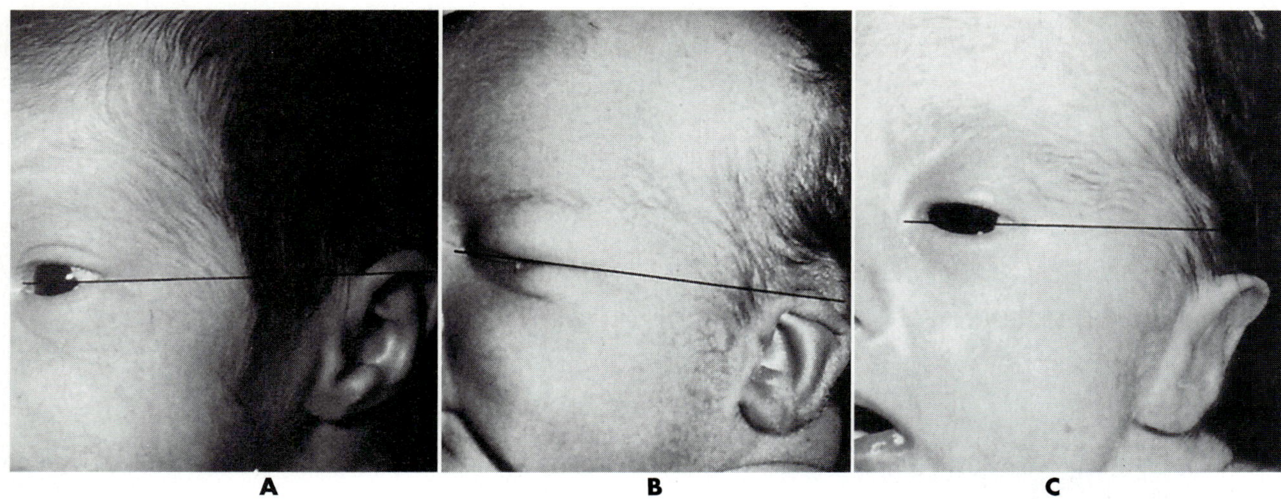

Fig. 16-7 Ear placement in relation to line drawn from inner to outer canthus of eye. **A,** Normal position; **B,** abnormally angled ear; **C,** true low-set ear. (Courtesy Mead Johnson, Evansville, IN.)

caused by erythromycin instillation and resolves within a few days. The reason for the eye irritation or conjunctivitis should be explained to the parents. It is important to note the time of onset of neonatal conjunctivitis to help determine its cause. Any exudate from the eyes that persists should be cultured to exclude bacterial conjunctivitis.

Ears

The ears may be folded and creased and may seem out of shape initially because of positioning while in the uterus. They soon return to their normal shape. Ear form and firmness of cartilage are indicators of maturity. The top (pinna) of the full term newborn's ear is firm, curved inward, and springs back quickly when folded and released. A line drawn from the inner to outer canthus of the eye to the occiput bone should intersect the top of the ear. Low set ears are characteristic of several chromosomal abnormalities and/or internal organ abnormalities (Fig. 16-7).

Nose

The nose should be assessed for patency, discharge, and septal deviation. If the infant breathes easily with the mouth closed, nasal patency is assured. Neonates are characteristically nose breathers and will sneeze occasionally to clear the nasal passages.

Mouth

The mouth can be easily visualized when the newborn is crying. The lips and mucous membranes should be pink and moist. The tongue should be freely movable and midline. Parents may be worried about the possibility of tongue-tie, or a restrictively short frenulum at the base of the tongue. Problems in food manipulation or speech because of this condition are rare.

Small white cysts—*Epstein's pearls*—on the hard palate are normal and will gradually disappear. An oral infection called *thrush* may be confused with Epstein's pearls. Thrush, or oral moniliasis, is caused by a fungus called *Candida (Monilia) albicans* that can be acquired from an infected vaginal tract during birth. The thrush coating on the tongue and cheeks looks something like milk curds (Fig. 16-8). It does not disappear when water is given to the infant as do milk curds. The white patches adhere to the mucous membrane, but gentle scraping with a tongue blade reveals a raw, red surface underneath.

The palate should be palpated with a gloved finger to ensure that it is intact. A cleft palate may be present in the absence of cleft lip. The gums of the newborn infant may appear somewhat jagged, and the rear gums may be whitish. Although the primary teeth are semiformed, they are not erupted. If a tooth is present at birth, it usually is an "extra," which has little root. If they are loose these so-called rice teeth are sometimes pulled to prevent aspiration.

Neck

The newborn's neck is short and creased. Because muscle tone is not well developed the neck muscles are unable to support the full weight of the head. The neck should be palpated for masses and inspected for webbing. Range of motion can be determined by fully extending the head in all directions.

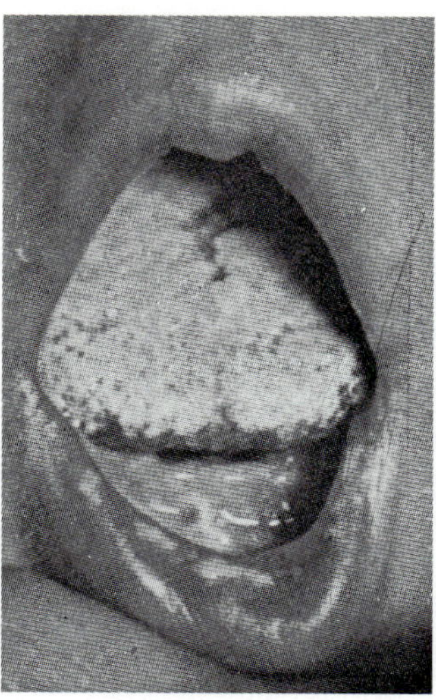

Fig. 16-8 Thrush (From Potter EL: *Pathology of the fetus and the newborn,* ed 3, Chicago, 1975, Mosby.)

The clavicles should be palpated for evidence of fracture which can occur during a difficult birth. The normal clavicle is straight and smooth. Palpation of a lump or grating sensation should be reported. The Moro reflex (see discussion under neurological assessment) should be elicited to evaluate equal movement of the arms. If a clavicle is fractured, the Moro response will be absent on the affected side.

Thorax

The chest is cylindric and the ribs flexible. The average chest circumference is 33 cm at the nipple line. The *xiphoid cartilage* at the end of the sternum is frequently visible in the newborn. As the infant gains weight, it will become less noticeable. The size of the areola and underlying breast tissue are indicators of maturity. The more immature the newborn, the less breast tissue and the smaller the areola. The breasts are frequently engorged in both females and males, a result of maternal hormonal influences that may persist for 2 weeks. Also the result of maternal hormones, the breasts may temporarily secrete small amounts of liquid known as *witch's milk.* The breasts should not be squeezed; this only increases the possibility of infection and tissue injury. Extra or supernumerary nipples are occasionally seen near the true nipples.

Heart and circulatory system

In fetal life the circulatory system serves also as a modified respiratory system, since oxygen is not obtained through the breathing of air into the lungs but through the umbilical cord vein. Carbon dioxide is eliminated through the two umbilical arteries. At birth, of course, this type of respiratory function ceases since the cord is cut or the placenta soon becomes detached. The fetal circulation, which is designed to channel blood flow to functioning organs and largely avoid the lung fields, is rerouted after birth. (See discussion of fetal circulation in Chapter 8.) The two fetal shunts that direct blood flow away from the pulmonary circulation normally close, as a result of changes in internal pressures, loss of the maternal oxygen source, and lung expansion (Fig. 16-9). The opening between the two atria of the heart, the *foramen ovale,* shuts, closing off the blood flow to the left atrium from the right heart and forcing more blood into the right ventricle. The *ductus arteriosus,* the fetal vessel between the pulmonary artery and the aorta, collapses, obliging the pulmonary artery to send its total contents to the lungs. When the cord is clamped and cut the two *umbilical arteries,* the *umbilical vein* and the *ductus venosus,* close and become ligaments.

The circulation of blood in the baby at birth is not at the same stage of development throughout the body. The hands and feet are typically acrocyanotic. At birth the neonate's body may be slightly blue because the fetal blood has a relatively low oxygen content, and a momentary disturbance of the placental circulation occurs before expansion of the lungs is possible. However, as soon as the airway is cleared and a healthy cry is elicited, the skin "pinks up" dramatically. Although significant, color is the least important of the characteristics evaluated for the Apgar score.

The nurse should listen to heart sounds throughout the entire heart region, below the left axilla, and below the scapula, preferably when the newborn is sleeping. The heart beat normally has a "tic toc" sound. A slur or slushing sound may indicate a *murmur.* Although approximately 90% of murmurs are transient and therefore considered normal, they should be further evaluated by a physician or nurse practitioner (Korones, 1986). Peripheral pulses (brachial, femoral, pedal) should also be palpated bilaterally for strength and equality.

Lungs and respiratory system

Although the fetus normally begins breathing movements in utero, the lungs serve no respiratory function because the oxygen supply is secured through the placental circulatory system from the mother. The birth process stimulates a series of events that transform the fluid-filled lungs into organs capable of gas exchange. Some of the lung fluid is squeezed out during the passage through the birth canal, and the rest is rapidly absorbed as the lungs fill with air. Initial breathing efforts are probably

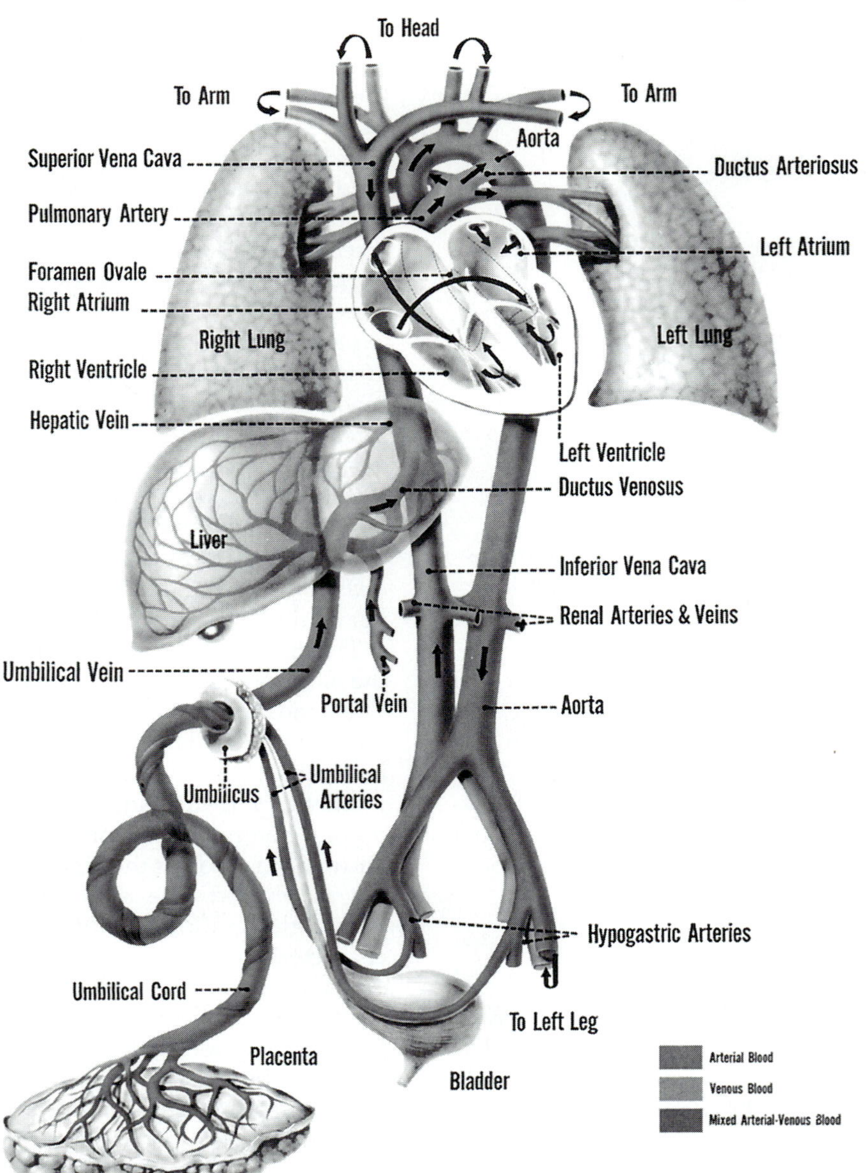

Fig. 16-9 Fetal circulation. *Before birth.* The foramen ovale and the ductus arteriosus act as bypass channels, allowing a large part of the combined cardiac output to perfuse body tissues without flowing through the lungs. The ductus venosis allows blood to bypass the liver. *After birth.* The foramen ovale closes; the ductus arteriosus closes and becomes a ligament; the ductus venosus closes and becomes a ligament; and the umbilical vein and arteries close and become ligaments. (Courtesy Ross Laboratories, Columbus OH.)

triggered by pressure changes in the chest cavity, the physical stimuli present at birth from cool air, noise, light, and handling, and the mild decrease in blood oxygen concentration as the cord is clamped and cut. Surfactant, a phospholipid which coats the lining of the alveoli in the lungs, reduces the surface tension of the lungs allowing expiration without lung collapse. Initially the newborn may need some assistance in clearing the upper airway because of thick mucous secretions.

The nurse should auscultate both the anterior and posterior chest. Lung sounds are louder in the neonate than in the adult because there is less adipose tissue. Lung sounds should be clear after the residual lung fluid has resolved. Cyanosis other than of the hands and feet, costal or substernal retractions, flaring nostrils, and expiratory grunts heard with or without a stethoscope all are possible signs of respiratory distress.

In the United States the most common cause of respiratory difficulty in the first few minutes or hours of birth has been the too liberal use of sedatives, tranquilizers, analgesics, and anesthetics during labor. These medications not only affect the mother but also cross the placenta to the baby, making the newborn sleepy, thus requiring stimulation to elicit spontaneous breathing. Because of this, these agents are used cautiously (see Chapter 12).

Abdomen

The newborn's abdomen is cylindrical and protrudes slightly. The abdominal muscles are relatively lax. There should be no distention or bulging. Few blood vessels should be visible in the healthy full-term infant. The nurse should listen for *bowel sounds* before palpating the abdomen because palpation may temporarily decrease bowel sounds. Bowel sounds should be present.

The abdomen should be gently palpated in all four quadrants to determine softness, tenderness, and masses. Palpation is best accomplished when the infant is quiet. The *liver* can usually be palpated between 1 to 2 cm below the right costal margin, and the *spleen* tip in the lateral upper left quadrant (Fig. 16-10). *Kidneys* are difficult to feel but are more easily felt before the intestines become filled with air and fluid from the first feeding. To palpate the kidney, the nurse places a finger underneath one flank to displace the kidney upward, then uses the fingers of the other hand to palpate the kidney from above. The kidney is felt as a firm oval mass between the nurse's fingers, about 1 to 2 cm above the umbilicus bilaterally.

Umbilical cord

Three blood *vessels* are found in the umbilical cord—one vein and two arteries. They are fairly easily seen in the cut umbilical stump. These vessels are counted at the time of admission. If only two vessels are found, there is an increased incidence of internal congenital defects such as malformation of the kidney or heart. The vessels of the umbilical cord are soon occluded by clot formation and shrinkage. However, if the cord is manipulated often, the clot may become dislodged, and bleeding through the cord stump may occur if the ligature or cord clamp is loose. Large cords that contain a great amount of gelatinous connective tissue, called *Wharton's jelly,* must be especially watched for bleeding, since the cord will shrink in diameter and the clamp or ligature may become ineffective. The cord has no sensory nerves; the newborn does not feel it when the cord is clamped or cut. The umbilical cord drops off in about 7 to 10 days, and the place of attachment heals shortly thereafter.

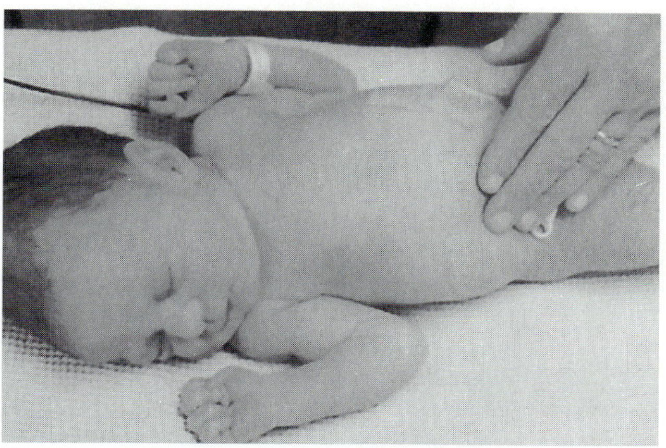

Fig. 16-10 Palpating infant's liver. (From Seidel HM et al, eds: *Mosby's Guide to physical examination,* ed 2, St Louis, 1991, Mosby.)

Elimination

The fetus has no need for a digestive system of its own. All its food is provided predigested by the placental circulation. A good share of the waste products created are eliminated through the same circulation. After birth, however, digestion and elimination are accomplished by the infant's systems.

Stools. The first stool of the newborn infant is *meconium,* a greenish black, tarry, odorless, but very tenacious material. It consists of old lining cells of the gastrointestinal tract, swallowed amniotic fluid debris, and early tract secretions. The first stool should appear in 24 to 48 hours. If it does not, malformation of the gastrointestinal tract is strongly suspected. It is the nurse's responsibility to monitor the frequency and character of infant stools. Meconium continues to be the normal stool for about 2 days, then the products of ingested milk begin to change the color of the stool. It becomes first brown and then yellow-green and more loose in consistency. These are the *transitional stools.* Later the stool will become yellow as more milk-product digestion takes place. The stools of *formula-fed* babies are characteristically pasty yellow-green, almost mustard-like in appearance with a distinct odor. The stools of *breast-fed* babies are yellow "cottage cheese" curds, noisy when passed, with a sweet odor. Normal stool patterns should be explained to the parents.

Urine. The newborn infant's renal system does not

A B

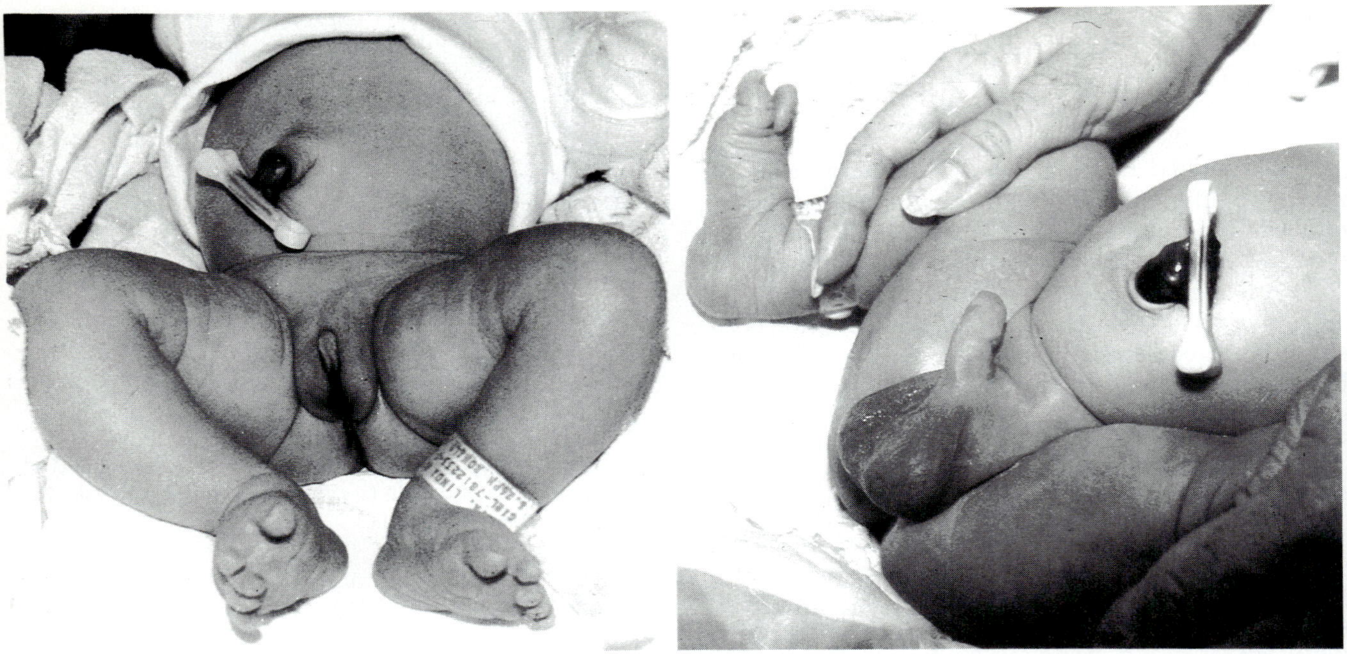

Fig. 16-11 **A,** Genitals in female term infant; **B,** genitals in male term infant. Uncircumcised penis. Rugae cover scrotum. Cord has been swabbed with ethylene blue to prevent infection. (From Bobak IM, Jensen MD: *Maternity and gynecologic care,* ed 5, St. Louis, 1993, Mosby.)

have the ability to concentrate urine to the degree of the older child or adult. Water is not reabsorbed as freely by the nephrons, and a newborn infant may become dehydrated rather easily. A newborn infant with profuse diarrhea or vomiting is in imminent danger of dehydration.

The first voiding usually occurs within 24 hours. If it does not the infant should be evaluated for adequacy of fluid intake and bladder distention. All infant voidings in the newborn period should be recorded. Although newborn infants may not void a large amount or often at first, it is important to note that they are able to void normally. Uric acid is found in relatively large amounts in the urine of the newborn infant. Occasionally this substance may "crystallize out" as it cools in the diaper, leaving a pink stain like "brick dust." The newborn's urine is often slightly cloudy because of mucous but clears with increased fluid intake.

External Genitalia

The genitalia of both the male and the female newborn may be edematous (Fig. 16-11). Breech infants may have particularly swollen genitalia because of prolonged pressure on the area.

Female infants

The labia majora, labia minora, clitoris, and vaginal opening should be visualized. The labia majora typically covers the labia minora in full term infants. In contrast, preterm infants have little adipose tissue in the labia majora, the labia minora is easily visible, and the clitoris prominent. Vaginal or hymenal tags that regress spontaneously may be evident. Smegma, a white cheese-like substance, is often present under the labia. White mucoid vaginal discharge, present in the first week of life, is the result of the withdrawal of maternal estrogen. If it is blood tinged it is referred to as *pseudomenstruation*. Usually only a few blood spots are seen on the diapers. This bleeding should not be profuse; any considerable blood loss may be an indication of hemorrhagic disease.

Male infants

The penis should be inspected to determine the placement of the urinary meatus—normally at the tip of the glans. *Hypospadias* refers to a condition in which the meatus is located on the ventral or lower surface. *Epispadias* refers to the placement of the urinary meatus on the dorsal or upper surface. Both can be surgically repaired.

The foreskin of the uncircumcised infant is normally tight. Few are retractable at birth, and only about 50% are retractable at 1 year. They should not be forced. True *phimosis* (inability to retract the foreskin at all) is rare and can be corrected by surgical removal (circumcision). In circumcised males the glans is exposed, slightly edematous and erythematous for a few days. A yellow exudate forms over the glans after circumcision. Parents should be educated that this exudate is part of the healing process and should not be washed off. Bleeding (larger than a quarter) or purulent discharge is abnormal.

In full term male infants the scrotum is relatively large and pendulous with many rugae. In contrast, the scrotum of the preterm infant is small, smooth, and shiny. The testes normally descend at about 36 weeks' gestation. The nurse should gently palpate the scrotum to determine that both testes are descended. The testes are palpated separately between the thumb and forefinger. Placing two fingers over the inguinal canal prevents the testis on that side from moving up into the canal during the examination. If the testes are not descended in a full term neonate, the nurse should notify the physician or nurse practitioner so that further evaluation can be done. A collection of fluid around the testes is known as *hydrocele,* is relatively common in newborns, and usually resolves spontaneously.

Anus

The anus should be inspected to verify that it is patent and has no fissure. Passage of the first meconium stool is the best indicator that there is no obstruction.

Extremities

The extremities should be inspected for deformities, *polydactyly* (extra digits), *syndactyly* (webbing), clubfoot, range of motion, and symmetry of motion. The nails usually extend beyond the fingertips in full term neonates. Hands should be inspected for normal (multiple) palmar creases. A single palmar crease, called a *simian line,* is sometimes indicative of Down syndrome. Plantar creases are reliable indicators of gestational age in the first 12 hours of life (Fig. 16-12). After that the skin dries and many superficial creases appear. The full term infant has multiple plantar creases, down to and including the heel, whereas the preterm infant has fewer creases, concentrated on the anterior portion of the foot.

The newborn's feet are frequently turned inward because of the intrauterine position ("positional" clubfoot). If the feet can be easily moved to midline, no treatment is necessary. If there is resistance, it may indicate a true clubfoot and further evaluation is indicated.

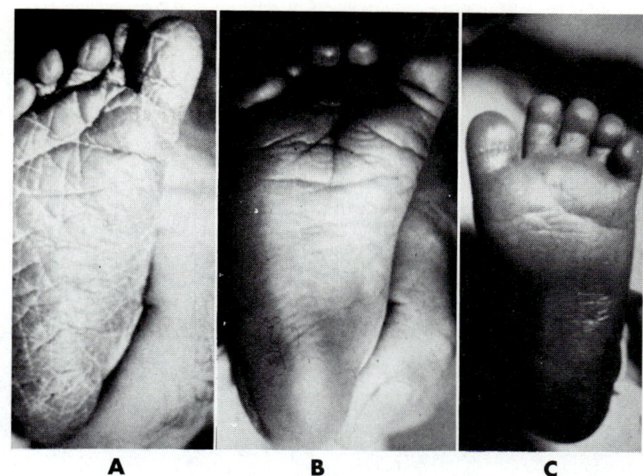

Fig. 16-12 Plantar creases. Infant's sole becomes more creased with maturity. **A,** Postterm; **B,** term; **C,** preterm. (From Dickason EJ, Silverman BL, Schult MO: *Maternal-infant nursing care,* St. Louis, 1994, Mosby.)

The legs and arms should be of equal length. The hips should be evaluated for dislocation by performing *Ortolani's maneuver.* The nurse places thumbs on the inner thighs and fingers on the outer aspect of the infant's leg. The knees are flexed, abducted, and pressed downward (Fig. 16-13). If a "clunk" is felt and there is resistance to abduction, a dislocation probably exists. The health care provider should be notified for further evaluation.

Back

With the infant in the prone position the nurse should inspect the back which should appear somewhat rounded. The spine, however, should be straight. The lumbar and sacral curves do not develop until the infant sits upright and walks. The sacrum and base of the spine should be inspected for tufts of hair or indentations that may indicate incomplete closure of the spinal column (spina bifida occulta).

Neurological Assessment

The neurological examination assesses the intactness of the newborn's nervous system. The nurse should begin by observing the state of alertness, posture, cry, quality of muscle tone and movement. The healthy full term newborn should have periods of full alertness, a flexed posture, lusty cry, strong muscle tone, and symmetrical movement of extremities.

The nervous system of the normal newborn infant is immature. The order of peripheral nervous system

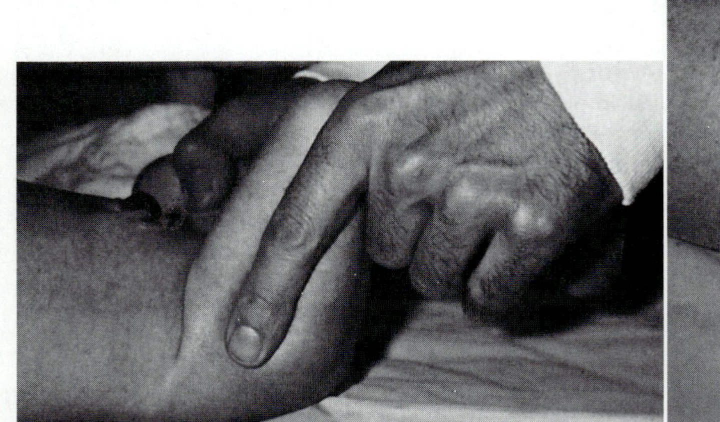

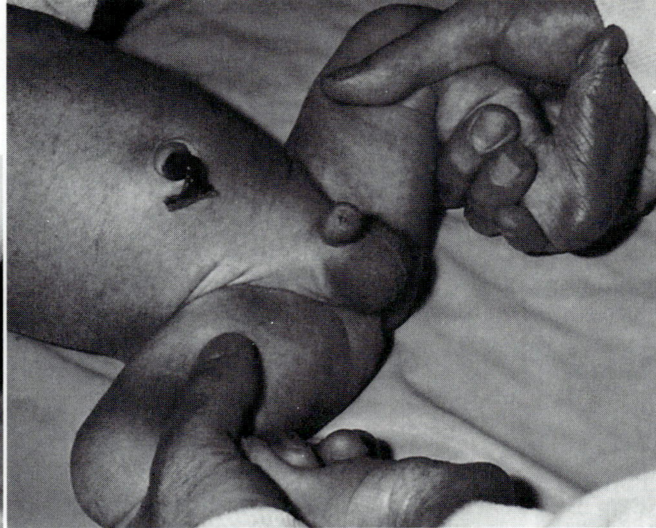

Fig. 16-13 Assessing for hip dysplasia (dislocation) using Ortolani's maneuver. **A,** Examiner's middle fingers are placed over greater trochanter and thumbs over inner thigh opposite lesser trochanter. **B,** Gentle pressure is exerted to further flex thigh on hip, and thighs are rotated outward. If hip dysplasia is present, examiner can feel head of femur slip forward in acetabulum and slip back when pressure is released and legs returned to their original position. A click or clunk is sometimes heard (Ortolani's sign). (Courtesy Mead Johnson, Evansville, IN.)

development and muscular coordination proceeds cephalocaudally, from the head to the arms and then the legs. Later, the fine motor activities of the hands and feet are perfected. Essential activities for maintenance of life and protection are largely reflexive in character—inborn reactions making life possible until the nervous system and associated muscles can mature. Inborn, or primitive, reflexes that normal newborn infants possess include the rooting, sucking, and swallowing reflexes employed in eating and the protective reflexes, such as coughing, sneezing, gagging, blinking, and perhaps crying. Other muscular reactions in newborn infants are also reflexive and some facilitate human interaction (grasping).

Rooting, sucking, and swallowing

The rooting reflex can be elicited by touching the side of the newborn's mouth or cheek. In response, the newborn turns toward that side and opens the lips. Inserting a gloved finger in the newborn's mouth should elicit the sucking reflex, which is strong in the full term newborn. Swallowing can be observed during an infant feeding.

Moro

The Moro reflex is normally strong during the first 8 weeks and then diminishes rapidly, disappearing completely by 6 months of life. When the infant's head is brought forward (about 30 degrees) and then allowed to fall back suddenly, abduction of the upper extremities at the shoulder, extension of the elbows, and opening of the hands follow (Fig. 16-14). The *startle reflex* initiated by a loud noise or sudden movement or jarring may be considered part of the Moro reflex consisting of flexion of the extremities and palmar grasping. These are two distinct movements, since one can occur without the other. When testing for the Moro reflex, make sure the infant's head is in midline position. The absence of the Moro reflex or an asymmetrical response in the newborn infant may indicate a fractured clavicle or neurological damage.

Grasp

The *palmar* grasp reflex is elicited by placing the nurse's finger in the newborn's palm. The neonate should grasp the finger firmly. The *plantar* reflex is elicited by placing the nurse's thumb against the ball of the foot (Fig. 16-15). The toes should curl down in response to the stimulation. The grasp reflexes should be symmetrical.

Babinski

When the nurse strokes the sole of the foot from the heel upward and across the ball of the foot, the newborn responds by dorsiflexing the big toe and fanning all toes (Fig. 16-16).

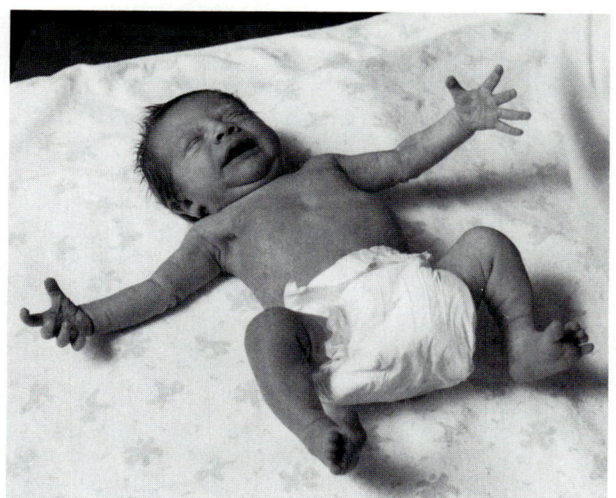

Fig. 16-14 Classical Moro reflex elicited when head was brought forward (30 degrees) and then allowed to fall back suddenly against a padded table. Head is in the midline; both arms are abducted at the shoulder, elbows are extended, and hands are opening.

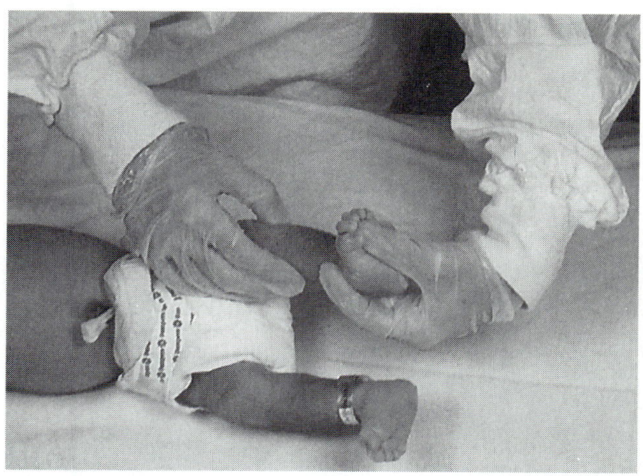

Fig. 16-15 Plantar reflex. Examiner presses against ball of foot. Toes curl down. (From Seidel HM et al, (eds): *Mosby's guide to physical examination,* ed 2, St. Louis, 1991, Mosby.)

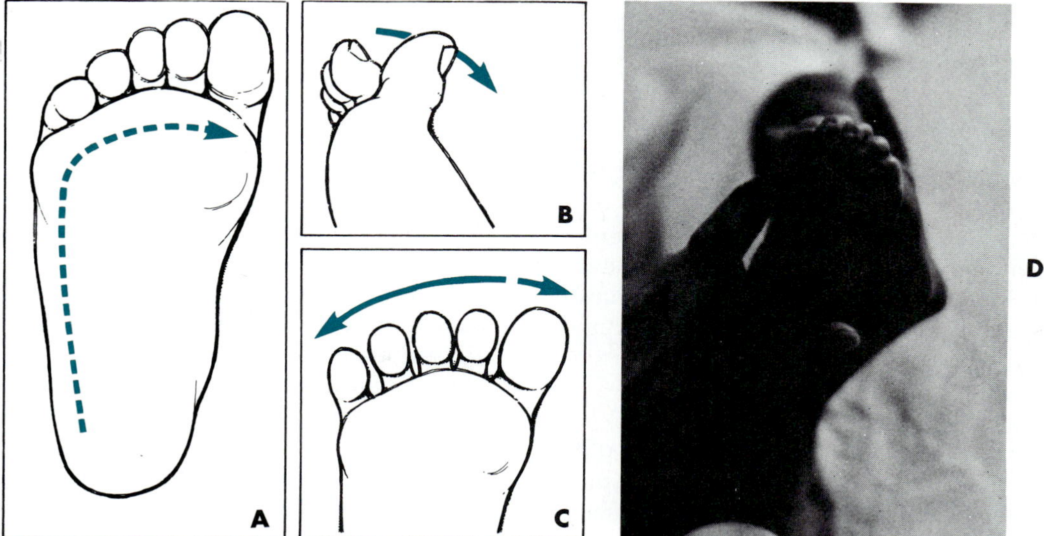

Fig. 16-16 Babinski's reflex. **A,** Direction of stroke. **B,** Dorsiflexion of big toe. **C,** Fanning of toes. **D,** Babinski's reflex in newborn. (From Whaley LF, Wong DL: *Nursing care of infants and children,* ed 4, St. Louis, 1991, Mosby.)

Tonic neck (fencer position)

With the infant in the supine position this reflex is elicited by turning the head to one side. In response, the arm and leg on the same side of the body will extend and the opposing arm and leg flex (Fig. 16-17). The fists shut and the toes curl. Although this reflex may be difficult to elicit in the first few days of life, once it appears it is commonly seen until the infant is about 4 to 6 months of age, disappearing before the infant can crawl.

Intellectual development is difficult to assess in the newborn, but it is reassuring when the primitive reflexes are present and symmetrical. There is cause for concern when an infant fails to fixate or focus briefly, sucks poorly, has poor muscle tone, is lethargic, or unresponsive to care.

Sensory capabilities

The immaturity of the nervous system is demonstrated by the involuntary movement, primitive re-

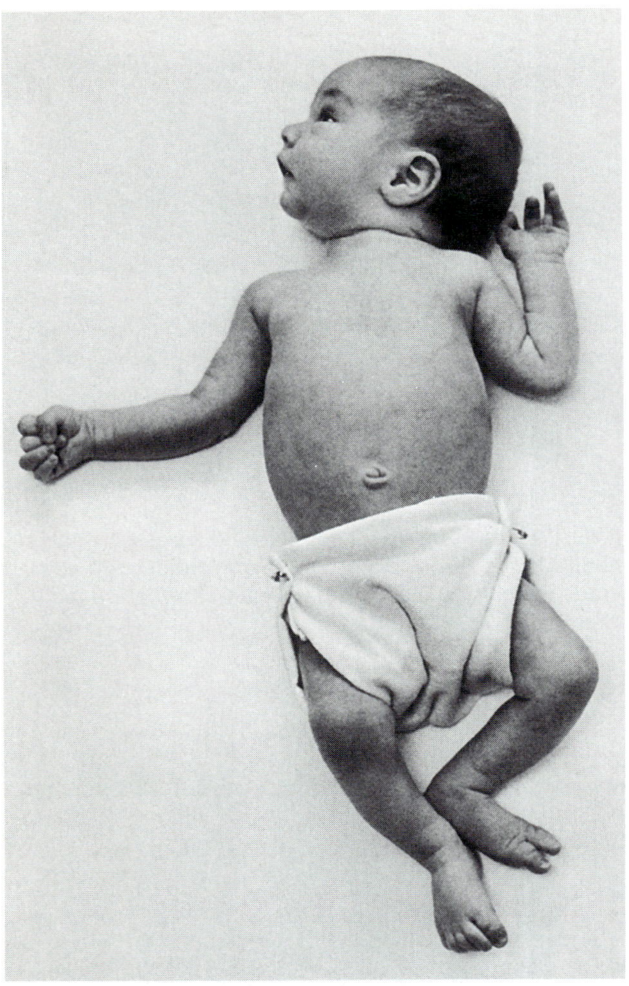

Fig. 16-17 Classic pose in spontaneous tonic neck reflex. (Courtesy Mead Johnson, Evansville, IN.)

flexes, and the unstable temperature regulation of the newborn infant. A newborn, however, has many sensory capabilities that if fostered will further neurological development. Nurses should educate parents about these capabilities and offer suggestions to further stimulate their development.

Sight. The infant can focus on objects (e.g., on a brightly colored ring) at 7 to 12 inches and visually follow the object to midline (Fig. 16-18). Newborn infants can see faces, shapes, and colors. They prefer faces and contrasting colors such as black and white. Vision improves at 2 months of age (Ludington-Hoe, 1983).

Hearing. The infant should respond to sound at birth and will respond to a loud noise with a startle reflex. If hearing function is questionable an audiological referral should be made. Infants respond to voices, particularly familiar ones, and like classical music (Brahms, Bach, Beethoven), bells, and chimes.

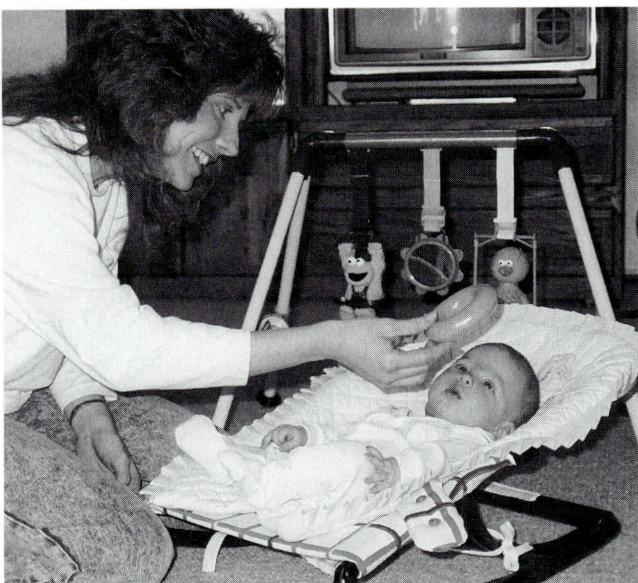

Fig. 16-18 Infant's ability to fixate and visually track brightly colored object.

Smell. The sense of smell is well developed. Newborns can smell breast milk and formula. Within a few days they show a preference for the smell of their own mother's breast milk over that of another nursing mother. They can also smell their parents' unique odor, perfumes, and colognes. Research suggests that they enjoy cooking odors and dislike strong odors such as cigars and cleaning fluids.

Taste. The taste buds are developed at birth. The newborn can taste sweet, bitter, sour, and salty and can discriminate between sweet and sour. Pacifiers and thumb sucking are means of self-consolation and stimulate saliva production, which helps digestion.

Touch. Cutaneous sensation is highly developed. The right side of the body is more sensitive to touch than the left side. Pressure, temperature, and pain are increasingly felt by the infant. The newborn reacts to cuddling, caresses, and skillful, gentle handling with greater relaxation and acceptance of care. Exposing the neonate to a variety of textures (silk, wool, etc.), and gentle massage are two other ways that parents can stimulate their infant's sense of touch.

GESTATIONAL AGE ASSESSMENT

The nurse must assess the gestational age of the newborn within the first few hours after birth in order that appropriate care be given to infants who are preterm, postterm, small for gestational age (SGA), or large for gestational age (LGA) (see Chapters 18 and 19 for discussion of the special needs of these infants). Traditionally the gestational age was

ESTIMATION OF GESTATIONAL AGE BY MATURITY RATING

Symbols: X - 1st Exam O - 2nd Exam

NEUROMUSCULAR MATURITY

	0	1	2	3	4	5
Posture						
Square Window (Wrist)	90°	60°	45°	30°	0°	
Arm Recoil	180°		100°-180°	90°-100°	$< 90^\circ$	
Popliteal Angle	180°	160°	130°	110°	90°	$< 90^\circ$
Scarf Sign						
Heel to Ear						

PHYSICAL MATURITY

	0	1	2	3	4	5
SKIN	gelatinous red, trans-parent	smooth pink, visible veins	superficial peeling &/or rash, few veins	cracking pale area, rare veins	parchment, deep cracking, no vessels	leathery, cracked, wrinkled
LANUGO	none	abundant	thinning	bald areas	mostly bald	
PLANTAR CREASES	no crease	faint red marks	anterior transverse crease only	creases ant. 2/3	creases cover entire sole	
BREAST	barely percept.	flat areola, no bud	stippled areola, 1–2 mm bud	raised areola, 3–4 mm bud	full areola, 5–10 mm bud	
EAR	pinna flat, stays folded	sl. curved pinna, soft with slow recoil	well-curv. pinna, soft but ready recoil	formed & firm with instant recoil	thick cartilage, ear stiff	
GENITALS Male	scrotum empty, no rugae		testes descend-ing, few rugae	testes down, good rugae	testes pendulous, deep rugae	
GENITALS Female	prominent clitoris & labia minora		majora & minora equally prominent	majora large, minora small	clitoris & minora completely covered	

Gestation by Dates ______________ wks

Birth Date __________ Hour __________ am pm

APGAR __________ 1 min __________ 5 min

MATURITY RATING

Score	Wks
5	26
10	28
15	30
20	32
25	34
30	36
35	38
40	40
45	42
50	44

SCORING SECTION

	1st Exam=X	2nd Exam=O
Estimating Gest Age by Maturity Rating	______ Weeks	______ Weeks
Time of Exam	Date ______ Hour ______ am pm	Date ______ Hour ______ am pm
Age at Exam	______ Hours	______ Hours
Signature of Examiner	______ M.D.	______ M.D.

Fig. 16-19 Newborn maturity rating and classification.

determined based on the mother's menstrual history. However, this method was frequently inaccurate. Gestational assessment tools currently in use involve the assessment of the newborn's physical and neuromuscular development. The Ballard tool (Fig. 16-19) is a simplified version of the Dubowitz tool and is frequently used by nurses in the hospital setting (Ballard et al., 1979). Each physical and neuromuscular finding is scored, and the total score is used to determine the gestational age. The physical items for the tool have been discussed in the physical assessment portion of this chapter. The neuromuscular maturity items are presented here.

Posture

The full term neonate's resting posture is fully flexed. Less mature newborns exhibit more extension of all extremities.

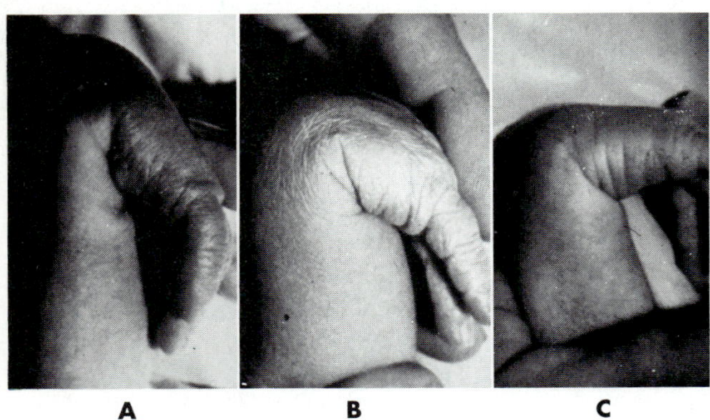

Fig. 16-20 Wrist flexion (square window). Flex the hand onto forearm and note the angle at which resistance is met. **A,** Postterm; **B,** term; **C,** preterm. (From Dickason EJ, Silverman BL, Schult MO: *Maternal-infant nursing care,* St. Louis, 1994, Mosby.)

Wrist flexion (square window)

The nurse flexes the infant's wrist toward the forearm and measures the angle between the fleshy portion of the palm and the forearm. The angle in the full term infant is approximately 0 degrees. A 90-degree angle is typical of infants under 32 weeks' gestation (Fig. 16-20).

Arm recoil

With the newborn in the supine position, the nurse fully flexes both elbows and holds that position for 5 seconds, then extends them and releases. A rapid return to the flexed position is typical of the full term infant. The more premature infant will demonstrate slower return.

Popliteal angle

With the newborn in the supine position, the nurse flexes the thigh on the abdomen. Then holding the knee with thumb and index finger, extends the leg with the index finger of the other hand placed behind the ankle. In the full term infant, there will be strong resistance to extension of the knee and the angle behind the knee will be less than 80 degrees. The angle is greater in premature infants and there is less resistance to extension.

Scarf sign

With the infant in the supine position, the nurse brings the arm across the chest as far as possible until resistance is felt (Fig. 16-21). The location of the elbow is noted in relation to the midline. In a premature newborn, the elbow can be drawn past the midline. The elbow cannot be drawn to the midline in the full term infant.

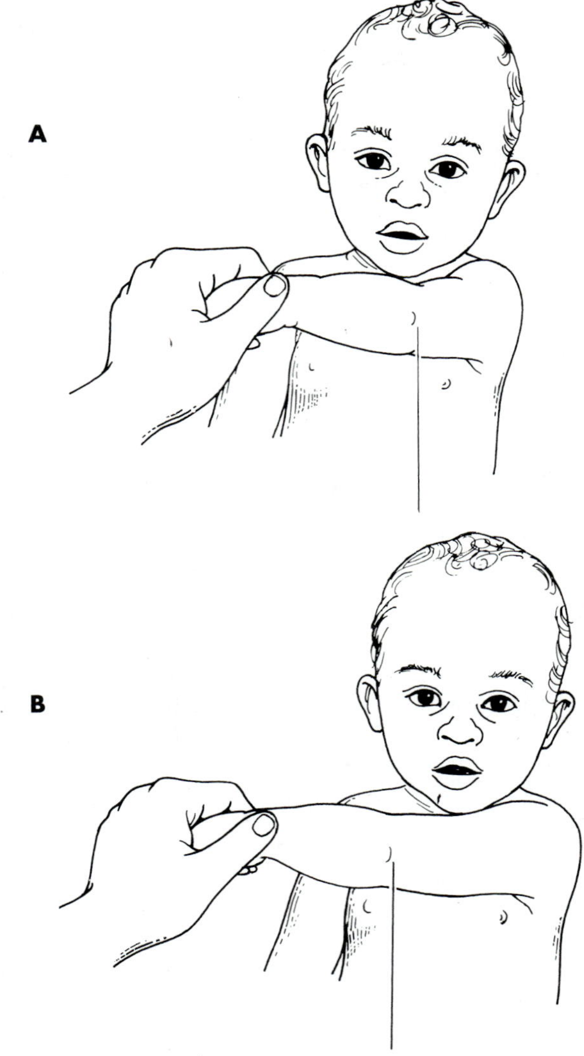

Fig. 16-21 Scarf sign. **A,** Term newborn; **B,** preterm newborn.

Heel-to-ear extension

With the neonate in the supine position and the hips flat on the mattress, the nurse brings the foot toward the ear on that side. The distance between the foot and the ear and the degree of extension at the knee are noted. The more premature the infant the less resistance will be noted, the closer the foot can be drawn to the ear, and the greater the knee extension.

BEHAVIORAL ASSESSMENT

Systematically assessing a neonate's behavioral patterns can help the nurse work with the parents to identify characteristic ways the infant responds to external and internal stimuli such as interesting objects, noise, and discomfort. The nurse should observe the newborn's sleep and awake patterns, the newborn's ability to self console, to be consoled by others, the newborn's ability to "tune out" or adapt to disturbing environmental stimuli, and the newborn's cuddliness and social behaviors such as smiling. Sharing this information with parents alerts them to when and how best to interact with and care for their baby.

A baby's level of consciousness ranges between deep sleep and crying (Table 16-1). Most infants move smoothly between these states. The so-called quiet-alert state affords an especially rewarding opportunity for parent-infant interaction. Although infants have a limited repertoire of behaviors, they do exhibit subtle cues indicating that they are ready for interaction or that they have had enough stimulation. The nurse should teach parents to be alert to these cues. Non-verbal cues such as eye widening and facial brightening indicate readiness for interaction. Subtle cues that signal the need for a "time-out" include such behaviors as turning away, falling asleep, hiccoughs, averting gaze, and yawning. Learning about their infant's unique behavioral patterns fosters the acquaintance and attachment process for parents. Parents who are sensitive to their infants' cues, who understand their infants' capabilities and foster those capabilities tend to have infants who are emotionally secure and socially competent.

◆ TABLE 16-1
Newborn Behavior States

State	Description	Characteristics
1	Deep sleep	Eyes closed, no eye movement under lids Respirations regular Occasional jerky movements at regular intervals
2	Light sleep	Eyes closed, rapid movement under lids Respirations irregular, occasional sucking movements Random but smoother movements
3	Drowsy	Eyes open or closed, eyelids fluttering Activity level variable, movements are smooth
4	Alert	Eyes open, bright look, attention focused on source of stimulation Minimal activity
5	Active	Eyes wide open, considerable activity Thrusting movements of arms and legs
6	Crying	Intense, difficult to break through High activity

Adapted from Brazelton TB: Neonatal behavioral assessment scale. In Clinics in developmental medicine, no. 50, London, 1973, MacKeith Press.

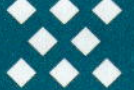

KEY CONCEPTS

1 The history, physical examination, gestational age assessment, and behavioral assessment are the components of a thorough newborn assessment.

2 The average male at birth weighs about 7½ pounds and is 20 inches in length. The average female newborn weighs about 7 pounds and is 19½ inches long.

3 Infants born vaginally in cephalic presentations usually undergo considerable head molding, which is caused by the compression of the head in the birth canal during labor. The phenomenon of overriding sutures occurs when the head, in response to the pressure of the cervix and bony pelvis, elongates and the skull bones overlap.

4 Two of the fontanels, where sutures cross or meet, can be felt and identified: the anterior diamond-shaped fontanel and the smaller triangle-shaped posterior fontanel just above the occiput. The larger fontanel closes at 9 to 18 months of age; the posterior fontanel closes by 6 weeks of age.

5 Common newborn skin conditions and manifestations include the following: vernix caseosa, an accumulation of old cutaneous cells mixed with an early secretion from the oil glands; lanugo, a relatively long soft growth of fine hair; erythema toxicum, red blotches that may become hive-like elevations; mongolian spots, blue-black colorations on the lower back, buttocks, and anterior trunk; petechiae, small blue-red dots on the body; and milia, small pinpoint white or yellow dots on the nose, forehead, cheeks, and chin.

6 Jaundice that is present before the newborn is 24 hours old is considered pathologic. Physiologic jaundice appears after 24 hours of age and is characterized by a rise in the serum bilirubin to a maximum level of 12 mg/100 ml.

7 The normal range of the newborn's vital signs are as follows: axillary temperature, 36.5° to 37.0° C (97.7° to 98.6° F); apical pulse, 120 to 160 beats per minute; respirations, 30 to 60 breaths per minute; and blood pressure 80-60/45-40 mm Hg.

8 Flaring of the nostrils, retractions—a sucking in of the chest wall in the rib or sternal area on

inspiration—and expiratory grunting are indications of respiratory distress.

9 The stools of formula-fed infants are characteristically pasty yellow-green, mustard-like in appearance, with a distinctive odor. The stools of breast-fed babies are yellow "cottage-cheese" curds, noisy when passed, with a sweet odor.

10 Maternal hormones crossing to the fetus may cause swelling of the infant's breasts, breast secretions, female pseudomenstruation, and swollen genitals.

11 Performing a gestational assessment assists the nurse in anticipating special problems associated with the transition to extrauterine life.

12 Inborn reflexes that newborn infants possess include the rooting, sucking, and swallowing reflexes employed in eating and the protective reflexes, such as coughing, sneezing, gagging, blinking, and possibly crying.

13 Parents who are aware of their infants' capabilities and methods for fostering them and are sensitive to infant cues are better able to facilitate healthy growth and development.

CRITICAL THOUGHT QUESTIONS 

1 Mr. and Mrs. Evers have just given birth to their first child. They are both African-American and are surprised at their newborn's light color. How would you explain this phenomenon? What other normal skin variation would you expect this baby to exhibit?

2 Compare and contrast physiological and pathological jaundice. Since many newborns are discharged before 24 hours, how would you teach parents to monitor their infants for evidence of physiological jaundice?

3 You have just done a behavioral assessment on the Garcia infant and noted that the baby is very fussy and difficult to console. How would you convey this information to the parents? Why is it of value?

4 New parents are discussing whether their infant can see, hear, and smell. What would you tell them? They express interest in ways they can enhance positive stimulation for the infant, such as mobiles or other crib toys. What suggestions would you make? Why?

5 The Green's are observing as you do a physical assessment of their newborn daughter. They seem anxious about what you are doing and have many questions. How would you handle this situation? Why?

REFERENCES

Ballard JL, Novak LK, Driver M: A simplified score for assessment of fetal maturation of newly born infants, *J Pediatr* 95(5):769-774, 1979.

Bobak IM, Jensen MD: *Maternity and gynecologic care,* ed 5, St Louis, 1993, Mosby.

Davis ME, Rubin R: *DeLee's obstetrics for nurses,* ed 7, Philadelphia, 1962, WB Saunders.

Dickason EJ, Silverman BL, Schult MO: *Maternal-infant nursing care,* St Louis, 1994, Mosby.

Korones SB: *High-risk newborn infants: the basis for intensive nursing care,* ed 4, St. Louis, 1986, Mosby.

Ludington-Hoe SM: What can newborns really see? *Am J Nurs* 83(9):1286-1289, 1983.

NAACOG, The Organization for Obstetric, Gynecologic, and Neonatal Nurses: *Neonatal thermoregulation: OGN nursing practice resource,* Washington, DC, February 1990, The Association.

NAACOG, The Organization for Obstetric, Gynecologic, and Neonatal Nurses: *Physical assessment of the neonate: OGN nursing practice resource,* Washington, DC, 1991, The Association.

Potter EL: *Pathology of the fetus and the newborn,* ed 3, Chicago, 1975, Mosby.

Seidel HM et al: *Mosby's guide to physical examination,* ed 2, St Louis, 1991, Mosby.

Smith DP et al: Comprehensive child and family nursing skills, St Louis, 1991, Mosby.

Whaley LF, Wong DL: *Nursing care of infants and children,* ed 4, St Louis, 1991, Mosby.

BIBLIOGRAPHY

Bowers AC, Thompson JM, Miller M: *Clinical manual of health assessment,* ed 4, St. Louis, 1992, Mosby.

Brazelton TB: Behavioral competence of the newborn infant, *Seminars in Perinatology* 3:35-44.

Broussard AB, Rich SK: Incorporating infant stimulation concepts into prenatal classes, *J Obstet Gynecol Neonatal Nurs* 19(5):381-387.

Dubowitz L, Dubowitz V, Goldberg C: Clinical assessment of gestational age in the newborn infant, *J Pediatr* 77(1):1-10.

Hopkins B, Westra T: Maternal expectations of their infant's development: some cultural differences, *Developmental Med Child Neurol* 31(3):384-390, 1989.

Johnstone HA, Marcinak JF: Candidiasis in the breastfeeding mother and infant, *J Obstet Gynecol Neonatal Nurs* 19(2):171-173, 1990.

Jones MB: A physiologic approach to identifying neonates at risk for kernicterus, *J Obstet Gynecol Neonatal Nurs* 19(4):313-318, 1990.

McClure VS: *Infant massage, a handbook for loving parents,* New York, 1989, Bantam.

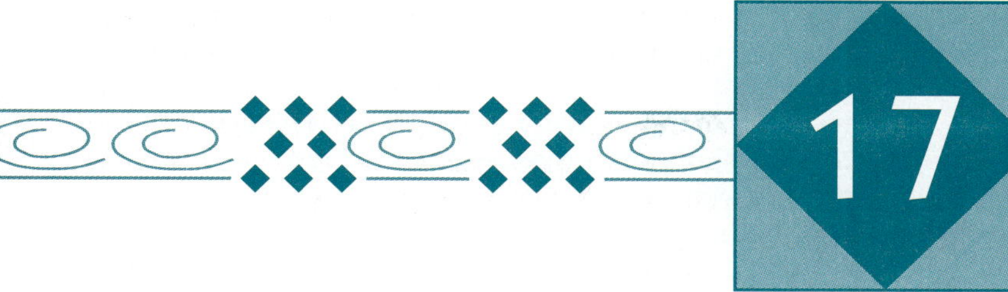
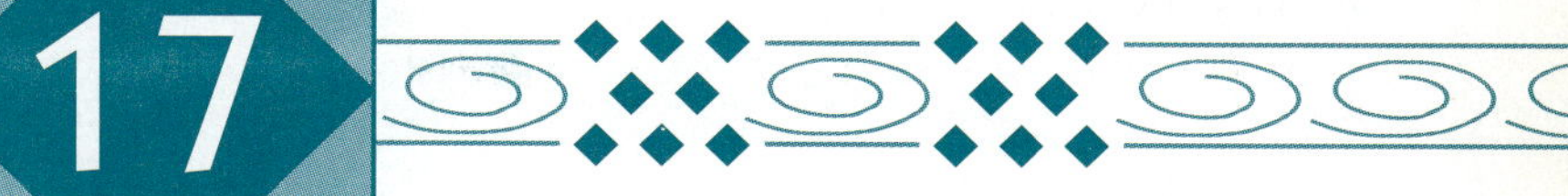

17

Care of the Normal Newborn

CHAPTER OBJECTIVES

After studying this chapter, the student should be able to:

1. List ten needs of the normal newborn.
2. Describe nursing measures to assist the newborn in maintaining effective respiration.
3. Explain why the newborn is more at risk for hypothermia than the adult.
4. Discuss the consequences of hypothermia.
5. Describe nursing measures to assist the newborn with thermoregulation.
6. Describe the signs of hypoglycemia.
7. Explain why the newborn is at risk for hemorrhage.
8. List at least six ways to protect the newborn from infection.
9. Demonstrate safe methods of lifting, carrying, and positioning an infant.
10. List the advantages of breast-feeding.
11. Explain dietary recommendations for the breast-feeding mother.
12. Develop a teaching plan incorporating basic techniques of breast-feeding.
13. Develop a teaching plan that incorporates the basic techniques of infant formula preparation and feeding.
14. Describe the methods of evaluating the nutritional status of an infant.
15. List five signs of dehydration in the infant that could indicate inadequate fluid intake.
16. Describe post-circumcision care according to circumcision technique.
17. Develop a discharge teaching plan that incorporates the six major areas for parent education.

PRIORITIES FOR CARE

The newborn assessment at delivery evaluates the neonate's initial adaptation to the extrauterine environment and determines whether the newborn is stable enough to remain with the parents or must be taken to the nursery for more careful observation. See Chapter 11 for immediate assessment and care of the newborn. Most normal newborns need not be separated from their parents unless they require special observation and/or treatment or if the mother is unable to care for her infant. In many hospitals a mother and her infant are seen as a unit and are cared for by one nurse. This is referred to as *mother-infant dyad* or *couplet care*. The neonate "rooms-in" with the mother and the father or a designated significant other has liberal visiting privileges and is encouraged to participate in infant care. Many centers permit healthy siblings and grandparents to see and hold the infant as well.

Whether or not the newborn remains with the parents or is transferred to a well-baby or admission nursery, all newborn infants have certain needs that must be met. Some of these needs take priority, some can be met simultaneously, and still others are important but can be met in a more leisurely fashion. The following are the primary needs of the newborn infant that dictate nursing care priorities:

1. Maintaining effective respiration
2. Thermoregulation
3. Assessment
4. Identification and security
5. Safe handling and positioning
6. Prevention of hemorrhage

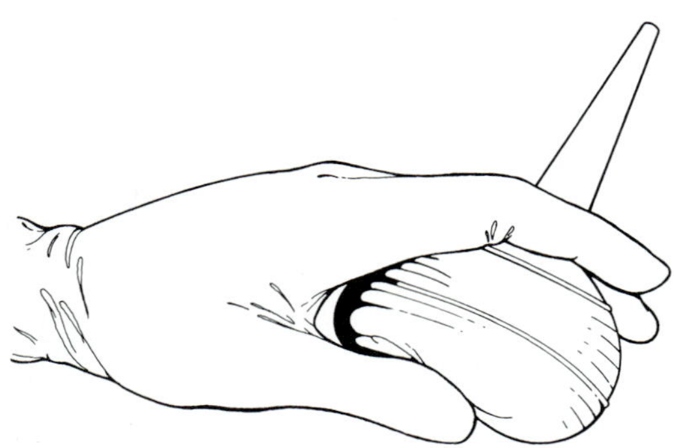

Fig. 17-1 Bulb syringe. Bulb must be compressed before insertion. (From Smith DP, et al: *Comprehensive child and family nursing,* St. Louis, 1991, Mosby.)

7 Protection from infection
8 Nourishment
9 Parent-infant interaction
10 Parent education

Maintaining Effective Respiration

Occasionally the neonate needs assistance to maintain a clear airway. Excess oral and nasal secretions can be gently suctioned with a bulb syringe (Fig. 17-1). The mouth should be suctioned *first.* Suctioning the mouth first prevents the newborn from aspirating oral secretions during the gasp response that occurs when the nares are suctioned. The bulb syringe is *first* compressed, then inserted in the mouth between the cheek and gums and compression gently released. Care should be exercised to avoid touching the back of the throat, which will stimulate the gag reflex. The bulb syringe should be kept with the crib and the parents taught how to use it. Wall suction (low-pressure setting) may be used for deeper mucus that cannot be removed with the bulb syringe or for suctioning stomach mucus and fluid.

The nurse should position the newborn on his or her side with a rolled blanket against the back for support. The newborn should never be left unattended in the supine position during the initial stabilization period because of the danger of aspiration from regurgitation of mucus or stomach fluid.

Neonates who have a low body temperature are likely to suffer respiratory complications because hypothermia causes increased oxygen consumption and tachypnea (rapid respiration). See discussion in the following section on thermoregulation.

Thermoregulation

Newborns may suffer from hypothermia not because they produce heat poorly but because they are vulnerable to heat loss. They lose heat easily because the body surface area is great in relation to weight, and they have relatively little subcutaneous fat to provide insulation; they have a poorly developed autonomic thermoregulatory response; are unable to produce heat by shivering; and experience greater evaporative heat loss because they have more body water per body weight than adults (NAACOG, 1990).

Maintaining body warmth in the postnatal period is critical to the well-being of an infant. The newborn does not raise or maintain body temperature by shivering but is aided in efforts to increase body temperature by a special tissue found only in neonates called *brown fat.* It is located principally between the scapulae, in the neck muscles and axilla, and around the kidneys and the adrenals. This tissue helps increase body heat by producing a chemical, noradrenaline, that increases the body's metabolic rate and stimulates brown fat to release glycerol and fatty acids to serve as fuel. Once used, supplies of brown fat are not replenished. Cold stress can result in hypoglycemia, hypoxia, and metabolic acidosis because of the metabolism of brown fat; pulmonary vasoconstriction because of the metabolic acidosis; and increased respiratory distress, because of hypoxia and acidosis (NAACOG, 1990).

Heat loss occurs when the infant's body heat is transferred to the surrounding environment. This may occur by: *evaporation* anytime the infant's skin is wet; by *convection* when the room is too cool or drafty, or when cold oxygen is blown on the infant's face; by *conduction* when the infant's skin is in direct contact with cold hands or objects; and by *radiation* when the infant's body heat is transferred to solid objects such as windows or walls that are near but not in direct contact with the infant's body.

For the first hour or so after birth if the newborn's temperature is stable, the infant is usually wrapped with warm blankets and given to the parents to hold (see Chapter 11). If the temperature is low or the mother very fatigued, the infant may be placed under a radiant warmer with a temperature sensor attached to the abdomen. The admission bath and shampoo should be delayed until after the temperature has stabilized (1 to 2 hours). To prevent heat loss, the bath can be done quickly under the warmer and the infant thoroughly dried. If not done under a warmer, the infant must be covered except for the body part being washed and dried. After the bath the axillary temperature is checked again. If it is within the normal range, the infant may be dressed, wrapped in a blanket, and placed in an open crib. After initial stabilization, the infant's axillary temperature is monitored according to the unit's protocol—usually every 4 to 8 hours. Axillary temperatures for the normal newborn should range between 36.5° to 37.0° C (97.7° to 98.6° F). See

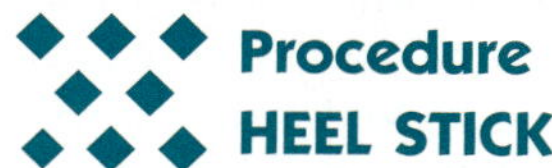

Procedure HEEL STICK

EQUIPMENT/SUPPLIES

- Chemical heat pad or cloth diaper or washcloth
- Gloves
- Alcohol swab
- Sterile gauze pads (2 to 3)
- Lancet (pediatric size)
- Glucose sensitive strip
- Portable glucose analyzer (optional)
- Adhesive bandage

STEPS

1. Warm neonate's heel for 5 to 10 minutes by wrapping the heel in a warm, moist cloth or using a specially designed chemical heat pad. Do not microwave moist cloth—severe burns can result.
2. Stabilize the neonate's foot with one hand.
3. With the other hand cleanse the heel with alcohol and blot dry with sterile gauze pad.
4. Using the lancet, puncture the selected site. Best site is the lateral aspect of the heel. Medial aspect of the heel is acceptable. (Fig. 17-2)
5. Wipe off the first drop of blood with sterile gauze.
6. Allow a large drop to form and fall onto the glucose-sensitive strip (avoid squeezing the heel).
7. Follow manufacturer's instructions for timing of test and interpreting results.
8. Apply pressure to the puncture site with a dry gauze pad to prevent additional bleeding.
9. Cover the puncture site with small adhesive bandage.

Nursing Alert

The nurse should be aware that because of the proximity to the axillary brown fat stores, axillary temperatures may remain high in the presence of cold stress.

nursing alert on p. 311. Other signs of hypothermia include acrocyanosis (after the first 12 hours), cool extremities, lethargy, apnea, and poor feeding. If hypothermia develops, the infant is returned to a preheated radiant warmer, undressed, and gradually rewarmed over a period of 2 or more hours. Rapid warming can result in apnea and acidosis (NAACOG, 1990).

The infant must be protected from drafts and from cold surfaces. Nursery or mother's room air temperature should be maintained at 24 to 26° C (75 to 79° F) with a relative humidity in the range of 35% to 50% for personnel comfort. Some infants are perfectly warm in only a cotton shirt and diaper, covered by a light cotton blanket. However, infants prone to low temperatures should be double wrapped and wear hats.

Newborn infants are also at risk for hyperthermia because they are not yet able to perspire effectively. Infants are sometimes overheated by overzealous nurses or parents who put too much clothing or bedding on or around them. Signs of hyperthermia include skin that is hot to touch and/or red in color, sweating (term infants), poor feeding, decreased tone and activity, weak cry, and apnea (NAACOG, 1990).

Assessment

The admission physical and gestational assessment is described in Chapter 16. The admission bath affords the nurse another opportunity to assess physical and behavioral adaptation to the extrauterine environment. The admission assessment and additional periodic assessments should be done in a draft-free area, and unless the infant is under a warmer, the nurse should expose only the body area being assessed and recover it before moving to the next area.

Although respiratory and thermoregulation problems are the most likely complications experienced by the normal newborn, it is also important for the nurse to monitor the newborn for signs of *hypoglycemia*. The brain depends on glucose for adequate functioning, and hypoglycemia can result in neurological impairment. Signs of hypoglycemia include jitteriness, lethargy, or temperature instability. If an infant exhibits these signs the nurse should perform a heel stick to obtain a drop of capillary blood, which is then placed on a glucose-sensitive strip. The strip is either visually read or a portable glucose analyzer is used to determine the glucose level. If the level is less than 40 to 45 mg/dL, a venous sample may be drawn to confirm the level. For stable infants treatment is feeding with 5% or 10% glucose water or formula. See Chapter 18 for discussion of infants most at risk for hypoglycemia. See accompanying box for heel stick procedure.

Many nurseries also obtain a heel stick blood sample to determine hematocrit. The normal hematocrit range is 45% to 65%. Higher levels should be vali-

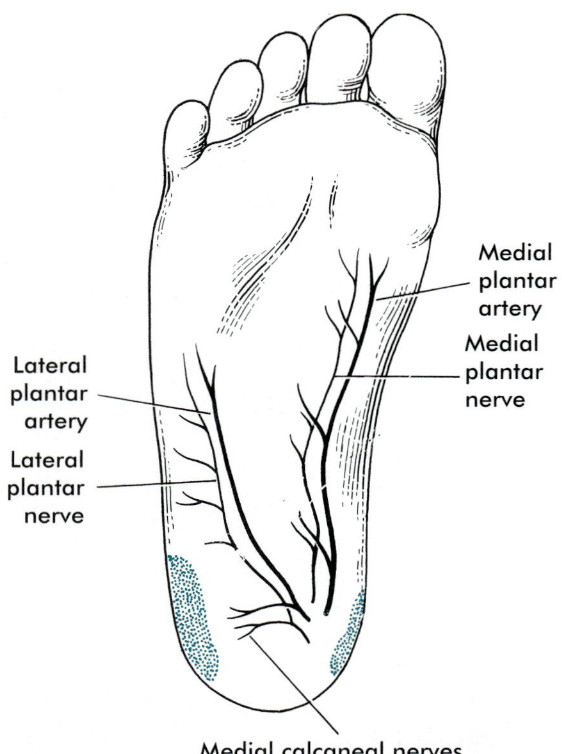

Fig. 17-2 Puncture sites (x) for heel stick samples of capillary blood.

dated by a venous sample because they may indicate *polycythemia* (increased number of erythrocytes), which can be caused by a large amount of placental blood being transferred to the neonate at birth or by hypovolemia.

The increased incidence of substance abuse also dictates the need for the nurse to be alert for signs of *neonatal abstinence syndrome* (withdrawal) after birth. The initial signs of abstinence syndrome include increased irritability, increased startle response, difficult to console, tremors, jitteriness, increased respiratory rate, and tachycardia. Most facilities have established guidelines for toxicology screening to detect drugs (including alcohol) in the newborn. The most common criteria for screening are a maternal history of substance abuse during the previous year, no prenatal care, and mothers and newborns exhibiting signs or symptoms of substance abuse or withdrawal.

If the infant is to be screened for drugs the nurse will need to collect a urine specimen. The sample should be fresh and examined within 1 hour of collection. Single-use urine bags are used to collect the sample (Fig. 17-3). The genitalia, perineum, and surrounding skin should be washed and dried before applying the bag so that the adhesive will stick. For girls, skin folds should be flattened and the bag applied starting just above the rectum and working upward to cover the vagina and urinary meatus. For boys, the penis and scrotum are covered and the adhesive flaps firmly attached to the surrounding skin.

Identification and Security

Matching identification bands are applied to the newborn's ankle and wrist at delivery, *before* the neonate is separated from parents and transferred to the nursery if that becomes necessary. Should bands become loose or one fall off, new bands can be applied *in the presence* of the parents. The newborn's bands match the ones applied to the mother and sometimes to the father (three or four matching bands). The nurse must always check the parent's matching band before leaving the baby with the parent (Fig. 17-4). Parents should be educated about the nurse's need to check identification bands and should also be cautioned not to give the infant to anyone who is not wearing appropriate picture identification. Infants should not be left unattended in the mother's room.

Safe Handling and Positioning

Handling and transporting young infants can sometimes be awkward for inexperienced student nurses and parents. Both need to be reassured of their ability to learn to care for their charges and to learn comfortable and safe methods of handling a newborn. Understanding certain principles will assist the caregiver in safe handling and carrying. The neonate has one continuous anteroposterior spinal curve and usually tries to maintain a flexed posture. The newborn has no real control of head movements, although in the prone position the infant may raise its head slightly and briefly.

Safe handling

Whenever the infant is lifted or transported, the head, which is large and heavy in relation to the rest of the body, must be supported for comfort and to prevent muscle strain. For safety all lifts must have at least two contact points so that if one fails, another is still available. Infants, even small ones, can be wriggly and sometimes slippery. Figure 17-5 illustrates one of the most common methods of lifting an infant. It is a good lift for placing the newborn on a scale or putting him into a tub. A neonate should not be lifted by the arms. When head stability is attained at about 3 months of age, the infant may be lifted by grasping the trunk with both hands under the arms.

Infants can be held and carried in many ways; some methods are more comfortable for the one who carries

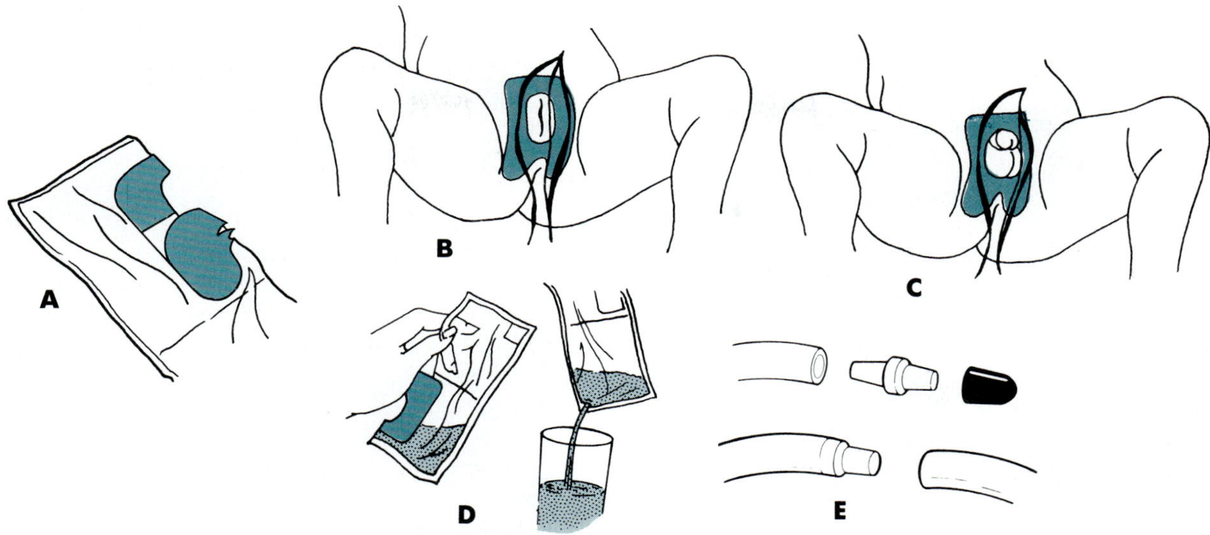

Fig. 17-3 Urine specimen collection. **A,** Protective paper is being removed from the adhesive surface; **B,** applied to girls; **C,** applied to boys; **D,** cut to drain urine; **E,** collection tube. (Courtesy Hollister, Chicago, IL.)

and others give the infant a greater sense of safety and support. The following three holds are the most commonly used in the United States: the traditional cradle hold (Fig. 17-6), the football hold (Fig. 17-7), and the shoulder hold (Fig. 17-8). The football hold should not be used to carry the neonate because the head is somewhat unprotected.

Safe positioning

A newborn infant should not be left alone flat on his back for the first few hours after birth because of the likelihood of regurgitation of mucus and stomach contents. The neonate may be propped with a rolled blanket along his back to maintain a side position. The American Academy of Pediatrics (AAP) recommends that parents do not place healthy infants in the prone position for sleep. The reason for this recommendation stems from study results that link the prone position with Sudden Infant Death Syndrome (SIDS). The AAP recommends that infants be placed on their sides or backs to sleep. Nurses must educate parents about the change in recommendations and the rationale for the change (Lerner, 1993).

Until the infant can change positions on her own, caregivers should vary positions. Always placing the neonate in the same position can distort the shape of the head or chest or cause localized baldness.

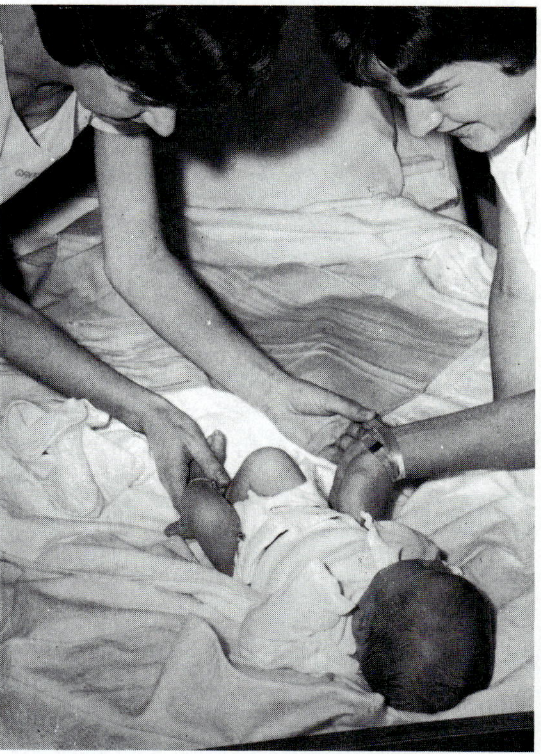

Fig. 17-4 Identification of neonate using double-banding technique. (Courtesy Grossmont Hospital, La Mesa, CA.)

Prevention of Hemorrhage

Intrauterine stores of vitamin K are depleted and the newborn's ability to produce vitamin K is still low, placing the neonate at increased risk for hemorrhage for 2 to 5 days after birth. To prevent bleeding 0.5 mg to 1 mg vitamin K (phytonadione) is given intramuscularly in the vastus lateralis or rectus femoris muscle

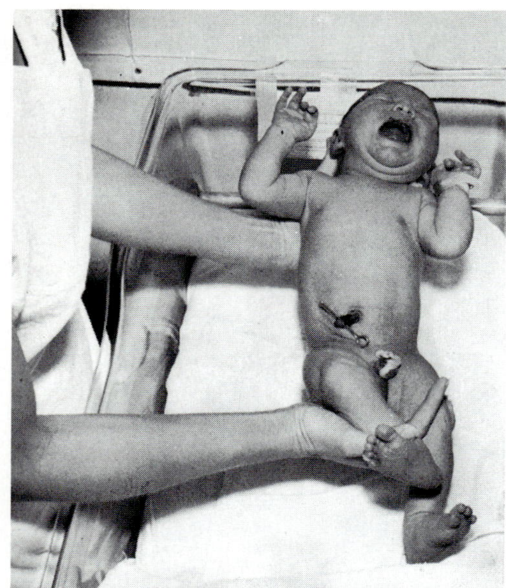

Fig. 17-5 One method of lifting newborn. Head and upper back are supported by one hand, legs by the other. Shown undressed to illustrate hand positions. (Courtesy Grossmont Hospital, La Mesa, CA.)

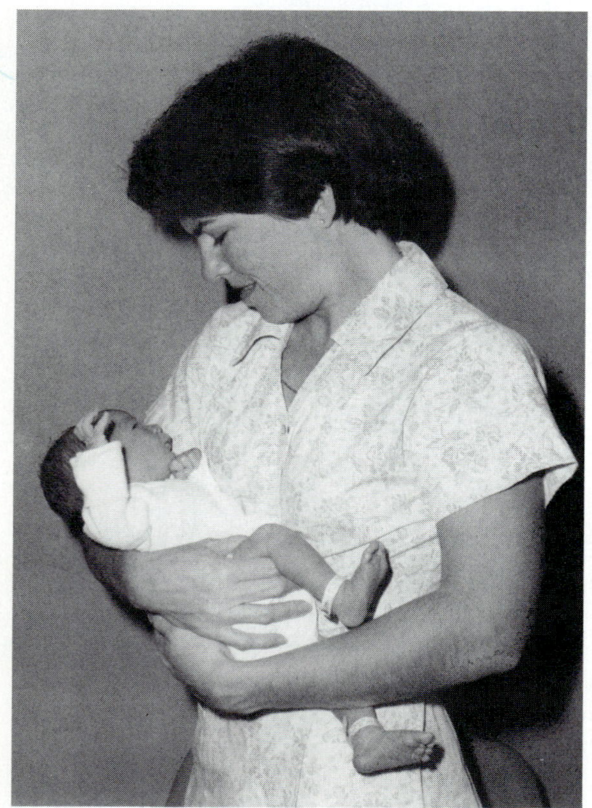

Fig. 17-6 Traditional cradle hold. Newborn unwrapped to illustrate hold. (Courtesy Grossmont Hospital, La Mesa, CA.)

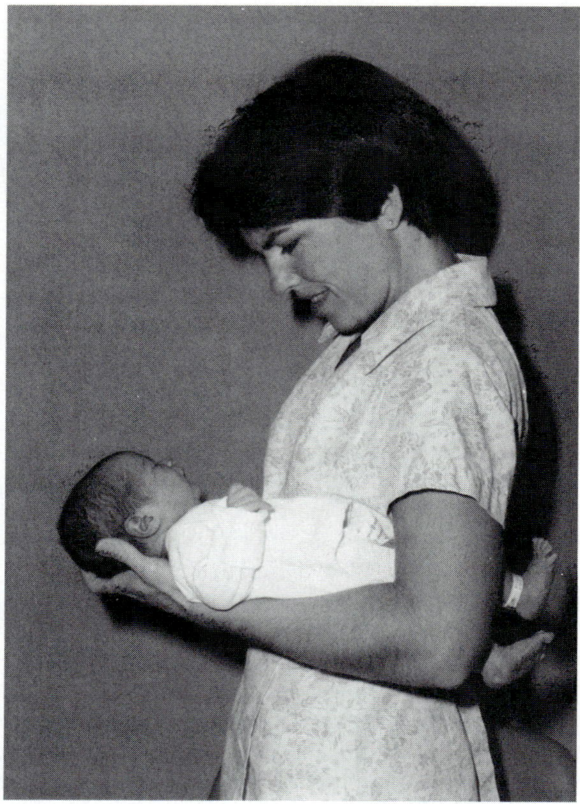

Fig. 17-7 Football hold. (Courtesy Grossmont Hospital, La Mesa, CA.)

of the anterior thigh (Fig. 17-9). It is usually given during the admission process. Vitamin K is especially important for those suffering from hemorrhagic disease of the newborn, infants born of complicated deliveries, or premature infants.

Although bleeding from a clamped cord is rare, the nurse should monitor the cord for bleeding. The nurse should also observe for bleeding (spots larger than a quarter on the diaper) after circumcision of the male infant. To decrease the possibility of increased cerebral pressure and subsequent intracranial bleeding, newborns are not placed in a head-down position for prolonged periods.

Protection from Infection

Because all newborns are at risk for nosocomial (hospital acquired) infections, protecting neonates from infection is a major responsibility of the nurses who care for them. Personnel should wash their hands, wrists and forearms with an antiseptic product such as povidone-iodine (Betadine) for 2 minutes, clean fingernails and wash hands again, before starting patient care. Hands should be vigorously washed with soap for 15 seconds before and after handling infants or

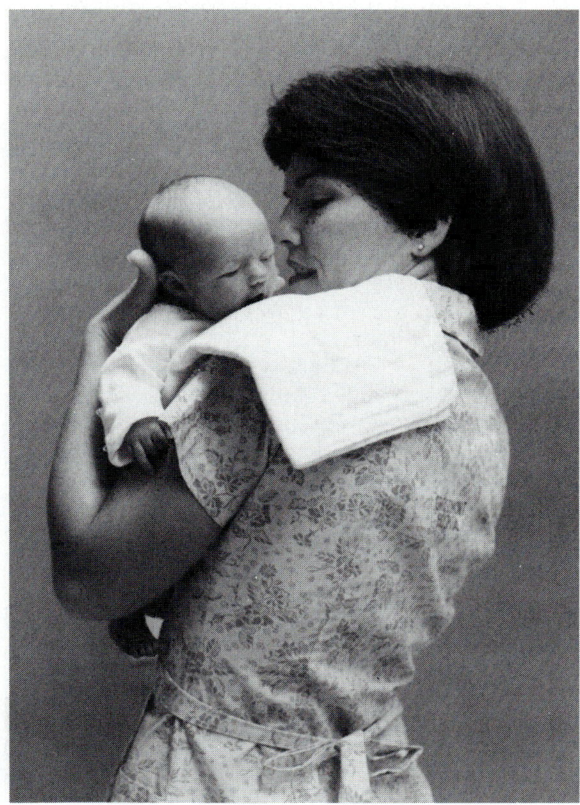

Fig. 17-8 Shoulder hold. (Courtesy Grossmont Hospital, La Mesa, CA.)

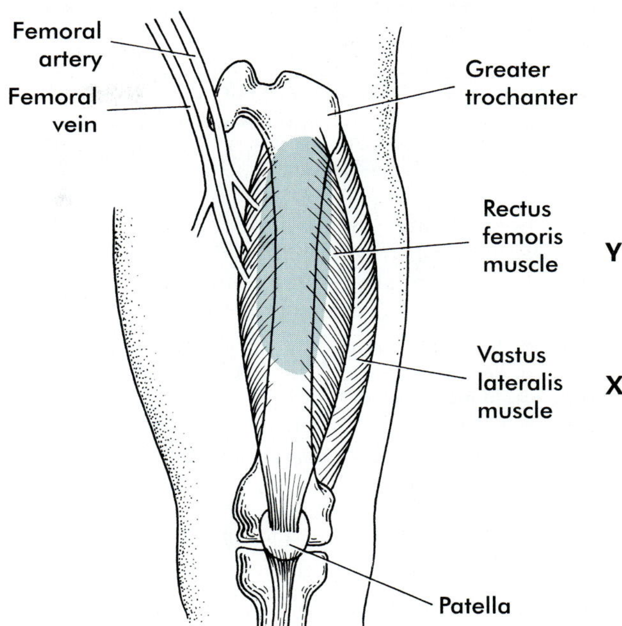

Fig. 17-9 Intramuscular injection sites, *X,* preferred site in vastus lateralis muscle; *Y,* alternate site in rectus femoris muscle.

contaminated objects (NAACOG, 1992). *Handwashing* after handling each infant is the single most effective means of preventing neonatal infection (Rush et al, 1990). Parents, visitors, and ancillary staff (e.g., x-ray personnel) should be taught the importance and technique of good handwashing before handling the infant in the mother's hospital room, in the nursery, or in the home. Research indicates that the use of cover gowns for parents and nurses caring for healthy newborns is not necessary (Rush et al, 1990). Personnel must also observe *universal precautions* when handling the newborn (see accompanying box). Hands should be washed after removing gloves.

Staff members should wear simple, hospital-supplied and laundered clothing, keep their fingernails short, restrict jewelry, and have yearly health maintenance examinations. They should also be vaccinated for hepatitis, rubella, and other communicable diseases. No personnel should assume responsibility of caring for newborns while suffering from an infectious disease.

The newborn's *skin* is a major barrier against entry of microorganisms. During admission and periodic assessments the nurse should observe for breaks in the skin that could predispose the infant to infection. The cord and circumcision site must also be watched for signs of infection. After the admission bath that removes amniotic fluid, maternal blood, and mucus, washing soiled areas with water and thoroughly drying should be sufficient to prevent infection during brief hospital stays. (See box on p. 316 for admission bath procedure.)

UNIVERSAL PRECAUTIONS

1. Wear gloves and gowns when handling the infant until after blood and amniotic fluid have been removed from the infant's skin (admission bath).
2. Wear gloves during the following procedures: venipunctures, heel sticks, starting IVs and discontinuing IVs, applying pressure after venipuncture or heel sticks, cord care, administering prophylactic eye medication, and suctioning the newborn.
3. Wear gloves when changing diapers and when collecting and testing urine or stool samples.
4. Take precautions to prevent injuries:
   - Needles should not be recapped, but placed directly into a puncture-resistant container.
   - Used heel stick lancets should be placed directly into a puncture-resistant container.

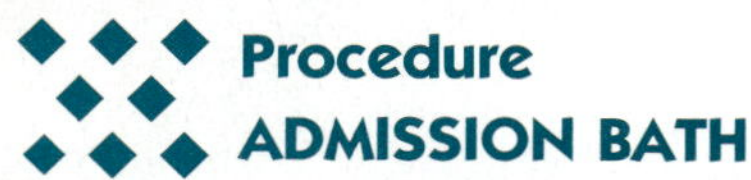

Procedure
ADMISSION BATH

EQUIPMENT/SUPPLIES

- Gloves
- Thermometer
- Basin of warm water (98° to 99° F)
- Mild soap or antibacterial product
- Paper mesh squares or soft washcloths
- Sterile cotton balls for eyes and cord
- Triple Dye, or 70% alcohol for cord care
- Applicators for cord care
- Two towels or soft blankets for covering and drying
- Small plastic comb
- Laundry hamper
- Diaper, shirt, blanket, and hat

STEPS

1 Take axillary temperature.
   a. Place a thermometer deep in the axilla while holding the arm gently but firmly against the chest. If using a glass thermometer, the time is 3 to 5 minutes.
   b. If the infant is cold, delay the bath until the temperature reaches the normal range.

2 Unless the newborn is under a radiant warmer, wrap the infant with a towel or blanket to prevent chilling. The area should be warm, without drafts.

3 Test water with inner wrist. It should feel pleasantly warm.

4 Wipe the eyes with cotton balls moistened with water, starting at the inner canthus and proceeding to the outer canthus.* This direction prevents drainage from the inner canthus of the eye from entering the lacrimal duct leading to the nose. (A clean cotton ball is used for each wipe.)

5 Clean the face with a paper mesh square or soft washcloth dipped in clear water. Avoid using soap because it is drying to the skin.
   a. If necessary, clear the opening of the nose with water-moistened, firmly twisted cotton balls.
   b. Gently wipe the external ears with water-moistened cotton balls but never probe the short ear canal with applicators.

6 Gently but firmly suds and rinse the head over the washbasin. (If the bath is not done under a radiant warmer, the head may be washed last to minimize heat loss. If so, use clean water.)
   a. Use the football hold to secure the infant, leaving one hand free to wash the head.
   b. Comb the hair and scalp to lift out particles of vernix and dried blood that are difficult to dislodge.

7 Continue the bath by washing, rinsing, and drying the neck, chest, arms, hands, abdomen, and back. If the bath is not done under the radiant warmer, take care to uncover only the body part being washed and dried and recover before moving to the next part.
   a. Support the shoulders with the hand to extend the neck and adequately clean neck creases.
   b. Vernix caseosa may be thick and difficult to remove, particularly from the creases. To avoid skin irritation remove only what wipes off easily.
   c. Place a dry folded towel under the washed portion of the infant and completely unfold it when the lower half of the body is clean.

8 Continue the bath, washing the legs, feet, and then the buttocks and perianal region. Special care should be taken in cleaning the genitalia.
   a. For females, separate the labia and gently wash downward from the pubic area to the anus. Use a clean cotton ball or portion of the washcloth for each stroke.
   b. For an uncircumcised male, pediatric urologists do not recommend attempting to retract the foreskin of the infant until about 5 months of age, since most are adherent. Gently wash the glans that is visible with a moistened cotton ball or washcloth.

9 Discard gloves; wash your hands and put on new gloves. Then with applicators and cotton balls, apply triple dye, alcohol, or other ordered antiseptic to the cord stump and the inner rim of the skin cuff surrounding the base of the cord.

10 Give the vitamin K injection. The hepatitis immunization may also be given at this time.

11 Repeat the axillary temperature. If in the normal range dress the infant in diaper and shirt and wrap in a blanket. For small infants or those otherwise at risk for low temperatures, add a hat.

12 Place the infant in its crib, propped on its side. Check the crib identification card against the infant's personal identification.

13 If the infant's temperature is low, he or she should be diapered and remain under or be returned to the preheated radiant warmer. The axillary temperature should be rechecked in 1 hour. If the temperature is in the normal range, the infant may be dressed and placed in its crib.

*The infant's bath should proceed from the cleanest to the dirtiest areas (head to perineum).

With discharge in less than 24 hours nurses see diaper rash less commonly than if stays are longer. Skin irritation from voiding and stool typically appears within 2 to 3 days of birth. Parents should be taught to change diapers frequently and thoroughly cleanse and dry the skin. An ointment such as A and D ointment may also help prevent diaper rash.

In the United States, protection from *eye* infections because of maternal gonorrhea or chlamydia is mandatory and involves the use of prophylactic eye medication. The prophylactic agent may be drops of silver nitrate, 1%, or an ophthalmic ointment containing tetracycline 1% or erythromycin 0.5%. Tetracycline and erythromycin are less irritating to the eyes than silver nitrate, which can cause a chemical conjunctivitis (American Academy of Pediatrics, 1991). Although the agent should be instilled shortly after birth, the Centers for Disease Control specify that a delay of up to 2 hours is acceptable. This delay may facilitate the initial parent-infant attachment by allowing the newborn unimpaired eye contact with the parents. The nurse should first cleanse the infant's face with water and dry it, then instill the eye medication. Wearing gloves, the nurse spreads the eyelids, exposing the conjunctival sac, and instills the medication. Care must be taken in administering the drops or ointment to avoid putting pressure on the eyeball itself. Occasionally shading the infant's eyes from the light will cause them to open spontaneously, making instillation comparatively easy. Parents should be told that the medication may cause some swelling and drainage within the next 24 hours.

The *umbilical cord* should be assessed for edema, erythema, and purulent discharge with each diaper change. The nurse should wipe the cord stump and the base of the cord with 70% isopropyl alcohol or Triple Dye, according to hospital protocol during each periodic assessment and with diaper changes to keep the area clean and promote drying. Folding the diaper down below the cord and positioning the infant on his side promotes drying. By 24 hours after birth the cord is usually dry and shriveled and the clamp can be removed. Student nurses should confer with the primary nurse before removing the clamp. The cord stump usually falls off within 1 to 2 weeks. Parents should be taught to clean the cord with alcohol soaked Q-tips and cotton balls at least 4 times a day until the stump falls off and the base is healed (up to 2 weeks). They should also be taught to examine the cord for redness, swelling, foul odor, or drainage and immediately report these signs to the physician or nurse practitioner.

After birth the infant should have her own individual crib, bath equipment, and supply of linen (Fig. 17-10). Infants should be bathed in their own beds and not on a common bathing table. The scale used for determining weight should be protected, balanced, and handled in such a way that no cross-infection can take place. Any instruments or appliances that must be used for more than one infant must be carefully disinfected or sterilized after use. This applies to stethoscopes, circumcision boards and instruments, and other equipment.

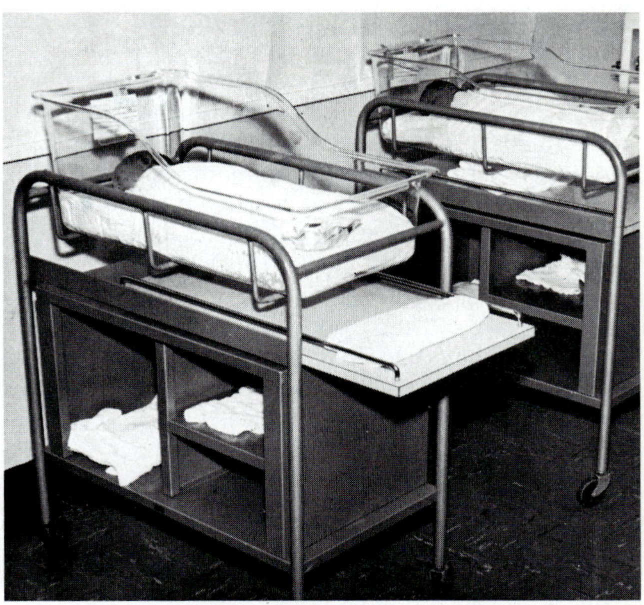

Fig. 17-10 Individual nursery units reduce possibility of cross-infection. (Courtesy Grossmont Hospital, La Mesa, CA.)

Professional organizations such as the AAP, hospital accreditation boards, and local public health and safety officials take an active part in making recommendations and requirements governing the construction, maintenance, and operation of the nursery, as well as other parts of the hospital. They are concerned about available floor space, distance between cribs, type of ventilation, control of temperature and humidity, provision for adequate lighting, safety of electrical appliances, elimination of possible fire hazards, appropriate dressing and handwashing facilities, and safe formula preparation.

NOURISHMENT

There are two ways of meeting the nourishment needs of infants—breast-feeding and formula-feeding.

Breast-feeding

Breast-feeding is the most universally recommended way of providing an infant with nourishment. For a healthy, full-term infant, breast milk is the only food needed for the first 4 to 6 months of life. A mother should carefully consider the advantages of breast-feeding when deciding how she will feed her infant. The father or other primary support persons will influence the mother's success. Therefore they should also be given information regarding the advantages of breast-feeding. Ideally, this decision is made prenatally. Once the decision to breast-feed is made, nurses have an important role to play in helping mothers identify and deal with barriers to successful breast-feeding. These barriers include: lack of consistent and accurate information about breast-feeding among health care professionals and the population in general; hospital practices oriented toward bottle-feeding, as well as conspicuous display of infant formula and formula advertising in hospitals and outpatient facilities; sexual connotations associated with the breast; misconceptions about dietary and other restrictions during breast-feeding; desire for rapid postpartum weight loss; lack of self-confidence; lack of flexibility in the workplace; and lack of role models and family support (American Dietetic Association, 1993).

Advantages

Putting the infant to breast contributes to the mother's well-being in that the stimulation of the infant's suckling causes the recently emptied uterus to contract and helps in the process of involution. A further benefit is the relaxing effect that prolactin, the milk-producing hormone, has on the mother. Breast-feeding also promotes the mother's feelings of closeness or attachment to the infant. The return of ovulation, and thus menstruation, may be delayed by breast-feeding. However, women should be counseled that breast-feeding is no guarantee that pregnancy will not occur. There is also some evidence that the risk of osteoporosis and breast cancer is lower in women who have breast-fed.

The infant also benefits from breast-feeding. The curd of human milk is softer than that of cow's milk and is easier for an infant to digest. It is also less likely to cause allergic reactions than commercially prepared formula. Although the iron content of breast milk is low, it is much better absorbed than the iron in formula. Human milk has more cholesterol than formula. This cholesterol is necessary for infants, aiding in the development of the nervous system and synthesis of hormones and bile acids. The infant receives immune factors through the breast milk, which help to protect against viral and bacterial diseases to which the mother has been exposed. Breast-fed babies have fewer respiratory tract infections, fewer alimentary tract disturbances, and fewer allergy problems. Obesity is also seen less often in children who have been breast-fed.

Breast milk is bacteriologically safe and always fresh. Therefore, when environmental hygiene is poor, breast-feeding is preferred over the likelihood of contaminated formula feedings.

Contraindications

Even though some mothers may want to breast-feed, occasionally the condition of the mother or infant makes it inadvisable. Maternal illness that is particularly protracted, severe, or contagious in nature may preclude breast-feeding. A mother who is HIV positive is at high risk for acquired immune deficiency syndrome (AIDS). The Centers for Disease Control recommends that HIV-positive women in the United States be advised not to breast-feed to avoid possible postnatal transmission to a newborn who may not be infected. An intravenous drug user should receive an HIV blood test before breast-feeding. Mothers who have newly diagnosed active tuberculosis should be separated from their newborn infants until they have received appropriate medications and are not contagious. The mother then will be individually evaluated regarding her health and the condition of her infant. To protect their milk supply these mothers need to be taught to pump and discard their milk until they are advised it is safe to begin breast-feeding. A woman with chronic cardiac or renal disease may be discouraged from nursing because of the physiological demands on her body. Maternal mental illness may also be a contraindication.

Other considerations

Most, if not all, drugs taken by the mother pass through the milk to the baby (Institute of Medicine, 1991). For example, the drug thiouracil used in treating hyperthyroidism actually becomes more concentrated in the maternal milk and may affect the infant. Some laxatives are as effective on the baby as on the mother and should be avoided or used only judiciously. Common laxatives to be avoided include cascara, emodium, anthraquinone, and aloes. Safe laxatives include magnesia, castor oil, mineral oil, bisacodyl (Dulcolax), senna phenolphthalein, non-prescription Ex-Lax, and stool softeners (Worthington-Roberts and Williams, 1993). Sedatives may produce drowsiness, anticoagulants may cause bleeding problems, and some antibiotics may cause allergic reactions in the infant. Nurses should counsel mothers to remind their health care provider that they are breast-feeding so that the safest option can be selected. Illegal drugs such as cocaine, amphetamines, heroin, and phencyclidine (PCP) all have negative effects on the breast-fed infant.

Concern has been expressed regarding the amount of DDT, PCBs, and other environmental contaminants found in some human milk samples. However, authorities do not recommend discontinuation of breast-feeding unless the levels are particularly high (Institute of Medicine, 1991).

A mother with severely cracked nipples, mastitis, or breast abscess is no longer required to terminate nursing. Many authorities recommend continuation of breast-feeding while antibiotics and other remedies are used. With proper initial management and frequent nursing such conditions are preventable.

Maternal diet

The breast-feeding mother must have a good diet to maintain her resources and provide sufficient nourishment for her infant. She produces about 25 ounces of milk daily when lactation is fully established. In the second half of the first year, production typically drops about 20%. The breast-feeding woman needs more *calories* than when she is not pregnant or breast-feeding. Some of these calories can come from the stores of maternal fat created during pregnancy. Therefore an additional 500 calories per day is adequate unless the mother is underweight or breast-feeding more than one infant. Breast-feeding mothers can expect a gradual loss of the weight gained during pregnancy. Severe calorie restriction, to lose weight rapidly, is likely to interfere with milk production and should be discouraged.

It is important that a lactating woman's diet incorporate adequate *calcium*. The Recommended Dietary Allowance (RDA) for lactating women is 1200 mg of calcium. Adequate calcium intake will protect her personal calcium supply and help to prevent *osteoporosis,* or weakening of the bony skeleton later in life. Calcium in the form of medication can be supplied if necessary, but a balanced diet containing calcium-rich foods will give her other healthful nutrients, benefit the entire family, and eliminate the need for medication.

The RDA indicates two different levels of nutritional requirements. These levels reflect the higher needs of the first 6 months of lactation compared with the reduced needs associated with the normal moderate decrease in milk production typical of the second 6 months. Only the recommendations for folate, iron, and vitamin B_6 are lower during lactation than during pregnancy (see Table 17-1). If lactating women ingest the minimum recommended servings from each food group in the Daily Food Guide (see Chapter 9) they will obtain the amounts of protein, vitamins, and minerals required for lactation.

In the past, women have been given lists of foods to avoid while breast-feeding. There is no scientific basis, however, for limiting foods to prevent gas in a breast-fed baby. Many babies are not affected by deviations in the maternal diet. However, although some infants do not seem to tolerate certain foods, no one food affects every infant. Examples of foods that have been reported to cause problems are vegetables, such as cabbage, brussel sprouts, asparagus, and onions, and fruits, such as prunes. By omitting the suspected food from her diet for a day or two and observing the infant's response, a mother can usually determine whether the infant is reacting to that food. Fussiness and jitteriness have been reported in infants whose mothers drink large amounts of caffeinated beverages (Hopkinson, 1987).

Some cultures advocate the addition of alcohol, usually beer or wine, to the breast-feeding mother's diet to increase milk production and promote a feeling of relaxation. It is true that a tense, worried mother may have difficulty in maintaining an adequate milk supply. However, alcohol passes into breast milk and its regular consumption should be discouraged while breast-feeding.

Nicotine contained in cigarette smoke is transmitted

◆ TABLE 17-1
Recommended Daily Dietary Allowances for Lactation

	First 6 Months	Second 6 Months
Energy (kcl)	+500	+500
Protein (gm)	65	62
Vitamin A (RE*)	1300	1200
Vitamin D (μg)	10	10
Vitamin E activity (mg αTE)†	12	11
Ascorbic acid (mg)	95	90
Folacin (mg‡)	280	260
Niacin (mg‡)	20	20
Riboflavin (mg)	1.8	1.7
Thiamine (mg)	1.6	1.6
Vitamin B_6 (mg)	2.1	2.1
Vitamin B_{12} (μg)	2.6	2.6
Calcium (mg)	1200	1200
Phosphorus (mg)	1200	1200
Iodine (μg)	200	200
Iron (mg)	15	15
Magnesium (mg)	355	340
Zinc (mg)	19	16

Modified from Food and Nutrition Board, National Research Council: *Recommended dietary allowances*, ed 10, Washington, DC, 1989, Government Printing Office.
*RE = retinol equivalent.
†α-Tocopherol equivalents: 1 mg d-α-tocopherol = 1 αTE
‡Although allowances are expressed as niacin, on average, 1 mg of niacin is derived from 60 mg of dietary tryptophan.

in breast milk. It's long-term effects on the infant are not clear. However, there is some evidence that it is associated with vomiting, diarrhea, rapid heart rate, and restlessness. There is also evidence that it may contribute to decreased milk production.

Maintaining lactation during separations or illness

Many mothers who work outside the home are successfully continuing to breast-feed. This requires some extra effort, because to maintain a milk supply the breasts must be stimulated and emptied every 3 to 4 hours. A breast-feeding mother may manually empty her breasts or use a manual or electric pump when separated from her infant. Some mothers elect to feed their infants with a combination of breast and formula. More employers are sensitive to the needs of breast-feeding mothers, providing quiet and clean environments for expressing and pumping.

Small premature infants usually do not have the strength to suckle at breast, but they do benefit from expressed maternal milk. For this reason, mothers of premature infants may wish to maintain their milk supply for the immediate use of the infant in the hospital (given by gavage) and for later use when the infant goes home. An infant with a cleft lip or palate can usually breast-feed, depending on the extent of the defect, but both mother and infant will require some extra support in getting started. Even if unable to suckle, the infant can still benefit from expressed milk.

Milk should be expressed into a hard plastic or glass container. The container should be labeled with the date and immediately immersed in a bowl of ice water for 1 to 2 minutes, then stored in the coldest part of the refrigerator or freezer. The best way to thaw frozen breast milk is to place it in the refrigerator for 12 to 24 hours. It can be thawed more quickly by swirling the container in a bowl of warm water. See accompanying box for recommendations for breast milk storage.

To be completely successful, most breast-feeding mothers must want to nurse, have supportive family members, and be convinced of its advantages. They also need prenatal instruction regarding the care and normal function of their breasts, as well as encouragement and assistance in the postpartum period. If a woman has flattened or inverted nipples, they may be treated during the prenatal period by using special breast cups, or suction. In some localities, groups of mothers particularly interested in promoting breast-feeding have formed organizations to help the new mother or mother-to-be. La Leche League International, founded in Illinois in 1956, is an organization that is dedicated to helping mothers successfully breast-feed.

BREAST MILK STORAGE

Room temperature	40 minutes
Refrigerator	48 hours
Freezer (separate refrigerator and freezer doors)	3 months
Deep freezer (-20° F)	12 months

(From California Department of Health Services, 1990)

Breast-feeding techniques and breast care

Some infants nurse well from the start; others take a little while to learn what they are supposed to do. With breast-feeding, however, the nurse and mother have some powerful allies—inborn reflexes and hunger. By using the newborn's own natural behaviors and reflexes the infant can be assisted to begin breast-feeding. In preparation for breast-feeding the mother first washes her hands. Then she and her infant should assume a comfortable position. The mother needs to be in good body alignment and well-supported in the position of her choice. If sitting up in bed or in a chair, she usually finds it more comfortable to place the infant on a pillow in her lap. This brings the infant closer to the breast with less strain. She may also lie on her side with her lower arm cradling the infant if the infant has no history of ear infections. Infants who are prone to otitis media should not be fed in the supine position.

To empty the breast effectively and to keep the nipple in good condition the infant must nurse with the areola in her mouth and not just the nipple. This is important because, if the infant is allowed to chew on the end of the nipple, painful, cracked, or fissured nipples may result. Sore nipples are the leading cause of women discontinuing breast-feeding. The following will help the infant to get a good latch. While in a comfortable sitting position the mother holds the infant using the cradle hold. The infant should then be turned onto his side so that his or her entire body faces the mother and the infant's lower arm can be tucked underneath him or her or around the mother's waist. In this position the infant does not have to turn his or her head or strain to reach the breast and is close enough to fit the open mouth well back onto the areola. Now the mother supports her breast, using her free hand, by placing her fingers under the breast and her thumb above. By lightly tickling the infant's lips with her nipple, the mother stimulates the infant to open his or her mouth. While the mouth is open wide, the mother quickly pulls the infant toward the breast. The tip of the infant's nose should touch her breast. If he or she needs more room to breathe, her thumb is there to gently

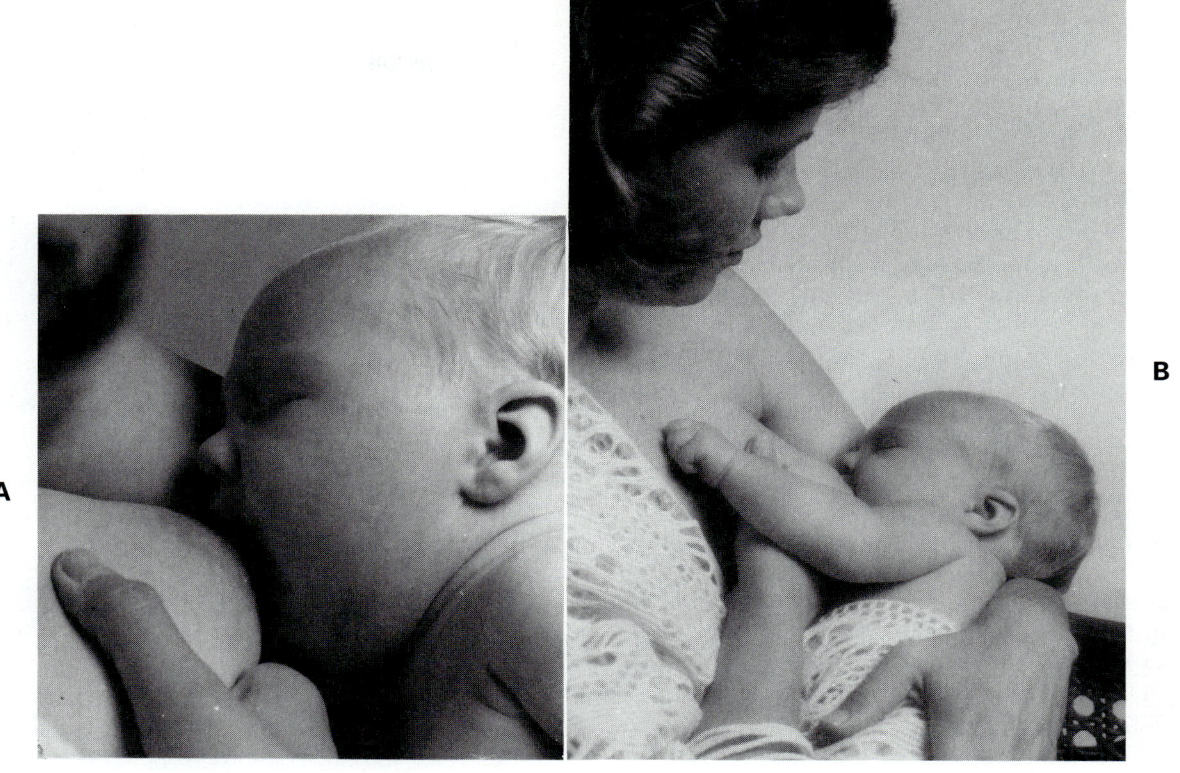

Fig. 17-11 **A,** Proper position of mother's hand on breast as she tickles baby's lips with nipple to initiate wide open mouth. **B,** Mother has pulled infant to breast and infant is latched on.

press the breast away from his or her nose (Fig. 17-11). Sometimes if the infant has difficulty getting started or is new at the breast, gently expressing a drop of milk on the tip of the nipple will give the infant the basic idea. If the breasts are engorged, expressing some milk before beginning to nurse will relieve tension of the breast and make it easier for the infant to grasp the areola.

The same steps apply to a mother who is breast-feeding lying down, except that the infant is placed on the bed lying on his or her side facing the mother. Varying positions (cradle, side-lying, football hold) varies the pressure points on the nipple and areola, helping to avoid soreness. The side-lying position and the football hold are usually more comfortable for the woman who has had a cesarean birth.

Initially the mother should alternate the breast she starts with—beginning with the one she left off with at the previous feeding. The infant is usually hungrier and nurses more vigorously at the first breast, often becoming satiated and falling asleep at the second. Alternating equalizes breast milk stimulation and helps to prevent nipple soreness. When removing the infant from the breast, the mother should be taught to gently pull down on the chin or insert a finger into the corner of the infant's mouth between the jaws to release them and break the suction. Failing to break the suction before removing the infant from the breast can cause nipple trauma.

Nipples should be air dried after feeding. Washing the breasts and nipples once a day with clear water is sufficient—soaps are drying and should not be used. Repeated washing of the nipple even with clear water removes the protective oils and predisposes it to cracking. Breast cream or ointments are not recommended. Gently rubbing a few drops of colostrum or breast milk on the nipple area after feeding will provide adequate lubrication and help decrease soreness.

The first few days the infant obtains an introductory milk, called *colostrum,* which has a laxative effect and contains protective antibodies. Maternal milk becomes complete several weeks later. The greatest aid to milk production is frequent stimulation and emptying of the breasts. If the breasts are not emptied, milk production may dwindle. For this reason mothers should be discouraged from introducing bottle feedings for the first couple of weeks or until the breast milk supply is well established. The ideal maternity accommodations for a nursing mother is the rooming-in plan or a modification of rooming-in. In this setting the infant may be put to the breast as desired and is not limited to the 4-hour feeding schedules followed by the few remaining hospitals that do not have family-centered care programs. Infants seem to do the best when allowed to feed on demand without limitations regarding frequency or length of feeding. Nursing infants are often fed every 2 to 3 hours when breast-feeding is initiated. The length of the feeding varies considerably from infant to infant and is usually somewhere between 10 to 30 minutes. Limiting the time the infant nurses at the breast is no longer considered effective in preventing sore nipples. It is generally recommended that a mother nurse from both breasts at each feeding. Perhaps the most important consideration is that the breast be emptied. If it is not emptied by the infant, the mother should empty it manually or with the aid of a pump to maintain milk production. For a brief presentation of breast anatomy and more details of breast care, see Chapter 13.

Breast-fed infants, like formula-fed infants, must be burped to remove swallowed air. The breast-fed infant should be burped between breasts and at the end of the feeding. Sitting the infant up or holding him or her over a protected shoulder while gently rubbing the back is effective for both breast and bottle-fed infants (Fig. 17-12 and Fig. 17-8).

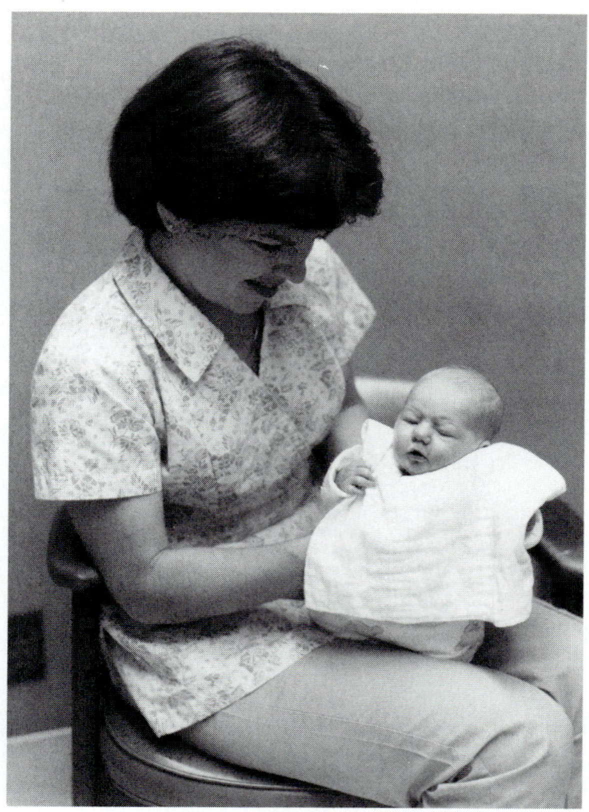

Fig. 17-12 Burping infant in the sitting position. (Courtesy Grossmont Hospital, La Mesa, CA.)

Formula Feeding

With present knowledge of nutrition and increased understanding of food processing and preservation, the formula-fed infant is not threatened with malnutrition or disease in developed countries. Although mothers should be told the advantages of breast-feeding, they should not be considered or made to feel like maternal failures if they cannot or choose not to breast-feed. To push a mother to breast-feed when she is not committed may lead to a cycle of rebellion, failure, and regret. Some have schedules that are difficult to combine with breast-feeding; some are concerned that their infants are not getting enough to eat; and some have been unsuccessful with breast-feeding in the past. For others the process of nursing is physically unattractive and they may lack support from their partners and other family members. Mothers who choose to bottle-feed should not be made to feel guilty by health care providers.

The primary health care provider should guide the selection of formula. The AAP recommends that nonbreast-fed infants receive iron-fortified formula during the first year of life. Numerous commercially prepared formulas that contain the necessary iron and vitamins are available. These come in liquid or powder form. Directions must be carefully followed, since some are ready to use and others must be diluted or mixed. Infants have developed mild to fatal illnesses because caretakers have prepared formula improperly. The cost differs with the type, form, and vendor. The less modification needed before use, the more expensive the product. A number of companies manufacture disposable prefilled nursing units, which are used by hospitals.

Preparation of formula

If the more costly ready-to-feed formula is not purchased, the most usual method of formula preparation uses tap water for dilution. The procedure for preparing formula is displayed in the box on p. 323. Special handling of infant formula is necessary because milk is an ideal medium for the growth of microorganisms. Organisms that are not compatible with the infant's digestive system may multiply rapidly in milk if it is improperly bottled or is left open to air and warmed for an extended period. Typhoid organisms were fairly common contaminants of milk and milk products before pasteurization. Because of the infant's susceptibility, disinfection or "sterilization" of the formula (aseptic or terminal methods) were considered necessary until the last decade. Now it is believed that in most instances a conscientious clean technique

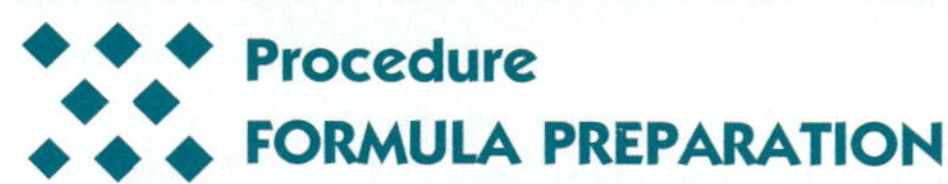

Procedure FORMULA PREPARATION

EQUIPMENT/SUPPLIES

Capped formula bottle
Nipple
Bottle brush
Soap or detergent
Sauce pan
Can opener
Spoon
Formula as prescribed: ready to use, liquid concentrate, powder

STEPS

1 Use a formula bottle that has been washed in the dishwasher or in warm, sudsy water, rinsed in *hot* water, and air dried.
2 Use a nipple that has been carefully washed and rinsed. Make sure that the nipple holes are open. Some references also recommend boiling the clean nipple 3 to 5 minutes.
3 Shake the formula can well (if liquid type); wipe off the lid before opening.
4 Measure the ingredients needed for one feeding into the bottle. Read the directions carefully. Be sure that you understand what dilution (if any) is to be made.
5 Add warm tap water to the bottle in the amount the directions indicate. Boil bottled water or well water for 5 minutes (neither contain chlorine and can become contaminated).
6 Mix with a clean spoon.
7 Unless you are planning to refrigerate the formula, feed *immediately;* do not save partially consumed bottles of formula from one feeding to the next or for more than an hour.
8 Prepared formula may be stored in the refrigerator for 48 hours.
9 Bring refrigerated formula to room temperature by placing the bottle in a warm pan of water. Do not microwave—hot spots can result.

is sufficient. Hospitals, however, usually use sterile precautions until an infant has reached 3 months of age. Plastic bottles used by older infants who hold their own bottle should be sterilized or discarded between patients.

Bottle-feeding techniques

Feeding an infant formula can be an enjoyable experience. The hands should be clean; the milk should be tepid (no sensation of hot or cold)—test on the inside of the parent's or nurse's wrist. Although experiments using cold formula for feeding the newborn have demonstrated no undesirable effects, even on premature babies, feedings are usually offered at room temperature. Many nurseries have discarded formula warmers because of problems with elevated bacterial count on the equipment. The rate of nipple flow should be almost one drop per second when the bottle is inverted. Nipple holes may be enlarged by a hot needle mounted on a cork. Vigorously sucking infants should be given a resistant nipple. Infants who tire easily and premature infants do better with a soft, pliable nipple.

Be sure the nipple is on top of the tongue, and do not push it too far back—it may stimulate the gag reflex. Infants seem to drink best when held closely at a 45-degree angle. Studies indicate that such positioning minimizes the possibility of retrograde infection through the eustachian tubes to the middle ear and also helps prevent aspiration. (Fig. 17-13) The neck of the bottle should always be tipped so that it is full of milk. The bottle should never be propped—the infant can choke. Air in the infant's stomach may cause pain, decrease appetite, or promote regurgitation. The infant should be burped after each ounce for newborns or halfway through and at the end of the feeding for older infants.

Newborns should be carefully observed before and during feedings for indications of any abnormality in the digestive or respiratory tracts. Prefeeding coughing, cyanosis, and excessive mucus may be associated with anatomical abnormalities. Regurgitation of a feeding through the nose and mouth should be reported at once. In some facilities, infants are offered water before the first breast or formula feeding to evaluate their ability to drink without difficulty.

After feeding, the infant may need to have his or her diaper changed. The infant should be propped on the right side to sleep. The amount taken should be recorded in the newborn's records. The newborn infant may take only 1 ounce per feeding the first day and 2 or 3 ounces per feeding on the second and third days. Bottle-fed newborns usually are fed every 3 or 4 hours. As the infant grows, the number of feedings decreases and the volume of feedings increases. See Table 17-2 for a typical pattern of infant feedings in the first year of life. This pattern may vary during growth spurts,

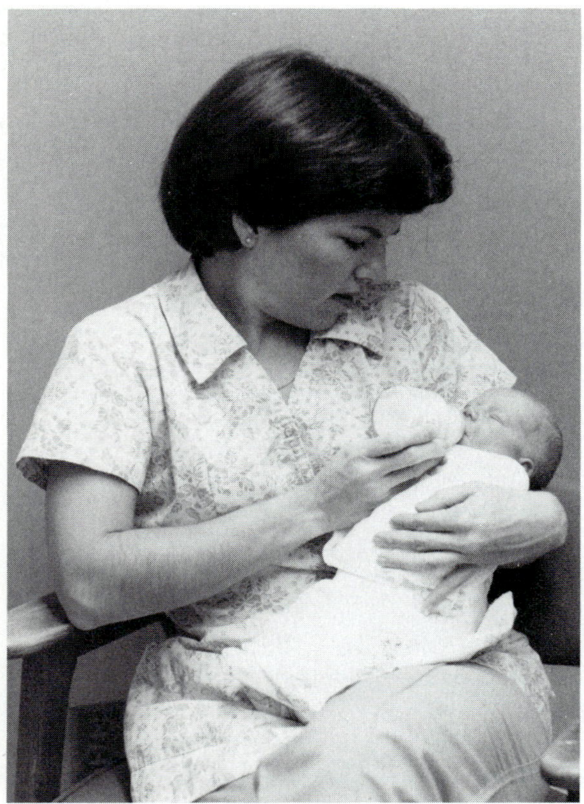

Fig. 17-13 Infant should be held for bottle-feeding. Nipple should always be full of formula and infant upright. (Courtesy Grossmont Hospital, La Mesa, CA.)

which usually occur at 6 and 12 weeks of age, at which time the infant may demand more frequent feedings. See nursing alert above right.

Evaluation of Infant Nutritional Status

There are numerous ways of judging whether a newborn infant, either formula-fed or breast-fed, is receiving enough to eat. The nurse should teach the parents to:

1 Observe behavior—does the infant seem content, or is the infant a short sleeper and irritable? (Note that infants cry for reasons other than hunger pangs; for example, if they are wet, too tightly bundled or too warm, have gas pains, or want to be held.) The infant should have vigorous activity and be generally happy.
2 Watch for signs of dehydration:
   a Fewer than 6 to 8 wet diapers per day
   b Dark, concentrated urine; dry, hard stools
   c Dry mucous membranes
   d Dry skin with little elasticity (poor turgor)
   e Watch for low-grade fever (Note that the most common cause of low-grade fever is dehydration, although the nurse should not overlook the possibility of infection.)
   f Elevated specific gravity (above 1.020)
   g In severe cases, sunken fontanels
3 Measure intake:
   a This is routine with bottle-fed infants.
   b If the infant is ill, measuring may be ordered for breast-fed infants. Breast-fed infants are weighed dressed and wrapped directly before the feeding and directly after the feeding, before any diapers are changed, with the same clothes and blankets (1 g = 1 ml).
   c Intake should be evaluated in terms of a 24-hour period and not individual feedings.
4 Measure weight gain:
   a This method is of little use currently because of the short hospital stays of most newborn infants in the United States.
   b All infants lose weight directly after birth, which should cause no concern unless the weight loss approaches 10% of the birth weight. Bottle-fed infants regain their birth weight more rapidly than most breast-fed infants.
   c After weight gain is reestablished, a gain of about 1 ounce a day is average, equaling about 6 ounces a week. At the end of 5 months most infants have doubled their birth weight.

Nursing Alert

Parents should be taught that infants should not be given honey until they are at least 18 months of age. Honey can cause botulism in younger infants.

Parent-Infant Interaction

Parents and infants both benefit from interacting with each other. The attachment process that begins in pregnancy continues in the early postpartum period and for several months thereafter. Interaction aids the parent-infant acquaintance process that evolves into a strong attachment. Parents need to learn to recognize infant cues that indicate a readiness for interaction and cues that indicate a need to stop the interaction to prevent overstimulation (see Chapter 16 for a discussion of infant cues). The full-term infant usually gives subtle but clear cues. Parents must also learn how to alleviate the infant's distress. Infant cues often provide clues to the source of discomfort or discontent. At other times, the parents must employ a trial-and-error method until they become more familiar with their

◆ **TABLE 17-2**
Typical Pattern of Daily Infant Feedings

Age	Number of Feedings	oz/ml Per Feeding	Total Volume (oz/ml)
First week	6 to 10	2 to 3/60 to 90	12 to 30/360 to 900
2 to 4 weeks	6 to 8	3 to 4/90 to 120	18 to 32/540 to 960
1 to 3 months	5 to 6	5 to 6/150 to 180	25 to 36/750 to 1080
3 to 7 months	4 to 5	6 to 7/180 to 210	25 to 36/750 to 1080
7 to 12 months	3 to 4	7 to 8/210 to 240	25 to 36/750 to 1080

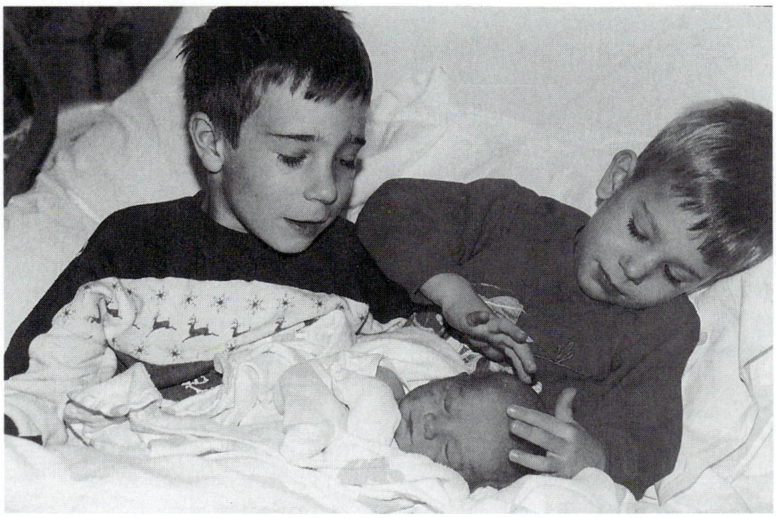

Fig. 17-14 Getting acquainted with a new baby brother.

infant's characteristic behavior patterns. Parents also need to provide situations that foster their young infant's optimal growth and development. Learning about infant capabilities and methods of providing appropriate sensory stimulation will help new parents foster their infant's innate abilities. Nurses have a major role to play in helping parents learn to read their infant's cues and respond appropriately and to learn appropriate ways to facilitate their infant's growth and development.

Fathers want to be involved not only in the preparation for parenthood and birth but also in the care and nurturing of the infant. Mothers must be helped to understand that just as they have many adjustments to make, so do new fathers. New fathers frequently report concerns for the health of their wives, concerns about changes in sexual practices and closeness as a couple, worries about increased financial responsibility, and like their partners, concerns about their competence in infant-care practices. If nurses and mothers encourage paternal involvement the father is more likely to take an active role in the care of his child. Nurses can facilitate the father's acquaintance process with the infant and his involvement by including him in all aspects of infant care and teaching.

If the newborn's siblings, grandparents, and other family members visit, they should be able to see and, after careful handwashing, to hold the infant and visit with the new mother (Fig. 17-14). For optimal development the newborn needs to develop primary and secondary attachments and parents need a social support network. The nurse can facilitate these family introductions to the new infant by organizing care around visits, and by including family members in teaching.

Parent Education

New parents will be less anxious if they are equipped with adequate knowledge of their child and child care. Although healthy newborns are often hospitalized less than 24 hours, it is the nurse's responsibility to initiate or build on teaching in the areas indicated in the box on p. 326. Additional

PARENT EDUCATION—NEWBORN CARE TOPICS

- Infant Care
  - Use of the bulb syringe
  - Temperature taking techniques and normal values
  - Positioning for feeding and sleeping
  - Safe handling and carrying
  - Signs/concerns which should be reported to the health care provider
  - Bathing and skin care
  - Cord care
  - Circumcision care
- Nutrition
  - Breast-feeding
  - Formula-feeding
  - Introduction of solids
- Elimination patterns
- Safety in the home and in the car (see Chapter 22)
- Importance of stimulation
- Developmental milestones (see Chapter 21)
- Possible sibling rivalry
- Available community resources

teaching can be initiated or reinforced in high school or college family education classes, prenatal and postnatal parent-education programs, home visits, clinic and office waiting rooms, and well-child visits. Three areas not discussed elsewhere are included in the following sections: bathing and skin care at home, circumcision care, and signs of illness to report to the health care provider.

Bathing and skin care

Bath time can be a pleasurable experience for parents and the infant. The nurse should educate the parents about bathing and skin care needs before discharge. The basic principles followed in the admission bath also apply in the home setting. In addition, parents should be aware of the following information. Infants do not need baths every day—parents can use common sense regarding bathing frequency. Usually two or three sponge baths per week until the cord falls off, then tub baths, is adequate. The infant's face and perianal area, however, do need to be washed with soap and water *every day.* A mild soap, such as Dove, is recommended. Highly perfumed soaps and deodorant soaps should be avoided because they can cause rashes. When the infant is bathed, the head should be thoroughly shampooed and rinsed well. Parents should pay particular attention to cleaning skin folds. Q-tips should not be used to clean the ears. Powders, cornstarch, and oils should be avoided because they tend to clog the pores and may cause rashes. Powders may also be inhaled. Bathing provides a good opportunity for parents to inspect the skin. They should be instructed to notify the health care provider if they observe redness, oozing, or foul odor from the cord and blisters or pustules on any area of the infant's skin.

Circumcision care

Circumcision involves the slitting or surgical removal of all or part of the foreskin, or prepuce, of the penis. Proponents of the procedure believe that it makes hygiene easier, decreases irritation of the area from an accumulation of cellular debris (smegma) under the foreskin, and may help to avoid urinary tract infections, sexually transmitted diseases, and cancer. Opponents state that circumcision is medically unnecessary and a possible source of infection, hemorrhage, and meatal stenosis. The outcome of this surgery depends on the skill and technique of the physician. In 1975 the American Academy of Pediatrics stated that there are no valid medical indications for circumcision in the newborn period. They revised that statement in 1988 to reflect the increased evidence that routine circumcision appears to reduce the incidence of urinary tract infections. Routine circumcision of all male infants, however, appears to be decreasing.

The circumcision of a Jewish infant has religious importance. Among Orthodox Jews it is undertaken by an ordained circumciser called a *mohel.* This ceremony, called the *brit* or *bris,* is usually performed at home on the eighth day of life. The child is then officially named.

Physicians usually have individual preferences regarding the technique used. Some prefer to use the Yellen (Gomco) clamp and others prefer the plastibell (Fig. 17-15 and Fig. 17-16). Local anesthetic (penile block) is being used more frequently as pain perception in infants is increasingly acknowledged. The equipment and procedure in the box on p. 328 are relatively standard.

After the procedure it is the nurse's responsibility to frequently check for edema and bleeding. Voidings, especially the first after the procedure, should be carefully noted and charted because there is a danger of urinary retention. The area should be kept clean; soiled or displaced dressings should be replaced with clean materials. The infant should be positioned on his side.

Circumcisions are usually performed shortly before the infant's discharge home. Thus the parents should be carefully instructed regarding observation and care of the area. The care differs only slightly, depending on whether the plastibell technique or Gomco clamp technique was used. Nurses should show

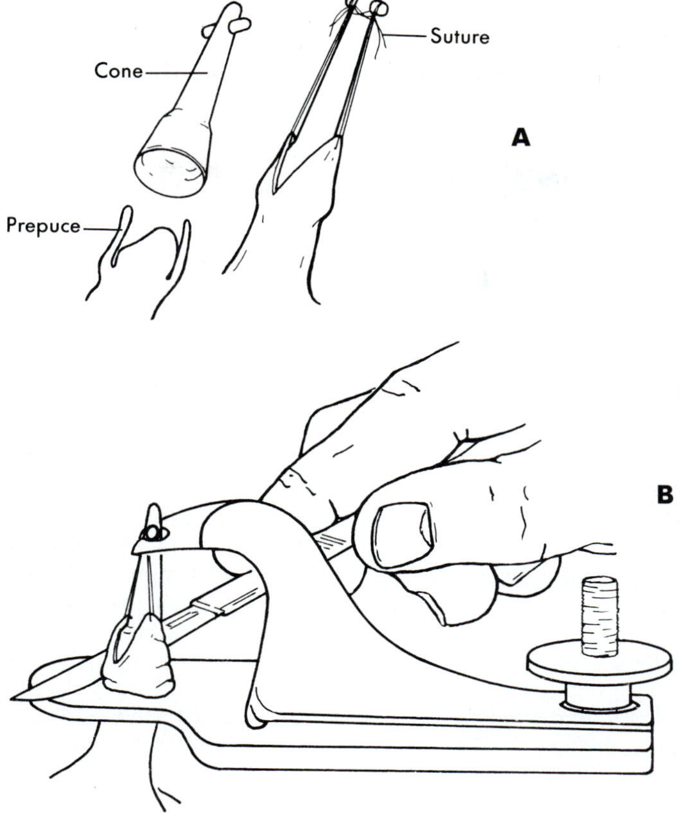

Fig. 17-15 Circumcision with Yellen clamp. **A,** Prepuce drawn over cone. **B,** Yellen clamp is applied, hemostasis occurs, then prepuce (over cone) is cut away. (From Bobak IM and Jensen MD: *Maternity and gynecologic care,* ed 5, St. Louis, 1993, Mosby.)

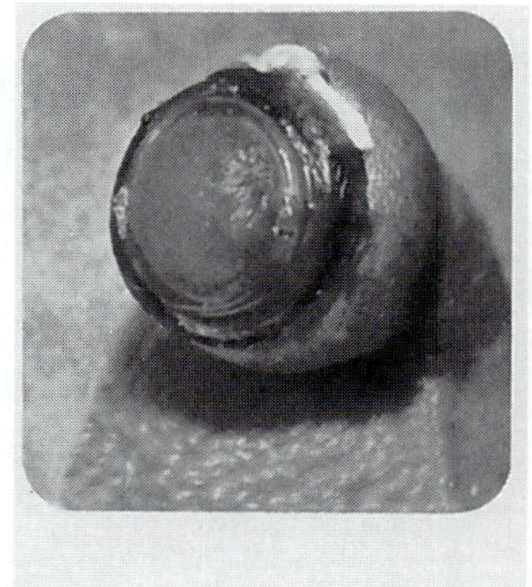

The plastic rim usually drops off 5 to 8 days after circumcision. No special dressing is required, and the baby can be bathed and diapered just as if he had not been circumcised. NOTE: A dark brown or black ring encircling the plastic rim is perfectly natural. This will disappear when the rim drops off.

A

B

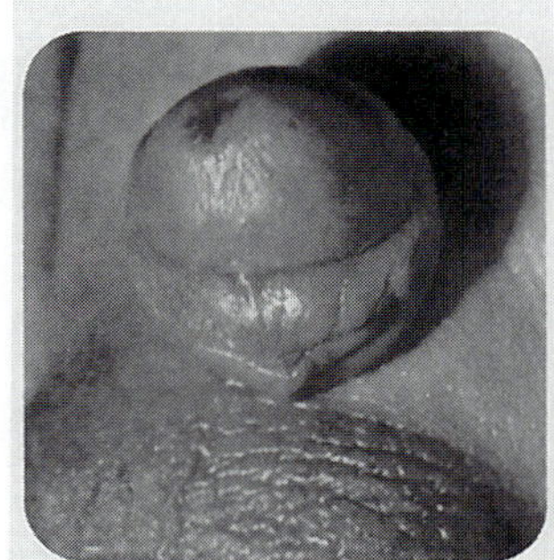

The result is a clean, well-healed line of excision.

Be sure to notify your doctor if healing does not proceed as described. Notify the doctor **immediately** if you should notice any unusual swelling, if the plastic ring has not fallen off within 8 days, or if the ring has slipped onto the shaft of the penis.

Fig. 17-16 Circumcision using Hollister plastibell. **A,** Suture around rim of plastibell controls bleeding. **B,** Plastic rim and suture drop off in 7 to 10 days. (Courtesy Hollister, Chicago, IL.)

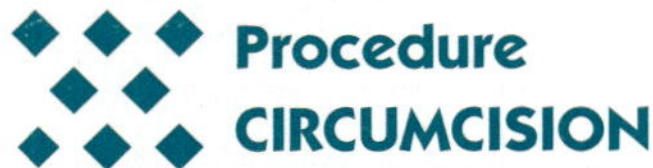

Procedure CIRCUMCISION

EQUIPMENT/SUPPLIES

- Sterile setup including
  a. One circumcision drape
  b. Two 4 × 4 squares (flats or gauze compresses)
  c. Four small hemostats (mosquito clamps)
  d. One Yellen (Gomco) clamp, 1.3 to 1.1 cm in diameter (or plastibell)
  e. One scalpel handle and added blade (or scissors if plastibell technique)
  f. One grooved director and probe
  g. One thumb forceps
- Sterile gloves, appropriately sized
- Antiseptic for skin preparation, such as povidone-iodine (Betadine)
- Dressing materials
  Petrolatum-impregnated gauze (if Gomco clamp technique is used)
- A circumcision board, diapers, and special restraining halter that ties over the board
- Lidocaine HCL 1% (Xylocaine), 1 ml, without epinephrine if anesthesia is used
- Syringe, 1 ml, with 27 gauge, 0.5 inch (1.2 cm) needle if anesthesia is used
- Bulb syringe

STEPS

1. Obtain a signed informed consent from parent before procedure.
2. Properly identify the infant. Check for possible reasons for not proceeding with the operation (presence of inflammation, tendency to bleed, genitourinary anomalies)
3. Clean diaper area.
4. Restrain the infant gently but firmly on a circumcision board. The infant may be covered to conserve body heat (Fig. 17-17).
5. Ensure good light. A stool or chair may be appreciated by the physician.
6. A pacifier helps to comfort the infant during the procedure.
7. After the procedure the infant should be removed from the circumcision board, diapered, comforted, and returned to his crib. The circumcision board should be disinfected and the equipment washed and sent for sterilization.

A 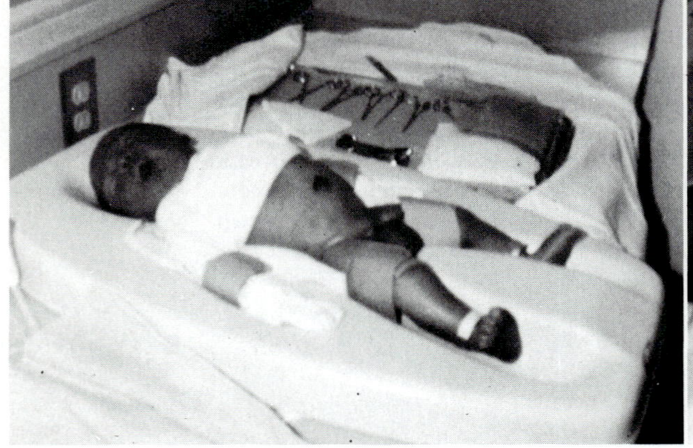

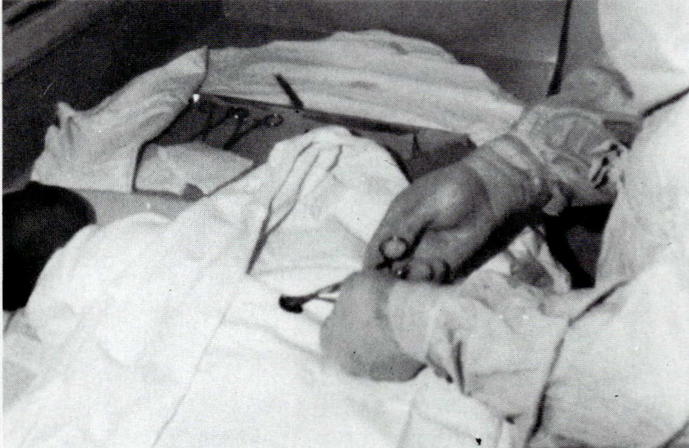 B

Fig. 17-17 **A,** Proper positioning of infant on circumcision board. **B,** Physician performing circumcision. Newborn is covered to prevent cold stress. (From Bobak IM and Jensen MD: *Maternity and gynecologic care,* ed 5, St. Louis, 1993, Mosby.)

the parent the area and discuss the care. If the *clamp technique* was used, the vaseline gauze dressing should be soaked off approximately 24 hours after the procedure. After it is removed the area is rinsed with warm water and gently dried whenever soiled. If the area is somewhat sticky, the parent can apply a small amount of vaseline to prevent sticking to the diaper. If the *plastibell technique* was used the area should be rinsed and gently dried when soiled. No vaseline is necessary. The plastibell will usually fall off within a

REFERENCES

American Academy of Pediatrics: *Report of the committee on infectious diseases,* ed 22, Elk Village, IL, 1991, The Academy.

American Dietetic Association, Position of The American Dietetic Association: Promotion and support of breast-feeding, *J Am Diet Assoc* 93(4):467-469, 1993.

Bobak IM and Jensen MD: *Maternity and gynecologic care,* ed 5, St Louis, 1993, Mosby.

Hopkinson JM: Maternal nutrition during lactation, *Nutrition and the MD* 13(2):1, 1987.

Institute of Medicine: *Nutrition during lactation,* Washington, DC, 1991, National Academy of Sciences.

Lerner H: Sleep position of infants: applying research to practice, *MCN* 18(5):275-277, 1993.

Nurses Association of the American College of Obstetricians and Gynecologists: *Neonatal thermoregulation: OGN nursing practice resource,* Washington, DC, February 1990, The Association

Nurses Association of the American College of Obstetricians and Gynecologists: *Neonatal skin care: OGN nursing practice resource,* Washington, DC, January 1992, The Association.

Rush J, Chiovitti R, Kaufman K, Mitchell A: A randomized controlled trial of a nursery ritual: wearing cover gowns to care for healthy newborns, *Birth,* 17(1):25-30, 1990.

Smith DP et al: *Comprehensive child and family nursing skills,* St Louis, 1991, Mosby.

Worthington-Roberts B and Williams SR: *Nutrition in pregnancy and lactation,* ed 5, St. Louis, 1993, Mosby.

BIBLIOGRAPHY

AAP Task Force on Infant Positioning and SIDS: Positioning and SIDS, *Pediatrics* 89(6):1120-1126, 1992.

Anderson PO: Drug use during breast-feeding, *Clin Pharmacy* 10:594-624, 1991.

Anderson PO: Medication use while breast feeding a neonate, *Neonatal Pharmacology Quarterly* 2(2):3-14, 1993.

Auerbach KG: Assisting the employed breast-feeding mother, *J Nurse Midwifery* 35(1):26-34, 1990.

Auerbach KG: The effect of nipple shields on maternal milk volume, *J Obstet Gynecol Neonatal Nurs* 19(5):419-427, 1990.

California Department of Health Services, Maternal and Child Health Branch, WIC Supplemental Food Branch: *Nutrition during pregnancy and the postpartum period: a manual for health care professionals,* Sacramento, CA, 1990, The Department.

Engel NS: Lidocaine dorsal penile nerve block for circumcision, *MCN* 14(5):311, 1989.

Hill PD: The enigma of insufficient mild supply, *MCN* 16(6):312-316, 1991.

Kearney MH and Cronenwett L: Breast-feeding and employment, *J Obstet Gynecol Neonatal Nurs* 20(6):471-480, 1991.

Lund MM: Perspectives on newborn male circumcision, *Neonatal Network* 9(3):7-10, 1990.

Mennella JA and Beauchamp GK: The transfer of alcohol to human milk: effects on flavor and infant's behavior, *N Engl J Med* 325(14):981-985, 1991.

Spiers PS and Gunteroth WG: Recommendations to avoid the prone sleeping position and recent statistics for Sudden Infant Death Syndrome in the United States, *Arch Pediatr Adolesc Med* 148(2):141-146, 1994.

Steihm ER and Vink P: Transmission of human immunodeficiency virus infection by breast-feeding, *J Pediatr* 118(3):410-411, 1991.

Walker M and Driscoll WJ: Sore nipples: the new mother's nemesis, *MCN* 14(4):260-265, 1989.

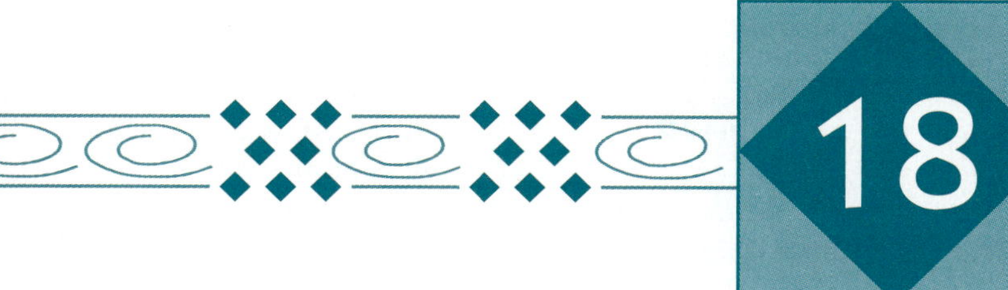
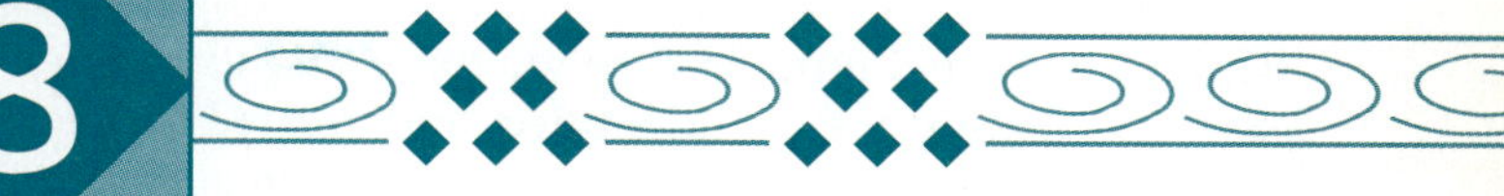

18

The Newborn with Special Needs

CHAPTER OBJECTIVES

After studying this chapter, the student should be able to:

1 Define these terms as they apply to the newborn: *preterm* or *premature, term, postterm, postmature, small for gestational age (SGA), appropriate for gestational age (AGA), large for gestational age (LGA),* and *low-birth-weight infants.*

2 List five factors that should be considered when determining the status of a small newborn.

3 Discuss the incidence of prematurity in the United States and its impact on infant mortality statistics.

4 Compare and contrast the appearance, and other characteristics, of the premature infant and the full-term infant in at least four ways.

5 Discuss the classification of hypoglycemia and the nursing assessment protocols related to this condition.

6 Identify three inborn errors of metabolism known to cause mental retardation, and note its incidence in the general population.

7 List six signs of increasing intracranial pressure in the infant.

8 Describe three types of shunts used to treat hydrocephalus.

9 Discuss the postoperative care of the infant who has undergone a shunt procedure, including observation, positioning, nutrition, and potential complications.

10 Describe a child with trisomy-21, including five characteristic signs.

11 Discuss the criteria used to determine the optimal time for the repair of a cleft lip (CL).

12 Describe the postoperative nursing care of children who have undergone cleft lip and cleft palate repairs and how they differ.

13 Define the following congenital abnormalities: *tracheoesophageal fistula (TEF), imperforate anus, omphalocele, hypospadias, syndactyly, polydactyly,* and *talipes equinovarus.*

14 Discuss the mechanism, prevention, and treatment of erythroblastosis fetalis associated with Rh incompatibility.

15 Compare the problems associated with the spinal abnormalities meningocele and myelomeningocele.

16 Describe maneuvers that assist in the identification of congenital dislocation of the hip (CDH).

17 Describe the most effective device for treating congenital dislocation of the hip (CDH) during infancy.

This chapter will help students recognize some of the more common conditions impacting infants with special needs and understand the underlying principles of optimal nursing care for these infants. Some of these conditions are identified and treated in the nursery and pose few subsequent problems. Other anomalies require long-term nursing and medical intervention.

Approximately 1 in 14 children is born with some kind of abnormality, causing disfigurement or resulting in physical or mental handicaps or a shortened life span. These problems may not be identified at birth.

The birth of a disabled or ill child is always a distressing time for the family. Feelings of failure, anxiety, guilt, frustration, anger, and exhaustion are common. Parents may at first be unable to believe that their child has special needs. When the realization comes, grief may be intense. Problems related to mobilizing the family to meet the unexpected demands created by hospital, physician, and multidisciplinary follow-up clinic visits may be intense. The extra financial burden can seem without end to often perplexed and unprepared parents.

term Any infant born between the beginning of the thirty-eighth week and the completion of the forty-second week of gestation, regardless of birth weight.

preterm or premature Any infant born before the completion of 37 weeks' gestation, regardless of weight.

postterm or postmature Any infant born after the end of 42 weeks' gestation, regardless of birth weight.

small for dates (SFD), small for gestational age (SGA), intrauterine growth retardation (IUGR) An infant whose rate of intrauterine growth was slowed and whose birth weight falls below the tenth percentile on the growth curve.

appropriate for gestational age (AGA) An infant whose weight falls between the tenth and ninetieth percentiles.

large for gestational age (LGA) An infant weighing more than 90% of babies of the same gestational age.

low-birth-weight infants An infant weighing less than 2500 gm, or 5½ lbs, regardless of gestational age.

very low-birth-weight (VLBW) An infant whose weight is less than 1500 gm. Approximately 34% of these children later experience school difficulty, including hyperactivity, as compared with 14% of the AGA group (McCormick, et al, 1990).

moderately low birth weight (MLBW) An infant whose birth weight is 1501 to 2500 gm.

ROLE OF THE NURSE

Although the nurse may not be in a position to mobilize all of the family and community resources to meet the child's needs, recognition of the stressors with which the family is coping is critical.

The nurse should know what information has been given to the parents regarding their child. The nurse should be supportive in allowing the parents to express themselves. Also the nurse should relay to the nurse coordinator or physician any problems that seem to be causing parental anxiety. It is important that the parents do not feel alone in adjusting to the reality of their child's disability. In an attempt to prevent such feelings the nurse can be a vital liaison between the family and health care providers, clergy, and community resource personnel. Guided participation in the care of their child and assistance in identifying a social-support network help to reduce feelings of isolation and augment effective coping strategies.

Neonatal Intensive Care Unit Nursing

Neonatal intensive care unit (NICU) nursing requires a highly specialized body of knowledge and clinical expertise that involves lengthy, supervised experience. An understanding of neonatal physiology and high-tech mechanical devices and the ability to recognize subtle physiological and behavioral deviations are essential. A student may not have the opportunity to be involved in the supervised nursing care of premature infants. Understanding the nature of the problems encountered in this setting, however, is an important foundation. The vocational nurse may collaborate with the registered nurse in a care partnership in the NICU setting.

Most premature infants are cared for in the NICU. Those infants who are not experiencing complications of prematurity may be cared for in the normal newborn nursery. Intensive care of the newborn is discussed in Chapter 19.

THE PRETERM (PREMATURE) INFANT

In the past the most common definition of prematurity was based on weight. Infants having a birth

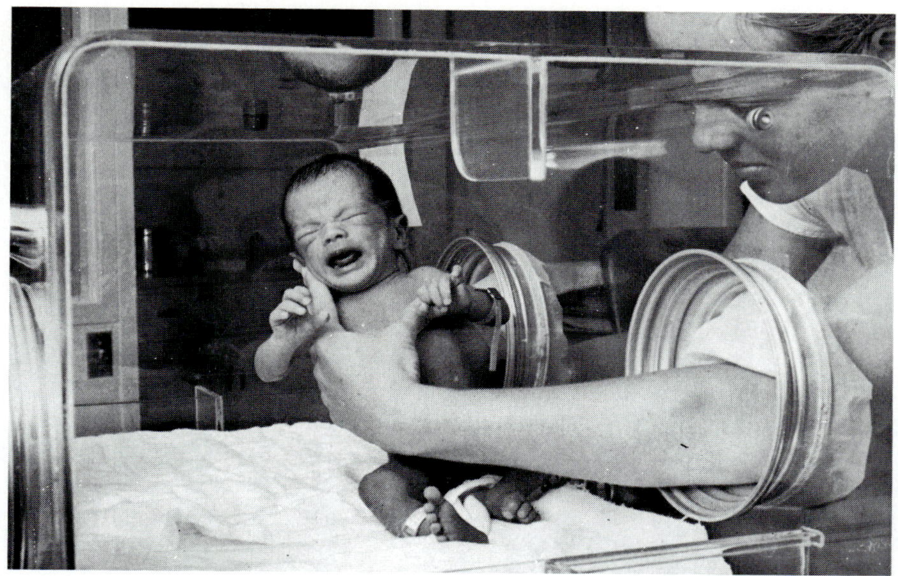

Fig. 18-1 This baby would have been premature by US standards if only birth weight was considered. However, Asian ancestry influenced his birth weight. He weighed less than 5½ lbs (2500 gm). (Courtesy UCSD Medical Center, San Diego, CA.)

weight under 5½ lbs (2500 gm) were considered premature. However, in reality some of these babies had completed a term gestation and were underweight because of genetic or intrauterine factors (Fig. 18-1). In fact the term *premature,* referring to the infant born before the end of the thirty-seventh week of gestation, has been replaced by the more descriptive adjective *preterm.* In this chapter the words *preterm* and *premature* are used synonymously. Infants who are small at birth for other reasons are referred to as *small for gestational age (SGA).* Infants may be of low-birth-weight because of an abbreviated gestation, unfavorable intrauterine conditions, or both (Fig. 18-2). The following is a more complete, newer classification of newborns based on gestational age (calculated from the first day of the last normal menstrual period) and birth weight (gestational age is 2 weeks longer than fertilization age).

In determining the status of the small infant, birth weight, heredity, length of gestation, clinical appearance, and behavior all must be considered. Although some infants cannot be classified as premature by the scale or calendar, they are judged underdeveloped and treated as "preemies."

The mortality percentages related to birth weight and gestational age have improved significantly because of prenatal care programs, the introduction of important new techniques in neonatal care, and an increased knowledge base among the members of health care teams. The survival of neonates with a gestational age of 26 to 27 weeks and weighing less than 750 gm is now a reality. However, prematurity remains the leading cause of neonatal mortality.

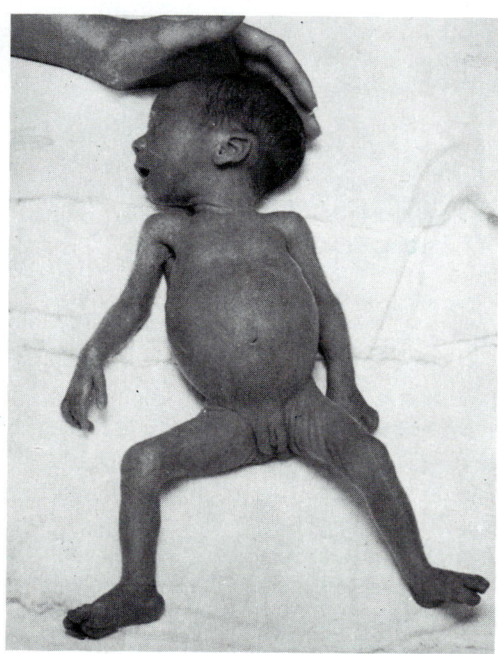

Fig. 18-2 Premature infant. (Courtesy Grossmont Hospital, La Mesa, CA.)

The incidence of prematurity in the United States varies with the population studied. In the general population, the prematurity rate approaches 7%. In the

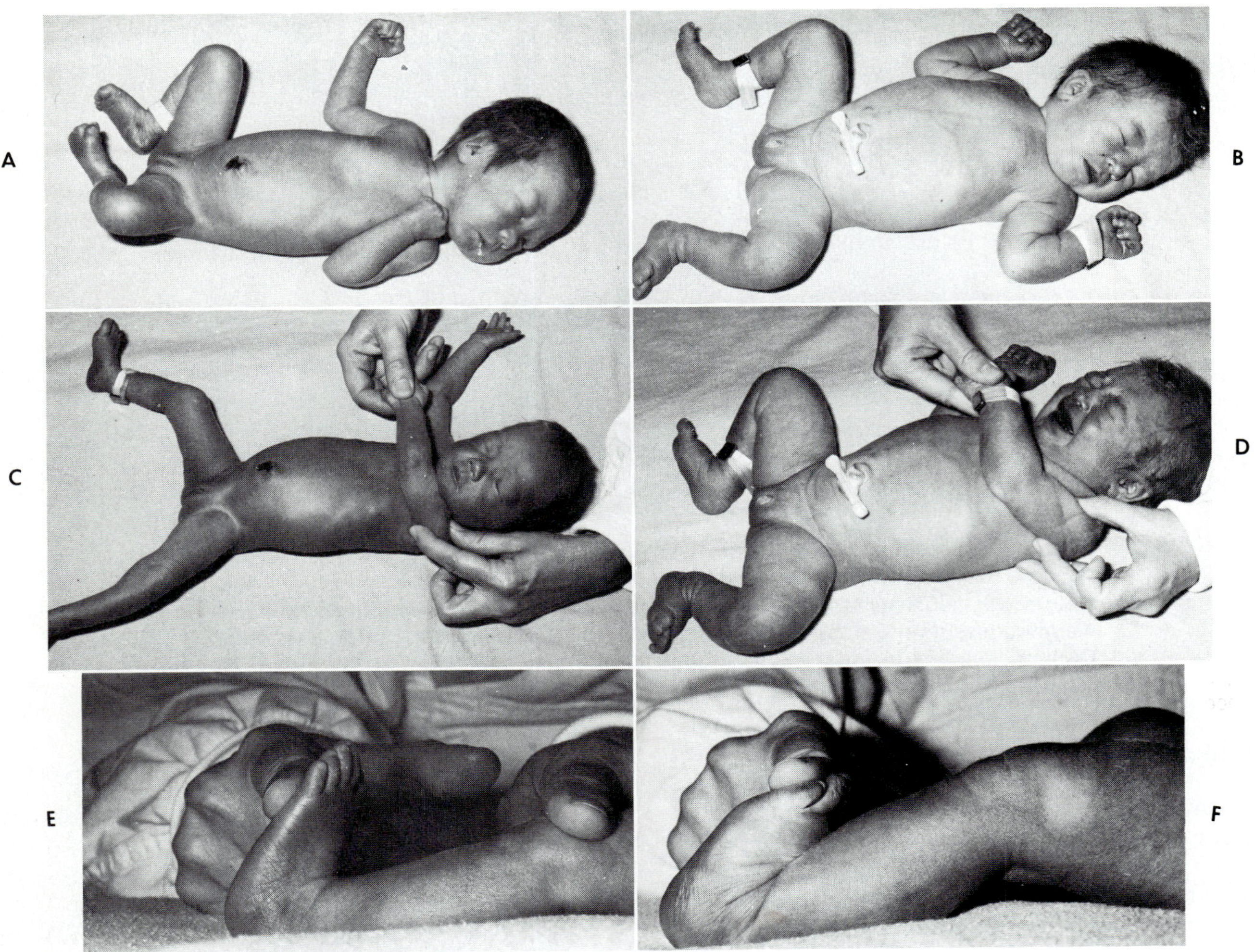

Fig. 18-3 Premature infant on left; mature infant on right. **A** and **B,** Typical body contours and postures. **C** and **D,** Scarf sign: immaturity seen when elbow passes midline. **E** and **F,** Prematurity is seen when heel cord is short and sole crease is scanty. (Courtesy Naval Hospital, San Diego, CA.)

African-American population the incidence of prematurity is 10% to 11%.

Etiology

The causes of low birth weight are not always known. Statistics recognize that low-birth-weight infants are more frequently born to mothers of a lower socioeconomic status. This incidence is related to a lack of prenatal care, infection acquired in utero, the obstetrical complications encountered, inadequate nutrition, and general health practices. Teenage mothers also have a higher rate of low-birth-weight infants. Multiple births are also associated with prematurity. Active and passive smoking by the mother are also important predictors of prematurity and low birth weight.

Appearance and Activity

The typical premature infant has a wrinkled appearance resulting from a lack of subcutaneous fat. The infant is covered with soft body hair called lanugo, the head and abdomen are relatively large, and the thorax is small. The skull has undergone little molding (Fig. 18-3). Respirations are usually irregular and apneic episodes (breathing pauses) up to 15 seconds in length are not unusual. Infants with breathing pauses greater than 15 seconds are carefully evaluated and are placed on cardiac monitors.

Premature infants may be surprisingly active. Their activity level and behavior patterns are often evaluated using a standardized screening tool. The infant's gestational age is determined within several hours of birth (Table 18-1).

♦ TABLE 18-1
Postnatal Estimation of Fetal Age Based on Signs of Maturity Assuming Normal Growth (Gestational Age)

	28 Weeks	32 Weeks	36 Weeks	40 Weeks
Skin	Thin, red, gelatinous	Smooth, dark pink; many vessels visible	Pink, tender; few vessels visible	Pale pink; no vessels
Breasts	Flat, areolae barely visible	Well-defined areolae	Areolae raised: 1 to 2 mm breast tissue	7 to 10 mm breast tissue
Sole creases	None	One anterior transverse crease	Creases on anterior two thirds of sole	Creases on heels
Ears	Pinna soft, flat; stays folded	Slight incurving at top; returns slowly from folding	Incurving upper two thirds; springs back from folding	Incurving to lobe; firm; stands out from head
Genitalia Male	Testes undescended; scrotum smooth	Testes high in canal; few scrotal rugae	Testes high in scrotum; more rugae	Testes low in pendulous scrotum; rugae complete
Female	Labia majora widely separated; clitoris, labia minora prominent	Labia majora and labia minora more equal in size	Labia majora becoming closer, nearly cover labia minora	Labia majora completely cover labia minora
Neurological posture	Hypotonic, arms and legs extended	Partial leg flexion	Froglike; flexion of all limbs	Hypertonic
Recoil	None	Partial leg recoil	Partial arm and leg recoil	Prompt recoil

Special Needs

Nutrition

Sucking and swallowing reflexes may be weak or absent in very small infants, necessitating feedings by gavage, insertion of a stomach tube, intravenous feedings, or all three of these methods (Fig. 18-4). Intravenous feedings are administered to infants weighing less than 1200 gm or those classified as "sick" prematures. These feedings may be given by umbilical catheter or peripheral veins.

After a period of evaluating an infant's tolerance to glucose water, oral feedings generally progress to formulas richer in calories than those fed to full-term infants. These calorie-rich formulas are necessary because of the premature infant's lack of nutritional reserves and a great need for rapid growth. Administering breast milk is optimal, based on the mother's health status. Immunological benefits, reduced incidence of allergic reactions, and the promotion of maternal-infant attachment are important advantages of breastfeeding.

To promote successful breastfeeding, the mother should be assisted with the proper neonate positioning and latch-on. If difficulties persist, the clinical nursing specialist or lactation consultant should be notified. The mother's milk may be pumped, labeled, and refrigerated in the nursery so that her milk may be used during her absence. Refer to Chapters 13 and 17 for additional information about breastfeeding.

Cultural aspects of lactation must also be considered when the patient's background differs from the nurse's. A thorough history should be obtained regarding the mother's traditions, desires, and preferences. Overgeneralizations regarding various ethnic groups should also be avoided.

The infant's diet is later supplemented with iron. The premature infant is also given vitamin E, which helps to protect lung structures, prevent eye problems, such as retrolental fibroplasia, and preserve red blood cell integrity.

Most premature infants are put on a 2- to 2½-hour feeding schedule. Nourishment is offered in very small amounts of 1 to 5 ml at a time, since the danger of overfeeding the premature infant is real. Overfeeding may increase abdominal distention, cause respiratory distress, and trigger vomiting, perhaps inducing aspiration. The infant must be burped frequently. If the mother chooses to bottlefeed or if her health status warrants bottlefeeding, both parents should be encouraged to feed the neonate. After a feeding the infant's head and chest are elevated by tilting the incubator mattress tray. To prevent emesis and aspiration a side-lying position is recommended.

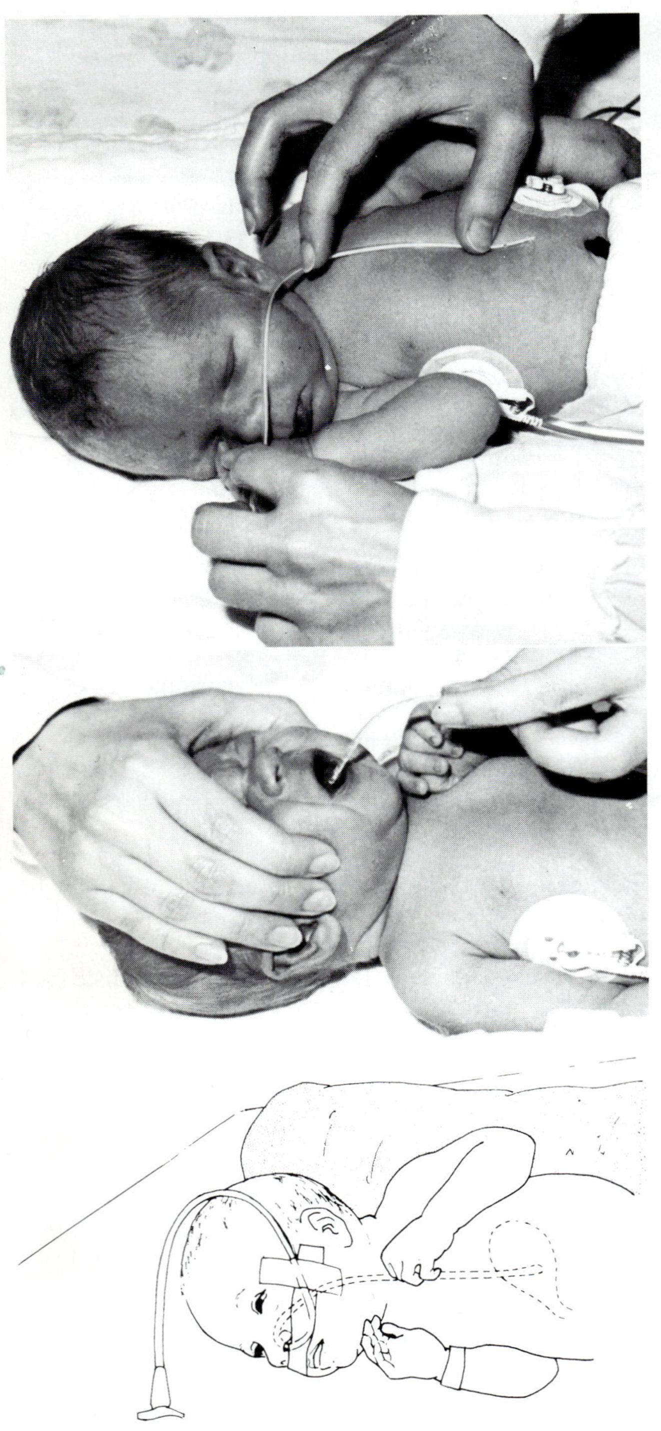

Fig. 18-4 Gavage feeding. (From Bobak IM, Jensen MD: *Maternity and gynecologic nursing,* ed 5, St. Louis, 1993, Mosby.)

Thermoregulation

The maintenance of body temperature is a challenge in the care of the premature infant. Because of the immaturity of the temperature-regulating center in the brain, stability may be difficult to sustain. The infant must be placed in a controlled thermal enviroment to assist in the maintenance of thermoregulation. Heart rate, respirations, and temperature are monitored closely with an alarm system that indicates when vital signs are above or below preset limits. It is essential to check vital signs periodically and compare them with the monitor readings. An open radiant warmer bed or an enclosed plastic incubator is used. Refer to Chapters 16 and 17 for additional information on regulating temperature.

Maintaining oxygenation

Oxygen levels above that of room air (21%) may be required to meet the infant's metabolic needs. The most accurate way to evaluate an infant's oxygen status is through the use of intermittent arterial blood gas determinations. Although some infants may approach oxygen toxicity levels when the environmental oxygen reaches 40%, others with diminished respiratory function will need higher levels of environmental oxygen to achieve correct blood concentrations. Environmental oxygen concentrations, together with blood gas analyses, are important. Monitoring these elements helps evaluate the infant's general condition in response to therapy and to prevent blindness or visual loss, called retrolental fibroplasia (RLF). RLF can be produced by extended exposure to high oxygen concentrations in the blood, causing the immature blood vessels in the retinas of the eyes to hemorrhage. The retinas partially or completely detach from the inner surfaces of the eyes' posterior chambers. The retinas then become fibrous masses behind the lenses, unable to receive visual stimuli.

Immaturity of the respiratory system is common in premature infants. Some of these infants require a ventilator to assist them with breathing. Failure of lung tissue to expand, or atelectasis, is frequently reported. Respiratory distress syndrome (RDS) is common in several neonatal disorders (e.g., hypoglycemia, hypovolemia, congenital heart disease, and cerebral hemorrhage). RDS is the most common cause of death in premature infants. The disorder is rare in infants of narcotic-addicted mothers or infants who have been subjected to intrauterine stress (maternal hypertension or preeclampsia). RDS is discussed further in Chapter 19.

Prevention of infection

Preemies are deprived of the antibody protection that crosses the placenta in the third trimester of pregnancy. They are also less prepared to manufacture their own antibodies. Thus they are at increased risk for infection. Handwashing is the best method of preventing infection. Refer to Chapters 19 and 31 for further information regarding the effect of infectious disease on the fetus and newborn.

Infant stimulation

Optimal interaction with the neonate occurs when the neonate is in the quiet/alert state. Overhandling of the infant should be avoided through observation of behavioral cues (e.g., crying, irritability, splaying of hands). Premature infants are particularly susceptible to injury at the time of birth and may have experienced an intraventricular hemorrhage (IVH) and resultant neurological sequelae. For further information regarding infant stimulation, refer to Chapter 16.

Assessment for neurological sequelae

A neurodevelopmental assessment is conducted periodically to evaluate neonate movement and tone, habituation, and reflexes. Cerebral palsy, a condition characterized by impaired movement and posture, is not diagnosed until later in infancy or toddlerhood. However, early abnormal neurological signs are often identified in the nursery. The majority of children with cerebral palsy were premature or had an anoxic event in the perinatal period. Mental retardation and lack of muscular coordination may result from brain injury or prolonged lack of oxygen caused by delayed or interrupted breathing at the time of or subsequent to birth. Neurological abnormalities may also be caused by bilirubin deposits in the brain tissue, resulting from the inability of the immature liver to handle red blood cell breakdown satisfactorily. Jaundice is a significant finding, and bilirubin levels must be carefully monitored. For additional information on hyperbilirubinemia, refer to Chapters 16 and 19.

Metabolic complications

The stressed neonate is at risk for a variety of complications related to physiological functioning. Fluid and electrolyte abnormalities, including hypoglycemia, are common.

Hypoglycemia. Hypoglycemia has four classifications. See the box above right for a list of these types.

Clinical manifestations. Signs may be vague, transient, or recurrent. Cerebral signs include a high-pitched cry, jitteriness, tremors, twitching, lethargy, convulsions, and coma. Noncerebral signs include apnea, cyanosis, sweating, rapid and irregular respirations, and refusal to eat.

Treatment and nursing considerations. Preventive treatment involves early feeding of normoglycemic infants and prevention of cold stress. When hypoglycemia is identified with a plasma glucose concentration less than 40 mg/dl, oral or IV glucose is administered. Nursing care protocols based on birth weight are identified in Table 18-2. The technique for obtaining a heel stick sample for testing capillary blood glucose is discussed in Chapter 17.

CLASSIFICATION OF HYPOGLYCEMIA

CLASS I
Early transitional:
Large or normal size infants who suffer from hyperinsulinism (see Chapter 19).

CLASS II
Classic transient neonatal:
Infants who suffered intrauterine malnutrition, which depleted fat and glycogen stores.

CLASS III
Secondary hypoglycemia:
A response to perinatal stresses that increase the infant's metabolic needs related to glycogen stores.

CLASS IV
Severe, recurrent hypoglycemia:
Caused by metabolic-endocrine or enzymatic defects.

Inborn Errors of Metabolism

Congenital hypothyroidism

Inadequate production of thyroid hormones may be due to congenital hypothyroidism, agenesis of the thyroid gland, or other genetic disorders of the thyroid. Delayed treatment of thyroid disorders results in irreversible mental retardation and developmental and physical disabilities.

Clinical manifestations. Clinical signs of hypothyroidism develop gradually in the infant and may not appear until the infant is several months of age or older.

Typically the affected baby has a large tongue that protrudes from the mouth, causing problems in feeding. Other manifestations in untreated children include a hoarse cry, dry skin, coarse hair, constipation, and growth retardation.

Diagnosis and treatment. The degree of mental retardation depends on the time of diagnosis and the initiation of treatment. If hypothyroidism is diagnosed early and hormone replacement therapy is initiated, the infant's growth usually progresses normally. Routine newborn screening occurs in all 50 states. Screening includes thyroxine (T_4) and thyroid-stimulating hormone (TSH) blood analyses. Early screening, diag-

◆ TABLE 18-2
Nursing Care Protocols

Age (hours)	Dextrostix	Hematocrit
I. LGA >4250 gm (9 lbs, 6 oz) and postterm >42 weeks by dates or assessment		
ASAP	X	—
1	X	—
3	X	—
6	X	X
9	X	—
12	X	—
24	X	—
II. SGA <2500 gm (send cord blood for IGM and urine for CMV)		
ASAP	X	—
1	X	—
3	X	—
6	X	X
9	X	—
12	X	—
24	X	—
III. Preterm by dates or assessment		
ASAP	X	—
1	X	—
3	X	—
6	X	X
IV. IDM		
ASAP	X	—
1	X	—
3	X	—
6	X	X
12	X (+ calcium level)	—
24	X	—
9	X	—
12	X	—
24	X	—

IGM,; CMV, cytomegalovirus; IDM, infant of a diabetic mother.

nosis, and treatment of hypothyroidism reduces the incidence of thyroid problems and resultant mental retardation.

Phenylketonuria

Phenylketonuria (PKU) affects 1 in every 10,000 to 15,000 live births and is a significant cause of mental retardation. This disorder primarily affects Caucasians and is rarely seen in people of African, Japanese, or Jewish descent. PKU is produced by an inherited error in the metabolism of an essential amino acid or protein (phenylalanine). PKU is an autosomal-recessive trait.

Diagnosis and treatment. Phenylalanine hydroxylase, which catalyzes the conversion of the essential amino acid phenylalanine to tyrosine, is absent in the liver of PKU-affected infants. Unless appropriate measures are taken, phenylalanine builds up in the bloodstream and after 1 to 3 months the toxic effects begin to produce brain damage. A high level of phenylalanine can be detected in the blood serum of the newborn infant. A few weeks are usually needed before urinary phenylketones present. The detection of PKU is achieved by mandatory screening of newborn blood. Measurement of blood phenylalanine (the Guthrie test) should be done after 72 hours of life. Because of early discharge from the hospital, however, the American Academy of Pediatrics and American College of Obstetricians and Gynecologists (1992) recommend that (1) the test be performed on all newborns before they leave the nursery, regardless of age, and (2) a repeat blood specimen be obtained by the third week of life from all infants in whom the initial specimen was taken within the first 24 hours of life.

Treatment of PKU is dietary. Phenylalanine cannot be eliminated because it is an esential amino acid for tissue growth. The criteria for dietary management include maintaining phenylalanine levels within a safe range and meeting the child's nutritional needs for optimal growth. Specially prepared milk substitutes, such as Lofenalac or PKU-1, are instituted to maintain plasma levels of phenylalanine between 2 and 8 mg/dl. Because of the low phenylalanine content of breast milk, total or partial breastfeeding may be allowed with close monitoring of phenylalanine levels. Mental retardation can be prevented without impairment of physical growth when dietary restriction of phenylalanine is initiated before the infant is 30 days old.

Nursing Alert

The sweetener aspartame (Nutrasweet) must be avoided because of its conversion to phenylalanine in the body.

Galactosemia

Galactosemia, a rare inherited disorder of carbohydrate metabolism, is another cause of mental retardation. In addition, it can produce a failure to thrive, liver disease, and cataracts in untreated children.

Diagnosis and treatment. This autosomal-recessive trait, in which an hepatic enzyme is absent, prevents the conversion of galactose to glucose. A galactose-free diet must be initiated immediately after birth. All milk and galactose-containing foods, including breast milk, must be eliminated from the diet. Strict adherence to the diet is critical for the first 7 to 8 years of life, followed by a modified regimen throughout life.

Nursing Alert

Many drugs, such as penicillin, contain lactose as fillers and must be avoided by children with galactosemia.

Birth Injuries

Birth injuries occur more frequently with breech presentation, when the infant is large, with the use of forceps, and if the practitioner is inexperienced. Normal variations of birth injuries, which are secondary to birth trauma and require no medical or nursing intervention, are discussed in Chapter 16.

Intracranial or intraventricular hemorrhage

The most common type of birth injury that produces serious trauma is intracranial hemorrhage or intraventricular hemorrhage (IVH). As noted previously, it is most often seen in premature infants but can be diagnosed in full-term babies as well.

Clinical manifestations. Signs of IVH manifest suddenly or gradually and may vary according to the location and extent of the hemorrhage. These signs include irritability, listlessness, cyanosis, marked irregular respiration, varying degrees of paralysis, and a lack of appetite. IVH also is evidenced in asymmetrical primitive reflexes including a poor sucking reflex, twitching, tremors, stupor, apnea, seizures, projectile vomiting, unequally dilated pupils, tense or bulging fontanels, separated sutures, and a high, shrill cry. These symptoms may arise from any etiology that increases pressure within the cranium, such as intracranial abscess, cerebral edema, tumors, or developing hydrocephalus.

Diagnosis. Diagnosis is usually made through the history and observation of the infant by computed ultrasonography or computed tomography (CT). The bleeding may be mild and stop spontaneously, thus the child recovers with few or no effects. Conversely, cranial pressure may be so intense that it must be relieved by aspiration of the subdural space or by surgery. Intense pressure may lead to permanent brain damage or death.

Treatment and nursing considerations. The infant is usually placed in an incubator with his or her head slightly elevated in an attempt to relieve pressure. Rarely, a spinal tap may be done to relieve pressure or as a diagnostic aid. Ventilatory support is provided and the acid-base balance is monitored closely. Vitamin K may be prescribed to relieve bleeding tendencies. Sedatives may be ordered to promote relaxation and prevent increased intracranial pressure. Anticonvulsants may also be ordered to prevent seizures. It is important for the nurse observing the infant to be able to assess and accurately describe the type of tremor, convulsion, or abnormal behavior pattern observed. A description of the part of the body affected, unilateral or bilateral, how long the episode lasted, and what event, if anything, occurred just before may help to localize the area of bleeding. Pressure-producing procedures, such as overstimulation or unnecessary suctioning, should be avoided.

Facial paralysis

Temporary or permanent facial paralysis may result from injury to cranial nerve VII during delivery. Facial paralysis may be caused by forceps pressure or pressure in the birth canal. Loss of movement on the affected side, inability to completely close the eye, drooping of a corner of the mouth, and the absence of a wrinkling forehead are observed (Fig. 18-5). This condition requires no medical intervention and usually disappears spontaneously within a few days to several months.

Erb Palsy (Erb-Duchenne paralysis)

Injury to the brachial plexus, the network of nerves that innervates the upper extremities, alters the normal

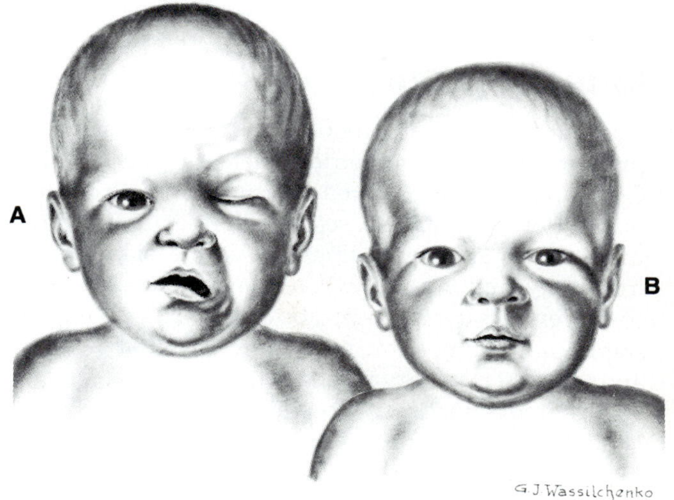

Fig. 18-5 **A,** Paralysis of right side of face 15 minutes after forceps delivery. **B,** Same infant 24 hours later. (From Wong D: *Essentials of pediatric nursing,* ed 4, St. Louis, 1993, Mosby.)

position of the arm, shoulder, and neck. The arm hangs limp and is internally rotated with the wrist pronated. With this condition the Moro reflex is asymmetrical. The infant cannot raise his or her arm. Treatment involves immobilizing the arm in an abducted, externally rotated position with flexion at the elbow. This injury is usually not permanent and resolves within 3 months.

HYDROCEPHALUS

Hydrocephalus is a condition caused by an imbalance in the production and absorption of cerebrospinal fluid (CSF) in the ventricular system. Prenatal diagnosis is having an impact on the prevalence of neural tube defects. The incidence of hydrocephalus, however, is currently 5.8 for every 10,000 births.

Types

Hydrocephalus has a variety of causes. The condition may result from an impairment of the circulation of CSF within the ventricular system. This may be a congenital, structural defect or may result from a space-occupying lesion within the ventricular system. This type of obstruction produces what is known as noncommunicative hydrocephalus (obstructive hydrocephalus), indicating that the impairment of flow is within the ventricular system. Occasionally the impairment is within the subarachnoid space; therefore CSF communicates from the ventricles to the subarachnoid space but cannot reach its primary sites of reabsorption in the arachnoid villi. This form of hydrocephalus is called communicating hydrocephalus, occurring subsequent to intracranial hemorrhage or infection.

Early Recognition and Treatment

Infants respond to mounting cerebrospinal fluid pressure by an asymmetrical increase in head size. Other manifestations noted shortly after birth include bulging of the fontanels, separation of cranial sutures, distended scalp veins, thinning of the skull bones, irritability, and vomiting. A downward displacement of the eyes (sclera visible above the iris) giving the pupils a "setting-sun" appearance, frontal bossing, and unequal pupillary response to light are later signs.

Early reduction in ventricular size is essential if the child is to have optimal neurological function and intellectual development. Hydrocephalus treatment is influenced by the degree of intracranial pressure, the level of obstruction, and any associated major congenital defects.

Hydrocephalus is usually treated by insertion of a tube or shunt that drains the ventricular fluid into a body space outside the skull. The well-being of the child depends on the continuous functioning of the shunt. The most commonly used shunt systems are the ventriculoperitoneal and lumboperitoneal shunts. When a ventriculoperitoneal or lumboperitoneal shunt can no longer function correctly, a ventriculoatrial shunt is used. Most shunt systems consist of a ventricular catheter, a flush pump, a unidirectional flow valve, and a distal catheter.

Ventriculoperitoneal shunt

A ventricular catheter is inserted into the lateral ventricle through a small burr hole. The distal catheter is passed beneath the skin, down the neck, and may tunnel across the front of the chest to enter the abdominal cavity. The ventriculoperitoneal (VP) shunt is the most commonly used shunt in infants because several inches of additional tubing can be placed in the abdominal cavity to allow for growth (Fig. 18-6).

Lumboperitoneal shunt

A proximal catheter is placed in the lumbar subarachnoid space. The distal catheter passes from the lumbar subarachnoid space to the peritoneum and empties into the peritoneal cavity, as does the ventriculoperitoneal shunt. The lumboperitoneal shunt is used

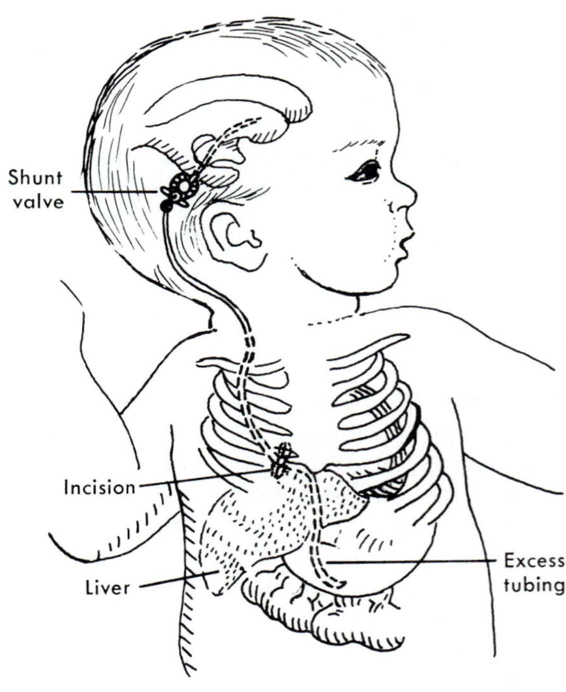

Fig. 18-6 Ventriculoperitoneal shunt drains cerebral spinal fluid from ventricles of brain into peritoneal cavity where it is absorbed.

with those forms of hydrocephalus in which there is a communication between the lumbar subarachnoid space and the ventricular system. The advantages of the lumboperitoneal shunt are that it avoids surgery in the cranium and it has a lower incidence of infection. It also requires less revision as the child grows. If the spinal subarachnoid space is spacious enough to accept shunt tubing, the lumboperitoneal shunt is used.

Ventriculoatrial shunt

The insertion of tubes and valves that allow one-way flow of fluid has led to the successful shunting of cerebrospinal fluid into the right atrium, and the peritoneal cavity. A burr hole is made in the skull, and a small tube is directed into the lateral ventricle of the brain. Through a small neck incision the cardiac tube is inserted into the right atrium by way of the internal jugular vein (Fig. 18-7). Both VP and ventriculoatrial (VA) shunts are connected to the reservoir behind the ear and are entirely covered with skin. Under normal operating conditions, CSF flow is unobstructed. The flushing devices differ with the various tubes used. In the Pudenz-Mishler double-lumen device, both the ventricular and distal tubes are flushed when the reservoir is compressed. Obstruction of the ventricular tube, the most common cause of shunt malfunction, may be cleared by occluding the easily felt distal catheter with finger pressure and compressing the reservoir. Thus the flushing device serves a dual purpose; it flushes and monitors the operation of the entire system.

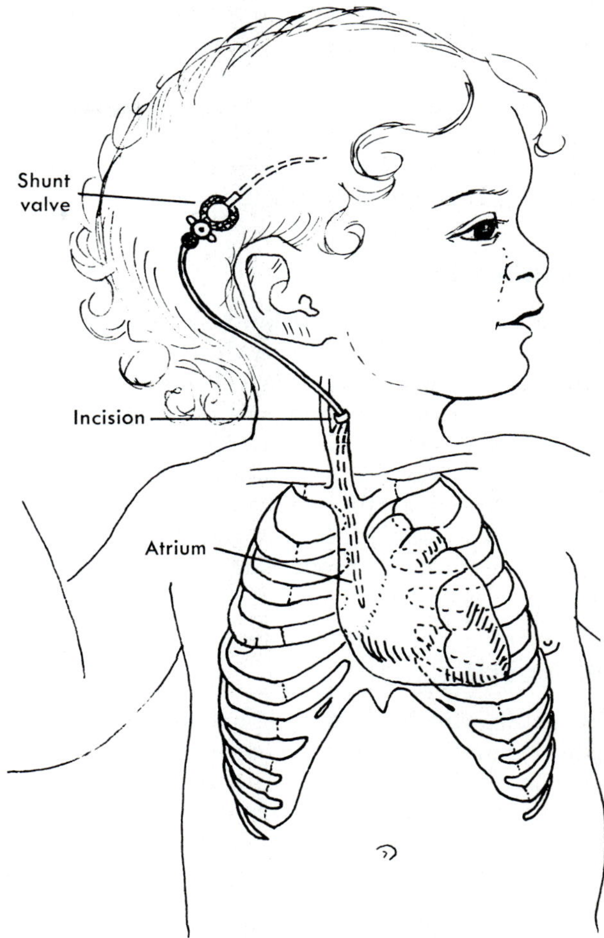

Fig. 18-7 Ventriculoatrial shunt drains cerebrospinal fluid from ventricles of brain to right atrium.

Nursing Alert

Intravenous infusions should not be placed in a scalp vein of a child with hydrocephalus if surgery is anticipated.

Postoperative care

When the infant is wide awake, dextrose in water is offered by mouth. If it is tolerated, breast milk or formula may be given. It is important that the nurse observes the baby before the shunting procedure to compare and evaluate his or her postoperative condition. To avoid respiratory complications the child must have a position change at least every 2 hours. The head should be placed to avoid pressure on the cranial wound, which might predispose the skin to breakdown. The fontanel should be less tense and slightly depressed. If the fontanels are sunken the child is kept flat. If the fontanels are full or bulging the head is elevated. Pulse and respiration determinations and pupil equality checks are done frequently. The nurse must constantly be alert for any signs of increased intracranial pressure, such as slowed pulse and respirations, lethargy, irritability, vomiting, and tense fontanels. Head circumference should be measured daily at the widest diameter. Any abnormalities detected during these observations, such as signs of faulty functioning of the flushing device or an elevated temperature indicating a postoperative infection, should be recorded carefully and immediately called to the attention of the attending physician.

Wide swings in body temperature, tremors or convulsions, lack of appetite, or vomiting may occur. The tension of fontanels and other signs of increasing intracranial pressure should be checked daily. Attention must be given to preventing pressure sores on the scalp by frequent turning and soft pillow supports. When not being supervised directly, the child should be positioned on his or her side, with the head turned to the side to prevent aspiration. Support for the head must always be given during feedings, and the nurse may find it more comfortable for the infant and for caregiving to support the head with pillows. After feeding and burping, overstimulation should be avoided to prevent vomiting. Malnutrition and infection are ongoing problems for these infants.

Complications

Shunt infection is the most serious complication and can occur at any time. Massive doses of intravenous antibiotics are then administered. Persistent infection, however, requires shunt removal. External CSF drainage is used until the CSF is sterile. Other problems include obstruction of the shunt system tubing by debris at the ventricular end, thrombus formation at the cardiac end, and adhesion formation at the peritoneal end. Methods of preventing these problems are currently being studied.

Prognosis

Surgically treated hydrocephalus with ongoing medical and neurosurgical management has a survival rate of approximately 80%, with the highest rate of mortality occurring within the first postoperative year. Of the survivors, one half have neurological disabilities and one third are neurologically and intellectually normal.

SPINA BIFIDA

Spina bifida is a term used to describe the more common congenital neural tube defects (NTD) (Figure 18-8). Spina bifida exists in varying degrees of severity. The term *spina bifida* simply means divided spine, or that a portion of the posterior wall of the spine is missing. Recent evidence supports the hypothesis that spina bifida is caused by an interaction of genetic predisposition with an essential nutrient deficiency (folic acid).

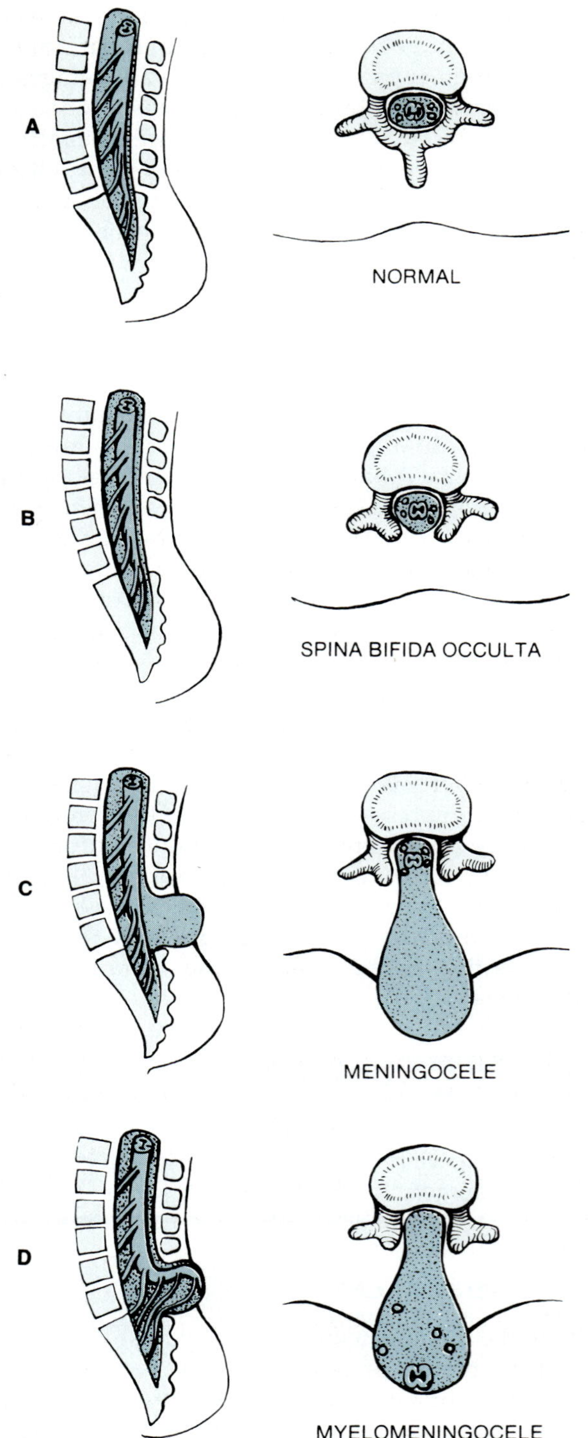

Fig. 18-8 Varying degrees of neural herniations through midline defects of the spine. (From Wong D: *Essentials of pediatric nursing,* ed 5, St. Louis, 1993, Mosby.)

Diagnosis

Spina bifida is identifiable in utero through analyses of amniotic fluid. Most states now require that the maternal alpha-fetoprotein (AFP) serum detection test be offered to women between 16 and 18 weeks' gestation.

Types

The defect may be so small that it offers no difficulty and is discovered only when an x-ray examination of the spine is done for other reasons. This type of defect is called spina bifida occulta or hidden divided spine. The spina bifida occulta detected by x-ray examination is without symptoms in 25% of the cases. However, there is a syndrome of spina bifida occulta in which not only this radiological abnormality is noted, but varying degrees of orthopedic deformities or urinary tract dysfunction are also seen. This is caused by pressure on the nerve roots on the lower part of the spine or pressure on the lower spinal cord itself. Such a condition is diagnosed with spinal ultrasonography in infancy.

Another form of this disorder is termed *spina bifida cystica* because it exhibits a cystlike structure. There are two kinds of spina bifida cystica. A meningocele involves a protrusion of only the covering meninges of the spinal cord and CSF. The child usually develops normal urinary and intestinal control and has no paralysis. The sac, until removed, is a cosmetic problem and its possible injury always poses the problem of infection of the nervous system. The second and more serious kind of spina bifida cystica is called myelomeningocele or meningomyelocele (Figs. 18-9 and 18-10). In this condition the meninges protrude through the spinal opening, and nerve tissues are also found in the herniated sac. Since spina bifida cystica occurs early in the pregnancy with a poor migration of the nerves involved in the defect, there are varying degrees of weakness of the legs, sensory disturbance, and impairment of rectal and urinary sphincter function. If the lesion is high in the spine the degree of paralysis is severe. If it is low, for instance, in the sacral spine only, the child has minimal weakness of the lower extremities but significant urinary and bowel control problems. Hydrocephalus is frequently seen in patients with myelomeningocele, depending on the position of the myelomeningocele in the spinal canal. Thus infants with myelomeningocele at a thoracic level have a 90% to 95% incidence of hydrocephalus. Those with a sacral myelomeningocele have a 45% incidence of hydrocephalus.

Nursing Considerations

The goals of nursing care of the child with myelomeningocele include preventing damage to the myelomeningocele sac, preventing complications, providing postoperative care, and providing education and support of the family.

Before surgery the sac, or mass as it is sometimes called, must be protected from injury and infection. To protect the sac, the child is positioned on his or her abdomen. To avoid putting strain or pressure on the sac, the nurse must be extremely careful in lifting the infant. Changing linens is best accomplished by two care providers. Slipping hands and forearms, palms up, under the infant's leg and chest area to grasp the opposite thigh, arm, and shoulder is a safe, effective way of lifting and supporting the infant. The other provider quickly changes the bed. A positioning device called a Bradford frame, a metal framework that rests on the bed and elevates the baby on a divided, padded canvas support, may be used. Diapering the infant is contraindicated before surgical repair and advanced healing. For feeding the infant's head is turned to one side.

Meticulous skin care must be given and pressure areas prevented. To prevent drying, a sterile, moist, nonadherent, saline dressing is applied over the defect. Moist dressings are changed every 2 to 4 hours. An antibiotic soak may also be used. A foam rubber ring with a hole large enough to surround the sac may be placed over the sterile compresses and anchored in place with strips of tape or bandage. A protective covering forms a roof over the opening and must not come in contact with the sac. The sac should be observed for variance in size and tenseness, as well as ulceration. Any leaking of fluid should be reported immediately. The frontooccipital circumference of a child with myelomeningocele is measured daily to detect a developing hydrocephalus. The sensation and movement of the lower extremities are evaluated while care is given.

Postoperative Care

Treatment depends on the size, location, and condition of the sac. Surgical closure is usually planned within the first 24 to 48 hours. Nursing care includes monitoring vital signs, monitoring intake and output, providing nourishment, and observing closely for signs of infection. After a surgical-flap procedure the prone position is maintained, at least until the sutures are removed. Some neurosurgeons allow a sidelying position, which facilitates feeding and allows some mobility.

Although surgery may not improve function, it improves the child's appearance and facilitates care. In these patients the effects of gravity, the lack of supportive muscles and uneven growth make a straight spine difficult to achieve. Other orthopedic anomalies may accompany this defect, including congenital hip dislocation or talipes equinovarus. This condition then requires additional, early intervention.

Complications

Urinary tract complications are frequently seen in the majority of these children with neurogenic bladders. The risks and consequences of inadequate blad-

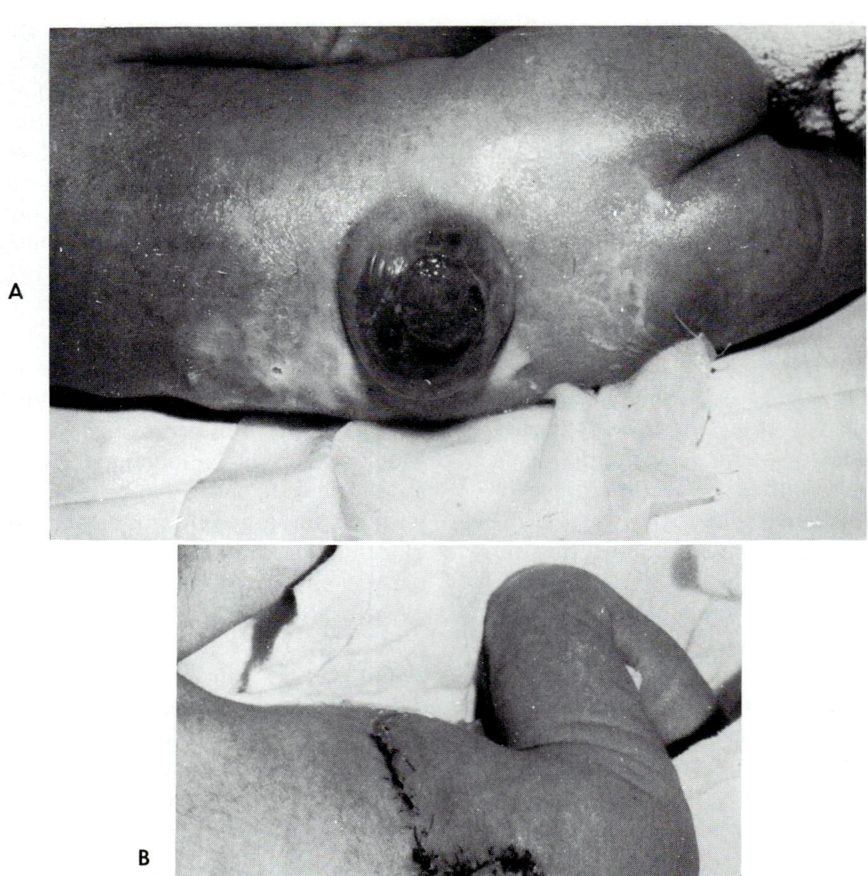

Fig. 18-9 **A,** Myelomeningocele before surgery (An antibacterial dressing was used.). **B,** Repair of same patient. (Courtesy Gleason MC, San Diego, CA.)

der drainage far exceed those of infection. Intermittent catheterization, several times a day, has become a standard intervention. Parents are taught clean, intermittent catheterization techniques when the child is diagnosed and the child is taught self-catheterization during the early elementary school years, if possible. This important technique provides continence, self-care, and improved self-esteem.

Long-term care

The care of a patient with spina bifida, complicated by a herniation of nerve tissue elements, continues for life. The child needs psychological and emotional support, as well as assistance in physical care. To meet the long-term specialized needs of these children and their families, many schools and communities have developed multidisciplinary educational programs and clinics.

Nursing Alert

If multivitamins containing folic acid are taken during the first six weeks of pregnancy, the occurrence of neural tube defects is reduced by 50%.

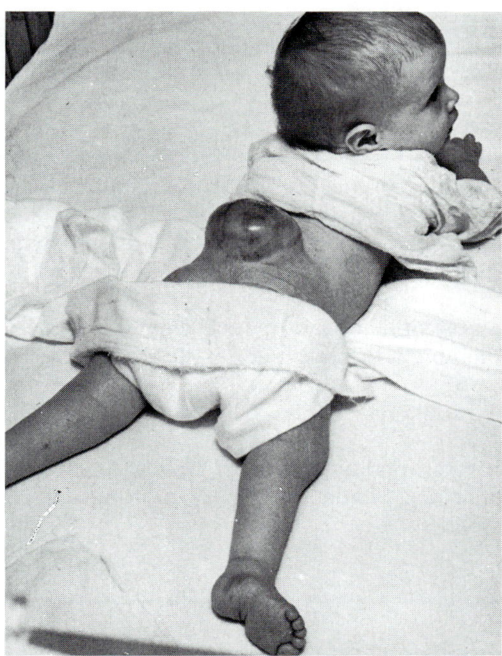

Fig. 18-10 This youngster's myelomeningocele was repaired shortly after photograph was taken. (Courtesy Children's Hospital and Health Center, San Diego, CA.)

KEY ELEMENTS OF FAMILY-CENTERED CARE

Recognizing that the family is the constant in a child's life, whereas the service systems and personnel within those systems fluctuate.

Facilitating parent/professional collaboration at all levels of health care, including care of an individual child; program development, implementation, and evaluation; and policy formation.

Honoring the racial, ethnic, cultural, and socioeconomic diversity of families.

Recognizing family strengths and individuality, and respecting different methods of coping.

Sharing with parents complete and unbiased information on a continuing basis and in a supportive manner.

Encouraging and facilitating family-to-family support and networking.

Understanding and incorporating the developmental needs of infants, children, and adolescents and their families into health care systems.

Implementing comprehensive policies and programs that provide emotional and financial support to meet the needs of families.

Designing accessible health care systems that are flexible, culturally competent, and responsive to family-identified needs.

From National Center for Family-Centered Care, Association for the Care of Children's Health, Bethesda, MD, 1990.

Developmental Disabilities

Several studies have indicated that approximately 15% of all infants manifest developmental delay. Developmental disabilities are associated with conditions such as prematurity, asphyxia, hydrocephalus, meningomyelocele, cerebral palsy, phenylketonuria, and mental retardation of an undefined origin. Delayed achievement of developmental milestones may occur in the fine motor, gross motor, language, and/or the personal-social areas. Emphasis is on early identification to minimize long-term problems and to foster optimal growth and development. The adoption of Public Law 94-142 (the Education of All Handicapped Children Act of 1975), Public Law 99-457 (the Education of the Handicapped Act Amendments of 1986), and the Americans with Disabilities Act (ADA) of 1990 have provided opportunities for normalization for children with special needs. These laws provide the right to equal educational opportunity. A multidisciplinary assessment and plan to meet the individual child's educational, developmental, and health care needs are provided with this legislation, thus allowing mainstreaming into the school setting and care in the home. As a result of this emphasis on family-centered care and empowering families, institutionalization of affected children is less common (see the box above right). The nurse assumes a primary role in the assessment, planning, and follow-up of the special needs of child and family.

Mental Retardation

Mental retardation affects approximately 2% of the general population. Good prenatal and delivery care helps prevent some of the possible causes (e.g., birth injury, asphyxia). Some types of mental retardation can be prevented through genetic counseling or treated with hormonal therapy or dietary supervision.

Approximately 15% of retardation instances result from brain injury associated with birth or from infection in utero. Another 5% are caused by chromosomal abnormality such as Down syndrome or specific single gene defects such as PKU. The remainder, or about 85%, result from unfavorable polygenetic combinations from the general gene pool. This group accounts for most of the milder forms of retardation. The more severe forms are usually caused by brain injury, chromosomal abnormalities, or single gene factors producing metabolical disorders.

◆ **TABLE 18-3**
Intelligence Classifications*

Classification	Intelligence Quotient (IQ)	Performance Level
Profound retardation	0-24	Unable to attend to personal needs; always requires supervision; 0- to 2-year-old intellectual ability.
Severe retardation	25-50	May be trained to meet personal needs but not self-sustaining; 3- to 7-year-old intellectual ability (trainable mentally retarded).
Moderately severe retardation	50-79	Self-sustaining in simple jobs with supervision; 8- to 11-year-old intellectual ability (educable mentally retarded).
Dull normal	79-89	Majority of the population.
Average	90-110	
Above average	110-130	
Gifted	130-150	May have problems in adjustment; emphasizing that both social competence and intellectual ability contribute to individual success in society.
Genius	150 and above	

*One of many classifications of intelligence used.

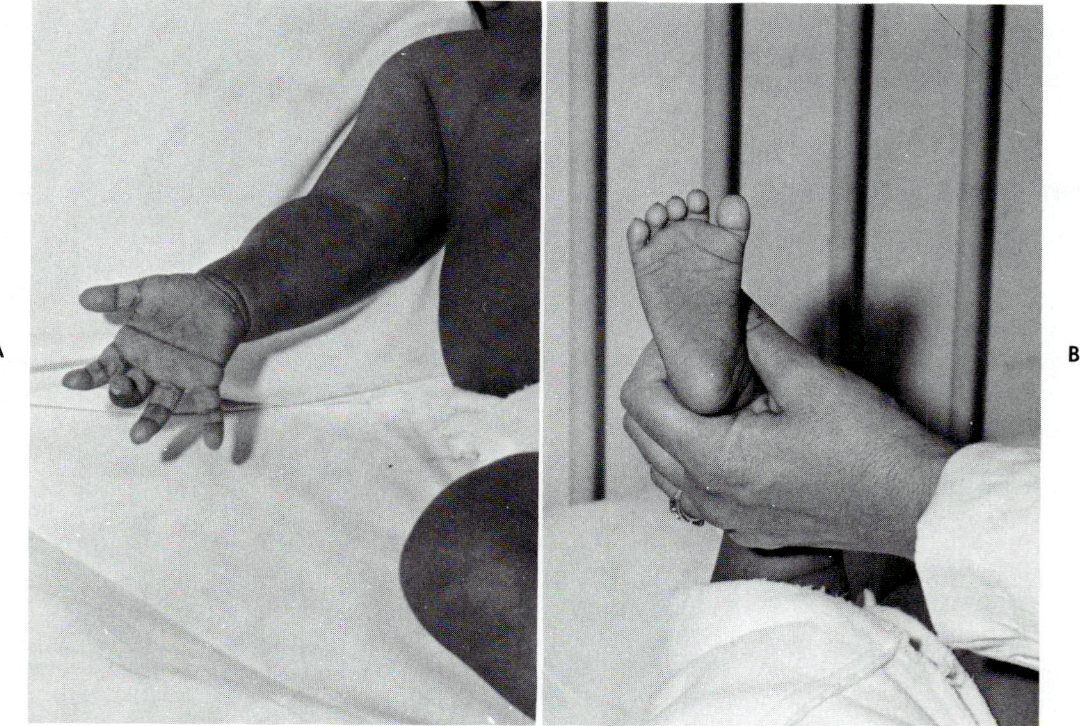

Fig. 18-11 **A,** Hand of infant with Down syndrome. Note deep, straight palmar crease (simian line). **B,** Same infant's foot. Note exaggerated space between big and little toes. (Courtesy Naval Hospital, San Diego, CA.)

Intelligence classification

Because of the many problems found in trying to determine a person's intellectual capacity by testing devices, the concept of IQ, or intelligence quotient, has lost much of its former significance. The mental age score attained by an individual in testing may be influenced by motivation and environment, as well as the test presentation itself. Nevertheless, IQ scores are still often obtained. They represent a special testing score (termed *mental age*), divided by the individual's chronological age, multiplied by 100. Table 18-3 demonstrates the ranges of IQ, indicating various degrees of intelligence.

Down syndrome

Down syndrome occurs in 1 in 650 live births. It is associated with certain physical characteristics. The most common type of Down syndrome, "standard trisomy 21," is associated with an abnormal chromosome count in all of the infant's body cells. Retardation ranges from very mild to profound. Trisomy 21 is found most often in the offspring of women over the age of 40. The translocation type of Down syndrome may be hereditary and occurs in younger women. For discussion of other genetic syndromes, refer to Chapter 20.

Clinical manifestations. Infants with Down syndrome are usually identified in the nursery, but some are diagnosed later. Characteristically, these infants are short; have relatively small skulls, flattened from front to back; low birth weight; and somewhat lethargic behavior. Typical signs of Down syndrome are exaggerated epicanthic folds, which make the eyes slant up and out; short hands and fingers with the little finger bent in (clinodactyly); a deep, horizontal crease across the palm (simian crease); and a large space between the great and small toes (Fig. 18-11). An ophthalmological examination of the eyes may reveal Brushfield spots, small white dots on the iris. Decreased muscle tone and excessive joint mobility are also significant findings (Fig. 18-12).

After the newborn period, other signs manifest themselves. These include delayed eruption of teeth, fissured tongue, and retarded intellectual and physical development. These infants often have congenital heart malformations, umbilical hernias, and duodenal atresia. Most children with Down syndrome have loving, affectionate personalities.

Nursing considerations. Family-centered care, empowerment of the family through education, and utilization of school, community, and health care resources often prevents institutionalization of children with Down syndrome.

CRANIOFACIAL AND DIGESTIVE ABNORMNALITIES

Craniosynostosis

Other rare congenital deformities of the skull may be evident at birth or soon after. The sutures of the skull may prematurely close (craniosynostosis), causing abnormal pressure on the brain; an asymmetrical, distorted appearance of the head; and possible mental retardation if unrelieved. This cranial deformity is managed with surgical release of the closed sutures.

Very rarely a child may be born without a developed brain and lack the typical cranial covering. This condition is termed *anencephaly* and is fatal.

Cleft Lip and Cleft Palate

Cleft lip (CL) and cleft palate are common congenital malformations. The incidence of CL with or without cleft palate is 1 in 1000 live births. The incidence of cleft palate alone occurs in 1 in 2500 live births. These facial malformations occur secondary to an interruption in embryonic development, causing a failure of the maxillary and median nasal structures to fuse. The cause appears to have a mixed genetic and environmental basis. CL is found more often in males, whereas females more often have cleft palates.

Clinical manifestations

CL may vary from a simple notching of the vermilion border of the lip to a deep cleft, extending through the lip to or into the nose. It may exist unilaterally or bilaterally (Fig. 18-13).

Treatment and nursing considerations

Special feeding problems are created by the CL and cleft palate deformities. The major problem, however, is the severe, emotional reaction of the parents to the infant's appearance. For this reason CL is usually repaired at 6 to 10 weeks of age. A second repair may be necessary when the child is 4 or 5 years of age to correct scar irregularities and nasal asymmetry.

A cleft palate may constitute a lack of fusion of only part of the hard or soft palate or may extend along the entire roof of the mouth. Cleft palate is repaired at about 12 to 18 months of age to take advantage of palatal growth.

Before discharge from the newborn nursery the parents must receive detailed instructions about the infant's care and have several opportunities to feed the infant with supervision. The infant with a cleft palate sometimes has difficulty sucking normally, since the child cannot create the necessary vacuum in the mouth. The child may be fed slowly with a rubber-tipped medicine dropper or syringe, no faster than the infant's capacity to swallow. A specially molded cleft palate nipple that makes effective sucking possible may be used. Occasionally, soft, long lamb's nipples are tried. The child may also be fed from the end of a small spoon. Sometimes the defect is so small that a regularly shaped, soft nipple may be used (Fig. 18-14). The infant is fed in an upright

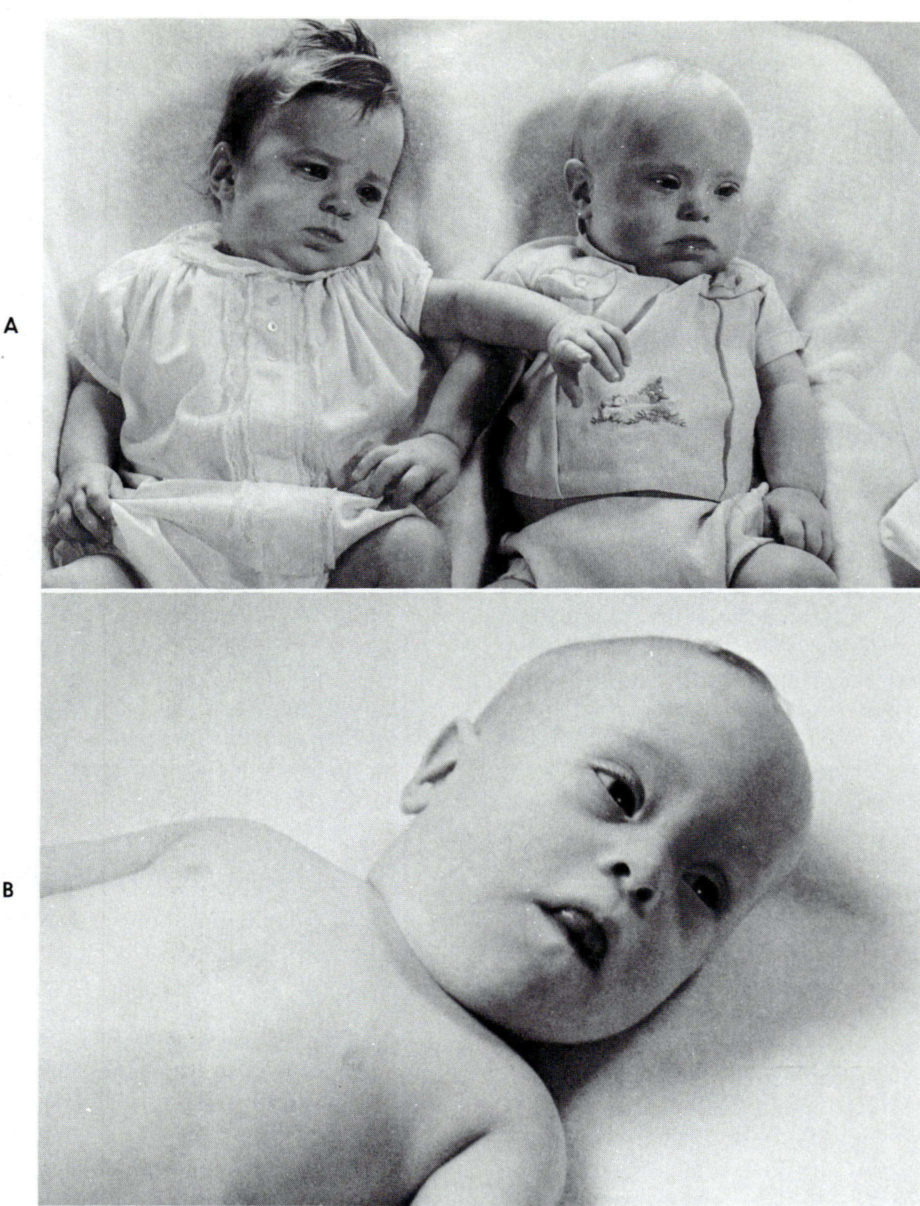

Fig. 18-12 **A,** These children are brother and sister (fraternal twins). Boy manifests Down syndrome; his sister is unaffected. **B,** Close-up of the male twin. Note the large tongue and the eyes typical of the syndrome.

position to help prevent aspiration and regurgitation through the nose. Since these infants swallow more air than usual, they should be burped frequently. This lessens the possibility of emesis or unattended "wet burps" and subsequent aspiration. Children with cleft palate are fitted early in life with a prosthesis to guard against nasal regurgitation, aid in the formation of speech patterns, and maintain anatomical relationships important to the final repair. The success of plastic surgery depends on the extent of the defect, the developmental stage of the individual, the repair techniques available, the skill of the surgeon, the standard of nursing care, and the involvement of the parents. A cleft palate is difficult to repair, and the child may have to undergo several procedures at different ages.

Postoperative care of the child with cleft lip

After surgery for CL the infant's arms should be restrained to prevent damage to the suture line. (Elbow

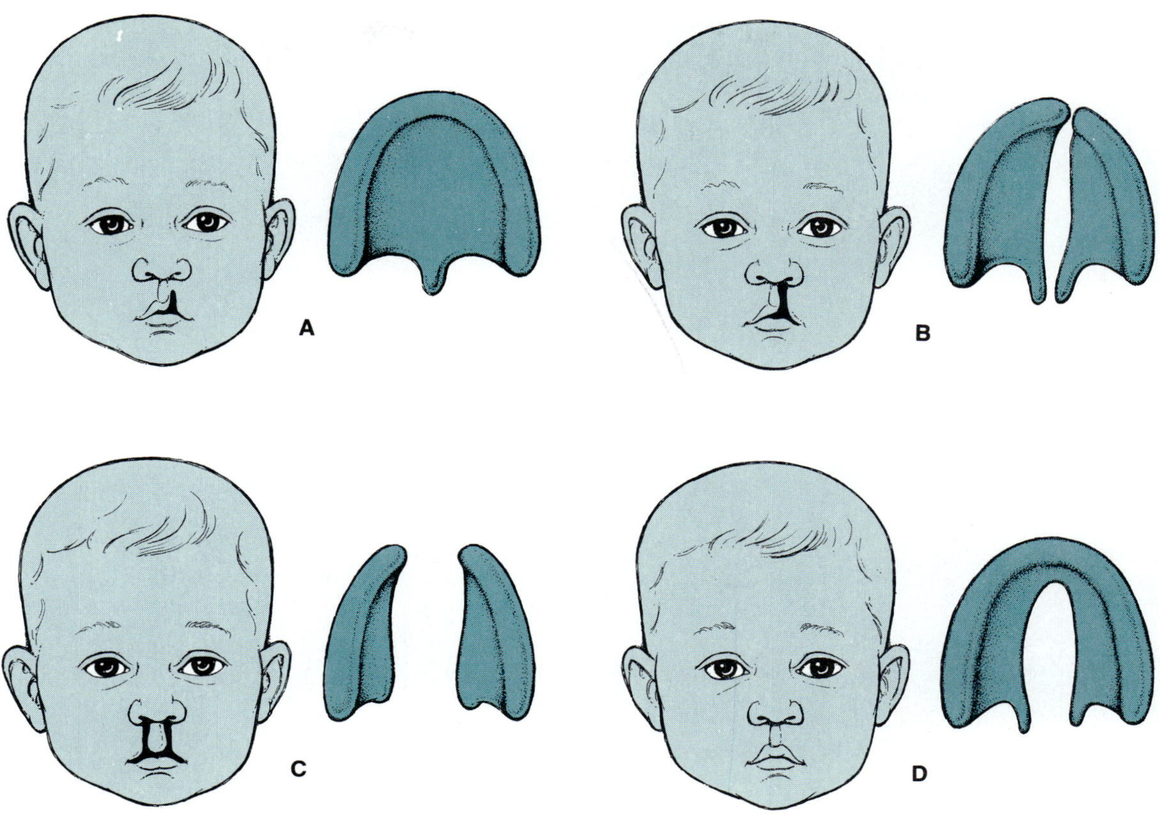

Fig. 18-13 Variations in clefts of the lip and palate at birth. **A,** Notch at vermilion border. **B,** Unilateral cleft lip and palate. **C,** Bilateral cleft lip and palate. **D,** Cleft palate. (From Wong D: *Essentials of pediatric nursing,* ed 4, St. Louis, 1993, Mosby.)

restraints may be used to prevent the infant from pulling on the suture lines.) At least every 2 hours, restraints should be removed one at a time to provide needed exercise and inspection of the arms. Placing the baby upright in an infant seat also helps protect the suture line from trauma.

The suture line should be kept clean and no crust should be allowed to form, since crusting can enlarge the scar. Various solutions are used for cleaning, depending on the surgeon's preference. Tightly wrapped, sterile cotton applicators saturated with warm, sterile water, or physiological saline solution may be gently applied to remove the blood or crust. Soaking the area for a brief period with a saturated applicator or sponge before any motion over the area is attempted helps considerably. Afterward the lip should be gently dried. An antibiotic ointment may then be applied to the suture line.

Every effort should be made to keep the child happy. A happy child cries less and puts less strain on the repair. The parents should be encouraged to cuddle the infant and participate in feedings with supervision. Water is offered first, and formula feedings soon follow. The child may be fed by a small medicine cup or a rubber-tipped medicine dropper and graduates to a soft nipple when sucking is allowed. Whichever method of feeding is used, the infant should be held in a sitting position, fed slowly, and carefully burped.

Postoperative care of the child with a cleft palate

A cleft palate is a more serious defect than CL, considering the impairment of function it produces. Not only is feeding difficult, involving possible problems of aspiration and dental placement, but speech is often nasalized. Infections of the respiratory tract and middle ear are common. The child who has undergone palate surgery is usually fed from a cup. Nothing is introduced into the mouth that may endanger the suture line, such as tongue depressors, straws, spoons, thermometers, or suction. Unless the child is old enough to understand and cooperate, arm restraints are necessary. The diet progresses slowly from clear liquid to full liquid. Infants over 6 months of age are slowly advanced to soft food over a period of approxi-

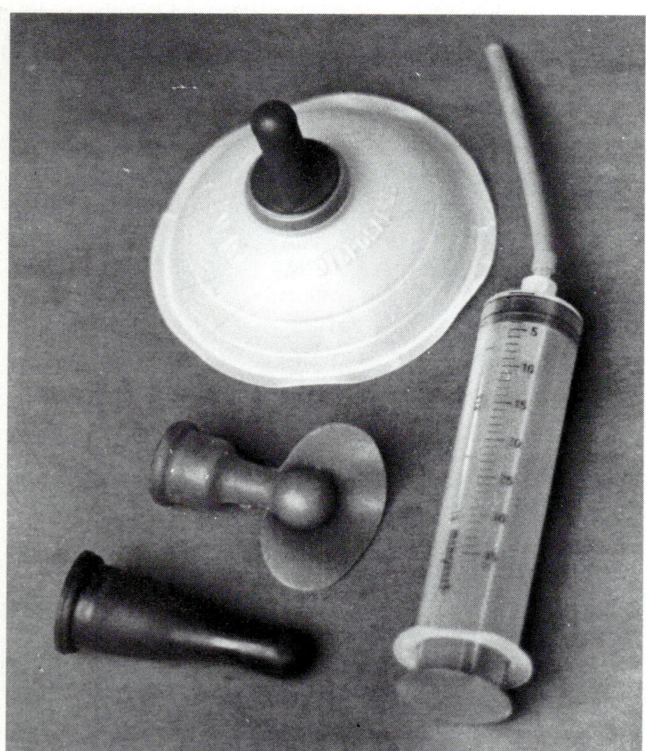

Fig. 18-14 Devices used to feed an infant with CL and cleft palate. *Clockwise,* Lamb's nipple, flanged nipple, special nurser, and syringe with rubber tubing. (From Wong D: *Essentials of pediatric nursing,* ed 4, St. Louis, 1993, Mosby.)

mately 2 weeks. The mouth should be rinsed with water at the end of a meal.

The problems of the child with CL, cleft palate, or both are so complex that a multidiciplinary team comprised of a nurse coordinator, plastic surgeon, pediatrician, orthodontist, speech pathologist, child psychologist, and medical social worker is optimal. Many hospitals, schools, and communities have parent groups that offer emotional and informational support to families, thus strengthening their coping strategies.

Other Digestive Tract Abnormalities

Serious abnormalities of the digestive tract require early diagnosis and treatment.

Esophageal atresia and tracheoesophageal fistula

Esophageal atresia refers to the congenital absence or closure of the esophagus at some point (Fig. 18-15). The upper portion usually ends in a blind pouch. Tracheoesophageal fistula (TEF) represents an open connection between the trachea and the esophagus. A frequent association exists between esophageal atresia

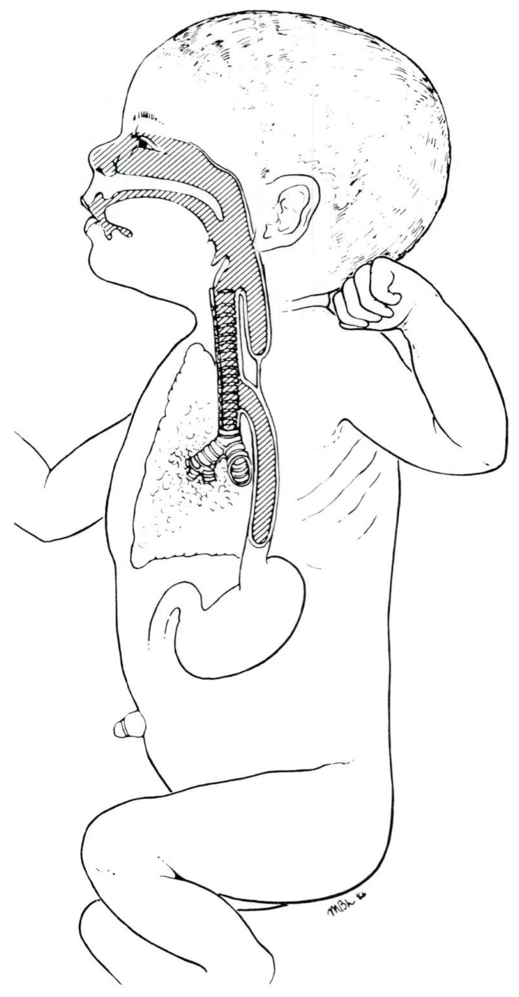

Fig. 18-15 Most common type of esophageal atresia involves upper esophageal segment, ending in a blind pouch and lower tracheoesophageal fistula.

and tracheoesophageal fistula as a result of the nature of embryonic development.

The three major types of gastrointestinal malformations are (1) tracheoesophageal fistula with esophageal atresia (80% to 95% of cases), in which the upper esophagus ends in a blind pouch and the lower esophageal segment connects with the trachea; (2) esophageal atresia alone; and (3) tracheoesophageal fistula alone. These anomalies are relatively common. About 25% of the infants with digestive tract abnormalities are premature. Another 25% usually have associated defects (congenital heart defects and gastrointestinal malformations, such as imperforate anus). Maternal polyhydramnios is frequently noted in these infants as a result of the inability of the fetus to dispose of swallowed amniotic fluid. These malformations are slightly more common in male infants.

Clinical manifestations. The infant with esophageal malformation usually cries at birth, breathes well, and has normal coloring. The diagnosis is suspected on the basis of clinical manifestations such as excessive salivation; frothing; drooling; the "3 Cs" of TEF, coughing, choking, and cyanosis; apnea; increased respiratory distress after feeding; and abdominal distention. Feeding is usually followed by the infant's aspiration of breast milk or formula into the lungs. This situation can lead to pneumonia and often to atelectasis. The pulmonary symptoms are caused by the drainage of secretions into the lungs from the stomach or mouth by way of an esophageal fistula or overflow from an esophageal pouch.

Diagnosis. Diagnosis can be made in the delivery room or nursery by the inability to pass a moderately stiff catheter into the stomach. X-rays positively confirm the diagnosis of an esophageal malformation. Films of the chest and abdomen, with the tube in place, will show the position of the upper blind pouch. Complete absence of air in the gastrointestinal tract confirms esophageal atresia without TEF.

Treatment. The treatment of esophagelatresia and TEF consists of prevention of pneumonia and surgical repair of the anomaly. For the infant with tracheoesophageal fistula a gastrostomy is performed as an emergency measure. This prevents over distention of the stomach with air, leading to regurgitation of gastric contents into the tracheobronchial tree. Since aspiration pneumonia is inevitable, broad-spectrum antibiotics are administered. Once the infant's condition is stable, usually within 7 to 10 days, surgical repair is done. A thoracotomy, the ligation (tying off) of the TEF and the connection of the esophageal segments, is performed. A staged procedure will be performed on less stable infants. If the esophageal segments are of insufficient length, requiring a colon interposition, the surgery will be delayed until the infant is 16 to 24 months of age.

Nursing considerations. Preoperative care is directed toward the prevention of aspiration and the stabilization of the infant. The infant's head is elevated 30 degrees to minimize reflux, and oxygen with warm, high humidification is administered to help relieve respiratory stress. Intermittent or continuous, gentle suction through an indwelling nasal catheter that extends to the end of the pouch is applied. The infant is handled minimally and oral fluids are withheld. Fluids are administered intravenously or via gastrostomy.

Postoperative care. Postoperative care includes support of the child and family; the warm, high humidification of the incubator; positioning; care of the surgical incision; and returning the gastrostomy tube to gravity drainage. When feedings begin through the gastrostomy 2 to 3 days postoperatively, the tube is elevated and secured at a point above the stomach. If gastrostomy feedings are well tolerated and the anastomosis is healing well, oral feedings are initiated on the tenth postoperative day.

Prognosis. The prognosis depends on the initial condition of the infant at the time of diagnosis, birth weight, degree of prematurity, and associated congenital anomalies. After the surgical repair is complete and recovery has taken place, these infants generally develop normally, with a 100% survival rate in uncomplicated full-term infants. The overall mortality rate is 10% to 15% in premature, low-birth-weight infants with congenital anomalies. Continued parental support and medical supervision is essential.

Imperforate Anus

In 1 in 5000 births the infant's rectum ends as a closed or blind pouch or connects to an adjacent canal (urethra, vagina) by means of a fistula (Fig. 18-16). Anorectal malformations are divided into the three categories of low anomalies, intermediate anomalies, and high anomalies.

Clinical manifestations

Imperforate anus is suspected if a newborn does not pass a stool within 24 to 36 hours of birth, or if meconium is excreted from a non-anal orifice.

Treatment

Successful treatment of simple anal stenosis is achieved by manual dilations initiated by the physician, continued by the nursing staff, and taught to the parents before discharge. The goal of surgical treatment of more complex anorectal malformations is reconstruction of an anus in the proper position. A temporary colostomy may be required.

Abdominal Hernias

Oomphalocele

Oomphalocele is an absence of the normal abdominal wall in the region of the umbilicus. This absence allows a portion of the intestinal contents to be clearly observed, virtually unprotected, and subject to herniation and strangulation. The defect may be small or large.

Treatment. The repair of oomphaloceles is usually considered a surgical emergency.

Diaphragmatic hernia

Another type of hernia, involving the abdominal contents and causing respiratory distress, as well as digestive problems, is the diaphragmatic hernia. In this condition an abnormally large opening is present in the

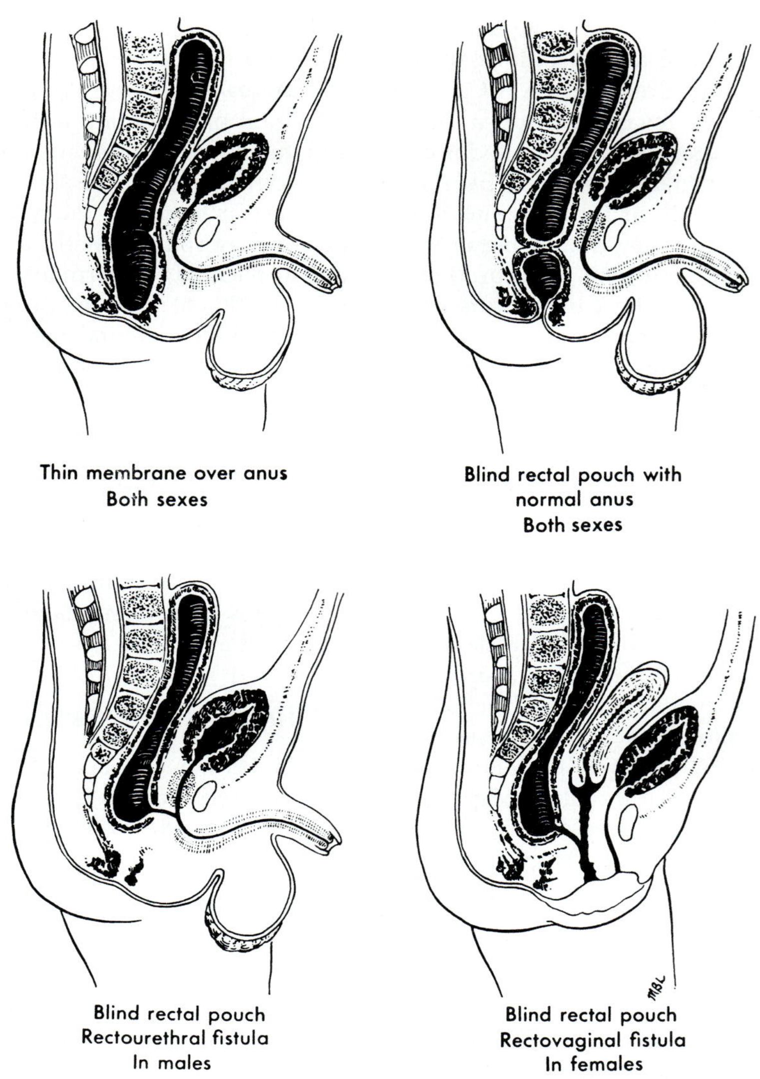

Fig. 18-16 Types of imperforate anus in the newborn infant.

diaphragm, allowing part of the contents of the abdominal cavity to displace upward into the chest. Sometimes the entire stomach, as well as portions of the intestine, are found in the thorax, crowding the heart and lungs.

Treatment. The treatment of diaphragmatic hernia is also a surgical emergency.

Congenital Heart Disease

The incidence of congenital heart disease (CHD) in children is 4 to 10 cases per 1000 live births. CHD is the major cause of death in the first year of life. Congenital cardiac conditions frequently stem from the persistence of some part of the fetal circulation pattern. The foramen ovale may fail to close, resulting in an atrial septal defect (ASD). The ductus arteriosus may persist, resulting in patent ductus arteriosus (PDA). However, structural deviations may exist in many different combinations (see Chapter 34). Improved pharmacological treatment and open-heart surgery, with the use of the heart-lung machine, offers hope for survival and the possibility of a normal life for most children with congenital heart defects.

Hemolytic Disease of the Newborn

A number of conditions can cause blood destruction in the fetus or newborn infant. Probably the most well-known cause is Rh-factor incompatibility, which may initiate an erythroblastosis fetalis condition. The Rh factor was first identified in the blood of Rhesus monkeys. Actually, the Rh factor has been found to be a group of related protein antigens, that under certain

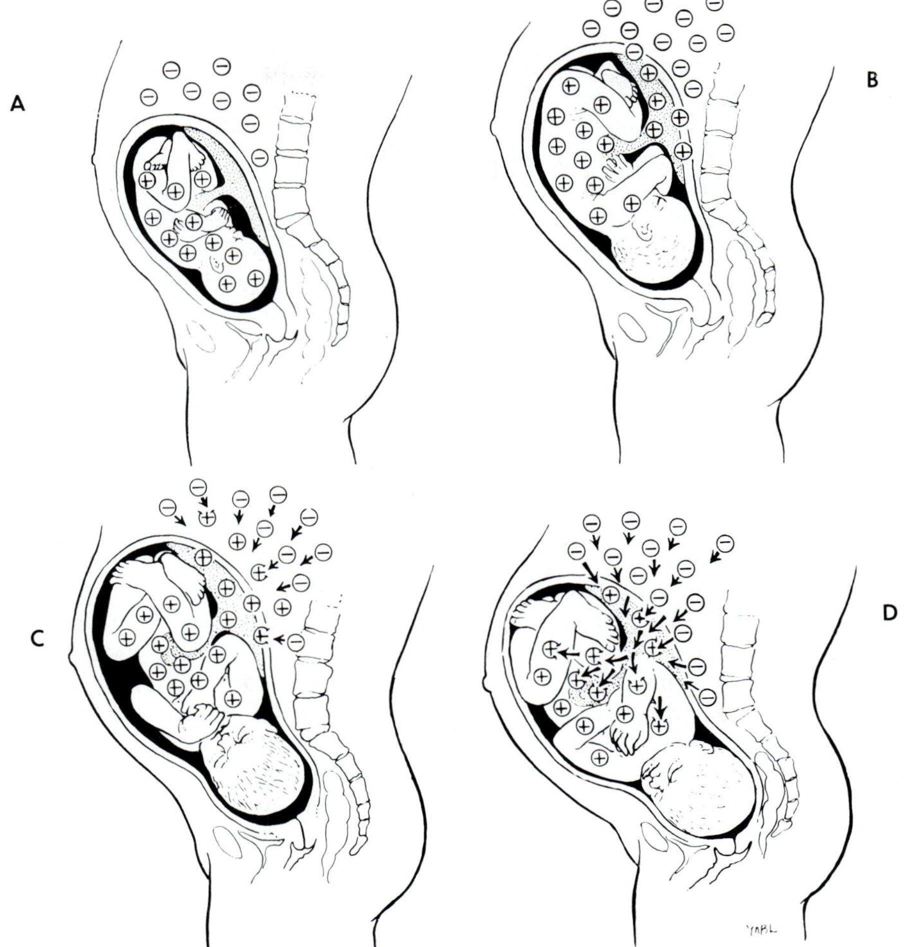

Fig. 18-17 Mechanism of erythroblastosis fetalis, which is caused by Rh incompatibility. **A,** Rh-positive child is carried by Rh-negative mother. **B,** Rh protein crosses placental barrier and invades mother's bloodstream. **C,** Mother's system manufactures antibodies to destroy foreign Rh protein. **D,** Antibodies cross back over placenta and destroy baby's blood cells, which are intimately associated with Rh protein.

conditions, may be capable of causing the formation of potentially dangerous antibodies. The two antigens that seem to cause clinical difficulty are D and its genetic variant D^m. Approximately 85% of the Caucasian population and 90% of non-Caucasians have these substances in their blood (Fig. 18-17).

Rh incompatibility

If both parents lack the Rh protein, no problem relating to their Rh factor exists for their offspring. However, if the father of the child is Rh positive and the child inherits Rh-positive blood from him, an incompatibility may occur.

Mechanism. Some of the fetus' blood cells carrying the Rh protein may pass through a microscopic tear in the placental barrier and reach the mother's bloodstream. The mother's body automatically manufactures protective antibodies designed to destroy the foreign protein in her body. These antibodies may enter the fetal circulation, where they destroy the Rh protein, or factor, and also destroy the red blood cells to which it is attached. The fetus suffers from the effects of anemia. In an effort to supply more red blood cells the child forces out into its bloodstream immature, inadequate forms of red blood cells called erythroblasts. For this reason, the resulting disease is termed *erythroblastosis fetalis*. In severe cases, congestive heart failure associated with enlargement of the spleen and liver occurs.

Shortly after birth, toxicity caused by the large amount of red blood cell breakdown products (mainly bilirubin) circulating in the infant's body may lead to a form of brain damage known as *kernicterus*. This condition causes neurological impairment such as spasticity, deafness, mental retardation, or death. One of the first clinical manifestations of Rh-factor sensitivity in the infant is the appearance of jaundice within 24 to 36 hours of birth. The infant with a more severe case may be lethargic, suck poorly, and manifest spasticity.

However, not all mothers with Rh-negative blood have affected infants. If the infant is also Rh negative, no problem arises. Sometimes the number of antibodies the mother has produced, in response to the infant's cells in her bloodstream, is so small that no damage to the infant is detected. Usually, trouble is not encountered until the second or third infant born to susceptible parents. After several pregnancies the titer (or strength) of antibodies in the blood usually increases greatly. This titer may be measured during pregnancy. The progress of the disease is also estimated by analyzing amniotic fluid aspirated from the sac surrounding the fetus. These tests allow the physician to evaluate the health of the fetus and plan for the birth and subsequent care.

Treatment. When the presence of erythroblastosis fetalis is determined in a newborn, an exchange transfusion is performed. The umbilical vein is used to achieve access to the infant's bloodstream by means of a polyethylene catheter. A carefully measured amount of blood is slowly withdrawn and discarded by a syringe equipped with a complex system of stopcocks. Then crossmatched, Rh-negative donor blood without an Rh antibody titer, warmed to room temperature, is slowly pushed by syringe back into the infant's body as a replacement. This process is repeated many times until complete replacement is estimated. During the procedure, close observation of the infant's vital signs and the blood-volume exchange is essential. The infant must be kept warm, and oxygen may be administered. This treatment may need to be repeated, but the results are usually highly successful. A child born in good condition and receiving prompt transfusions when needed has an excellent prognosis.

Intrauterine transfusion of the fetus, who shows signs of distress, is available in research centers. The procedure is not without risk; however, outcomes are improving.

Infants with hyperbilirubinemia are exposed to fluorescent light to reduce the amount of circulating bilirubin. The naked infant is positioned under the light with protective eye shields in place. The infant is turned periodically to increase body surface exposure and is given increased fluids.

Prevention. For the Rh-negative mother who has never been sensitized (formed detectable levels of Rh antibodies) because of a previous contact with the Rh protein, protection is available. When properly used, it is essentially 100% effective in preventing the detrimental effects of Rh incompatibility. Passive immunization or ready-made antibody protection, given within 72 hours of the birth of an Rh-positive infant or abortus, destroys the invading Rh protein and inhibits the natural formation of the mother's antibodies. This special, passive immunization, Rh-immune globulin, first marketed as Rho-Gam, unfortunately does not aid Rh-negative women who have already actively developed their own immunization against the Rh factor.

Rh-immune globulin must be administered to the woman at risk *after each exposure* to Rh-positive blood. In certain instances, fetal-to-maternal hemorrhages take place that are too large for the normal dose of 300 μg of Rh-immune globulin to provide adequate protection. The number of fetal cells in the maternal circulation can be estimated by the use of the Kleihauer-Betke test, or the more recent commercially available Fetaldex technique. The dosage is increased as necessary. In an effort to protect Rh-negative women who have unknown antepartal bleeds that may cause early sensitization, obstetrical care providers may administer the immune globulin to all Rh-negative women at 28 weeks' gestation, as well as after amniocentesis and birth.

A mechanism similar to the Rh problem but usually of a less serious nature can operate when the mother has type O blood and the baby has type A, B, or AB. Such a situation is called ABO incompatibility.

Hypospadias

Hypospadias is a common malformation of the urinary system and is found in male infants. The urethral opening is located behind the glans penis or anywhere along the ventral surface of the penile shaft. The presence of hypospadias, coupled with other irregularities of the external genital organs, lead to confusion in determining the gender of the infant. Genetic studies and exploratory procedures may be necessary.

Treatment

The surgical repair of hypospadias by the extension of the urethral canal is recommended before the oedipal period (age 3 to 6 years), during which children demonstrate a strong concern about the genital area and its appearance. Performing this surgery when the child is 2 to 2½ years of age is optimal, as it preceeds the oedipal stage when these fears and anxieties

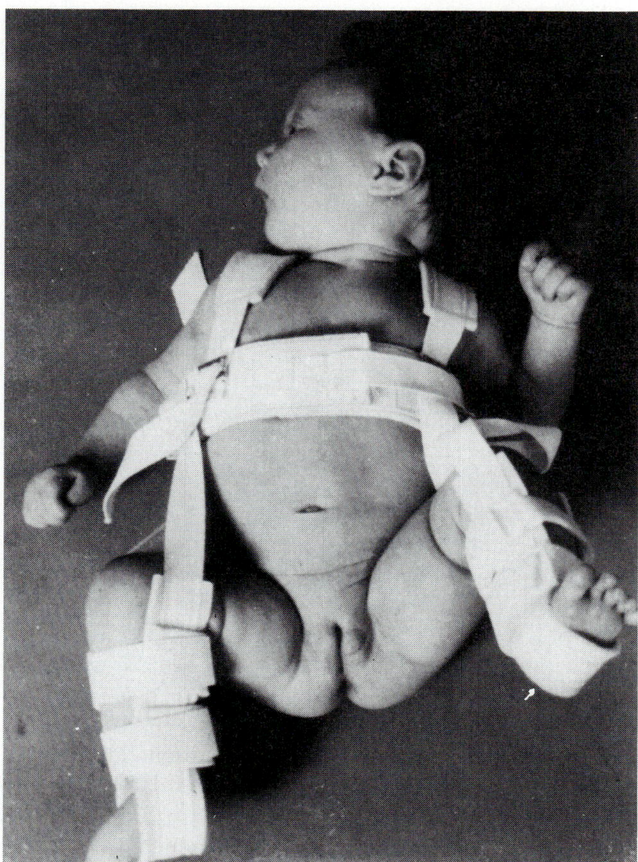

Fig. 18-18 Pavlik harness is recommended in treatment of congenital subluxation or dislocation of hip in newborns or infants up to 8 months. Chest halter is positioned at nipple line and fastened with Velcro closures. Leg and foot are placed in stirrups and fastened by Velcro closures. Front stirrup straps are connected to halter. Straps are adjusted so that hip is flexed beyond a right angle. (From Wong D: *Essentials of pediatric nursing,* ed 4, St. Louis, 1993, Mosby.)

develop. Minor positional deviations of the urethral meatus may noyt require treatment.

Orthopedic Abnormalities

Orthopedic abnormalities are common in the newborn nursery. The earlier they are treated, the better the prognosis.

Fractures

Fractures may occur during the birth process. The most frequently broken bone is the clavicle, or collarbone. It usually heals without treatment. Fractures of long bones secondary to the birth process are rare. All broken bones normally heal rapidly during infancy. For further information regarding fractures, refer to Chapter 32.

Congenital dislocation of the hip

Two main types of congenital dislocations of the hip (CDH) include (1) teratological, which develops during life in utero and is commonly associated with other orthopedic problems, and (2) typical, which occurs just before, during, or shortly after birth. Typical dislocations are probably caused by the softening effects of the maternal hormone *relaxin* on the infant's ligaments and the stress of labor and birth. The hip joints of every newborn should be examined within 24 hours of birth for congenital dislocation. Infants can usually be treated successfully by simple manipulation. CDH appears at the rate of 1.5 cases per 1000 live births. The disorder affects females eight times more frequently than males. Dislocation, or luxation, is present when the femoral head is completely displaced from the socket, or acetabulum. Subluxation, or partial displacement, is more common, occurring in approximately 1 in 60 births. A subluxated hip may become completely dislocated during an infant's care unless certain types of maneuvers are avoided. Infants should never be lifted by their feet for diapering. Their legs should never be pulled, nor should their hips be completely extended when wrapped in a blanket. Since hip problems may be missed on the initial examination, these precautions should apply to the care of all infants. Barring complications, the subluxated hip of 88% of the affected newborns becomes normal by 2 months of age.

Clinical manifestations. Physical findings of CDH that the nurse can detect include asymmetry of the thigh folds, limited abduction of the affected hip, and shortening of the femur when the knees and hips are flexed at right angles and when abduction is attempted with the child lying supine on a firm table. The diagnosis is usually confirmed by x-ray examination.

Treatment. Since the hip socket becomes progressively more distorted if reduction is delayed, the goal of treatment is the immediate return of the femoral head to the acetabulum. A normal hip joint can be obtained when treatment is begun in the first few weeks of life. Reduction of the hip is not difficult and involves maintenance in a stable position of flexion and abduction. Semirigid abduction devices are more practical and preferred for treatment of infants with CDH. The best and most popular device for treating CDH is the Pavlik harness (Fig. 18-18). This device allows flexion and abduction but prevents extension or adduction. The child's orthopedic condition is frequently evaluated on an outpatient basis. Early treatment may reduce therapy to approximately 3 months' duration. If the child's x-ray film indicates normal location of the hip at 2 years of age, the condition may be considered cured. Treatment after 6 months of age varies. It may involve traction for a few weeks followed by casting or operative reduction. However, when CDH is first diagnosed at 2 years of age, the outcome is seldom optimal. In children over 8 years, even the most extensive operative procedures cannot produce a functionally satisfactory hip. Approximately one third of the degenerative hip joint disease cases found in adults is caused by the residual effects of CDH. In adults, such conditions may be helped by a total hip arthroplasty.

Clubfoot (Talipes Equinovarus)

Clubfoot is the most common congenital anomaly of the lower extremity. In the most common form of this condition (talipes equinovarus), the anterior half of the foot is adducted and inverted. The medial border of the foot is concave, the lateral border is convex, and the heel is drawn up (Fig. 18-19). The cause of clubfoot is unknown, but it has been postulated that it results from arrested or abnormal development of a particular part of the germ plasm during embryonic life. One or both feet may be involved. This anomaly is twice as common in males as in females.

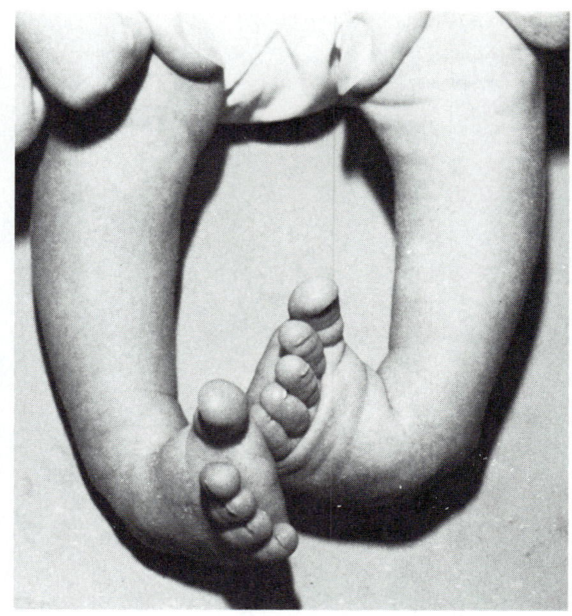

Fig. 18-19 Talipes equinovarus. (Courtesy McDade WC, San Diego, CA.)

The feet of the newborn infant must be carefully evaluated. Not all apparent deformities are true clubfoot. Some distortions are simply caused by intrauterine positions and are not real, structural differences. The feet, in this case, can be corrected to a neutral position in all elements of the deformity by manipulation during examination. A true clubfoot cannot; however, both need careful follow-up.

Treatment. The treatment of talipes equinovarus should be started as soon as the infant's condition is stable. Treatment may be divided into the three stages of (1) correction, (2) maintenance of correction, and (3) long-term follow-up. Correction usually consists of stretching and strapping or casting. Casting is changed as often as every 3 to 7 days over a period of approximately 10 weeks. Follow-up must continue for several years, after completion of active treatment, to prevent recurrence of the deformity and a less than satisfactory outcome. Surgery is often necessary to fully correct the deformity.

Syndactyly and polydactyly

Syndactyly, or webbing of the fingers or toes, is an anomaly that usually responds well to surgical separation. Syndactyly may accompany another digital abnormality termed *polydactylism,* or the presence of extra fingers or toes. These extra digits may have no bony connection with the hand or foot. For polydactylism, a ligature is tied around the fleshy digit, circulation is obstructed, and the digit soon drops off. When a bony connection exists, surgery is necessary.

KEY CONCEPTS

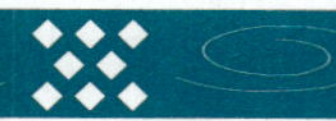

1. In determining the status of the small infant, birth weight, heredity, length of gestation, clinical appearance, and behavior must all be considered.
2. The incidence of prematurity in the United States varies with the population studied; in general, it approaches 7%. Prematurity accounts for approximately two thirds of infant mortality.
3. The typical, premature infant lacks subcutaneous fat, is covered with lanugo, has a relatively large head and abdomen, a small thorax, little molding of the skull, irregular respirations, and may be surprisingly active.
4. Sucking and swallowing reflexes may be weak or absent in very small infants, necessitating supplemental nutrition. The danger of overfeeding is real.
5. Special needs of the premature infant may include

maintenance of body temperature, provision of the appropriate level of oxygen, protection from injury and infection, assistance with respiration, and stimulation when the infant is in the quiet/alert state.

6 The most common type of serious birth injury is intracranial hemorrhage. Symptoms include irritability, listlessness or cyanosis, marked irregular respiration, varying degrees of paralysis, lack of appetite or poor sucking reflex, tremors, convulsions, projectile vomiting, unequally dilated pupils, tense or bulging fontanels, and a high and shrill cry.

7 Hydrocephalus results from the accumulation of abnormally large amounts of cerebrospinal fluid within the cranium. Three types of shunts used for treatment are ventriculoperitoneal, lumboperitoneal, and ventriculoatrial. Infection is the most common complication after shunting.

8 Mental retardation affects approximately 2% of the general population. Causes include birth injury, infection in utero, chromosomal abnormalities, and unfavorable polygenetic combinations.

9 Infants with Down syndrome are characteristically short; have relatively small head circumference, flattened from front to back; usually have low birth weights; and exhibit lethargic behavior. Reliable signs include exaggerated epicanthic folds; short hands and fingers with the little finger bent in; a deep, horizontal crease across the palm; and a large space between the great and small toes.

10 Spina bifida is a genetic condition in which a portion of the posterior wall of the spine is missing. A meningocele presents a cosmetic problem and possible injury of the sac poses the problem of infection of the nervous system. A myelomeningocele results in varying degrees of weakness of the legs, sensory disturbance, and impairment of rectal and urinary sphincter function.

11 Cleft lip and palate occurs in 1 of 1000 live births. Cleft palate alone occurs in 1 of 2500 live births. A cleft lip is usually repaired when the infant is 6 to 10 weeks of age. Cleft palate is repaired at 12 to 18 months of age.

12 Nursing care after cleft lip surgery includes restraining the infant's arms, cleaning the suture line, careful feeding, and keeping the infant as happy as possible. After cleft palate surgery, the child is usually fed from a cup. Nothing is introduced into the mouth that may injure the suture line. Arm restraints may be necessary. The mouth is rinsed with water after each meal.

13 Tracheoesophageal fistula causes an open connection between the trachea and esophagus. A gastrostomy is performed as an emergency measure. Surgical repair is done after the infant's condition has stabilized.

14 An infant with imperforate anus may require a temporary colostomy before the surgical creation of a normally placed, functional rectal opening.

15 Oomphalocele and diaphragmatic hernia are both considered surgical emergencies.

16 Hypospadias is a fairly common malformation of the male urinary system. Surgical repair is accomplished before the child reaches the oedipal stage.

17 Rh-factor incompatibility may initiate an erythroblastosis fetalis condition. This occurs only when the fetus of an Rh-negative woman inherits Rh-positive blood from the father. Treatment involves an exchange transfusion. Administration of Rh-immune globulin prevents the detrimental effects of Rh incompatibility in the newborn. It must be administered to the woman at risk after each exposure to Rh-positive blood.

18 The two main types of congenital dislocations of the hip are teratological and typical. They can usually be successfully treated by simple manipulation. Reduction of the hip involves maintaining a stable position of flexion and abduction.

19 To avoid completely dislocating an unidentified subluxated hip, infants should never be lifted by their feet for diapering, their legs should never be pulled, nor should their hips be completely extended when wrapped in a blanket.

20 Treatment of clubfoot may be divided into the three stages of correction, maintenance of correction, and long-term follow-up.

CRITICAL THOUGHT QUESTIONS

1 Regarding fetal growth and development, why is length of gestation a more significant measure of maturity than size or weight?

2 With technological advances, it is now possible to save many infants with abnormalities who would formerly not have survived. Many of these infants will have developmental disabilities and require special care. What significance does this have for family-centered nursing care?

3 Amniocentesis and ultrasound enable the physician to detect abnormalities before birth. As a nurse, how would you respond and provide care to parents

who know before delivery that the child will not be normal?

4 Hemolytic disease in the newborn is most often related to blood incompatibilities. Which combinations are most likely to cause hemolytic problems? What diagnostic tests are used to monitor the fetal/neonatal condition? What can be done to prevent these problems?

BIBLIOGRAPHY

American Academy of Pediatrics and American College of Obstetricians and Gynecologists: *Guidelines for perinatal care,* ed 3, Evanston, IL, 1992, The Academy.

American Academy of Pediatrics, Committee on Genetics: Maternal phenylketonuria, *Pediatrics* 88(6):1284-1285, 1991.

Brown D: Feeding the low-birth-weight infant. In Burg FD, Ingelfinger JR, Wald ER, editors: *Gellis and Kagan's current pediatric therapy,* Philadelphia, 1993, HD Saunders.

Feigin FD, Adcock LM, Miller DJ: Postnatal bacterial infections. In Fanaroff A, Martin R, editors: *Neonatal-perinatal medicine,* ed 5, St. Louis, 1992, Mosby.

Fisher C: The abnormal infant: protecting yourself against blame, *RN* 53(4):69, 1990.

Jackson PL: Primary care needs of children with hydrocephalus, *J Pediatr Health Care* 4(2):59, 1990.

Heyerdahyl S, Kase B, Lie S: Intellectual development in congenital hypothyroidism, *J Pediatr* 116(6):850-857, 1991.

Holzman I: Meconium aspiration syndrome. In Burg FD, Ingelfinger JR, Wald ER, editors: *Gellis and Kagan's current pediatric therapy,* Philadelphia, 1993, HD Saunders.

Kennard JJ: Cocaine use during pregnancy: fetal and neonatal effects, *J Perinat Neonat Nurs* 3(4):53-63, 1990.

Lynch ME: Iatrogenic hazards, adverse occurrences, and complications involving NICU nursing practice, *J Perinat Neonat Nurs* 5(3):78-86, 1991.

Manqurten HH: Birth injuries. In Fanaroff A, Martin R, editors: *Neonatal-perinatal medicine,* ed 5, St. Louis, 1992, Mosby.

Morin FC: Treatment of respiratory distress syndrome. In Burg FD, Ingelfinger JR, Wald ER, editors: *Gellis and Kagan's current pediatric therapy,* Philadelphia, 1993, HD Saunders.

Nora JG: Perinatal cocaine use: maternal, fetal, and neonatal effects, *Neonatal Intensive Care* 4(2):68-77, 1990.

Novak JC: Facilitating nurturant fathering behavior in the NICU, *J Perinat Neonat Nurs* 4(2):68-77, 1990.

Polin RA, Schneiderman R: Birth injuries. In Burg FD, Ingelfinger JR, Wald ER, editors: *Gellis and Kagan's current pediatric therapy,* Philadelphia, 1993, WB Saunders.

Robinson T: Discharge teaching in the NICU, *Neonatal Network* 10(4):77-78, 1991.

Rovet JF: Does breast-feeding protect the hypothyroid infant whose condition is diagnosed by newborn screening? *Am J Dis Child* 144:319-323, 1990.

Rowe MA: Asphyxiated infants: pathophysiologic consequences, parenting, and nursing management, *Neonatal Network* 8(4):7-10, 1990.

Schaming D, et al: When babies are born with orthopedic problems, *RN* 53(4):62, 1990.

Silverman RA: Hemagiomas and vascular malformations, *Pediatr Clin North Am* 38(4):811-834, 1991.

Taft LT: Cerebral palsy. In Green M, Haggerty RJ, editors: *Ambulatory pediatrics,* Philadelphia, 1990, WB Saunders.

Wennberg RP: Hemolytic diseases of the neonate. In Burg FD, Ingelfinger JR, Wald ER, editors: *Gellis and Kagan's current pediatric therapy,* Philadelphia, 1993, WB Saunders.

Wong D: *Essentials of pediatric nursing,* ed 4, St. Louis, 1993, Mosby.

Zuckerman B, Frank D: "Crack kids:" not broken, *Pediatrics* 89(2):337-339, 1992.

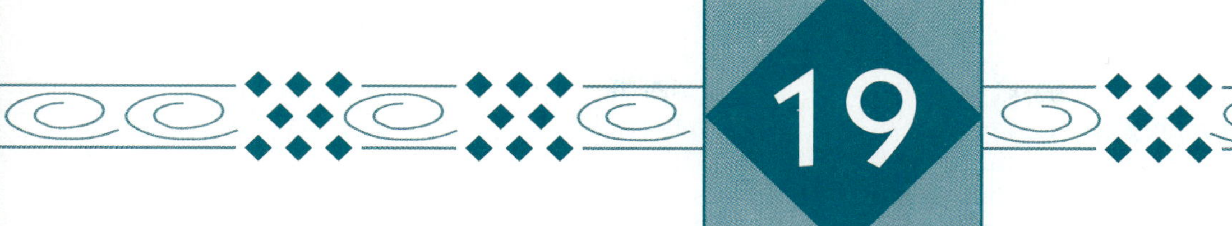

19 Intensive Care of the Newborn

CHAPTER OBJECTIVES

After studying this chapter, the student should be able to:

1. State the main objective of neonatal intensive care units (NICUs).
2. Discuss common diagnoses encountered among the newborns admitted to an NICU.
3. List five responsibilities of a comprehensive, regional, perinatal center.
4. Discuss four ways that health care personnel can reduce the anxiety of parents whose infants are transferred to a regional NICU.
5. Identify at least six maternal-risk factors that correlate with potential neonatal difficulty.
6. Discuss the potential for increased heat loss by the premature neonate.
7. Describe how output is monitored (measured and analyzed) for the NICU patient.
8. Enumerate five types of analyses of the nurse caring for a newborn who is receiving oxygen-enriched ventilatory support.
9. Explain the increased fluid needs of the premature or low-birth-weight infant.
10. Discuss four methods of monitoring the hydration of a low-birth-weight infant.
11. State two reasons why overfeeding a premature infant may be particularly dangerous.
12. Discuss two methods used to evaluate the infant's ability to digest what is offered.
13. Describe four methods of providing nourishment to NICU patients.
14. Discuss methods of maintaining a patent airway and avoiding further respiratory problems for the infant receiving ventilatory assistance.
15. Discuss three problems associated with the use of umbilical catheters.
16. Indicate the major developmental problem associated with respiratory distress syndrome (RDS) and its prenatal assessment of risk.
17. Identify normal values for pH, Po_2, and Pco_2 in arterial blood after the first few hours after birth.
18. Indicate three nursing considerations when caring for an infant receiving phototherapy.
19. Discuss the infections identified by the acronym *TORCHES* and their impact on the fetus.
20. Describe three aspects of the treatment and nursing care of the newborn infant undergoing withdrawal symptoms because of prenatal, maternal drug addiction.
21. Discuss prenatal education for the prevention of fetal alcohol syndrome.
22. Describe methods of assessment and the potential problems of infants of diabetic mothers.

NEONATAL INTENSIVE CARE UNIT

Neonatology, the study and treatment of the newborn, has rapidly become a highly specialized area of pediatrics. Continuing advances in detection, prevention, and treatment of disorders of the newborn have led to the development of specialized neonatal units with highly trained personnel. In general, basic nursing courses do not prepare nurses to work in the neonatal intensive care unit (NICU). However, with advanced coursework, education, and orientation, selected nurses may work in these specialized units. Students may have a period of observation and closely guided participation during their obstetrical or pediatric experiences. This chapter is designed to help students better understand the types of patients, conditions, and procedures they may encounter, and to help nurses better comprehend the perinatal histories of NICU graduates.

Objectives and Characteristics

The main objective of the NICU is to provide the earliest and highest degree of medical and nursing care for the infant at risk so that each infant attains the best possible outcome. As neonatal mortality is reduced, continuing efforts must also be made to decrease the incidence of long-term problems, such as chronic lung disease, intestinal disorders, and neurodevelopmental delay. Awareness of the causes and prevention of residual damage is therefore necessary for the NICU nurse.

Prematurity and its various complications are the most frequently encountered problems in the NICU. Other common diagnoses include birth defects, infection, jaundice, hypoglycemia, and perinatal asphyxia. Furthermore, since many hospital recovery rooms are not equipped and staffed to care for small infants, the NICU must provide postoperative care for neonates recovering from general anesthesia and various surgical procedures.

NICU patients require many types of specialized care to meet their needs. Mechanical ventilation, intravenous fluid therapy, continuous monitoring of vital signs, body temperature regulation, and feeding require specially trained physicians and nursing personnel, as well as sophisticated biomedical equipment. The NICU nurse must become comfortable with handling tiny, fragile infants and be proficient with the high-tech equipment used in their care.

The Regional Perinatal Center

Because intensive care facilities are very expensive and are seldom necessary in smaller, general hospitals, the concept of the regional, perinatal center has evolved. In addition to the NICU, such a center provides an obstetrical-perinatal service for both outpatient and inpatient care of high-risk mothers and their unborn babies. The center usually serves a defined geographical region, accepting referrals of patients with complicated conditions from other hospitals. It often operates a newborn transport system to bring critically ill neonates born elsewhere to the NICU.

Other responsibilities of the comprehensive, perinatal center include the supervision of continuing education for health professionals of the region, long-term follow-up of infants treated in the NICU, and ongoing research in perinatal-neonatal medicine. Many perinatal centers are associated with schools of nursing, medicine, and other health professions.

Neonatal Transport

When neonatal problems are anticipated, the mother should be transferred to the perinatal center for delivery, if possible. Such an "in utero transport" is not only safer for the infant but also prevents the undesirable separation of mother and baby. However, since many infants with serious problems are born at hospitals without NICU facilities, the regional center must be able to provide safe, immediate transfer to the NICU when necessary. The neonatal transport team usually consists of a pediatrician or a neonatal nurse clinician or practitioner, a respiratory therapist, and one or more NICU staff nurses. Reliable ambulance, helicopter, or airplane service is necessary. Special equipment is needed, including a transport incubator capable of maintaining the infant's body temperature, a portable monitor, an intravenous infusion device, and ventilation equipment to provide care in transit (Fig. 19-1).

Assessment

The newborn infant must be evaluated quickly. A nursing and medical assessment, laboratory tests, and x-rays are commonly performed. Other specialized procedures, such as intubation, umbilical catheterization, chest tube placement, administration of antibiotics, glucose, or fluids, as well as warming may also be required. Infants should always be adequately stabilized before departing for the NICU.

Before the transport team leaves the referring hospital, they should talk with the infant's parents, telling them about the child's condition and what will be done in the NICU. Visiting hours should be discussed and telephone numbers given, as well as directions to the NICU. If at all possible, both parents should be allowed to see and handle the infant, and a photograph of the

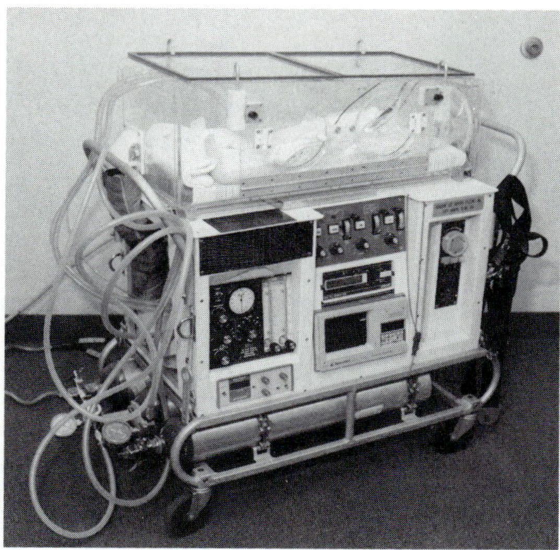

Fig. 19-1 Infant transport incubator equipped with built-in ventilator, cardiorespiratory and blood pressure monitor, intravenous infusion pump, and trancutaneous Po_2/Pco_2 monitor. (Courtesy John Wimmer, MD, East Carolina University.)

baby should be provided. The parents should be encouraged to visit their infant as soon and as frequently as possible.

Supportive Care of the Parents

Separation of an infant from its parents in the immediate postpartum period, although necessary to provide adequate treatment for critically ill babies, is disruptive to the establishment of normal parent-infant interaction. For this reason the NICU personnel must be extremely supportive of the parents and make every effort to help them adapt to this stressful situation. Visiting should be restricted only when absolutely necessary (e.g., while procedures are performed, while the medical staff is making rounds, or during emergencies). Parents should be encouraged to touch and hold their infant as much as possible. They should also help with bathing, feeding, giving vitamins, and other daily routines as soon as the infant's condition permits. Special consideration to facilitating fathering and mothering is critical (Novak, 1991).

Preparation for discharge should begin as soon as the infant is physiologically stable to provide a smooth transition from the NICU to the home environment. Parents must be taught infant CPR, since premature infants are at greater risk for apnea (breathing pauses) and bradycardia (heart rate below 100 beats per minute), and for sudden infant death syndrome (SIDS). Special procedures (e.g., gastrostomy feedings, care of equipment such as cardiac monitors) and general infant care classes must be initiated early so that the discharge-planning process is not rushed.

Ominous terms such as *brain damage, cerebral palsy,* and *blindness* should not be used. Parents whose children have suffered setbacks should be informed and counseled appropriately. The practice of telling them to "expect the worst" can severely interfere with the parent-infant attachment process. Most patients cared for in the NICU survive with few, if any, permanent disabilities. Therefore most parents may be reassured. Open lines of communication between the parents and staff should provide parental awareness of the child's progress and alleviate unfounded apprehension. Parents often describe the NICU experience as an "emotional roller coaster." Primary care nurses provide the informational and emotional support that buffers this traumatic experience.

Staffing in the NICU

Because of the critical nature of the NICU patient's condition, constant vigilance is necessary to anticipate crises, to prevent them, if possible, and to be prepared when they occur. Early detection of deterioration improves the chances for successful intervention. The nurse works closely with a neonatal nurse practitioner and physician who are always available.

Since potentially life-threatening conditions may be heralded by subtle changes in the patient's behavior or appearance, the nurse must develop astute observational skills. A clear understanding of each infant's disease process is imperative, and preparation must be made for any emergency situation that might result from the disease itself or from the treatment (e.g., a pneumothorax that develops in an infant receiving mechanical ventilation). The nurse must also be familiar with the biomedical equipment, such as monitors and ventilators, and be able to interpret alarms and recognize malfunction quickly.

The ideal nurse-patient ratio is 1:1 for infants who are critically ill or in an immediate postoperative phase (Fig. 19-2). The average ratio is 1:2 for most sick infants and up to 1:4 during the convalescent phase. Some hospital settings provide a separate, intermediate-care unit where the staffing ratio can be increased.

Nursery personnel may use a separate cover-gown technique for each infant. Handwashing is of major importance. Meticulous handwashing before and after handling any infant or piece of equipment is imperative. Caps and masks are not used. Cover gowns may be worn by physicians, parents, and other personnel. In some hospitals, persons may freely enter the NICU without gowning or handwashing as long as no infant or equipment is handled.

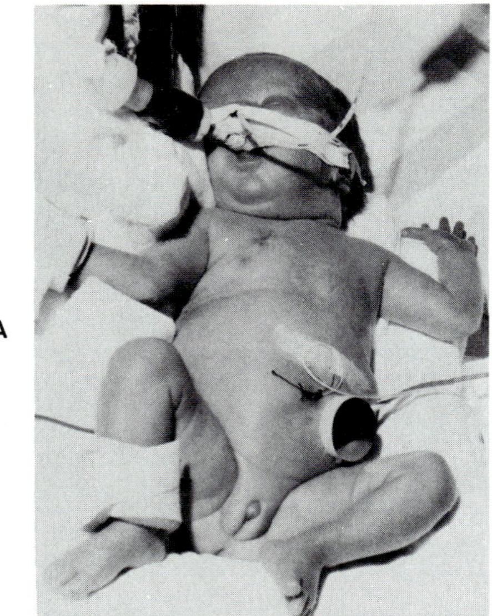

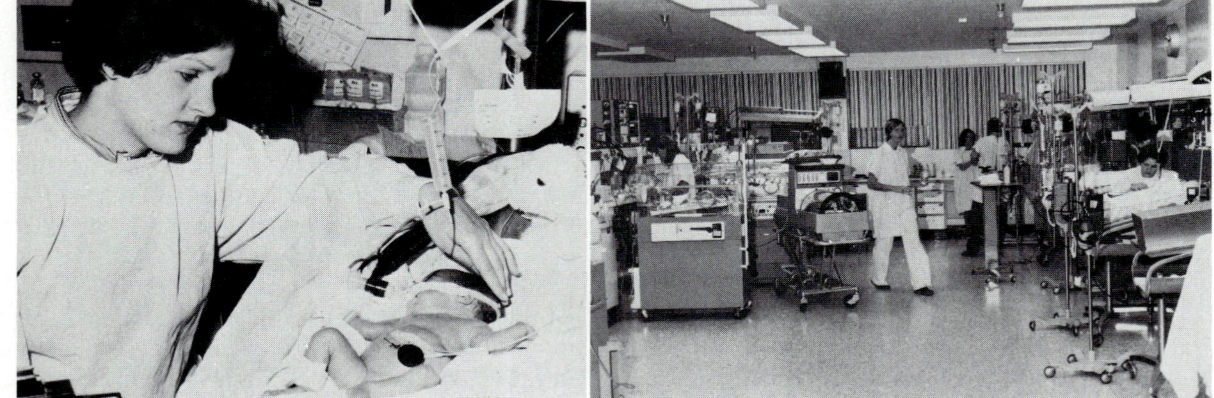

Fig. 19-2 Neonatal intensive care unit or special care nursery from three perspectives. **A,** This tiny infant was 1 month old when photograph was taken. Born weighing 2¼ lbs (1022 gm), she was first ventilated mechanically because of respiratory distress syndrome. A heat sensor and umbilical catheter are present. She had patent ductus arteriosus repair when 6 days old. **B,** Mother came in almost every afternoon. She progressively participated in care of her daughter as child improved. **C,** One corner of a busy NICU, showing mother with her baby. (Photograph by Bob Burgen; courtesy Children's Hospital and Health Center, San Diego, CA.)

THE CRITICALLY ILL NEONATE

Anticipation of the Need for Care

Prompt recognition and treatment of a sick infant are of utmost importance in obtaining the best possible outcome. The majority of patients are the products of a relatively small number of high-risk pregnancies. Therefore knowledge of predisposing factors often allows anticipation and early treatment when appropriate, including transfer of the mother to the perinatal center for delivery. An increased incidence of neonatal complications is seen in infants whose mothers have any of the following risk factors: (1) lack of prenatal care, poor nutrition, or other socioeconomic problems; (2) previous history of obstetrical complications, such as spontaneous abortion, stillbirth or neonatal death, premature delivery, prolonged infertility, pregnancy-induced hypertension (PIH), placenta previa, placental abruption, or blood group incompatibilities; and (3) medical illnesses, such as diabetes mellitus, cardiac or renal disease, infection, alcoholism, or drug addiction. Complications of labor and birth may also adversely affect the infant. These conditions include premature labor, premature rupture of membranes, abnormal presentation or fetal size, meconium staining of amniotic fluid, and inappropriate maternal analgesia or anesthesia. Multiple births place the infant at greater risk for complications. A pediatrician will attend the birth, and a period of observation in the NICU may be necessary.

Maintenance of Body Temperature

Attention to temperature regulation is an important part of the nursing care of sick neonates. Many neonates, especially low-birth-weight, premature infants, have difficulty maintaining body temperature. They have thin skin that is not insulated by the subcutaneous fat characteristic of full-term infants. Small babies also have an increased proportion of body surface area to body mass and immature central nervous system temperature-regulation centers. For these reasons, neonates have increased heat loss caused by conduction, convection, radiation, and evaporation. Keeping the infant's environmental temperature in the neutral thermal range allows normal body temperature to be maintained with the least expenditure of energy. This decreases the baby's requirements of oxygen, calories, and fluid. It is an extremely important measure, particularly in the small, premature infant with little reserve capacity.

Skin temperature is continuously monitored by a sensor attached to the baby's chest or abdomen (Fig. 19-2, *A*). Axillary and/or rectal temperature should be checked with a thermometer and recorded periodically. Fluctuations in temperature or discrepancies between skin and core temperature may indicate infection or other problems. The situation should be reported promptly.

Radiant warmer beds provide easy access to infants requiring frequent intervention and close observation. Treatments, procedures, and nursing care can be performed without disturbing the thermal environment. The bed can be tilted up or down. Special enclosed infant care units (incubators) are used for infants who need to be isolated.

Monitoring the NICU Patient

Heart rate and respirations are monitored continuously by an electronic cardiorespiratory monitor with audible alarms for apnea, tachypnea, bradycardia, and tachycardia. Blood pressure is measured by the Doppler method, by a standard infant blood pressure cuff, or by means of a pressure transducer connected to an in-dwelling arterial catheter (usually umbilical). Pulse oximeters may be used to monitor oxygen saturation, and transcutaneous oxygen and carbon dioxide monitors may be helpful with patients with respiratory problems. With each voiding the infant's urine is measured and tested for blood, glucose, protein, pH, and specific gravity. Urine output can be measured using disposable diapers, which are weighed (in grams) before and after the infant has voided. Alternatively, plastic urine collection bags can be used, but they may cause skin trauma and collection is sometimes difficult, (especially from females). Stools should be described and checked for occult blood. Accurate intake and output charts must be maintained and must include blood withdrawn for diagnostic tests. Daily weights should also be recorded. Small infants with fluid balance problems are weighed every 12 hours.

Infants with respiratory problems require particularly careful observation. The oxygen content of the inspired air-oxygen mixture ideally should be monitored continuously or checked hourly. For patients receiving ventilatory support (either continuous positive airway pressure or mechanical ventilation) the ventilator settings, endotracheal tube position, and infant respirations and breath sounds must be assessed. The chest should be transilluminated periodically to detect pneumothorax if this complication is likely. Equipment malfunction occasionally occurs and must be detected and corrected quickly. Although all the modern, highly developed equipment currently used in the NICU is a great asset, *the nurse is the most important and accurate monitor* of the infant's condition, and the tendency to rely totally on mechanical devices must be avoided.

Fluid Therapy and Feeding

The fluid requirements of the newborn are highly variable and depend on many factors. In the healthy full-term infant an intake of 75 to 90 ml/kg/24 hr is usually adequate during the first 24 to 48 hours of life, increasing to about 150 ml/kg/24 hr over the next few days. The premature infant, however, has increased insensible water losses and may normally require 140 to 160 ml/kg/24 hr. Water losses are also increased by tachypnea, abnormal gastrointestinal losses, administration of a concentrated solution (either orally or intravenously), and fever. The open-radiant warmer bed further increases evaporative loss of water, as does the use of phototherapy for hyperbilirubinemia. Thus a small infant in whom several of these conditions are present may need an intake of 200 ml/kg/24 hr or even more. On the other hand, fluids should be restricted in some cases, depending on the infant's particular problems. The most important aspect of fluid therapy management is constant monitoring of the infant's state of hydration and appropriate readjustment of fluid intake. This is accomplished by following serial weights, intake and output, urine specific gravities (normal range 1.002 to 1.010), and serum electrolytes.

Caloric requirements are also somewhat variable and are higher in the low-birth-weight infant (120 to 150 cal/kg/24 hr) than in the full-term infant (110 to 130 cal/kg/24 hr). Increased metabolic rate, for any reason, increases caloric requirements. Various diseases, environmental temperature above or below the neutral thermal environment, and increased physical activity all increase the infant's needs.

Fluids are given intravenously to small, sick infants. Since volumes are relatively small and must be measured precisely, automatic infusion pumps with safety features to prevent accidental fluid overload are used. Fluids may be given through a peripheral vein, an umbilical arterial catheter (if one is needed for blood gas sampling), or a central venous line.

Tube feedings are begun with stable infants who are unable to take the breast or bottle, usually because of prematurity, respiratory, or neurological difficulties. Orogastric or nasogastric tubes can be used for either intermittent or continuous feeding. Longer tubes can be passed through the stomach into the small intestine for continuous infusions, called transpyloric or nasoduodenal feeding. Initially, small amounts of diluted formula or breast milk are given. If these early feedings are well tolerated, the concentration and volumes are gradually advanced. Excessive feeding may cause regurgitation and aspiration or intestinal complications. Feeding intolerance is recognized by aspirating the stomach contents before giving feedings or periodically when feedings are continuous. Changes in abdominal girth, bowel sounds, and stool patterns are also assessed.

Nipple feedings may be attempted in the vigorous infant with intact gag and suck reflexes. The breastfeeding mother is encouraged to begin nursing as soon as the infant's condition permits. Until then, she may express milk manually or with an electric or manual breast pump, freeze it, and bring it to the nursery, where it is stored to give to the infant at a later time.

Infants in whom intestinal feeding must be delayed for long periods are begun on parenteral (intravenous) hyperalimentation, which provides carbohydrates, fat, protein, vitamins, and minerals. Central venous catheters may be inserted for this purpose, or peripheral veins can be used. Complications may occur including sepsis (with central catheters), metabolic imbalance, and liver toxicity. Successful management requires a team effort involving the nurse, physician, and pharmacist.

Airway Maintenance

Infants requiring ventilatory support are unable to clear secretions from their lungs and airways by normal mechanisms. Endotracheal tubes must therefore be suctioned to prevent airway occlusion. Atelectasis must be performed to minimize the risk of respiratory infections. The frequency of this suctioning depends on the disease process and the amount and type of secretions present, ranging from every 2 hours in those with copious secretions to every 6 to 8 hours in patients with scant secretions.

Suction of the endotracheal tube should be performed with a sterile technique. The length of the suction catheter inserted should be no greater than the length of the endotracheal tube to minimize trauma to the tracheobronchial epithelium. The suctioning should be as gentle as possible and continued for no longer than 5 to 10 seconds, after which the catheter should be withdrawn and the baby ventilated briefly to allow for recovery before continuing suction. Small amounts (0.5 to 1 ml) of saline may be injected into the endotracheal tube to thin secretions if necessary. The infant should, of course, be monitored carefully during the suctioning procedure, ideally with a continuous transcutaneous blood gas reading or oximeter.

Infants with excessive secretions, such as those with pneumonia or meconium aspiration, may benefit from chest physiotherapy (CPT) before airway suctioning. Percussion or vibration should be done for 1 to 2 minutes, either manually or with a portable vibrator. CPT should not be done on small, premature infants with respiratory distress syndrome in the first few days of life. The therapy may increase the risk of intracranial hemorrhage if done too early in the premature infant's life. Fortunately, these patients do not usually have a significant amount of secretions.

Infants with respiratory disease or neurological impairment should not be maintained in a flat supine position for extended periods of time. Their position should be alternated every few hours to prevent pooling of secretions in any one area of the lungs. A specific position may be indicated in cases of unilateral atelectasis (collapse of alveoli) or other localized problems.

Care of the Umbilical Catheter

Umbilical arterial catheters (UACs) are normally used in the NICU for monitoring arterial blood gases and aortic blood pressure in critically ill patients requiring ventilatory support. Umbilical venous catheters are used for exchange transfusions, emergency administration of fluids, medications, or blood, or occasionally for monitoring of central venous pressure. Either umbilical arterial or venous catheters may lead to serious complications if proper precautions are not observed. Hypovolemic shock or death may result from sudden blood loss if the catheter is accidentally removed or if loose connections at the stopcock or extension tubing allow leakage. Infection or emboli may be introduced with careless withdrawal of blood samples, administration of medications, or changing of tubing. Finally, clot formation in the aorta or other major arteries may lead to infarction of the kidneys, intestines, or lower extremities.

Most NICUs have written policies and procedures regarding the use and care of UACs. These policies provide details, such as how to draw blood samples, how to connect and calibrate blood pressure monitoring equipment, and how to infuse various fluids and medications. Vasoconstrictive drugs, such as epinephrine, should never be given via the UAC. Hypertonic substances should be diluted or infused very slowly. Difficulty drawing blood, changes in the blood pressure tracing, and discoloration, coolness, or loss of pulses in the legs may indicate serious UAC complications. Immediate removal may then be necessary.

COMMON PROBLEMS ENCOUNTERED IN THE NICU

Respiratory Distress Syndrome

Respiratory distress syndrome (RDS), or hyaline membrane disease, is the most common problem in the NICU. Before recent advances in ventilator management, RDS was the leading cause of neonatal mortality (Fig. 19-3). It is most frequently seen in infants of less than 36 weeks' gestation, although occasionally a near-term baby is affected.

Etiological factors

The cause of RDS is somewhat controversial, but it is definitely a developmental disease (related to natural, maturational changes) with many contributing factors. Biochemical lung maturity, marked by the appearance of adequate amounts of surface-active phospholipid compounds in alveoli, is important in preventing RDS.

These surface-active compounds, collectively referred to as surfactant, begin to appear in the fetal lung early in development but are usually not fully mature until approximately 36 to 37 weeks' gestation. Surfactant opposes the natural tendency of alveoli to collapse completely at the end of each expiration, and thereby keeps the lung partially expanded at all times.

Infants in whom surfactant is deficient must completely reexpand their lungs with each breath, greatly increasing the work of breathing. Extreme stiffness of the lungs (decreased compliance) and progressive atelectasis result. This condition leads to hypoxia, fatigue, and decreased ventilation, all of which cause acidosis. The acidosis further decreases the lung's ability to synthesize surfactant and decreases pulmonary blood flow, thus worsening the RDS and creating a vicious cycle.

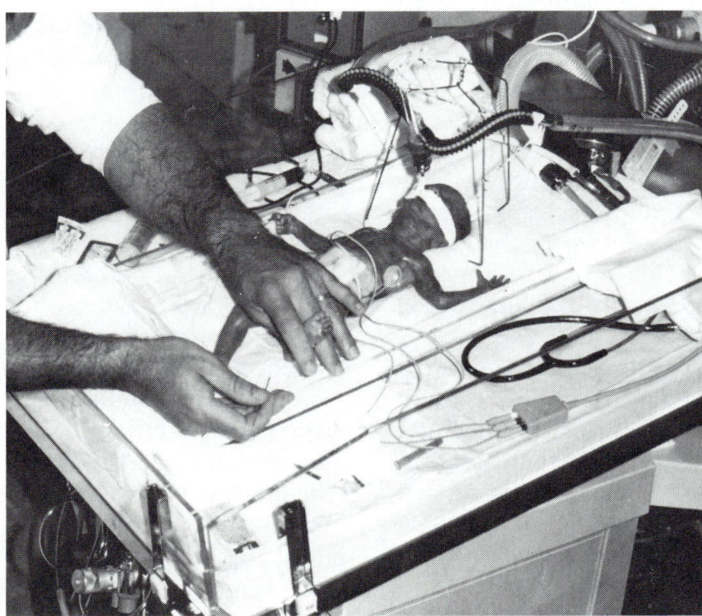

Fig. 19-3 Blood gas determination for a premature infant with respiratory distress syndrome. (Courtesy Louis Gluck, MD, University of California, San Diego Medical Center.)

The amount of surfactant in the lungs normally increases significantly at approximately 33 to 34 weeks' gestation. Certain factors, such as chronic placental abruption, prolonged rupture of membranes, maternal hypertension, and possibly maternal narcotic drug use, induce earlier surfactant appearance and therefore protect the infant from RDS. On the other hand, maternal diabetes and erythroblastosis fetalis appear to delay lung maturation. Perinatal asphyxia also worsens RDS.

Clinical manifestations

The onset of symptoms often occurs in the delivery room where the baby has low Apgar scores and requires assistance in establishing respirations. In other cases the infant may initially appear normal but begin to have expiratory grunting and nasal flaring in the first few hours of life (usually less than 6 hours). Respiratory distress becomes increasingly obvious in room air with progressive tachypnea, retractions, and cyanosis. A chest radiograph is diagnostic, revealing characteristic granular density, air bronchograms, and diminished lung volume. Arterial blood gases show hypoxia and usually a combined metabolic and respiratory acidosis.

Treatment and nursing considerations

Treatment with various types of surfactant preparations has decreased the incidence and severity of RDS. The treatment of RDS is aimed at supporting the infant by assisting oxygenation and ventilation until the infant's lungs produce adequate surfactant (usually within 2 or 3 days). The measures used depend on the severity of the disease. Mild- to moderate-cases are treated with increased concentrations of environmental oxygen, usually given by hood. More severely affected infants require continuous positive airway pressure (CPAP) to prevent the atelectasis that occurs at the end of expiration. This in turn improves oxygenation. This pressure is usually applied through nasal prongs or an endotracheal tube.

If the infant develops hypoxia, respiratory failure, or recurrent apnea despite CPAP and oxygen, mechanical ventilation is instituted with an infant respirator. Appropriate adjustments must be made for respiratory rate, expiratory and inspiratory pressures, and concentration of oxygen.

Extracorporeal membrane oxygenation (ECMO) uses cardiopulmonary bypass for the purpose of oxygenation of the infants blood outside the body through a membrane oxygenator. The oxygenator serves as a mechanical lung to decrease the workload of the infant's lungs and heal the injury caused by barotrauma and hyperoxia during ventilation. ECMO has been successful in treating acute and chronic respiratory disease, including persistent pulmonary circulation and meconium aspiration syndrome.

It must be remembered that all of these forms of treatment carry certain risks to the infant. High concentrations of inspired oxygen and ventilator pressures are known to be damaging to the lungs. High arterial P_2 (exact critical levels are unknown) in the retinal arteries can cause blindness in premature infants. Infants receiving increased pressure therapy (CPAP or mechanical ventilation) are at risk for pneumothorax and cardiovascular disturbances. Endotracheal intubation predisposes the infant to infection, and the tube itself may become occluded with secretions. Because of these potential complications, the infant with RDS must be carefully evaluated, and the risks of therapy balanced against the benefits.

General supportive measures, such as proper regulation of fluids, acid-base status, and thermal environment, are of great importance in the infant with RDS. An umbilical artery catheter is often used for frequent arterial blood gas sampling and blood pressure monitoring, as well as for administration of parenteral fluids and medications. Antibiotics are not effective against the disease itself but are used as a prophylactic measure. Transfusions may be necessary if blood drawn for testing has been extensive.

Complications

Aside from the risks of therapy previously mentioned, the complications of RDS include intracranial hemorrhage, patent ductus arteriosus (PDA), hypoglycemia, hypocalcemia, and hyperbilirubinemia. Intracranial hemorrhage is more common in infants of less than 32 weeks' gestation and is a major cause of death and disability. The onset of symptoms resulting from PDA usually coincides with the recovery phase of RDS. Typical congestive heart failure may occur with an enlarged heart and tachycardia. More often, however, an infant who has been improving clinically simply stops making progress and becomes dependent on oxygen, CPAP, or the ventilator. Fluid restriction and diuretics may be beneficial and often the PDA closes spontaneously. Some patients, however, require pharmacological closure with indomethacin or surgical ligation.

Prevention of RDS

Prenatal assessment of lung surfactant maturity can be done by performing an amniocentesis and analyzing surfactant in the amniotic fluid. The lecithin/sphingomyelin (L/S) ratio compares the content of lecithin, an important surfactant, with sphingomyelin, an inactive phospholipid. An L/S ratio of 2.0 usually indicates lung maturity, as does the presence of another important compound, phosphatidyl glycerol (PG). Elective delivery (cesarean section or induction) should be delayed until the studies indicate lung maturity to minimize the risk of RDS. In some cases the administration of glucocorticoids to the mother 48 to 72 hours before delivery may stimulate fetal lung maturity and therefore decrease the risk of RDS.

Meconium Aspiration

Staining of the amniotic fluid with meconium, the stool of the fetus, occurs in approximately 10% to 15% of all births. It may indicate intrauterine distress, and in some instances the infant may make gasping respiratory efforts before the head is delivered, and thus aspirate the meconium into the lungs. Although normal amniotic fluid is usually harmless to the lungs, the particles of meconium produce obstruction of the airways and cause respiratory difficulty. The infant may be vigorous and breathing easily. If significant intrauterine asphyxia has occurred, however, the infant will be depressed and require assistance in establishing respirations.

Treatment and nursing considerations

Intubation and direct tracheal suction are performed to remove as much meconium as possible before the use of positive pressure ventilation. Ideally this prevents forcing meconium from the airway into the lungs and reduces the severity of the disease. Suctioning of the infant's oropharynx after delivery of the head but before delivery of the shoulders and chest also minimizes the inhalation of meconium. Respiratory distress occurs in about 15% of meconium-stained infants and varies from mild to severe. In most cases, distress resolves within 48 hours. Occasionally, ventilatory assistance must be continued for longer periods. Treatment also consists of oxygen, CPT and suction, and generally supportive measures. Antibiotics are used, and mechanical ventilation is sometimes necessary for severe cases. Pneumothorax is a common complication.

Pneumothorax

Approximately 1% of all newborns develop pneumothorax (free air in the pleural space). The majority of them remain asymptomatic and the condition resolves without treatment. Pneumothorax usually occurs spontaneously as a result of the high intrathoracic pressures that infants generate when expanding their lungs with the first few breaths. Other cases may be caused by positive pressure ventilation or aspiration of meconium or blood. Premature infants are more susceptible to pneumothorax than are full-term infants.

Clinical manifestations

Clinical signs of pneumothorax include tachypnea, tachycardia, cyanosis, shifting of the cardiac impulse, decreased blood pressure, and irritability. Transillumination of the chest is significantly increased by a tension pneumothorax. The diagnosis is confirmed by chest radiograph.

Treatment and nursing considerations

Treatment of the infant with pneumothorax depends on the severity of the symptoms. The infant with mild or no signs needs only careful observation. If severe distress is present, the pneumothorax should be aspirated by needle and a chest tube inserted into the pleural space. The chest tube is usually connected to suction with a water seal. Follow-up radiographs are indicated to determine the position of the chest tube and reexpansion of the lung. Patency of the tube must be maintained by prevention of kinking, clotting, and looping. The chest tube can usually be removed within a few days, as the respiratory status improves.

Hyperbilirubinemia

Hyperbilirubinemia occurs in normal newborns and is often exaggerated in the premature or sick neonate. Bilirubin, most of which is formed from the breakdown of hemoglobin, is taken up by liver cells, where it is modified and excreted through the bile ducts into the intestine. This process is delayed in newborns, leading to so-called physiological hyperbilirubinemia.

Hyperbilirubinemia is considered to be pathological if the serum bilirubin level exceeds 12 mg per 100 ml, or if obvious jaundice appears in the first 24 hours. The most common cause is hemolytic disease (e.g., Rh or ABO blood group incompatibility of the fetus and mother). Other causes include polycythemia, excessive bruising, hemolytic anemias, sepsis, intrauterine viral infection, and metabolic disorders.

Clinical manifestations

Jaundice or a yellow discoloration of the skin and sclerae is the major clinical manifestation of hyperbilirubinemia. The intensity of the jaundice is unrelated to the level of hyperbilirubinemia.

Treatment and nursing considerations

Hyperbilirubinemia is treated with phototherapy and, in severe cases, exchange transfusions. Phototherapy breaks down bilirubin in the skin. Infants receiving this treatment wear a diaper and eye shields. The infants must periodically be turned to ensure total skin exposure. The child should be given increased fluids to compensate for evaporative fluid loss associated with the treatment.

In an exchange transfusion, the infant's blood is replaced, ideally removing much of the excess bilirubin. The objective of the treatment is the prevention of kernicterus, a neurological condition caused by the deposit of bilirubin into the basal ganglia of the brain. Hearing loss may result from bilirubin toxicity of the auditory nerve. The exact serum bilirubin level at which damage occurs varies widely, depending on the maturity and clinical condition of the infant. A sophisticated hearing assessment is conducted by the audiologist in the NICU using the brainstem auditory evoked response screening (BAERS). This accurate screening tool is used for most NICU patients before discharge.

Neonatal Sepsis

The newborn infant with neonatal sepsis has immature immunological responses and, therefore has increased susceptibility to infection (e.g., bacterial, viral). Once an infection is acquired, it may quickly invade the bloodstream (neonatal sepsis or septicemia) and lead to meningitis, pneumonia, a urinary tract infection, osteomyelitis, or other complications. Certain factorspredispose infants to infection, including prematurity, prolonged rupture of membranes, maternal infection, difficult labor with fetal distress, and special procedures such as resuscitation, intubation, and umbilical or central vein catheterization.

Group B streptococcal infections have most often been identified in the past years. Many other bacteria may also cause sepsis, including other streptococci, *Staphylococcus, listeria,* and Gram-negative organisms. In long-term NICU patients, *Staphylococcus epidermidis* has become the most common pathogen. Less common bacteria, such as *Citrobacter, Serratia,* and *Pseudomonas,* or viruses may also be encountered in the NICU. Fungal infections, usually *Candida albicans,* are commonly seen.

Clinical manifestations

Presenting signs of neonatal sepsis are respiratory distress with grunting and tachypnea, poor feeding, vomiting, lethargy, temperature instability, jaundice, and apnea.

Treatment and nursing considerations

Early treatment of neonatal sepsis is of extreme importance in obtaining a favorable outcome. Once infection is suspected, cultures should promptly be taken of blood, urine, spinal fluid, stool, tracheal aspirate, and additional sites as indicated. Broad-spectrum therapy, usually involving a combination of two antibiotics, such as ampicillin and gentamicin, should be started immediately. Therapy may be changed later when the results of cultures are obtained and sensitivities of the particular organism(s) are known. As always, good and frequent handwashing is critical.

Intrauterine Infection

Although the fetus is protected by the mother from many infectious diseases, some microorganisms have the ability to cross the placenta and cause significant damage. If a pregnant woman becomes infected at a time when her fetus is susceptible, intrauterine infection may result. These infections are commonly referred to as the **TORCHES** (*TO*xoplasmosis, *R*ubella, *C*ytomegalovirus, *HE*rpes, and *S*yphilis), although other agents are also now known to cause fetal infection, including chlamydia and HIV.

Rubella (German measles) is probably the best-known and most-feared intrauterine infection. Rubella infection occurs in up to 50% of fetuses of mothers who acquire the disease during the first 8 weeks of pregnancy. The fetal-infection rate then declines and is very low after the first trimester. Affected infants have demonstrated a variety of manifestations from the most severe congenital rubella syndrome (intrauterine growth retardation, cardiac defects, cataracts, deafness, anemia, jaundice, and mental retardation) to the apparently normal newborn with only mild hearing loss. Diagnosis can be confirmed by viral cultures of the infant's pharynx, urine, or stool and by antibody titers of the mother and infant. Immunization programs to prevent infection of pregnant women are of the utmost importance, since no specific treatment exists.

Cytomegalovirus (CMV) is the most common intrauterine infection and, like rubella, may have a variety of effects on the infant. Most infants are asymptomatic, but others may have microcephaly, growth retardation, hepatitis, low platelet count, seizures, and pneumonia. Diagnosis is confirmed by cultures and by antibody studies.

Toxoplasmosis, a protozoan disease that may be contracted by the ingestion of raw meat or food contaminated with cat feces, is relatively uncommon in the United States. It may be entirely asymptomatic in the infected mother. It primarily affects the fetal central nervous system and may cause mental retardation, blindness, deafness, convulsions, and hydrocephalus. These infants should be treated with sulfadiazine and pyrimethamine, although much of the damage is probably irreversible.

Congenital syphilis is most likely if maternal infection occurs in the latter part of pregnancy, or if infection is acquired during the birth process. Infected infants usually appear normal in the immediate postpartum period, although prematurity and stillbirths sometimes result. Most cases of congenital syphilis exhibit a typical rash, profuse nasal discharge, radiographical defects of the long bones, and hepatitis in early infancy. Congenital syphilis is most often detected by screening for maternal disease with routine serological testing on all pregnant women. Treatment with penicillin eradicates the disease, although mental retardation and other sequelae may not be totally prevented.

An important sexually transmitted bacterium, *Chlamydia trachomatis* may also be acquired by the infant during birth. Conjunctivitis or pneumonitis can result during the first few weeks of life. Other organisms known to infect fetuses include the hepatitis B virus and HIV, the virus that causes acquired immune deficiency syndrome (AIDS). Infants with these illnesses do not usually become symptomatic in the neonatal period. The herpes simplex virus may be transmitted from maternal, genital infections to the infant during birth and cause a rapidly fatal illness. As screening techniques and virology studies become more sensitive and widespread, knowledge of these fetal infections will increase, as will their relative importance in NICU patients.

Intraventricular Hemorrhage

Intraventricular hemorrhage (IVH) is a hemorrhage into and around the ventricles of the brain. It is caused by vessels ruptured as a result of an event that increases cerebral blood flow to an area of the brain. It is most common in premature infants.

Clinical manifestations

Signs of IVH include evidence on cranial ultrasonography and/or CT scan, asymmetrical primitive reflexes and deep tendon reflexes, a tense and bulging anterior fontanelle, deterioration in condition, twitching, stupor, apnea, and seizures.

Treatment and nursing considerations

The therapeutic management of neonates with IVH includes the maintenance of oxygenation, ventilatory support, suppression or prevention of seizures, and the regulation of fluid and electrolyte balance. The nurse must prevent increased intracranial pressure through pain control, avoidance of over-stimulation and unnecessary suctioning, and elevation of the head of the bed. Provision of informational and emotional support for the family is essential.

Perinatal Substance Abuse

The increasing use of cocaine, especially "crack," by pregnant women has elevated the number of premature deliveries and fetal deaths. Such mothers may have placental detachment (abruption), causing significant maternal bleeding and hypoxia in the infant. Infants of these mothers may die or suffer brain damage. Others are exposed to the risks normally associated with premature birth.

Infants whose mothers are addicted to heroin, barbiturates, amphetamines, or other drugs inherit the drug dependence. These babies usually appear normal at birth but begin to show signs of withdrawal after 8 to 12 hours.

Clinical manifestations

Extreme irritability, constant crying, jitteriness, poor feeding, emesis, diarrhea, respiratory distress, and seizures may occur in the infants of substance-abusing mothers.

Treatment and nursing considerations

Signs of substance exposure are alleviated by administration of paregoric, phenobarbital, or tranquilizers (chlorpromazine, diazepam) and by keeping the infant well wrapped in a quiet, dimly lighted environment. Intravenous fluids may be necessary to prevent dehydration or hypoglycemia. Medication is gradually decreased and discontinued over several days.

Fetal Alcohol Syndrome

Fetal alcohol syndrome has been well documented in infants born to mothers who drink alcohol during pregnancy. These infants may exhibit intrauterine growth retardation, microcephaly, mental deficiency, cardiac defects, and characteristic anomalies of the face and extremities. Lesser effects may occur in babies born to moderate drinkers and may be difficult to recognize, although intellectual impairment may result. These infants may experience withdrawal symptoms similar to those of infants of drug-addicted mothers.

Infants Born to Diabetic Mothers

Infants born to diabetic mothers (IDMs) are predisposed to a number of neonatal disorders. Late intrauterine fetal deaths occur more commonly in diabetic mothers. Their pregnancies must be monitored carefully by the physician. Maternal blood glucose should be controlled as closely as possible, and the fetus should be evaluated frequently for abnormalities of growth and signs of distress. IDMs are at increased risk for RDS, especially if delivered prematurely. Amniocentesis is, therefore, usually performed to assess fetal lung maturity and help determine the optimum time for delivery.

When maternal diabetes is poorly controlled the mother's hyperglycemia promotes fetal insulin secretion. These secretions lead to excessive growth and deposition of fat. The infants may be very large (10 or more pounds) and have a higher incidence of hypoglycemia at birth because of the abrupt removal of the mother's glucose supply and the continued production of insulin by the infant. Blood glucose should be checked frequently in these infants and in any infant judged to be large for gestational age (see Chapter 18).

Mild maternal diabetes may have gone undetected. Early institution of feedings may prevent hypoglycemia in the child, or intravenous glucose water may be necessary. IDMs are also susceptible to hypocalcemia, hyperbilirubinemia, polycythemia, congenital anomalies, and renal vein thrombosis, especially if the mother's diabetes is not well controlled.

Infants born to mothers with severe or long-standing diabetes suffer intrauterine growth retardation and are usually small, rather than large, for their gestational age. Their lungs appear to mature early, and they may be protected from having RDS. The severity and duration of the mother's diabetes and her control during pregnancy are the most important factors influencing the infant's problems.

Necrotizing Enterocolitis

Necrotizing enterocolitis is an acute, sometimes fatal, intestinal disorder in the newborn and is most commonly seen in the small, premature infant. The cause of necrotizing enterocolitis may be because of ischemia (inadequate blood flow to the gut) or pathogenic bacteria. Such ischemia may damage the intestine and increase susceptibility to infection and possible harmful effects of digestive enzymes.

Clinical manifestations

Clinical signs of necrotizing enterocolitis include abdominal distention, vomiting, diarrhea with blood in the stool, apnea, lethargy, hypothermia, and shock. Positive diagnosis is established by abdominal radiographical examination. This examination may show air in the intestinal wall or free air in the peritoneal cavity.

Treatment and nursing considerations

Initial treatment of necrotizing enterocolitis consists of nasogastric suction, intravenous fluids, antibiotics, and transfusions. Serial abdominal radiographs are performed at frequent intervals to detect progression of the disease or perforation of the bowel, either of which is an indication for surgery. During surgery the areas of necrotic bowel are resected and a colostomy is usually performed. Anastomosis of the intestine is then done as an elective procedure after the infant has recovered.

Postmaturity

Postmature infants are those who are born after 42 or more weeks' gestation. They have dry, parchmentlike skin, long fingernails, and a wide-eyed, alert expression. Meconium staining of the skin is common, and meconium aspiration occurs more frequently than with normal-term infants. Mortality of the postmature infant is nearly twice as high as that of the full-term infant. Postmature infants have diminished glycogen stores and are therefore susceptible to hypoglycemia. They should be fed early and have periodic blood-glucose determinations.

KEY CONCEPTS

1 The main objective of the NICU is to provide the earliest and maximum degree of medical and nursing care for the infant at risk so that each infant attains the best possible outcome.

2 Newborns may be admitted to the NICU with problems such as prematurity and its various complications, birth defects, infection, jaundice, hypoglycemia, or perinatal asphyxia.

3 The comprehensive, regional perinatal center provides an obstetrical-perinatal service for outpatient and inpatient care of high-risk mothers and their fetuses. These centers often operate a new-

born transport system, supervise continuing education for health professionals in the region, provide long-term follow-up of infants treated in the NICU, and is responsible for ongoing research in perinatal-neonatal medicine.

4 Health care personnel can reduce the anxiety of parents whose infants are transferred to a regional NICU by encouraging them to touch and hold their infant, and by involving them as much as possible in daily routines such as feeding and bathing. Parents should be kept informed of their child's progress and counseled appropriately.

5 An increased incidence of neonatal disease is seen in infants whose mothers have risk factors such as lack of prenatal care, poor nutrition or other socioeconomic problems, previous history of obstetrical complications, and medical illnesses. Complications in labor and delivery that may signal potential neonatal problems include premature labor, premature rupture of membranes, abnormal presentation or fetal size, multiple births, meconium-stained amniotic fluid, and inappropriate maternal analgesia or anesthesia.

6 Small, premature infants have difficulty maintaining body temperature because they have thin skin that is not insulated by the subcutaneous fat characteristic of full-term infants, an increased proportion of body surface area to body mass, and immature central nervous system temperature regulators.

7 The NICU infant's intake and output must be carefully measured and charted. Output includes urine, stool, and blood withdrawn for diagnostic tests. Urine can be measured using disposable diapers or plastic collection bags and is tested for blood, glucose, protein, pH, and specific gravity. Stools should be described and checked for occult blood.

8 When caring for an infant receiving oxygen-enriched ventilatory support the nurse should frequently monitor the oxygen content of the air-oxygen, the mixture, the ventilator settings, the endotracheal tube position, and the infant's respirations and breath sounds.

9 The premature or low-birth-weight infant experiences increased water losses as a result of tachypnea, abnormal gastrointestinal losses, administration of a concentrated solution, fever, the use of an open-radiant warmer bed, and phototherapy. The infant's state of hydration is monitored by following serial weights, intake and output, urine specific gravities, and serum electrolytes.

10 Overfeeding a premature infant may cause regurgitation and aspiration or intestinal complications. Feeding intolerance can be evaluated by aspirating the stomach contents before giving feedings or periodically when feedings are continuous, and by watching for changes in abdominal girth, bowel sounds, and stooling patterns.

11 Nourishment can be provided to newborns through nipple feeding, orogastric or nasogastric tubes, transpyloric or nasoduodenal feedings, or parenteral hyperalimentation.

12 The patency of the airway of infants receiving ventilatory support can be maintained by suctioning endotracheal tubes, injecting small amounts of saline into the tube to thin secretions, and by administering chest physiotherapy before airway suctioning.

13 Infants with respiratory disease or neurological impairment should not be maintained in a flat supine position for extended periods of time. These infants should be repositioned every few hours to prevent the pooling of secretions in the lungs.

14 If proper precautions are not observed, the use of umbilical catheters may result in hypovolemic shock or death from sudden blood loss, infection or emboli, or clot formation leading to infarction of the kidneys, intestines, or lower extremities. Indications of possible complications include difficulty in drawing blood, changes in the blood pressure tracing, and discoloration, coolness, or loss of pulses in the legs.

15 Infants with RDS lack biochemical lung maturity marked by the appearance of adequate amounts of surface-active phospholipid compounds in alveoli. Prenatal assessment of lung surfactant maturity can be done by performing an amniocentesis and analyzing surfactant in the amniotic fluid.

16 Respiratory distress occurs in about 15% of meconium-stained infants and varies from mild to severe. Distress usually resolves within 48 hours.

17 Clinical signs of pneumothorax include tachypnea, tachycardia, cyanosis, shifting of the cardiac impulse, decreased blood pressure, and irritability. The diagnosis is confirmed by chest radiograph.

18 Hyperbilirubinemia is treated with phototherapy and, in severe cases, exchange transfusions. Infants receiving phototherapy usually wear only an abbreviated diaper and eye shields. They must be periodically turned to ensure proper skin exposure and should be given additional liquid to compensate for evaporative fluid loss.

19 Certain factors predispose infants to infection, such as prematurity, prolonged rupture of membranes, maternal infection, fetal distress during labor, and certain special procedures.

20 If a pregnant woman becomes infected with certain microorganisms, it is possible for them to cross the placenta and infect the fetus. These

infections are known as the **TORCHES** (*TO*xoplasmosis, *R*ubella, *C*ytomegalovirus, *HE*rpes, and *S*yphilis). Chlamydia and HIV and may also be transmitted to the neonate.

21 An infant who has inherited the mother's drug dependence usually begins to show signs of withdrawal after 8 to 12 hours. Treatment includes the administration of paregoric, phenobarbitol, or tranquilizers, and keeping the infant well wrapped in a quiet, dimly lit environment.

22 An infant born to a mother who drinks alcohol during pregnancy may exhibit intrauterine growth retardation, microcephaly, mental deficiency, cardiac defects, and characteristic anomalies of the face and extremities.

23 The severity and duration of the mother's diabetes and her diabetic control during pregnancy are the most important factors influencing problems in the infant. Problems may include RDS, hypoglycemia, hypocalcemia, hyperbilirubinemia, polycythemia, congenital anomalies, and renal vein thrombosis.

24 Necrotizing enterocolitis is an acute, sometimes fatal, intestinal disorder most commonly seen in the small, premature infant.

25 Infants born after 42 or more weeks' gestation are considered postmature and have nearly twice the mortality rate as that of the full-term infant.

CRITICAL THOUGHT QUESTIONS

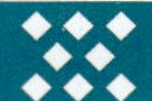

1 Neonatal intensive care units are usually located in major medical center. What plan of care is recommended if a high-risk birth is anticipated? What if there is no warning and birth occurs at a location some distance from the nearest NICU?

2 Why is respiratory distress syndrome a major concern in the premature infant? What observations indicate respiratory distress? What diagnostic tests are normally performed? What is the typical treatment of an infant with RDS? What are the treatment risks?

3 Infections acquired before or after birth place the neonate at increased risk. Identify those infections most likely to be contracted before birth. What can be done to reduce this risk? Identify those infections most likely to be contracted at or after birth. What can be done to reduce this risk?

4 Fetal problems related to the life habits or addictions of the mother, such as alcohol or drug abuse, are becoming increasingly common. The newborn becomes the victim of the mother's problem. What do you think should be done in these situations? How can you recognize fetal alcohol syndrome or drug withdrawal in the newborn? What special care will the infant need? Does the mother require special care? Should other social service agencies be included in the plan of care?

REFERENCES

American Academy of Pediatrics and American College of Obstetricians and Gynecologists: *Guidelines for perinatal care,* ed 3, Elk Grove Village, IL, 1992, The Academy.

Beckholt AP: Breast milk for infants who cannot breastfeed, *J Obstet Gynecol Neonatal Nurs* 19(3):216, 1990.

Bobak IM, Jensen MD: *Maternity and gynecologic care.* St. Louis, 1993, Mosby.

Brazelton TB: *Neonatal behavioral assessment scale,* ed 3, Philadelphia, 1990, JB Lippincott.

Cunningham N, Hutchinson S: Neonatal nurses and issues in research ethics, *Neonatal network* 8(5):29-48, 1990.

Damato EG: Discharge planning from the NICU, *J Perinatal Neonatal Nurs,* 5(43):47-50, 1991.

Edgehouse L, Radzyminski SG: A device for supplementing breast-feeding, *MCN* 15(1):34, 1990.

Fanaroff AA, Martin RJ: *Neonatal-perinatal medicine: diseases of the fetus and infant*, St. Louis, 1992, Mosby.

Gordin PC: Assessing and managing agitation in a critically ill infant, *MCN* 15(1):26, 1990.

Harrison LL: Teaching stimulation strategies to parents of infants at high risk, *MCN* 14(2):125, 1989.

Ioli J, Klaus MH, Fanaroff AA: *Care of the high-risk neonate,* Philadelphia, 1993, WB Saunders.

Kimble C: Nonnutritive sucking: adaptation and health for the neonate, *Neonatal Network,* 11(3):29-33, 1992.

Korones SB, Lancaster J: *High-risk newborn infants: the basis for intensive nursing care,* ed 5. St. Louis, 1993, Mosby.

Merenstein GB, Gardner SL: *Handbook of neonatal intensive care,* St Louis, 1989, Mosby.

Novak J: An ethical decision making model for the NICU, *J Perinatal Neonatal Nurs,* 1(3):57-67, 1988.

Novak J: Facilitating fathering. In Craft M, Denehy J: *Nursing interventions with infants and children,* Philadelphia, 1991, WB Saunders.

Polin RA, Fox WW: *Fetal and neonatal physiology,* Philadelphia, 1992, WB Saunders.

Ryan P, Cote-Arsenault D, Sugarman L: Facilitating care after perinatal loss, J Obstet Gynecol Neonatal Nurs 29(5):385-389, 1991.

Richardson M: Giving surfactant to premature infants, *Am J Nurs* 90(3):59, 1990.

Thomas KA: How the NICU environment sounds to a preterm infant, *MCN* 14(4):249, 1989.

BIBLIOGRAPHY

Substance Abuse

Centers for Disease Control: Progress toward achieving the 1990 national objectives for the misuse of alcohol and drugs, *MMWR* 39(15):256, 1990.

House MA: Cocaine, *Am J Nurs* 90(4):41, 1990.

Lindmark B: Maternal use of alcohol and breast-fed infants, *N Engl J Med* 322(5):338, 1990.

Little RE, et al: Maternal alcohol use during breast-feeding and infant mental and motor development at one year, *N Engl J Med* 321(7):425, 1989.

O' Doherty N: *Atlas of the newborn*, ed 3, Hingham, MA, 1992, Kluwer Academic.

Povenmire KI, House MA: Recognizing the cocaine addict, *Nursing '90* 20(5):46, 1990.

Wong D: *Whaley and Wong's essentials of pediatric nursing*, St. Louis, 1993, Mosby.

Circumcision

Anderson GF: Circumcision, *Pediatr Ann* 18(3):205, 1989.

Engel NS: Lidocaine dorsal penile nerve block for circumcision, *MCN* 14(5):311, 1989.

Feeding

La Leche League International: *The womanly art of breast-feeding*, ed 5, New York, 1992, New American Library.

Nice FJ: Can a breast-feeding mother take medication without harming her infant? *MCN* 14(1):17, 1989.

Pipes PL: *Nutrition in infancy and childhood*, ed 5, St Louis, 1993, Mosby.

Tiedje LB, Collins C: Combining employment and motherhood, *MCN* 14(1):23, 1989.

Walker M, Driscoll JW: Sore nipples: the new mother's nemesis, *MCN* 14(4):260, 1989.

Williams KM, Morse JM: Weaning patterns of first time mothers, *MCN* 14(3):188, 1989.

Woldt EH: Breastfeeding support group in the NICU, *Neonatal Network* 9(5):53-56, 1991.

Temperature Maintenance

Greer PS: Head coverings for newborns under radiant warmers, *J Obstet Gynecol Neonatal Nurs* 17(4):265, 1988.

Prematurity

Wink DM: Better breast milk for preemies, *Am J Nurs* 89(1):48-50, 1989.

Infections and Infection Control

American Academy of Pediatrics/American College of Obstetricians and Gynecologists: *Guidelines for perinatal care*, ed 3, Elk Grove Village, IL, 1993, The Academy.

Crow S: Calling in sick: how to decide, *Nursing '90* 20(3):63, 1990.

Hammerschlag MR, et al: Efficacy of neonatal ocular prophylaxis for prevention of chlamydial and gonorrheal conjunctivitis, *N Engl J Med* 320(12):769, 1989.

Jackson MM: Infection prevention and control for HIV and other infectious agents in obstetric and gynecologic and neonatal settings, *NAACOG Clinical Issues* 1(1):115, 1990.

Lynch P, et al: Implementing and evaluating a system of generic infection precautions: body substance isolation, *Am J Infect Control* 18(1):1, 1990.

Abnormalities of the Newborn

Avery ME, Taeusch HW: *Diseases of the newborn*, ed 6, Philadelphia, 1992, WB Saunders.

Campbell JR: Inguinal and scrotal problems in infants and children, *Pediatr Ann* 18(3):189, 1989.

Crocker AC: The causes of mental retardation, *Pediatr Ann* 18(10):623, 1989.

Fisher C: The abnormal infant: protecting yourself against blame, *RN* 53(4):69, 1990.

Jackson PL: Primary care needs of children with hydrocephalus, *J Pediatr Health Care* 4(2):59, 1990.

Schaming D, et al: When babies are born with orthopedic problems, *RN* 53(4):62, 1990.

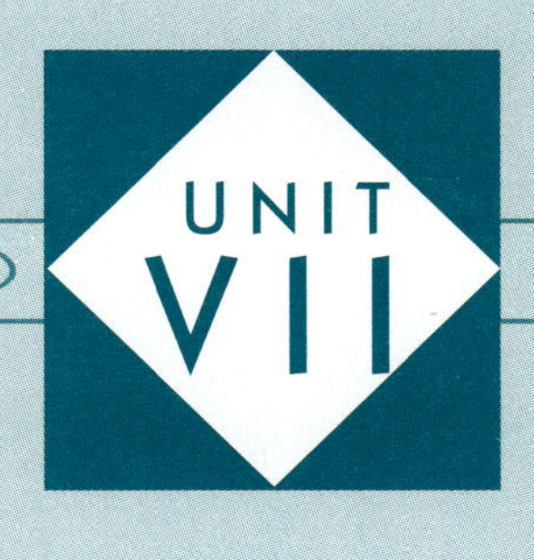

DEVELOPMENTAL HEALTH PROMOTION

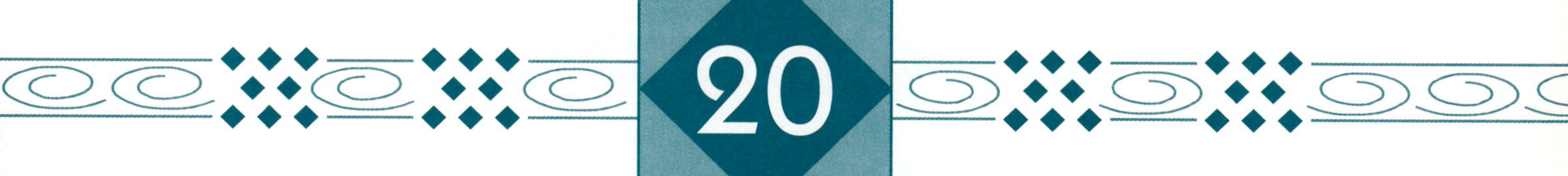

20

Genetic and Environmental Factors

CHAPTER OBJECTIVES

After studying this chapter, the student should be able to:

1. Define the following terms: *growth, development, maturation, genes, chromosomes, karyotype, genogram, pedigree, consanguinity,* and *heterozygous* and *homozygous inheritance.*
2. State five principles of growth and development.
3. Identify the periods of greatest physical growth during an individual's life span.
4. Explain the mechanism of autosomal-dominant inheritance, give one example, and construct a "probability box."
5. Explain the mechanism of autosomal-recessive inheritance, give one example, and construct a "probability box."
6. Explain why X-linked recessive disorders are usually expressed by only the male child. Cite one example.
7. Discuss the role of the genetic counselor and the techniques they use to assist families.
8. Discuss the purpose of the US Human Genome Project.
9. Discuss two diagnostic methods that are commonly used in first trimester genetic screening.
10. List five examples of prenatal, natal, and postnatal environmental influences on a child.
11. Demonstrate the use of the measurement called *percentile rank* on the NCHS growth charts. State what this ranking indicates.
12. Explain different methods of evaluating growth. Indicate which of these methods is considered the best for assessing a child's general growth progress.
13. Trace the average height growth in children from birth through the first year, second year, preschool period, and from 6 to 10 years of age.
14. Indicate the intervals at which a child's birth weight usually doubles and triples.
15. Identify centers of ossification that can be evaluated for bone-age studies in children.
16. Discuss the normal progress of dentition in children. State which teeth usually appear first and second and the age at which the eruption of all 20 primary teeth is customarily complete.
17. Explain what is meant by cephalocaudal and proximodistal development.
18. State the normal sequence of prehension and the typical timetable cited for these accomplishments.
19. Trace the normal locomotion sequence, starting with head and chest elevation and ending with walking alone.
20. Describe the process of habituation and its posssible role as a predictor of intelligence.
21. Describe three styles of parenting. Discuss the possibility of a parent using more than one style.
22. Discuss the **PET** approach to parenting.
23. List six techniques used to shape behavior and moral values.

The terms *growth* and *development* are closely related and are sometimes used interchangeably. Increases in structure (growth) are accompanied by increases in function (development). As children grow in size, they mature mentally, emotionally, and socially.

As growth and development continue, various levels of maturity are observable. Maturation is the process in which inherited tendencies begin to unfold, independent of any special practice or training. All children have their own patterns of growth and develoment.

CONCEPTS OF GROWTH AND DEVELOPMENT

As children grow, they are constantly changing physically and developmentally. This continuous period of change is the main distinction between the child and the adult. Growth is exhibited by all healthy children, although it may be impaired by malnutrition and disease. Child growth and development characterize pediatrics as a specialty.

Every nurse who cares for children must have a basic understanding of the stages of human growth and development. Such an understanding helps when evaluating the physical, intellectual, emotional, and social behavior of the dynamic child (Table 20-1). Developmental assessment is an important component of the nursing process. For additional information regarding developmental assessment, refer to Chapter 21.

Some children mature rapidly. Other children who are slower physically, mentally, and emotionally are called late maturers. A wide range of normal varations exist in the growth and development rates of children. Whereas one child walks at 12 months of age, another may be 15 months old when first steps are taken. Each child matures physiologically and developmentally at his or her own rate.

The overall acquisition of developmental milestones is similar in different cultures. Thus some generalizations can be made concerning growth and development. Recognizing the unique child rearing characteristics of various cultural and ethnic groups, however, specific variations are highlighted. This discussion of growth and development follows the child through an orderly sequence, beginning with the prenatal phase and continuing through infancy, childhood, and adolescence.

Nursing Alert

Overgeneralizations regarding various ethnic and cultural groups should be avoided.

Principles

The normal growth and development of a child through the prenatal period, infancy, childhood, and adolescence are guided by certain basic principles. Growth and development (1) are self-fueling, ongoing processes that require physical and psychological energy; (2) occur in an orderly sequence, although the sequence is not a smooth continuum but is characterized by a series of lulls and spurts; (3) progress at highly individualized rates from child to child; (4) vary at different ages for their specific structures; and (5) represent a total process involving the whole child where all areas of development are interrelated.

Orderly sequence

Growth and development occur in an orderly sequence and are continuous. The sequence of development is the same for all children. Some children, however, do things earlier than others. Children

◆ TABLE 20-1
Progressive Stages of Development

Stages of Life	Divisions of Life Stages	Chronological Age
Prenatal		
Conception to birth	Germinal	Conception to 10 days' gestation
	Embryonic	10 days to 2 months' gestation
	Fetal	2 months' gestation to birth
Infancy		
Birth to 1 year	Newborn (neonate)	Birth to 1 month
	Infancy	1 month to 1 year
Childhood		
1 to 12 years	Toddler	1 to 3 years
	Preschool	3 to 6 years
	School	6 to 10 years
	Preadolescence (puberty)	10 to 12 years
Adolescence		
12 to 19 years	Early adolescence	12 to 16 years
	Late adolescence	16 to 19 years

generally creep before they stand and stand alone before they walk. Average children talk before they read and usually read before they can write. One child reads at 4 years of age and another reads at 6 years of age. What happens at one stage influences what happens during the next stage. Each stage in the development of an individual is an outgrowth of an earlier stage. During the first year of life, babies coo then babble. As they grow, they begin to say simple words. The toddler uses words in phrases, and the preschooler uses words in short sentences. No child speaks clearly before babbling. Each stage in the sequence of development can be anticipated.

Continuity

Growth and development continue from the moment of conception until the individual reaches maturity. At no time, however, is growth even and regular. Lulls and spurts occur within the development of a child, even though no real interruptions occur until growth is completed. Growth is greatest during the prenatal period and remains rapid during infancy and early childhood. The rate is slow but constant in middle childhood. A spurt occurs during early puberty and then tapers off in the latter part of puberty.

Differences in growth rates

All children have their own unique growth timetables. A child who develops rapidly during the early years of life will continue to develop rapidly. Whereas one child may sit unaided at 6 months of age and walk alone at 9 months of age, his or her sibling may sit unaided at 8 months of age and walk alone at 15 months of age. Thus within the same family siblings demonstrate unique individual differences.

Variation of growth rates

Not all parts of the body mature at the same time. The brain attains its physical adult size when the child is about 6 or 7 years of age. It does not, however, complete mental maturation until many years later. Different phases of physical and mental growth occur at their own individual rates, and maturity is reached at different times.

Growth and development as a total process

Children grow physically, mentally, socially, and emotionally at the same time. The child simultaneously develops as a whole being. Changes in interest and cognitive development are closely related to development in walking and talking. Growth is a total process involving the whole child, not just the body, mind, and emotions individually. One aspect of the child cannot be considered in isolation. All areas of child development are interrelated. The interrelated history of the whole child and his or her environment is a foundation for understanding the child's present needs.

GENETIC AND ENVIRONMENTAL FACTORS

Every child's growth and development (pattern, rate, rhythm, and extent) are governed by genetic and environmental forces. Within the broad categories of genetic and environmental influences are many overlapping and diverse factors. These factors include gender differences, endocrine gland function, ethnic and cultural factors, cellular mutations, other inherited strengths and weaknesses, psychological and cultural milieu, nutritional and physical advantages or disadvantages, and concurrent malformation or disease. For decades the controversy raged regarding the respective importance of genetics and environment, or "nature versus nurture." Most experts believe this theory to be a futile argument, acknowledging that both are critically important. These experts propose a newer, dynamic, and interactional understanding of child development.

Genetic Influences

One fourth of all hospitalized children have diseases or defects with underlying genetic components. The science of genetics is based on principles of inheritance, which were first described in the mid-1880s by the Augustinian monk and scientist, Gregor Mendel. Mendel's law explains certain aspects of gene activity in humans during the formation of gametes (eggs and sperm) and during fertilization (the union of an egg and spermatazoan).

Genes, the hereditary elements, are defined lengths of deoxyribonucleic acid (DNA). They are located in structures called chromosomes, which are found in every cell's nucleus. DNA consists of pairs of four nucleotide bases: adenine (A), guanine (G), cytosine (C), and thymine (T), found in a double-helix formation. DNA directs the assembly of amino acids into proteins essential for normal functioning. When cells divide the DNA duplicates itself and passes on its genetic code to the next generation of cells. Twenty-three chromosomes from each parent, combine to make a total of 46 at fertilization. Each of the 22 chromosomes donated by one parent has a microscopically similar counterpart that is donated by the other parent. These chromosomic counterparts, called autosomes, can be paired whether the developing individual is a boy or a girl. Each pair of autosomal chromosomes is different in its genetic content and appearance. Two other, different chromosomes, labeled X and Y, determine the gender of the child. These chromosomes are called sex chromosomes. Each parent donates only one. The mother is able to contribute only an X chromosome, whereas the father may give to his child either an X or a Y chromosome. Infants having an XX inheritance are girls; those with XY are boys.

The three known general pathways involved in the etiology of genetic disease are (1) Mendelian patterns of inheritance involving only one or two defective genes, (2) multifactorial disorders related to multiple gene defects and environmental factors, and (3) gross genetic imbalances caused by chromosomal abnormalities. Defects in chromosomal structure or numbers can be considered packaging defects. The chromosomes are the "packages" that carry the genes from generation to generation. Defects in individual genes—the contents of these packages—are not evident on inspection of the chromosomes themselves. They are revealed by disease and abnormality in the affected person.

A brief discussion of the various modes of inheritance provides an understanding of the basic characteristics associated with each inheritance pattern.

Mendelian disorders may be subdivided into four distinct patterns of inheritance. Each pattern involves one or two defective genes. To observe the distribution pattern of a specific trait in a family, it is essential to have detailed background information on the child's relatives. The construction of a chart that uses standard symbols to designate family members, their relationships, and other pertinent information is called a pedigree, genogram, or family tree. Pedigrees are valuable in demonstrating the various modes of inheritance for a given disorder in a particular family. For disorders with more than one mode of transmission, reviews of genograms may establish the specific type of transmission. For example, a disorder called retinitis pigmentosa may be recessive, autosomal-dominant, or sex-linked. A genogram is helpful in determining the type of inheritance patterns present.

Two terms often used to describe an individual's gene inheritance are *heterozygous* and *homozygous*. When a specific gene that controls a certain characteristic is contributed by one parent and a nonmatching gene for that characteristic is donated by the other parent, the inheritance for that trait is said to be heterozygous. If both parents donate matching genes, the inheritance is said to be homozygous.

Autosomal-dominant inheritance

An autosomal-dominant genetic disorder expresses itself even though the defect is limited to a single gene on one of two paired autosomal chromosomes. Usually one parent has a single gene defect that dominates its normal gene partner (heterozygous dominant inheritance). Since the parent may give either the normal or abnormal gene to the offspring, each of that parent's children has a 50% chance of being affected. Male and female children are affected equally. If the offspring does not inherit the dominant gene, that person will not transmit the trait or disorder. Usually the first affected individual in a family represents a new mutation. This genetic change, depending on the individual's reproductivity, may either be transmitted to the next generation or will end with the original person affected (Fig. 20-1).

Autosomal-recessive inheritance

Autosomal-recessive disorders are expressed only when the individual has two affected paired genes for the particular disorder (homozygous inheritance). Since both parents contribute one gene for each trait, these disorders are inherited from both parents. Most often, the parents are carriers of one abnormal gene that is dominated by its normal paired gene. The parents have an essentially normal appearance. As a result, they are unaware of the gene's presence until an offspring inherits both genes and is affected. It should be emphasized that the probability of having a child with an autosomal-recessive disorder increases when the parents share a common ancestor, thus sharing a common gene pool. This is referred to as *consanguinity*. Males and females are affected with equal frequency. Each child has a 25% chance of being affected, a 50% chance of being a carrier, and a 25% chance of not inheriting the gene from either parent. Affected children whose mates do not carry this gene will have unaffected children who will all be carriers of the gene (Fig. 20-2).

X-linked inheritance

Each individual has two sex chromosomes that differ from the autosomal chromosomes in that they are not alike in both genders (males = XY, females = XX). A female may be homozygous for genes located on the two X chromosomes, but a male can only be heterozygous because he carries only one X chromosome.

X-linked recessive inheritance

X-linked recessive inheritance involves genes located on the X chromosome. The defective X-linked

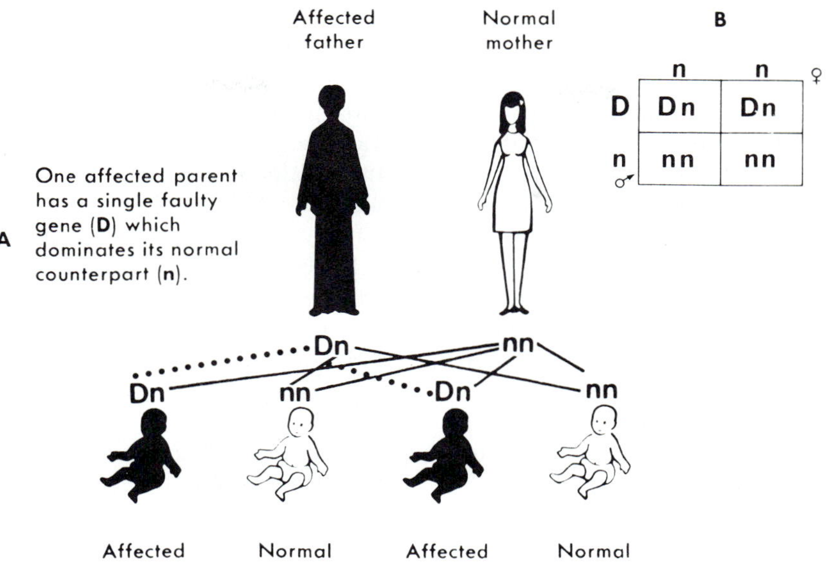

Fig. 20-1 **A,** Dominant inheritance. (From The National Foundation—March of Dimes, 1990.) **B,** Different methods of expressing the probability of dominant inheritance outlined in **A.**

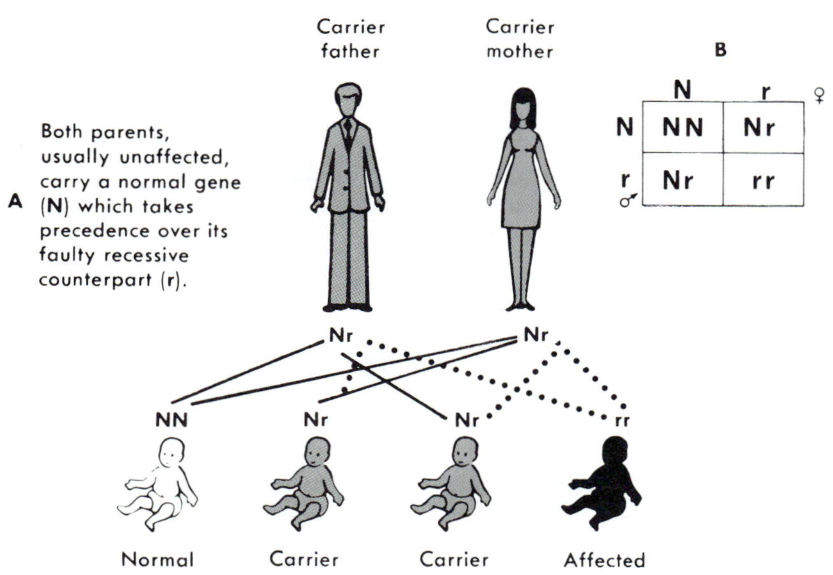

Fig. 20-2 **A,** Recessive inheritance. **B,** Different methods of expressing the probability of recessive inheritance outlined in **A.** (**A,** From The National Foundation—The March of Dimes, 1990.)

gene of an affected male must come from his mother, who is a carrier, since fathers give male offspring only a Y chromosome. A recessive X-linked gene in a female is usually matched by a normal, dominant gene on the paired X chromosomes. Therefore the disorder is not expressed. However, a male who inherits a recessive, X-linked gene on his one X chromosome is always affected, because there is never a matching gene on the Y. Females affected with an X-linked recessive disorder are rare because they must carry affected genes on both their X chromosomes. Each male child of a female carrier has a 50% chance of being affected; each female offspring has a 50% chance of being a carrier. No male-to-male transmission occurs, but the female offspring of an affected male all will be carriers. This happens because they inherit the father's only X chromosome with the defective recessive gene. Transmission occurs from one generation to the next, with only males affected in the majority of families. A generation may be skipped if only females inherit the recessive gene and the males are unaffected (Fig. 20-3).

X-linked dominant inheritance

In X-linked dominant disorders, females are affected if they carry a single abnormal gene on one of their X chromosomes. The inheritance pattern of an X-linked dominant trait resembles autosomal-dominant inheritance with one exception—the trait is transmitted from an affected male to all of his daughters but not to his sons. An affected female's offspring have a 50% chance of being affected, whether male or female. In X-linked dominant disorders, usually twice as many females as males are affected.

Multifactorial inheritance

Multifactorial disorders result from an interaction between multiple defective genes and environmental influences. A thorough analysis of the family genogram does not reveal a distinctive mode of inheritance as with Mendelian patterns of inheritance. However the increased incidence of such disorders in relatives of affected persons, especially in identical twins, yields

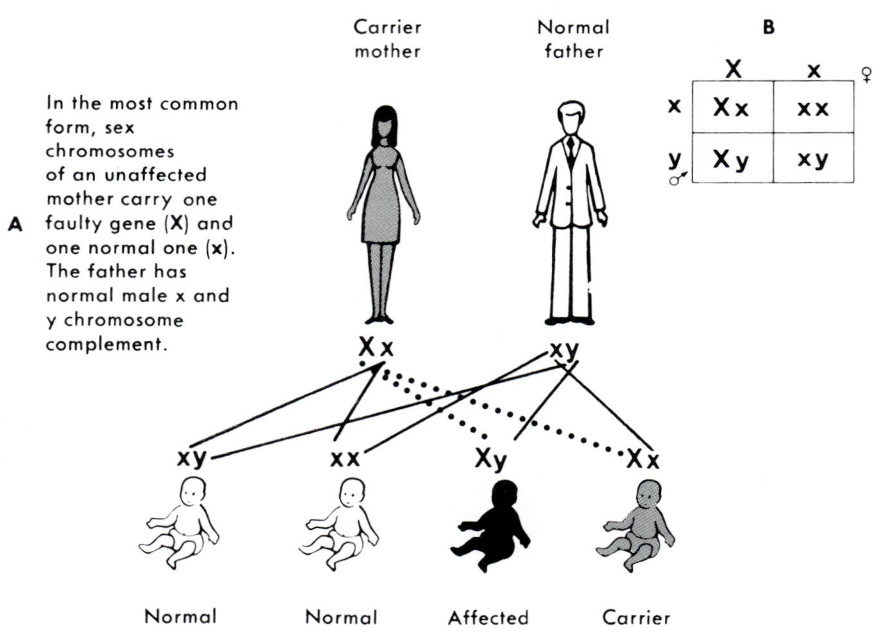

Fig. 20-3 **A,** X-linked inheritance. **B,** Different methods of expressing the most common form of X-linked inheritance outlined in **A.** (**A,** From the National Foundation—The March of Dimes, 1990.)

evidence of a genetic factor. The recurrence risk for the disorder depends on the number of affected persons within a family, how closely related they are to the person seeking genetic counseling, and the gender of the affected persons. It has been established that certain multifactorial disorders are more likely to occur in one gender than in the other. A genogram demonstrates which people within a family are affected so that the recurrence risk can be established.

Chromosomal abnormalities

Accurate identification of each chromosome is accomplished using a special straining technique that produces a characteristic banding pattern for each chromosomal pair. The standard, systematized arrangement of chromosomes is called a karyotype. It is an orderly arrangement of an individual's autosomal and sex chromosomes, according to size, shape, and banding pattern, as they appear in cutouts of photographic enlargements (Fig. 20-4). Chromosomal disorders can be diagnosed in a cytogenetics laboratory by examining the chromosomal pattern of cells derived by a culture of any of several body tissues. A leukocyte culture obtained from a blood sample is most often used. Syndromes are now being identified that are associated with specific chromosomal abnormalities. Chromosomal abnormalities result from various failures in the production of ova and sperm within the two gonads (meiosis) and from abnormal segregation of chromosomes during the first several mitotic divisions of body cells (mitosis). This latter cause results in cells with different chromosomal numbers within one individual, a condition called mosaicism.

One kind of chromosomal change that may be inherited involves the transfer of material between two chromosomes, called a translocation. In a balanced translocation, all of the chromosomal material is present in the cell, although not located in its normal position. An unbalanced translocation occurs when a portion of the chromosomal material has been lost or additional material has been gained. This unbalanced condition is usually associated with serious defects in the individual. A parent carrying a balanced translocation, though normal, is at risk of having offspring with an unbalanced translocation. The genogram may be used to help identify those persons at risk for carrying a balanced translocation. It is recommended that such persons undergo a chromosome analysis (karyotype). Should they carry the translocation, each pregnancy may be monitored by means of amniocentesis. The parents then have the option of either

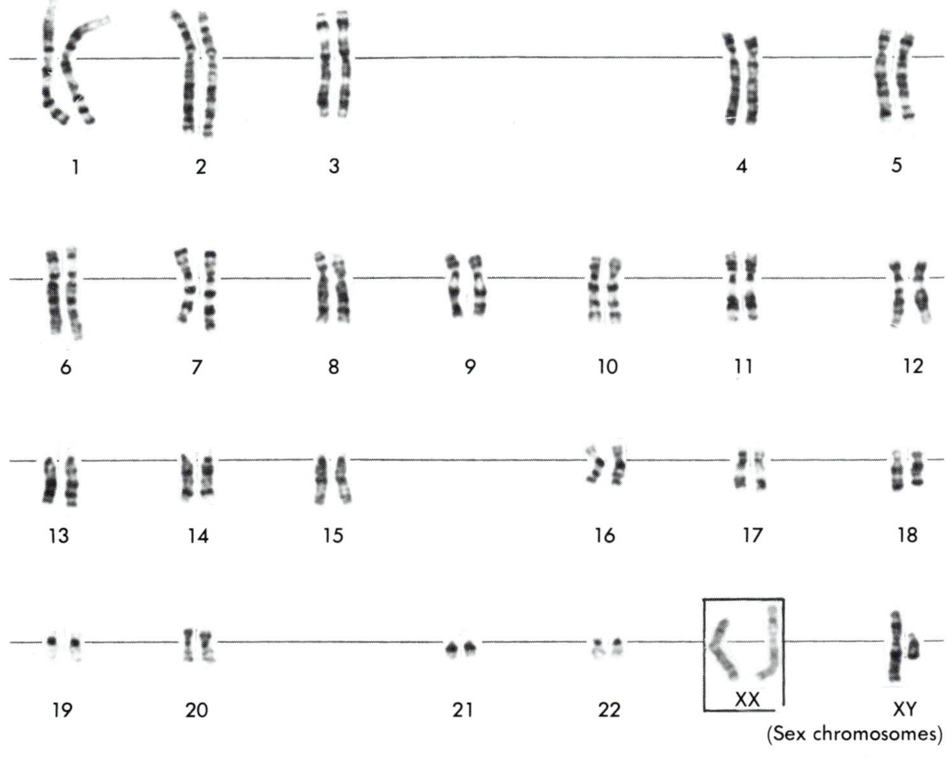

Fig. 20-4 High-resolution, G-banded human karyotype (male). *Inset* shows XX pair from normal female. (From Bradshaw C, UCSD Medical Genetics, La Jolla, CA.)

continuing or terminating the pregnancy if the fetus is found to have an unbalanced chromosomal pattern.

Another chromosomal abnormality is related to nondysjunction of the chromosomes. This abnormality occurs when a chromosomal pair does not separate normally during either formation of the sex cells in the ovary or testes (meiosis) or when the body cells divide (mitosis). If the gamete carrying the extra chromosome was fertilized the offspring would then have a total chromosomal count of 47 rather than 46 per cell. This phenomenon is often related to advanced maternal age. The most common disorder resulting from this process is one type of Down syndrome (Trisomy 21). An extra chromosome at the number 21 position produces mental retardation and other physical deviations in the child. Previously, 50% of infants with Trisomy 21 were born to mothers over 35 years of age. However, now only 20% of infants with Trisomy 21 are born to women in that age group. This is in large part because of the availability of prenatal diagnosis.

The most common chromosome abnormality is simply a change in the total chromosome number. In general a reduction of the total number of autosomal chromosomes is incompatible with the reproduction of human life. An increase in the total number of autosomes results in multiple physical abnormalities, mental retardation, and often a limited life span. Numeric disorders of the sex chromosomes may also be present. One condition, characterized by a complete chromosome loss (45 instead of 46), that is compatible with reproducing life is Turner's syndrome. This syndrome is coded as 45 XO, indicating that one X chromosome is missing (Table 20-2).

◆ TABLE 20-2
Patterns of Inheritance and Common Disorders

Autosomal-dominant inheritance	Achondroplastic dwarfism Huntington's chorea Neurofibromatosis
Autosomal-recessive inheritance	Albinism Cystic fibrosis Phenylketonuria Sickle cell disease Tay-Sachs disease
X-linked recessive inheritance	Duchenne's muscular dystrophy Hemophilia Hurler's syndrome
X-linked dominant inheritance	Vitamin D-resistant rickets
Multifactorial inheritance	Cleft lip, cleft palate Clubfoot Congenital heart disease Dislocated hip Pyloric stenosis Spina bifida Anencephaly
Chromosomal abnormalities	Klinefelter's syndrome (XXY) Trisomy 13 Trisomy 18 Trisomy 21 (Down syndrome) Turner's syndrome (XO)

The Human Genome

The US Human Genome Project has been initiated with the purpose of creating a complete map and sequence of all three billion base pairs of DNA that make up the human genetic complement. An estimated 50,000 to 100,000 genes exist. About 1500 genes have been mapped to specific chromosomes and chromosome regions. Six hundred or more genes have had the DNA sequenced. The ultimate goal of this project is to provide information to help understand genetic disease in general. Initially, single gene disorders will be evaluated. As more information accumulates, however, multifactorial diseases will be better understood and hopefully treated. Predictive and preventive medicine based on the identification of susceptibility to disease is now used as a result of this project.

Prenatal Diagnosis

Genetic screening is now available for certain defects by determining the parental carrier status. Simple blood studies can reveal whether one or both parents carry a defective gene, such as the sickle cell trait. It can then be predicted that if both parents carry the sickle cell trait, their unborn child has a 25% chance of having sickle cell disease. Such carrier testing is available for other genetic diseases such as Tay-Sachs and thalassemia.

Parents often wish to know prenatally whether a fetus is affected or not. Some disorders such as neural tube defects, which involve incomplete development of the brain or exposed spinal cord, can be screened by measuring the amount of α-fetoprotein (AFP) in the mother's blood. If the AFP is elevated, the client is referred for diagnostic testing, which may include ultrasound and amniocentesis.

Amniocentesis is usually performed at 16 weeks, although prenatal diagnosis centers now offer early amniocentesis between 10 and 14 weeks. Another technique, chorionic villi sampling, provides an alternative approach to prenatal diagnosis. At the tenth to eleventh week of pregnancy, a transcervical or transabdominal approach is used to obtain extraembryonic, placental tissue. This tissue is genetically identical to fetal tissue. Chromosome or DNA analysis can then be performed on this tissue or on amniotic cells obtained through amniocentesis.

Direct DNA analysis or the use of specific genetic markers found in DNA material is now available for the prenatal diagnosis of such disorders as cystic fibrosis, Duchenne's muscular dystrophy, Huntington's chorea, sickle cell anemia, and other genetic diseases. Health care providers have an obligation to inform couples with at-risk pregnancies that genetic prenatal diagnosis for certain conditions is available.

Genetic Counseling

Although individual birth defects may seem relatively rare (4% to 5% of all births), the total number of families affected is well into the millions. About 250,000 American babies are born each year with mild- to severe-physical or mental defects. With each passing year, more disorders are identified as genetic problems, thereby increasing the known incidence of hereditary disease.

A genetic counselor is a health professional who is capable of communicating to the parents the magnitude and implications of and the alternatives for dealing with the risk of hereditary disorders occurring within a family. Unfortunately, most genetic counseling is initiated by the birth of a child with a genetic disorder. Caring, understanding, and emotional and informational support are necessary to effectively communicate with the child's parents and extended family.

The implications and options related to the possible genetic disorder are thoroughly discussed with the parents. Using genograms, modern laboratory detection techniques (e.g., blood tests, enzyme assays, amniocentesis, chorionic villi sampling, and chromosome analysis), and knowledge of basic laws of heredity and incidence statistics, a genetic counselor can often predict the probability of the recurrence of a given abnormality in a family. The primary aim is to prevent genetic defects. When that is not possible, the aim is to keep their damaging effects to a minimum. Genetic counseling is an important component of preventive medicine. It involves the delivery of genetic information, such as diagnosis, prognosis, presentation of odds for recurrence, and the effect of genetic diseases on the family. It is a field with its own growing body of knowledge. Because a wide range of laboratory resources and multidisciplinary approaches are required, genetic counseling is normally only available in larger medical centers. A list of genetic counseling centers throughout the United States is sent to health care providers or to the general public, free on request, from the Professional Educational Department of the National Foundation—March of Dimes.

Environmental Influences

The environment is an important influence on health outcomes. Examples of environmental factors include the family composition, interrelationships, culture and ethnicity, socioeconomic status, the degree and type of stimulation offered by the primary caregivers, health habits (e.g., nutrition, exercise, smoking, exposure to drugs and alcohol), stressors and coping strategies, disease, mass media, and exposure to environmental toxins. A strong, healthy, happy child adapts to the environment and is better equipped to cope with daily stressors.

Home and family

For optimal development a child needs a family environment that is loving, accepting, and understanding. A healthy home environment provides the growing child with more than physical necessities. It provides positive parental role models and fosters self-respect, thus building the child's self-esteem. The family provides a framework that assists the child in developing inner self-control through loving discipline. This environment allows the child to seek new experiences and enjoy new opportunities and challenges. The emotional nurturance provided in the home is as important as the provision of physical care. Lack of a trusting, primary attachment can result in failure to thrive.

Nursing Alert

Sadness, withdrawal, loss of appetite, failure to gain weight, abnormal sleep patterns, regressive behaviors, frequent temper tantrums, and persistent respiratory tract infections may indicate a stressful home environment.

Nutrition

The growing child is vulnerable to many nutritional inadequacies. Disturbed patterns of skeletal development caused by the lack or overabundance of one nutrient exemplify the need for balance. A lack of protein during the prenatal period and early infancy may limit the number and size of brain cells. A well-balanced diet is essential for the development of normal bones and teeth, healthy skin, resistance to disease caused by dietary deficiency and infections, and general physical well-being. Clarification of the nutritional needs of children, the general abundance of high-quality foods, and government programs have improved the overall nutritional status of infants and children. Despite these positive factors, nutritional inadequacies may occur as a result of poor dietary habits, food fads, or tension centering around mealtime and the feeding situation. Overnutrition presents more problems in the United States than does undernutrition. A severe form of protein deprivation known as kwashiorkor, however, is common in the underdeveloped countries of South America and Africa. Kwashiorkor is found among children under 4 years of age. It typically manifests itself after the child is weaned, because of the birth of a younger sibling. Characteristically, these children have delayed growth and skeletal development. For more information regarding nutritional needs, refer to Chapter 22.

Disease

Illness is both a physical and a psychological stressor for the young child. Prolonged illness causes a decrease in the rate of growth and height, as well as a decreased ability to function. Any disease that interferes with physical activity and metabolic processes over a long period of time deters normal growth and development. Although minimal slowing of the growth rate may occur during a minor illness, a subsequent growth spurt compensates for the temporary setback.

Uncontrolled diabetes always results in retarded growth in both height and weight. Congenital heart disease associated with hypoxia hampers growth, as do malabsorption syndromes such as cystic fibrosis and celiac disease. Growth and development are interdependent and represent a continuous process of interactions between genetic potential and the environment. Factors influencing overall development include heredity, neuroendocrine factors, interpersonal relationships, nutrition, socioeconomic status, stress, disease, and the mass media. A child's heredity and home, school, and community environment influence the realization of optimal physical, social, cognitive, and emotional growth.

> **Nursing Alert**
>
> The average American child spends more time watching television than engaging in any other activity, with the exception of sleeping. (25 hours per week for 2 to 5 year olds; 22 hours per week for 6 to 12 year olds; 23 hours per week for 12 to 17 year olds). The nurse should assess the amount of time spent watching TV and playing video games and suggest growth-promoting alternatives.

PHYSICAL GROWTH

Growth describes a change in quantity. It occurs when cells divide and synthesize new proteins. Although all phases of growth are continuous and take place concurrently, the main aspects of growth and development are presented in separate discussions in this chapter. Physical growth may be divided into four, well-defined periods:

1. The very rapid growth during infancy.
2. The slow, steady growth during childhood years.
3. The growth spurt during puberty.
4. The decreasing growth and attainment of maximum height during adolescence.

The greatest increase in extrauterine growth occurs during the early part of infancy. Small, steady gains continue during slower growth periods. This general pattern of growth is characteristic of all the body systems, with two exceptions. The nervous system grows rapidly during infancy, decelerates, and, after puberty, ceases growing. The reproductive organs, however, grow very slowly until sexual maturation, which occurs during the pubertal growth spurt.

Tables of average height and weight are commonly used to show what a boy or girl of a particular age should approximate. In the course of development, observable trends in height and weight imply that one can draw certain conclusions regarding these aspects of growth. Growth norms can be successfully determined for a group of children and may serve as a point of reference for making comparisons. However, any table of averages should be interpreted with caution. The value of the growth charts is the establishment of a baseline measurement for the child and a method of recording ongoing serial, comparison measurements.

> **Nursing Alert**
>
> The accuracy of US growth charts in evaluating the growth of children from various cultural and ethic groups is a present concern. Generally, however, these growth charts can be used as a reference guide for all racial and ethnic groups. Nurses must avoid unnecessarily alarming parents with the use of these charts. An evaluation of two to three consecutive measurements gives the health care provider a clearer picture of the child's growth pattern.

Although these tables may accurately state averages, they do not necessarily state what is desirable for individuals. Growth charts for infants and children in the United States have been constructed to show weight, length, the weight for various lengths, and head circumference. (For the full set of growth charts see Appendix B.)

Nursing Alert

For proper use of the NCHS growth charts, recumbent length should be recorded on growth charts for children from birth to 36 months. Stature should be recorded on the growth charts for children 2 to 18 years of age.

Clinical use of these charts can immediately show how the growth of any child ranks in comparison with the rest of the US child population of the same age and gender. The primary use of these charts is to detect nutritional and growth disturbances clinically.

Height

Infants average approximately 20 inches in length at the time of birth. During the first year of life the child grows approximately 10 inches. Five inches are added to a child's height during the second year, and the child grows 3 inches per year during the preschool period. From the sixth to the tenth year of life the annual height gain is reduced to approximately 2 inches. The maximum growth in height occurs during the pubertal period at the approximate time of sexual maturity. Growth in height reaches a peak for boys at approximately 14 years of age, and approximately a year earlier for girls. Growth in height ceases sometime before the child reaches his or her twenties. Puberty occurs at a wide range of ages. An early pubertal growth spurt is associated with an early cessation of growth. Individuals who experience puberty late in life tend to grow for a longer period of time.

Weight

At birth an infant weighs approximately 7½ to 8 lbs. The infant's weight doubles by the fourth or fifth month of life. By the child's first birthday his or her birth weight has approximately tripled. A sharp drop in the rate of gain occurs after the first year. During the preschool years a child's weight rises slowly, averaging approximately 5 lbs each year. During school years the gaining of weight slightly increases. Weight varies more than height, since it is readily susceptible to external factors, such as dietary intake.

Generally, boys are taller and heavier than girls, except in the years preceding puberty. A rapid gain in weight usually occurs in both genders during puberty, corresponding closely with the gain in height. Girls begin their preadolescent growth spurt at approximately 10 to 12 years of age, 2 years earlier than boys. In addition, girls typically reach their adult proportions sooner than boys.

Body Proportions

Distinct changes in body proportions occur between birth and maturity (Fig. 20-5). The small child not only differs from the adult in size but also in proportion. At birth the child's head is relatively large, comprising approximately one fourth of the total body length. The adult, however, has a head measuring approximately one eighth to one tenth of the body length. An infant's arms and legs are relatively short. During infancy the trunk is longer than the extremities. The midpoint of the total length of an infant is at the umbilicus. In the adult, the length midpoint is at the symphysis pubis.

During puberty, adult proportions are attained. The characteristic mature body shape for each gender becomes differentiated at this time. The straight leg-lines of the young girl become curved by 15 years of age. Her hips grow wider, whereas her shoulders remain narrow. The boy's shoulders become broader, whereas his hips remain narrow. Body proportion and build, or physique, are unique to the individual. Within the individual's own general pattern—slender, stocky, or muscular—each child's growth is relatively constant.

Bone Formation

During the early days of fetal development, bones are comprised of simple, connective tissue. Later, this tissue becomes cartilage. By the end of the fifth month of gestation, mineral salts, especially calcium phosphate, are deposited in the cartilage, causing it to harden. Cartilage is gradually replaced by bone, completing the process called ossification. During the early years of life, cartilage persists between the diaphysis (shaft) and the epiphyses (ends) of the long bones. Bones grow in length through a continual thickening of the epiphyseal cartilage.

As the child grows, changes occur in the texture, size, and shape of the "old" bone, and the new bone appears. Bone development continues in an orderly sequence and is complete by the third decade of life.

Bone age can be determined by x-ray examination of certain joints. The information gained in this examination is compared with a standard age measurement. The x-rays are studied to detect the appearance of new bone, changes in the contour of the ends of bones, and the union of the epiphyses with the bone shaft.

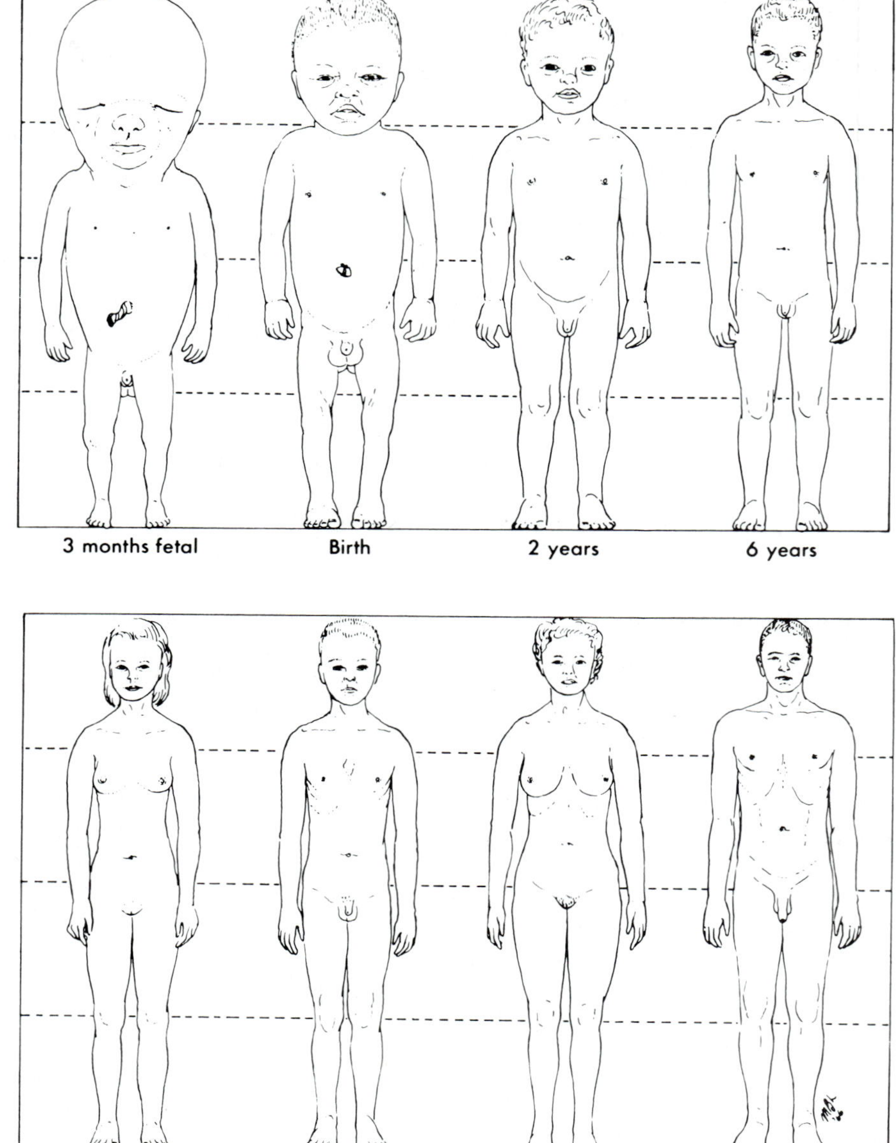

Fig. 20-5 Changes in body proportions from fetus to maturity.

Growth of the long bones is complete when the epiphyses and diaphyses are fused. Bone development of the hand and wrist is a good index of the individual's progress in total skeletal growth. Since boys lag behind girls in bone development at all ages, separate standards are used for each gender.

At birth the ends of the arms (epiphyses) are not yet developed, and the carpal bones are not yet present (Fig. 20-6). Shortly after birth the carpal bones and epiphyses gradually appear. Changes in the size and contour of the ends of bones continue throughout the school years. Bone development of the wrist and hand is complete at the seventeenth year of life for girls and 2 years later for boys.

Tooth Formation

The foundation of a child's tooth structure is formed early in fetal life (Fig. 20-7). At birth, all of the primary (deciduous or baby) teeth and the first permanent teeth (6-year molars) are developing within the child's jaw. Individual dentition is widely varied.

It is not always possible to predict exactly when a child's first tooth will erupt. It is, however, possible to

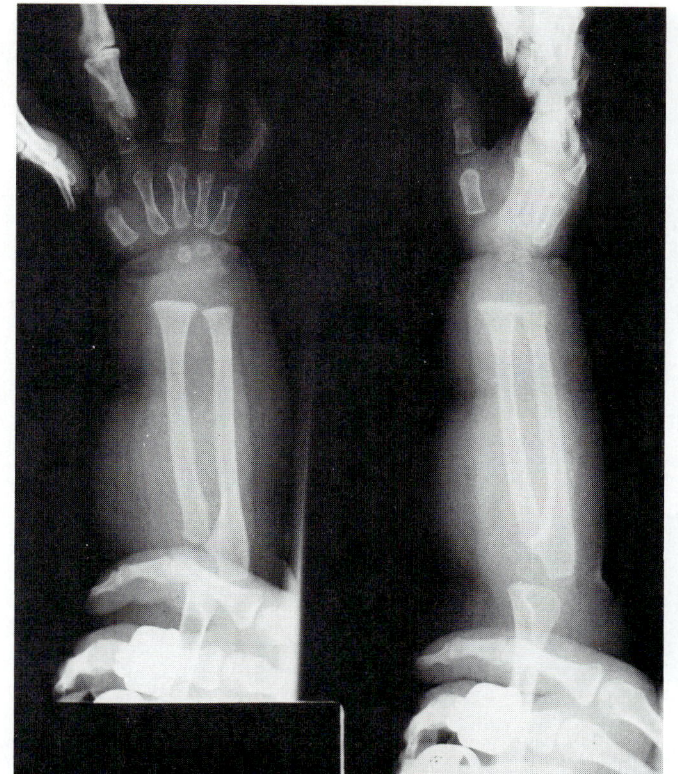
A

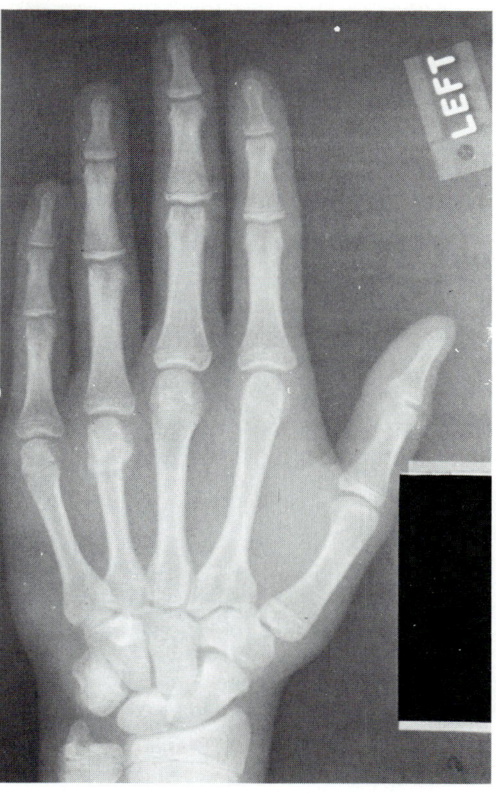

B

Fig. 20-6 X-rays illustrating bone age in children. **A,** Eight-month-old child (note the complete ossification in adult fingers holding the child's arm). **B,** Fourteen-year-old child with epiphyses visible. (From Whaley L, Wong D: *Nursing care of infants and children,* St. Louis, 1991, Mosby.)

predict with some accuracy which teeth will erupt first (Table 20-3). The two lower, central incisors usually appear first, between 5 and 7 months of age. The upper, central incisors appear next. Most children have a total of six teeth at 1 year of age and all 20 primary teeth by 2½ years of age. Wide variation occurs between individuals in the pattern of tooth shedding and permanent tooth eruption. Before the appearance of the first molars (6-year molars), all permanent teeth are growing and maturing. During this time the roots of the primary teeth are disappearing through the process of resorption. Only the crowns of the primary teeth are left when the permanent teeth below are ready to erupt. The loose crowns then drop out. The care and preservation of the primary teeth are important. Unless they are beyond repair, primary teeth should not be extracted. They contribute in large measure to proper alignment and good health of the permanent teeth.

Tetracycline, a broad-spectrum antibiotic has an adverse effect on newly formed bones. This drug stains developing teeth with a yellow-brown material. Tetracyclines also cross the placenta during pregnancy. After the fourth month of gestation the primary teeth of the developing fetus are also affected.

Nursing Alert

Discoloration of the teeth may be prevented by avoiding the use of Tetracycline during pregnancy and the first 12 years of life.

MOTOR DEVELOPMENT

As their bodies grow, children acquire the ability to function in increasingly complex ways. Motor changes accompany physical growth. Motor abilities involve various types of body movements that result from the coordinated activity of nerves and muscles. Maturation of the nervous system and learning skills are interrelated in the acquisition of motor abilities.

Motor development is the process of learning, controlling, and integrating muscular responses. Great advances in body control and locomotion are accom-

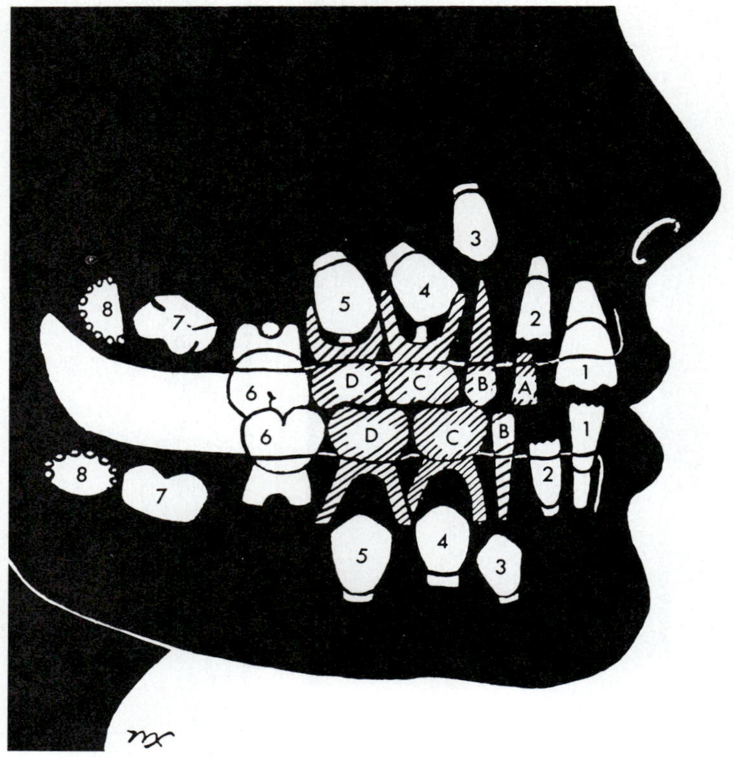

Fig. 20-7 Illustration of a seven-year-old child with good occlusion. Primary teeth: *A,* lateral incisors; *B,* cuspids; *C,* first molars; and *D,* second molars. Permanent teeth: *1,* central incisors; *2,* lateral incisors; *3,* cuspids; *4,* first bicuspids; *5,* second bicuspids; *6,* first molars; *7,* second molars; and *8,* site of wisdom teeth.

◆ **TABLE 20-3**
Typical Pattern of Dentition

Teeth	Lower (Mandibular) Appear at Age	Upper (Maxillary) Appear at Age
Primary		
Central incisors	5 to 7 months	6 to 8 months
Lateral incisors	12 to 15 months	8 to 11 months
Cuspids (canines)	16 to 20 months	16 to 20 months
First molars	10 to 16 months	10 to 16 months
Second molars	20 to 30 months	20 to 30 months
Total per jaw—10		
Total—20		
Permanent		
Central incisors	6 to 7 years	6 to 7 years
Lateral incisors	7 to 9 years	8 to 9 years
Cuspids (canines)	8 to 11 years	11 to 12 years
First bicuspids	10 to 12 years	10 to 11 years
Second bicuspids	11 to 13 years	10 to 12 years
First molars (6-year molars)	6 to 7 years	6 to 7 years
Second molars (12-year molars)	12 to 13 years	12 to 13 years
Third molars (wisdom teeth)	17 to 22 years	17 to 22 years
Total set—32		

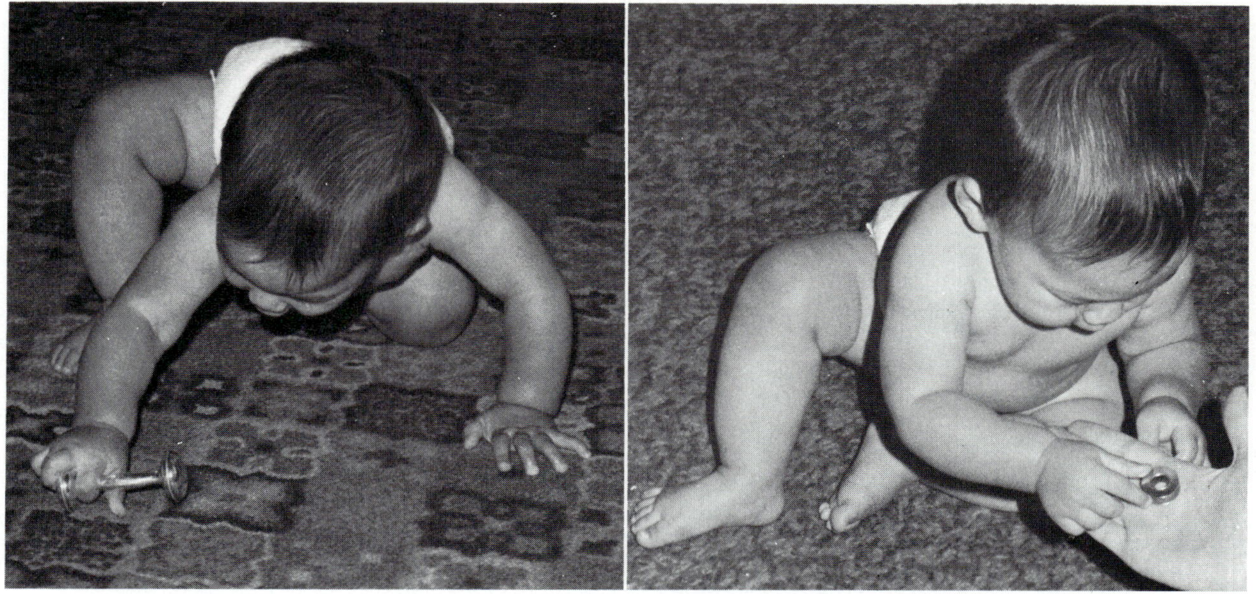

Fig. 20-8 **A,** Crude pincer grasp at 8 to 10 months. **B,** Neat pincer grasp at 10 to 11 months. (From Wong D: *Essentials of pediatric nursing,* ed 4, St. Louis, 1993, Mosby.)

DEVELOPMENT PROGRESSION IN GRASPING

12 weeks	Looks at a cube.
20 weeks	Looks at and approaches a cube.
24 weeks	Looks at and crudely grasps a cube with the whole hand.
36 weeks	Looks at and deftly grasps a cube with the fingers.
52 weeks	Looks at, grasps a cube with the use of the forefinger and thumb, and deftly releases it.
15 months	Looks at, grasps, and releases a cube to build a tower made of two cubes.

plished during the first 2 years of life. The child, who at first was an uncoordinated infant, is soon able to sit, stand, walk, reach, and grasp. Like other phases of growth, motor development unfolds in an orderly sequence that is closely related to the maturation of the nervous system. It follows a definite sequence. Characteristically, this development begins in the child's head region and moves down toward the feet (cephalocaudal). Development also tends to proceed from the center of the body toward the extremities (proximodistal). At first, motor response to stimulation is diffuse, involving the whole body. As maturation continues the response becomes more specific and may involve only the withdrawal of the foot. The sequence of motor development is similar for all children. The rate at which the development progresses, however, varies with each child. Prehension and locomotion provide examples of the usual sequences in the course of motor development.

Prehension

The ability to oppose the thumb to the fingers in picking up an object is preceded by reaching, grasping, and raking movements. Early attempts in reaching also involve eye-to-hand coordination. Effective use of the hands in picking up small objects or for grasping is called prehension. The developmental sequence proceeds from the eye-to-hand coordination required in grasping to the child's reaching without looking, from large muscle activity of the arms and shoulders to the fine muscle activity of the fingers, and from a crude pawing closure to a closure of the fingertips that is more refined. The norms for prehension are presented in Fig. 20-8.

Locomotion

The ability to walk alone is also gradually attained after developments that begin during the first days of life (Fig. 20-9). Moving from place to place and walking are examples of gross motor skills. Complete establish-

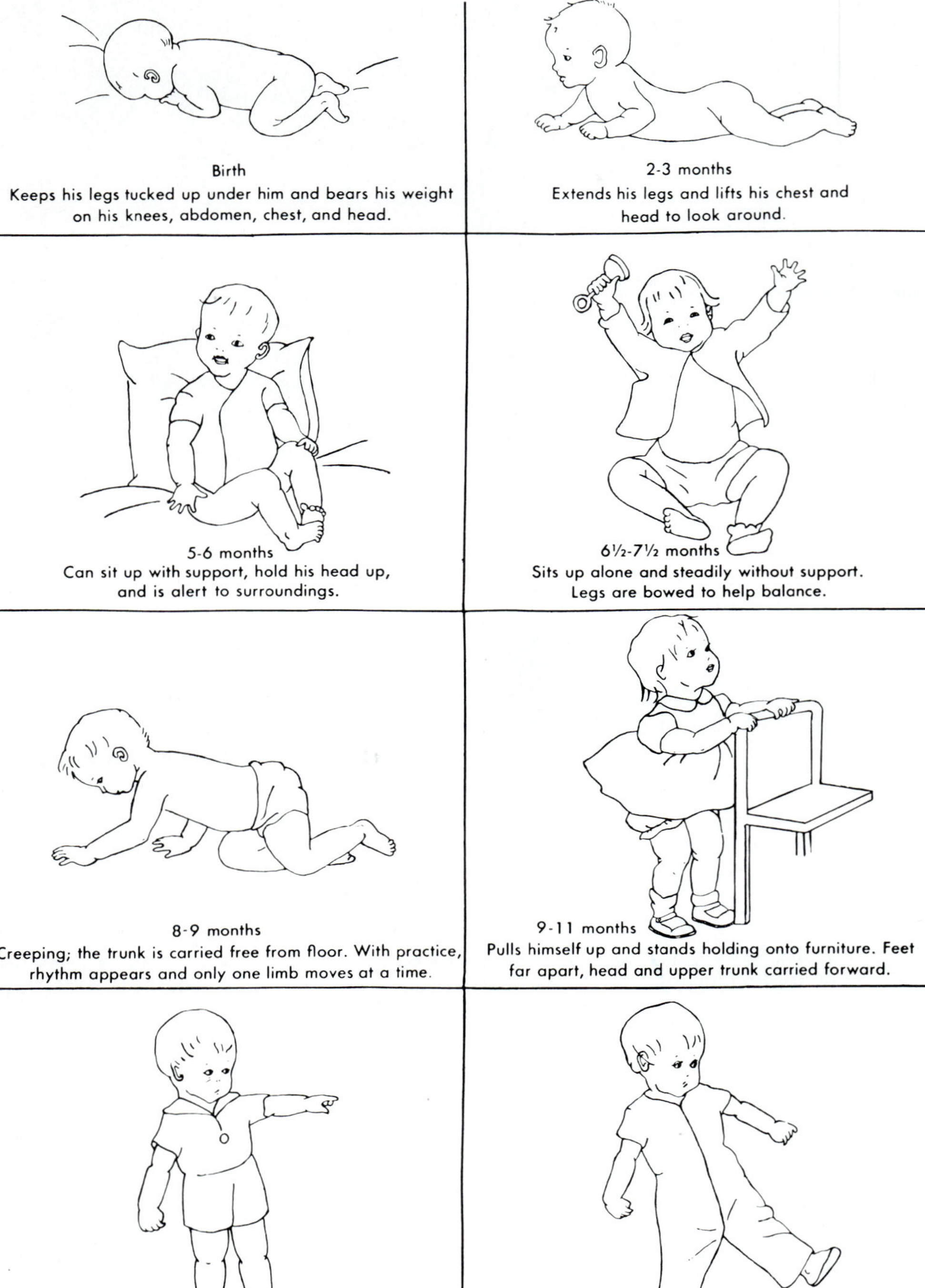

Fig. 20-9 Motor development milestones, emphasizing average age of attainment.

THE MOTOR SEQUENCE (FIG. 20-9)

AGE (months)	ACTIVITY
½ to 1	Lifts head.
2 to 3	Raises chest.
3 to 4	Turns from side to back.
5 to 6	Sits with support.
6 to 7	Rolls from back to abdomen.
6½ to 7½	Sits alone.
8 to 9	Creeps.
9 to 11	Pulls self up.
11 to 12	Walks with help.
12 to 14	Walks alone.

ment of these skills is usually accomplished during the first year for early walkers and after approximately 15 months for those children who mature later. The walking sequence begins when the baby is able to hold its head up. The sequence is half accomplished when the baby can sit alone. When an infant is able to change from a prone to a sitting position, he or she begins to creep. Infants usually creep to an object or person and pull themselves up to a standing position. Gradually the infant stands alone and walks independently.

Prehension and locomotion develop independent of any teaching. Each skill follows an orderly, sequential course, the rate of which may be affected by environmental factors. As each skill develops the opportunity to use and practice it is necessary. The child needs adequate space for play and exploration, as well as toys that promote the development of fine motor and gross motor skills.

INTELLECTUAL DEVELOPMENT

Cognition refers to the process by which individuals become acquainted with the world. Children are born with inherited potential for intellectual growth. They must develop this potential, however, through interactions with the environment. Intelligence influences the overall development of the child. Intelligence is defined as the ability to reason abstractly, think in a logical manner to solve problems, and achieve goals. It affects the child's observation, thought, and understanding.

Many changes take place in the intellectual lives of children as they develop from infancy to adulthood. At birth the centers of higher intellectual activity in the brain are not fully developed. The sensory acuity necessary for these higher intellectual functions is also immature. The world of the newborn infant consists of experiences acquired through physical contact with the environment and through the sensations that originate within the child's own body. New experiences expand cognitive development and are interpreted in the light of previous experience.

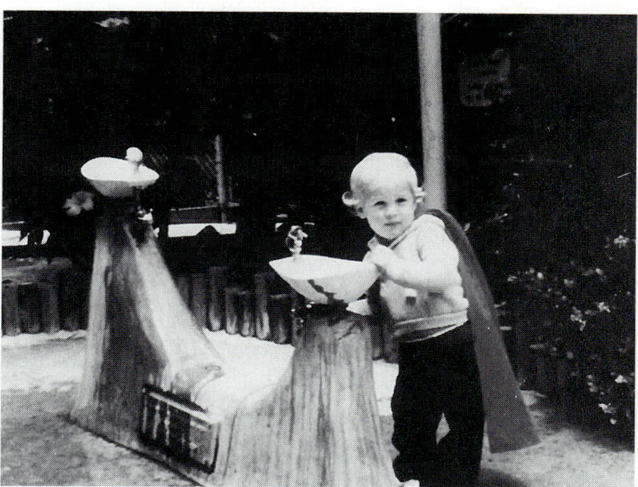

Fig. 20-10 The stage of magical thinking.

Habituation is defined as the period of time that elapses between the infant's initial response to a repeated visual or auditory stimulus and the cessation of that response. The duration of a child's response is measured by observation or a skin electrode and an assessment of motor activity. The ability to adapt to external stimuli or habituate is a predictor of normal neurological function. In toddlerhood, children exhibit the ability to imagine and to engage in make-believe activities. This ability aids children in exploring the real world, organizing experiences, and solving problems. Through make-believe, children are able to participate in a wider range of experiences and to partially overcome their own limitations (Fig. 20-10). Such fantasies are a necessary and normal part of learning. Language, morals, and spiritual development also emerge as cognitive development progresses.

As growth proceeds, the ability to concentrate develops. The child's attention span is likely to be longer during activities that a child chooses. The development of a child's ability to reason is gradual and continuous. Young children are concerned with events related to their own immediate experience and well-being. As they grow, they become increasingly able to conceptualize and shape abstract thought processes. Such changes can be noted in the language children use, in the interest and ability they eventually display in facing social issues, and in their ability to relate to events in the world beyond their immediate experience. Reading to children from early infancy onward, providing safe, developmentally appropriate stimulating toys, and the opportunity for consistent interaction with caring adults will promote the child's cognitive development and emotional growth.

EMOTIONAL GROWTH

The reaction that accompanies either the satisfaction or frustration of a basic need may be termed an *emotion*. Another way of describing an emotional response is to define it as a psychological reaction caused by internal or external stimuli. Although emotions are not identical to basic drives, they are related. The basic drives can be physical, social, intellectual, or personal. Emotional experiences include feelings, impulses, and physiological reactions. When children lack a quality, interpersonal relationship with a primary attachment figure, they experience emotional deprivation. Emotional deprivation leads to developmental retardation.

All emotions cause a physical response. Just as no two people think or act alike, however, no two people react to the same emotion in the same way. For example, in response to fear, one person may feel anxious and still another depressed. As soon as one begins to experience an emotion, physiological changes take place. Manifestations of these changes include facial expressions, smiling, cooing, laughter, crying, and an alteration in vital signs.

Emotions appear early in life. Even during the first days of life the infant's need to satisfy his or her physical needs is accompanied by an emotional response. The infant usually reacts by crying or kicking. Soon the infant finds stimulation pleasant or unpleasant. When the infant is hungry or uncomfortable, an unpleasant state results. The child reacts by crying or restlessness. When the infant's wants are satisfied, a pleasant state of well-being results. It is expressed by cooing, gurgling, or sleep. Thus the emotional responses of the infant are initially stimulated by physiological needs. An infant's pleasant responses to attention reward the caregiver. Ideally, both infant and parent satisfy each of their needs through these encounters, and their attachment to each other is strengthened.

Through a combination of maturation and learning, more specialized responses soon occur. By the end of the first year, emotions of fear, rage, excitement, anger, and joy become recognizable. Facial expression, vocalization, and body movement become part of the child's emotional repertoire. Changes in emotional expression continue throughout childhood.

Love

Love is the most important of all the emotions, since it is the foundation on which all positive relationships are built. A child's first love is focused on the mother or primary caretaker. The child's capacity for affection and love develops gradually from this early association. During the normal course of development, children transfer a part of their affection to others who share their pleasures and achievements. These early relationships are the basis of the child's ability to develop relationships throughout life.

Fear

Fear is naturally aroused when infants experience any startling, sudden occurrence, such as a loud noise, an unexpected jarring, or a fall. They characteristically respond to these threats to their security with crying and general body distress. The young child also acquires other fears that are associated with objects and persons in their immediate environment. As children become older, fearful responses become increasingly specific. They are expressed by withdrawal from the fearful situation. Later, children learn to avoid situations that cause anxiety.

Once a child becomes afraid in a certain situation, repetition of the same or similar situation usually reproduces fear. However, if the boy or girl learns that the situation is not truly hazardous, the fear diminishes or disappears. Parents and other adults should not laugh at or ridicule a child's fears—identified or unnamed as they may be—but should help the child to understand the situation or thing that is frightening. Reasonable fear is a valuable safeguard against many dangers. Fear acts as a check on behavior. A person may be driven to action by anger, hate, or jealousy. His or her conduct is held within reasonable bounds through the fear of consequences.

Anger

Anger denotes a variety of emotional states, ranging from turbulent rage to milder forms of resentment. In infancy, anger arises primarily through the interference with body movement or the lack of gratification of basic needs such as feeding. Crying, screaming, biting, hitting, and kicking are physical expressions of anger. In early childhood, anger may take the form of numerous acts of disobedience and resistance. Preverbal children may express their anger in the form of a temper tantrum. These negative behaviors occur more often when a child is hungry or tired. When children learn to talk, they gain command of new ways to express their anger. Children may find outbursts of anger useful for attracting attention to themselves and for obtaining a desired end. Feelings of anger may be frightening to the child. Young children need to be reassured that these angry feelings are very common.

PARENT GUIDELINES: USING TIME-OUT

Select an area for time-out that is safe, convenient, and unstimulating but where the parent can monitor the child, such as the bathroom, hallway, or laundry room.

Determine what behaviors warrant a time-out.

Make sure children understand the "rules" and how they are expected to behave.

Explain to children the process of time-out:

When they misbehave, they will be given *one* warning.

If they do not obey, they will be sent to the place designated for time-out.

They are to sit there for a specified period of time.

If they cry, refuse, or display any disruptive behavior, the time-out period will begin *after* they quiet down.

When they are quiet for the duration of the time, they may then leave the time-out area.

A rule for the length of time-out is *1 minute per year of age;* use a kitchen timer with an audible bell to record the time rather than a watch.

Implement time-out in a public place by selecting a suitable area or explain to children that time-out will be spent immediately on returning home and mark their hand with a felt-tip pen as a reminder.

(From Wong D: *Essentials of pediatric nursing,* ed 4, St. Louis, 1993, Mosby.)

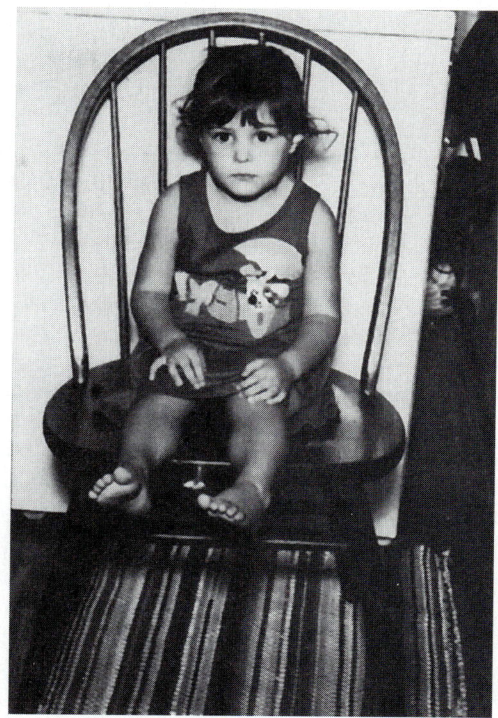

Fig. 20-11 Time-out is the most effective disciplinary strategy for young children. (From Wong D: *Essentials of pediatric nursing,* ed 4, St. Louis, 1993, Mosby.)

However, they also need to be guided toward more appropriate means of expressing anger. Children are likely to feel more secure when behaviors, such as acting out, hitting, and biting are firmly limited by adults. Parents can also aid in anger-management by maintaining poise and self-control, refusing to be manipulated by theatrical displays of emotion (temper tantrums). This reaction is best accomplished by leaving the child and the scene of the display, if possible. Following through with a clearly defined "time-out" period as soon as possible is helpful. See the box above and Fig. 20-11 for a discussion of this technique. Providing regular and healthy meals, daily exercise, uninterrupted naptimes, and quality time with parents will diminish the frequency of negative outbursts.

Jealousy

Jealousy is an emotional response comprised of anger, fear, and love. It is an emotion that, in general, seems to arise when people threaten to take something away, share something, or interfere with something the child feels is a personal belonging. In the young child, jealousy tends to develop when the child is threatened by possible loss of love. For example, children become jealous as a result of the presence of a newborn brother or sister initiating sibling rivalry. Because of the mother's preoccupation with the new infant the older child may equate this loss of time and attention with a loss of love. The child may see the younger sibling as an unwanted competitor and become jealous. The child's physical reaction may be either aggression toward or competition with the new baby. Thus the jealous child may hit the baby or return to infantile habits to gain the attention desired. A negative reaction may consist of withdrawal from competition or repression. For example, a child may sulk or refuse meals. The form of jealous expression varies with age. Behavior caused by such personal envy gradually becomes less direct and less openly violent; it is more subtle but no less real.

The factors precipitating emotions and the reaction patterns they elicit have typical stages of development. Emotional responses not only vary in form and intensity from person to person but also from age to age. The emotions identified previously and the reactions they stimulate are closely related to the person's maturity and life experience. Emotions always find an outlet; if the most desired expression is blocked, another less desirable emotion is substituted. This theory has many practical applications and is basic to the understanding of many behavior problems and the concept of psychosomatic illness. Teaching children and families to problem-solve and engage in healthy, open communication patterns, rather than "acting out" or "stuffing" (suppressing) feelings, is extremely important.

SOCIAL BEHAVIOR AND MORAL VALUES

The child's immediate environment is provided by their parents or significant caretakers and is of immense importance to their physical, intellectual, and emotional well-being. The environment is an important influence in the formation of a child's personal sense of worth, behaviors, and moral values. Children also acquire moral reasoning in a developmental sequence.

Family Functioning

In most cultures the child's principal provider of nurturance is the family. However, the makeup of the family unit varies greatly among different cultural and ethnic groups, regions, and socioeconomic conditions. In the mid-twentieth century the typical American family was described as "nuclear." This means that the family consisted of a mother, father, and children. At times, other members, such as grandparents, aunts, and uncles, may have joined the household. Family roles were less flexible. Only 12% of middle-class mothers worked outside the home and most were the children's primary care givers. Conversely, the male parent was the primary source of family income.

Today the typical American family unit is more diverse. Approximately 80% of American mothers work outside the home. The nuclear family is much less common. A family is whatever the client considers it to be. Male or female single-parent families are increasing, as are blended or adoptive families. Members of some family structures find it more difficult to provide or obtain the appropriate skills or assistance needed to function adequately.

The family may be functionally defined as a special grouping, usually of biologically related persons bound by ties of intimacy and caring whose commitments usually have included provisions for the following:

1. Physical safety, growth, and development.
2. Emotional and social support, and family life skill practice.
3. Teaching of ethical and spiritual concepts, community responsibilities, and world views.
4. Assistance with role definition, career exploration, development of independence, establishment of separate residence, and self-realization.

Through the years, as society has changed, the expectations and functions of families have changed. As the more basic needs of survival and education are met or provided by society, less critical but important considerations are often emphasized. Conversely, if basic needs are not being met by the family or community resources, family dysfunction and societal strain become apparent.

An assessment by the nurse of the family composition, cohesiveness, adaptability, and ability to meet health-related physical or psychological needs is critically important. The nurse functions as an important member of a multidisciplinary team in the provision of family-centered care.

Parenting

Child rearing is a developmental stage in the adult life cycle for which most individuals are not prepared. Role modeling is a critical factor in the enactment of the parenting role. With societal changes, however, models from the mid-twentieth century are not always relevant to the challenges of today. Requests for parent education programs are common. Through effective nurturant parenting a child is introduced to the responsibilities and rituals of social groups. The child is then assisted in becoming a productive member of one of these groups.

Parenting, by no means an exact science, does include a number of skills that can be learned. Many parents are unaware of community resources available for this purpose. Classes may include identifying social support networks, dealing with stress, effective coping strategies for issues related to discipline, anticipatory guidance for developmental milestones, learning how to plan and prepare relatively inexpensive and nutritious meals, designing a balanced budget, and using community resources.

Three main styles of parenting have been identified as authoritarian/autocratic, permissive/laissez-faire, and authoritative/democratic (Table 20-4). Most parents mix styles of parenting depending on the situation in which they are involved. The parenting style, however, is only one factor. The parents should be able to provide emotional support and their expectations of the child's behavior and the parental reactions to it should be consistent and child-appropriate, benefiting

◆ **TABLE 20-4**
Three Main Styles of Parenting

Style	Description
Authoritarian/Autocratic—Emphasizes obedience and respect of parental role.	Characterized by rather rigid, clearly defined rules. Negative reinforcement is more frequently applied for noncompliance than rewards granted for compliance.
Permissive/Laissez-faire—Emphasizes relative freedom from parental restraint and direction.	Characterized by lack of or few defined limits. Parent is more likely to use reasoning to guide child, and few punitive measures are applied. Child may learn consequence of action the hard way, and may have difficulty fitting into the structured environment of school, etc.
Authoritative/Democratic—Emphasizes rational issue-related guidance.	Characterized by input from both parent and child for problem solving. Rules tend to be flexible depending on situation. This style encourages development of analysis and responsibility.

the family as a whole. "Consistent" in this context means predictable or equitable. For example, the child's knowledge of dependable follow-through by the parent regarding behavior and expected consequences, rather than blanket uniformity in the treatment of all children or lack of recognition of extenuating circumstances is vital. Some parents use a certain parenting pattern, even if it is ineffective or abusive, because it is all they know. It was "modeled" for them by their own parents.

An authoritative/democratic parenting style is generally considered to be the most effective. This style involves seeking input from both the child and the parent in problem-solving and encouraging analysis and self-discipline. The methods endorsed are initially more time-consuming but are usually deemed more productive in the long run. Thomas Gordon has explored and refined this style in his Parent Effectiveness Training **(PET)** programs. His training has promoted the use of techniques that assist family communication and conflict resolution. The **PET** approach is valuable in shaping interactions within the family. Some of these techniques are noted later in this unit (Gordon, 1989).

One of the tasks of parenting has been described as moving the child's focus from the pleasure principle to the reality principle. In other words, as children grow, they must be taught that the immediate gratification of desires is not always wise or possible. Everyone, from time to time, is forced to wait for certain experiences or rewards. Children must be helped to develop self-control and an awareness of the kinds of situations that interrupt plans or make it impossible to do just what one wants to do at the time one wants to do it. It should also be observed that certain preparations may be necessary to be able to enjoy pleasurable outcomes.

Undoubtedly, part of the reality principle that will be discovered in this process is that parents are not "all-knowing" or without flaws. Therefore parents should feel free to communicate that they too are still learning and growing. Although parents may view child rearing as an endurance contest at times, with knowledge and support parenting can be rewarding and pleasurable.

Communication

Communication is necessary for any relationship to endure. Many factors influence this process. Communication is critical to healthy family functioning. Communication may be verbal, nonverbal, or abstract. Verbal communication is comprised of speech and language, whereas nonverbal communication includes body language, such as a caress, a smile, a nod, or a reaction. Abstract communication includes artistic expression, play, photographs, and symbols. Effective communication is an ability to say what is meant. It also involves an ability to listen attentively to what is being said to determine the meanings of others.

Parents are advised to listen to their children intently, empathetically, without unnecessary interruptions, comments, interpretations, or evaluations. Interruptions may sidetrack children, causing them to stop a discussion. The result is a premature closing off of communication and a stifling of what could be an important and gratifying trust-building experience for both parent and child. In **PET,** Thomas Gordon lists four basic listening skills necessary for effective communication.

1 Passive listening (silence).
2 Use of acknowledgment responses (e.g., "oh!," or "uh-huh").
3 Door openers (e.g., "Would you like to talk about it?").
4 Active listening—the most useful tool when used appropriately (when a conversation is not forced, privacy is respected, sufficient time is available, and the technique is not overused).

Active listening is a supportive communication technique that reflects the child's feelings back to him or her. It is used to indicate the acceptance of a child with a problem. Active listening allows the child's emotional release and sharing, helping the child discover an effective answer to his or her problem, and allowing the parent to view the difficulty and dynamics of the solution. By feeding back the information that the child shares the parent's perceptions are verified, helping the child express and organize his or her thoughts.

An active listening dialogue:

TOM: (an angry high school freshman arriving home): I never want to go back to Mr. Blake's English class again!

PARENT: You're upset about Mr. Blake's English class?

TOM: Yes. I tried really hard on that theme last week, I spent a lot of time. I got a "C–". Jerry wrote his in 45 minutes, it was only 1½ pages long, and got an "A"!

PARENT: You're frustrated because you spent more time and effort than Jerry and didn't get as good a grade as he did.

TOM: You got it! I don't understand why—guess I'll ask Mr. Blake.

For the parent who is having a problem with the behavior of a child, **PET** recommends I-messages. I-messages include the following three elements: (1) the parent's feelings regarding the behavior, (2) a nonblameful description of the specific behavior, and (3) the tangible (concrete) effect of the behavior on the parent. Because they share feelings and consequences without depreciating or "putting the child down," I-messages may achieve results without producing negative confrontations. They give the child data instead of blame. I-messages do *not* spell out the specific solution to avoid the described consequences. The solutions are generated by the child and may be very creative and quite acceptable. An example of a problem-identifying I-message would be a parent stating "I get upset when I can't hear my friend on the telephone because there is so much commotion and noise in the room; trying to hear her with all that noise wastes my time and energy."

I-messages may also be used to express positive feelings regarding a child's activities and are superior to ordinary praise, which the child may construe as manipulative. Such an I-message would be a parent stating "When you come in and hug me after school, it feels so good—the rest of my housework seems easier!"

If a problem is not solved through active listening or I-messages, conflict-resolution is advocated. This is a method of cooperative problem solving, which is designed to meet the needs of both parties with a no-lose or win-win result.

Parental Expectations

If parents are to be successful in teaching family life skills and social values, communication with children should be developmentally appropriate. This requires the provision of anticipatory guidance (see Chapter 22). However, not all children grow at the same rate or respond in the same way to the same stimuli. In addition to a child's calendar age, his or her abilities and previous experiences will also affect the communication level. Usually parents are sensitive to differences in a child's skills, temperament, and personality. Parents are aware of the child's interests and dislikes, as children are aware of the differences in their care givers.

Consistency in parenting and caregiving is ideal. It is, however, difficult and unrealistic in all situations. Each parent must identify their differences in patience and tolerance and support one another in a way that the child will not find it profitable to play one parent against the other, thus precipitating a power struggle. Parents must develop a mutual disciplinary plan to avoid confusing the child.

Role Modeling

The day-by-day life example (model) presented by the care givers is probably the most effective communication technique known. "Do as I say, not as I do" is *not* effective modeling. A thoughtful, courteous parent is much more likely to raise a thoughtful, patient child, willing to talk about and resolve problems rather than act out frustrations with negative behaviors.

In some families an adult male or female may not be present to serve as a positive role model for the children. In this situation, special efforts should be made to ensure that boys and girls have healthy relationships with healthy adults of both genders. Role modeling is one of the goals of organizations such as Big Sisters, Big Brothers, and various youth associations sponsored by churches, synagogues, and other community groups.

Through the years, many approaches have been advocated to promote constructive behavior and instill worthy moral values in each developing generation of society. Current literature reveals a wide range of sometimes conflicting suggestions in regard to the best guidance and preparation of future generations. These suggestions include personal health maintenance, environmental modifications, clarification of parent-child communications and mutual expectations, and possible techniques of control or negotiation to achieve the goals desired.

This last category, exploring techniques of negotiation, is particularly controversial. For example, some parents feel that negotiations may be inappropriate or too time-consuming. They find reward systems too complex, too difficult to maintain, and bordering on bribery. Others conclude that listening techniques and mutual problem-solving may take longer to implement but will result in better self-discipline and effective problem-solving skills. Some parents are satisfied with a system of rewards for specific behaviors. If parents use money as a reward (a variable allowance), they may believe that the technique is very helpful in teaching how to use money, as well as habits of charity and thrift. The final technique listed—that of applying limited physical punishment—causes the most comment and objection. Corporal punishment most often takes the form of spanking, resulting in a decrease in the behavior. This approach, however, teaches children that violence is acceptable. It is estimated that approximately 85% of parents in the United States have used some type of physical punishment while childrearing. The impulsive escalation of such techniques often results in parental rage and physical harm to the child.

An explanation of desired behaviors and assurance of the parents'continuing love is extremely important in any effective method of punishment. Most experts view time-out as the best form of punishment. The home environment is the developmental site of the child's basic moral and spiritual concepts. The family's religious beliefs, culture, and ethnicity are critical factors, whereas the school and community contribute as well. The parents' behavior and modeling strongly influence the child. "What they are speaks so loud that the child does not hear what they say" is an applicable statement. Physical growth, psychological development, social skills, and moral sensitivity do not proceed independently of one another. It is the blending of genetic and environmental factors that will determine the child's development.

KEY CONCEPTS

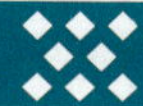

1 A child's normal growth and development are guided by certain basic principles. Growth and development occur in an orderly sequence; are, although continuous, characterized by lulls and spurts; progress at highly individualized rates; vary at different ages for specific structures; and represent a total process involving the whole child.

2 Every child's growth and development are governed by genetic and environmental forces. A child's cellular inheritance and early embryonic growth will affect the pattern of growth and development.

3 The three major types of genetic problems are (1) Mendelian patterns of inheritance involving only one or two defective genes, (2) multifactorial disorders related to multiple gene defects and environmental factors, and (3) gross genetic imbalances caused by chromosomal abnormalities.

4 The genetic counselor uses various genetic information to determine the probability of the occurrence of a given abnormality in a family. The goal of genetic counseling is to prevent genetic defects or reduce their damaging effects.

5 Environmental factors that influence a child's growth and development include the following: family composition and interrelationships, culture and lifestyles, stimulation, health habits, nutrition, and malformation or disease.

6 Physical growth may be divided into four periods: (1) rapid growth during infancy; (2) slow, steady growth during childhood; (3) the growth spurt during puberty; and (4) decreasing growth and attainment of maximum height.

7 Growth norms serve as a point of reference for evaluating the growth of an individual child. Since these averages do not necessarily reflect what is desirable for each individual a child's general progress should be evaluated by drawing comparisons over time.

8 Growth can be measured by the level of bone formation. Bone development continues in an orderly sequence and bone age can be determined through the x-ray examination of certain joints.

9 Dentition is widely varied. Patterns of tooth shedding and permanent tooth eruption also vary. Most children have six to eight teeth at 12 months of age and all 20 primary teeth by 30 months of age.

10 Motor development proceeds in an orderly sequence. The rate of motor development, however, varies with each individual child. Prehension and locomotion provide examples of the usual se-

quences in the course of fine motor and gross motor development.

11 Intelligence influences the overall development of the child. Intelligence strongly influences the level of difficulty at which the child is able to function efficiently and the scope of his or her activities. Many changes take place in the intellectual lives of children during their development from infancy to adulthood.

12 The factors precipitating emotions and the reaction patterns they initiate have typical stages of development. Emotional responses vary in form and intensity from person to person and from age to age. Significant emotions include love, fear, anger, and jealousy.

13 The immediate environment of children, provided by their parents or caretakers is of immense importance to the child's physical, intellectual, and emotional well-being. It is important for the nurse to assess the structure of the family, its composition, and its ability to meet health-related physical or psychological needs.

14 Three main styles of parenting have been identified: (1) authoritarian/autocratic, (2) permissive/laissez-faire, and (3) authoritative/democratic. Most parents combine these styles, depending on the specific situation.

15 Communication is critical to healthy family functioning. PET indicates that active listening is the most useful tool for parents attempting to communicate with their children.

16 I-messages are recommended for parents having a problem with a child's behavior. I-messages include the parent's feelings regarding the behavior, a nonblameful description of the behavior, and the tangible effect the behavior is having on the parent.

17 Many approaches have been advocated to promote constructive behavior and instill worthy moral values. Techniques include personal health maintenance, modifications of environment, clarification of parent-child communications and mutual expectations, and techniques of control or negotiation to achieve desired goals.

CRITICAL THOUGHT QUESTIONS

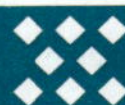

1 What are the principles of growth and development as described in this chapter? What impact do these principles have on the nursing process?

2 Carrier testing is available for which autosomal-recessive conditions? What are the ethical issues involved in this technology?

3 Describe a situation in which genetic testing is advisable. What is the role of the genetic counselor in this situation?

4 Environment plays a significant role in the growth and development of an infant. Identify and discuss those factors in the home environment which you feel will have a major impact. As a nurse, what can you do to promote a healthy home environment?

5 If physical, motor, intellectual, and emotional growth and development all unfold in an orderly sequence, why is each child so different? What steps can be taken to diminish the frequency of a child's negative outbursts?

REFERENCES

Gordon T: *Teaching children self-discipline at home and at school,* New York, 1989, Times Books-Random House.

Novak J: Multiple role women and their spouses: variables influencing family functioning. *Dissertation Abstracts,* 1989, University of Michigan.

Wong D: *Essentials of pediatric nursing,* ed 4, St. Louis, 1993, Mosby.

BIBLIOGRAPHY

Parenting Classics

Brazelton TB: *Toddlers and parents,* New York, 1974, Delta.

Brazelton TB: *Working and caring,* Menlo Park, CA, 1985, Addison-Wesley.

Dixon SD, Stein MT: *Encounters with children: pediatric behavior and development,* St. Louis, 1992, Mosby.

Dobson D: *Dare to discipline,* Wheaton, IL, 1970, Tyndale House.

Elkind D: *The hurried child-growing up too fast, too soon,* Menlo Park, CA, 1988, Addison-Wesley.

Ginott HG: *Between parent and child,* New York, 1961, Macmillan.

Grossman ER: *Everyday pediatrics,* Philadelphia, 1994, WB Saunders.

Howe J: *Parenting and functions of the family.* In Scipien GM, et al, editors: *Pediatric nursing care,* St. Louis, 1990, Mosby.

Kutner L: *Parent and child,* New York, 1991, Avon.

Leach P: *Your baby and child,* London, 1978, Albert Knopf.

Leman K: *Keeping your family together when the world is falling apart,* New York, 1993, Dell.

Spock B: *Dr. Spock on parenting,* New York, 1988, Simon & Schuster.

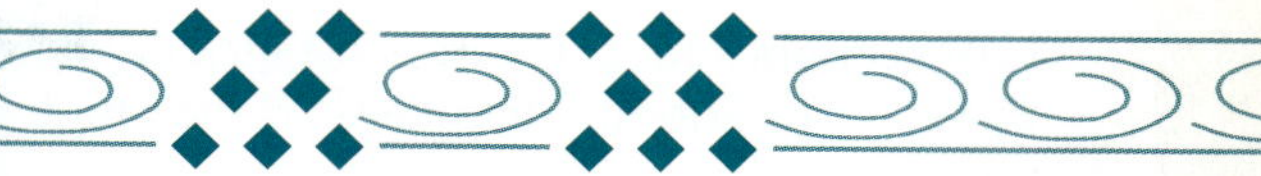

21

Developmental Assessment

CHAPTER OBJECTIVES

After studying this chapter, the student should be able to:

1. Indicate the average, daily weight gain of an infant during the first 6 months of life and his or her growth in height during the first year.
2. Discuss five topics related to anticipatory guidance for parents of children of the following ages: 2 weeks, 2 months, 5 months, 10 months, 16 months, 30 months, 3 years, 4 years, 5 years, 10 years, and 15 years.
3. Explain the significance of the following words or phrases and identify the age group(s) they describe: separation anxiety, crawling, creeping, parallel play, ritualism, imaginary friend, hero worship, and peer pressure.
4. Identify the average ages for the following infant behaviors: fixates and follows, raises head, disappearance of Moro, rooting, asymmetrical tonic neck reflexes, sleeps 8 to 10 hours through the night, rolls from abdomen to back, sits with support, rolls from back to abdomen, crawls, has pincer grasp, says "ma-ma," stacks two blocks, and walks unassisted.
5. Describe primary tooth eruption and when a complete set of primary (deciduous, baby) teeth appears.
6. Indicate when the following skills usually appear: kicks ball, throws ball overhand, bowel training established, brushes teeth, buttons and unbuttons clothes, uses one foot per step when going down stairs.
7. Describe the main purpose of the Denver II, or Denver Developmental Screening Test II (DDST-II).
8. Identify four developmental tasks of adolescence.
9. Identify the key components of an adolescent health history.

In caring for children, one must have an awareness of the approximate ages at which the child is capable of various activities and functions. The caregiver should also be aware of the different types of behavior children are likely to display at each stage of development. This information assists the nurse in fostering the child's growth and development while caring for him or her in health and illness. Many books have been written that describe the physical, motor, and psychological changes that take place as an individual goes through the process called *growing up.* Table 21-1 identifies the developmental characteristics of certain ages. The stages of psychosocial development as identified by the psychoanalyst Erik Erikson are discussed in Chapter 1. This table also offers anticipatory guidance for the various stages of growth to help parents provide for the needs of the child. The nurse must remember throughout the nursing process that a child's understanding is influenced by previous experience, ethnicity, intellect, development, and educational levels. The performance times noted are averages only. An allowance must be made for individual differences. Chapter 22 offers a more detailed list of developmental expectations related to nutrition.

This chapter also includes a discussion of the Denver II Developmental Screening Test (DDST-II) and the Prescreening Developmental questionnaire, both of which are often used to evaluate young children.

◆ TABLE 21-1
Ages and Stages of Maturation

Infancy (0 to 1 yr)—newborn (birth to 1 mo) (see Fig. 21-1)

Physical growth	***Motor development***	***Language development***	***Anticipatory guidance***
Average weight: 7½ lbs (3.4 kg) Gains 1 oz/day (5 to 7 oz weekly for first 6 mo) Average height: 20 inches (grows 10 inches during first year) Head circumference: 13 to 14 in (33 to 35.5 cm)	Readily assumes fetal position Primitive reflexes: Rooting, sucking, tonic neck, grasp, plantar, and Moro reflex present Raises head but not stable Turns head from side to side	Cooing	*Development:* Early evening crying Sneezing normal Sleeps 20 hrs/day Unless family bed is desirable maintain in crib Will sleep through the night when doubles birth weight or reaches 13 to 14 lbs Regards faces Will eat every 2½ to 4 hrs Breast-fed infants eat more often *Safety:* Burp well Prevent suffocation in crib Position on side or back Car safety restraint *Stimulation*: Colorful hanging toys Talk to infant Use of touch *Feeding practices:* Hold while feeding *Diaper care:* *Bathing:* Use mild soaps (no lotion or powder) *Immunizations:* Infant series

A
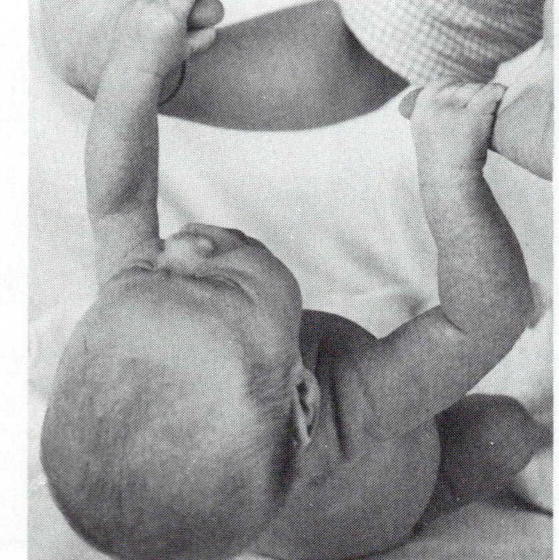
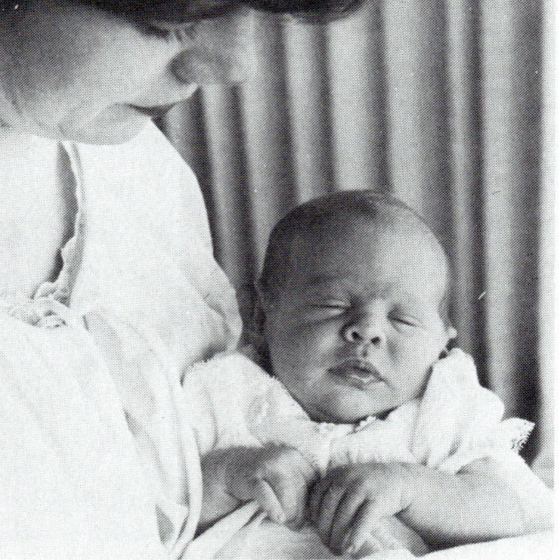
B

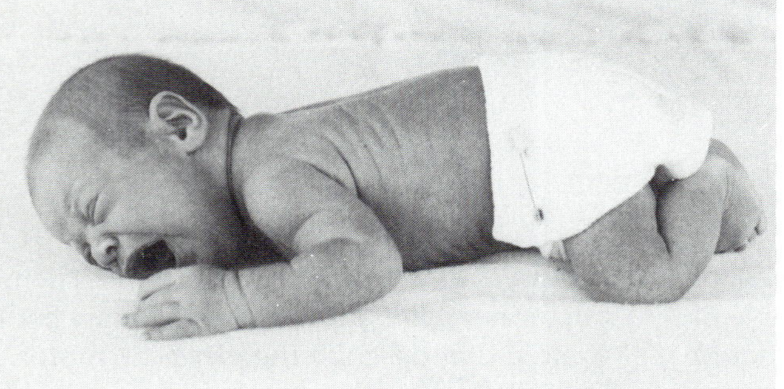
C

Fig. 21-1 Newborn infant. **A,** Grasp reflex is strong; **B,** sleeps 20 hours a day; **C,** readily assumes fetal position.

◆ TABLE 21-1
Ages and Stages of Maturation—cont'd

Infancy (0 to 1 yr)—1 to 3 mo (see Figs. 21-2 and 21-3)

Physical growth	***Motor development***	***Language development***	***Anticipatory guidance***
Posterior fontanel closes at 3 mo Grows in height about 1 inch/mo Head circumference increases 1 to 2 cm/mo	Activity diffuse and random Specific reflex activities May initiate facial expressions Cries with tears at 2 mo; can hold rattle Raises head 45 degrees 3 mo—raises head 90 degrees Will attempt to roll over	Cooing, laughing, squealing	*Development:* Head control increasing, alert, likes to look around Follows objects 180 degrees 8 to 12 wks—may sleep 6 to 8 hrs through night *Safety:* See Newborn Prevent falls Car safety restraint Approved pacifier (one piece to prevent choking) *Stimulation:* Infant seat Mobile Talk to and touch infant Musical toys *Feeding practices:* May "spit up" approximately 1 tbsp *Other:* Thumbsucking Immunizations Taking temperature

Continued.

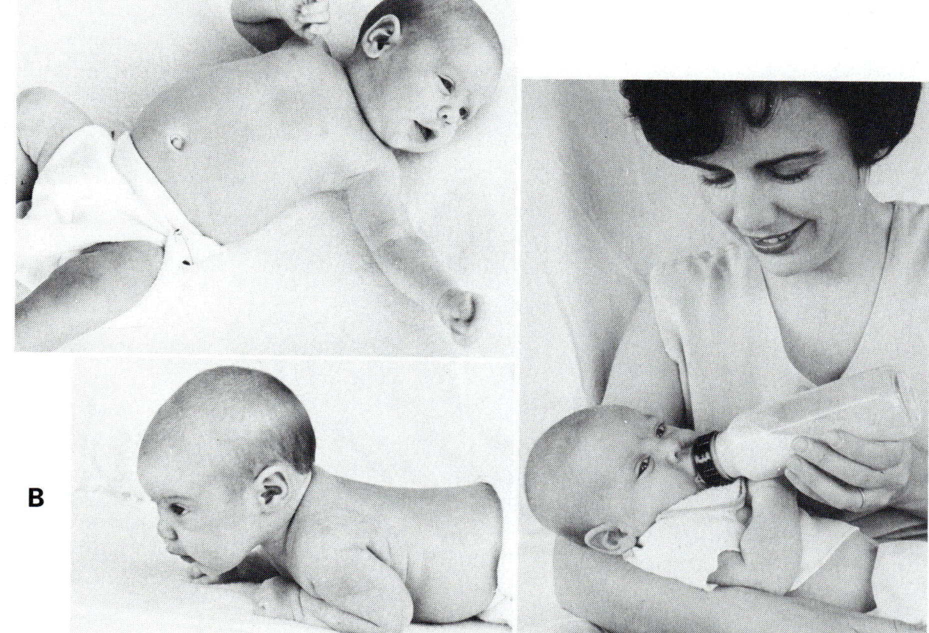

Fig. 21-2 Infant at 1 month. **A,** Tonic neck posture readily assumed; **B,** lifts and turns head when prone; **C,** held while feeding.

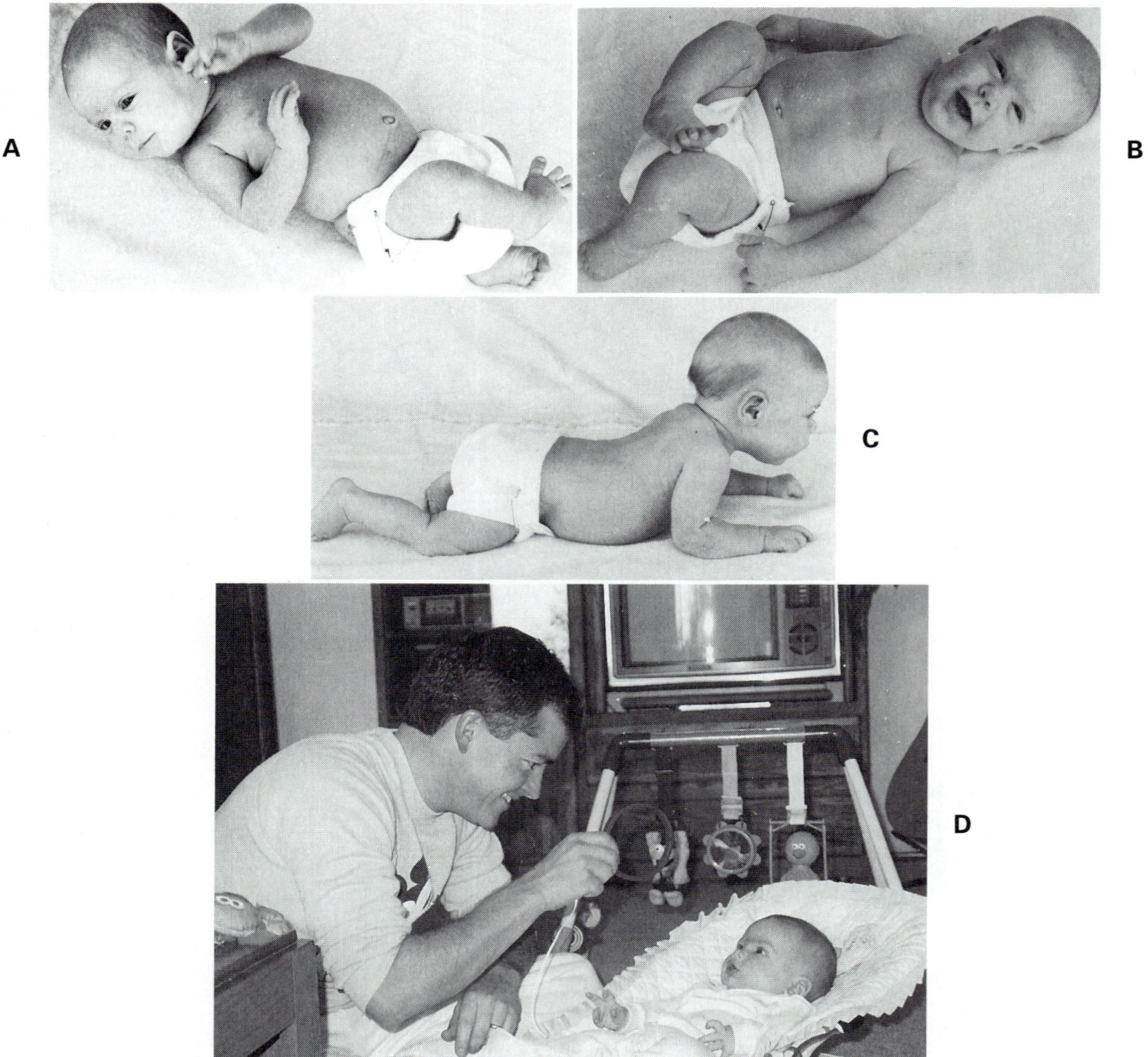

Fig. 21-3 Infant at 2 months. **A,** Activity diffuse and random; **B,** sociable smile appears; **C,** raises head 45 degrees; **D,** eyes follow objects.

◆ **TABLE 21-1**
Ages and Stages of Maturation—cont'd

Infancy (0 to 1 yr)—3 to 6 mo (see Figs. 21-4, 21-5, and 21-6)

Physical growth	*Motor development*	*Language development*	*Anticipatory guidance*
Birth weight doubled by 5 mo Head circumference increases 1 cm/mo until age 12 mo	3 to 4 mo—purposefully turns from back to side Reaches out at objects 4 mo—rooting, palmar grasp, and Moro reflex disappear 5 mo—rolls from abdomen to back 6 mo—asymmetric tonic neck reflex absent—must disappear before infant can crawl 6 mo—sits with support Best toys are rattles	Sociable smile, squeals, coos Imitates several tones 5 mo—understands name and babbles vowel-like sounds Responds to human sound more definitively Daily reading promotes language development	*Development:* Spitting up Teething Sleeps 8 to 10 hrs through night. Will awaken for social stimulation by 6 months. Unless parents desire a family bed, they must avoid overstimulation at bedtime. (Feeding, changing, safety checks only). Maintain in crib. If removed from crib for play, undesirable pattern may be established. *Safety:* Prevent falls and burns Car safety restraint *Stimulation:* Play-yard observation Vocal interaction Games Toys to mouth, grab and touch *Feeding practices:* Introduce cereal and cup at 5 to 6 mo (see Table 18-1) *Immunization:* DPT, OPV, HIB

Continued.

A 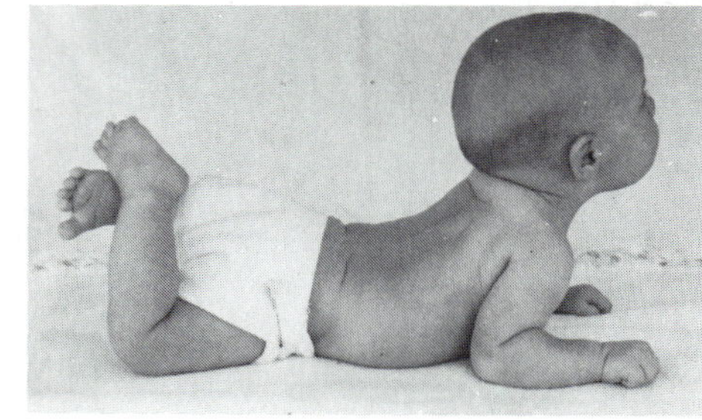

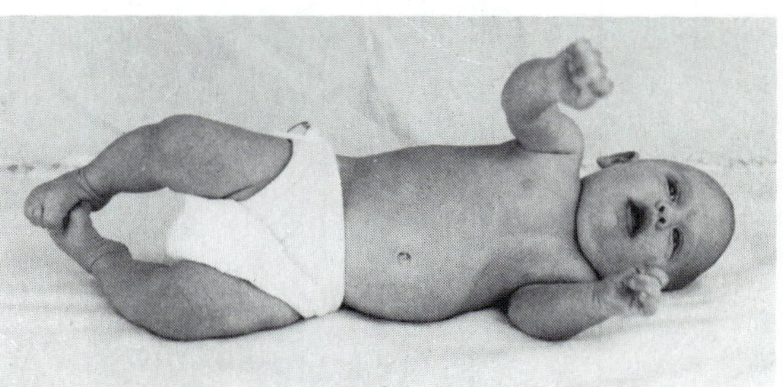 B

Fig. 21-4 Infant at 3 months. **A,** Raises head when prone, supports self on forearms; **B,** turns from back to side.

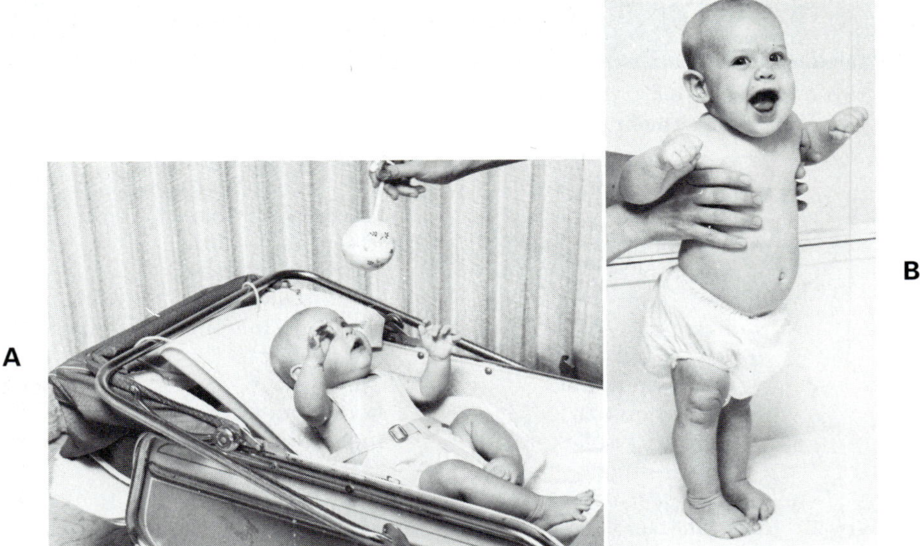

Fig. 21-5 Infant at 4 months. **A,** Reaches and grasps at objects; **B,** pushes with feet when held erect.

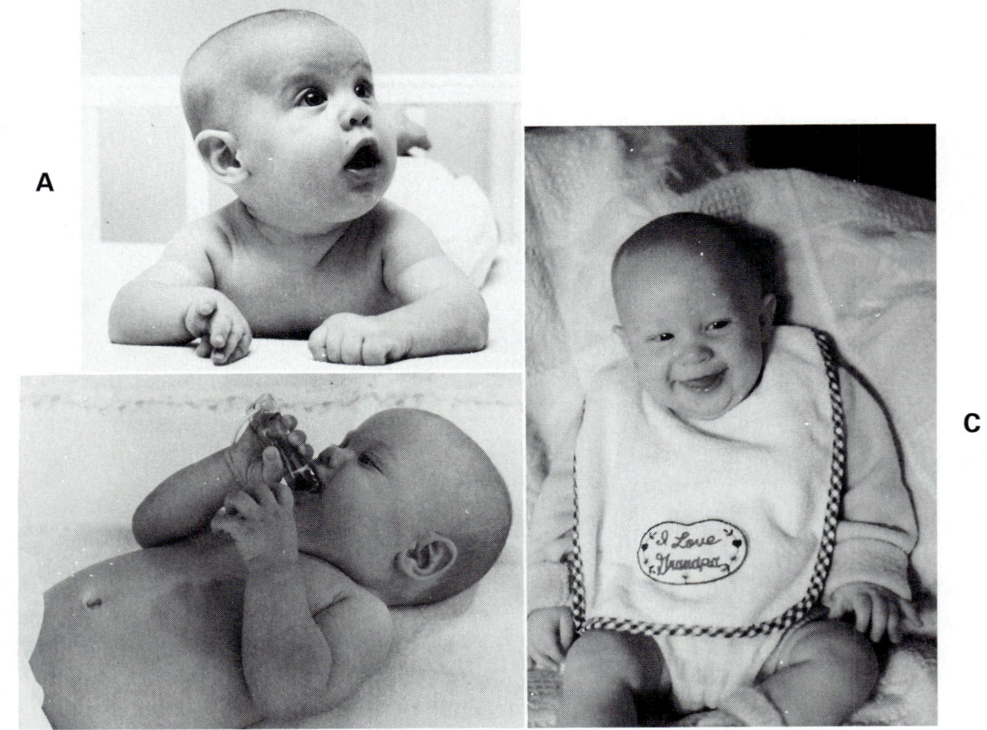

Fig. 21-6 Infant at 5 months. **A,** Understands name and babbles; **B,** manipulates and chews small objects; **C,** very sociable.

◆ **TABLE 21-1**
Ages and Stages of Maturation—cont'd

Infancy (0 to 1 yr)—6 to 11 mo (see Figs. 21-7, 21-8, 21-9, 21-10, and 21-11)

Physical growth	*Motor development*	*Language development*	*Anticipatory guidance*
First primary teeth appear 6 mo—lower central incisors 7½ mo—upper central incisors 10 mo—upper lateral incisors	Gross Motor: 6 mo—rolls from back to abdomen 6½ to 7½ mo—sits alone 9 mo—creeps 10 mo—pulls self to stand 9 to 12 mo—may begin cruising, walking Rejects confinement or restraint Fine Motor: Crude pincer grasp, picks up small object using thumb and finger in opposition	Can grunt, growl, and gurgle; says "da-da," "ma-ma," and "ba-ba" Read to child daily to promote language development	*Development:* Puts everything in mouth 7 to 9 mo—fear of strangers Special blanket or toy Dentition and dental care *Safety:* Discipline—begin setting safe limits Prevent burns, poisoning, ingestion of small objects, falls, drowning Child-proof home Car safety restraint *Stimulation:* Motion, nesting, and cuddle toys, stacking by 12 mo., offer Cheerios to promote fine motor development Peek-a-boo; pat-a-cake Kitchen utensils *Feeding practices:* Finger foods, cup 12 mo—wean from bottle, no bottles in bed or supine breast-feeding ad lib

Continued.

A

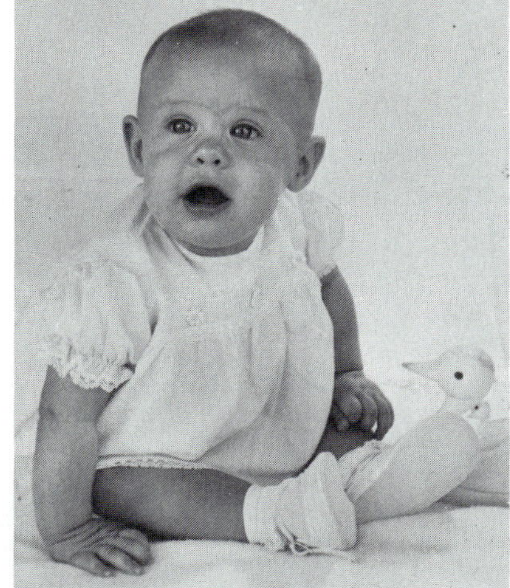

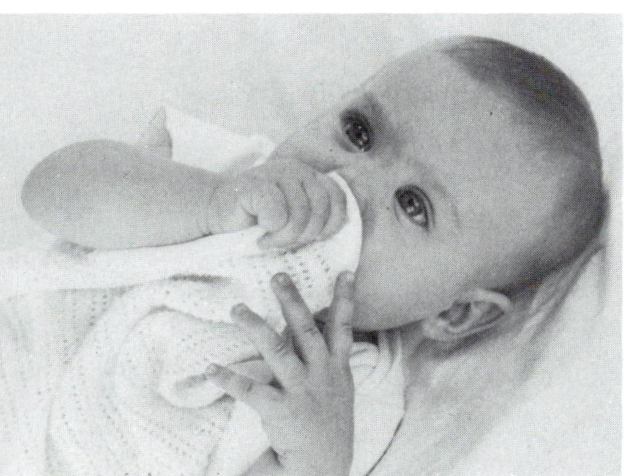

B

Fig. 21-7 Infant at 6 months. **A,** Sits alone, leaning forward on one hand; **B,** sleeps with favorite blanket and thumb in mouth.

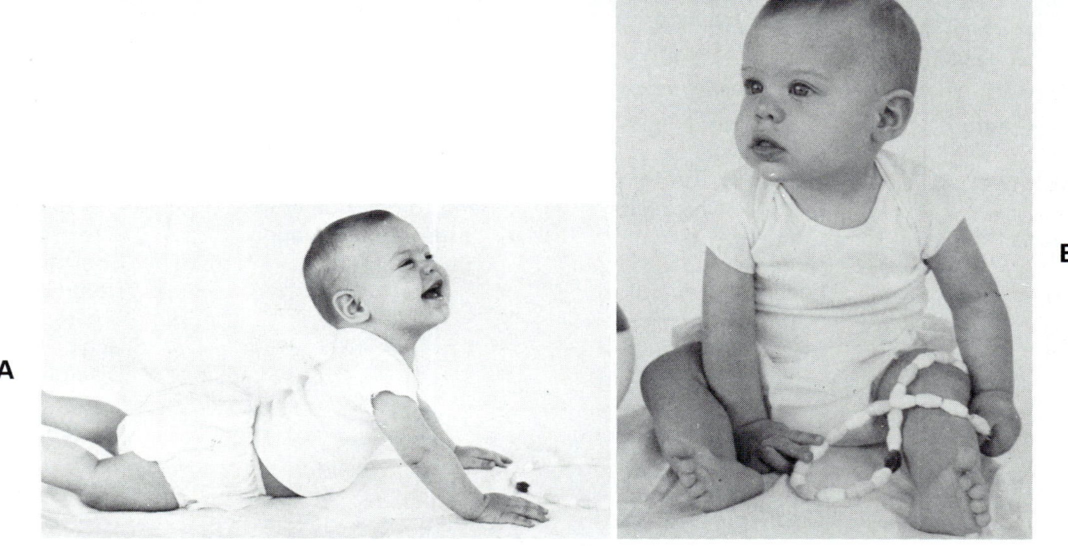

Fig. 21-8 Infant at 7 months. **A,** Propels self forward on abdomen (crawling); **B,** sits alone without support.

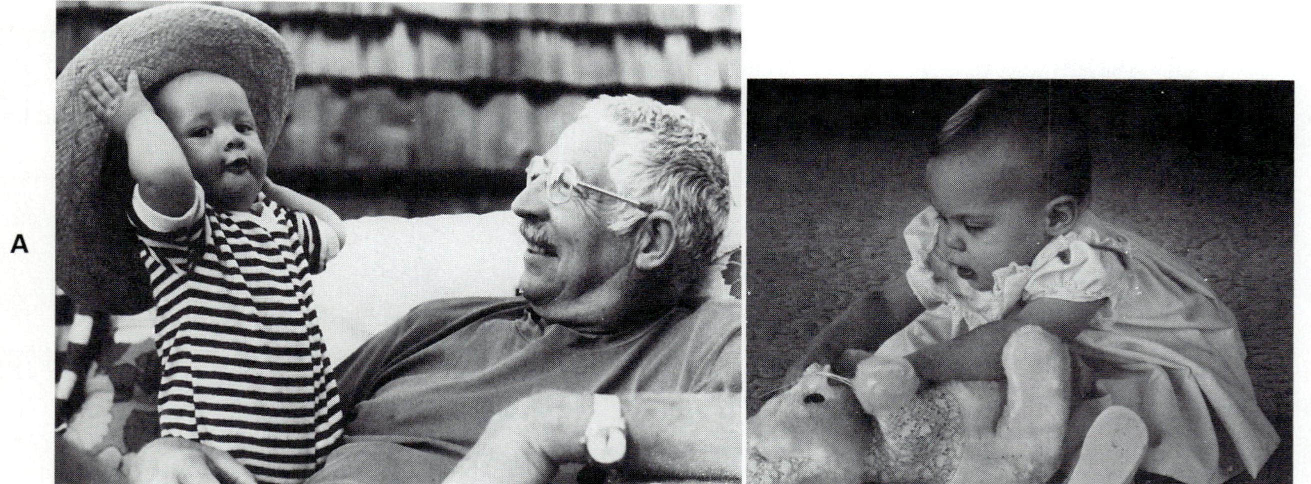

Fig. 21-9 Infant at 8 months. **A,** Babbles, gurgles, loves to play with familiar adults (may experience stranger anxiety); **B,** can lean forward and straighten up.

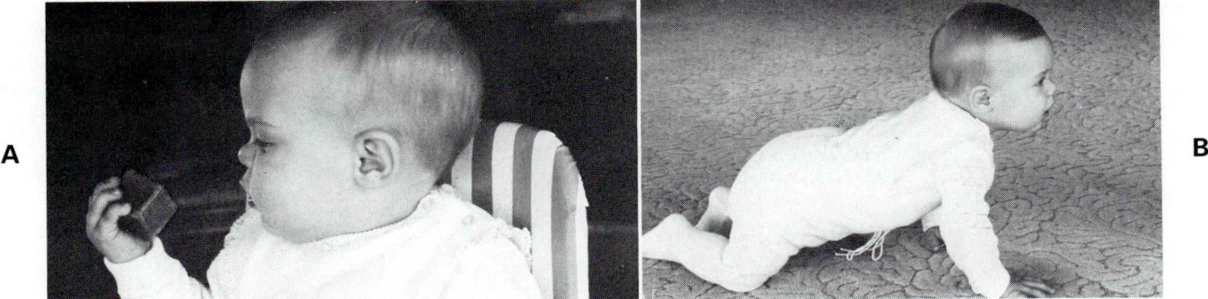

Fig. 21-10 Infant at 9 months. **A,** Grasps small objects; **B,** propels self forward on all fours, trunk above and parallel with floor (creeping).

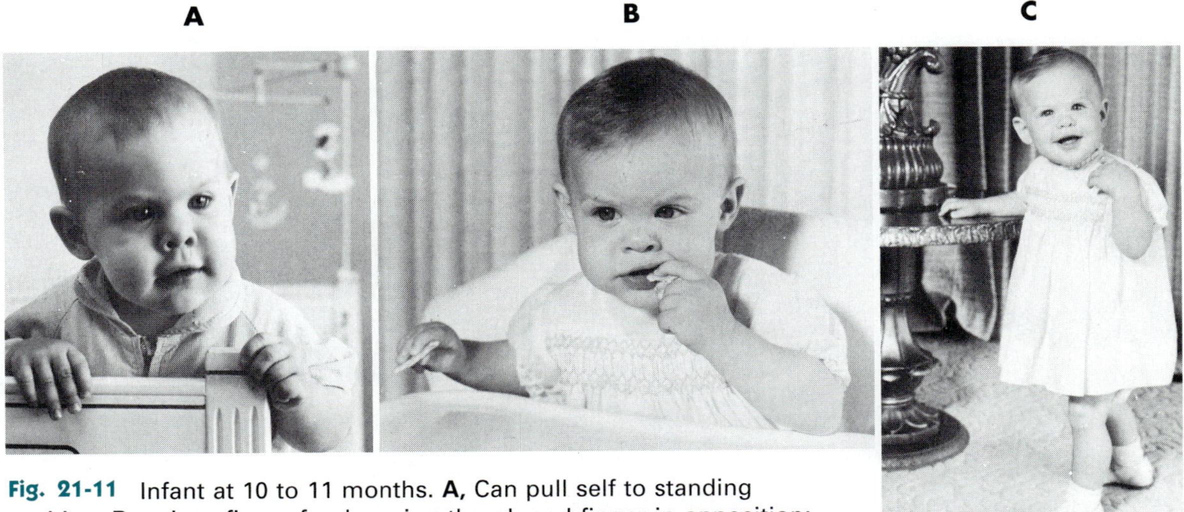

Fig. 21-11 Infant at 10 to 11 months. **A,** Can pull self to standing position; **B,** enjoys finger foods, using thumb and finger in opposition; **C,** cruises around, holding on to furniture.

◆ **TABLE 21-1**
Ages and Stages of Maturation—cont'd

Infancy (0 to 1 yr)—12 mo (see Fig. 21-12)

Physical growth	***Motor development***	***Language development***	***Anticipatory guidance***
Birth weight tripled; height 29 to 30 in Six to eight teeth	Gross Motor: Walks alone with wide stance and short steps Fine Motor: Picks up small objects with forefinger and thumb Drinks from cup with ease	Says "ma-ma," "da-da," and "ba-ba" plus other words such as "no-no" and "bye-bye" Read to child daily	*Development:* Negativism begins Likes to explore Plays spontaneously One to two naps/day May cooperate in dressing Gives a kiss *Safety:* See precautions for 6 to 11 mo *Stimulation:* Stacking toys Push and pull toys *Feeding practices:* Three meals/day Nutritious snacks Begin weaning from bottle

A

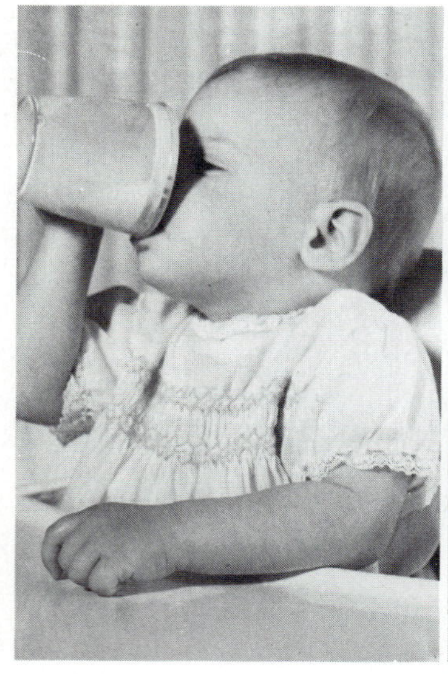

B

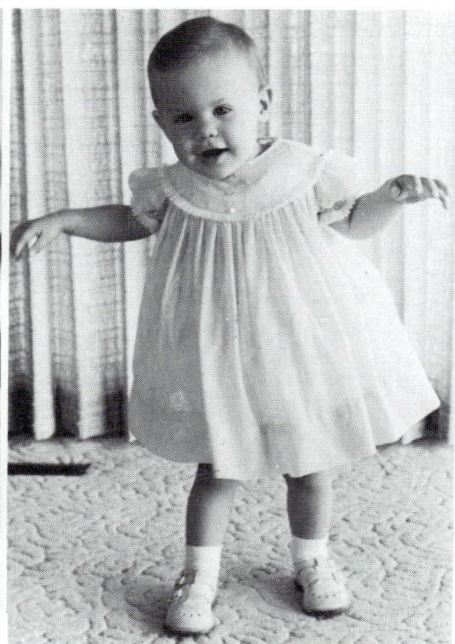

C

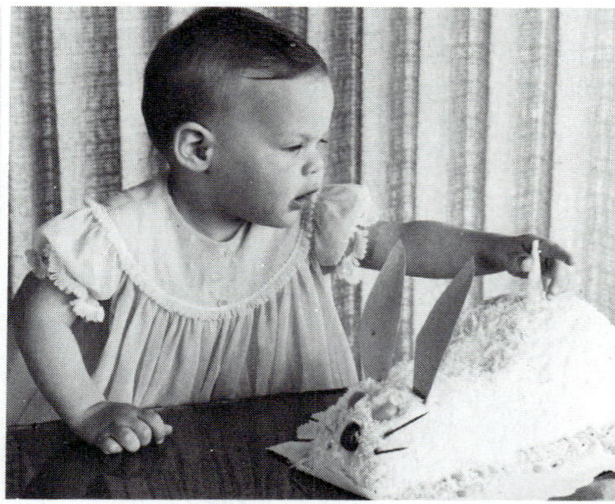

Fig. 21-12 Infant at 12 months. **A,** Drinks from cup with ease; **B,** walks alone with wide stance and short steps; **C,** has good finger-thumb opposition.

◆ **TABLE 21-1**
Ages and Stages of Maturation—cont'd

Toddler (1 to 3 yr)—15 to 18 mo (see Figs. 21-13 and 21-14)

Physical growth	*Motor development*	*Language development*	*Anticipatory guidance*
Growth rate slows Abdomen protrudes eight to twelve teeth Anterior fontanel closed	Walks well without support Builds a tower of 2 to 4 blocks Uses spoon but spills Can throw object Ceaseless activity Walks upstairs holding on Need for active mastery of newfound motor skills	Vocabulary of 6 to 18 words; follows simple commands Uses jargon that will develop into sentences Daily reading promotes language development	*Development:* Toilet training— Girls may show signs of readiness by 18 to 24 mo Boys by 30 to 36 months. Discuss how to prevent unrealistic expectations by parents. May be assertive and independent Anger and temper tantrums occur in preverbal children, fatigue and hunger are contributing factors Sleep—unless family bed is desired, maintain in crib during the night after a brief safety check Ritualistic behavior Takes off shoes and socks Can climb into everything *Safety:* Water safety Lock medications Toddler immunizations *Stimulation:* Enjoys coloring, spontaneous scribbling Moves from solitary to parallel play (playing alongside other children) Turns pages of book *Feeding practices:* Small servings Decrease in appetite Totally weaned from bottle to prevent caries and infection. Note: Bottle becomes source of infection once child is ambulating. Breastfed toddlers often nurse at bedtime and on awakening in morning. *Continued.*

A

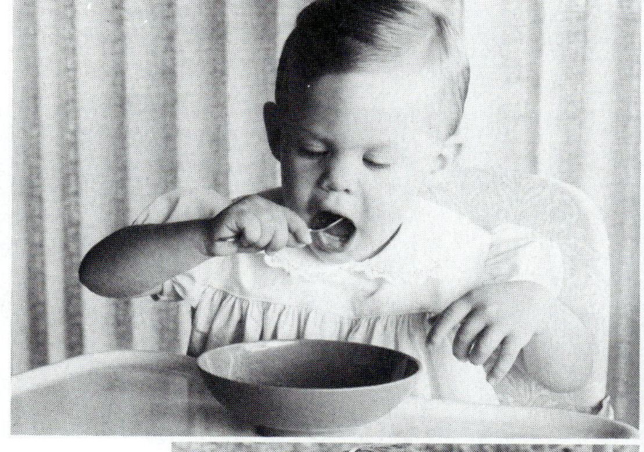

B

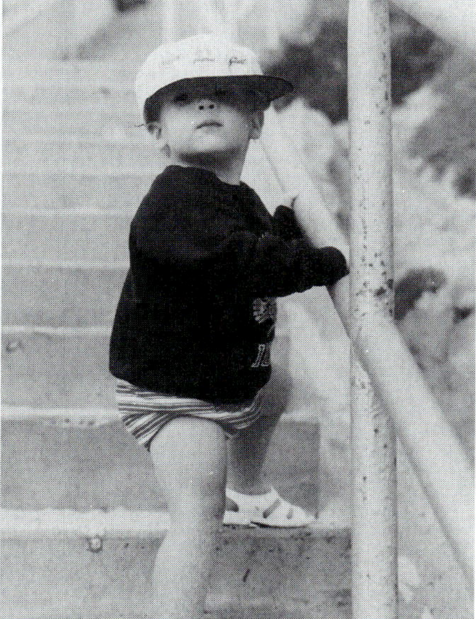

C

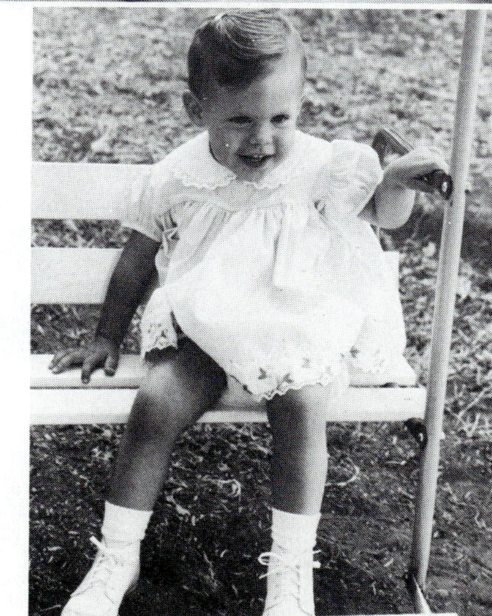

Fig. 21-13 Toddler at 15 months. **A,** Uses spoon but spills; **B,** walks upstairs holding onto railing; **C,** plays outside.

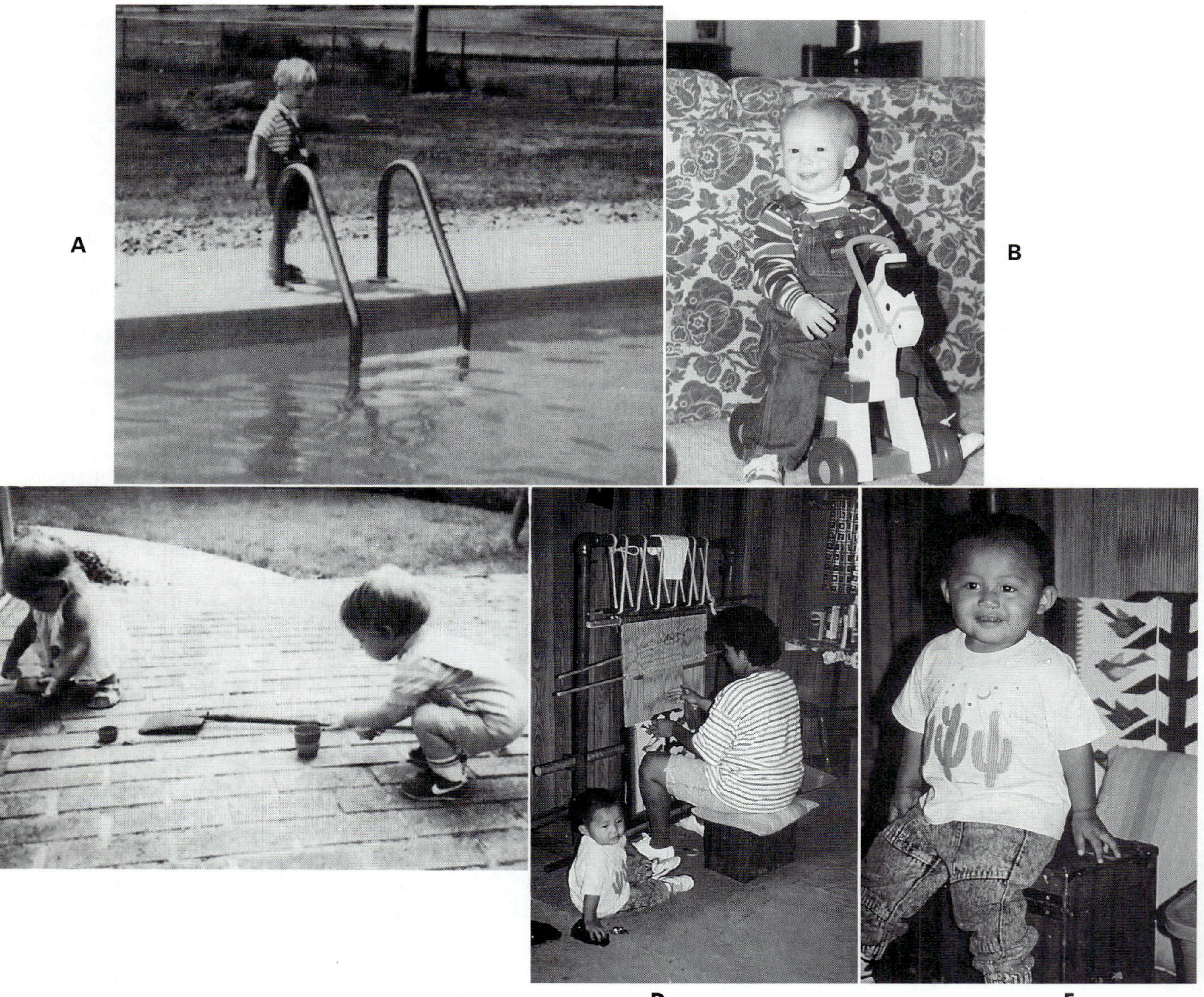

Fig. 21-14 Toddler at 18 months. **A,** Needs close supervision near water, since drowning is the second leading cause of death in boys aged 1 to 4 years; **B,** loves riding toys; **C,** moves from solitary to parallel play; **D,** enjoys security of spending time with parent; **E,** negativism subsides as verbal skills increase. (**A,** and **C,** from Wong D: *Essentials of pediatric nursing,* ed 4, St. Louis, 1993, Mosby).

◆ TABLE 21-1
Ages and Stages of Maturation—cont'd

Toddler (1 to 3 yr)—24 mo (see Fig. 21-15)

Physical growth	***Motor development***	***Language development***	***Anticipatory guidance***
Grows 3 to 5 in during second year Gains 5 lbs in second year Weighs 26 to 28 lbs Sixteen teeth	Gross Motor: Walks up and down stairs alone Runs without falling Opens door Kicks ball Throws ball overhand Overestimates own capabilities Fine Motor: Copies lines Scribbles Stacks blocks	Names familiar objects; says simple phrases; has vocabulary of 300 words; "me" and "mine" dominate	*Development:* Bowel control may be achieved (girls earlier than boys) Has difficulty sharing Dressing ability increases Thumbsucking and temper tantrums decrease Bedtime rituals important Discipline—safe limits must be set; define unacceptable behavior *Safety:* Set limits See previous precautions Continue to childproof Avoid food that may be aspirated *Stimulation:* Will advance to cooperative play over next 12 mo Picture book, stories Begins to imitate doing household tasks *Feeding practices:* Dexterity increases Appetite fluctuates Feeds self

Continued.

A 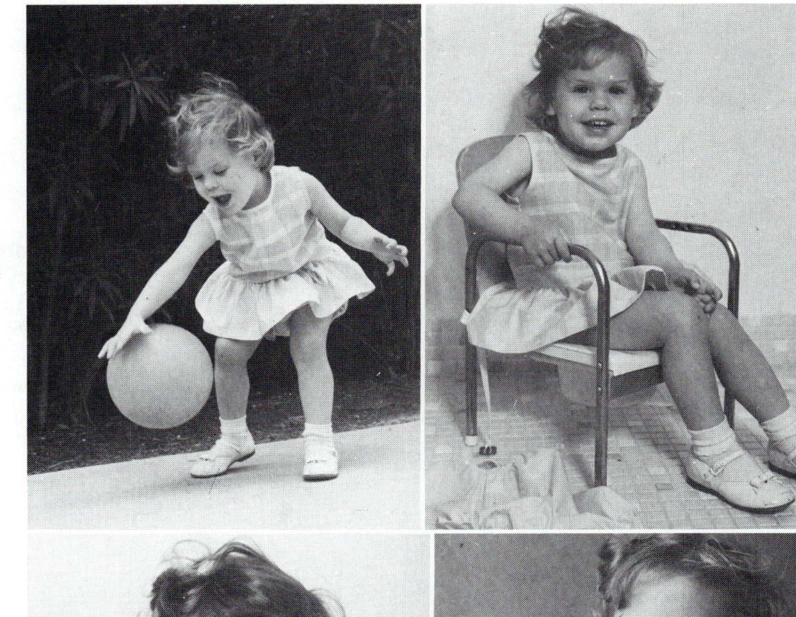 B

C 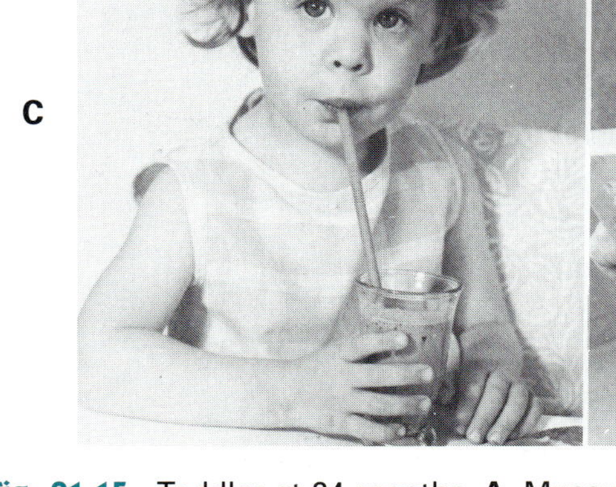

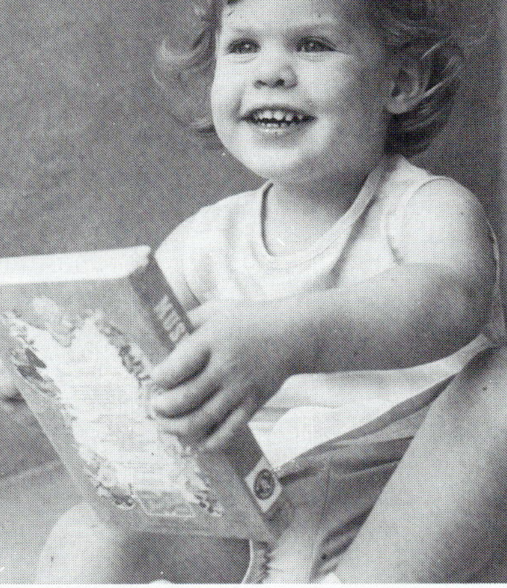 D

Fig. 21-15 Toddler at 24 months. **A,** Muscular coordination greatly advanced; **B,** verbalizes toileting needs (girls average 6 months earlier than boys); **C,** drinks from straw; **D,** enjoys picture books.

◆ **TABLE 21-1**
Ages and Stages of Maturation—cont'd

Toddler (1 to 3 yr)—30 mo (see Fig. 21-16)			
Physical growth	***Motor development***	***Language development***	***Anticipatory guidance***
Complete set of 20 primary teeth Slow, steady growth	Gross Motor: Jumps with both feet Walks on tiptoes Fine Motor: Undresses self easily Builds tower of eight blocks	Says full name; sings; begins to express needs verbally	*Development:* Loves routine Magical thinking Bladder training improves Washes and dries hands Make first dental appointment *Safety:* Prevent burns, falls, drownings, ingestions Provide stimulation in car seat to help keep content, secure *Stimulation:* Exposure to other children Coloring, fingerpainting, games, cooking group Short attention span *Feeding practices:* Definite likes and dislikes Food jags (prefers 1 to 2 foods) common Avoid engaging in battle *Other:* Sexual curiosity

A

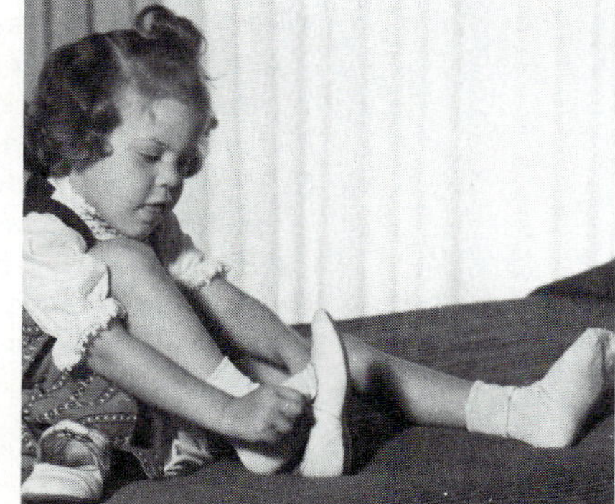

B

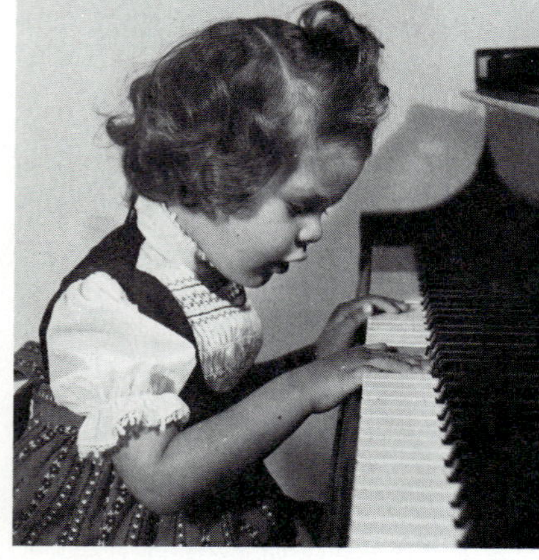

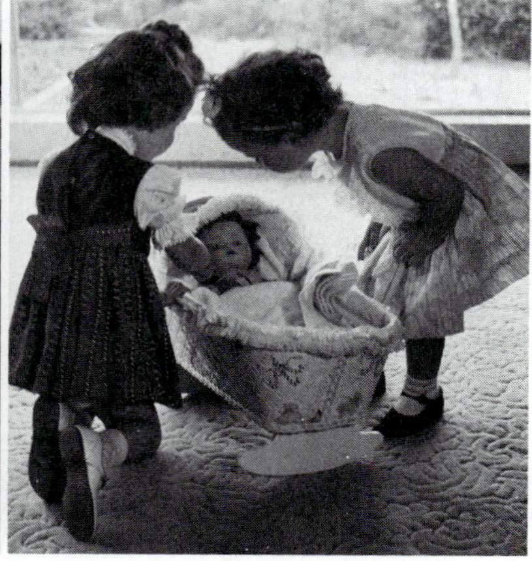

C

Fig. 21-16 Toddler at 30 months. **A,** Can put shoes on; **B,** attempts to sing simple songs; **C,** enjoys playing with others.

◆ **TABLE 21-1**
Ages and Stages of Maturation—cont'd

Preschool (3 to 6 yr)—3 yr (see Fig. 21-17)

Physical growth	Motor development	Language development	Anticipatory guidance
Relatively slow growth; gains about 5 lbs; height increases average of 3 in/yr	Gross Motor: Uses stairs with alternate feet Hops on one foot Rides tricycle Fine Motor: Strings large beads Copies cross and circle Loves art projects	Has vocabulary of 900 words or more Knows two to three colors May talk with imaginary playmate	*Development:* Can brush teeth May display sibling rivalry Bladder control usually achieved Interest in sexuality Needs 12 hr sleep a day Allow independence within limits of safety *Safety:* Child overestimates capabilities—set safe limits Water-safety, swimming lessons are advised *Stimulation:* Cooperative play Desires constant activity Resents interference with play or possessions Climbing activities essential Wagons, tricycles, other riding toys and boats enjoyed *Feeding habits:* Food "jags" common; may not like "mixtures" (i.e., casseroles) Regularity of mealtime important Teach dental prophylaxis

Continued.

A
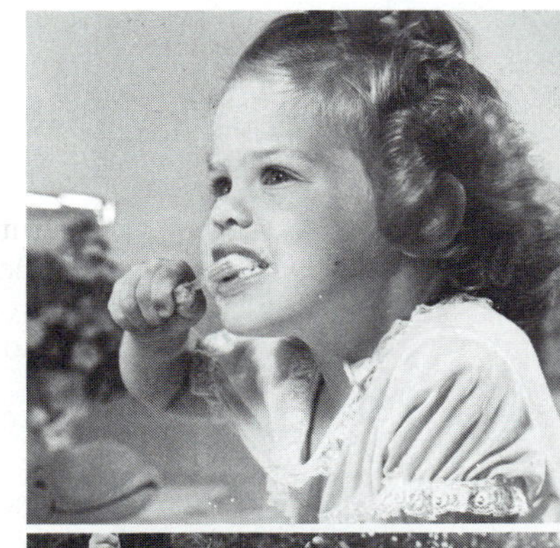

B
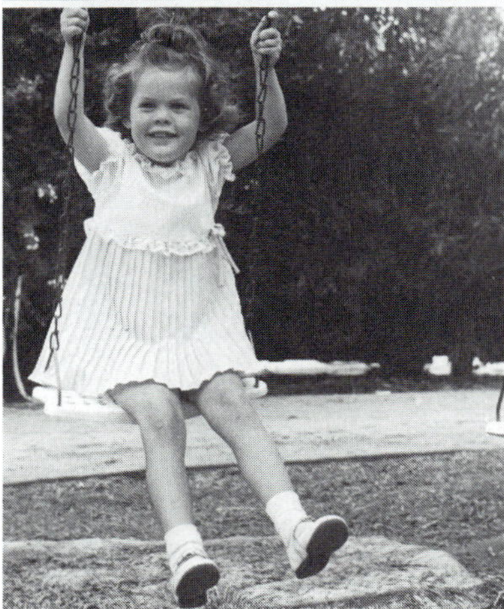

C
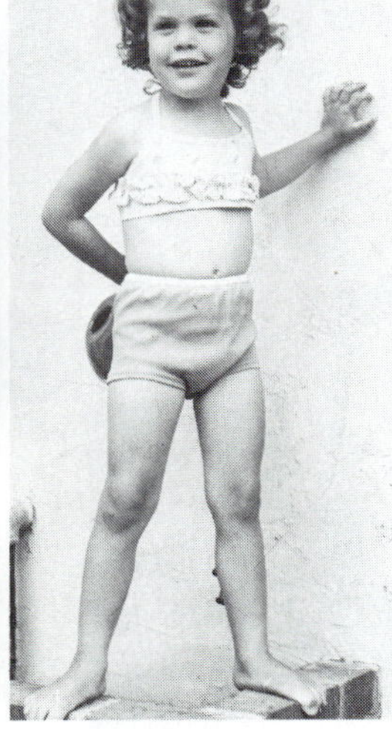

Fig. 21-17 Preschooler at 3 years. **A,** Can brush teeth and wash hands; **B,** can pump swing with legs; **C,** knows own age and sex and has good balance.

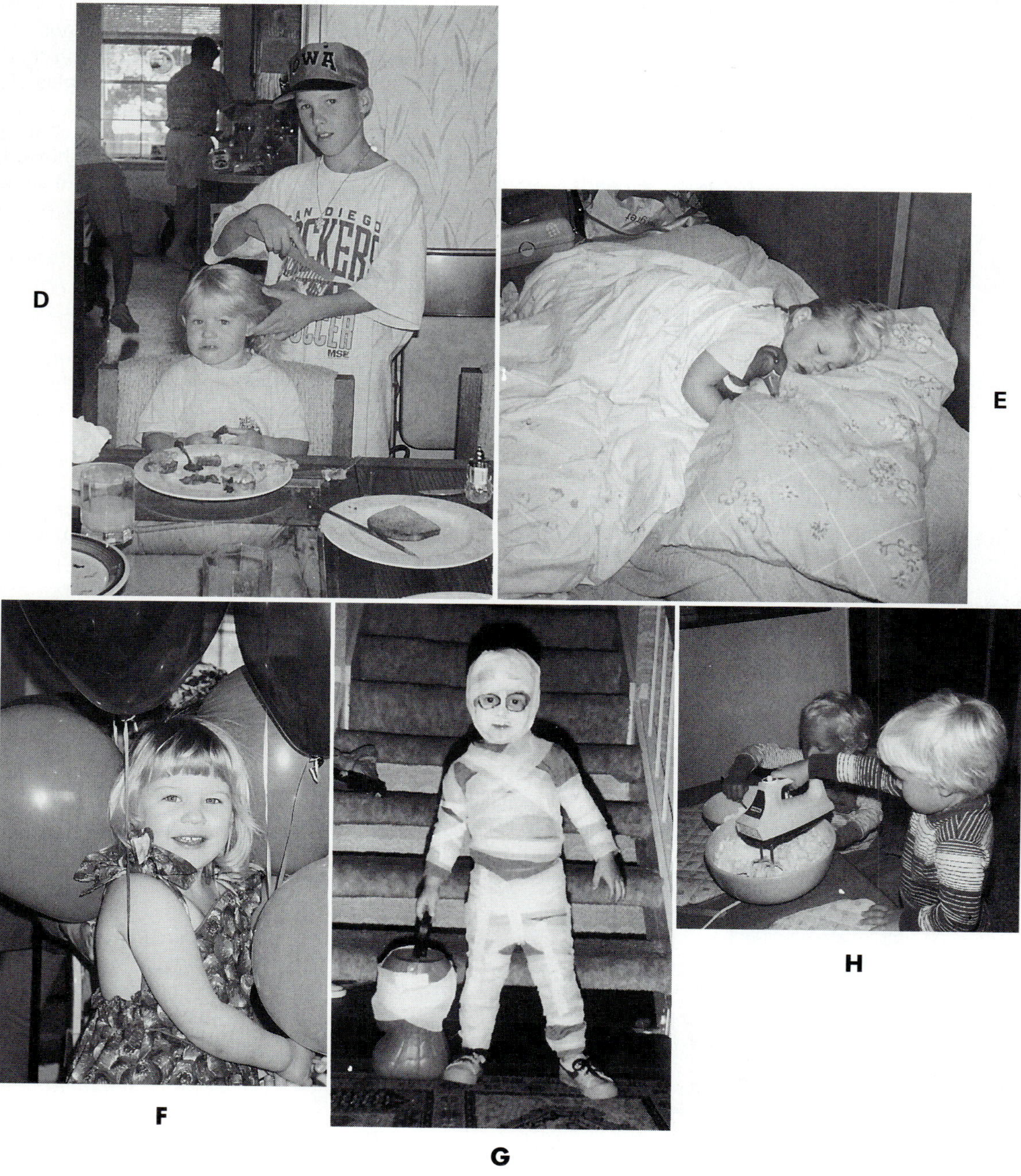

Fig. 21-17 (cont'd) **D,** Loves attention from older children; **E,** sleeps with favorite toy; **F,** loves parties and socializing; **G,** period of magical thinking begins; **H,** parents encourage initiative within a safe environment. (Courtesy Michael Clement, MD, Mesa, AZ.)

◆ **TABLE 21-1**
Ages and Stages of Maturation—cont'd

Preschool (3 to 6 yr)—4 yr (see Fig. 21-18)

Physical growth	*Motor development*	*Language development*	*Anticipatory guidance*
Height 39 to 41 in Weight 35 to 40 lbs Continued relatively slow growth at rate of 3 year old	Gross Motor: Uses one foot per step when going down stairs Climbs, runs, and jumps well Fine Motor: Increasing finger dexterity Buttons and unbuttons clothes Copies square	Vocabulary of 1500 words Can explain own drawing; knows several colors; repeats rhymes and songs Asks many questions Begins to identify words Loves hearing books read aloud	*Development:* Magical thinking Sexual curiosity Continues becoming more self-sufficient Knows own age *Safety:* May use seatbelt when weight reaches 40 to 50 lbs Teach safety precautions (i.e., cross streets on signals only. Hold hand of adult). Avoid hot radiator and stove, coffee/tea pots and cups Water-safety, swimming lessons are advised *Stimulation:* Moves from cooperative play with one child to small group play—plan projects accordingly Assess school readiness *Feeding practices:* Offer nutritious, between-meal snack *Immunizations:* Preschool series

Continued.

A

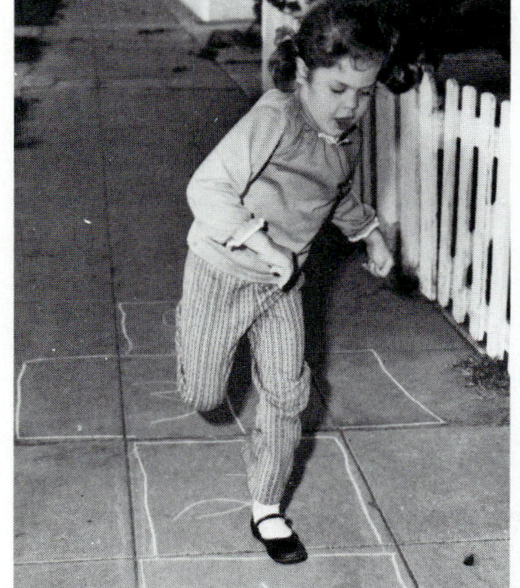

B

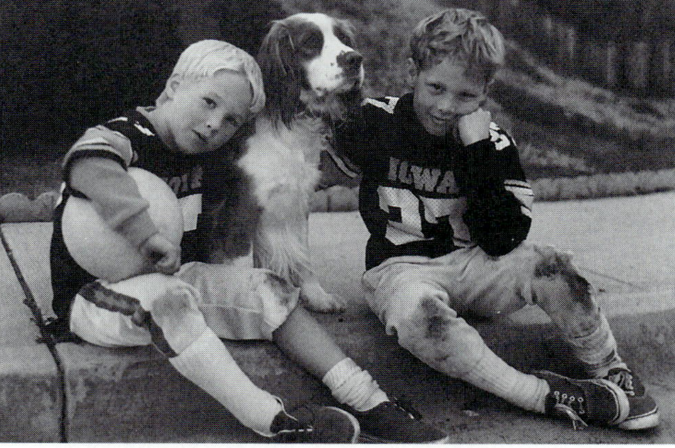

Fig. 21-18 Preschooler at 4 years. **A,** Hops on one leg; **B,** Enjoys playing with older siblings and pets.

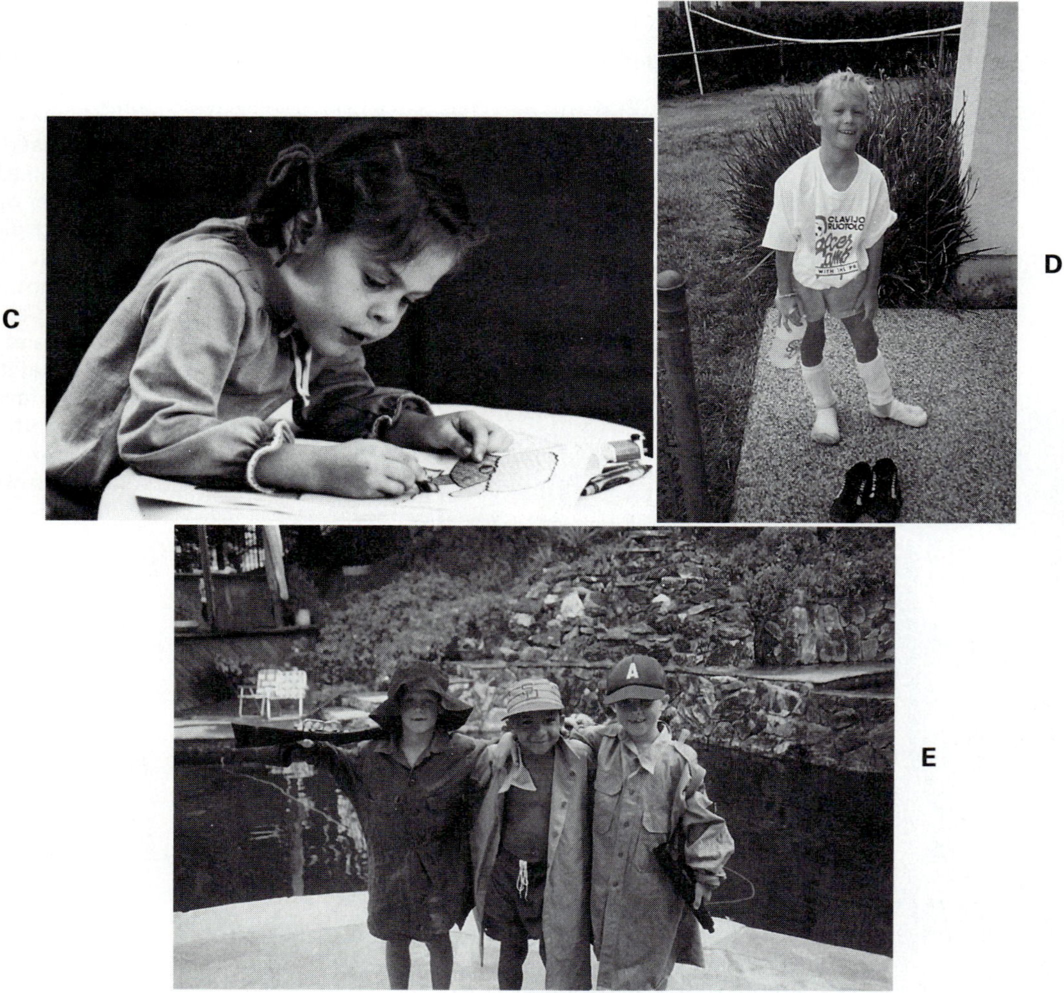

Fig. 21-18 (cont'd) **C,** Has increasing fine motor skills; **D,** needs good hydration for sports and begins to develop a sense of self-care; **E,** period of magical thinking continues.

◆ TABLE 21-1
Ages and Stages of Maturation—cont'd

Preschool (3 to 6 yr)—5 yr (see Fig. 21-19)			
Physical growth	***Motor development***	***Language development***	***Anticipatory guidance***
Height 43 to 45 in Weight 40 to 45 lbs May lose lower central incisors	Gross Motor: Good muscular coordination; can hop, skip, run, and catch ball Climbs on jungle gym Handles tricycle well Needs rest periods Fine Motor: Brushes teeth Plays board games Copies triangle	Names all primary colors and coins Talks in sentences; talks constantly	*Development:* Prints Dresses and undresses without assistance Sensitive to praise *Safety:* Reinforce safety precautions (bike helmet, seat belts, stranger awareness, pool safety) *Stimulation:* Enjoys group activities, conformity, rules *Feeding practices:* Likes finger foods (i.e., carrot sticks, peeled apples, bananas) Teach importance of preventing caries Flouride

Continued.

A

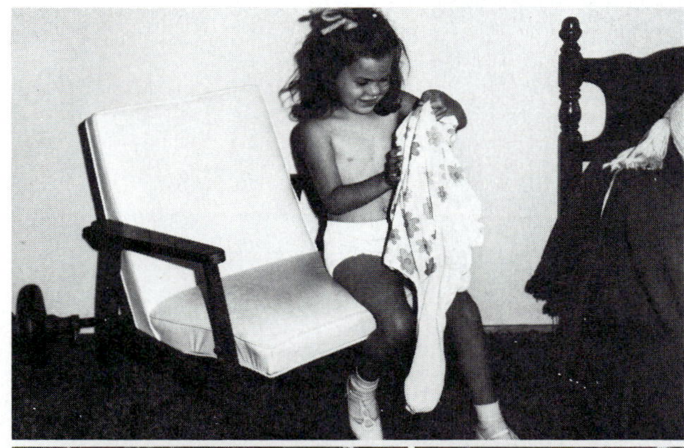

B

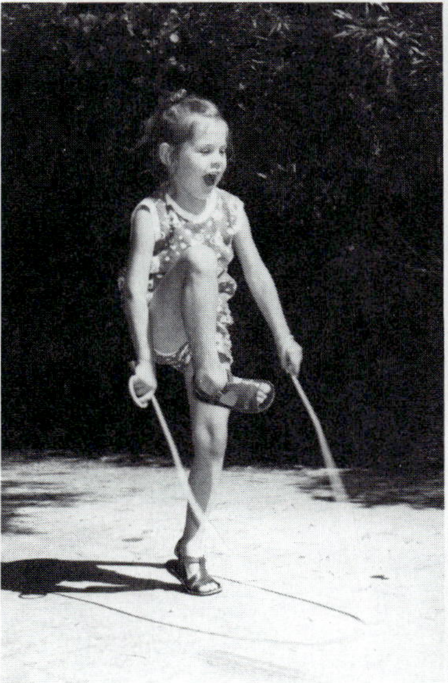

C

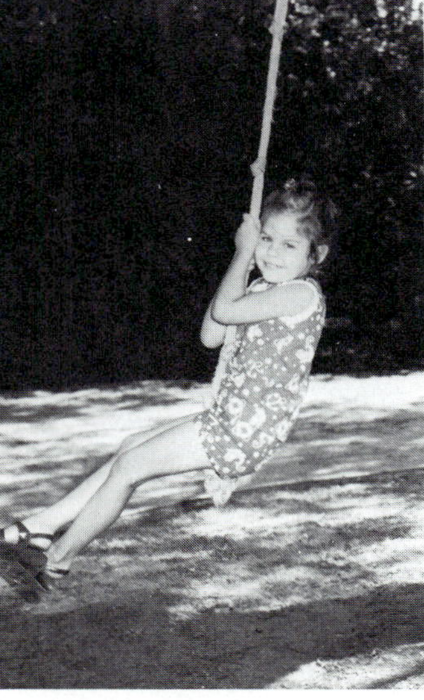

Fig. 21-19 Preschooler at 5 years. **A,** Dresses and undresses without help; **B,** can jump rope; **C,** has good muscular coordination.

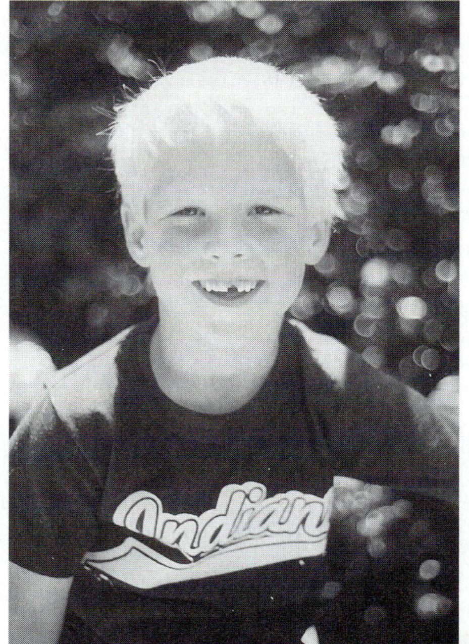

D

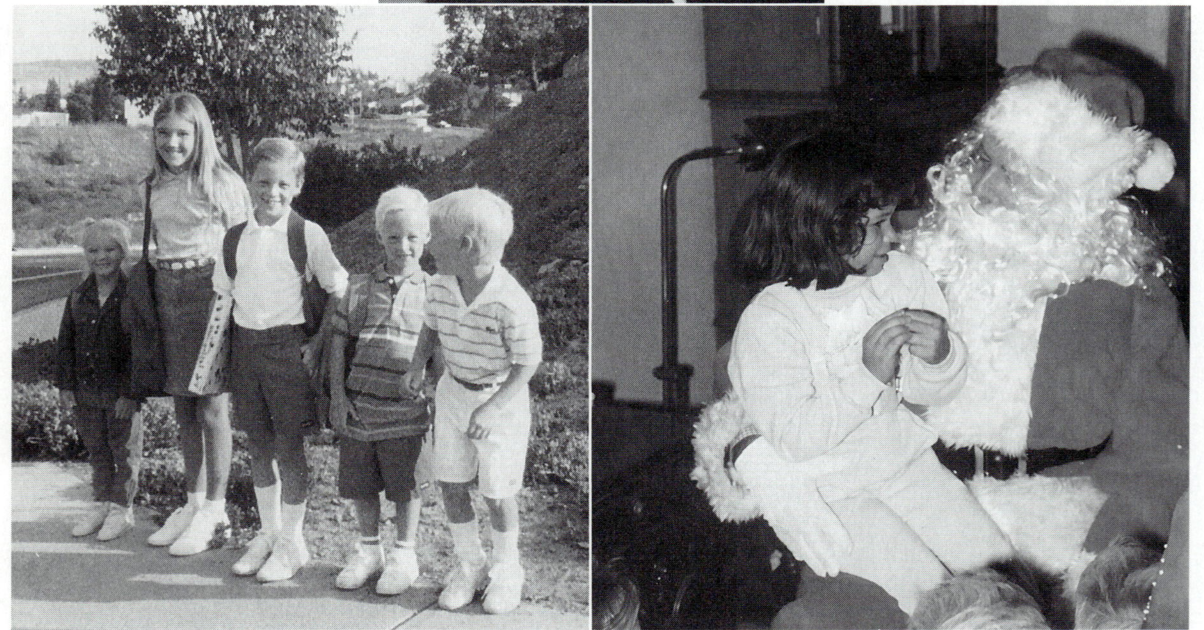

E

F

Fig. 21-19 (cont'd) **D,** Loses first deciduous tooth; **E,** off to kindergarten with older siblings; **F,** magical thinking and "belief in Santa" waxes and wanes.

◆ **TABLE 21-1**
Ages and Stages of Maturation—cont'd

School age (6 to 10 yr)—6 and 7 yr (see Figs. 21-20 and 21-21)			
Physical growth	***Motor development***	***Language development***	***Anticipatory guidance***
6-yr molars; first permanent teeth Annual growth of 2 in Height 47 to 48 in Weight 50 to 51 lbs Loses upper incisors	Gross Motor: Good balance Advanced throwing Roller skates Swims Enjoys outdoor sports; can ride bicycle, swim, jump rope, walk straight line Fine Motor: Penmanship readable Increased dexterity Ties shoes	Vocabulary of 2500 words Reads and writes Counts May tell time	*Development:* Can bathe self Modest; curious Conscious of rules Household chores important Begins to write Allow independence *Safety:* Teams, clubs, gangs, hero worship pronounced *Feeding practices:* Influenced by peers Nutritious snack *Immunizations:* Tuberculosis screening annually *Other:* Assess school performance Parental involvement critical

Continued.

A

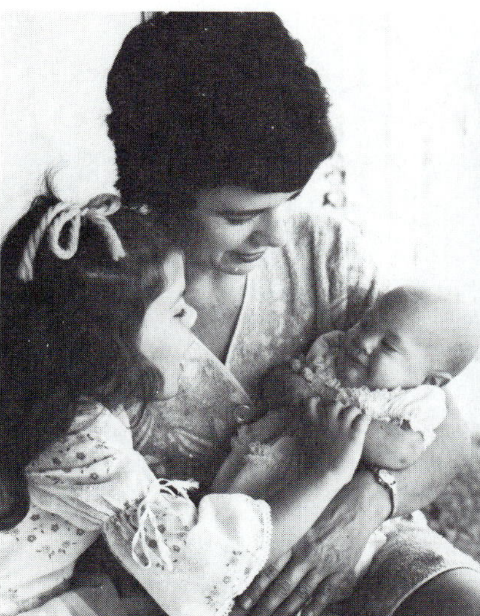

B

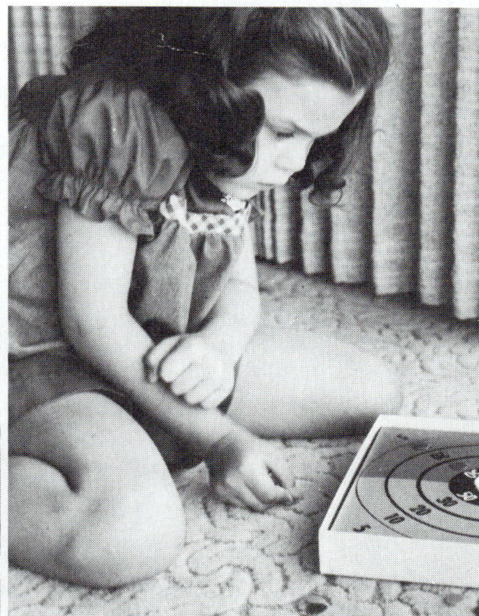

C

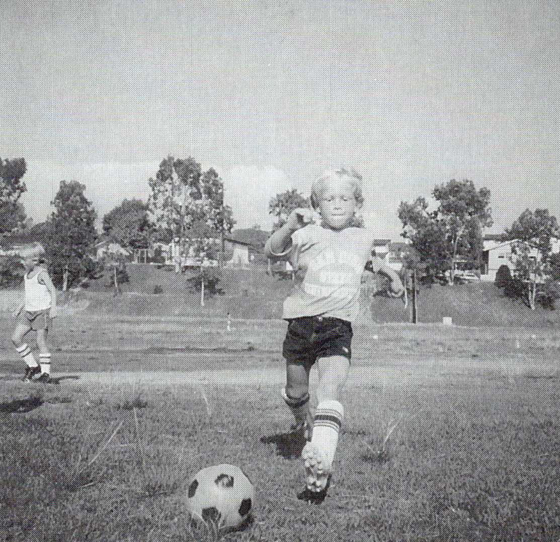

D

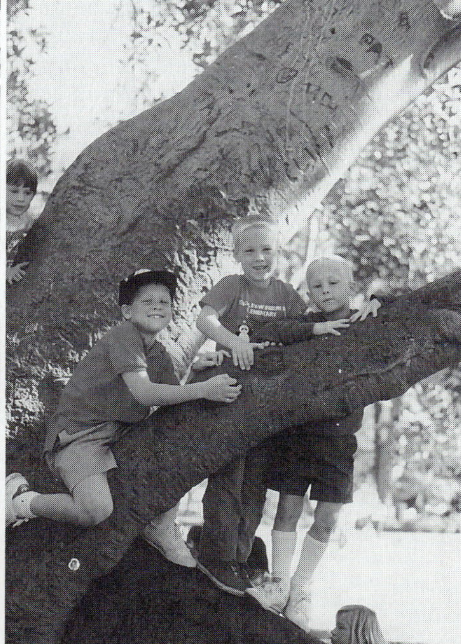

Fig. 21-20 School age—6 years. **A,** Helps with younger children; **B,** has increased interest in games and team sports; **C,** coordination improves tremendously; **D,** tree climbing a favorite pastime.

B

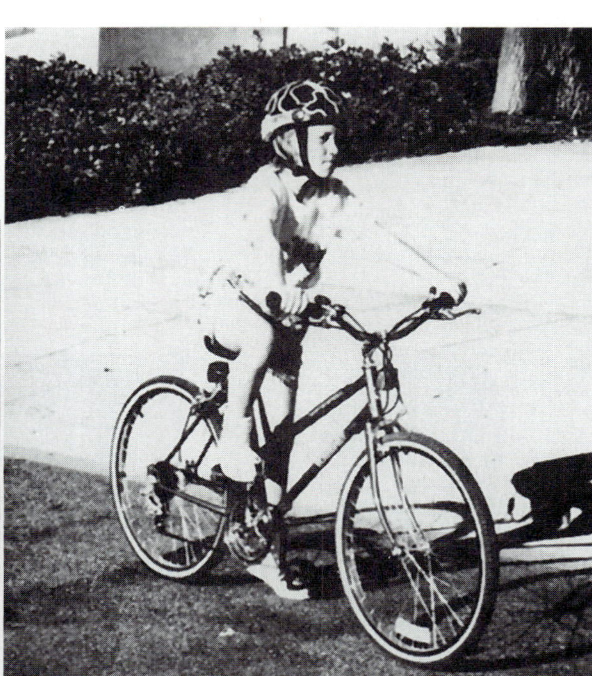

A

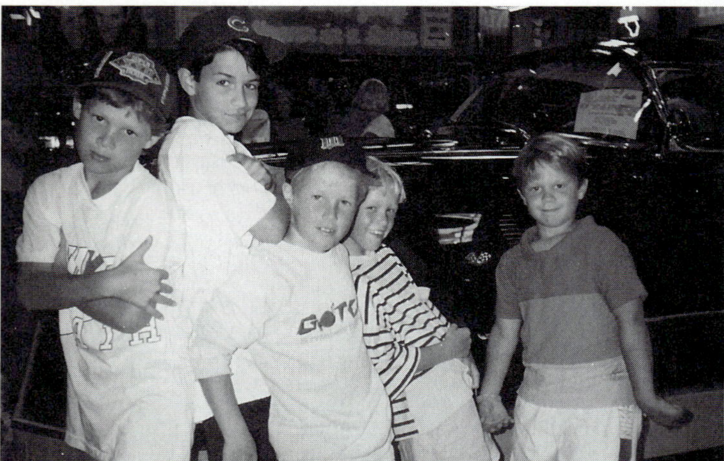

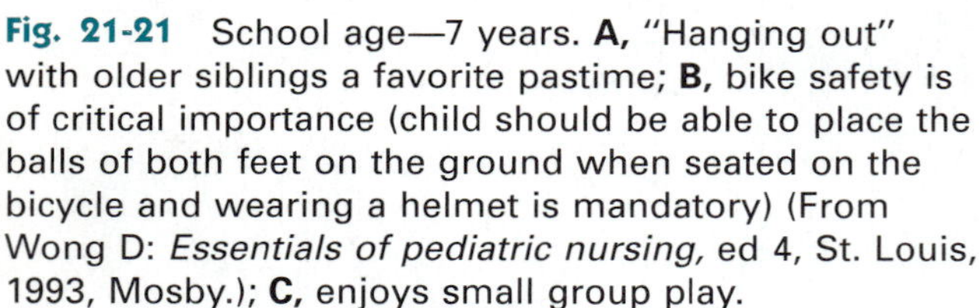

Fig. 21-21 School age—7 years. **A,** "Hanging out" with older siblings a favorite pastime; **B,** bike safety is of critical importance (child should be able to place the balls of both feet on the ground when seated on the bicycle and wearing a helmet is mandatory) (From Wong D: *Essentials of pediatric nursing,* ed 4, St. Louis, 1993, Mosby.); **C,** enjoys small group play.

C

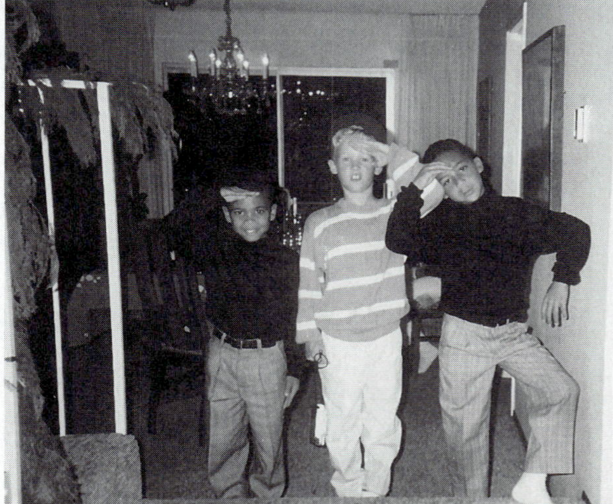

◆ **TABLE 21-1**
Ages and Stages of Maturation—cont'd

School age (6 to 10 yr)—8 and 9 yr (see Figs. 21-22 and 21-23)

Physical growth	*Motor development*	*Language development*	*Anticipatory guidance*
Gradual increase in size—steady growth	Gross Motor: Movements more graceful; able to accomplish more Fine Motor: Complex skills	8-yr—tells days of week 9-yr—tells months of year Enjoys puns, jokes, and stories Reading may be an enjoyable pastime and should be encouraged	*Development:* Enjoys solitary and group play Bicycles and skates are enjoyed Competitive sports valued; importance of exercise Prefers own gender; peer group important Favorite television shows Continues to enjoy stories May enjoy collections *Feeding practices:* Afternoon snacks Teach importance of good nutrition; allow time for adequate breakfast May have problems with manners and mealtime punctuality Good appetite *Education:* Substance abuse DARE program (Drug awareness Resistance education)

Continued.

A

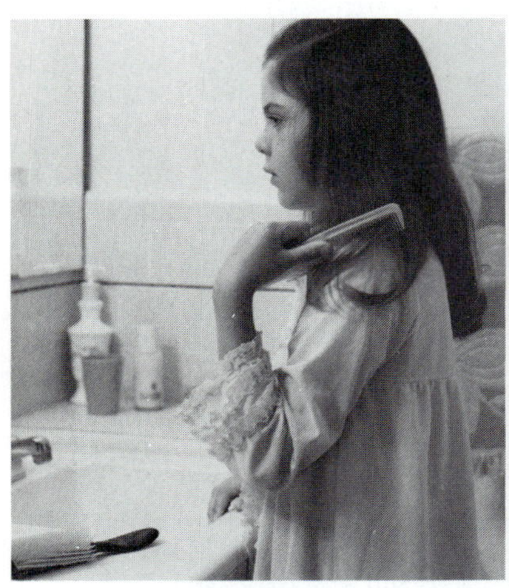

B

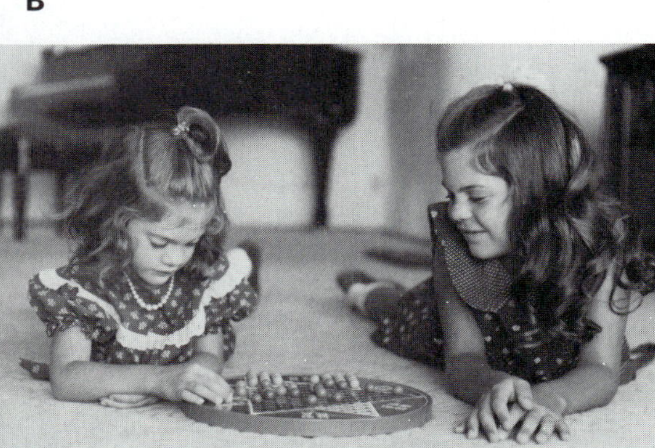

Fig. 21-22 School age—8 years. **A,** Increasing self-care; **B,** satisfaction gained helping younger sister learn.

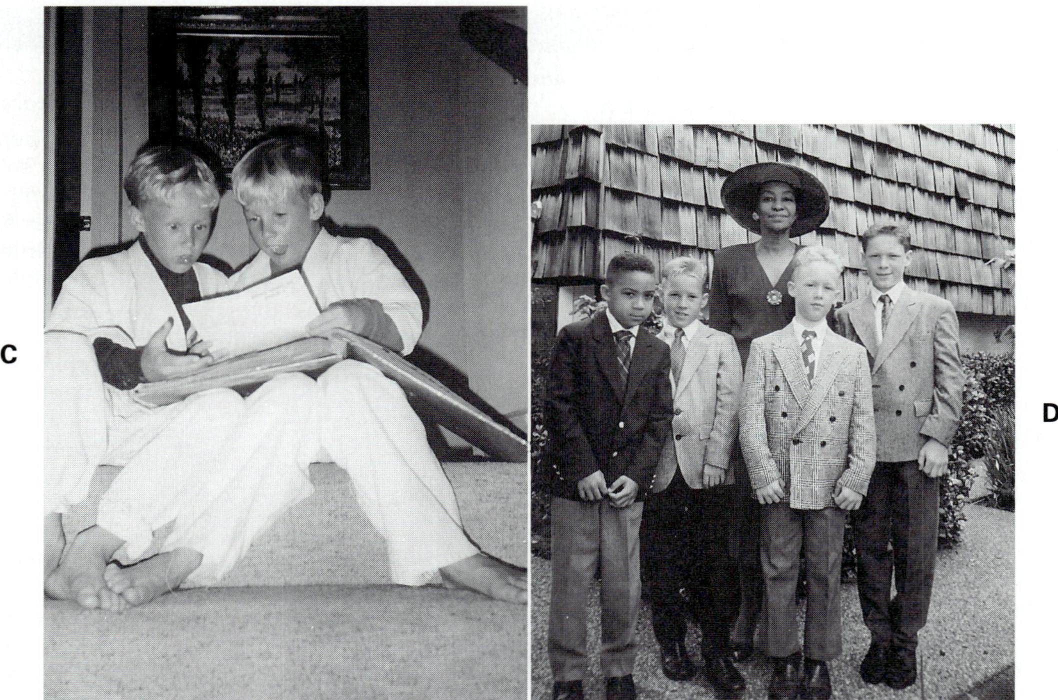

Fig. 21-22 (cont'd) **C,** Enjoys memorabilia; **D,** enjoys special holidays with extended family.

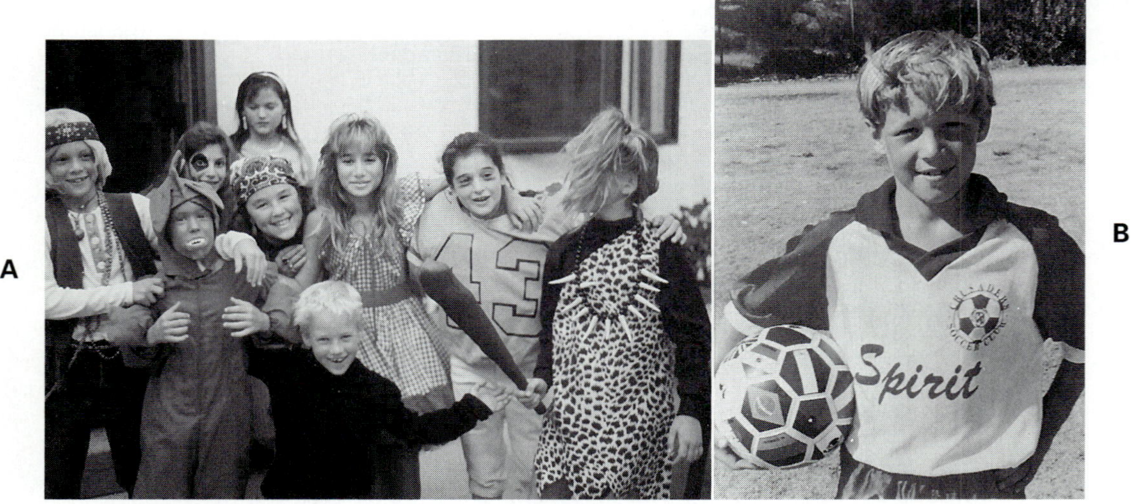

Fig. 21-23 School age—9 years. **A,** Enjoys Halloween; **B,** may select a favorite sport.

◆ **TABLE 21-1**
Ages and Stages of Maturation—cont'd

Preadolescence (10 to 12 yr) (see Figs. 21-24 and 21-25)

Physical growth	*Motor development*	*Language development*	*Anticipatory guidance*
Appearance and development of secondary sexual characteristics Pubescent growth spurt; 2 yrs earlier for girls Girls may show widening of hips, budding breasts, pubic hair, menses (average age is 12.3 yrs) Boys ahead of girls in physical strength and endurance; boys increase in muscle mass and bone size especially shoulder girdle and ribs; penis and scrotum enlarge	Gross Motor: Poor control will ensue if body framework and muscular development are out of proportion in their rate of growth Posture may be poor Fine Motor: Steady progress	Vocabulary increases; language reflects increasing ability to think introspectively and abstractly	*Development:* Four basic tasks of preadolescence and adolescence: Emancipation from parents and other adults Development of healthy self-concept Beginning acquisition of skills for future Understanding psychosexual differences *Possible problems:* Obesity caused by inactivity and ravenous appetite Poor nutrition (fad diets); need for increased protein Acne associated with hormonal changes Poor self-image (changing body image) Peer pressure; ambivalence toward parents and other adults Lack of sexual identity Adolescent pregnancy Sexually transmitted diseases Injuries Substance abuse prevention *Adolescent:* Health history acronym "HEADS" Home environment Education Activities (extracurricular peer group) Drug use Sexuality

Continued.

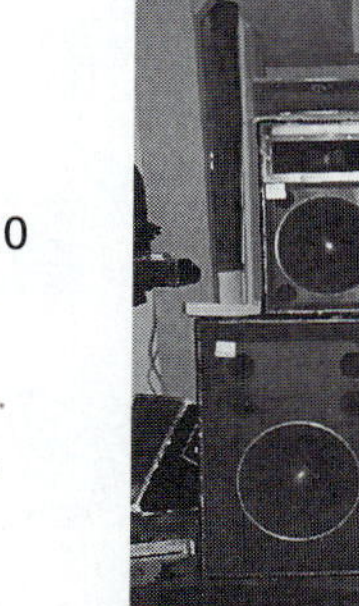

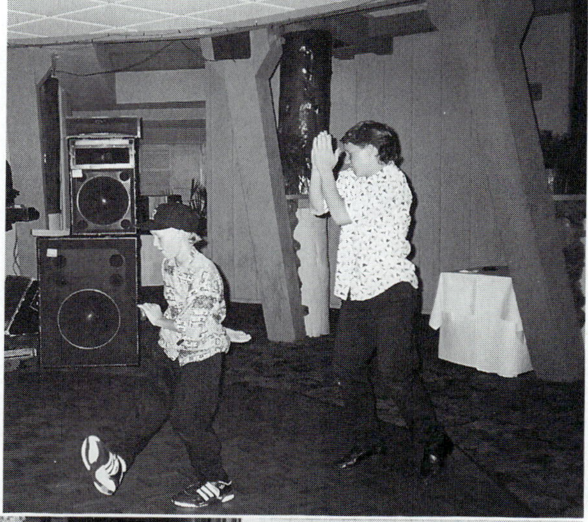

A

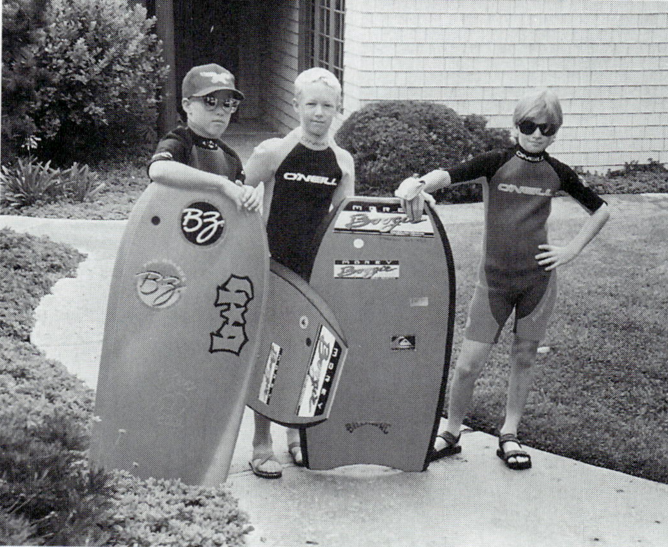

B

Fig. 21-24 Preadolescence—10 years. **A,** Listens to music and may love to dance; **B,** enjoys adventure (water safety rules and supervision are essential).

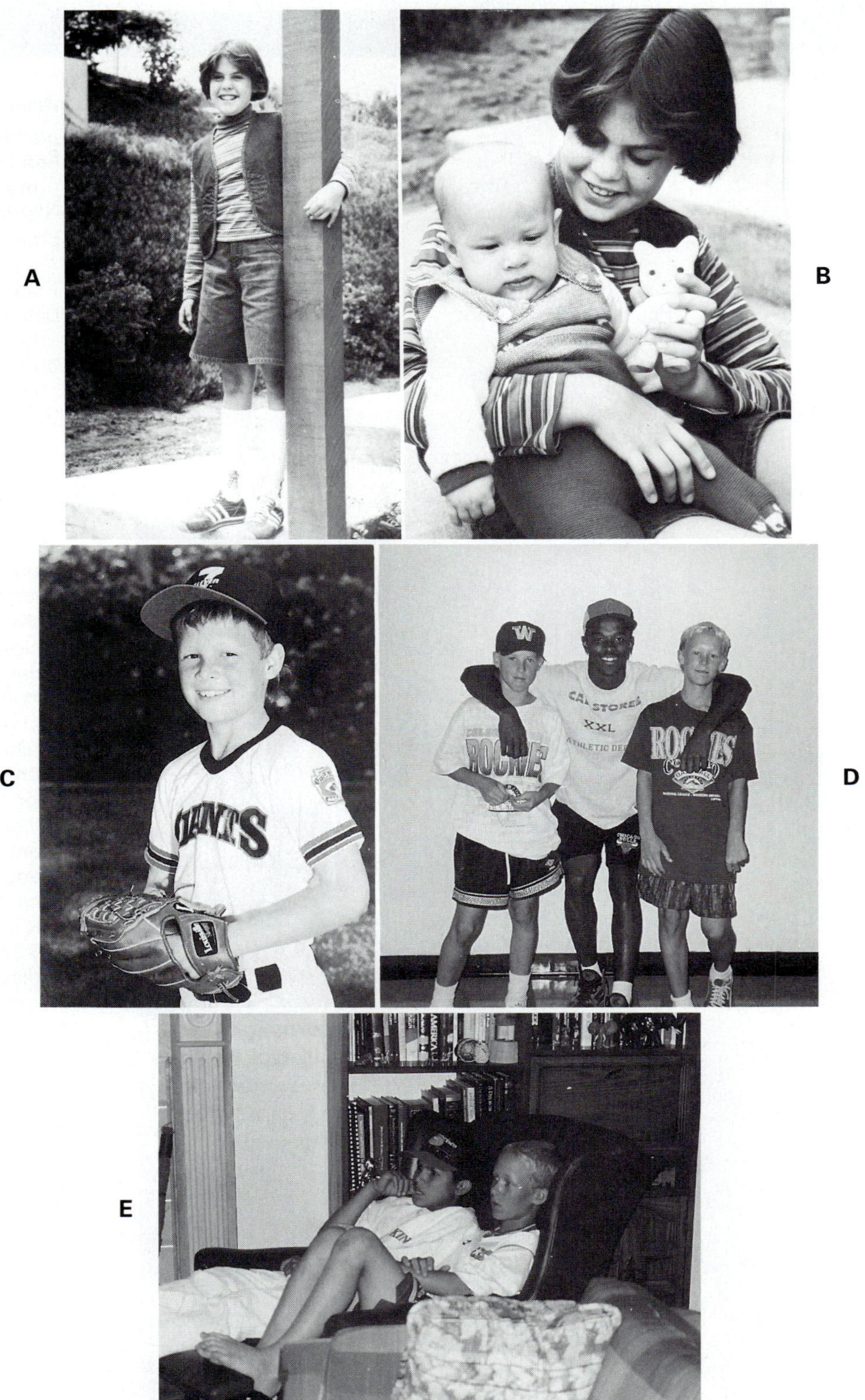

Fig. 21-25 Preadolescence—11 years. **A,** Growing up; **B,** babysitting a favorite pastime; **C,** Little League; **D,** hero worship; **E,** time spent in front of the television needs to be monitored.

◆ **TABLE 21-1**
Ages and Stages of Maturation—cont'd

Adolescence (12 to 19 yr)—early adolescence (12 through 15 yr) (see Figs. 21-26, 21-27, and 21-28)			
Physical growth	***Motor development***	***Language development***	***Anticipatory guidance***
Wide individual variability as to onset and rate of growth Girls: growth spurt between 10 and 14 yr, gain 2 to 8 in (5 to 20 cm) in height, 15 to 55 lbs (7 to 25 kg) in weight; menarche occurs 2 yr after pubescent changes Boys: growth spurt at 12 to 16 yr, gain 4 to 12 in (10 to 30 cm) in height and 15 to 65 lbs (7 to 30 kg) in weight Growth of pubic, axillary, and upper lip hair; facial appears 2 yr after pubic hair	Wide individual variability Hands and feet out of proportion; self-conscious, awkward	Increased vocabulary influenced by attainment of intellectual maturity Talkative but not communicative; giggly	*Development:* See preadolescent section Needs parental respect and acceptance Preparing for difficult decisions of late adolescence (i.e., continuing education, work, military service, dating, intimacy, marriage, financial responsibilities, political and religious affiliations) *Feeding practices:* Fad diets common Teach food guide pyramid *Teaching:* Girls: breast self-examination (BSE) monthly after age 16 yr Boys: testicular self-examination (TSE) monthly after age 14 yr

Continued.

B

A

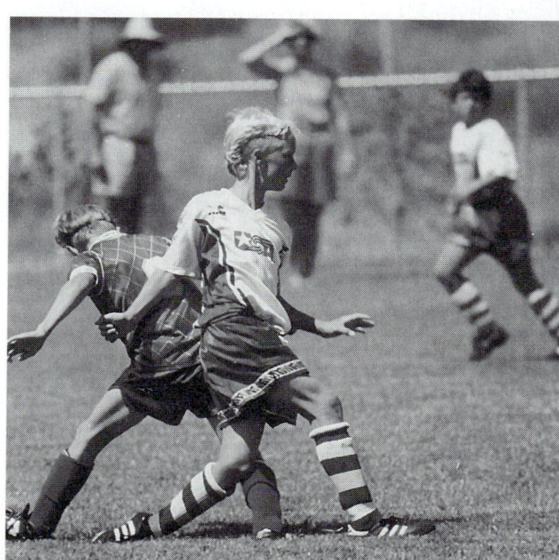

C

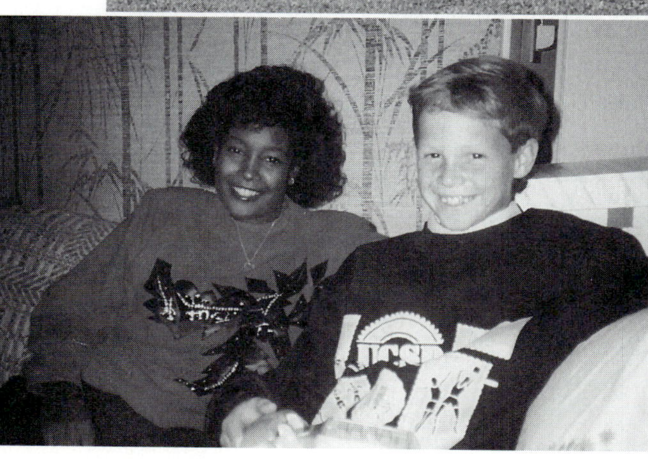

D

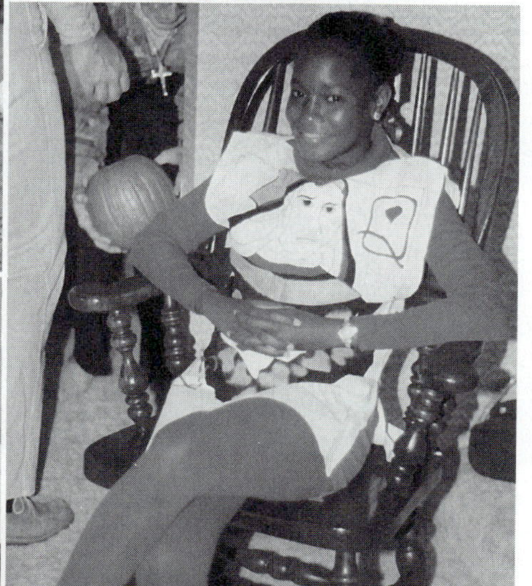

Fig. 21-26 Early adolescence—12 to 15 years. **A,** Good coordination; **B,** moving toward maturity at 13 years of age; **C,** chooses best friend and confidant; **D,** continues to love costume parties.

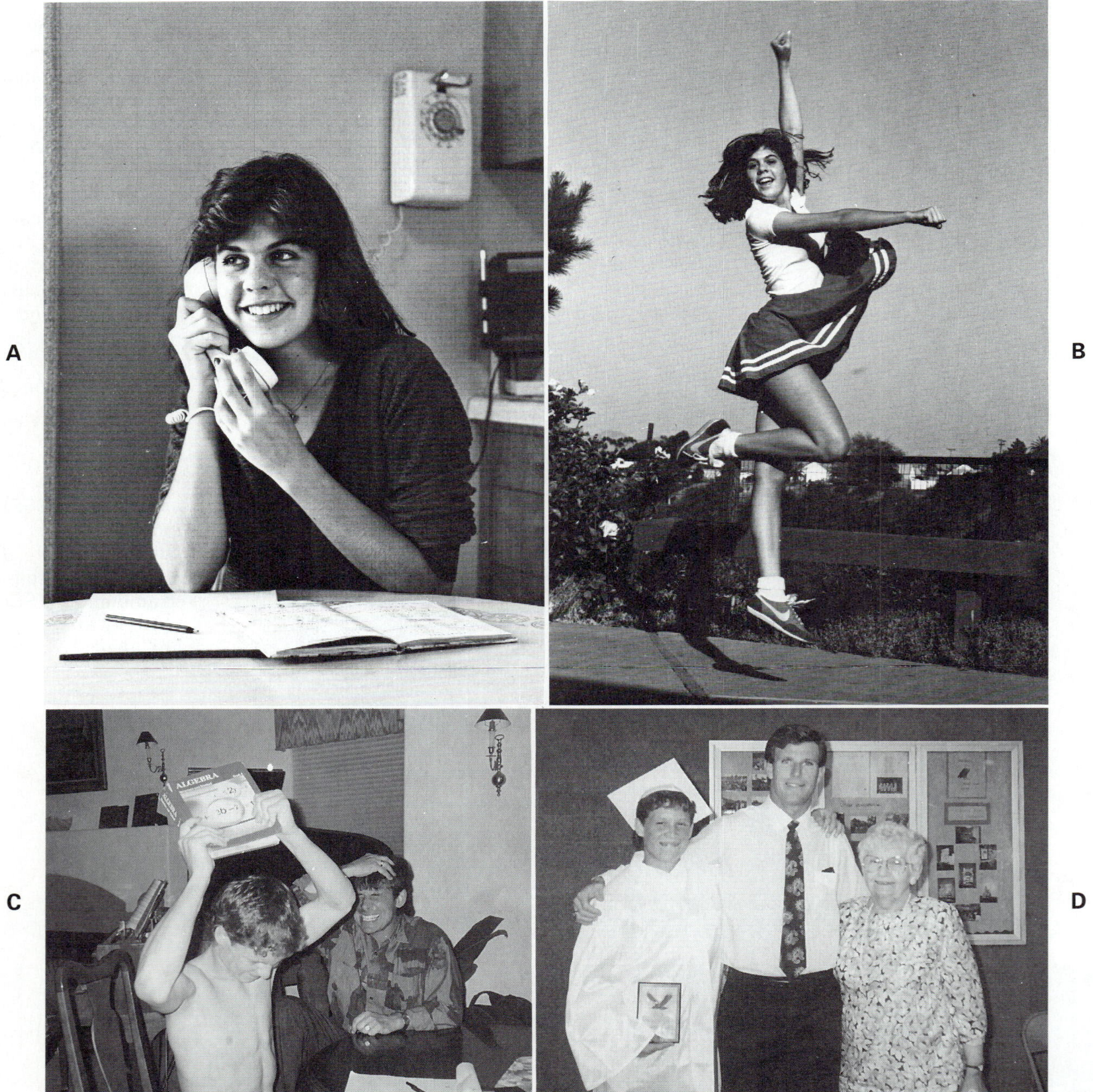

Fig. 21-27 Early adolescence—14 years. **A,** The telephone becomes a favorite pastime; **B,** athletic ability highly prized; **C,** homework becomes more of a challenge; **D,** middle-school graduation.

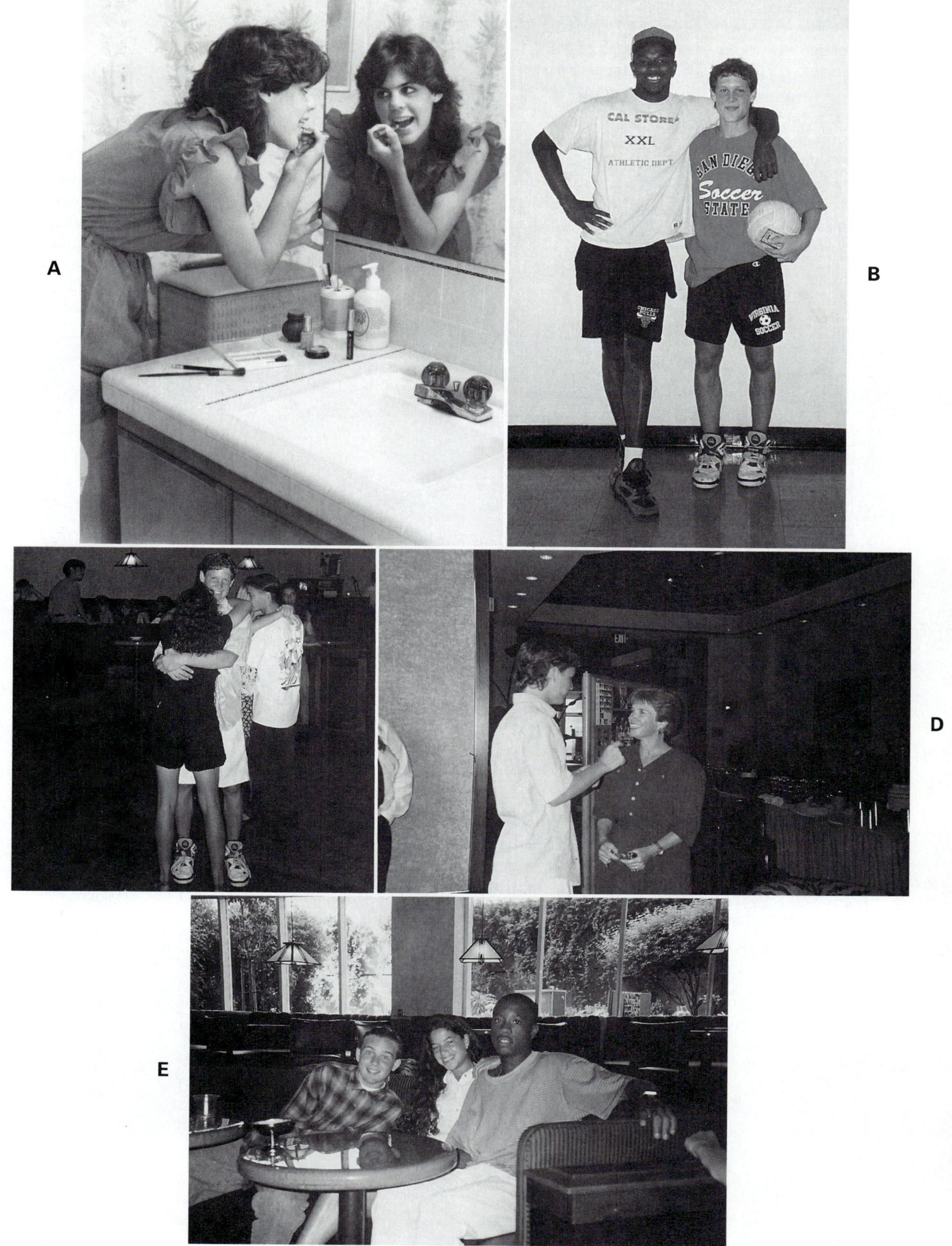

Fig. 21-28 Mid-adolescence—15 years. **A,** Experiments with cosmetics; **B,** first real job as a camp counselor; **C,** first love; **D,** favorite teacher or mentor an important influence; **E,** peer group important.

◆ **TABLE 21-1**
Ages and Stages of Maturation—cont'd

Late adolescence (16 to 19 yr) (see Figs. 21-29, 21-30, 21-31 and 21-32)

Physical growth	*Motor development*	*Language development*	*Anticipatory guidance*
Adult size and proportion usually attained Spermatogenesis established by 17 yr; slow, continuous growth in height ceases at 18 to 20 yr in boys and at 16 to 17 yr in girls	Gross Motor: Improvement in coordination; strength and athletic ability highly prized Social and sporting activities emphasized Fine Motor: Adult level	Abstract thought evident	Dominant developmental thrust Establishment of ego identity: "Where do I fit in this world?" Increased concern for philosophical and religious questions Due to wide variability, refer to early and mid-adolescent tables.

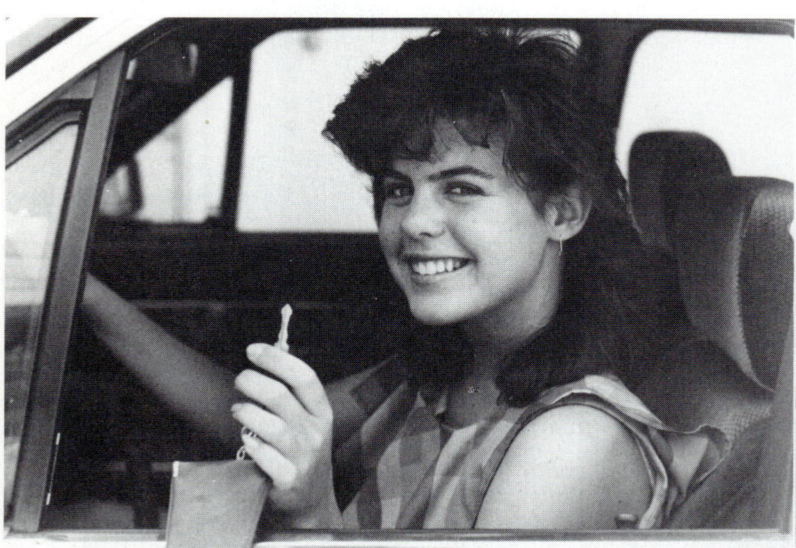

Fig. 21-29 Mid-adolescence—16 years. The long-awaited driver's license.

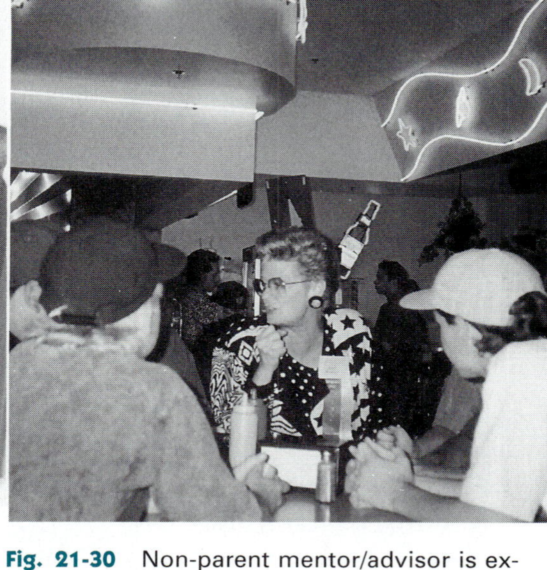

Fig. 21-30 Non-parent mentor/advisor is extremely important.

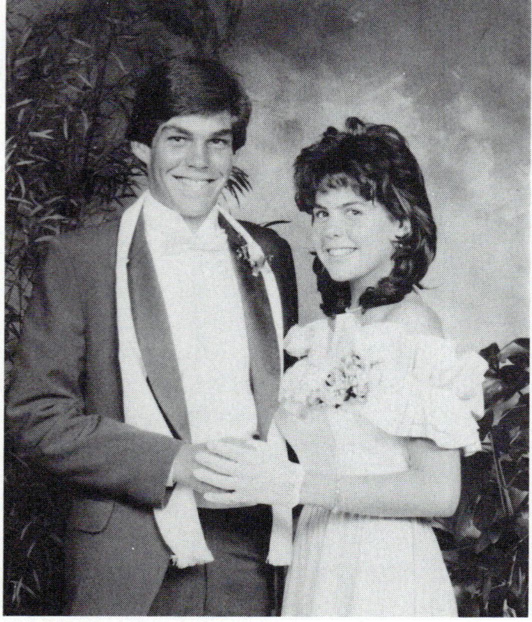

Fig. 21-31 Late adolescence—17 years. Junior prom.

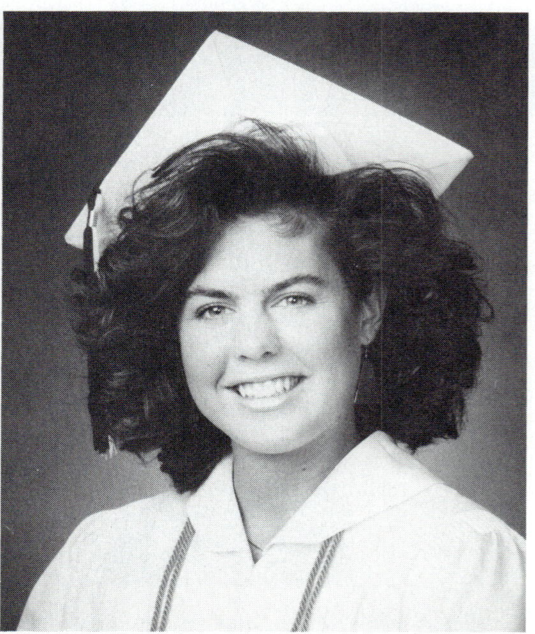

Fig. 21-32 Late adolescence—18 years. High School graduation.

◆ **TABLE 21-2**
Developmental Assessment

Assessment Tool	Functions Studied
Amiel-Tison	Neurological assessment.
Ballard Scale	Gestational age.
Brazelton Neonatal Behaviorial Assessment Scale	Newborn behavior and neurological assessment.
Dubowitz Assessment of Gestational Age	Gestational age.
Dubowitz Neuromaturational Assessment	Neurological assessment.
Carey Temperament Questionnaire	Temperament.
Denver II	Fine and gross motor, perceptual, cognitive, language, and social skills.
Knoblock Revised Developmental	Fine and gross motor, personal, social, and language assessment.
PEER	Preschool readiness.
Anna Freud's Lines of Development	Play, body functions and social development.
Mahler's Stages of Attachment	Development of attachment to others and a sense of identity.

THE DENVER II DEVELOPMENTAL SCREENING TEST (DDST-II)

One of the most widely used screening tools for assessing a young child's developmental level is the Denver Developmental Screening Test (DDST). The DDST detects developmental delays through infancy and the preschool years. It evaluates the child's achievement in four major areas of development: gross motor, fine motor adaptive, language, and personal-social. The DDST was originally standardized on a large cross section of the 1967 Denver population and has undergone two revisions since the establishment of its original form. A lack of sensitivity in identifying children with speech and language delays, as well as an inability to identify general delays in children from diverse cultures and lower socioeconomic groups, were weaknesses of the original tool. The latest, major revision is the Denver II, which differs from the first DDST in items included in the test, the test form, and the interpretation of scoring. The Denver II includes many more language items and a reduction in the total amount of report items. From a pool of 336 items, a final selection of 125 items was made on the basis of eight criteria. Many items that were previously tested by parental report now require examiner observation. The test items are displayed on a form appropriate to certain ages, corresponding to the American Academy of Pediatrics recommended health maintenance visits (Fig. 21-33, *A*). For other specific differences between the DDST and the Denver II, review the Denver II Screening Manual. The test is administered with ease and speed, lending itself to serial evaluations on the same test sheet. The directions for the administration of the Denver II are on the reverse side of the test sheet (Fig. 21-33, *B*).

Nursing Alert

Allowances are made for infants who were born prematurely by subtracting the number of weeks of prematurity from their present chronological age. The child is then tested at the level of their adjusted age. For example, a 20-week-old infant who was born 8 weeks early is tested at the 12 week adjusted age level.

A simpler, related preliminary screening instrument, designed to identify those children who require screening with the Denver II, is the Revised Denver Prescreening Developmental Questionnaire (R-PDQ) of 1986. The R-PDQ facilitates periodical development screening of all children. The R-PDQ is a parent-answered prescreening test, which consists of 105 questions arranged in chronological order, ranging from children aged 3 months to 6 years. Parents respond to age-appropriate questions, answering with a "yes" or "no" on the appropriate form (orange for children aged 0 to 9 months; purple for children aged 9 to 24 months; gold for children aged 2 to 4 years; and white for children ages 4 to 6 years). Children who have no age-appropriate delays are considered to be developing normally. Children who have one delay should be scheduled for re-screening in 1 month. If, on rescreening, the child has one or more delays, he or she should be screened with the Denver II as soon as possible. Also, children having two or more delays on their first R-PDQ should be screened with the Denver II as soon as possible. Since development is a dynamic process that may be retarded at various ages, developmental screening should be repeated periodically for every child.

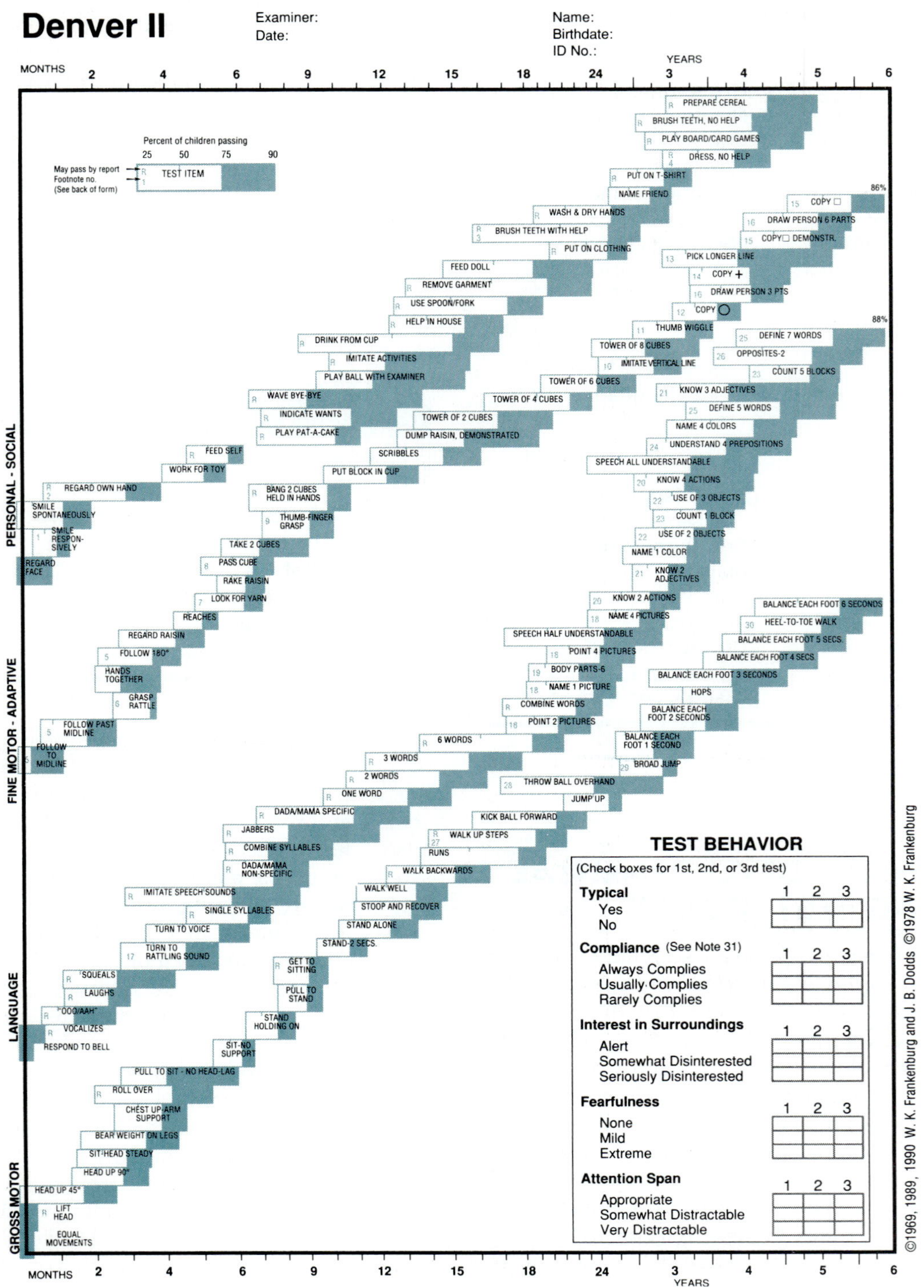

Fig. 21-33 **A,** Denver Developmental Screening Test sheet.

DIRECTIONS FOR ADMINISTRATION

1. Try to get child to smile by smiling, talking or waving. Do not touch him/her.
2. Child must stare at hand several seconds.
3. Parent may help guide toothbrush and put toothpaste on brush.
4. Child does not have to be able to tie shoes or button/zip in the back.
5. Move yarn slowly in an arc from one side to the other, about 8" above child's face.
6. Pass if child grasps rattle when it is touched to the backs or tips of fingers.
7. Pass if child tries to see where yarn went. Yarn should be dropped quickly from sight from tester's hand without arm movement.
8. Child must transfer cube from hand to hand without help of body, mouth, or table.
9. Pass if child picks up raisin with any part of thumb and finger.
10. Line can vary only 30 degrees or less from tester's line.
11. Make a fist with thumb pointing upward and wiggle only the thumb. Pass if child imitates and does not move any fingers other than the thumb.

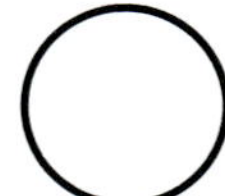

12. Pass any enclosed form. Fail continuous round motions.

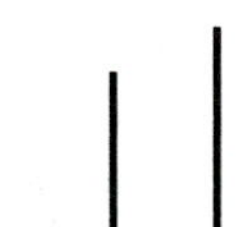

13. Which line is longer? (Not bigger.) Turn paper upside down and repeat. (pass 3 of 3 or 5 of 6)

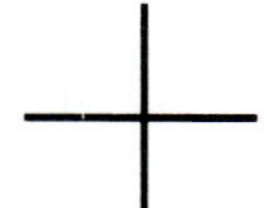

14. Pass any lines crossing near midpoint.

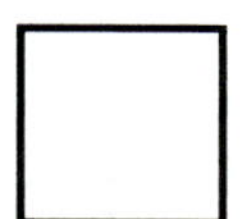

15. Have child copy first. If failed, demonstrate.

When giving items 12, 14, and 15, do not name the forms. Do not demonstrate 12 and 14.

16. When scoring, each pair (2 arms, 2 legs, etc.) counts as one part.
17. Place one cube in cup and shake gently near child's ear, but out of sight. Repeat for other ear.
18. Point to picture and have child name it. (No credit is given for sounds only.) If less than 4 pictures are named correctly, have child point to picture as each is named by tester.

B

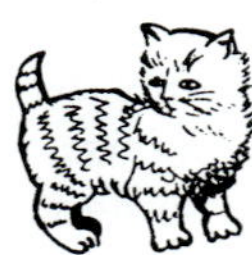 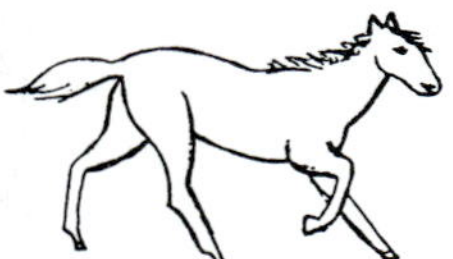 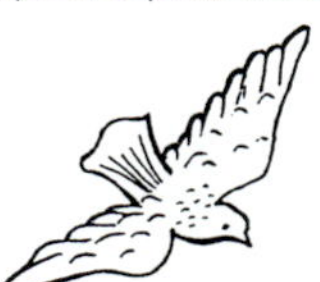 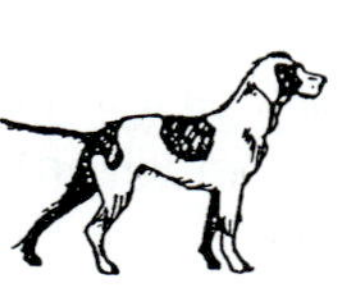 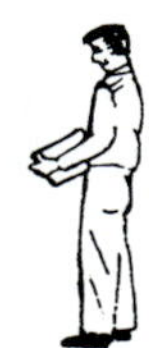

19. Using doll, tell child: Show me the nose, eyes, ears, mouth, hands, feet, tummy, hair. Pass 6 of 8.
20. Using pictures, ask child: Which one flies?... says meow?... talks?... barks?... gallops? Pass 2 of 5, 4 of 5.
21. Ask child: What do you do when you are cold?... tired?... hungry? Pass 2 of 3, 3 of 3.
22. Ask child: What do you do with a cup? What is a chair used for? What is a pencil used for? Action words must be included in answers.
23. Pass if child correctly places and says how many blocks are on paper. (1, 5).
24. Tell child: Put block **on** table; **under** table; **in front of** me, **behind** me. Pass 4 of 4. (Do not help child by pointing, moving head or eyes.)
25. Ask child: What is a ball?... lake?... desk?... house?... banana?... curtain?... fence?... ceiling? Pass if defined in terms of use, shape, what it is made of, or general category (such as banana is fruit, not just yellow). Pass 5 of 8, 7 of 8.
26. Ask child: If a horse is big, a mouse is __? If fire is hot, ice is __? If the sun shines during the day, the moon shines during the __? Pass 2 of 3.
27. Child may use wall or rail only, not person. May not crawl.
28. Child must throw ball overhand 3 feet to within arm's reach of tester.
29. Child must perform standing broad jump over width of test sheet (8 1/2 inches).
30. Tell child to walk forward, → heel within 1 inch of toe. Tester may demonstrate. Child must walk 4 consecutive steps.
31. In the second year, half of normal children are non-compliant.

OBSERVATIONS:

Fig. 21-33 (cont'd) **B,** reverse side of test sheet.

Test Materials for the Denver II

The screening manual is designed to teach those performing the screening test the step-by-step procedures for administration and interpretation of the test. The manual also contains data on the level at which 25%, 50%, 75%, and 90% of children performed on various items at different ages.

The Denver II test kit contains a new screening manual that lists step-by-step instructions for teaching adults the administration of the test, and a test of proficiency to determine if the adult is able to properly administer and interpret the test. Test items include a small plastic doll, a toy feeding bottle, and a plastic cup with a handle. Other items used in both the Denver II and the DDST include ten 1-inch square, colored, wooden blocks; a box of raisins; a red, yarn pom-pom; a rattle with a narrow handle; a clear glass bottle with ⅝-inch opening; a bell; a tennis ball; the test form; and a red pencil.

A videotape is available to give adults an overview of how to administer and interpret the Denver II properly. It is suggested that this videotape be viewed before studying the Denver II Screening Manual.

1. Fig. 21-32 provides an overview of the test and is not complete.
2. The Denver II is not an intelligence test. It is intended as a screening instrument for use in clinical practice to note whether the development of a particular child is within the normal range.
3. The test materials and the training materials are available through Denver Developmental Materials, Inc., P.O. Box 6919, Denver, CO 80206-0919, (303) 355-4729.

Parents can provide a healthy and happy environment in which children can grow, develop, and reach their optimum developmental potential. The provision of developmentally appropriate toys, encouragement of safe exploration, acceptance of individual differences, self-esteem building experiences, and loving care will enhance the child's capacity for healthy growth and development.

KEY CONCEPTS

1. Development at a given age may be measured by physical growth, motor development, and language development. Each stage presents basic psychosocial challenges. Anticipatory guidance identifies the needs of the child at each stage and assists in the development of parenting skills.
2. During infancy (birth to 1 year) the child grows and develops rapidly. By 1 year of age the child has six to eight teeth and his or her birth weight has tripled. The majority of children walk alone, pick up small objects, drink from a cup, and say several simple words at this age. The basic psychosocial challenge is the development of trust versus mistrust. Anticipatory guidance includes developmental milestones, safety, sleep patterns, stimulation, optimal nutrition, bathing, and immunizations.
3. The growth rate of children slows during toddlerhood (1 to 3 years of age). By the age of 3 the child can run and climb stairs, string large beads, throw a ball, ride a tricycle, has a vocabulary of 900 words, knows their full name, and begins to express his or her needs. The basic psychosocial challenge during this period is autonomy building versus shame and doubt. Anticipatory guidance includes developmental milestones, safety, sleep patterns, stimulation, optimal nutrition, immunizations, child-centered toilet training, and sexual curiosity.
4. The average preschooler (3 to 6 years of age) weighs 40 to 45 pounds and is 43 to 45 inches tall by the age of five. The child has increasing fine motor skills and good muscle coordination. The child uses a 1500-word vocabulary in sentences, asking numerous questions. The child's basic psychosocial challenge is initiative versus guilt. Anticipatory guidance includes development milestones, magical thinking, fears, sexual curiosity, safety, immunizations, stimulation, assessment for school readiness, and optimal nutrition.
5. Steady growth is seen in the school-aged child (6 to 10 years of age). Balance and fine motor skills are well-developed. The child can count, read, write, and has a 2500-word vocabulary. His or her basic psychosocial challenge is industry versus inferiority. Anticipatory guidance includes developmental milestones, safety, stimulation, optimal nutrition, team sports and other group activities, and the importance of parent involvement in the child's school experience.
6. Preadolescence usually occurs between 10 to 12 years of age. This period involves a growth spurt and the appearance and development of secondary, sexual characteristics. Poor motor control may ensue if body build and muscular development are disproportional to their rate of growth. Anticipa-

tory guidance includes developmental challenges, safety issues, peer influence, the importance of continued parent involvement and monitoring, and identification of potential problems.

7 During adolescence (12 to 19 years of age), adult size and proportion are usually attained. Motor development varies widely and coordination generally improves. Intellectual maturity is attained. Basic psychosocial challenges include identity development versus role confusion and intimacy versus isolation. Anticipatory guidance includes immunization, optimal nutrition, exercise, stress management, peer pressure, career and vocational guidance, self-care to include testicular self-examination (TSE) or breast self-examination (BSE), as well as those which were introduced during preadolescence.

8 The Denver II Developmental Screening Test evaluates the child's achievement in four major areas of development: gross motor, fine motor adaptive, language, and personal-social.

9 The child's capacity for healthy growth and development are enhanced by developmentally appropriate toys, encouragement of safe exploration, acceptance of individual differences, self-esteem building experiences, and a loving, caring family.

CRITICAL THOUGHT QUESTIONS

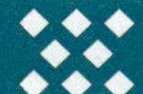

1 The Denver II Developmental Screening Test is a helpful tool in the assessment of a child's developmental level. Describe the tool and the necessary precautions for administration. What are the dangers of administering any developmental assessment tool?

2 Discuss the anticipatory guidance that the nurse should provide to parents at their child's 6-month "well child" medical visit. How might the nurse evaluate parental understanding of this teaching?

3 Observe a toddler. How would you compare and contrast your observations with the stage of development described in Erikson's work? Refer to Chapter 1 for additional content.

4 Safety is an important topic during a child's life span. The safety concerns related to children change greatly as the child moves from one stage to another. What are the major safety concerns for the infant through adolescent, and what are effective teaching approaches?

REFERENCES

Dixon S and Stein M: *Encounters with children,* ed 2, St Louis, 1992, Mosby.

Frankenburg WK, et al: The Denver II: a major revision and restandardization of the Denver Developmental Screening Test, *J Pediatrics* 89(1):91-97, 1992.

Simeonsson RJ and Simeonsson NE: Developmental assessment. In Hoekleman RA, et al, editors: *Primary pediatric care,* ed 2, St Louis, 1992, Mosby.

Wade GH: Update on the Denver II, *Pediatric Nursing* 18(2):140-141, 1992.

Whaley L and Wong D: *Nursing care of infants and children,* St Louis, 1992, Mosby.

Wong D: *Whaley and Wong's essentials of pediatric nursing,* ed 4, St Louis, 1993, Mosby.

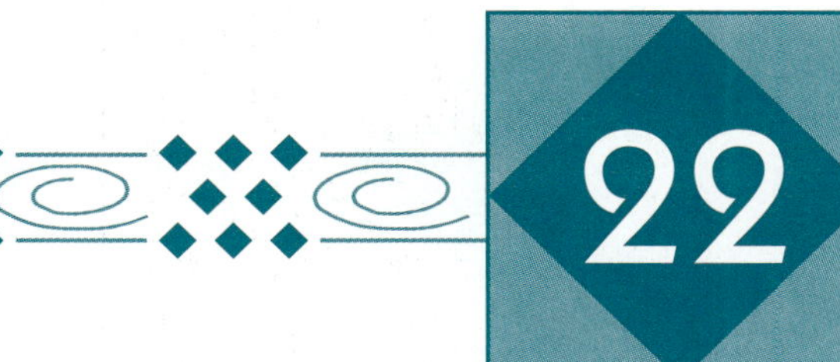
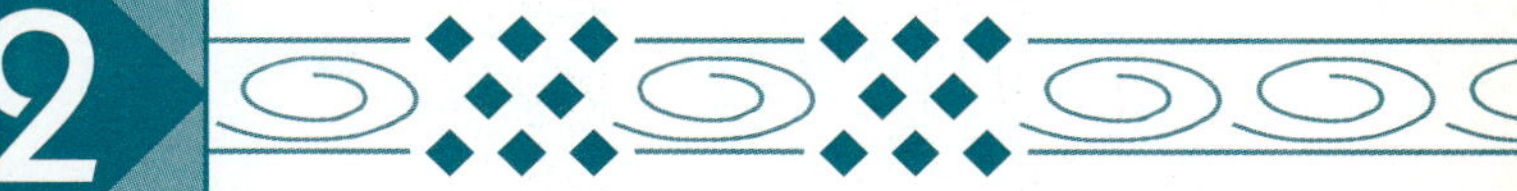

22

Child Health Promotion

CHAPTER OBJECTIVES

After studying this chapter, the student should be able to:

1. Describe the important characteristics of breast milk and the nurse's role in the promotion of breastfeeding.
2. Indicate the recommended feeding practices for formula-fed infants, the type and amount of fluid intake, typical hunger patterns, the need for vitamins, and the use of skim and whole milk.
3. Discuss neuromuscular indicators for the introduction of solids and the typical sequential development of skills that lead to successful self-feeding.
4. Explain the main reason why an infant needs more calories per kilogram of weight than an older child.
5. Discuss the effect of minerals, iron, calcium, and fluoride on growth.
6. Outline the recommended active-immunization schedule for normal infants and children from birth to 16 years of age, including protection against nine different infectious diseases.
7. Describe the impact of injuries on the pediatric population, and state three principles of injury prevention.
8. List six different methods of poison prevention.
9. Discuss the use of syrup of Ipecac, when its use is contraindicated, the method of administration, and the recommended dose for children over 1 year of age.
10. Identify six physical and behavioral signs of child maltreatment.
11. Discuss the mandatory reporting laws for health care providers when child maltreatment is suspected or confirmed.
12. Identify the important components of primary, secondary, and tertiary prevention of child maltreatment.

Health promotion is a principal component of any system of child health supervision. Child health maintenance or "well-child care" is designed to promote health, prevent disiease, and provide anticipatory guidance for developmental and parenting issues. Records of the child's individual and family health history are maintained, and height, weight, and blood pressure are plotted in graph form. The roles of individual health care providers, nurse practitioners, and physicians must be closely integrated with community programs including public health initiatives, school health curriculum, parent education programs, and health education topics covered by the mass media.

Since healthy newborns are usually discharged within 24 hours of delivery, infants are scheduled to visit the nurse practitioner or physician within 1 week for well-child care. Visits are then scheduled monthly for the first 6 months, and every other month until the first birthday. Two to four visits should be

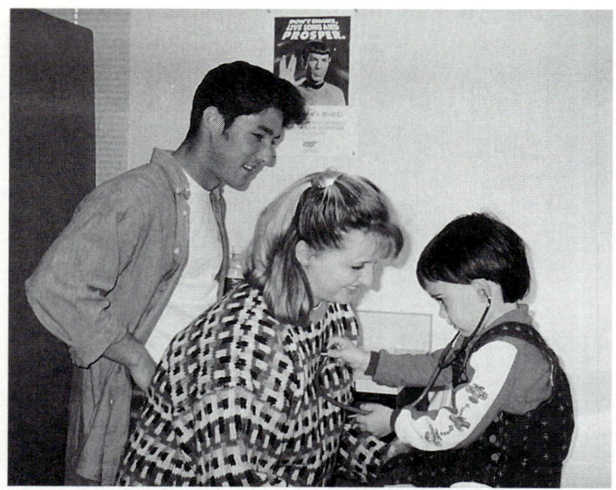

Fig. 22-1 Two year old being examined by nursing students.

made during the second year, and visits should be yearly thereafter (Fig. 22-1). Special attention should be directed toward assessment of family relationships and stressors, detection of language delay, questionable hearing loss, visual deficit, orthopedic abnormality, or other developmental delay. The first visit to a dentist should be initiated before the child's third birthday. Dental care at home should begin when dentition occurs.

School-age children in the United States usually receive more consistent health supervision than do preschool children because of the activities of the school nurse, public health nurse, requirements for participation in organized sports, and state-supported programs. School-age children should have annual health screenings (Fig. 22-2).

The following topics of study are fundamental to child health promotion: nutritional guidance, immunization schedules, child safety, and injury prevention. Other important areas of child health promotion are highlighted in the anticipatory guidance section of Chapter 21.

NUTRITIONAL GUIDANCE

The discussion of optimum nutrition should begin prenatally with the decision of feeding method. For the first 6 months of life the most desirable and complete diet is human milk (see the box on p. •••). Commercially prepared formula is an acceptable alternative for women who choose not to breastfeed or who have a medical contraindication, such as human immunodeficiency virus (HIV).

During the second 6 months, human milk or formula continues to be the primary source of nutrition.

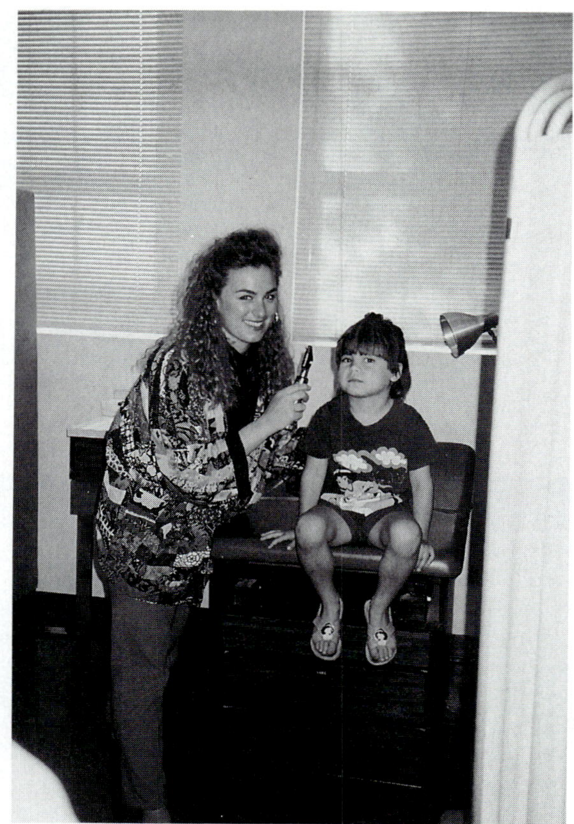

Fig. 22-2 Five year old receiving her kindergarten assessment.

The attainment of developmental milestones, however, readies the infant for the introduction of solid foods. Infants and toddlers accept solid foods and feed themselves as their neuromuscular development progresses. Several studies indicate that infants and children select food of the right type at the right time and in the right amounts, if it is available to them from the beginning of the self-feeding process (Fig. 22-3).

Physiological Readiness

Hunger vs. appetite

Infants have a rhythmic pattern of hunger contractions, characterized by discomfort, restlessness, and crying. The rhythm of hunger contractions differs in each infant, but they usually reappear every 3 to 4 hours and more frequently in breast-fed babies. Infants should be fed according to their hunger rhythms, since rigidly prescribed feeding schedules ignore these hunger patterns. The normal infant's nutritional needs can be met for the first 12 months by breast-feeding or iron/vitamin-fortified formula plus flouride. The Committee on Nutrition of the American Academy of Pediatrics urges that "all bottle-fed infants be given an

ADVANTAGES OF HUMAN MILK VS COW'S MILK

Contains adequate (not excessive) protein; has greater quantities of certain amino acids, including cystine and taurine

Contains more lactalbumin (produces easily digested curds) than casein (produces large, hard curds)

Contains more lactose, which in the gut stimulates growth of microorganisms, which synthesize some B vitamins and produce organic acids that may retard growth of harmful bacteria

Contains more monounsaturated fatty acids, which enhance absorption of fat and calcium

Contains adequate (not excessive) minerals with exception of fluoride (low in both)

Amounts of iron and zinc are low but more readily absorbed

Contains less calcium and phosphorus but a more favorable ratio of the minerals, which prevents excessive calcium excretion

Contains adequate amounts of vitamins A, B complex, and E; vitamin C content depends on maternal intake; vitamin D is low but more readily absorbed (vitamin C, D, and E are low in cow's milk, but K is higher)

Contains growth modulators that modify growth or maturation

Offers several immunological benefits: contains various immunoglobulins (Ig), especially IgA; macrophages; granulocytes; T- and B-cell lymphocytes; and other factors that inhibit bacterial growth

Has laxative effect

Is economical, readily available, and sanitary

Has psychological benefits of close bond between infant and mother during feeding

From Wong DL: *Whaley and Wong's essentials of pediatric nursing,* ed 4, St Louis, 1993, Mosby.

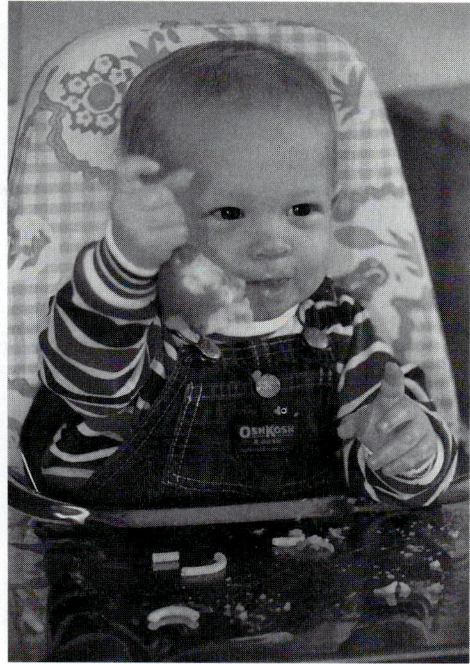

Fig. 22-3 Ten month old enjoying finger foods.

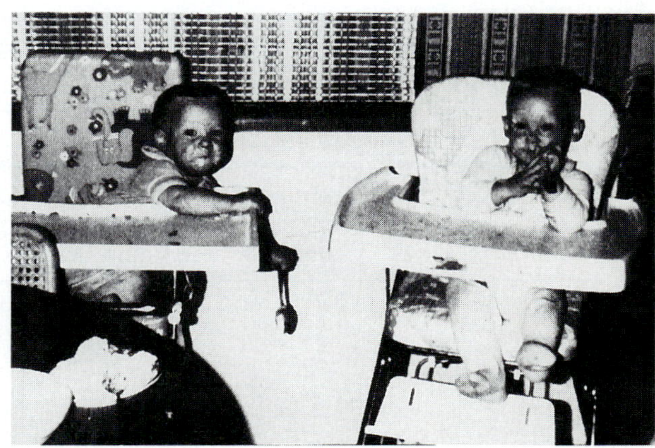

Fig. 22-4 Siblings begin to influence food preferences.

iron-fortified formula for at least the first 12 months of life." The amount of breast milk or formula consumed varies from day to day. In general, however, most infants take 2½ ounces of formula per pound of body weight, distributed over a 24-hour period. After solid foods are introduced, when the infant is about 5 to 6 months of age, this amount decreases. When sucking stops and the healthy infant falls asleep the hunger-appetite mechanism has been satisfied. The infant should not be forced to finish the bottle before sleeping.

During infancy, hunger prompted by physiological needs chiefly controls food intake. Before 6 months of age an infant's diet is primarily comprised of human milk or formula. However, in the latter half of the first year, appetite preferences related to taste, texture, appearance, and culture become important. Parental and sibling diet strongly influence the child's eating habits (Fig. 22-4). By 12 months of age the infant shows definite preferences and dislikes. If feeding has been a positive experience, the infant's appetite will be a physiological index of nutritional needs. If an infant refuses an essential food item, it should not be forced. Reintroduction of the food at a later time is preferable.

Breast or formula feeding should be continued through the first year of life (Fig. 22-5). Whole milk may be introduced in the second year of life. Skim milk

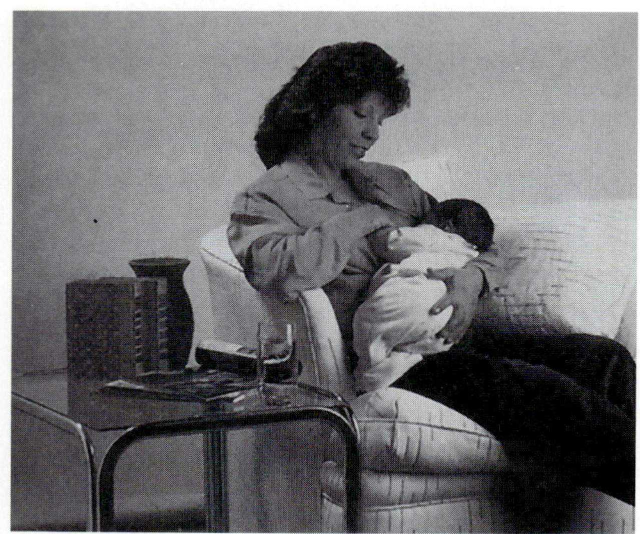

Fig. 22-5 Breastfeeding mother and child. (From Dickerson EJ, et al: *Maternal and infant nursing,* St. Louis, 1994, Mosby.)

should be avoided until after the second birthday, unless prescribed by the pediatrician, since skim milk is not nutritionally sound for infants. Skim milk provides an inadequate intake of fat, fatty acids, calories, and protein in excess of four times the estimated requirements.

Developmental Readiness

Protrusion reflex

The protrusion reflex manifests itself when the infant pushes out solid food placed on the anterior third of the tongue. This response, common during the first 10 weeks, disappears by the fourth month of life. It does not interfere with the baby's breast or bottle feeding, since the nipple empties into the back of the mouth. However, it makes early feeding of solid foods difficult. The disappearance of the protrusion reflex and the development of the ability to sit with minimal support are the neuromuscular indications for the introduction of semisolid food. There appears to be no advantage in introducing solids (baby foods) during the first 6 months of life (Table 22-1).

◆ TABLE 22-1
Feeding for the First 12 Months of Life

Month 1	2	3	4	5	6	7	8	9	10	11	12
Breast milk: Nutritionally sound, believed to provide immunity, facilitates a close mother-infant relationship, decreases allergies, decreases incidence of dental caries and malocclusion. Formula: 24-32 oz/24 hr: well tolerated when breast milk is not available											
				Iron fortified rice cereal: source of calories, iron and fiber; avoid wheat products first 12 months of life.							
					Strained vegetables: source of calories, fiber, iron, vitamins A and B, and minerals. Introduce yellow vegetables before green.						
						Strained fruits: source of calories, iron, fiber, vitamin C, and minerals. Will offset constipating effect of cereals.					
							Plain lowfat yogurt: excellent source of calcium, phosphorus, vitamin B, and protein. Meats: source of protein, calories, iron, and vitamins. Finger foods: assists in teething and fine motor coordination				

Acceptance of the spoon is an important learning process that proceeds slowly. New food should be offered while the infant is hungry, rather than after being satiated from milk intake. However, hungry babies may refuse new foods because of their urgent desire for milk and a low-frustration tolerance.

Self-feeding

If an infant is given the opportunity, self-feeding skills will develop in the second 6 months of life. A healthy 6 month old can put his or her hands around a supported bottle and guide it to his lips. It is important, however, to also begin offering juice, breast milk, or formula from a cup at this time. By 6 to 7 months of age an empty plastic cup may be placed on the infant's tray for practice. A 7 month old may hold the formula bottle unassisted. At 8 months a baby can feed him or herself crackers. Chewing motions appear at about 8 or 9 months of age and are the neuromuscular indications that solid foods can be introduced, whether teeth are present or not. The self-feeding of finger foods begins with the development of the pincer grasp at 9 to 10 months of age. If finger foods are not offered to the older infant, the acquisition of this self-feeding skill and other fine motor skills may be delayed. Chopped foods should be introduced gradually. If undigested food appears in the stool, one should wait a week and try again. At 10 months of age the infant can begin to practice with a spoon. By 12 months he or she can use a cup well. By 18 months of age the child can use a spoon skillfully. Skillful self-feeding is usually accomplished between 12 and 18 months and combines feeding skills using the spoon, hand, or cup. Several foods are not recommended for children 12 to 24 months of age because of possible aspiration or poor digestibility. These include hot dogs, corn, leafy vegetables, cucumbers, chocolate, olives, peanut butter, uncooked onions, baked beans, and grapes. Nuts and popcorn should not be offered until the child is 4 years of age. In addition, children should always be seated when eating to prevent aspiration. Mealtime should be a pleasant, relaxed experience for the child and the entire family (Fig. 22-6).

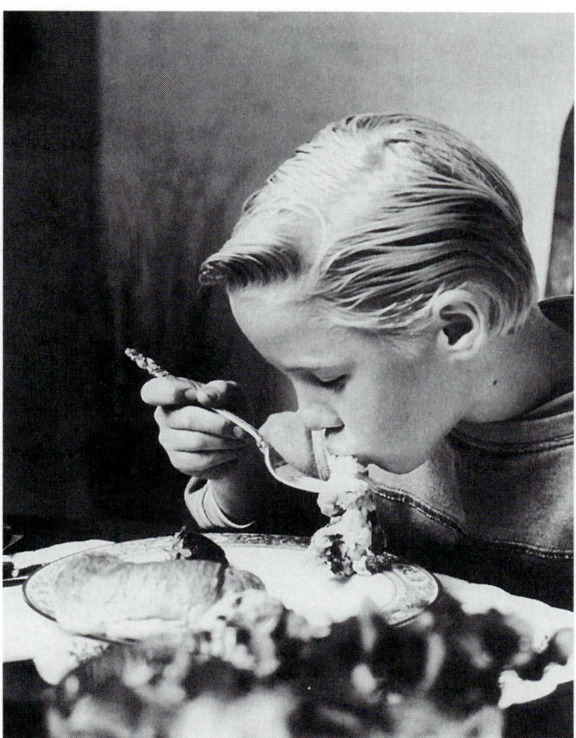

Fig. 22-6 Seven-year-old enjoying a meal reflecting parental preferences.

Nursing bottle caries

Nursing bottle caries, or *nursing bottle syndrome*, refers to the decay of the upper anterior primary teeth resulting from bottle feeding of high carbohydrate fluids (Figs. 22-7 and 22-8). This devastating condition, which may occur as early as 9 to 10 months, is attributed to bottle propping at night and at naptimes. When a nipple filled with a sugar-sweetened beverage remains in the child's mouth the flow of saliva is minimized and, therefore, cannot neutralize juice acidity or the acidity developed in the bacteria-laden plaque. Both of these acid sources promote decalcification of tooth enamel. The result is painful, unattractive, and severely damaged carious teeth. Any child with caries of the anterior teeth, especially the maxillary anterior teeth, should be referred for pediatric dental evaluation and treatment.

Nursing bottle caries can be prevented. Juices should be offered from a cup rather than a bottle. Well-child assessments should include appropriate counseling regarding the adverse effects of using a bottle at naptime or during the night, proper techniques of tooth brushing, restricting intake of sucrose-containing carbohydrates, and giving the appropriate daily fluoride dose.

Basic Nutrition Concepts (Table 22-2)

Optimal nutrition is a key component of child health promotion. The identification of nutrient imbalance is a primary nursing goal. What and how children eat later in life is established during infancy. Studies have shown that obesity may be associated with an increase in adipose fat cell number (hyperplasia) and in cell

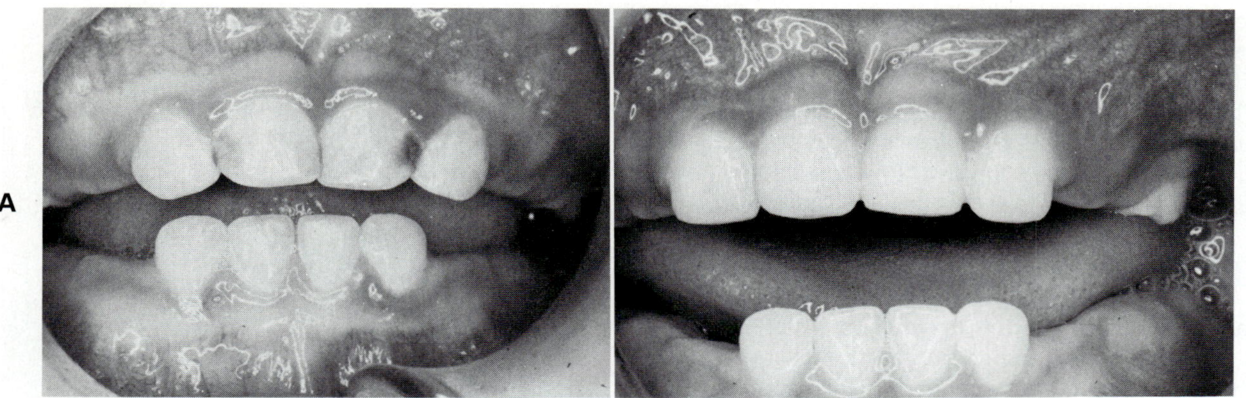

Fig. 22-7 **A,** Decayed teeth (nursing bottle caries evidenced at 9 months of age); **B,** teeth returned to normal health and function through aesthetic restoration. (Courtesy Barry H. Gruer, DDS, MS, San Diego, CA.)

◆ TABLE 22-2
Clinical Signs of Nutritional Status

	Good	Poor
General appearance	Alert, responsive	Listless, apathetic, cachexic
Hair	Shiny, lustrous; healthy scalp	Stringy, dull, brittle, dry, depigmented
Neck (glands)	No enlargement	Thyroid enlargement
Skin (face and neck)	Smooth, slightly moist; good color, reddish pink mucous membranes	Greasy, discolored, scaly
Eyes	Bright, clear, no fatigue circles beneath	Dryness, signs of infection, increased vascularity, glassiness, thickened conjunctiva
Lips	Pink color, moist	Dry, scaly, swollen, angular lesions (stomatitis)
Tongue	Pink color, surface papillae present, no lesions	Papillary atrophy, smooth appearance; swollen, red, beefy (glossitis)
Gums	Pink color; no swelling or bleeding, firm	Marginal redness or swelling, receding, spongy
Teeth	Straight, no crowding, well-shaped jaw, clean, no discoloration	Unfilled caries, absent teeth, worn surfaces, mottled, malpositioned
Skin (general)	Smooth, slightly moist, normal color	Rough, dry, scaly, pale, pigmented, irritated, petechiae, bruises
Abdomen	Flat	Swollen
Legs, feet	No tenderness, weakness or swelling; good color	Edema, tender calf, tingling, weakness
Skeleton	No malformation	Bowlegs, knock-knees, chest deformity at diaphragm, beaded ribs, prominent scapulae
Weight	Normal for height, age, body build	Overweight or underweight
Posture	Erect, arms and legs straight, abdomen in, chest out	Sagging shoulders, sunken chest, humped back
Muscles	Well developed, firm	Flaccid, poor tone; undeveloped, tender
Nervous control	Good attention span for age, does not cry easily, not irritable or restless	Inattentive, irritable
Gastrointestinal function	Good appetite and digestion; normal, regular elimination	Anorexia, indigestion, constipation or diarrhea
General vitality	Good endurance, energetic, sleeps well at night, vigorous	Easily fatigued, no energy, falls asleep in school, looks tired, apathetic

From Williams SR: *Nutrition and diet therapy,* ed 7, St Louis, 1993, Mosby.

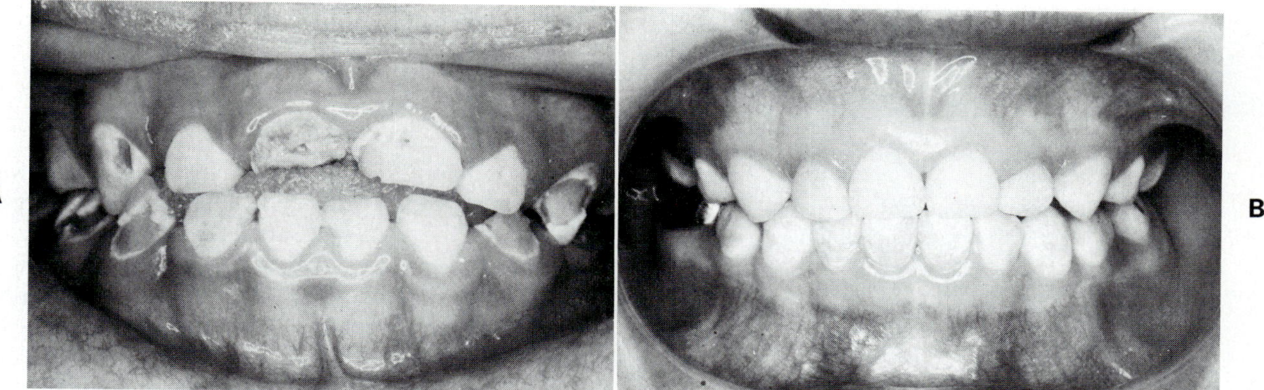

Fig. 22-8 **A,** Severe caries that began with overretention of bottle; **B,** complete restoration of primary teeth, providing child a means for mastication, speech, and improved aesthetic appearance. (Courtesy Barry H. Gruer, DDS, MS, San Diego, CA.)

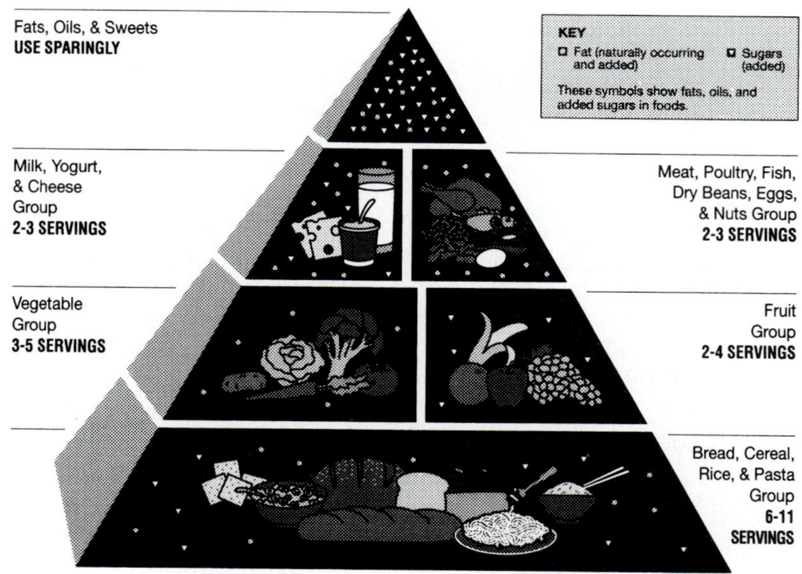

Fig. 22-9 Food guide pyramid: a guide to daily food choices. (Courtesy, USDA, 1992.)

size (hypertrophy) or with only an increase in the size of the cell. The number of adipose cells in children who became obese in the first year of life is higher than in those who became obese in later childhood. Dieting in later life can reduce cell size but not the cell number that was established in childhood. If food is used as a reward or punishment it will have life-long consequences. Thus early feeding practices are of utmost importance. For US Department of Agriculture recommended servings, refer to the Food Guide Pyramid: a guide to daily food choices (USDA, 1992) (Fig. 22-9). The Food Guide Pyramid replaces the basic four food groups and is recommended for use after the age of 2 years. (See the box on p. 446.)

All systems and tissues in the body depend on proper nourishment for their existence and maintenance. This nourishment is obtained from the foods

FOOD GUIDE PYRAMID: SAMPLE SERVING SIZES

BREAD, CEREAL, RICE, AND PASTA GROUP
- 1 slice of bread
- 1 ounce of ready-to-eat cereal
- ½ cup of cooked cereal, rice, or pasta

VEGETABLE GROUP
- 1 cup of raw leafy vegetable
- ½ cup of other vegetable, cooked or chopped raw
- ¾ cup of vegetable juice

FRUIT GROUP
- 1 medium apple, banana, or orange
- ½ cup of chopped, cooked, or canned fruit
- ¾ cup of fruit juice

MILK, YOGURT, AND CHEESE GROUP
- 1 cup of milk or yogurt
- 1½ ounces of natural cheese
- 2 ounces of processed cheese

MEAT, POULTRY, FISH, DRY BEANS, EGGS, AND NUTS GROUP
- 2-3 ounces of cooked lean meat, poultry, or fish
- ½ cup of cooked dry beans, 1 egg, or 2 tablespoons of peanut butter count as 1 ounce of lean meat

Courtesy USDA, 1992.

each individual eats and drinks. Food must perform the following three functions within the body:

1. Provide heat and energy.
2. Build and repair body tissues.
3. Regulate body processes.

Substances essential to perform these vital functions include the following:

1. Oxygen.
2. Water.
3. Carbohydrates.
4. Proteins.
5. Fats.
6. Minerals.
7. Vitamins.
8. Fiber.

Oxygen

Oxygen is so vital to the activity of the body cells that, without it, life would cease. The natural source of oxygen is fresh air. Through the activity of the respiratory system, oxygen enters the circulating blood, which carries it to every living cell.

Water

Second only to oxygen, water is necessary for life. Without water, death ensues in just a few days. The body of the infant contains proportionately more water (75% to 80% of body weight) than the adult (60% to 65%). The adult value is reached at about 12 years of age. Water is a basic constituent of all cells and is a major component in blood, lymph, and spinal fluid, and the various body excretions such as urine and sweat. In infancy, considerable water is lost through the kidneys and skin. To keep pace with normal fluid losses the infant must receive an equal fluid intake. The infant is subject to conditions causing water loss, notably fever, vomiting, and diarrhea. Unless water intake is increased during illness, symptoms of dehydration and its consequences appear rapidly (see Chapter 26).

Carbohydrates

Carbohydrates serve as the body's primary source of heat and energy. Examples of carbohydrate-rich foods include grains, fruits, vegetables, and sweets. Excess carbohydrates are primarily stored in the liver and muscles as glycogen. Alternatively, they are converted in the liver to glucose when carbohydrate is not available in the food consumed. Since immediate heat and energy requirements have priority over tissue growth and repair the body is also capable of using tissue fat and protein to furnish its energy needs. It is therefore important to have sufficient carbohydrates in the diet to meet these needs adequately, thus sparing protein for its primary use of building and maintaining tissues. The waste products of carbohydrate metabolism are excreted from the body in the form of carbon dioxide and water.

Protein

Protein requirements are greatest during infancy. Every living cell and almost all body fluids contain protein. Protein is necessary for the growth, repair, and maintenance of all body tissues. Immune bodies, which help the body resist infection, contain protein. Enzymes and hormones also include protein in their composition.

Amino acids are the building blocks of which proteins are constructed and the end products of protein digestion. Of the 80 amino acids found in nature, 20 are necessary for human metabolism and growth. Essential amino acids are provided by food, whereas nonessential amino acids are provided by the body.

> **Nursing Alert**
>
> Arginine, an amino acid of less importance to the adult, cannot be formed quickly enough to supply the demand in growing infants. Commercially prepared formulas must be evaluated for the presence of arginine.

Proteins are divided into two groups: complete and incomplete. The complete proteins contain essential amino acids. A dietary supply of these amino acids is necessary because they cannot be synthesized by the body. Proteins from animal sources such as meats, poultry, fresh eggs, milk, and cheese provide the essential amino acids. Gelatin is 100% protein from an animal source but is not a complete protein.

Incomplete proteins are found in vegetables and grains. They contain many amino acids, but not all of the essential ones. When protein intake is insufficient the result is a slower rate of growth and an increased susceptibility to malnutrition and bacterial infections. A closely monitored lacto-ovo-vegetarian diet that includes milk, eggs, and fish is a healthy diet. A strict vegetarian diet, however, does not ensure adequate nutrition for infants and children.

When an incomplete protein is the only source of protein, malnutrition and rickets may result (Dagnelie, et al., 1990). Children may receive adequate amounts of protein in meat, poultry, fish, milk, eggs, tofu, and other soy products. The overall protein value is improved when both animal and vegetable proteins are eaten together. Amino acids pass through the intestinal wall and portal vein into the blood, then through the liver into the general circulation, from which they are absorbed by the tissues according to what is needed by the specific tissue. If amino acids are not metabolized, they may be converted into urea (Thomas, 1993).

Finally, it is important to note that essential amino acids work together. New tissue cannot be formed unless all the essential amino acids are present in the bloodstream throughout the day. Human milk is believed to contain an ideal pattern of amino acids and is of high biological value.

Fats

Certain fatty acids found in dietary fats are necessary to maintain good nutrition. These essential fatty acids permit normal growth and the health and maintenance of normal skin. Fat also provides the vehicle of absorption of the fat-soluble vitamins A, D, E, and K. Unless dissolved in fats, these vitamins cannot be retained in the body in adequate amounts. Fats are found in both animal and vegetable foods. Fat contributes approximately 40% of the calories in human milk. Egg yolks, butter, meat, soybean oil, cottonseed oil, corn oil, and olive oil are good sources of essential fatty acids. One of these sources must be included in the daily diet, since the essential fatty acids cannot be synthesized from other fats. The waste products of fat metabolism, like those of carbohydrate metabolism, are carbon dioxide and water.

If fat intake is inadequate the child may not receive the essential fatty acids required to prevent the formation of certain types of skin lesions or to promote optimum myelinization of the brain. Brain cells reach adult numbers late in infancy. Brain size by cell enlargement is completed by 2 years of age. Thus skim milk is an inappropriate food source during the first 2 years of life. Overall brain growth is 90% complete by 6 years of age.

Energy requirements

To meet the individual's energy requirements the body must be supplied with fuel in the form of sufficient amounts of food. To determine how much food a child needs, it is necessary to know the child's metabolic rate, or rate of heat production. The unit of heat in metabolism is called a *kilo-gram calorie.* It may be defined as the amount of heat needed to raise the temperature of 1 kilogram of water 1° C. A person's basal metabolic rate (BMR) is described as the minimum amount of heat produced by body cells when the body is at rest, with only vital processes, such as circulation and respiration, functioning. Several factors—size, age, gender, hormonal levels, and body temperature—influence the BMR. The total metabolic rate of a person represents the total amount of heat produced by the body in a given time (usually 24 hours) under normal conditions. The total metabolic rate of a child represents the amount of food the body must burn, not only to keep alive and awake, but also to continue physical activity, to support growth, to supply specific dynamic action (ingestion and assimilation of food), and to replace calories lost (Fig. 22-10).

Total energy expended determines the need for calories. The fuel values of energy-producing foods are as follows:

Carbohydrates	4 cal/gm
Protein	4 cal/gm
Fats	9 cal/gm

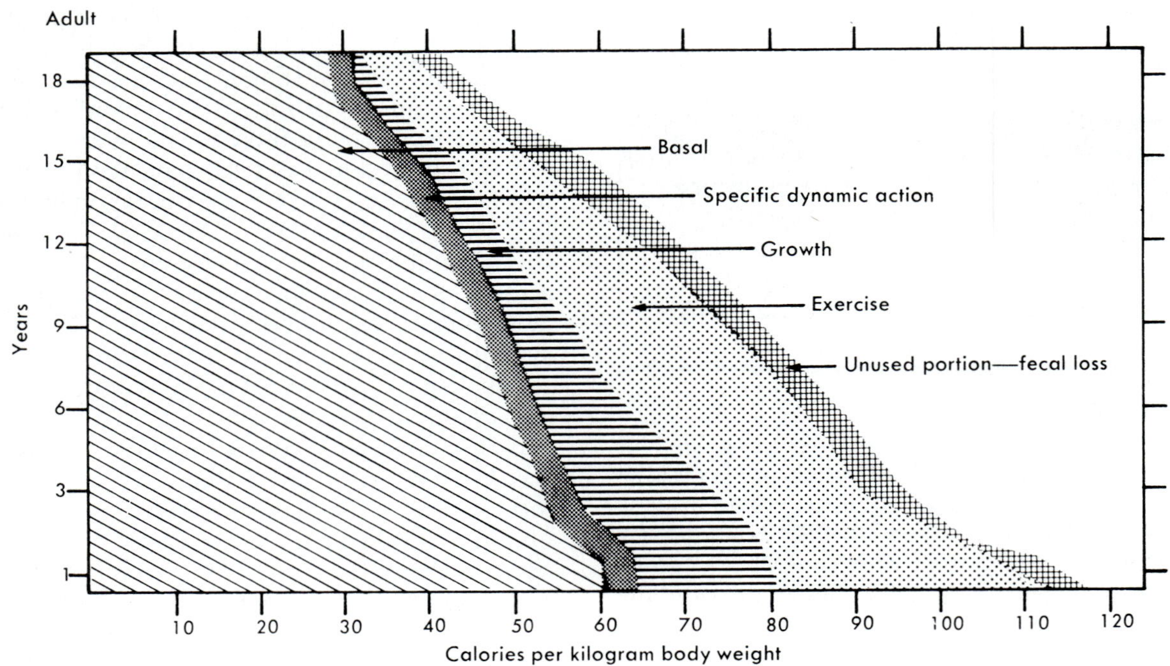

Fig. 22-10 To determine the total caloric requirements of a child, multiply his or her weight in kilograms by the number of calories for age.

The average distribution of calories in a well-balanced diet is as follows:

	Infant	*Child*
Carbohydrates	29% to 58%	50%
Protein	7% to 16%	15%
Fat	35% to 55%	<35%

If the number of grams of carbohydrate, protein, and fat in a food is known, the caloric value can be determined by multiplying each by the appropriate fuel value.

When food is not available the body's nutritional reserves and tissues are used to meet its need for caloric energy. Carbohydrates stored as glycogen in different body organs are used first, followed by fat deposits. Fat in the extremities is usually used first, followed by fat in the trunk. Fat in the cheek pads of young children disappears last, thus indicating malnutrition.

Minerals

Inadequate nutrition is most often seen as a mineral deficiency, such as iron-deficiency anemia, failure to thrive, and, less commonly in the United States, vitamin deficiency. A number of minerals are essential nutrients. Those with a daily requirement greater than 100 mg include calcium, phosphorus, magnesium, potassium, sodium, chloride, and sulfur. Trace minerals, having a requirement of less than 100 mg include iron, fluorine, iodine, zinc, copper, and selenium.

Mineral balance regulation is a complex process. Often one mineral is combined with another to complete a reaction. For example, in the bones, calcium, phosphorus, and magnesium function, together with sufficient vitamin D, for the proper use of calcium. Most minerals are readily obtained from a well-balanced diet. Calcium, iron, and zinc deficiency, however, require special attention. Excessive mineral intake may cause interactions which result in mineral deficiencies or excesses. As an example, excessive amounts of zinc can result in a copper deficiency. However, large amounts of minerals may be lost through vomiting and diarrhea. There is also concern now that excess intake of sodium, which may result from the addition of salt to baby foods in the home, predisposes some infants to hypertension.

Calcium. Large amounts of calcium are required for many vital functions in the body. Calcium is essential for normal heart action and is an important element in the blood-clotting mechanism. Calcium, in combination with phosphorus, is critical to the development and maintenance of bones and teeth. It is also necessary for normal musculoskeletal contraction and nerve conduction. When a diet is calcium-deficient the blood uses the calcium in the bones to maintain its normal composition. Bowed legs (genu varum) and rickets may result from calcium deficiency. Ongoing calcium

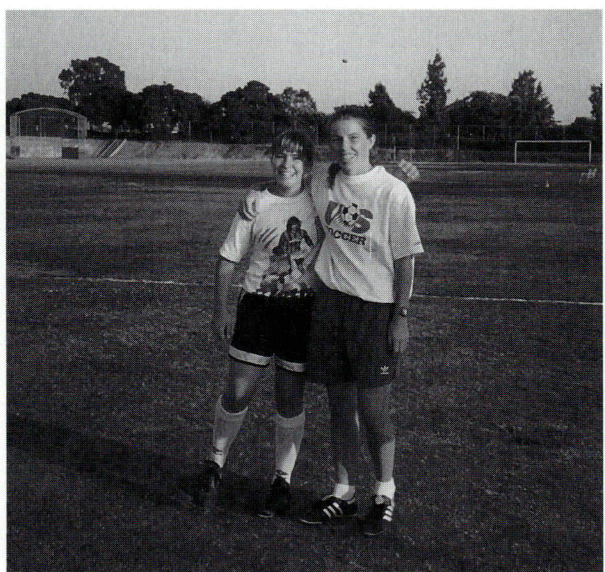

Fig. 22-11 Female athletes are at an increased risk for iron-deficiency anemia.

deficiency places the child at greater risk for osteoporosis later in life. Untreated hypocalcemia may cause neonatal tetany, crying, muscle twitching, convulsions, coma, or death. Dairy products, egg yolks, sardines, and dark green, leafy vegetables are good calcium sources. Lactose-free products are available for those children who are lactose-intolerant, to provide the calcium needed.

Iron. One of the most vital elements in the body is iron. It is a component of hemoglobin, the oxygen bearing element in the blood. Iron is required for growth, and the need for iron varies with the rapidity of growth at different periods of infancy and childhood. It is an essential part of several proteins and enzymes.

In the United States, 30% of children between the ages of 6 and 30 months from lower socioeconomic backgrounds and 5% from upper middle-class families of the same age group suffer from iron-deficiency anemia. Iron deficiency leads to the development of anemia, or insufficient hemoglobin for the needs of the body. Mild anemia may be asymptomatic, thus its identification relies on routine laboratory screening during a well-child visit. Moderate-to-severe iron deficiency results in muscle weakness; easy fatigability; pale mucous membranes and skin; and central nervous system manifestations, such as headaches, dizziness, irritability, and slowed thought processes. The peak incidence of iron-deficiency anemia occurs in the 6- to 24-month-old infant and in pubertal female athletes after the onset of menses (Fig. 22-11).

◆ **TABLE 22-3**
Current Fluoride Dosage Recommendations

Fluoride Content of Drinking Water (ppm)	Daily Dosage (F ion)		
	Birth to Age 2 (mg)	Age 2-3 (mg)	Age 3-14 (mg)
Less than 0.3	0.25	0.50	1.00
0.3 to 0.7	0	0.25	0.50
Over 0.7	Fluoride dietary supplements unnecessary		

Approved by the Council on Dental Therapeutics of the American Dental Association.

Cow's milk does not contain sufficient iron. When the calcium stores present at birth become depleted (at 4 to 7 months of age), iron-deficiency anemia develops unless a supplement is given. Iron-fortified formula and supplementation of iron-fortified cereal after 6 months help ensure an adequate iron status in both breast-fed and bottle-fed infants. Iron-rich foods include liver; red meat; poultry; shellfish; whole grains; enriched cereals and breads; dark-green, leafy vegetables; potatoes; dried fruits; molasses; and egg yolks.

Nursing Alert

Because of its oxalate content, spinach is not a good source of iron and calcium. Oxalates interfere with mineral absorption.

Fluoride. Fluoride is an essential mineral found in minute quantities in many foods. The main role of fluoride in the body lies in its ability to reduce the incidence of dental caries. Public water fluoridation is the most economical and effective preventive measure against dental caries. Fluorides act to inhibit the demineralization of tooth enamel and its ultimate carious destruction. Fluoridated drinking water, which contains one part per million (1 ppm), reduces caries by 50% to 60%. The additional use of topical fluoride can contribute to a further decline in caries by 20% to 30%. Since municipal water fluoridation is not available to all children, various dietary alternatives are suggested. Fluoride drops or chewable tablets should be prescribed when drinking water contains less than 0.8 ppm fluoride (Table 22-3). If community water is not sufficiently fluoridated, naturally fluoridated water or supplemental fluoride should be prescribed and given

◆ TABLE 22-4
Significant Vitamins

Vitamin	Function	Effects of Deficiency
A	Promotes good eyesight Aids in maintaining resistance to infections Maintains skin integrity Helps form and maintain mucous membranes Helps in formation of bones and teeth	Nightblindness Frequent infections Dry, rough skin, and papular eruptions Burning, itching eyes Retarded growth, thin and defective tooth enamel
B complex B_1 (thiamin)	Aids in maintenance and function of nervous system Regulates appetite, normal digestion Promotes feeling of general well-being	Beriberi Listlessness, fatigue, and irritability Anorexia, vomiting, and diarrhea Generalized weakness; gross symptoms of neuromuscular, digestive, and cardiovascular impairment
B_2 (riboflavin)	Aids in eye adaptation to light Provides essentials for metabolism of carbohydrate, fat, and protein Necessary for normal growth	Photophobia, impairment of visual acuity, cataracts Impaired formation of blood cells Anemia
Niacin (nicotinic acid)	Essential for normal function of digestive tract and nervous system	General poor health Gastrointestinal changes—loss of appetite, nausea, vomiting, abdominal pain, red tongue, ulcers and fissures of tongue Dermatitis Nervous system manifestations—headaches and dizziness, impairment of memory, and neurotic symptoms
C (ascorbic acid)	Important role in formation, maintenance, and repair of teeth, bones, and blood vessels Facilitates absorption of dietary iron Maintenance of normal blood hemoglobin levels	Scurvy Loose teeth, faulty bones, slow growth Weakness and irritability Delayed healing of wounds Cutaneous hemorrhages
D	Enhances absorption of calcium and phosphorus Plays a vital role in formation of normal bone Promotes tooth development	Rickets Retarded growth and lack of vigor Variety of bone deformities—large head, pigeon chest, kyphosis, and curved long bones Teeth erupt late and decay early
E (tocopherol)	Production of RBCs and protection from hemolysis Muscle and liver integrity Coenzyme factor in tissue respiration Minimizes oxidation of polyunsaturated fatty acids and vitamins A and C	Hemolytic anemia from hemolysis caused by shortened life of RBCs, especially in premature infants

on a daily basis from 2 weeks of age until eruption of all permanent teeth. Precaution should be taken to prevent an excessive intake of fluoride, which produces mottling of tooth enamel (dental fluorosis). Continuous, systemic concentrations of fluoride greater than 2 ppm may produce a brown stain on teeth, which is of aesthetic concern, although the strength of the teeth is not diminished.

Vitamins

Fat-Soluble	Water-Soluble
A	C
D	B Complex
E	Thiamin (B_1)
K	Riboflavin (B_2)
	Niacin
	Folic acid
	Pyridoxine (B_6)
	Biotin
	Pantothenic acid
	Cyanocobalamin (B_{12})

Vitamins are organic compounds found in minute quantities in foods. They participate as catalysts in almost all metabolic processes and are vital to growth and good health. Vitamins A and D are the only two vitamins stored in the body. Excessive intake of these two vitamins results in toxic manifestations, such as skin lesions, liver enlargement, and bone spurs. Any vitamin may be lacking, causing disturbances in the pattern of growth, metabolism, and development of the child.

The best sources of vitamins are found in natural foods. A well-balanced diet containing daily food choices in the amounts suggested in the Food Guide Pyramid ensures an adequate supply of vitamins (see Table 22-4). For children who are "picky eaters" or in the midst of a food jag a daily children's multivitamin may be beneficial.

Recent research suggests that the antioxidant group of vitamins (vitamin A in the form of beta carotene, vitamin C, and vitamin E) may have a protective effect against many forms of cancer. The ingestion of oxidants or free radicals through food or environmental exposure causes chemical reactions, resulting in cellular damage. As a result of this important research, modifications of the recommended daily allowance (RDA) of the antioxidant vitamins are expected (Dudek, 1993).

Prevention of Atherosclerosis and Coronary Heart Disease

Atherosclerosis, which leads to coronary heart disease, has its origins in childhood. The Committee on Nutrition of the American Academy of Pediatrics (AAP), the American Heart Association, and the National Institutes of Health Consensus Conference on lowering blood cholesterol to prevent heart disease have recommended a "prudent" diet for children who are older than 2 years of age. Unfortunately, there is no consensus on what defines a prudent diet for children. General recommendations emphasize substituting polyunsaturated and monosaturated fat for saturated fats, reducing total fat, dietary cholesterol and salt, and avoiding obesity through a healthy diet and exercise (Williams, 1993).

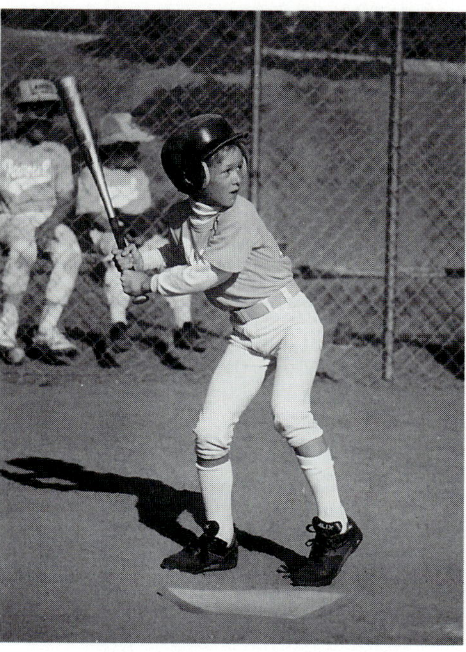

Fig. 22-12 For the prevention of coronary artery disease, regular physical activity should be initiated in early childhood.

The long-term effects of breast-feeding on cholesterol metabolism are not due to the differences in cholesterol intake between formula-fed and breast-fed infants. Rather, researchers believe that the fatty acid composition, immunoglobulins, and hormones in breast milk may have a long-term beneficial effect on cholesterol homeostasis.

Many proponents of early cholesterol screening recommend that the screening should be universal, beginning between age 2 and 5 years. Others recommend testing only those children whose first-degree (parents or siblings) or second-degree relatives (grandparents, aunts, uncles) have a history of stroke, atherosclerosis, or coronary heart disease under 65 years of age, or a positive family history of elevated cholesterol.

Most researchers agree that a total lifestyle approach is optimal and that anticipatory guidance, related to all risk factors, must begin in childhood. Recommendations include advocating smoking prevention and cessation; yearly monitoring of blood pressure beginning at age 3; promoting regular physical activity and monitoring fat intake to maintain ideal body weight; reducing stress; and increasing high density lipoproteins (HDLs) thought to be protective against coronary artery disease (Fig. 22-12).

◆ **TABLE 22-5**
Food and Nutrition Board, National Academy of Sciences—National Research Council Recommended Dietary Allowances,[2] Revised 1989
(Designed for the maintenance of good nutrition of practically all healthy people in the United States)

Category	Age (years)	Weight[b] kg	Weight[b] lb	Height[b] cm	Height[b] in	Protein (g)	Fat-soluble Vitamins: Vitamin A (μg RE)[c]	Vitamin D (μg)[d]	Vitamin E (mg α-TE[e])	Vitamin K (μg)
Infants	0.0-0.5	6	13	60	24	13	375	7.5	3	5
	0.5-1.0	9	20	71	28	14	375	10	4	10
Children	1-3	13	29	90	35	16	400	10	6	15
	4-6	20	44	112	44	24	500	10	7	20
	7-10	28	62	132	52	28	700	10	7	30
Males	11-14	45	99	157	62	45	1000	10	10	45
	15-18	66	145	176	69	59	1000	10	10	65
	19-24	72	160	177	70	58	1000	10	10	70
Females	11-14	46	101	157	62	46	800	10	8	45
	15-18	55	120	163	64	44	800	10	8	55
	19-24	58	128	164	65	46	800	10	8	60

[a]The allowances, expressed as average daily intakes over time, are intended to provide for individual variations among most normal persons as they live in the United States under usual environmental stresses. Diets should be based on a variety of common foods to provide other nutrients for which human requirements have been less well defined.

[b]Weights and heights of Reference Adults are actual medians for the US population of the designated age, as reported by NHANES II. The median weights and heights of those under 19 years of age were taken from Hamill et al. (1979). The use of these figures does not imply that the height-to-weight ratios are ideal.

[c]Retinol equivalents. 1 retinol equivalent = 1 μg retinol or 6 μg β-carotene.

[d]As cholecalciferol. 10 μg cholecalciferol = 400 IU of vitamin D.

[e]α-Tocopherol equivalents. 1 mg d-α tocopherol = 1 α-TE.

[f]1 NE (niacin equivalent) is equal to 1 mg of niacin or 60 mg of dietary tryptophan.

The nurse in a variety of health care settings has a unique opportunity to assess family history, provide anticipatory guidance, plan and implement education programs, and encourage lifestyle changes, thus reducing the incidence of coronary artery disease.

Digestion refers to those processes that prepare food for assimilation into the bloodstream. *Metabolism* refers to all the changes that occur in the use of those nutrients by the cells and the generation of heat and energy (Table 22-5). Amino acids, essential fatty acids, vitamins, and minerals are used primarily for cell growth and repair. They are also used in the formation of enzymes, hormones, and other body substances. Carbohydrates and fats are used primarily for caloric energy to supply fuel to keep the body warm and mechanical energy for performing the body's work. When caloric needs are not met by fats and carbohydrates, protein is then used for energy. Adequate intake of carbohydrates and fats spares protein for cell growth. Thus the diet must contain a balance of all six substances—carbohydrates, fats, proteins, vitamins, minerals, and water. Each one plays a vital role in the processes of growth and development (Table 22-6).

Research is currently underway in an effort to determine any dietary modifications that will help to further decrease the incidence of high blood pressure, cardiovascular disease, cancer, and other chronic diseases.

IMMUNIZATION

The most routine procedure in preventive pediatrics is immunization, a process through which a person is able to build up defenses against certain infectious diseases. When individuals can resist a certain disease, they are said to be immune. They are immune because

Water-soluble Vitamins							Minerals						
Vitamin C (mg)	Thiamin (mg)	Riboflavin (mg)	Niacin (mg NE)[f]	Vitamin B_6 (mg)	Folate (μg)	Vitamin B_{12} (μg)	Calcium (mg)	Phosphorus (mg)	Magnesium (mg)	Iron (mg)	Zinc (mg)	Iodine (μg)	Selenium (μg)
30	0.3	0.4	5	0.3	25	0.3	400	300	40	6	5	40	10
35	0.4	0.5	6	0.6	35	0.5	600	500	60	10	5	50	15
40	0.7	0.8	9	1.0	50	0.7	800	800	80	10	10	70	20
45	0.9	1.1	12	1.1	75	1.0	800	800	120	10	10	90	20
45	1.0	1.2	13	1.4	100	1.4	800	800	170	10	10	120	30
50	1.3	1.5	17	1.7	150	2.0	1200	1200	270	12	15	150	40
60	1.5	1.8	20	2.0	200	2.0	1200	1200	400	12	15	150	50
60	1.5	1.7	19	2.0	200	2.0	1200	1200	350	10	15	150	70
50	1.1	1.3	15	1.4	150	2.0	1200	1200	280	15	12	150	45
60	1.1	1.3	15	1.5	180	2.0	1200	1200	300	15	12	150	50
60	1.1	1.3	15	1.6	180	2.0	1200	1200	280	15	12	150	55

antibodies are present that injure or destroy the disease-producing agent or neutralize its toxins. Active immunization (artificial) is achieved when certain substances called *antigens* are injected into the body to stimulate the production of antibodies. Childhood immunization provides protection against nine major diseases. Recommendations for immunizing infants, children, and adults are governed by the Advisory Committee on Immunization Practices (ACIP) of the US Public Health Service and the AAP.

Provisional data for 1993 indicate that the number of reported cases of congenital rubella syndrome, diphtheria, measles, polio, rubella, and tetanus were at or near the lowest levels ever. However, decreases in morbidity and mortality can be sustained only by achieving and maintaining high vaccination levels among children aged 0 to 2 years. Immunization is the best and the cheapest method of preventing illness.

In 1993, President Clinton set forth the Childhood Immunization Initiative (CII), a comprehensive national response to undervaccination. The goals of CII are to eliminate indigenous cases of six vaccine-preventable diseases by 1996 (e.g., diphtheria and Hib disease among children aged <5 years; measles, mumps, polio, rubella and tetanus among children aged <15 years), increase vaccination coverage levels to at least 90% among 2-year-old children for each of the vaccinations recommended routinely (Table 22-6), and establish a vaccination-delivery system that maintains and further improves high-coverage levels.

Because the mechanisms for developing immunity are immature in infants, children are highly susceptible to some infections. The protection they have against infection is obtained from the mother, if she is immune. Any passive immunity acquired from the mother lasts approximately 4 to 6 months after birth and may protect the child against diphtheria, tetanus, measles,

◆ TABLE 22-6
Recommended Schedule for Routine Active Vaccination of Infants and Children*

Vaccine	At Birth (Before Hospital Discharge)	1-2 Months	2 Months†	4 Months	6 Months	6-18 Months	12-15 Months	15 Months	4-6 Years (Before School Entry)
Diphtheria-tetanus-pertussis§			DTP	DTP	DTP			DTaP/DTP¶	DTaP/DTP
Polio, live oral			OPV	OPV	OPV**				OPV
Measles-mumps-rubella							MMR		MMR††
Haemophilus influenzae type b conjugate									
HbOC/PRP-T§,§§			Hib	Hib	Hib		Hib¶¶		
PRP-OMP§§			Hib	Hib			Hib¶¶		
Hepatitis B***									
Option 1	HepB	HepB†††				HepB†††			
Option 2		HepB†††		HepB†††		HepB†††			

*See table for the recommended immunization schedule for infants and children up to their seventh birthday who do not begin the vaccination series at the recommended times or who are less than 1 month behind in the immunization schedule.

†Can be administered as early as 6 weeks of age.

§Two DTP and Hib combination vaccines are available (DTP/HbOC [TETRAMUNE]; and PRP-T [ActHIB, OmniHIB], which can be reconstituted with DTP vaccine produced by Connaught).

¶This dose of DTP can be administered as early as 12 months of age provided that the interval since the previous dose of DTP is at least 6 months. *Diphtheria and tetanus toxoids and acellular pertussis vaccine (DTaP) is currently recommended only for use as the fourth and/or fifth doses of the DTP series among children aged 15 months through 6 years (before the seventh birthday).* Some experts prefer to administer these vaccines at 18 months of age.

**AAP recommends this dose of vaccine at 6-18 months of age.

††The AAP recommends that two doses of MMR should be administered by 12 years of age with the second dose being administered preferentially at entry to middle school or junior high school.

§§HbOC: [HibTITER] (Lederle Praxis). PRP-T: [ActHIB, OmniHIB] (Pasteur Merieux). PRP-OMP: [PedavaxHIB] (Merck, Sharp, and Dohme). A DTP/Hib combination vaccine can be used in place of HbOC/PRP-T.

¶¶After the primary infant Hib conjugate vaccine series is complete, any of the licensed Hib conjugate vaccines may be used as a booster dose at age 12-15 months.

***For use among infants born to HBsAg-negative mothers. The first dose should be administered during the newborn period, preferably before hospital discharge, but no later than age 2 months. Premature infants of HBsAg-negative mothers should receive the first dose of the hepatitis B vaccine series at the time of hospital discharge or when the other routine childhood vaccines are initiated. (All infants born to HBsAg-negative mothers should receive immunoprophylaxis for hepatitis B as soon as possible after birth.)

†††Hepatitis B vaccine can be administered simultaneously at the same visit with DTP (or DTaP), OPV, Hib, and/or MMR.

From Immunization Practices Advisory Committee (ACIP) Centers for Disease Control, *MMWR* 43 (RR-1):9, 1994.

♦ **TABLE 22-7**
Recommended Accelerated Immunization Schedule For Infants and Children <7 Years of Age Who Start the Series Late* or Who Are less than 1 Month Behind in the Immunization Schedule† (e.g., Children for Whom Compliance With Scheduled Return Visits Cannot Be Assured)

Timing	Vaccine(s)	Comments
First visit		
(≥4 months of age)	DTP§, OPV, Hib¶,§, Hepatitis B, MMR (should be given as soon as child is age 12-15 months)	All vaccines should be administered simultaneously at the appropriate visit.
Second visit (1 month after first visit)	DTP§, Hib¶,§, Hepatitis B	
Third visit (1 month after second visit)	DTP§, OPV, Hib¶,§	
Fourth visit (6 weeks after third visit)	OPV	
Fifth visit (≥6 months after third visit)	DTaP§ or DTP, Hib¶,§, Hepatitis B	
Additional visits		
(Age 4-6 yrs)	DTaP§ or DTP, OPV, MMR	Preferably at or before school entry.
(Age 14-16 yrs)	Td	Repeat every 10 yrs through-out life.

DTP Diphtheria-tetanus-pertussis

DTaP Diphtheria-tetanus-acellular pertussis

Hib Haemophilus influenzae type b conjugate

MMR Measles-mumps-rubella

OPV Poliovirus vaccine, live oral, trivalent

Td Tetanus and diphtheria toxoids (for use among persons ≥7 years of age)

*If initiated in the first year of life, administer DTP doses 1, 2, and 3 and OPV doses 1, 2, and 3 according to this schedule; administer MMR when the child reaches 12-15 months of age.

†See individual ACIP recommendations for detailed information on specific vaccines.

§Two DTP and Hib combination vaccines are available (DTP/HbOC [TETRAMUNE]; and PRP-T [ActHIB , OmniHIB] which can be reconstituted with DTP vaccine produced by Connaught). DTaP preparations are currently recommended only for use as the fourth and/or fifth doses of the DTP series among children 15 months through 6 years of age (before the seventh birthday). DTP and DTaP should not be used on or after the seventh birthday.

¶The recommended schedule varies by vaccine manufacturer. For information specific to the vaccine being used, consult the package insert and ACIP recommendations. Children beginning the Hib vaccine series at age 2-6 months should receive a primary series of three doses of HbOC [HibTITER] (Lederle-Praxis), PRP-T [ActHIB, OmniHIB] (Pasteur Merieux; SmithKline Beecham; Connaught), or a licensed DTP-Hib combination vaccine; **or** two doses of PRP-OMP [PedvaxHIB] (Merck, Sharp, and Dohme). An additional booster dose of any licensed Hib conjugate vaccine should be administered at 12-15 months of age and at least 2 months after the previous dose. Children beginning the Hib vaccine series at 7-11 months of age should receive a primary series of two doses of an HbOC, PRP-T, or PRP-OMP-containing vaccine. An additional booster dose of any licensed Hib conjugate vaccine should be administered at 12-18 months of age and at least 2 months after the previous dose. Children beginning the Hib vaccine series at ages 12-14 months should receive a primary series of one dose of an HbOC, PRP-T, or PRP-OMP-containing vaccine. An additional booster dose of any licensed Hib conjugate vaccine should be administered 2 months after the previous dose. Children beginning the Hib vaccine series at ages 15-59 months should receive one dose of any licensed Hib vaccine. Hib vaccine should not be administered after the fifth birthday except for special circumstances as noted in the specific ACIP recommendations for the use of Hib vaccine.

From Immunization Practices Advisory Committee (ACIP) Centers for Disease Control, *MMWR* 43(RR-I):10, 1994.

♦ TABLE 22-8
Recommended Immunization Schedule for Persons ≥7 Years of Age Not Vaccinated at the Recommended Time in Early Infancy*

Timing	Vaccine(s)	Comments
First visit	Td†, OPV§ MMR¶, and Hepatitis B**	Primary poliovirus vaccination is not routinely recommended for persons ≥18 years of age.
Second visit (6-8 weeks after first visit)	Td, OPV, MMR††,¶, Hepatitis B**	
Third visit (6 months after second visit)	Td, OPV, Hepatitis B**	
Additional visits	Td	Repeat every 10 years throughout life.

MMR Measles-mumps-rubella

OPV Poliovirus vaccine, live oral, trivalent

Td Tetanus and diphtheria toxoids (for use among persons ≥7 years of age)

*See individual ACIP recommendations for details.

†The DTP and DTaP doses administered to children <7 years of age who remain incompletely vaccinated at age ≥7 years should be counted as prior exposure to tetanus and diphtheria toxoids (e.g., a child who previously received two doses of DTP needs only one dose of Td to complete a primary series for tetanus and diphtheria).

§When polio vaccine is administered to previously unvaccinated persons ≥18 years of age, inactivated poliovirus vaccine (IPV) is preferred. For the immunization schedule for IPV, see specific ACIP statement of the use of polio vaccine.

¶Persons born before 1957 can generally be considered immune to measles and mumps and need not be vaccinated. Rubella (or MMR) vaccine can be administered to persons of any age, particularly to nonpregnant women of childbearing age.

**Hepatitis B vaccine, recombinant. Selected high-risk groups for whom vaccination is recommended include persons with occupational risk, such as health-care and public-safety workers who have occupational exposure to blood, clients and staff of institutions for the developmentally disabled, hemodialysis patients, recipients of certain blood products (e.g., clotting factor concentrates), household contacts and sex partners of hepatitis B virus carriers, injecting drug users, sexually active homosexual and bisexual men, certain sexually active heterosexual men and women, inmates of long-term correctional facilities, certain international travelers, and families of HBsAg-positive adoptees from countries where HBV infection is endemic. Because risk factors are often not identified directly among adolescents, universal hepatitis B vaccination of teenagers should be implemented in communities where injecting drug use, pregnancy among teenagers, and/or sexually transmitted diseases are common.

††The ACIP recommends a second dose of measles-containing vaccine (preferably MMR to assure immunity to mumps and rubella) for certain groups. Children with no documentation of live measles vaccination after the first birthday should receive two doses of live measles-containing vaccine not less than 1 month apart. In addition, the following persons born in 1957 or later should have documentation of measles immunity (i.e., two doses of measles-containing vaccine [at least one of which being MMR], physician-diagnosed measles, or laboratory evidence of measles immunity): a) those entering post-high school educational settings; b) those beginning employment in health-care settings who will have direct patient contact; and c) travelers to areas with endemic measles.

From Immunization Practices Advisory Committee (ACIP) Centers for Disease Control, *MMWR* 43(RR-I):11, 1994.

and poliomyelitis. Because such passive protection varies greatly among infants and no passive immunity exists against pertussis (whooping cough), immunization should be initiated as early as possible. Combined antigens reduce the number of injections, enhance the action of each, and establish a desired immunity within the first 6 months of life.

Hepatitis B vaccine is given to the newborn, before discharge. Other immunizations are begun when the infant is 2 months of age (Tables 22-7 to 22-11). A "triple toxoid" of diphtheria, tetanus, and pertussis antigens in one injection, as well as a *Haemophilus influenzae* b conjugate vaccine and a concurrent dropper of oral polio vaccine are given. The "triple toxoid" DTP is given three times, not less than 1 month apart. The necessity of preventing the high mortality from pertussis (whooping cough) in infancy is the main reason for early initiation of the DTP immunization.

◆ TABLE 22-9
Summary of Recommendations of Advisory Committee on Immunization Practices for Tetanus Prophylaxis in Routine Wound Management—United States, 1991

History of Adsorbed Tetanus Toxoid (Doses)	Clean, Minor Wounds		All Other Wounds*	
	Td†	TIG	Td†	TIG
Unknown or <3	Yes	No	Yes	Yes
≥3§	No¶	No	No**	No

*Such as, but not limited to, wounds contaminated with dirt, feces, soil, saliva; puncture wounds; avulsions; and wounds resulting from missiles, crushing, burns, and frostbite.

†For children <7 years old, DTP (DT, if pertussis vaccine is contraindicated) is referred to tetanus toxoid alone. For persons ≥7 years of age, Td is preferred to tetanus toxoid alone. Diphtheria and tetanus toxoids and acellular pertussis vaccine (DTaP) may be used instead of DTP for the fourth and fifth doses.

§If only 3 doses of *fluid* toxoid have been received, then a fourth dose of toxoid, preferably an adsorbed toxoid, should be given.

¶Yes, if more than 10 years since last dose.

**Yes, if more than 5 years since last dose. (More frequent boosters are not needed and can accentuate side effects.)

From Immunization Practices Advisory Committee (ICAP) Centers For Disease Control. *MMWR* 41(SS-8):7, 1992.

After the initial series of immunizations, recall or booster doses are given to stimulate high antibody levels and maintain maximum immunity. Children who have received three doses of triple toxoid (DTP), three doses of *Haemophilus influenzae* b (HIb) vaccine, and two doses of oral polio vaccine (OPV) should be given a booster dose at 12 to 15 or 18 months of age (see Table 22-6). Subsequent booster doses are recommended between 4 and 6 years of age. Active, up-to-date immunization produces a degree of resistance in children comparable to that which follows the natural infection.

For a more detailed discussion of this procedure, refer to the American Academy of Pediatrics Red Book (1994).

Pertussis Vaccine

Routine vaccination with a combined diphtheria tetanus and whole-cell pertussis vaccine (DTP) has been highly effective. Combined diphtheria tetanus and acellular pertussis (DTaP) vaccines are now available. Although mild systemic reactions such as fever, drowsiness, fretfulness, and anorexia occur frequently after both vaccines (DTP and DTaP), they are less common after the DTaP vaccine. These reactions are self-limited and can be managed with symptomatic treatment.

After the initial three-dose series of whole-cell DTP vaccine, the DTaP vaccine may be used as the fourth and/or fifth doses of the recommended series.

◆ TABLE 22-10
Adverse Events Occurring Within 48 Hours of DTP Immunizations

Event	Frequency*
Local	
Redness	1/3 doses
Swelling	2/5 doses
Pain	1/2 doses
Mild/moderate systemic	
Fever 38° C (100.4° F)	1/2 doses
Drowsiness	1/3 doses
Fretfulness	1/2 doses
Vomiting	1/15 doses
Anorexia	1/5 doses
More serious systemic	
Persistent, inconsolable crying—duration, 3 hours	1/100 doses
High-pitched, unusual cry	1/900 doses
Fever 40.5° C (105° F)	1/330 doses
Collapse (hypotonic-hyporesponsive episode)	1/1,750 doses
Convulsions (with or without fever)	1/1,750 doses
Acute encephalopathy†	1/1,110,000 doses
Permanent neurological deficit†	1/1,310,000 doses

From *MMWR* 34:411, 1985.

*Number of adverse events per total number of doses regardless of dose number in DTP series.

†Occurring within 7 days of DTP immunizations.

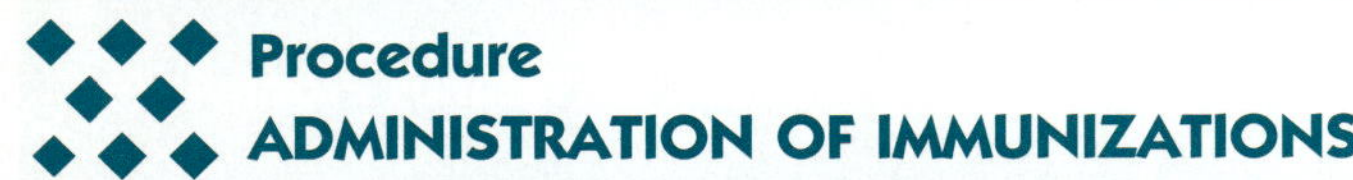

Procedure ADMINISTRATION OF IMMUNIZATIONS

INSTRUCTIONS

1. A separate, sterile needle and syringe, preferably disposable, should be used for each injection.
2. Preferred sites for subcutaneous and intramuscular injections include the anterolateral aspect of the upper thigh and the deltoid muscle of the upper arm. Each injection should be given at a different site.
3. A 1-inch needle (22-gauge) is the preferred length for intramuscular injections.
4. The infant or child should be adequately restrained before an injection.
5. Toxoids and vaccines (antigens) containing alum are given intramuscularly, preferably into the midlateral/anterolateral thigh or deltoid muscles.
6. The package insert should be read before administration of the immunization.
7. Patients and parents should be informed of any possible side effect or adverse reaction. They should be counseled regarding the benefits of the vaccine and the risks of the disease.
8. Systemic reactions such as fever, rashes, and arthralgia subside within 48 hours and are controlled by symptomatic measures and antipyretics.
9. Tylenol 10-15 mg/kg may be given after the injection. This dosage may be repeated as needed *not more than five times at 4-hour intervals* without medical consultation.
10. Premature infants should be given the same dosage and indications as for normal, full-term infants.

PRECAUTIONS

1. Immunization should not be delayed because of the presence of a mild illness, with or without a fever.
2. Caution should be exercised if a child has a history of any of the following events occurring within 48 hours of a previous dose of vaccine containing the pertussis component: temperature of 40.5° C (105° F) not resulting from another identifiable cause, collapse or shock-like state, persistent and inconsolable crying lasting 3 hours, or seizures with or without fever occurring within 3 days of vaccination.
3. Nonprogressive, neurological disorders *do not* constitute a valid reason for deferring or withholding routine immunization. However, if the child has an evolving neuropathic process, DTP administration should be decided on an individual basis.

CONTRAINDICATIONS

1. Anaphylactic-like reactions (e.g., generalized urticaria or hives, swelling of the mouth and throat, difficulty breathing, hypotension and shock) to the vaccine or vaccine constituent (e.g., if the individual is allergic to eggs or neomycin).
2. Moderate-or-severe illness, with or without a fever.
3. DTP or DTaP should not be repeated if encephalopathy (e.g., major alterations in consciousness, unresponsiveness, or seizures that persist without recovery within 24 hours) occurred within 7 days of administration of the previous dose.
4. Immunization procedures are deferred during the administration of steroids, irradiation, and anticancer drug therapy because antibody response is depressed or abnormal. Immunizations should also be deferred if the child has recently received (within 12 weeks) immune globulin, plasma, or blood.
5. Infants, children, and other household contacts with individuals with an immunological deficiency should not receive oral poliovirus vaccine, since the polio viruses are transmissible to the immunocompromised individual.
6. Live virus vaccines against measles, rubella, and mumps are *not* given to pregnant women or patients with a generalized malignancy.

For a more detailed discussion of this procedure, refer to the American Academy of Pediatrics Red Book (1994).

Rubella (German Measles) Vaccine

The principal objective of rubella (German measles) vaccination is to prevent congenital rubella infection (CRI) (Fig. 22-13). CRI can result in miscarriage, abortion, stillbirth, and congenital rubella syndrome (mild-to severe-multiple organ congenital anomalies, such as heart defects, hearing loss, and cataracts) in infants.

This can best be achieved by eliminating the transmission of the virus among children, who are the primary sources of infection for susceptible pregnant women. All children aged 12 to 15 months should receive the live rubella virus vaccine. Unless there is an epidemic, it is not recommended for younger infants because of possible interference in active antibody formation by persisting maternal rubella antibody. Children of pregnant women may be given the rubella vaccine, since the vaccine virus is not communicable.

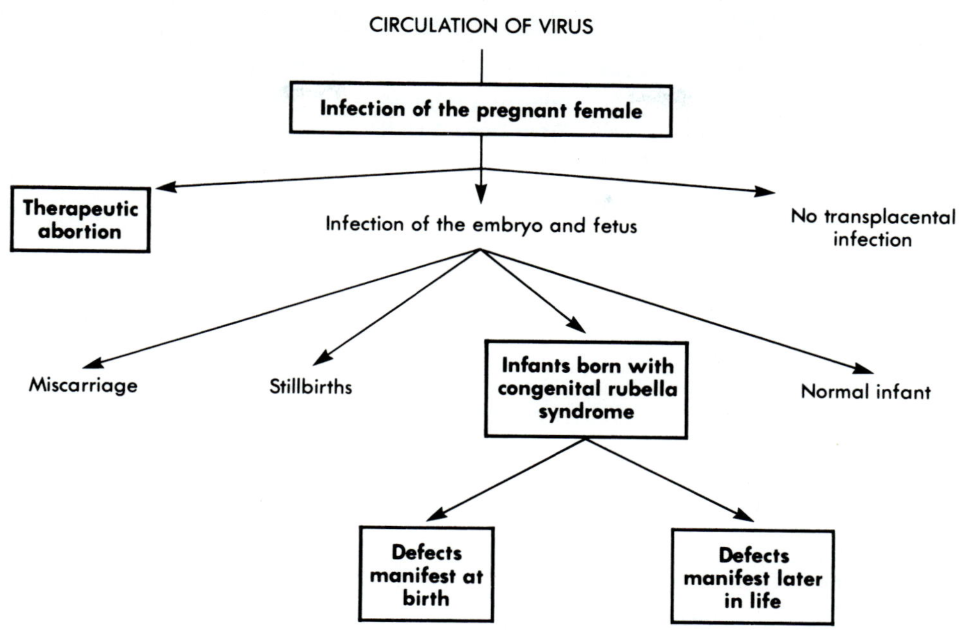

Fig. 22-13 The occurrence and monitoring of congenital rubella infection (CRI) and congenital rubella syndrome (CRS).

However, the mother's immunization with a live virus vaccine during pregnancy should be avoided because of possible risk to the fetus.

Mumps Virus Vaccine

The principal objective of the mumps vaccine is prevention of mumps in preadolescent males and young male adults. Live attenuated mumps virus vaccine is recommended for all susceptible children aged 12 to 15 months and especially for preadolescent males and men who have not had the disease. MMR is the vaccine of choice for persons likely to be susceptible to mumps (as well as measles and rubella). The vaccine should not be given to pregnant women.

Measles (Rubeola) Vaccine

Measles (rubeola) is often a serious disease. It is frequently complicated by middle ear infection or bronchopneumonia. Encephalitis occurs in about 1 of every 1000 reported cases. Survivors of this complication often have permanent brain damage and mental retardation. Death associated with complications occurs in 1 of every 1000 cases, and the risk of death is greater in infants and young children. Because of recent outbreaks a routine two-dose measles vaccination schedule is now recommended (see this schedule in Table 22-12). Revaccination is recommended for persons who received the measles vaccine before 1980. Measles antibodies develop in at least 95% of susceptible children vaccinated at 15 or more months. Measles vaccine produces an inapparent or mild, noncommunicable infection. Because measles is often a severe disease with frequent complications, the live measles vaccine may be given as early as 6 to 9 months of age if exposure of the infant is probable. A second dose must be given at approximately 12 to 15 months of age.

School-entrance laws require documentation of measles immunity at the time of entry into kindergarten or first grade. The existence of these regulations, requiring immunity to measles documentation before children are allowed to enter kindergarten or first grade, has been shown to correlate with reduced incidence of measles.

Smallpox Vaccine

Global eradication of smallpox was declared in 1980 by the World Health Organization (WHO). Smallpox vaccine is currently indicated only for laboratory workers directly involved with smallpox viruses.

Haemophilus Influenzae Type B Conjugate Vaccine

Haemophilus influenzae type b (Hib) is one of the major causes of serious systemic disease among infants and young children, especially those younger than 18 months. It is the leading cause of bacterial meningitis, and the *Haemophilus* species is the most common cause

◆ **TABLE 22-11**
Minimum Age for Initial Vaccination and Minimum Interval Between Vaccine Doses, By Type of Vaccine

Vaccine	Minimum Age for First Dose*	Minimum Interval From Dose 1 to 2*	Minimum Interval From Dose 2 to 3*	Minimum Interval From Dose 3 to 4*
DTP (DT)†	6 weeks§	4 weeks	4 weeks	6 months
Combined DTP-Hib	6 weeks	1 month	1 month	6 months
DTaP*	15 months			6 months
Hib (primary series)				
HbOC	6 weeks	1 month	1 month	¶
PRP-T	6 weeks	1 month	1 month	¶
PRP-OMP	6 weeks	1 month	¶	
OPV	6 weeks§	6 weeks	6 weeks	
IPV**	6 weeks	4 weeks	6 months††	
MMR	12 months§§	1 month		
Hepatitis B	birth	1 month	2 months¶¶	

DTP Diphtheria-tetanus-pertussis

DTaP Diphtheria-tetanus-acellular pertussis

Hib *Haemophilus influenza* type b conjugate

IPV Inactivated poliovirus vaccine

MMR Measles-mumps-rubella

OPV Live oral polio vaccine

*These minimum acceptable ages and intervals may not correspond with the optimal recommended ages and intervals for vaccination. See tables 22-3 to 22-5 for the current recommended routine and accelerated vaccination schedules.

†DTaP can be used in place of the fourth (and fifth) dose of DTP for children who are at least 15 months of age. Children who have received all four primary vaccination doses before their fourth birthday should receive a fifth dose of DTP (DT) or DTaP at 4-6 years of age before entering kindergarten or elementary school **and** at least 6 months after the fourth dose. The total number of doses of diphtheria and tetanus toxoids should not exceed six each before the seventh birthday (*14*).

§AAP permits DTP and OPV to be administered as early as 4 weeks of age in areas with high endemicity and during outbreaks.

¶The booster dose of Hib vaccine, which is recommended after the primary vaccination series should be administered no earlier than 12 months of age **and** at least 2 months after the previous dose of Hib vaccine (Tables 22-3 and 22-4).

**See text to differentiate conventional inactivated poliovirus vaccine from enhanced-potency IPV.

††For unvaccinated adults at increased risk of exposure to poliovirus with <3 months but >2 months available before protection is needed, three doses of IPV should be administered at least 1 month apart.

§§Although the age for measles vaccination may be as young as 6 months in outbreak areas where cases are occurring in children <1 year of age, children initially vaccinated before the first birthday should be revaccinated at 12-15 months of age and an additional dose of vaccine should be administered at the time of school entry or according to local policy. Doses of MMR or other measles-containing vaccines should be separated by at least 1 month.

¶¶This final dose is recommended no earlier than 4 months of age.

of invasive infections including septicemia, pneumonia, epiglottitis, cellulitis, arthritis, osteomyelitis, and pericarditis. The mortality rate from Hib meningitis is 5% to 10%. Even when antibiotic treatment is provided, neurological sequelae are observed in at least 25% to 35% of survivors. A primary series of one of the licensed Hib conjugate vaccines beginning at 2 months of age, and continuing at 4 months, 6 months, and a booster dose at age 12 to 15 months is recommended routinely for all infants. A new combined diphtheria/tetanus toxoids and whole-cell pertussis vaccine (DTP) and Hib conjugate vaccine has been licensed, allowing simultaneous administration (e.g., fewer separate injections).

Hib vaccine is not recommended for children over the age of five, except for those at risk. Children who

◆ TABLE 22-12
1989 Recommendations For Measles Vaccination

Routine childhood schedule, United States	
Most areas	Two doses*† first dose at 15 months second dose at 4-6 years (entry to kindergarten or first grade)‡
High-risk areas§	Two doses*† first dose at 12 months second dose at 4-6 years (entry to kindergarten or first grade)‡
Colleges and other educational institutions post-high school	Documentation of receipt of two doses of measles vaccine after the first birthday† or other evidence of measles immunity.¶
Medical personnel beginning employment	Documentation of receipt of two doses of measles vaccine after the first birthday† or other evidence of measles immunity.¶

From *MMWR* 38:4, 1989.

*Both doses should preferably be given as combined measles, mumps, rubella vaccine (MMR).

†No less than 1 month apart. If no documentation of any dose of vaccine, vaccine should be given at the time of school entry or employment and no less than 1 month later.

‡Some areas may elect to administer the second dose at an older age or to multiple age groups.

§A county with more than five cases among preschool-aged children during each of the last 5 years, a county with a recent outbreak among unvaccinated preschool-aged children, or a county with a large inner-city urban population. These recommendations may be applied to an entire county or to identified risk areas within a county.

¶Prior physician-diagnosed measles disease, laboratory evidence of measles immunity, or birth before 1957.

attend day-care facilities and children with certain chronic conditions, such as sickle cell disease and antibody deficiency disease, are at increased risk of *H. influenzae* infections (Fig. 22-14).

Hepatitis B Vaccine

Most persons with hepatitis B acquire the infection as adolescents or young adults. However, efforts to vaccinate persons in these groups have had limited success. The acute and chronic consequences of hepatitis B virus (HBV) infections are major health problems in the United States. Each year nearly 5000 people die from chronic liver disease and approximately 1.25 million people with chronic HBV infections are potentially infectious to others.

Infants and young children become infected with HBV through a variety of ways, but the infection is generally asymptomatic. However, the risk of sequela is great and not seen until adulthood. Therefore hepatitis B vaccine is recommended for all infants. Immunization with haptatitis B vaccine is the most effective means of preventing HBV infection and its consequences. A recommended series of three intramuscular doses of HBV induces a protective antibody response in greater than 95% of infants, children, and adolescents.

Passive Immunity

Immune globulin (human) (IG), formerly called *immune serum globulin* or *gamma globulin,* is an antibody-rich fraction of pooled plasma from normal donors. It confers temporary immunity that is attained in approximately 2 days and lasts from 1 to 6 weeks. The large, viscous dose should be divided and given intramuscularly in two different sites with an 18– or 20–gauge needle. IG is limited in supply and has been clearly documented to be helpful in the prevention or modification of measles and viral hepatitis A (HAV), and in the treatment of certain antibody deficiencies. IG does not transmit HBV, HIV, or other infectious diseases.

Specific Immune Globulins (Human)

Special preparations of specific immune globulin are obtained from a preselected human donor pool

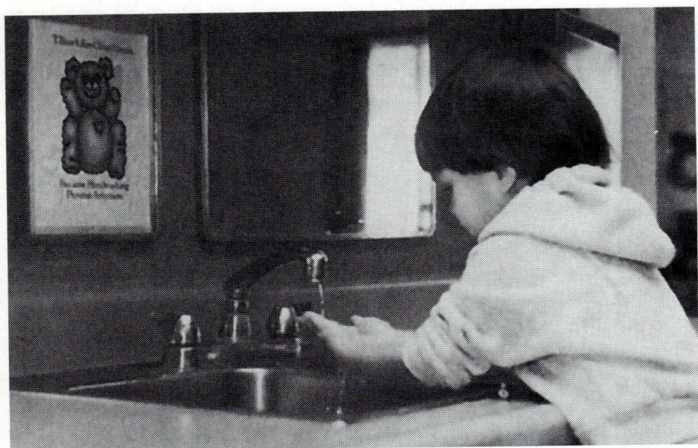

Fig. 22-14 Thorough handwashing is the single most effective method of preventing infection (From Wong DL: *Essentials of pediatric nursing,* ed 4, St. Louis, 1993, Mosby.)

and include hepatitis B immune globulin (HBIG), varicella zoster immune globulin (VZIG), rabies immune globulin (RIG), and tetanus immune globulin (TIG).

Immune Globulin Intravenous (Human)

Immune globulin intravenous (IGIV) is derived from a similar pool to that of the IG pool but is prepared to be suitable for intravenous use. Indications for use include replacement therapy in antibody deficiency disorders, idiopathic thrombocytopenic purpura, Kawasaki's disease, premature infants, and AIDS. IGIV should be used only when its efficacy has been established. The instructions given in the package insert should be followed.

EDUCATION AND ANTICIPATORY GUIDANCE

Parents should be educated about the benefits and risks of each immunization their child is to receive. The nurse and physician are responsible for informing the parents regarding the nature, prevalence, and risks of the infection or disease that is being prevented or modified. Verbal statements should be reinforced with written documents (Fig. 22-15).

Every child should be immunized against preventable, contagious diseases. The nurse can reinforce the importance of continuing the immunization program and inform parents about the need for immunization. The nurse must elicit from the caretaker information regarding allergies and reactions to previous immunizations. During the administration of the immunizations the nurse's calm, matter-of-fact, positive attitude is most effective.

Record Keeping

An ongoing, written immunization record should be given to the parents. The date and time of the next appointment should be clearly understood (see Fig. 22-11). The following information regarding the immunization should be entered into the patient's medical record, as well as the parent's record.

1 Date: month, day, and year of vaccination.
2 Name of the vaccine/immunization.
3 Manufacturer, lot number, and expiration date of the vaccine.
4 Site and route of administration.
5 Name, address, and title of nurse administering the vaccine.

The National Childhood Vaccine Injury Act (1986) requires that the information listed above and any events occurring after the vaccine be recorded on the patient's permanent medical record. The law stipulates that children who are inadvertently injured must go through a compensation system before attempting to sue either the manufacturer or the person who gave the vaccine. The system is designed to ensure fair compensation to children and to provide protection from liability for vaccine manufacturers and providers. It is also important to record all immunizations received on the patient's WHO immunization record, clinic folder, and hospital record, if one exists. Immunization status is reviewed at the time of each health assessment, illness, or injury. It is equally worthwhile to inquire about the current status of the parents' immunizations.

Immunization is a major component of child health promotion and primary prevention. An initial overview of the immunization schedule is presented in prenatal classes. New parents are very concerned about "doing what is right" for their child. Before going home from the hospital the parents are reminded about the immunization program. Although immunizations are usually given by the primary health care provider, parents should be informed regarding community resources where free immunization services are available.

CHILD SAFETY AND INJURY PREVENTION

Successful prevention and treatment of infectious diseases and nutritional disorders have resulted in a significant decrease in child mortality. The greatest

◆ **TABLE 22-13**
Accidental Death in Children, 1993*

Type of Accident	0 to 4 Years	5 to 14 Years	15-24 Years	Total
Motor vehicle	1000	2000	10600	13600
Drowning	700	500	900	2100
Fires, burns	850	350	200	1400
Firearms	40	180	550	770
Falls	90	80	230	400
Suffocation by ingestion of objects	140	30	30	200
Poisoning (solids/liquids)	40	30	280	350
Poisoning (gases/vapors)	40	30	110	180
Other	500	400	1000	1900
TOTAL	3400	3600	13,900	20,900

Data from the National Safety Council: Accident facts, 1993, pp. 4, 5.

*Deaths per 100,000 population in each age group.

threat to the health and well-being of the child today is injury. Injuries are responsible for more than 50% of childhood fatalities. An estimated 8000 to 12,000 children under 15 years of age die annually in the United States from injuries (Table 22-13). Injuries kill more children than the next six leading causes of childhood death combined. Nurses play a primary role in the provision of anticipatory guidance regarding child safety and injury prevention. See Chapter 1 for specific information regarding causes of death in selected age groups.

The magnitude of this problem is further identified by the fact that 19 million children suffer nonfatal injuries every year. Many of these children are crippled or disabled for life. In 1990 over 550,000 children were treated in hospital emergency rooms for toy-related injuries. Of course, not all childhood injuries are brought to the attention of medical and nursing personnel.

An additional 25% of children up to 14 years of age have significant but unreported injuries. Thus the conservative figure of 19 million childhood injuries indicates that a serious national problem exists.

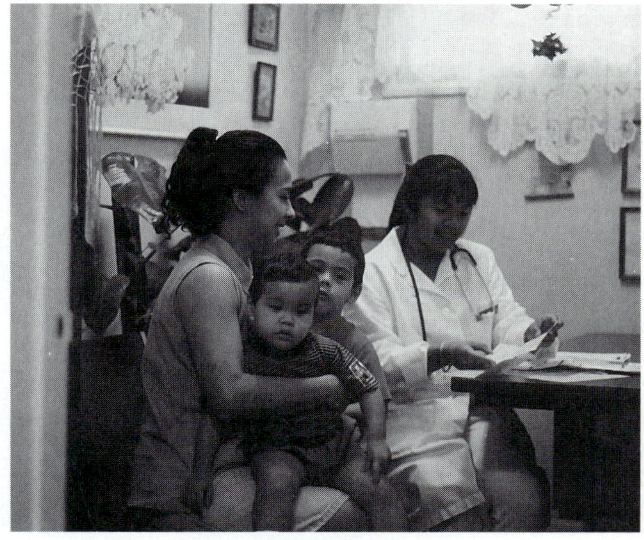

Fig. 22-15 Immunizations should not be given without follow-up instructions for parents.

Injuries

Few people know what "injury" really means except that it represents the leading cause of death in the United States before age 55, the largest cause of years of potential life lost, and a cost of several hundred billion dollars annually. *Injury* is a term not yet widely understood, probably because the word accident has been used to describe many injuries. However, most injuries are preventable, thus *not* accidental.

Common childhood injuries include lacerations, blows from objects, animal bites, and injuries related to motor vehicles. Motor vehicles are the major cause of death from injury. Also ranked among the leading causes of fatal injuries are firearms, drownings, fires, and ingestion of objects (see Table 22-13).

Certain factors seem to be influential in causing childhood injuries: (1) approximately one half of all fatalities occur in children under 5 years of age; (2) boys at all ages have more accidents than girls; (3) the non-Caucasian population has a considerably higher incidence of accidents than does the Caucasian population; (4) most injuries occur during the spring

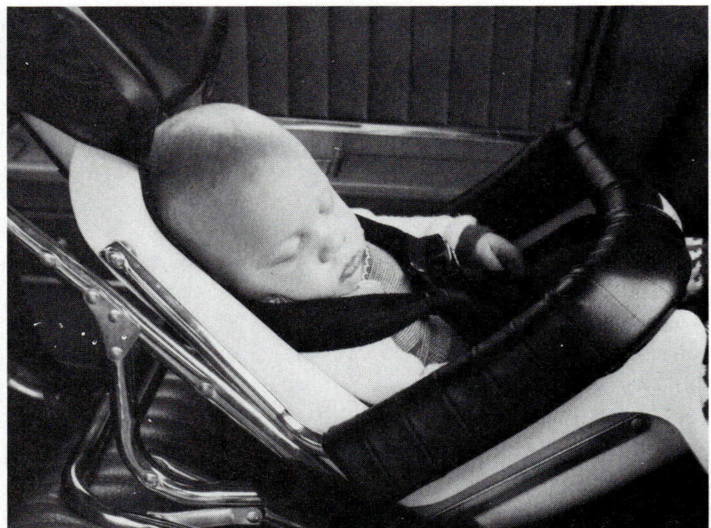

Fig. 22-16 Correct use of an infant car carrier. Children weighing less than 40 pounds (18.8 kg) need special safety restraints designed to distribute crash forces over a large body area. All car occupants should ride restrained. Infants and young children should be restrained in the back seat. Purchasing and properly using crash-safe automotive restraints are the keys to prevention or reduction of severe injuries. (For information and evaluation of restraints, contact Physicians for Automotive Safety, 50 Union Avenue, Irvington, NJ, 07111.)

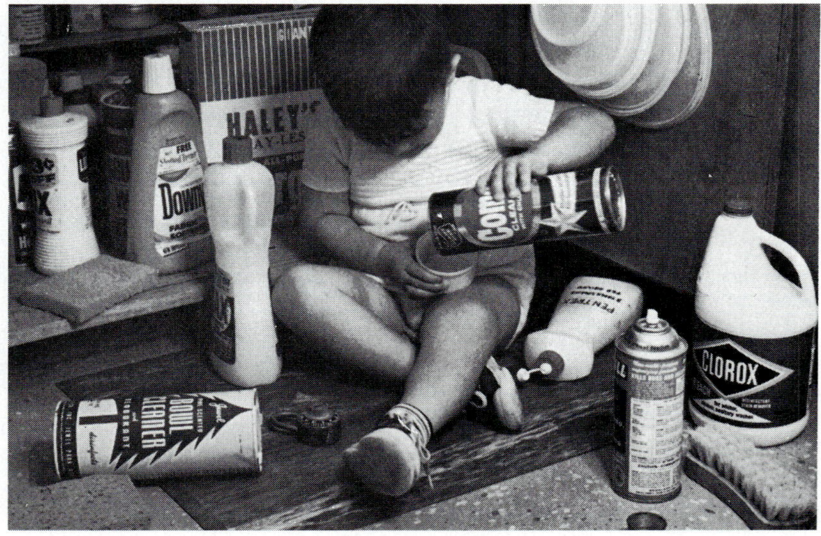

Fig. 22-17 Young children may eat and drink anything, regardless of taste. Keep household poisons in a *locked* cupboard.

and summer months; (5) a higher percentage of injuries occurs in the home, especially during the preschool period; (6) the child between 1 and 2 years of age is most vulnerable to injuries of all sorts; and (7) some children are accident-prone. Combinations of certain personality characteristics and environmental influences predispose a child toward repetitive injuries.

Injury prevention

Good safety habits could eliminate many of the causes of injury. Safeguarding the lives of children depends on injury prevention (Figs. 22-16 to 22-22). Continued emphasis has been placed on two particular approaches to injury prevention: (1) the elimination of specific environmental hazards peculiar to different age groups and (2) supervision of small children by

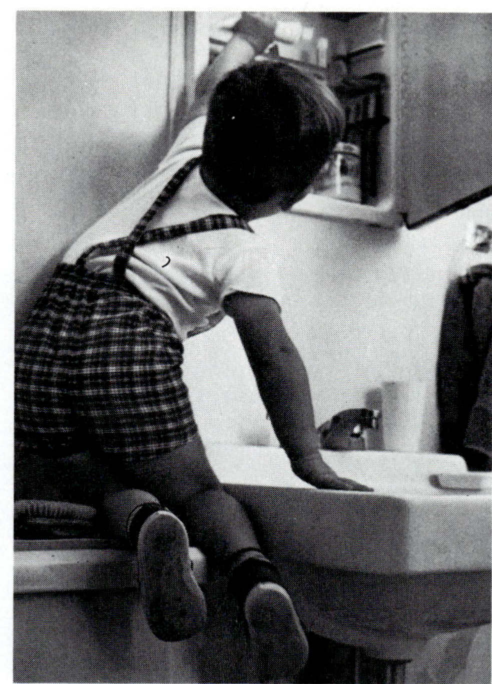

Fig. 22-18 Keep medicine in a locked cabinet.

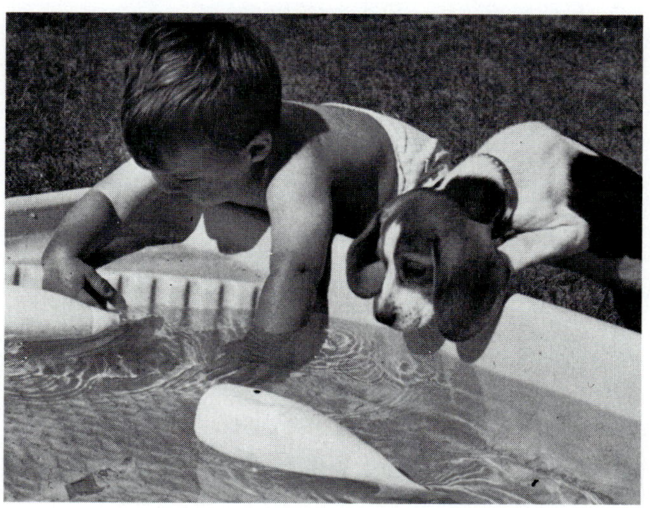

Fig. 22-19 Even shallow water is dangerous for an unattended child.

adults that is to be gradually replaced by the child's training for safety. Recent data reveals a continued increase in the actual number of injuries.

Vital statistics in the United States indicate the number of children injured and the kinds of situations causing the injuries. However, they do not provide sufficient detail about each individual case to fully describe the complete situation of each event. This lack

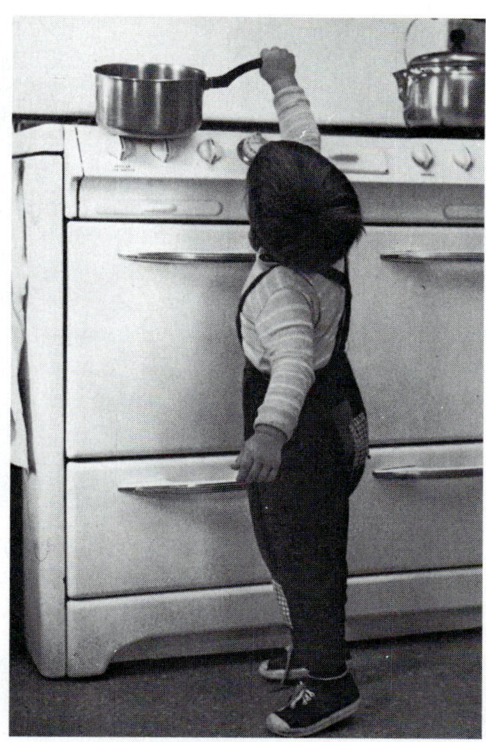

Fig. 22-20 Always turn handles of pots and pans to the back of the stove.

of information prevents making valid conclusions concerning injury causation and prevention in childhood. Often, vital information is not recorded. This is undoubtedly why specific recommendations for the prevention of certain injuries have not always been effective.

To date, no single approach to injury prevention has been formulated. The widespread misinterpretation that injuries happen by chance is reflected in the use of the unscientific term *accident*. Accident implies that the event was unpredictable. However, most accidents are predictable and preventable.

Injuries are the result of a large number of complex mechanisms. Like other illnesses, effective intervention programs must be developed through systematic investigation. To understand the nature and cause of injuries, several factors must be considered simultaneously. These factors include the host (the child who is affected), the agent (the object that is the direct cause), and the environment (the situation in which the injury takes place). This is the epidemiological approach to the study of injuries.

Although a great deal remains to be learned about the interaction of these major factors the existing knowledge has led to the following new principles aimed at injury prevention: (1) control of the agent

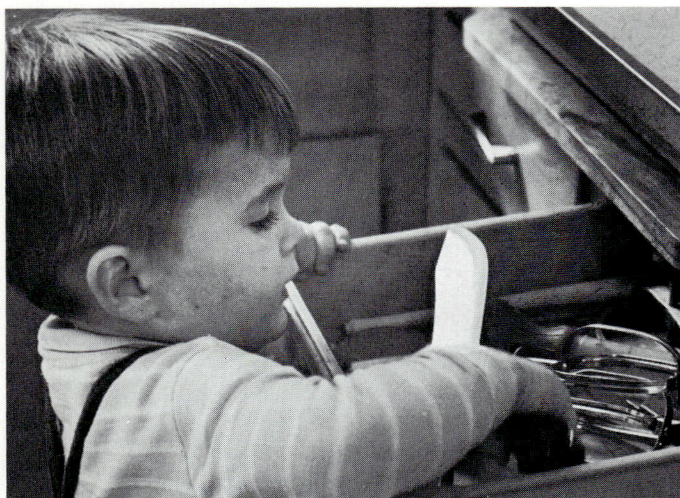

Fig. 22-21 Keep sharp objects out of the reach of children.

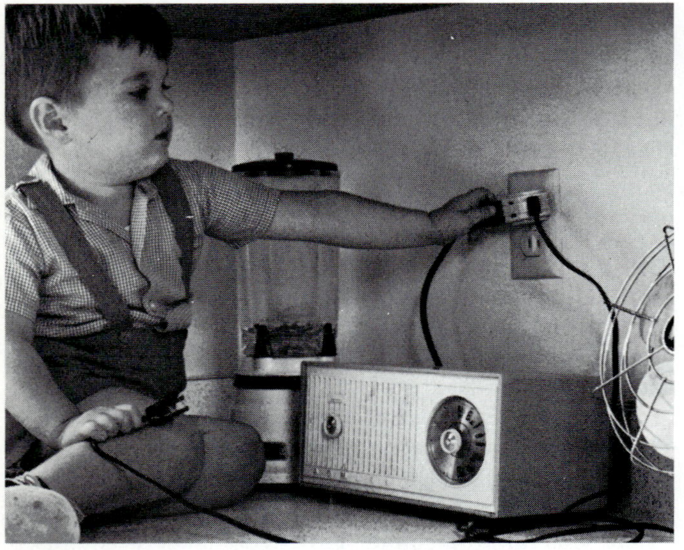

Fig. 22-22 Disconnect appliances not in use. Cover outlets with plastic plugs to prevent burns and electrocution.

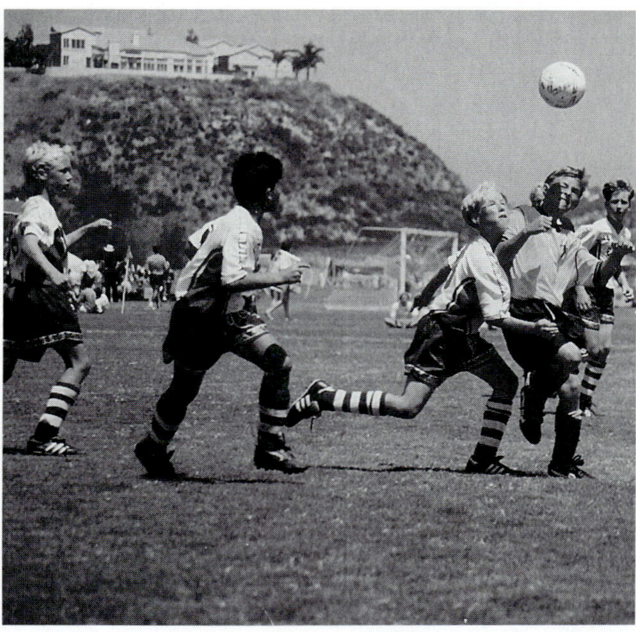

Fig. 22-23 With 11 million children playing soccer nationwide the incidence of injury during athletic competition and the incidence of injury resulting from overuse has steadily risen.

whenever possible (for example, use of child-protective caps on medicine-bottles and household products); (2) recognition and protection of a vulnerable host (young, inquisitive children, especially those with a history of injuries); (3) control of the environment or milieu by offering consistent discipline within a safe environment. Control of each factor can lead to control of the injury itself.

Sports participation. Serious injury can also result from sports participation during recreational sports and organized athletic competition (Fig. 22-23).

Nursing Alert

As a result of a higher level of competition at an earlier age, an increasing incidence of overuse injuries and other types of sports injuries are being seen in school-age children. Nurses play a role in advising parents regarding the selection of developmentally-appropriate athletic and recreational programs.

EDUCATION AND ANTICIPATORY GUIDANCE

All parents should be made aware of the dangers confronting children at each stage of their development (Table 22-14). Parents need to fully realize that normal children explore their environment and often do not have the cognitive ability to understand the consequences of their actions. Parents should know that fatigue, hunger, family discord, and anxiety increase the likelihood of an injury. A wise and loving parent knows that discipline is a fundamental prerequisite for injury prevention. Consistent discipline within a safe environment becomes the only reliable method of ensuring the child's protection. Parents must screen child care providers, coaching staffs, and camp personnel to ensure that safety and injury prevention is a top priority for those individuals who supervise their children.

All children and families should be instructed in safety. Community educational efforts aimed at injury prevention should include information on CPR; fire and burn prevention, including flame-retardant clothing, smoke detectors, fire escapes and drills; water safety; toy safety; approved automobile restraint devices; and the use and proper storage of potentially toxic household chemicals, medicines, cosmetics, tools, equipment, and firearms. The important influence of the media on child behavior should also be discussed, and participation in community education and intervention programs should be encouraged

The Injury Prevention Program (TIPP)

Anticipatory guidance for injury prevention should be an integral part of child health care. Recently the AAP initiated The Injury Prevention Program (TIPP), which is considered one of the most useful and practical approaches to preventing injuries in children. TIPP consists of a series of easy-to-use patient information handouts and questionnaires, designed for parents and for children through the age of 4 years. These materials provide the practitioner with printed, approved guidelines for injury prevention, organized according to the child's age and stage of development. TIPP is now considered a significant part of anticipatory guidance, which is recognized as being as much a part of routine health supervision as the history and physical examination.

Poison Ingestion

The most frequently ingested poisons include cosmetics, cleaning products, plants, analgesics (acetaminophen), mutivitamins with iron, cough and cold preparations, and birth control pills. Parental negligence may be directly responsible, as 90% of poisonings occur in the home. Approximately 10% occur in the home of grandparents or friends, the school setting, or in a health care facility. Most accidental poisonings in childhood are entirely preventable.

Each year, several hundred children die as the result of poisoning, and an estimated 500,000 to 2 million children are involved in poisoning incidents. A large number of accidental poisonings occur in children under 4 years of age, the "age of curiosity." These children are not selective about what they ingest. A number of nonfatal poisoning victims are left with permanent disabilities such as esophageal stricture or hepatic or renal damage.

Emergency supportive treatment

All poisonings in childhood are treated as an emergency. Supportive and symptomatic treatment should be initiated immediately, even though the specific poisonous substance may not be known.

POISON PREVENTION

Check the child's breathing. Ensure that there is a clear airway and fresh air is available. CPR or mouth-to-mouth resuscitation may be lifesaving. Initiate immediate irrigation and dilution of highly corrosive substances associated with dermal or ocular exposure. In the event of caustic ingestion, immediate administration of water or milk to irrigate or dilute the poison has been advised. After first aid has been administered, call the Poison Control Center or physician immediately and bring the child and the poisonous substance to a hospital emergency room.

Immediate management

The following immediate action should be taken in the case of poisoning:

1 Identify and remove the poison.
2 Administer the antidote.
3 Administer other supportive treatment.

Removal of poison. In most cases the immediate necessity is to empty the child's stomach, even if hours have passed since the ingestion. If not contraindicated, emesis should be induced if possible. After prevention, removal is the most important aspect of poison management. However, emesis should *not* be induced in the event of ingestion of corrosives (lye or strong acids), strychnine, or hydrocarbons (kerosene, gasoline, fuel oil, paint thinner, and cleaning fluid). Emesis

◆ TABLE 22-14
Injuries Common at Various Stages of Development

Typical Behavior	Type of Accident	Precaution and Safety Education
Infant		
Sleeps most of time	Suffocation	Use a firm mattress, no pillow; destroy plastic covers and filmy bags
Wiggles and rolls	Falls	Never leave child unattended on a surface such as a table or sofa; keep crib bars up
Helpless in water	Drowning	Never leave alone in bathtub or near pools
Sucks on objects	Choking, ingestion of foreign objects	Keep small objects out of reach, especially pins or other sharp objects; buy toys too large to swallow
	Poisoning	Keep medicines and poisons in a locked cabinet
Toddler		
Roams all over house Climbs into things	Falls	Use gates on stairways; keep windows and doors locked; fence yard
Takes things apart	Cuts	Provide large, sturdy toys without sharp edges or small removable parts; keep sharp instruments and knives out of reach
Curious about everything	Burns	Needs constant supervision; never leave hot coffeepot or running water unattended; turn pot handles inward; keep matches locked up; treat flimsy clothing with fire-retardant (7 oz borax, 3 oz boric acid, 2 qt hot water)
Pokes and probes with fingers	Electric shock	Keep electrical appliances out of reach; cap unused light sockets with safety plugs
Chews everything	Poisoning	Keep medicines, cosmetics, and household poisons out of reach
	Ingestion of foreign objects and aspiration	Keep small objects such as coins, beans, needles, pins, jewelry, and doll's eyes out of reach
Enjoys playing in water	Drowning	Keep away from unattended pools and ponds; stay with child while in bathtub; fence in bodies of water
Rides tricycle	Motor vehicle accidents	Be firm and instruct child to keep clear of driveways and out of streets
Likes to ride in car and wants to go everywhere with mother		Instruct child in proper car safety; keep car doors locked and use safety belts or other approved restraints; never allow child to sit or stand in front seat of a car or allow child to put hands or head out of window
Preschooler		
Ventures into neighborhood		Teach child safety rules and demonstrate principles by good example; enforce obedience Do not overprotect—preschoolers can begin to protect themselves, and overprotection deprives them of experience they need in growing up and learning independence
Inquisitive	Burns	Teach children danger of open flames and hot objects
Rides bicycle Plays ball	Motor vehicle accidents	Instruct them in proper traffic safety rules—look both ways before crossing street, walk, never run across street, go with traffic light and walk in crosswalk, and never dart into street to go after a ball

Continued.

◆ TABLE 22-14
Injuries Common at Various Stages of Development—cont'd.

Typical Behavior	Type of Accident	Precaution and Safety Education
Preschooler—cont'd.		
Climbs trees and fences	Falls	Teach them good footing and proper handholds when climbing
Enjoys playing in water	Drowning	Begin swimming instruction; never let child play around unsupervised pools
Plays rough; runs up and down stairs	Blows; cuts	Check play areas for hazards
		Store dangerous tools and equipment in a locked cupboard
	Poisoning	Teach child not to taste unidentified foods, especially berries
		Lock up poisons; store in labeled bottles
		Discard old medicines down drain before putting containers in trash
Early school age, 6 to 9 year		
Adventurous	Motor vehicle accidents	Needs intensive instruction in safety rules
Will try anything	Drowning	Encourage swimming safety
Loyal to friends	Falls	Point out importance of fun and not getting hurt
		Needs to know consequences for failing to follow rules
	Burns	Teach child to avoid smoldering fires; bottles and cans may explode and cause fatal injuries
		Teach child danger of matches and fires
		Teach proper use of chemistry sets
	Firearms	Point out serious consequences of playing with dry ice, fireworks, and other hazardous materials
Late school age, 10 to 14 year		
Rides bicycle constantly	Motor vehicle accidents	Enforce safety rules; explain reasons for them
Plays away from home, often in hazardous places	Drowning; burns; explosions	Know where child is at all times
Has lots of energy and enjoys strenuous play, sport injuries	Sprains; concussions	Point out importance of safe play; developmentally appropriate athletic programs
Enjoys working with power tools	Lacerations	Show children how to work around house safely (they should not use power tools unless tools are in good condition and they have knowledge of their use and safety); use proper equipment and keep it in good condition
Curious about firearms	Gunshot wounds	Lock up firearms and ammunition in separate locations
Increased availability of firearms		Monitor activities and peer group
		Increase parental involvement in all levels of education

also should not be initiated if the child exhibits a decreased level of consciousness or is convulsing.

Administration of 15 ml of syrup of Ipecac, followed by 1 cup of water is the most effective way to induce emesis in a child over 12 months of age. The dose may be repeated once in 20 minutes if vomiting has not occurred. The child's head and shoulders should be lowered to prevent aspiration of the vomitus. A subcutaneous injection of apomorphine is sometimes used in the hospital in lieu of syrup of Ipecac. An antidote such as naloxone (Narcan) must be given after vomiting has occurred to counteract the depressant effects of the apomorphine. Packaged in 1 fluid oz containers, syrup of Ipecac may be sold without a prescription. Parents should be carefully counseled at the 6 month well-child visit concerning poison prevention. Information regarding syrup of Ipecac should be emphasized so that parents may have it available for use if necessary. The shelf life of this product is 18 months. Therefore a new bottle should be purchased and the old bottle should be discarded at the appropriate time.

Gastric lavage is usually reserved for use when emesis is contraindicated or for the child who has not vomited after two doses of syrup of Ipecac. A gastric tube with a large lumen is inserted, and the stomach contents are aspirated first and then irrigated with copious amounts of physiological saline. Because of the time lapse in getting to the hospital and because the stomach normally traps material inaccessible to the lumen of the tube, chemical emesis is favored over gastric lavage. Specific measures can be instituted as soon as the particular poison is identified. In most cases of acute poisoning the physician can identify the agent by a quick history of the incident or by the label on the container. The poison container should always be brought to the hospital with the child.

POISON PREVENTION

The following recommendations should be explained to parents and other child care providers:

1 Household products and medicines should be kept out of reach and sight of children, preferably in a locked cabinet or closet. When a caretaker leaves the room however briefly, containers of such products should be moved to a safe place.
2 Medicines should be stored separately from other household products and kept in their original containers—*never* in cups or soda bottles.
3. All products should be properly labeled, and the label should be read before use.
4. A light should be turned on when one gives or takes medicine.
5. Since children tend to imitate adults, adults should avoid taking medications in their presence. Medicines should not be drunk from the bottle.
6. Medicines should be referred to by their correct names and *never* referred to as candy.
7 Medicine cabinets should be cleaned out periodically. One should discard old medicines by flushing them down the drain, rinsing the container with water, and discarding it.
8 Household substances in child-resistant packaging should be used. Prescription medicines should be contained in safety packaging. Safety features should be carefully resecured after use.

Poison Control Centers

Information about poisons and emergency treatment of poison ingestion may be obtained immediately by telephoning the nearest Poison Control Center. More than 250,000 toxic or potentially toxic trade name products are on the consumer market. Federal law requires that the ingredients of drugs, pesticides, and caustic products be clearly stated on labels. However, many household products frequently involved in accidental ingestions are not required to be so labeled. To assist health care providers with the problem of identification, Poison Control Centers have been established in key areas of the United States. These centers are usually associated with medical schools or large hospitals equipped with laboratories, library, house staff, and faculty. They are available to dispense information 24-hours a day. They also serve as treatment centers and are actively engaged in programs of public education to prevent poisoning. Parents should be instructed to keep the Poison Control Center number on their telephone. Callers may receive first-aid instruction and are advised to call the physician at once.

Administration of antidotes

Antidotes should be given immediately after emesis or lavage to render any remaining poison inert or prevent its absorption. Specific antidotes are not available for all poisons. Among the few available antidotes is dimercaprol (BAL, British antilewisite), which is a good antidote for arsenic, mercury, antimony, and lead poisoning.

Activated charcoal is a powerful physical antidote that adsorbs most poisons to itself. It effectively reduces the absorption of most substances. It should not be used with other substances, such as syrup of Ipecac, that may interfere with its adsorptive capacity or with which it may interfere. Large doses of adsorbent should be used. Optimal adsorption occurs when charcoal is administered in doses 5 to 10 times the amount of the ingested substance. Activated charcoal is usually administered in water and is available in 6- to 8-oz containers, to which water can be added. The antidote should be put in the Levin tube before the tube is removed from the stomach. The specific antidote is given, if one is available.

Overtreatment by emetics, sedatives, and stimulants is dangerous and should be avoided. Overtreatment may result in more harm than the ingestion of the poison. Keep the patient comfortable, warm, and dry.

Acute salicylate (aspirin) poisoning

Until recently, salicylate intoxication was the most common cause of poisoning in children. The decreased incidence of salicylate poisoning is attributed to safety packaging of aspirin including a limited number of baby aspirins per bottle, and increased public awareness of the contraindications of salicylate use in childhood. Approximately 50% of all hospitalizations for salicylate poisonings are caused by therapeutic misuse of aspirin, usually by a poorly informed parent.

Clinical signs. Clinical signs of salicylate poisoning include hyperpnea, with an increase in respiration depth, followed by severe acidosis, electrolyte imbalance, and dehydration. Other common symptoms include restlessness, extreme thirst, high temperature (usually 103° F or higher), profuse sweating, oliguria, tinnitus, tremors, delirium, convulsions, and coma. Cerebral hemorrhage may occur.

Treatment. The treatment for acute salicylate poisoning is always immediate emesis. Parents should attempt to induce vomiting as soon as the discovery is made. The physician or nearest Poison Control Center should be called for emergency instructions. The child is usually ordered to the hospital. The parents are requested to bring with the child any implicated container, loose pills, and, sometimes, the material vomited.

Emesis may be induced with syrup of Ipecac in the emergency room. After evacuation of the stomach, activated charcoal is administered. A blood specimen is immediately ordered to determine the level of salicylate intoxication (30 mg/100 ml invariably is associated with symptoms). Peak levels are usually reached about 90 minutes after ingestion. Treatment of salicylate intoxication is aimed at correcting electrolyte imbalance. Measures are taken to promote the rapid excretion of salicylates in the urine. Parenteral fluids are given both to combat dehydration and to facilitate prompt excretion of salicylates from the body.

Nursing care. Nursing care for salicylate poisoning is supportive. Fever may be reduced by cool sponges, hourly urinary output is recorded, and pH of the urine is tested with Nitrazine paper. Accurate hourly output notations help determine amounts of parenteral fluids necessary. Temperature, pulse, and respiration are checked every 15 minutes until stable; oxygen is given as necessary. Exchange transfusions or dialysis may be considered in severe, life-threatening intoxication.

Substance Abuse

Drug abuse is a growing social and personal problem in the United States. The average age of substance abuse victims is steadily dropping. The term *drug dependence* includes *addiction* (which implies tissue dependence, tolerance, and withdrawal symptoms) and *habituation* (which specifies the continuing nature of the drug-taking and implies psychological rather than physiological dependence). One may become addicted to heroin and other opium derivatives (narcotics), habituated to barbiturates, dependent on any of these or on psychedelic drugs (lysergic acid diethylamide [LSD] or mescaline), amphetamines, alcohol, marijuana, or tobacco.

The subject of drug abuse cannot be treated in detail in this text. However, students should acquire a beginning knowledge regarding assessment and treatment of this problem. Because of the severity and widespread nature of substance abuse, pediatric nurses will encounter this problem in a variety of settings.

Drug reactions vary. A heroin overdose produces a severe depression, whereas an amphetamine overdose results in hyperactivity and overstimulation. Violent psychological reactions, varying from hallucinations to severe psychoses (paranoia) may result from LSD use. A recent upsurge in the use of LSD (acid) is occurring. Phencyclidine (PCP or angel dust) and concentrated cocaine ("crack") abuse are also common. The severe impact of cocaine abuse is noted in pediatrics, with the birth of babies to addicted mothers or with the sequelae of abuse and neglect stemming from the parent's addiction.

Assessment

Nurses should be alert for any unusual behavior not typical of the individual or age group. Such signs include abnormal dilation of the pupils, excitability, talkativeness, profuse perspiration, staggering, mental confusion, disturbances in perception, and general personality changes. The nurse can best assist these patients initially by using a calm, supportive manner and a quiet atmosphere, carefully attempting to ground the patient in reality. Sincere concern by the nurse may help to motivate the child to willingly participate in rehabilitation. Care of the parent-child unit may mandate that the addicted parent obtain treatment.

Child Maltreatment (Nonaccidental Injury)

The term *child abuse* includes many types of physical, sexual, mental, and emotional molestation, injury, and neglect. Hundreds of children are killed annually, and thousands of others are permanently harmed at the hands of adults, usually their parents.

Affected children commonly manifest abrasions, lacerations, burns, skull fractures, intracranial bleeding, and multiple long bone fractures in various stages of healing, as well as personality disturbances and mental impairment. One type of child abuse in which the victim is characterized by severe physical injury and neglect was in the past called the *battered child syndrome.* Neglected, nonaccidentally injured children brought to the hospital are typically under 3 years of age and frequently are boys. Many times they are born out of wedlock, unwanted, mentally retarded, or physically malformed. The children are often too young or too afraid to talk.

The parents of these children are described as emotionally immature and unready to accept the responsibilities of parenthood. Child abuse occurs in all socioeconomic levels, but often the parents are burdened by adverse social conditions, financial strain, social isolation, and personal frustration. Some have reversed roles with their children, expecting the child to provide love, gratification, and fulfillment to meet their own needs. Most of these parents were abused themselves. They are repeating familiar parental behavior experienced in childhood and have not learned different coping mechanisms. Repeated abuse occurs in over 70% of abuse cases. Prompt and early recognition of child abuse may break the vicious cycle before permanent injury or death of not only the involved child but also his or her siblings results.

Recognition

When first admitted to the hospital, neglected and nonaccidentally injured children typically shut their eyes, turn their heads away, and cry irritably, in contrast to well-nurtured children who characteristically cry loudly and reach out for their parents. The skillful observer may recognize the difficulty when parents offer no reasonable explanation regarding the character, circumstances, or nature of the trauma sustained. The signs may be obvious or more subtle. Keen observation on the part of the health caregiver is critical.

Suspicion should always be aroused when any of the following are noted: extreme uncleanliness, malnutrition, multiple soft tissue injuries or burns in various stages of healing, and illness obviously caused by a lack of medical attention. Often the behavior of the child indicates that he or she has no real expectation of being comforted or helped.

Actual case presentation: A 2½-year-old boy entered the hospital to have his "right leg pain" assessed. He weighed 19 pounds, one front tooth was missing, a fingernail had been forcefully removed, his head and face were covered with skin lesions, and his right femur was broken. The only information offered by his mother was, "He was very clumsy and stumbled in the yard." Two weeks passed before he would turn to look at anyone. His parents visited once in a period of 2 months.

Protection

As part of public comprehensive child welfare services, most communities have established " protective services" for neglected and abused children. The purpose of a protective service is not only to provide care and protection for the child, but also to help parents who "want to be good" but for some reason are unable to assume their proper role. Why else do parents bring their neglected and battered children to the hospital? They always run the risk of punishment. Could an abused or neglected child be their way of actually asking for help? The emergence of self-help parent groups such as Parents Anonymous, as well as nationwide "hot lines," are a direct outgrowth of parents' need for help and anonymity.

Management of this serious problem may range from professional counseling and the introduction and explanation of various community services involved in child care (e.g., crisis nurseries and lay therapists [parent aides who may serve as role models and friends])—to criminal court action. Juvenile courts have power over "neglected children" but do not use criminal sanctions against the parents. However, when the case is reported, prosecuting agencies may institute criminal charges. According to recent studies, criminal prosecution is a poor means of preventing child abuse. Usually, criminal proceedings divide the family and cause parents to hate their children. Legal action is advisable only when all other means of protection and prevention have failed.

Reporting

Because parental neglect and abuse may be difficult to understand, the problems may go unrecognized. Children may recover from their injuries and go home, only to be battered again. The alert nurse is usually the first to suspect that a child has been abused. The nurse should carefully chart what observations and *report* the situation to the physician or child-protective services. Every state requires that nurses and physicians report suspicions to the police department or to the appropriate child-protection service in the community. After a written report has been submitted the case is carefully investigated. The person participating in good faith in making a report is immune from civil or criminal liability. Willful refusal to report child neglect or abuse is a violation of the law.

Prevention of Child Maltreatment

Nurses have the opportunity to observe the parent-child interaction in a variety of health care settings. Therefore, they may identify high-risk infants and children and potentially abusive parents. Prevention of child abuse is categorized as primary, secondary, and tertiary. Primary prevention includes methods that reduce the incidence of abuse in the general population before an abusive occurrence (e.g., public education regarding child-rearing practices, that promote improved parenting skills, and the identification of community resources and support networks). Secondary prevention focuses on the population who have been identified as high risk for child maltreatment. These interventions focus on protecting the infant's health and safety and the enhancement of healthy family functioning. Tertiary prevention or treatment involves situations where abuse has occurred. The goal is to prevent repeated abuse and its harmful effects on the child and family.

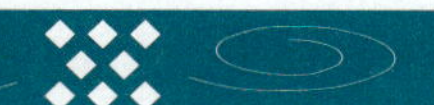

KEY CONCEPTS

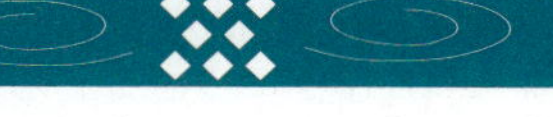

1 The normal infant's nutritional needs can be adequately met for the first 6 months by breastfeeding or iron-fortified formula plus vitamins. Cereal, fruits, vegetables, yogurt, meats, and finger foods are added gradually between 5 and 12 months of age (Winick, 1990).
2 Self-feeding is usually accomplished between 12 and 18 months of age.
3 All systems and tissues in the body depend on proper nourishment for their existence and maintenance. Food must perform three functions within the body: (1) provide heat and energy, (2) build and repair body tissues, and (3) regulate body processes. The following substances are essential to perform these functions: oxygen, water, carbohydrates, proteins, fats, minerals, vitamins, and fiber.
4 To determine how much food a child needs to meet energy requirements, it is necessary to know the child's metabolic rate.
5 The main role of fluoride is its ability to reduce the incidence of dental caries. If community water is not fluoridated, fluoridated water or supplemental fluoride should be given daily from birth until the eruption of all permanent teeth.
6 Iron is one of the most vital elements in the body and is required for growth.
7 Relatively large amounts of calcium are required for many vital functions in the body.
8 Vitamins act as catalysts in almost all metabolic processes and are vital to growth and good health.
9 Atherosclerosis, which leads to coronary heart disease, has its origins in childhood. A total lifestyle approach for health promotion and disease prevention is optimal.
10 With the exception of the Hepatitis B vaccine (HBV), immunizations begin when the infant is between 8 and 12 weeks old. Active, up-to-date immunization produces a degree of resistance in children, comparable to that which follows a natural infection.
11 All children between 15 months of age and puberty should receive the live rubella virus vaccine. A live attenuated mumps virus vaccine is recommended for all susceptible children over 15 months of age, especially preadolescent males and men who have not had the disease.
12 A routine, two-dose measles (rubeola) vaccination schedule is now recommended. A live measles vaccine may be given as early as 6 to 9 months of age, if exposure of the infant is probable. A second dose must be given at approximately 15 months of age.
13 *Haemophilus influenza* type b (Hib) conjugate vaccine is routinely recommended for all children at 2, 4, 6, and 15 months of age.
14 Human immune globulin has been clearly documented to be helpful in the prevention or modi-

fication of measles and viral hepatitis A, and in the treatment of certain antibody deficiencies.

15 The greatest threat to the health and well-being of children today is childhood injury. Continued emphasis has been placed on two particular approaches to injury prevention: (1) elimination of specific environmental hazards peculiar to different age groups; and (2) supervision of small children by adults, gradually to be replaced by training for safety.

16 Anticipatory guidance for injury prevention should be an integral part of child health care.

17 Childhood poisonings are preventable. Parents should be informed of precautions to reduce the risk of poisoning.

18 All childhood poisonings are treated as an emergency. Supportive and symptomatic treatment should be initiated immediately. The Poison Control Center or physician should be notified and specific measures instituted as soon as the particular poison is identified.

19 The most common substances ingested by children include cosmetics, cleaning products, plants, analgesics, cough and cold preparations, multivitamins, and birth control pills.

20 Salicylate (aspirin) intoxication is a cause of accidental poisoning in children. The treatment of acute salicylate poisoning is always immediate emesis. Nursing care is supportive.

21 Substance abuse by school-age children and adolescents is a major and growing problem in the United States. Nurses should be alert for any unusual behavior not typical of the individual or age group.

22 Prompt and early recognition of child abuse is essential to prevent permanent injury or death. Management of this serious problem may range from professional counseling and referral, to various community services, to criminal court action.

23 Every state requires that nurses and physicians report suspicions of child abuse to the police department or to the appropriate child protection service in the community.

CRITICAL THOUGHT QUESTIONS

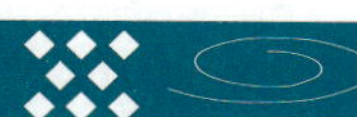

1 What are the important components of a comprehensive nutritional assessment and its implications for current and future health?

2 The parents of a 6 month old are attempting to initiate solid foods. Discuss the order in which solid foods should be introduced, and some of the concerns related to introduction of solids such as protrusion reflex, aspiration, allergies, and nutritional adequacy. How would you explain all of this to the parent?

3 Discuss the importance of immunizations and which immunizations are recommended for infants and children. How often are boosters required for tetanus? Where are immunizations available in your community?

4 Injuries are the leading cause of morbidity and mortality in children. What are the major types of injuries that occur at different ages and why?

5 You are working in a public school as part of a health screening team. You observe that one of the children has several bruises visible on his arms and face. What would you do with this information?

6 What is the primary, secondary, and tertiary prevention of child abuse?

REFERENCES

Dagnelie P et al: High prevalence of rickets in infants on macrobiotic diets, *Am J Clin Nutr* 51:202-208, 1990.

Advisory Committee on Immunization Practices (ACIP), Centers for Disease Control, *MMWR* 39:232, 1990.

American Academy of Pediatrics: *Report of the committee on infectious diseases,* ed 22, 1994, The Academy.

Dudek S: *Nutritional aspects of nursing care,* Philadelphia, 1993, JB Lippincott. US Dept of Agriculture: *Food guide pyramid: a guide to daily food choices,* Washington, DC, 1992, The Department.

Thomas CT: *Taber's cyclopedic medical dictionary,* ed 17, Philadelphia, 1993, FA Davis.

Williams SR: *Nutrition and diet therapy,* ed 7, St Louis, 1993, Mosby.

Winick M, editor: Nutrition, *Pediatr Ann,* 19(4):(entire issue), 1990.

Wong S: *Essentials of pediatric nursing,* St Louis, 1993, Mosby.

BIBLIOGRAPHY

Safety/Injury Prevention

The American Academy of Pediatrics: *Guidelines for health supervision,* Elk Grove Village, IL, 1992, The Academy.

Robitaille Y et al: Evaluation of an infant car seat program in a low-income community, *Am J Dis Child* 144(1):74, 1990.

Shovin JT et al: Near drowning: neurological evaluation is

your guide to managing near-drowning victims, *Am J Nurs* 89(5):680, 1989.

Thomson R: Helping to prevent accidents in the home, *Nurs Stand* 4(16):28, 1990.

Wintemute GJ, Wright MA: Swimming pool owners' opinions of strategies for prevention of drowning, *Pediatrics Immunization*, American Academy of Pediatrics: *Report of the committee on infectious diseases*, ed 23, Elk Grove Village, IL, 1994, The Academy.

Barness LA, ed: *Pediatric nutrition handbook*, ed 3, Elk Grove Village, IL, 1993, American Academy of Pediatrics.

Centers for Disease Control: Protection against viral hepatitis (ACIP), *MMWR* 39(RR-2):1, 1990.

Centers for Disease Control: Tetanus 1987-1988, *MMWR* 39(3):37, 1990.

Salerno MC, Jackson MM: What does the "national childhood vaccine injury act" require of nurses? *Am J Nurs* 88(7):1019, 1988.

Child Maltreatment

Aiken MM: Documenting sexual abuse in prepubertal girls, *MCN* 15(3):176, 1990.

Bullock LF, McFarlane J: The birth weight/battering connections, *Am J Nurs* 89(9):1153, 1989.

Chadwick D: *Color atlas of child sexual abuse,* St Louis, 1989, Mosby.

Daro D, McCurdy K: *Current trends in child abuse reporting and fatalities: results of the 1991 fifty state survey,* Chicago, 1992, National Committee for Prevention of Child Abuse.

Fontana VJ: *Save the family, save the child,* New York, 1992, Mentor.

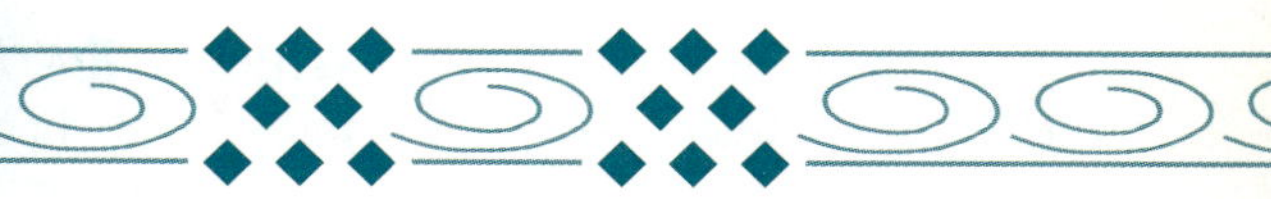

23

Diagnostic Tests Used in Child Health

CHAPTER OBJECTIVES

After studying this chapter, the student should be able to:

1. Describe the components of a typical complete blood count and urinalysis.
2. Identify what size of needle should be used for routine blood draws. State why smaller gauge needles should be avoided.
3. Discuss some of the advantages and disadvantages of the following equipment used to obtain venous blood specimens: winged infusion or scalp vein needles, eccentric tip blood-drawing syringes, and Vacutainer devices.
4. Identify special needs for capillary blood collection, the sites of choice, and the devices used.
5. Indicate which specimen tubes of blood must be inverted four to six times immediately after collection and which should be left undisturbed.
6. Describe how to collect a clean-catch midstream urine specimen.
7. Discuss comfort and safety measures for the infant undergoing a percutaneous bladder aspiration (bladder tap).
8. Describe how to initiate and collect timed urine and stool specimens.
9. Describe one of the correct methods of holding a young child during a lumbar puncture.
10. Discuss universal precautions and their relevance for specimen collection.

Diagnostic tests may involve the services of the clinical laboratory, the x-ray department, the operating room suite, or other specialized areas of health care facilities. Tests may also be performed in the nursing unit. The nurse needs to know the purpose of the test, whether patient preparation is necessary, the general procedure followed during the test, its effect on the patient, and the necessity for follow-up care.

APPLICATION OF UNIVERSAL PRECAUTIONS

The concept of universal precautions is a nursing care standard that is a result of the dangers of blood-borne diseases and frequent exposure of health care personnel to potentially contaminated body fluids. This precautionary approach assumes that every patient may be infected. Appropriate protective measures should be used while performing procedures involving possible exposure. Special signs appear in the rooms of all patients indicating what measures should be taken. The use of gloves, masks, gowns, or goggles may be necessary. For example, using gloves for a phlebotomy is required in most institutions. Strict adherence to universal precautions must be maintained at all times with every patient. Refer to Chapter 31 for an in-depth discussion of universal precautions as related to the prevention of transmission of infectious disease.

The tests described in this chapter are arranged in

table form and are grouped as follows: blood analysis, urine analysis, stool analysis, miscellaneous specialized tests, and x-rays. Diagnostic tests commonly performed in child health settings are described. Diagnostic tests used in obstetrics are discussed in Chapter 4. The norms of each test may differ from one hospital or clinic to another, even though automated or computerized laboratory techniques are used. Thus the nurse must consult the institutional procedure manual before administering any test.

BLOOD ANALYSIS (Table 23-1)

General Considerations

Most hospitals and clinics use specialists—phlebotomists—who are usually considered a part of the laboratory department. The phlebotomist's skills include a variety of specialized techniques for all types of blood specimen collection. However, the nurse, the licensed technologist, or the physician may collect specimens for testing purposes, depending on the needs of the individual patient. For instance, in many outpatient clinics or convalescent facilities the nurse is responsible for collection of specimens to be sent to a reference laboratory. In some states, regulations require that nurses and other personnel obtain a "blood-drawing certificate," indicating successful completion of an educational program that includes both theory and clinical experience.

Some blood specimens for chemical analysis must be collected after a period of fasting. Nurses should be aware of the test procedures that require fasting before blood withdrawal and take appropriate measures to ensure that such requirements are met. Orders for laboratory specimens to be drawn in the morning does not necessarily mean that food or fluids must be withheld from the patient. Individual tests differ. Water may be allowed in normal amounts for fasting patients for laboratory procedures. Blood specimens used for determining therapeutic drug levels are sometimes drawn at specific times, after the administration of a drug (e.g., gentamicin or tobramycin). Often two specimens—a "peak" and a "trough"—are collected to determine drug levels in the blood. It is extremely important for the nurse to indicate exactly when the drug was administered so that testing is accurate. The following blood specimens are frequently obtained.

Venous Blood Sites

Adults

Most blood specimens are obtained by venipuncture, allowing the relative ease of collecting large amounts of blood. The amount of blood to be drawn and the sites for collection may differ depending on the laboratory requirements and hospital policies. The most common site is the antecubital space. The back of the hand and the veins on the lower arm may be considered as alternative sites. The type of procedure to be used in collection depends on the expertise of the health care provider in obtaining such specimens.

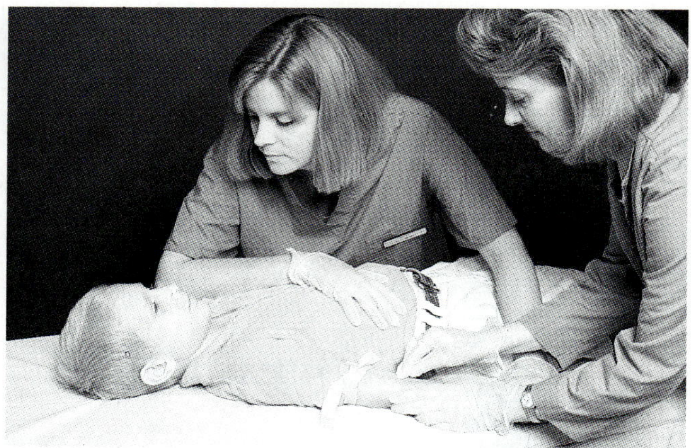

Fig. 23-1 Restraining child for extremity venipuncture. (From Wong D: *Essentials of pediatric nursing,* ed 4, St Louis, 1993, Mosby.)

Children—2 years or older

A venipuncture is usually performed if capillary puncture is impractical or unfeasible, because of the minimum amount of blood needed or the patient's status. Most often the antecubital area is used for the procedure, since the veins tend to be larger and closer to the surface. Veins in the ankle or the top of the foot may also be used. Policies and procedures of the individual facility should be used as guidelines.

Infants and children under 2 years

The physician may use jugular veins if large amounts of blood must be obtained in emergencies or cannot be obtained elsewhere. Often the placement of an intravenous (IV) device is a consideration. The IV insertion may be coupled with simultaneous blood collection. The nurse must be acquainted with the minimum amounts of blood needed for specific tests and the proper use of color-coded tubes for specimen collection (Fig. 23-1).

Equipment

Equipment varies with the procedure selected and the patient's condition (Fig. 23-2).

Tourniquet. Disposable, rubber tourniquets are

Text continues on p. 488.

◆ **TABLE 23-1**
Tests of Blood Specimens

Test	Purpose and Rationale	Preparation of Patient and Specimen	Special Considerations	Normal Value
Albumin, globulin, total protein, and A/G ratio (usually performed together)	To aid in diagnosis or evaluation of treatment of many diseases, including those of liver and kidney Blood may contain excessive globulin when albumin is abnormally displaced or lost, causing change in blood protein and A/G ratio	Fasting patient Specimen—minimum 3 ml clotted blood (red top tube); pediatric collection may be capillary blood in Microtainers		Adults: A/G ratio—1.5-2.5:1 Total protein 6-8 g/dl Newborn: lower levels
Antistreptolysin O titer (ASOT or ASO titer)	To aid in diagnosis of suspected rheumatic fever, although not specific for this disease Indicates antibodies formed from recent streptococcal infections	Nonfasting patient Specimen—minimum 3 ml clotted blood (red top tube)		<160 Todd units for 2- to 4-yr old 170 to 330 Todd units for school-age child
Arterial blood gases (ABGs)	To evaluate respiratory exchange and acid-base balance	Specimen—1 ml from arterial puncture or arterial line collected in heparinized syringe Blood gas evaluation may be performed by capillary collection in the nursery by use of special pipets Some facilities perform tests for venous blood gases as well	Place syringe (or capillary tube if from capillary draw) containing specimen in ice immediately and transport for analysis	P_{CO_2} 35-45 mm Hg P_{O_2} 75-100 mm Hg pH 7.35-7.45 Arterial, capillary, and venous blood have different normal values

Continued.

◆ TABLE 23-1
Tests of Blood Specimens—cont'd.

Test	Purpose and Rationale	Preparation of Patient and Specimen	Special Considerations	Normal Value
Bleeding time "Simplate"—disposable, controlled device and modification of Ivy bleeding time	To determine time needed for constriction of small blood vessels To evaluate patient's status when excessive bleeding might be a problem; frequent "T and A" screen To assist in diagnosis of bleeding disorders	Blood pressure cuff is applied and 40 mm Hg is maintained by placing a hemostat between bulb and cuff Incision device is placed laterally about 4 inches below antecubital area and triggered; stop watch is set Drops of blood are removed by allowing filter paper below area to absorb blood	Exact procedure necessary or results invalid Bleeding time is interval between triggering of device until bleeding ceases	Usually up to 11 minutes; Simplate (G-D) 2.75-8 minutes
Bilirubin serum—direct (conjugated)	To determine bilirubin levels; to prevent kernicterus	Blood must be collected from a heel puncture; two full microblood sampling tubes (size 0.3 ml) are collected	2 to 5 days after delivery	0.0-0.2 mg/dl
Blood counts Differential smear; "diff"—part of complete blood count (CBC)	Counts types of white blood cells (WBCs) present expressed as percentage with 100 WBCs counted Evaluates types, and abnormalities of WBCs, red blood cells (RBCs), and platelets (thrombocytes)	Nonfasting patient Uniform, thin smear made from capillary blood test Some smears made from anticoagulant tube (purple top) may show cell distortion	Morphology of WBCs, RBCs, and platelets is noted (size, shape, abnormalities)	Percentage patterns vary with age Adult: Neutrophils—50%-65%, increased during infections; eosinophils—1%-6%, increased in allergic conditions and parasitic infections; basophils—0%-1%, increased in some blood disorders; lymphocytes—25%-40%, increased in some viral and most bacterial infections; monocytes—0%-5%, increased during some infections Children: varied normal patterns according to age and maturity of child

			Infant: percentages of lymphocytes and neutrophils reversed Adult: Male—37%-49% Female—36%-46% Child (2-6 months of age): may be as low as 35% Newborn: 45%-65%
Hematocrit (Hct) or packed cell volume (PCV)—part of CBC	To determine relative percentage of RBCs in plasma Reliable screening test for certain anemias, hemorrhage, dehydration	Nonfasting patient Specimen—3 ml minimum venous blood; anticoagulant tube (purple top) may be performed by nurse, rather than in laboratory "Crit" centrifuge used with red top (heparinized) capillary tubes to collect capillary blood Height of RBC column is read on special graph and recorded as percent of total	
Hemoglobin (HgB or Hb)—part of the CBC	To determine amount of hemoglobin in RBCs available for transport in oxygen-carbon dioxide exchange Hemoglobin levels are proportional to red color in blood	Nonfasting patient Specimen—3 ml venous blood anticoagulant tube (purple top) Capillary collection by use of Microtainer	Newborn: 14.5-22.5 g/dl 2 mo: 9-14 gm/dl 6-12 yr: 11.5-15.5 g/dl Adult: Male—13-16 g/dl Female—12-16 g/dl Below 11—g/dl-iron deficient
Lead—whole blood	To rule out lead poisoning	Screen annually at well child visit	<10 μg/dl
Platelet count (thrombocyte)—not part of CBC	Platelets necessary for proper clotting To aid in diagnosis of diseases of clotting and bleeding To determine bleeding potential before surgery	Nonfasting patient Specimens—may be from 3 ml minimum anticoagulant (purple top); special capillary blood collection in infants usual; not done from blood smear	Methods and thus normal values may differ Usually 150,000-450,000/ mm^3

Continued.

◆ **TABLE 23-1**
Tests of Blood Specimens—cont'd.

Test	Purpose and Rationale	Preparation of Patient and Specimen	Special Considerations	Normal Value
Red blood cell count (erythrocyte or RBC)—part of CBC	To aid diagnosis of anemia type or effects of disease on blood cells RBCs carry O_2 to tissues and CO_2 from tissues Elevated counts indicate dehydration, cardiopulmonary problems, specific disease processes (e.g., polycythemia vera); low counts indicate anemias (cause usually needs more study)	Nonfasting patient Specimen—3 ml minimum venous blood; anticoagulant tube (purple top); special capillary collection by Microtainers		Adult: Male—4.5-5.5 million/mm^3 Female—4.1-5.1 million/mm^3 Child: usually 4.5-6 million/mm^3 Newborn: has higher RBC count than adult
White blood cell count (leukocytes or WBCs)—part of CBC	WBCs combat infectious organisms Blood levels usually elevated in bacterial infections and some viral infections High in most leukemias, other blood diseases	Nonfasting patient Specimen—3 ml minimum venous blood; anticoagulant tube (purple top) Special capillary collection by Microtainers		Adult: range usually 4,500-11,000/mm^3 Newborn: WBC averages 20,000/mm^3 at birth with counts as high as 38,000/mm^3 considered normal Infants: count usually falls with age and approaches adult values by age 3 yrs
Blood culture	To identify microorganisms that may be circulating in bloodstream Antibiotic sensitivity tests may be done if organism present Special media available emitting low-level radioactivity if organisms present; saves time in diagnosis	Nonfasting patient Specimen—special venous blood culture media; often performed when temperature spikes present Drawn under strict aseptic conditions before administration of antibiotics Requires laboratory incubation at 37° C (98.6° F) for organisms to grow	Area of collection must be cleansed with iodine preparation using careful aseptic technique Preliminary reports may be available in 36 hr Specimen may be collected aerobically or anaerobically (with or without air)—check with hospital procedure manual	Negative culture

Blood sugar (blood glucose)	To aid in determination of abnormal glucose metabolism; hyperglycemia or hypoglycemia caused by diabetes mellitus or insulin treatment as well as other diseases	Random, fasting, or timed specimens, depending on patient's needs and diagnosis Timed postprandial (after eating) tests are common Specimen—3 ml minimum venous blood; anticoagulant tube (gray top tube) Capillary collection may be done by Microtainer or even "crit" tubes if performed "stat"	Portable glucose monitors using special strips increasingly used by patients and staff Usually capillary blood and dipstick for Glucometers and Dextrometers	65-110 mg/dl fasting (Orthotoluidine method) but normals depend on timing
Blood grouping (ABO grouping)	To determine blood group for possible transfusion or maternal-newborn studies and ABO incompatibilities	Nonfasting patient Exercise extreme care in specimen/patient identification and collection Specimen—most often minimum 5 ml in clot tube (red top tube); rarely, additive tube, (purple top) is requested		Four main blood types found in US population: A—38% B—12% AB—5% O—45%
Rh factor (Rh_0 or RhD)	To determine blood type for possible transfusion and for maternal-newborn studies; identify high-risk mothers at beginning of prenatal care Although other Rh subgroups are potential problems, the most common source of difficulty is RhD (Rh_0)	Nonfasting patient Extreme care exercised in patient/specimen collection and ID Most often 5 ml clotted blood (red top tube) Rarely an additive tube (purple top tube) requested Usually performed concurrently with blood grouping		85% of Americans Rh+ (positive); 15% of Americans Rh– (negative)

Continued.

◆ TABLE 23-1
Tests of Blood Specimens—cont'd.

Test	Purpose and Rationale	Preparation of Patient and Specimen	Special Considerations	Normal Value
Blood urea nitrogen (BUN)	To determine kidney disease or urinary obstruction Urea, a waste product of protein metabolism, normally excreted by kidney; if urinary system fails, blood urea levels will be elevated	Fasting patient Specimen—3 ml minimum clotted venous blood in clot tube (red top) Capillary blood may be collected in Microtainer		7-20 mg/dl (depending on method)
Coombs' test	To monitor level of antibody formation in Rh-negative mother initiated by Rh factor from fetus entering mother's blood To help determine Rh status of unborn infant To determine need for prophylactic administration of RhoGAM to mother before delivery To assess need for treatment of newborn including blood replacement transfusion	Nonfasting patient Specimen—usually 5 ml clotted blood (red top tube) obtained from mother by venipuncture May be obtained from newborn as cord blood, by arterial line, or by venipuncture	Direct or indirect Coombs' test may be ordered, depending on purpose Mother's blood before childbirth—indirect Infant cord blood—direct	If direct Coombs' test negative and baby Rh_o (RhD) positive or D^u positive and mother is negative, mother is immune globulin candidate
C-reactive protein (CRP)	To aid detection of inflammation and tissue breakdown Nonspecific test, often for diagnosis of rheumatic fever and infarctions	Serum from a red top vacuum tube or capillary blood in a Microtainer, depending on specimen needs		Normally, no C-reactive protein present

Glucose tolerance test (GTT)	To aid in determination of abnormal glucose metabolism To plot a "metabolic curve" up to a period of 5 hrs, using blood glucose and urine glucose over required time to diagnose specific diseases	Fasting patient (high CHO diet 1 day before for validity) Specific dose of glucose given orally after fasting; blood and urine specimens obtained Specimens obtained at exact intervals (usually ½ hr, 1 hr, 2 hr, 3 hr, etc). after administration of glucose Normal amounts of water given to ensure collection of urine specimens Specimens—3 ml minimum venous blood in anti-coagulant tube (gray top) at precise times For children microtainers may be used "Crit" tubes (red top) are sometimes used when specimens are to be analyzed immediately	Adults: Prepared dose of either 75 or 100 g/dl water Commercial preparations made to resemble soft drinks Children: Dosage calculated according to body weight in lesser amounts of water Comparison with standard curves indicates various diseases Diabetes mellitus and liver and kidney diseases may be diagnosed	Peak of not more than 150 mg/dl blood and a return to below fasting level after 2 hours Glycosuria is abnormal
PKU (test for phenylketonuria)	To identify early excessive amounts of phenylalanine in infant for prevention of mental retardation by use of restrictive diet Metabolic disorder that requires adherence to restrictive diets throughout life	Capillary blood obtained 72 hr to 7 days after birth (should be after infant has ingested milk) Mothers birthing at home are urged to have baby tested at a specific time Requires saturation of five "dime-sized" circles on special paper with capillary blood; blood must saturate both sides of paper before examiner proceeds to next circle	Many states mandate test performance If tested before 24 hrs or elevated result, repeat test before 3 weeks of age Phenylalanine is not present in urine until third day in milk-fed babies	1.2-3.4 mg/dl phenylalanine level in serum. Above 8 mg/dl blood diagnostic of PKU

Continued.

◆ TABLE 23-1
Tests of Blood Specimens—cont'd.

Test	Purpose and Rationale	Preparation of Patient and Specimen	Special Considerations	Normal Value
Sedimentation rate (ESR, Sed rate)	To aid in detection of inflammation and tissue breakdown Nonspecific test; if rate is elevated, may point to rheumatic fever activity, arthritis, infections, infarctions, and cancer Usually elevated during pregnancy	Nonfasting patient Specimen—3 ml minimum venous blood in anticoagulant tube (purple top) Blood placed in a calibrated thin tube and level of plasma separation from cells in exactly 1 hr is expressed in mm/hr	Some methods provide a "correction factor" for anemia patients	Adults: Male—0-10 mm/hr Female, 0-20 mm/hr Children under 12 years; usually 0-20 mm/hr (Wintrobe)
Serology test for syphilis—STS (RPR, VDRL, TPI, ABS)	To aid in detection of syphilis Legally require before marriage in most states; routine test in prenatal examinations Performed on infants whose mothers show reactive result to test to detect congenital syphilis	Nonfasting patient Specimen—serum from 5 ml clotted blood tube (red top)	Reactive results should be handled discreetly Occasionally persons show reactive results throughout life when screening tests are performed, although not communicable after treatment	Nonreactive Because occasionally false positives may result from screening with RPR and VDRL tests, confirmatory tests are performed
T_4 (thyroxine) assay	Adult: to identify thyroid abnormalities Infant: to identify congenital hypothyroidism and prevent mental retardation	Specimen—5 ml minimum venous blood in clot tube (red top) Infant: cord blood or capillary blood collected in two blue top "crit" tubes	All infants should be screened T_4 levels of 4 μg/dl or less are tested for thyroid-stimulating hormone (TSH) TSH levels greater than 25 μg/dl are diagnostic for congenital hypothyroidism	After 1 month 4-11 g/dl 5 days—1 month 14-21 μg/dl Birth—4 days 14-23 μg/dl Cord blood 8-12 μg/dl

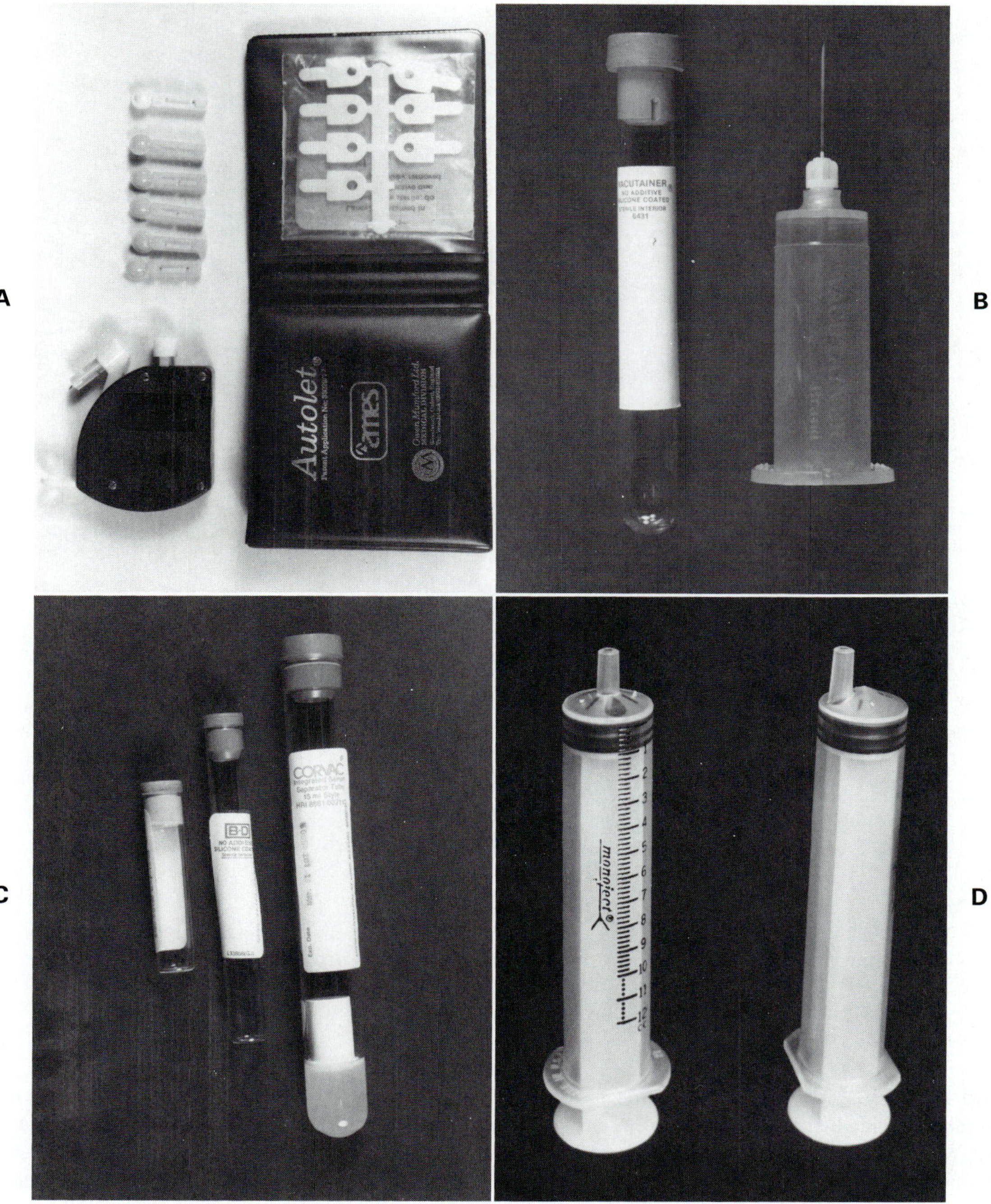

Fig. 23-2 **A,** Automatic capillary puncture device (Autolet) used by diabetic patients and nurses to secure small amounts of blood. Presterilized disposable blades encased in plastic are inserted before triggering. **B,** *Left to right,* 7-ml vacuum tube; vacutainer needle holder (shield) with multidraw needle in place. After penetration of vein, vacuum tube is pushed against needle within holder, causing rapid flow of blood specimen into tube. **C,** Three of several sizes of vacuum tubes used for blood collection. *Left to right:* 2- and 4-ml (used for pediatric specimens) and 15-ml tube containing serum separation material. **D,** *Left to right,* center tip syringe; eccentric tip blood-drawing syringe, which permits angle of entry at 0 to 10 degrees.

Continued.

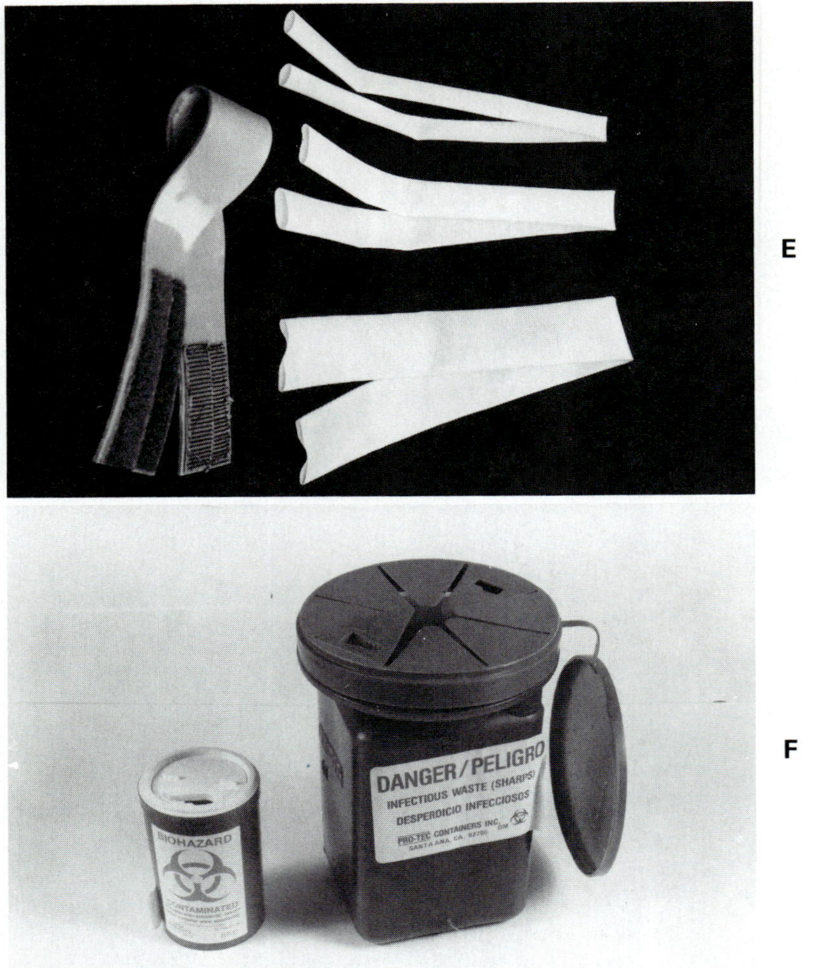

Fig. 23-2 cont'd **E,** Various tourniquets used to restrict venous blood return in preparation for venipuncture; three sizes of Penrose drains and one Velcro type. **F,** Containers used for disposal of "sharps" (needles, syringes, Butterflies, lancets, razors) before autoclaving and discarding. Note the symbol for a biological hazard.

recommended for most drawing procedures, since the amount of tension may be quickly and easily regulated. The wider, Velcro-type tourniquet is costly and more difficult to adjust. However, it is preferred by some health care personnel. Blood pressure cuffs are often used for difficult draws from infants and young children, reducing discomfort and trauma, as well as improving vein distension.

Antiseptic sponges. Current methods recommend presterilized, individually packaged alcohol preps rather than nonsterile cotton balls doused with alcohol. Alcohol is a frequently used washing, degreasing, and dehydrating antiseptic. When sterile collection of a *specimen* is important (e.g., for blood cultures), preparations containing povidone-iodine (Betadine) or chlorhexidine gluconate (Hibiclens) are often recommended. The nurse should inquire whether allergies to iodine exist before applying povidone-iodine.

Needles. Needle size is important in obtaining the best possible specimens with minimum trauma to the patient. Since blood-drawing procedures depend on specific patient and specimen needs, the choice must be carefully evaluated. Twenty- to 22-gauge needles should be used for most blood draws. A needle smaller than 22 gauge should not be used, with the exception of the 23 gauge TW (thin wall). Even if veins seem small and a preliminary evaluation might indicate the need for a smaller needle, reduced sizes should be avoided. The specimen obtained with a smaller needle will yield erroneous results because of undesirable hemolysis of red blood cells or small clots in the specimen itself. Also, the proper amount of blood may not be obtained because the system tends to occlude or "clot off."

Hypodermic needles. Hypodermic needles are used in conjunction with a tip syringe to make a complete unit for difficult draws. Usually a 1-inch, regular bevel needle is desirable, since penetration of a ½-inch needle into the vein is necessary to prevent hematoma formation.

Winged infusion devices. Winged infusion devices (butterflies or scalp-vein needles) are especially useful in drawing blood from pediatric patients, as well as adults with small or "difficult" veins. Most often a ¾-inch long, 23-gauge TW needle is used because it has the interior capacity of a 22 gauge. Its design includes two plastic wings that, when squeezed together, allow a flattened penetration. The needle is attached to a plastic tube. This tube is supplied with an adaptor where a syringe may be connected to provide suction. It is particularly helpful in properly filling pediatric-sized vacuum tubes (pedi-tubes). A syringe is attached to the adaptor at the end of the tubing and, after entry into the vein, the syringe plunger is pulled to begin the fill. Only 10- to 12-ml syringes may be used. Smaller syringes do not provide enough suction. Larger syringes fill too slowly, allowing the blood to clot before completion or causing the vein to collapse as a result of excessive suction. After obtaining the desired amount of blood, the butterfly needle is removed from the vein and inserted through the rubber top of a pedi-tube. The vacuum within the pedi-tube pulls the specimen from the syringe and into the tube. When larger tubes of blood are necessary a 20-gauge needle should be placed on the syringe after removing the butterfly adaptor, creating a greater suction that will not hemolyze the blood as it passes through the needle into the tube. By intermittently relaxing the pull on the syringe plunger during the draw the vein does not collapse and sufficient amounts of blood are secured. The flat entry of the butterfly needle causes less pain when hand veins or other superficial or small veins must be used. Children find this device less painful and threatening. It doesn't look as if they are getting a "shot," and, once placed, it is stable and needs no taping or support for blood collection. The butterfly is taped if it is to be used for IV administration after the blood collection is completed. A care partner is needed to comfort and assist the child, as well as to maintain position and keep the child still during the procedure.

Vacutainer-type needles. Vacutainer-type multi-draw needles are used for most adult blood collection. The procedure should be limited to adults and should be used only in the antecubital area and where no identifiable patient problem exists. Other procedures are better choices for collection from the back of the hand and the lower arm. Children find vacutainer needles intimidating, because the insertion and removal of tubes cause stress and sometimes pain. A special gasket on the portion of the needle entering the collection tube prevents regurgitation of the blood into the needle holder when the tubes are changed. This permits collection of sequential color-coded tubes without contamination of the reusable needle holder. However, the following limitations do exist with vacutainer needles: because the constant suction tends to cause small veins to collapse, it is undesirable for other locations such as the hand, wrist, or foot; because the angle of entry is greater than with other devices, more pain may result from draws where bony structures are close to the vein; hematomas may occur more frequently because the greater angle of entry may also be associated with accidental transection of the vein.

Vacutainer needle holders (shields). Plastic vacutainer needle holders or shields allow the use of a two-way needle, which is screwed into the shield. When the vacuum tube is inserted into the shield after the venipuncture, the stopper is penetrated and the blood flows into the tube. The shield (needle holder) does not become contaminated and can be used again. At some clinical facilities, however, the custom is to discard the needle holder after completion along with the needle.

Syringes. True blood-drawing syringes have an eccentric tip, permitting a flat angle of entry into the vein. They also have a very tight barrel-to-plunger fit, producing more efficient suction and specimen collection. Although a 20-ml size is available, the 12-ml size syringe tip is the most versatile and is compatible with pediatric-sized collection tubes.

Vacuum tubes. All manufacturers of vacuum tubes abide by uniform color coding of stoppers. The colors indicate the presence or absence of certain additives in the tubes. Since it is extremely important to choose the correct size and color for any given testing procedure a collection manual should be checked before use. The necessity of knowing the type of specimen to be collected (serum, plasma, or whole blood) and the specific color to be used cannot be overemphasized. The size of the tubes are 2, 3, and 4 ml in the pedi-tube sizes and 5, 7, 10, and 15 ml in regular sizes. Selecting the proper size tube and filling it adequately is necessary for accurate testing. Partially filling tubes is to be avoided; results of these tests are often erroneous. A much better procedure is to select a smaller tube and fill to the vacuum rather than put a small amount of blood in a larger tube.

Aftercare. After removal of the needle the puncture site should be elevated while firm digital pressure is applied for approximately 2 minutes to avoid hematoma formation. A Band-Aid or 2 × 2-inch sterile gauze square is usually recommended to keep the puncture site clean. The latter is often wrapped with an adherent stretch material. The use of such a material will help avoid a tape allergy reaction and skin injury at removal.

Disposal containers for "sharps" and other materials. Extreme care is needed in handling materials contaminated with blood or other bodily secretions. Needles are dangerous if not handled and disposed of properly. A needle cutter should never be used. Most hospital rooms have a disposable sharps container mounted on the wall at the patient's bedside.

Although universal precaution guidelines do not recommend recapping needles, this procedure is sometimes necessary when a needle must be covered promptly to provide safety when a disposal unit is not in immediate reach. The following is a suggested safe alternative to leaving needles uncapped.

1 Place the proper size needle cover on a flat surface with the open end toward you.
2 With your dominant hand holding the venipuncture device and your other hand behind your back, insert the needle into the cover, raising your hand to "scoop up" the cap. Hold the covered device in an upright position.
3 Use your nondominant hand to grasp the needle cover from the sides *(not over the tip)* to pull the cap down tightly.

In blood drawing areas, phlebotomy trays with rigid, puncture-resistant disposal containers for sharps are mandatory. An entire syringe and needle set-up or butterfly device is carefully inserted into the container. In many facilities the Vacutainer needle holder (shield) is reused, making it necessary to unscrew the needle and dispose of it separately. The tight fit of the contaminated needle and the needle's location make it too dangerous to remove with one's fingers. Some health facilities use special "sharps" disposal containers, equipped with plastic grippers to hold the needle while the shield is twisted off. At other facilities, employees use hemostats or small forceps to unscrew a needle after use. Some use the one-handed capping method, allowing a needle to be safely unscrewed with its cap tightly in place. Other materials contaminated with blood are placed in a special plastic bag labeled "biologically contaminated." See the symbol for biological hazards (Fig. 23-2, *F*). All of these items are then autoclaved before disposal.

Capillary Blood

Sites

In adults and older children the fingertip is frequently selected as the site for drawing capillary blood. In normal-sized children aged 6 months to 3 years the tip of the great toe may be considered. In infants the inner and outer sides of the plantar surface of the heel is the area of choice. The midplantar surface is avoided, since scar tissue formation may later interfere with walking. In rare cases the earlobe is used for small specimen collection.

Equipment

The "Autolet," or other trigger devices, are sometimes used when only a few drops of blood are needed. A sterile lancet may be used and is a satisfactory means of collecting capillary blood. It has a deeper predetermined depth of puncture. These "stickers" must be placed promptly into a special waste receptacle. Allowing them to become covered with paper tissues or bedding in cribs or Isolettes is dangerous. If a second "stick" is needed a fresh lancet should be used.

Collection devices include capillary tubes, Microtainers, and particular solutions for dilution of blood samples. Special slide preparations and certain specimen collection papers may be needed for specific tests.

Arterial Blood

Arterial blood specimens are primarily used for arterial blood gas (ABG) determinations and are taken from either the brachial or the radial arteries. The angle of entry is 45 to 90 degrees. The procedure is very different from venipuncture. A 22-gauge needle is fastened to a heparinized blood gas syringe. On completion of the collection the syringe and needle are immediately immersed in a cup of ice and taken at once to be analyzed. ABG analysis is not limited to arterial sources. In special care nurseries, capillary collection may be appropriate. Venous blood gas analysis is still performed in many facilities, although arterial collection is preferred. Special certification is required for arterial blood collection.

Nursing Considerations

Nursing care during specimen collection may consist of simply explaining the procedure to a child and helping in support and restraint. The qualified nurse may be responsible for the actual collection, depending on the certification needed and the hospital policy.

Blood specimens must be collected, labeled, transported, and checked into the laboratory properly. When actually drawing specimens the nurse must immediately invert those tubes containing anticoagulants four times to ensure mixture with the anticoagulant—*the nurse should never shake specimens.* Those tubes containing no anticoagulant (red top tubes) are allowed to clot, undisturbed, for ½ hour at room temperature. Labeling of the specimen with a stamped label is the responsibility of the person collecting the specimen. In smaller facilities a clearly printed, hand-prepared label may be acceptable. Labeling must be done in the prescribed manner before the specimen is removed from the patient's presence. Date, time of specimen collection, and phlebotomist's initials should also be on the label.

Written requisitions must accompany every laboratory specimen. It is imperative to check the patient's identification number with that on the requisition and on the labels made for the collection tube. The patient or parent is asked to spell their name to ensure correct identification.

URINE ANALYSIS

General Considerations

Urine specimens, except for bladder taps, are obtained by the nurse (Table 23-2). Specimens may be ordered with regulations concerning the preparation of the patient or the timing of the specimen collection. For a routine voided specimen, no special preparation is needed. The patient is asked to void into a clean container. Since children and some adults do not understand the word "void," terminology in accord with the age, education, and ethnicity of the patient should be selected. The patient should be told not to put toilet paper in with the specimen. If the patient is menstruating, a routine voided specimen will be of only limited value. A "clean catch" may be ordered or the test deferred until later.

For a voided "clean-catch midstream specimen,"

Text continues on p. 495.

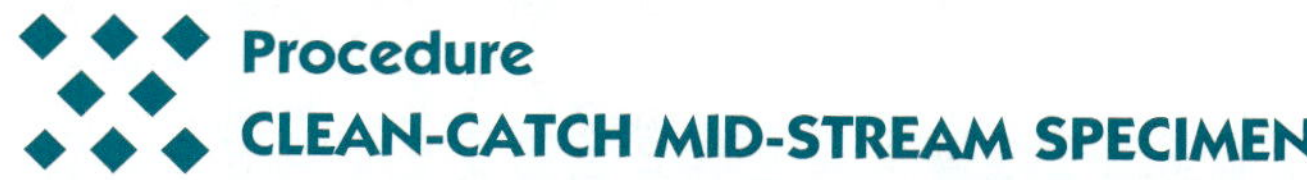

Procedure
CLEAN-CATCH MID-STREAM SPECIMEN

EQUIPMENT/SUPPLIES

- Six or more sterile cotton balls or sterile wash packets, gauze compresses, or four povidone-iodine prep packets if patient is not allergic to iodine.
- Povidone-iodine solution in squeeze bottle or bowl if sterile wash packet is not used (or four povidone-iodine prep packets), other antiseptic or soap solution.
- Water for rinsing the area.
- Paper bag or other waste receptacle.
- Sterile collecting container with a tight-fitting lid.
- Clean gloves.

PROCEDURE

For female patients the perineum is carefully cleansed with an appropriate product. The labia are retracted, and each cotton ball compress or preparation is used only once, moving from front to back. After cleansing with the antiseptic the area is rinsed with sterile water using compresses, cotton balls, or an irrigation technique. The labia are kept retracted if possible. After the urinary stream begins the collecting bottle is positioned to collect an adequate specimen and removed before the stream slows. Older patients may be able to carry out the procedure alone with proper instructions. Gloves are omitted if the patient collects the specimen. Younger patients may find it difficult to void when directed. Little girls may be washed off and placed directly on a sterile bedpan if unable to void with the labia retracted. Infants and toddlers must be "taped" for a specimen using a sterile plastic bag that adheres to the perineum with an adhesive. If the patient is well hydrated the request for a specimen is more easily fulfilled. A midstream collection kit includes everything necessary for the collection of sterile specimens. For male patients the glans penis is washed with antiseptic solution, and the foreskin, if present, is retracted to ensure proper cleansing (unless the infant is under 5 months of age). When the patient begins to void the container is positioned to collect an adequate specimen and removed before the stream dwindles. Older boys and young men may also desire to carry out the procedure unassisted.

To obtain a "three-glass specimen" (male patients) the glans penis is cleansed. Three sterile urine specimen bottles are labeled no. 1, no. 2, and no. 3. The patient begins the urine stream, voiding approximately 20 ml in bottle No. 1. Without interrupting the urine stream, he voids approximately 100 ml into bottle no. 2. Without interruption, he continues to collect the specimen in No. 3 until his bladder is empty. Assistance may be needed.

Catheterized specimen collection is used much less frequently because of the danger of infection. The female catheterization technique is described in Chapter 13. The urethra of the female infant curves downward. The catheter, therefore, should be inserted in a slightly downward direction.

A percutaneous bladder aspiration (bladder tap) specimen is usually obtained by a physician. If possible the patient is given some fluid approximately 20 minutes before the tap. The patient is placed in a supine position on a firm surface. The abdominal area is cleansed with an antiseptic. The puncture is made above the pubis with a 22-gauge (1-inch) or 21-gauge (1½-inch) needle with a 5- or 10-ml syringe attached to aspirate a specimen in a sterile manner. With female infants the labia are tightly closed, or pressure may be placed on the urethra to prevent voiding before the aspiration. The procedure should be delayed if the infant voids just before the specimen is scheduled to be taken. Afterward, pressure is applied digitally with a gauze sponge over the tap site. The site is then covered with an adhesive bandage.

◆ **TABLE 23-2**
Tests of Urine Specimens

Test	Purpose and Rationale	Preparation of Patient and Specimen	Special Considerations	Normal Value
Routine urinalysis				
Acetone* (to detect ketonuria)	To determine presence of ketones in urine, a possible sign of developing acidosis found as a result of diabetes mellitus, starvation, vomiting and diarrhea, or prolonged protein diet	One drop of urine placed on Acetest tablet, and after 30 sec color change compared with scale; or dipstick analysis (Diastix) may be performed	Though uncommon, urine specimens of diabetics may be free from sugar but contain acetone. This is usually the result of other concurrent problems	No acetone present normally
Albumin* (to detect albuminuria)	To detect loss of plasma albumin through kidney May indicate kidney disease, heart failure, drug poisoning, or toxemia of pregnancy	Dipstick analysis	Often done in conjunction with urine glucose test in prenatal checkups	Usually no albumin present; however, orthostatic or postural albuminuria sometimes occurs in absence of disease Albuminuria is common finding in newborn infant
Blood, occult*	To determine presence of free hemoglobin (hemolyzed cells) or intact RBCs	Dipstick analysis	Infections, injury, neoplasms, calculi—usual causes; hemolytic diseases also may cause presence	Normally none present
Glucose*	To detect presence and/or amount of glucose in urine, caused by diabetes mellitus; liver and kidney disease	Clinitest—follow directions issued with Clinitest tablets *carefully*; the 5-drop and/or 2-drop method may be ordered, depending on patient's condition; not specific for glucose, since other "reducing sugars" may give false-positive results	When performing Clinitest, observe reaction—rapid passage through green, tan, orange, and finally to dark shade of greenish brown indicates amount of glucose is over 2% in 5-drop method; continue testing with 2-drop method, which indicates up to 5% glucose	No glucose present Clinitest sensitive to other simple sugars (lactose, pentose); confirmation test done by dipstick if Clinitest positive
		Dipstick is specific for glucose—thus avoids false-positive results. May be used qualitatively for screening and positive color change noted without specific timing; precise timing must be done on second evaluation as a quantitative test	Do not touch tablets; store away from heat and sun; keep in dry place; replace lid tightly and immediately. Watch for "blue color and stickiness" in the tablet, invalidating results	

Gross appearance (color, clarity, odor)	To aid in estimation of degree of hydration and ability of kidneys to concentrate or dilute urine		Turbidity does not always indicate pathology; confirmation of cause of turbidity by microscopic examination	Color may depend on amount of hydration or medication given—may change greatly from one time interval to next Smoky urine may indicate hematuria
Cells (microscopic analysis)	RBCs and WBCs found in urinary tract disease in large amounts	Need 12 to 15-ml specimen of urine; sediment examined microscopically after centrifugation	Presence of a few RBCs or WBCs in voided specimen of mature female has little significance, since these results may be caused by vaginal contamination Recheck by clean-catch if large numbers present	Occasional red blood cell A few white blood cells (0-5) in female; 0-2 in male A moderate number of epithelial cells is inconsequential for females
Casts (microscopic analysis)	Casts usually represent abnormal sediment in urine; may be formed of several substances passing relatively slowly through tubules; presence usually indicates kidney disease	Specimen of urine sediment examined microscopically after centrifugation	Several types of casts; meaning differs with each type	Rare hyaline cast may be present; other types indicate pathologic conditions
Bacteria (microscopic analysis)	If large number present in fresh or refrigerated voided specimen, midstream clean-catch specimen may be ordered for culture	Specimen should be observed soon after collection or stored in refrigerator	Freshly voided specimens should be refrigerated within minutes to avoid bacterial growth	A few bacteria in voided specimen insignificant, especially in female patient No bacteria in catheterized or midstream clean-catch specimen
Specific gravity (sp gr)	To measure density of urine as compared with distilled water High specific gravity may occur in albuminuria, glycosuria, and dehydration Low specific gravity may reflect kidney's inability to concentrate urine or overhydration	Tested with a urinometer (calibrated float) or refractometer (TS meter or total solid meter) that needs only 2 drops and is more accurate than urinometer (Fig. 23-3) Be sure to clean and dry urine chamber of refractometer immediately after use; dipstick now also available	Detects presence of many dissolved substances, but does not identify them Also indicates patient's ability to concentrate or dilute urine when monitored with fluid intake/output records	Adult: 1.003-1.030 Newborn (after ingestion of milk): 1.002-1.010

Continued.

◆ TABLE 23-2
Tests of Urine Specimens—cont'd.

Test	Purpose and Rationale	Preparation of Patient and Specimen	Special Considerations	Normal Value
pH	To determine acidity or alkalinity of urine To differentiate acid urine from alkaline amniotic fluid to detect ruptured bag of waters	Strip of Nitrazine paper is dipped into urine, placed in a baby's diaper, or dampened by vaginal drainage; color change compared with scale Other dipsticks available Result <7 = acid Result >7 = alkaline (7 = neutral pH)	pH should be measured quickly because urine becomes alkaline on standing Sometimes alkaline urine is needed to keep excreted substances soluble (during sulfadiazine therapy or blood or tissue destruction), and therapy is directed to this end Acid pH is encouraged (medication or diet ordered to alter pH to kill bacteria requiring alkaline environment)	4.5-7.5 (urine is usually acid, but pH may vary, depending on diet, patient's condition, and age of specimen)
Vanillylmandelic acid (VMA—not a routine urine test)	To aid diagnosis of neuroblastoma and follow the response of therapy Urine measurements of vanillylmandelic acid (VMA)	24-hr urine specimen collected in refrigerated brown bottle with preservative hydrochloric acid; 2 days before collection diet restricted by elimination of bananas, ice cream, foods containing vanilla flavoring, and so on; no vigorous exercise on day before collection	Certain drugs interfere with test, discontinue 2 days before test Check hospital manual	0.5-7.0 mg/24 hr

*The dipstick analysis has become the routine screening procedure for the tests indicated. These strips also provide other essential information to the clinician not detailed here.

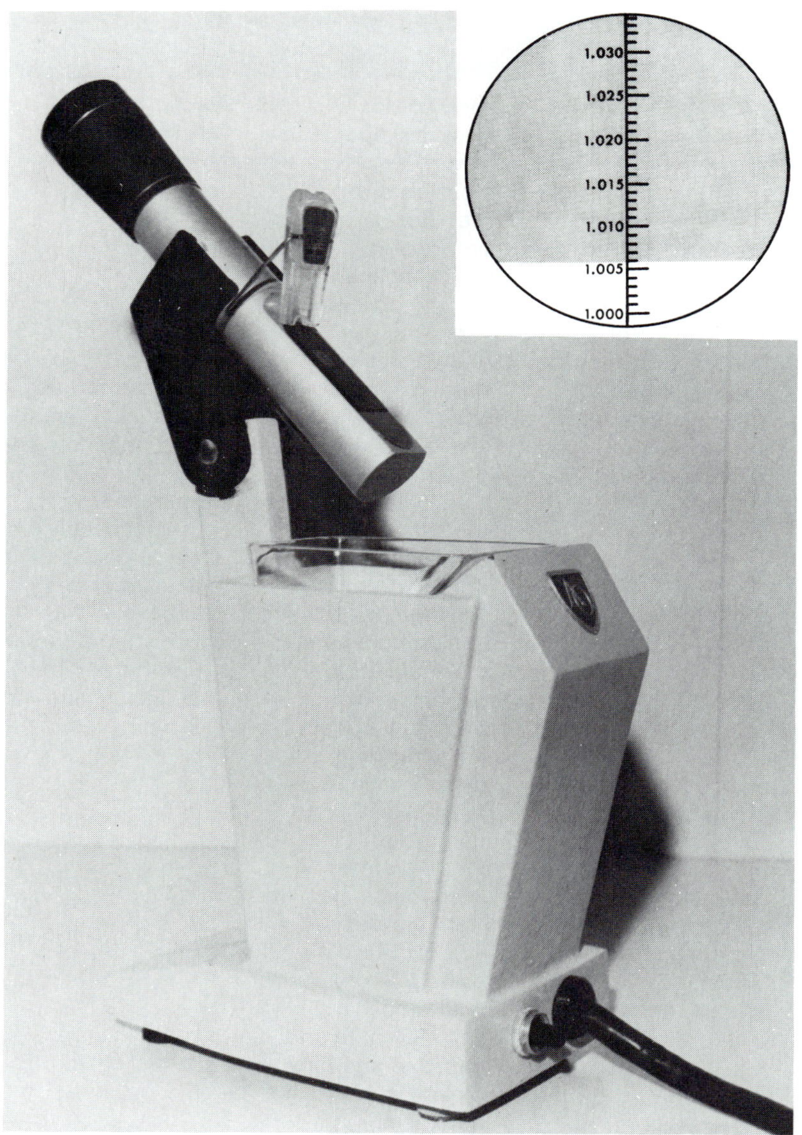

Fig. 23-3 One type of total solids (TS) meter or refractometer. *Inset,* What is seen on specific gravity scale with specific gravity of 1.006.

special preparations are made before the specimen is collected.

Timed specimens (the most common is a 24-hour collection) usually consist of voided urine, although it may involve drainage from a urinary catheter. To begin the specimen collection the patient empties his bladder and the time is noted. This first urine specimen is discarded. A large collection bottle of the type approved by the laboratory is labeled with the patient's name, the name of the health care provider, and the time the urine specimen was voided. This constitutes the beginning of the test. All voided specimens for the ordered period are collected in this single large collection bottle. Even if a special preservative is used the bottle is usually kept in a refrigerator or in a basin of ice unless instructed otherwise by the laboratory. At the exact end of the timed testing period the patient empties his or her bladder again. This specimen is added to the total collection. The total specimen is then sent to the laboratory. Since this specimen represents the total urine output of a patient within a known period the collection *must* begin with an empty bladder. The 24-hour urine specimens are more difficult to obtain in pediatrics.

◆ TABLE 23-3
Tests of Stool Specimens

Test	Purpose and Rationale	Preparation of Patient and Specimen	Special Considerations	Normal Value
Fat determination	To confirm diagnosis of steatorrhea (excess fat in stools), signs of celiac syndrome	Patient on normal diet 2 or 3 days before test Timed specimen usually ordered		Between 15% and 25% of weight of fecal sample
Occult blood	To detect presence of fecal blood, which is changed by process of digestion	Usually three random specimens used If test is positive, patient is placed on meat-free diet for 3 days and another specimen obtained. Positive findings may indicate presence of an ulceration/neoplasm in gastrointestinal tract; further testing procedures may be indicated	Diet containing meat may sometimes cause positive result, depending on method used Hematest tablets or Hemoccult prepared packets with developer are available Various amounts are reported as trace, 1^+, 2^+, 3^+, and 4^+	No occult blood
Ova and parasites	To aid in diagnosis of parasites or their eggs	Testing requires a fresh, warm specimen		
Timed stool specimen	To determine amount of certain substances excreted in feces in given time	Patient should not void or place tissues in bedpan with stool Determine date and approximate time of previous defecations; this will be start of test collection; refrigerate total specimen until complete and then take to laboratory		

Routine urine specimens should be properly collected, free of fecal material, labeled, transported, and checked into the laboratory with the proper requisitions. Urine specimens should be sent promptly to the laboratory unless protected from deterioration by refrigeration or a preservative.

Urine for culture may be obtained by midstream clean-catch or catheterization. Replace the lid immediately after collection and ensure that the inner sides of the container are not touched. This type of specimen should *not* be refrigerated but should be sent immediately to the laboratory.

STOOL ANALYSIS

General Considerations

Stool specimens are obtained by the nurse (Table 23-3). They may be obtained by collection from a bedpan or diaper for limited testing or by rectal swabs.

◆ **TABLE 23-4**
Miscellaneous Specialized Tests

Test	Purpose and Rationale	Preparation of Patient and Specimen	Special Considerations
Electrocardiogram (ECG or EKG)	To aid in determination of irregularities in electrical impulses controlling heart action and to help diagnose certain types of heart damage	Usually no special preparation except simple explanation; no pain involved Leads positioned on limbs and chest by technician	ECG on infant or child uses tiny electrodes often in place over long periods
Electroencephalogram (EEG)	To aid in determination of abnormalities in brain waves Useful in diagnosing convulsive disorders, brain tumors; estimating cerebral activity	Simple explanation Young children need to be sedated before test Testing takes about 1 hr; no pain involved Electrodes placed on scalp with adhesive substance by special technician in quiet atmosphere May need shampoo before and after test	
Fetal lung maturity Foam stability test (Shake test); positive result usually indicative of fetal lung maturity L/S (lecithin/sphingomyelin) ratio; 2:1, or 2, usually indicative of fetal lung maturity	To detect presence of surfactants denoting fetal lung maturity or possibility of respiratory distress syndrome	Amniocentesis necessary to secure sample of amniotic fluid for analysis	Used to best advantage to determine time of elective cesarean procedures
Lumbar puncture	To obtain cerebrospinal fluid specimens for cell count, protein and sugar content, culture, or Gram stain Spinal fluid glucose lowered in cases of meningitis Spinal fluid protein elevated in meningitis or subarachnoid hemorrhage WBC count moderately increased in encephalitis; greatly elevated in most cases of meningitis	Inform child just before procedure Positioning: place child on side with knees drawn up sufficiently to arch back, or in sitting position with spine curled forward to increase the space between vertebrae for needle insertion (Fig. 23-4) Child must be supported and maintained in position throughout procedure	Three specimens properly labeled, transported, and checked into the laboratory immediately Normal value in children: Pressure 70-200 mm of water Cell count 0-8 WBCs (under 5 yr) and 0-5 WBCs (over 5 yr), 0 RBCs Protein total 15-40 mg/dl Glucose 50-90 mg/dl

Continued.

◆ **TABLE 23-4**
Miscellaneous Specialized Tests—cont'd.

Test	Purpose and Rationale	Preparation of Patient and Specimen	Special Considerations
Sweat test	To help detect cystic fibrosis Abnormal amount of sodium chloride present in perspiration of affected persons Positive sweat chloride 60 mEq/L or higher Positive sweat sodium usually 10 mEq/L higher than sweat chloride	Pilocarpine iontophoresis: an electric current via attached electrodes drives pilocarpine into skin of forearm, stimulating local sweat production in about 5 min; a specimen of perspiration is then absorbed into gauze or filter paper; typical time for sweat collection is 30 minutes; sample is weighed and analyzed	
Magnetic resonance imaging (MRI)—No x-rays used; no risks of ionizing radiation	A combination of a strong magnetic field and radio frequency waves plus computer technology produce diagnostic images The interior of certain body parts can be studied from many angles with excellent imagery MRI is used most frequently for discovery or evaluation of CNS abnormality	Ask patient to void before Patient placed in tunnel-like body scanner with a special call button No movement allowed during scan Restless or claustrophobic patients may be sedated All metal objects (hairpins, belt buckles, snaps, zippers, coins, credit cards, jewelry, etc.) should be removed if possible: those that cannot be must be evaluated by radiologist before the scan Infusion pumps cannot be used in scanning room	Noninvasive technique; no known side effects Contrast media (if used) does not contain iodine Adverse reactions rare—consist of headache Objects containing iron may be affected by the magnet; patients with pacemakers, Holter monitors, shrapnel, etc., are not candidates for test Machine makes loud knocking sound; ear plugs may be offered

The specific procedure may be confirmed by contacting the laboratory.

Procedure

The stool specimen should be placed, with tongue blades, inside a properly labeled, clean, disposable, wide-mouthed container with a tight-fitting lid. The specimen must *not* be contaminated with urine. The specific test must be clearly indicated on the requisition, since many tests may be performed on the specimen. The entire specimen need not be sent to the laboratory unless a timed specimen is ordered or the reason for the stool collection is the

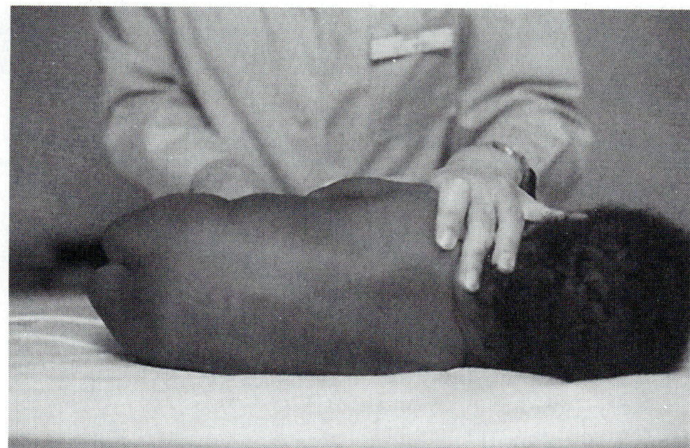
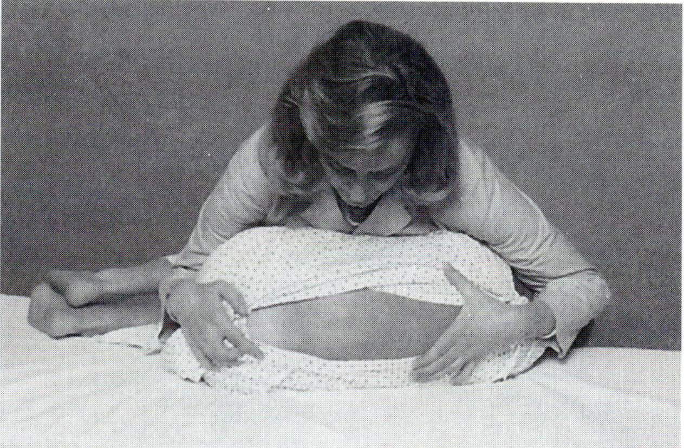
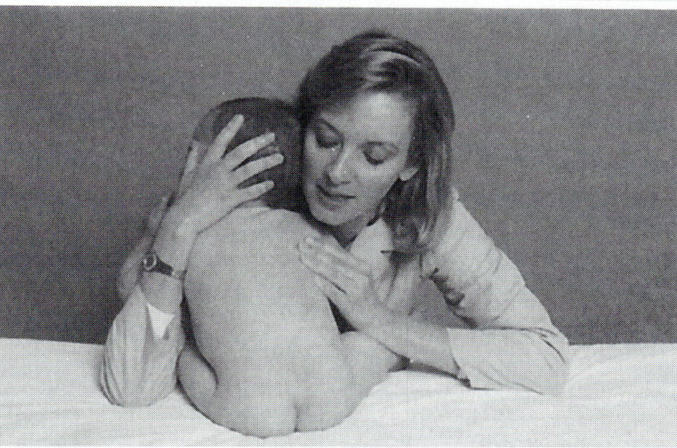

Fig. 23-4 Restraining a small child or infant for lumbar puncture. When an older child (2 to 3 years of age) is positioned, child's head may be tucked under elbow, and nurse may have to lean over the child to maintain positioning. (From Wong D: *Essentials of pediatric nursing,* ed 4, St. Louis, 1993, Mosby.)

detection of a tapeworm head (scolex). Specimens for ova and parasites should be sent to the laboratory soon after collection. If transport will be delayed, approximately 2 ml of stool specimen should be placed in polyvinyl alcohol (PVA) solution and the container sealed tightly. The balance of the specimen can go in a carton to the refrigerator to be sent to the laboratory when possible.

SPUTUM ANALYSIS

Occasionally, sputum specimens are requested for culture and sensitivity studies, cell analysis, Gram stain, or wet mounts. These specimens are usually difficult to obtain from young children. Even older children and adults, however, may find it difficult to produce sputum which originates in the bronchial tree. Specimens are best secured from cooperative patients after undergoing an IPPB treatment or chest therapy (cupping, vibration, and postural drainage).

For those who cannot cooperate the use of a sterile specimen trap connected to a suction apparatus has been helpful. Avoid saliva if possible. It is better to obtain scant material from lower areas than greater volume contaminated by saliva. For additional information on specialized tests and radiologic examinations, refer to Tables 23-4 and 23-5.

◆ TABLE 23-5
X-ray Tests

Test	Purpose and Rationale	Preparation of Patient and Specimen	Special Considerations
Barium enema* (BE)	To aid in diagnosis of lower bowel pathology by outlining colon with radiopaque material May be part of treatment for intussusception	Cathartics and cleansing enemas may be ordered on previous day or morning of test Clear liquid diet may be given 1 day before test until test completion Barium enema given in x-ray department when patient is under fluoroscope; examination takes 1 to 2 hr Enema or cathartic may be ordered after radiographs completed to remove contrast media	Note and record patient's bowel movements after procedure
Computed tomography (CT scan)*	To provide a visual display of abnormal tissue within skull; useful in diagnosing brain tumors	Possible IV injection of radioactive isotope	If isotope used, patient should be NPO Allergy to iodine may alter technique used
Cystogram*	To aid in diagnosis of urinary obstruction or other abnormality by visualization of bladder, ureter, and urethra with radiopaque material during filling and emptying of bladder	Urethral catheter inserted before procedure Bladder emptied Radiopaque material injected into bladder and radiograph taken Catheter removed	
Voiding cystourethrogram*		Radiographs taken during voiding process	
Ciné cystourethrogram	To determine whether reflux appears or increases at voiding pressure	Continuous fluoroscopic pictures taken during voiding process	
Gastrointestinal series (GI series)*	To aid in diagnosis of stomach and small bowel disease by outlining areas with radiopaque material	Night before test, patient may have light supper No food, fluids, or medications per orders X-ray department gives oral barium under fluoroscope Patient remains NPO per orders If 24-hr studies ordered, no enema or cathartic given until studies completed Check for enema or cathartic orders when test completed	

◆ **TABLE 23-5**
X-ray Tests—cont'd.

Test	Purpose and Rationale	Preparation of Patient and Specimen	Special Considerations
Intravenous pyelogram (IVP)*	To detect kidney or urinary disease by intravenous dye injection followed by abdominal radiographs	Cathartic or enema ordered on day before test Patient may eat light dinner with little fluid Fluids, food, and medications withheld after midnight Radiographs of abdomen taken before and after intravenous injection of dye by physician Fluids usually forced after completion of test to rid patient of residual contrast media	Allergy to iodine is contraindication to routine technique
Renal ultrasound	Noninvasive method of detecting genitourinary abnormality without radiation	None	None

*If the nurse is holding or positioning the child during the x-ray procedure, a lead apron must be worn.

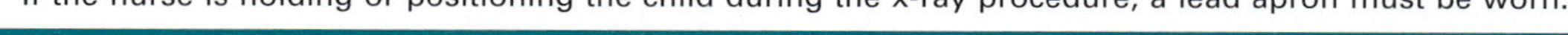

KEY CONCEPTS

1 Nurses should know the purpose of each diagnostic test, what patient preparation is necessary, the general procedure followed during the test, its effect on the patient, the follow-up care needed, and the importance of universal precautions.
2 Components of a typical complete blood count (CBC) include a hematocrit (Hct), hemoglobin (Hgb), white blood cell count (WBC), red blood cell count (RBC), and differential blood smears (diff).
3 The following types of blood specimens are frequently obtained: venous, capillary, and arterial. Most blood specimens are obtained by venipuncture.
4 Sites for venipuncture vary according to the patient's age and the amount of blood to be drawn. Equipment also varies but usually includes a tourniquet, antiseptic sponges, needles, syringes, gloves, and vacuum tubes.
5 Needle size is important to obtain the best possible specimens with minimum trauma to the patient. Only 20- or 22-gauge needles should be used for most blood draws. Smaller needles may result in a specimen that yields erroneous results because of unwanted hemolysis of red blood cells or small clots in the specimen itself. Also the proper amount of blood may not be obtained because the system tends to occlude or "clot off."

6 Winged infusion devices (butterflies or scalp-vein needles) are especially useful in drawing blood from pediatric patients. This is because the flat entry causes less pain, children feel less threatened because the device does not resemble a "shot," and, once placed, no taping or support is needed for blood collection.

7 Vacutainer-type needles, which are used for most adult specimens, should not be used for pediatric patients.

8 True blood-drawing syringes have an eccentric tip, permitting a flat angle of entry into the vein, and a tight barrel-to-plunger fit, producing more efficient suction and specimen collection.

9 It is extremely important to select the correct size vacuum tube with the appropriate color-coded stopper for any given testing procedure.

10 Extreme care should be used when handling materials contaminated with blood or other body secretions. Needles are especially dangerous if not handled and disposed of properly. Universal precautions should be observed.

11 The tip of the finger or great toe is frequently selected as the site for drawing capillary blood in children, depending on their age. In infants the inner and outer sides of the plantar surface of the heel are the areas of choice. A sterile lancet is the most satisfactory means of collection.

12 Arterial blood specimens are primarily used for arterial blood gas (ABG) determinations. The procedure is very different from venipuncture and requires special certification.

13 Blood specimens must be collected, handled, labeled, transported, and checked into the laboratory properly.

14 Specimens containing anticoagulants must be immediately inverted four times to ensure mixture. Those containing no coagulant are allowed to clot undisturbed for ½ hour at room temperature.

15 Routine urinalysis includes acetone, albumin, occult blood, glucose, gross appearance, cells, casts, bacteria, specific gravity, and pH.

16 Urine specimens may be obtained in various ways. Orders may regulate the preparation of the patient or the timing of the specimen collection.

17 For a routine voided urine specimen the patient simply voids into a clean container. For a clean-catch midstream specimen the perineal area or glans penis is first carefully cleansed. The specimen is then collected after the urinary stream begins, with the specimen container being removed before the stream slows.

18 A percutaneous bladder aspiration (bladder tap) specimen is usually obtained by a physician. In preparation the patient is placed in a supine position on a firm surface and the abdominal area is cleansed with antiseptic. After the procedure, pressure is digitally applied with a gauze sponge over the tap site. The site is then covered with an adhesive bandage.

19 Timed specimens must begin with an empty bladder. The first specimen, therefore, is discarded. All voided specimens for the ordered period are then collected in a single, large collection bottle, which is usually kept in a refrigerator or a basin of ice between urine additions.

20 Tests of stool specimens include fat determination, occult blood, ova and parasites, and a timed stool specimen evaluation.

21 Sputum specimens are requested for culture and sensitivity studies, cell analysis, Gram stain, or wet mounts. These specimens are difficult to obtain from young children.

22 Other specialized tests include: electrocardiogram, fetal lung maturity, lumbar puncture, sweat test, and magnetic resonance imagery (MRI).

23 X-ray tests include barium enema, brain scanning, voiding cystourethrogram, cystourethrogram, gastrointestinal series, and intravenous pyelogram.

CRITICAL THOUGHT QUESTIONS

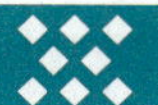

1 Collection of blood samples from children requires variable techniques. Which sites are used for venipuncture? Why are these sites recommended? What unique precautions must be taken when drawing blood from an infant or child?

2 How does the preparation of a pediatric patient for diagnostic tests differ from the preparation of an adult? Are the normal values for blood-based tests the same as they are for adults or do they differ?

3 Obtaining a urine specimen from an infant or child can present a significant challenge. What equipment is used to obtain urine specimens? What are the special challenges involved in collection of a 24-hour specimen?

4 What special considerations and precautions are involved in a lumbar puncture of an infant or child? How is the child positioned and restrained for this procedure?

5 X-ray diagnostic tests can be frightening and confusing to a child and family. How would you provide informational and emotional support?

REFERENCES

Behrman RE, et al, editors: *Nelson textbook of pediatrics,* ed 14, Philadelphia, 1992, WB Saunders.

Fischback R: *Laboratory screening and diagnostic procedures,* ed 5, Philadelphia, 1993, JB Lippincott.

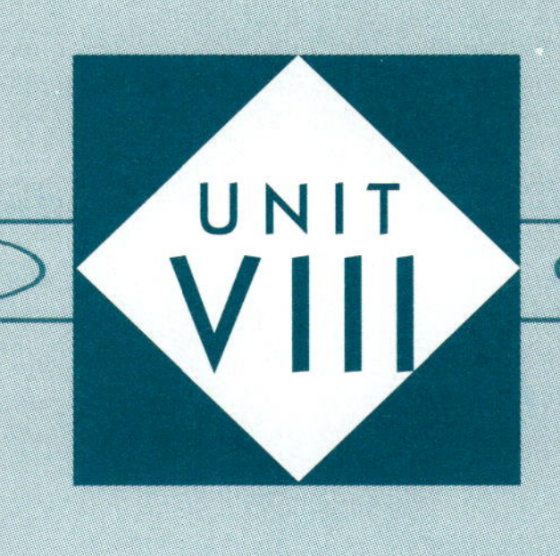

THE HOSPITALIZED CHILD AND FAMILY

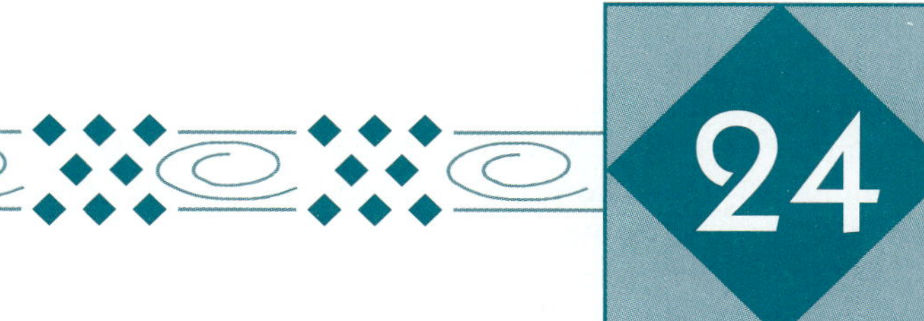

24

The Hospitalized Child

CHAPTER OBJECTIVES

After studying this chapter, the student should be able to:

1 Discuss factors that influence the child's reaction to hospitalization.
2 Describe methods that pediatric units and care givers use to reduce stress for the child and family when hospitalization is necessary.
3 Explain the three phases of separation anxiety.
4 Discuss three nursing principles that help children cope with hospitalization and explain how they may be implemented.

PREPARATION FOR HOSPITALIZATION

During the last two decades, a growing body of research has addressed the issue of the preparation of the child and family for hospitalization. Although a great deal remains to be learned, health care providers recognize that old approaches were unnecessarily traumatic for all concerned. Attempts have been made to shorten hospitalization, use special parent-care units, or avoid admission altogether by relying on day surgery departments designed for minor operations and recovery. When properly prepared and supported, families will assist the child in coping with the stress of hospitalization.

The Parents

Illness and hospitalization are frequently the first crises that children face with their families. Because children have few coping strategies to resolve the stress of hospitalization, it is critical to offer parents informational support so that they can provide emotional support for their child. They must receive sufficient information regarding the reason for hospitalization and the proposed treatment. It is also necessary for parents to have some understanding of the tests and treatments given to their child and the risk and discomfort involved.

Children's reactions to illness and hospitalization are influenced by parental reactions, the child's developmental level, previous illness experience, previous separations or hospitalizations, coping strategies, the seriousness of the diagnosis, and available support systems (Wong, 1993).

A child's morale will reflect parental attitudes and expectations. When parents are inadequately prepared, they cannot adequately prepare their child. It is extremely important that the parents have accurate information about the child's illness; confidence in their health care provider's recommendations; and knowledgeable, caring, and supportive nursing care.

The Siblings

A child's hospitalization is a stressful experience for the entire family. Siblings should receive accurate information regarding the need for the ill sibling's hospitalization. The siblings of the hospitalized child experience fear, worry, and loneliness. Siblings may use fantasy to substitute for a lack of knowledge about hospitalization, and what a child creates to substitute for reality can often be more frightening than the truth. When the situation is explained in a developmentally appropriate way, children can usually understand and cope with potentially serious situations. Open communication and education of all family members help to minimize the well siblings' misconceptions and fantasies about the ill child.

Sibling rivalry may be intensified because of the shift of family attention. When parents spend most of their time with the ill child, as they often do, the well siblings begin to develop feelings of rejection, abandonment, anger, and jealousy. Siblings should be encouraged to discuss their feelings with parents, and parents should be encouraged to help each child identify an extended family member or friend to be their support person during parental absence (Rollins, 1992).

Sibling visitation increases the parent's awareness of the changes older siblings are experiencing but not those of younger siblings. Parents often have a tendency to include older siblings in most aspects of the ill child's care, whereas younger siblings are given toys to occupy their time or sent to the playroom (Craft, 1991). Because most young children learn best through direct experience, they benefit by seeing the ill child in the hospital setting and using role play to help them understand and cope with the hospitalization.

The Child

For optimum coping, children should be told the reasons for their hospitalization in a developmentally appropriate way. The truth is less frightening to youngsters than the scenarios their imaginations invent. Children who are not given accurate information often believe that they are being punished for unacceptable behavior. Children must have confidence in their parents, health care providers, and other authority figures to feel secure in the hospital environment. The basis for a trusting relationship is initiated during the first year of life and strengthened or diminished through each stage of development. An honest, caring approach to the child and family is critical for the preservation of a trusting relationship during this stressful time.

Telling children about surgery is a highly individual matter and depends on the child's age, developmental level, temperament, culture, and ethnicity. A brief, simple explanation of what is wrong and what must be done to change or improve the situation helps the child develop effective coping strategies. A detailed explanation of the operation is not necessary and may confuse the child. Developmentally appropriate preoperative teaching helps to relieve tension and speed recovery, thus shortening the hospital stay. Pediatric units in hospitals throughout the United States have developed methods to prepare parents and children for hospitalization and various surgeries. Colorful booklets and pamphlets, telephone calls, hospital tours, preadmission orientation parties, movies, puppet shows, teaching dolls, and the use of educational television have lessened the trauma of hospitalization. Advising parents of procedures and inviting children and their parents to visit the hospital before admission help children to know what to expect (Fig. 24-1). Allowing the child to share in planning for a hospital stay or helping to pack a suitcase may be helpful.

Children should know in advance what the hospital is like. They should be told simply and in a matter-of-fact manner about such things as the differences between hospital beds and beds at home, use of the bedpan and urinals, bed baths, special classrooms, the playroom, and the food service (Fig. 24-2).

It is not always possible, necessary, or desirable for children to know everything that will happen. They need to know enough to assure them that what happens is according to plan and that their parents will be at their side whenever possible. When parents cannot be there, health care providers will provide a secure environment until their discharge.

Before admission parents will complete a health history information sheet including the child's diet, developmental level, temperament, habits, skills, likes, dislikes, fears, need for special blanket or toy (transitional object), and family composition. This information assists the staff in individualizing care.

Liberal visiting hours that include sibling visitation, rooming-in facilities, and appropriate parent participation in care make it much easier for parents to continue their supportive role and help counteract any sense of isolation or desertion the child may feel. No matter how well children are prepared for hospitalization, however, they may still cry at the prospect of separation and painful treatments. For an in-depth discussion of pediatric pain management, refer to Chapter 27.

The nurse should explain to the parents that separation anxiety is a normal reaction, and they should be encouraged to stay with their child when possible. Usually the parents' presence helps the child to cope with each stressor and greatly reduces the risk of long-term emotional trauma.

Nursing Alert

Some nonpharmacological techniques for the management of pain include: relaxation (holding, rocking, deep-breathing, massage), distraction (play, music, television, blowing bubbles), and guided imagery (help child to recall in detail a highly pleasurable real or pretend experience).

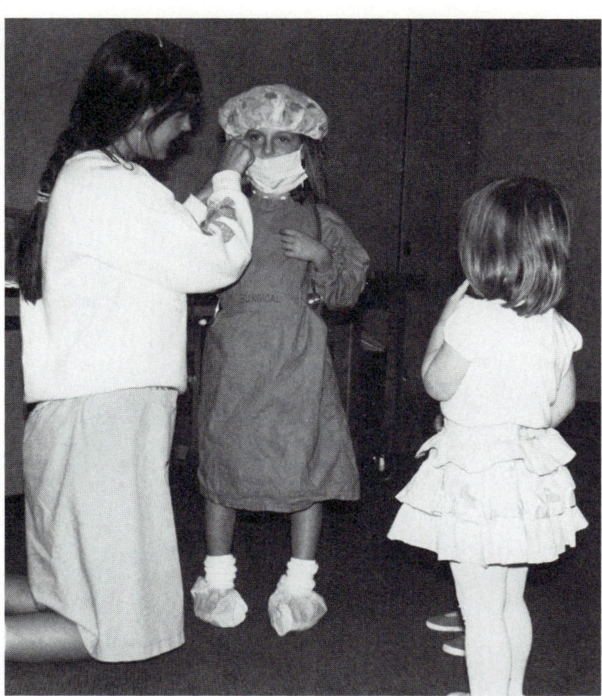

Fig. 24-1 Inviting children and their parents to visit the hospital before admission helps them know what to expect.

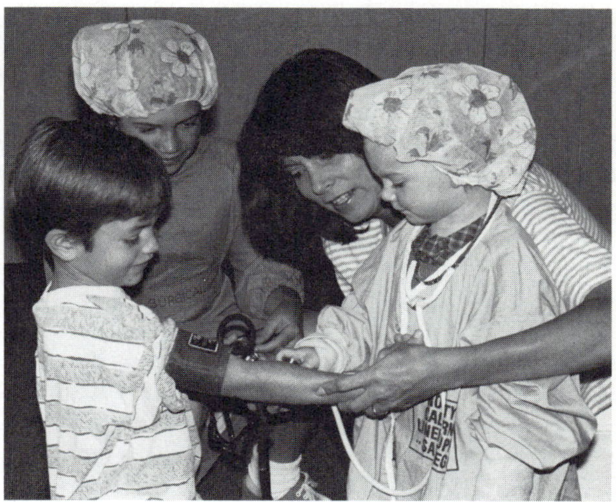

Fig. 24-2 A child who knows in advance what will happen is less likely to be shocked when facing the situation directly. (Courtesy Children's Hospital and Health Center, San Diego, Calif.)

AGE AND DEVELOPMENTAL NEEDS

The child's age and stage of development at the time of illness or hospitalization are prime factors in understanding the significance of the illness in the child's life. In addition, children come to the hospital with their own unique personalities, past experiences, and methods of dealing with anxiety. The nurse can encourage emotional growth by accepting these children as they are and by assisting them to continue in their present stage of development. For example, often young children are expected to conform to hospital rules by staying in cribs when they have had the run of the whole house before hospitalization. Unless acutely ill, a child may refuse to stay in bed. The nurse should not arbitrarily urge the child to "stay there." Children should not be confined to their cribs unless ambulation is contraindicated. For the toddler, limited mobility may lead to anxiety and hostility. When the basic motor urge is thwarted, the child becomes frustrated and angry and may regress or withdraw.

In general, when a child must be hospitalized, flexible and adaptive arrangements become necessary both to help maintain the family integrity and to respect the needs of the child and other members of the family. The nurse must try to provide the physical and social environment appropriate for the child's continuing development.

> **Nursing Alert**
>
> Risk factors that increase a child's vulnerability to hospitalization include: "difficult" temperament, lack of fit between child and parent, age between 6 months and 5 years, male gender, below average intelligence, and multiple stresses, such as repeated hospitalizations (Wong, 1993).

The Infant

During the first year of life, infants develop trust by having their needs met in a consistent, satisfying manner. Rooming-in accommodations are most desirable for the hospitalized infant and parents. The repetition of the same feeding routine, basic physical care by the parent or the same care provider provides a sense of security and trust that is vital to optimum development. An infant younger than 4 to 6 months of age may be content in the hospital, provided that the parent or nurse adequately fulfills these needs. By the time the child has reached the second half of the first year, however, the attachment to the parent or primary care giver is well established, and separation will be difficult.

When parents of a young child are unable to come to the hospital for prolonged periods, the hospitalized child is exposed to additional traumatic factors resulting in frustration of those inborn needs that are normally met in a family environment. Hospitalization interrupts the parent-child relationship and arouses the fear of desertion. As a result, the child may fail to thrive physically, socially, and psychologically. In extreme situations such as institutionalization, maternal deprivation may be manifested as a general marasmus or wasting away.

The Toddler

Considerable evidence has shown that under certain circumstances children may view hospitalization as desertion by their parents and thus may be profoundly affected by their hospital experience.

Children between 7 months and 4 years of age are most likely to suffer separation anxiety, with a peak incidence between 18 and 24 months. *Separation anxiety* tapers off beyond 5 years but never disappears entirely during childhood. Separation anxiety is characteristic of all young children who have established a healthy parent-child relationship.

The phenomenon of "settling in," or adjustment to hospitalization and separation, is deceptive. Children younger than 4 years of age experience three phases in the process of settling into the hospital: protest, despair, and denial. These emotional phases may not be as severe when pediatric policies are more enlightened, but they are probably still present. At first young children *protest* the separation (Fig. 24-3). They cry, scream, shake the crib, throw themselves around, avoid and reject strangers, cling to the parent, and are alert for any signs of the parent's return. The nurse may pick up the child and try to quiet him or her, but this approach is not successful. Telling children to stop crying only conveys to them that they are not understood and adds to their feelings of helplessness. This phase may last from hours to days.

During the phase of *despair* the child becomes depressed, sad, apathetic and withdrawn, signs often mistaken for acceptance (Fig. 24-4). Instead of crying loudly, the child sobs softly or is uncommunicative. The hope of parent's return fades, but the wish remains. During this quiet stage, distress seemingly has lessened, and the nurse presumes that the child is "settling in." When the parents arrive, the child may turn away and cry aloud. These children do not understand why they are in the hospital. They reject their parents in the same way that their parents seem to have rejected them. Parents spend most of the visiting time trying to get the child to respond to them more normally, and just as the child brightens up, the parents must leave again. Children crying when their parents arrive and depart may lead the nurse to mistakenly think that the child is better off without the parents.

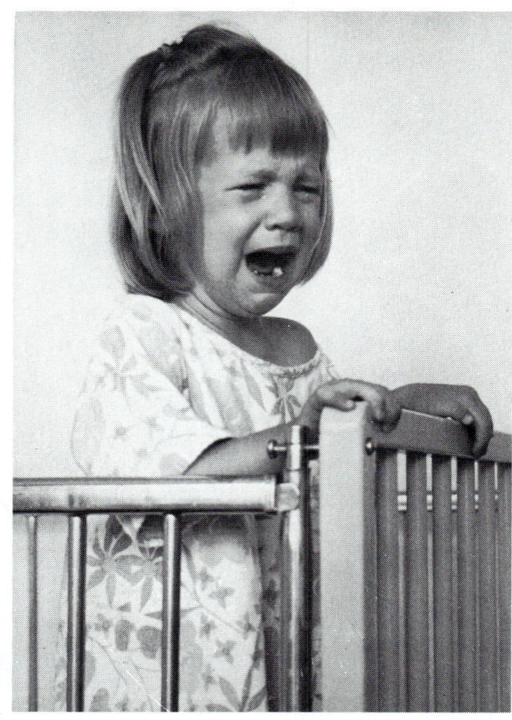

Fig. 24-3 Phase I: protest. First day after admission, child (2½ years old) cries aloud for "Mama," shakes the crib, and is alert for signs of her mother's return. (Courtesy Children's Hospital and Health Center, San Diego, Calif.)

The child may regress to an earlier behavior such as use of the bottle, use of the pacifier, bed-wetting, or thumb-sucking. The nurse, understanding the reason for these behaviors, can be of great help to parents who dread coming back because they anticipate their child's distress. The parents need to realize how much their child needs them, and they should be encouraged to stay with the child when possible. When they leave, they should be sure to tell the child when they will come back. It is unfair for parents to tell their child that they are going for a cup of coffee when they are actually leaving for the night. Children may lie awake all night awaiting their parent's return.

If the hospitalization is prolonged, the stage of *detachment* follows despair. Children begin to show more interest in the surroundings, are more responsive to nursing attention, interact with strangers, and appear happy. They may deny the need for their parents. When their parents visit, they may seem hardly to know them, may be happy and cheerful throughout the visit , and may even wave good-bye (Fig. 24-5). Psychologists have explained this phenomenon as the inability of young children to tolerate the intensity of distress, which causes them to repress the need for their parents. After these young children

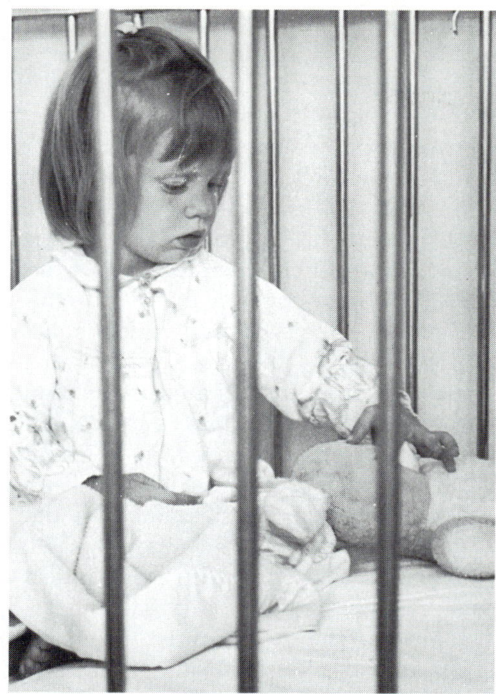

Fig. 24-4 Phase II: despair. Four days after admission, child has become apathetic and withdrawn. She does not understand why her mother has left her or why she is in the hospital. (Courtesy Children's Hospital and Health Center, San Diego, Calif.)

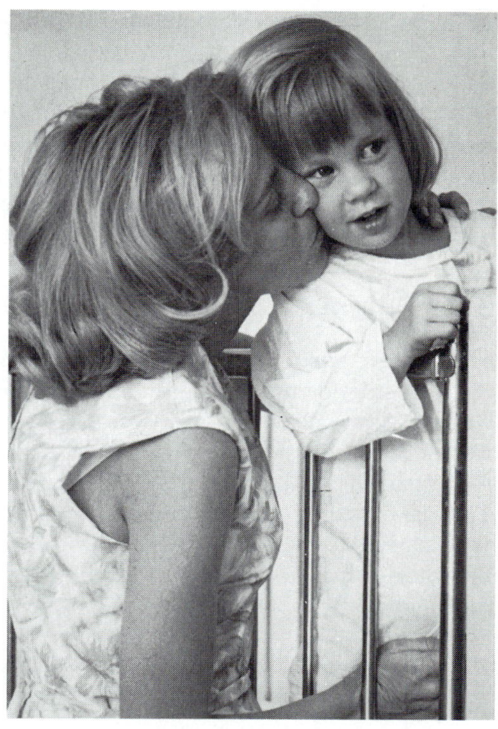

Fig. 24-5 Phase III: denial. Eight days after admission, the child cannot tolerate her intensity of distress so she represses need for mother. When her mother comes, she seems hardly to know her and is happy and cheerful. (Courtesy Children's Hospital and Health Center, San Diego, Calif.)

return home, however, they often demonstrate their disturbed feelings by regressive, clinging behavior. This reaction suggests that the behavior exhibited in the hospital was a superficial adjustment to loss.

The Preschooler

The preschooler demonstrates separation anxiety to a lesser degree than the toddler. The focus has changed from earlier separation fears and loss of love to physical integrity. Belief that illness is punishment for wrongdoing and fears of mutilation are expressed in the art and verbalization of the preschooler. The child is particularly sensitive to surgical procedures and bodily intrusion such as rectal temperatures, injections, and blood tests. If immobilized or confined, feelings of frustration and despair occur, which are often manifested by social withdrawal.

Preschool children struggle to understand and to assimilate the illness experience. Routine hospital procedures can be overwhelming. The taste of medicine, painful injections, radiography, and other hospital procedures are frightening. At times, parents are the only acceptable buffer between the child and the stress of hospitalization. The only really effective way to ease psychological distress is to provide overnight facilities for parents so that they can be with the sick child as often as possible. Without parental support, even if the child has been prepared, the preschooler finds hospitalization a terrifying experience.

The School-aged Child

School-aged children worry about having to give up their independence. To these children, health care providers are all-powerful. School-aged children ask questions about the disease process and its treatment. They are very aware that they are different and that uncontrollable things are happening to their bodies through illness or surgery. The child may experience self-blame for the illness and often perceives treatments and procedures as punishment. Imagination persists strongly throughout the school years. Like the preschooler, the school-aged child often fantasizes. Fears of mutilation influence the degree of emotional reaction. Nurses who encourage open communication and demonstrate caring and understanding are able to establish rapport with most school-aged children.

School-aged children cope fairly well if their illnesses are short and if they have supportive care providers who strengthen their coping strategies. These children have learned to rely on other adults and their peers when away from home through their school experience. They can understand that hospitalization is a temporary situation and that their parents may not be able to be with them at all times.

The Adolescent

Adolescents are particularly affected by the confinement and dependency inherent in hospitalization. The typical adolescent needs for independence, copious quantities of food, physical activity, and a peer group are hard to supply in a hospital setting. Adolescents may be more concerned about their separation from their usual activities and their peers than the absence of their parents. Thus the illness or accident is seen as a source of alienation. The teen may be afraid that illness or surgery will produce a permanent disability that will interfere with future participation in school, sports, social activities, and intimate relationships.

Illness and hospitalization at a time when the individual is dealing with major developmental tasks of independence, sexual identity, peer relations, and future job and career goals create additional stress. Although hospitalization may impede the accomplishment of developmental tasks, it may in some instances aid in their accomplishment. Whether hospitalization is ultimately a positive or negative experience for the adolescent is influenced by the knowledge, understanding, interest, and sensitivity of the health care providers (Craft and Denehy, 1991).

PLANNING NURSING CARE

While hospitalized, children should continue to grow physically, emotionally, intellectually, and socially in spite of illness. Three principles for nursing of children may be suggested to encourage their growth.

Maintain a Basic Sense of Trust

Whether well or sick, a child needs to feel secure. Maintaining a sense of trust is crucial. Experiences associated with the fulfillment of basic needs are prime sources for development and support. Parents are best able to fulfill their child's basic needs and give a quality of care that enhances trust and a feeling of security.

A sense of trust should be established between the nurse and the parent and child during the admission process. When admitting the child to the hospital, the nurse routinely checks the pulse, respiration, and temperature. During this procedure the nurse explains to the child what is being done and answers the parents' questions. Parents judge the nurse's ability to care for their child at this time.

When parents perceive the nurse as knowledgeable, caring, and gentle, a trusting relationship develops. Fears of their child's hospitalization subside, and they begin to trust and have faith in the nurse. Parents become relaxed and may even talk about their many difficulties. Worries about an operation, the cost of surgery, and uncertainty of the child's recovery are some of the problems they face. Although it is not always possible to remove all anxieties, the nurse can assist parents step-by-step to solve the concrete problems they face each day. Taking time to listen to them and to answer their questions often relieves many fears. Frequent rounds, easy availability, and a willingness to help and explain make parents more comfortable. The parents' feelings of confidence and trust carry over to the child. Gradually, as the child's health stabilizes, the nurse must provide sensory experiences and a safe environment for increasing mobility.

Protect from Fear, Frustration, and Pain

Children often are afraid of hospitals and fear what nurses and doctors might do to them. Parental threats of sending the child to the doctor as punishment confuse the child and help develop the idea that illness may be a punishment. The necessary diagnostic measures and treatment procedures may cause great apprehension and physical discomfort. The nurse can readily see from the responses of many children that illness imposes difficult emotional adjustments to unpleasant and painful experiences.

Unpleasant experiences can be minimized by giving the child every opportunity to talk about fears. Questions should be answered truthfully, simply, and patiently. Preparing the child emotionally for a procedure is helpful; however, a child should not be told of unpleasant procedures too far in advance to avoid activating fantasies and fears.

Because children are interested only in that which will affect them, information about a treatment must be focused on how they will feel and what they may do during the procedure. A painful procedure should be explained just before it is performed. Telling the child that the injection will hurt does not necessarily result in acceptance, but the fact that the nurse has been truthful demonstrates that she or he understands the patient's reactions. Honest explanations lessen a child's fears and strengthen trust and confidence in the nurse.

Protection against pain and feelings of distress promote constructive use of the hospital experience. Friendly and comforting hands, answering a child's cry, not forcing the child to eat, and not waking the child from sleep all are sound nursing decisions that enable the child to use inner strengths to get well.

Facilitate Social Contacts and Communication

Children who are hospitalized for a long time often become overdependent. The hospital stay may lessen initiative because satisfaction is gained from the nursing care. Physical restoration from illness is not enough. Adverse effects of extended hospitalization must be offset by educational opportunities in the hospital that provide experiences for growth and development. Often a child is socially immature because of the protective hospital environment. To combat the isolation illness may inflict, the child needs to be provided with experiences that are as comparable as possible to those experienced outside the hospital, the world of home, schoolwork, and recreation. These experiences include activities suitable to physical condition, which provide the companionship of children of the same age. A well-rounded program of guidance, instruction, and recreation will promote self-esteem and self-respect, encourage initiative, and help fulfill the needs of the whole child.

Self-care

Teaching the child self-care promotes independence and self-esteem in the hospital setting and in the home environment (Orem, 1991). It may be easier for the nurse to provide the care needed; however, teaching self-care and using a collaborative approach for the overall plan of care will be more productive and rewarding. For example, during the early morning period, which is a busy time in the hospital, many children can be taught to take care of their personal hygiene. Success is a strong incentive for every child, and the child who experiences success develops increased self-esteem and self-confidence.

With each assessment the nurse is confronted with questions about illness, body concept, and nursing and medical procedures. One essential aspect of a constructive hospital experience is to create a balanced, emotional climate in which it is possible to learn by asking questions. The nurse is uniquely qualified to educate the child and family about the human body and specific illnesses. Talking with the child and answering questions may calm specific fears and contribute to long-range education and development.

Instruction

The public school system is responsible for providing education for all children, including children in the hospital for extended periods. Pediatric hospitals should supply adequate space for educational facilities. The schoolroom should be large enough to accommodate a group of children in beds, wheelchairs, or carts. The nurse should arrange routine procedures and treatments to allow adequate time for a consistent educational program.

Play

Play is an integral part of the hospitalized child's plan of care. Play offers the child an opportunity for creative expression, diversion, and effective coping. In the hospital a supervised play program provides a warm, friendly atmosphere that will help the child continue to grow and develop. In larger hospitals a child-life specialist may coordinate the play program. A place to play, suitable materials, and other youngsters to play with are what children need. Because play is a child's way of learning, toys, materials, and equipment are learning tools. Paints, modeling clay, dolls, blocks, games, books, and toys are some of the materials with which children rebuild the world to their size—a world they bring with them of people, special belongings (e.g., blanket or toy), and feelings. Children play wherever they are. A child's play is his or her occupation just as surely as teaching may be the child's parent's occupation.

A play program should be designed to help buffer the effects of separation from family, feelings of isolation, and painful or frightening experiences such as intrusive procedures. Play promotes healing and helps the child to cope with stressful experiences. Children who fear treatments are helped to release their pent-up feelings in their use of dolls and other toys.

Case Presentation: Janie, age 5 years and confined to the hospital for chemotherapy, picked up her doll and said, "Don't cry Janie. It isn't your fault. Mommy is going to come every day to take care of you." Janie continued to role-play her fears, anxieties, and painful procedures throughout her hospitalization. Her transition after discharge seemed smooth and uneventful to her parents. Janie's use of her doll seemed to be an effective coping strategy.

The attitudes and feelings that children reveal in their play are full of meaning. Every opportunity should be afforded the hospitalized child to use play and other expressive activities to lessen stress, thus promoting healthy resolution of the negative aspects of the hospital experience.

PROLONGED HOSPITALIZATION

Long-term hospitalization imposes numerous anxieties on children of all ages. During a serious illness, even older children have a great need for their parents and can tolerate their absence only for short periods. They need to know that their parents will be there when they need them most and that they are loved and missed (see Chapters 20 and 21).

This discussion has highlighted the emotional and informational needs of the hospitalized child and family. It is reassuring to note that most children are able to survive the event of hospitalization without long-term negative effects. Nurses play a critical role in helping the child and family adapt to the hospital environment and cope with this family crisis.

KEY CONCEPTS

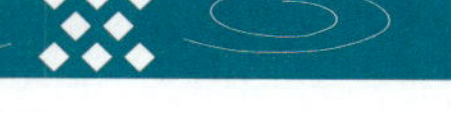

1 Three principles for the nursing care of sick children are suggested to encourage their growth: (1) maintain a basic sense of trust; (2) protect them from fear, frustration, and pain; and (3) facilitate social contacts and communication with the outside world.
2 A well-rounded program of guidance, instruction, and play promotes self-respect, encourages initiative, and helps fulfill the needs of the whole child.
3 It is imperative that parents are prepared for their child's hospitalization because they are best able to help prepare the child.
4 Siblings should be provided explanations about the hospitalization, should be allowed to communicate their feelings, and should be encouraged to visit their brother or sister.
5 In preparing for hospitalization, children should be provided with truthful explanations in keeping with their level of understanding, should be allowed to visit the hospital, and should be involved with planning for their stay.
6 The age of the child and stage of development at the time of hospitalization are prime factors in understanding its significance.
7 Children between 1 and 4 years of age are most likely to suffer when parent-child separation occurs. The three phases of separation anxiety are protest, despair, and detachment.

CRITICAL THOUGHT QUESTIONS

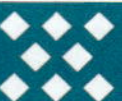

1 Regarding ages and stages of development, describe fears experienced by hospitalized children in each of these stages.
2 What techniques would you use to explain the hospital and hospital procedures to children in each of these stages?
3 How could you help reduce a parent's anxiety regarding the need to hospitalize a child?
4 Separation of parent and child is difficult, particularly if the child is ill. What are hospitals in your area doing to reduce this trauma for both parents and children?
5 Many young children who have been previously toilet trained experience bedwetting when they enter the hospital. Why does this regressive behavior occur? How would you explain this behavior to a parent?

REFERENCES

Craft M: Sibling reactions to hospitalization. In Craft M and Denehy J: *Nursing interventions with infants and children,* Philadelphia, 1991, WB Saunders.

Gillis A: Hospital preparation: the children's story, *Child Health Care* 19(1):19-27, 1990.

Orem D: *Nursing: concepts of practice,* ed 4, St Louis, 1991, Mosby.

Rollins J: Supporting the child. In Smith DP, et al, editors: *Comprehensive child and family nursing skills,* St Louis, 1991, Mosby.

Wong D: *Whaley and Wong's essentials of pediatric nursing,* ed 4, St Louis, 1993, Mosby.

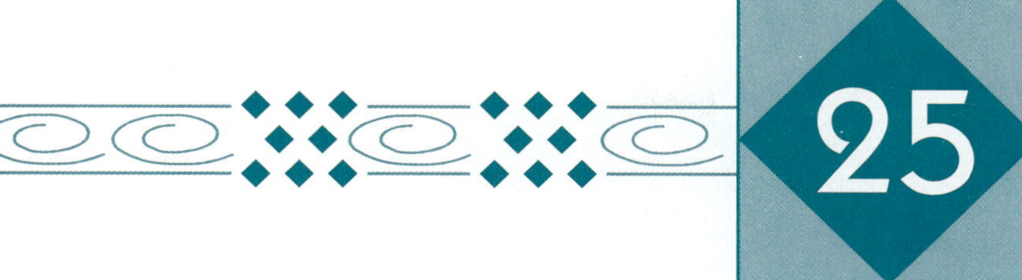

25

Hospital Admission and Discharge

CHAPTER OBJECTIVES

After studying this chapter, the student should be able to:

1. Describe the role of the pediatric nurse and discuss necessary qualifications.
2. Make a pediatric admission checklist that could be used to record the nursing assessment.
3. State how to properly select a blood pressure cuff.
4. Explain three ways in which an infant's blood pressure may be obtained.
5. Determine whether a pulse, respiratory rate, or blood pressure is within normal limits for a certain age group.
6. Describe how to obtain a urine specimen from an infant or toddler.

Hospitalization of a child may be a planned event with an orientation party or visit in advance of the admission. For many families, however, hospitalization comes as an abrupt, unscheduled, and frightening experience. A smooth admission process completed by a caring and knowledgeable nurse eases the family's transition into the hospital setting. The nurse ministers to the needs of both the child and family during the initial assessment. If the nurse gains the trust of the parent or guardian through the provision of informational and emotional support, anxiety will subside and the child's coping mechanisms will be strengthened (Fig. 25-1).

Equally important to the admission process is discharge planning. Discharge planning should begin as soon as the child is stabilized or the treatment is administered so that it is not a hurried, last minute effort. The following discussion is intended to help the nurse provide optimum care in both situations.

ADMISSION

Admitting nurses should first introduce themselves to both the new patient and the parents. In many hospitals, identification of the patient is accomplished through use of a bracelet, which should be checked for accuracy. The parent's surname may be different from the child's. This should be clearly noted to understand the family composition and prevent embarrassing incidents. To help the staff know their patients better, many pediatric departments send out questionnaires to the parents of prospective patients requesting helpful information regarding the developmental milestones attained, habits, likes, and dislikes of the child. Nicknames and special vocabulary used by the child are also recorded. Information regarding transitional objects such as special blankets or toys is also helpful.

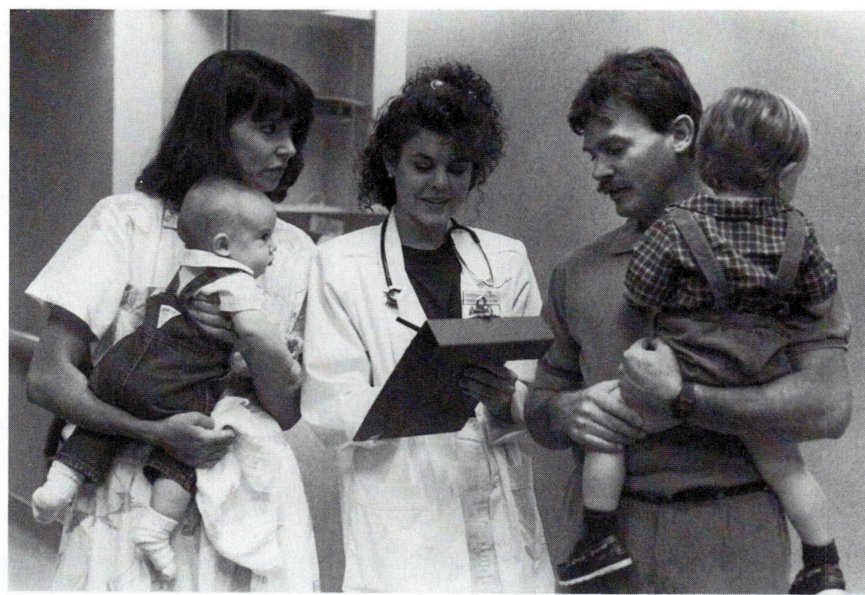

Fig. 25-1 Family accompanies infant to hospital for day surgery.

Qualifications of a Pediatric Nurse

The pediatric nurse should feel comfortable with children and should gain great satisfaction in promoting their health. Children can readily detect when nurses genuinely care. Conversely, they know when nurses are insincere. Those who find it difficult to work with children because of inexperience can learn to function successfully in a pediatric area if they are motivated, caring professionals. If their discomfort persists however, they may consider a different specialty. The pediatric area is emotionally taxing, since it is challenging to see a child and family suffer and to experience grief and loss; however, the vast majority of hospitalized children regain their health status.

With technological advances, health care providers in the pediatric setting confront ethical, legal, and philosophical issues created by complex circumstances. The nurse must be familiar with standards of care, hospital policies, and available resources.

Nursing care and effective communication must be based on accurate information gained from the patient assessment, medical record, primary nurse, clinical nursing specialist, nurse practitioner, nurse manager, nursing supervisor, or attending physician. Patient information is private and should be shared only with those directly involved with the child's care. Curious bystanders should not be given diagnoses, progress reports, or other information.

Finally, the pediatric nurse should be knowledgeable about child growth and development, family health promotion, common pediatric diagnoses, and the nursing process.

Parent-Nurse Partnership

For optimum child health promotion, the nurse and parents collaborate in the care of the child. The nurse has the advantage of practical and theoretical knowledge; however, the parents know their child best and are thus the experts. The goals of the pediatric nurse and the child's parents should be the same—to develop each child's optimum health potential. The family learns from the nurse, and the nurse learns from the family. The nurse is not a parent substitute, except in the parent's absence.

For the admission process parents may assist by undressing the child, positioning the child for temperature readings, helping with feedings, and providing comfort. After the admission the amount of parent participation in the care of the child depends on the child's health status and the parent's motivation and desire to be involved. Extensive, unrelieved participation at the bedside may produce an exhausted, worried parent, thus defeating the purpose. Instead, mutual participation enhances learning, strengthens the assessment, and prevents legal complications of parental care. The shared decision making of parent-nurse collaborative partnerships allows the nurse to provide more individualized care while increasing parental knowledge of their child's diagnosis and plan of care.

Some parents are unable to provide care for their hospitalized child due to lack of transportation, distance, or the need to care for other children. Others do not wish to participate. Occasionally, children may be more relaxed when the mother and father do not participate. Children may sense parent anxiety caused by possible feelings of guilt, inadequacy, or frustration, which may in turn cause them to be anxious. In certain cases the child may be confused about the role of the parent when the parents are at the bedside and the nurse must minister to the child. In this situation, asking the parents to take a break until the procedure is completed may benefit both parent and child. For the most part, however, the presence of parents is comforting to the child.

The liberal visiting privileges currently extended to parents in pediatric hospitals are designed to ease tensions, not create them. Nurses must be nonjudgmental regarding parent involvement and time spent at the bedside.

Orientation

If the circumstances of hospital admission and the patient's age and condition permit, the child and parents should be oriented to the unit and introduced to other children. Sharing information related to safety, such as the call system in the bathroom, is essential. The parents should be introduced to key personnel and shown where such conveniences as the public telephone, rest rooms, public dining area, and waiting rooms are located. Many children receive a simple toy such as a hand puppet or coloring book at the time of admission, which helps to entertain and to pass the difficult periods of waiting for examination or surgery. The nurse should be sure the child has something appropriate at the bedside for diversion. A safe transitional object (toy, blanket, or pacifier) may be brought from home. The nurse should make sure that any clothing or personal toys kept at the hospital are carefully labeled. In most cases the use of the child's own clothes, with the exception of bathrobes and slippers, is discouraged because of the high incidence of loss in the hospital laundry, despite attempts by the staff to avoid such confusion. The nurse should communicate with children at their developmental level for special introductions, serious talks, or mutual enjoyment.

Nursing Procedures

Patients are usually admitted directly to their own units. During the admission it is customary to secure the following:

1 Pertinent information regarding the child's family composition, habits, vocabulary, possible allergies, normal diet, history of childhood illnesses, current immunization status, and exposure to contagious diseases such as chickenpox, strep throat, tuberculosis, hepatitis, or human immunodeficiency virus. A brief description of current health problems, any ongoing treatment or medication schedules, and the child's preparation for hospitalization should be included. This type of information may be obtained on a form filled out by the parent while the admission is in progress, if it was not secured, before the actual hospitalization.

2 Height, weight, and, if less than 2 years of age, head circumference
   a. Infants are routinely weighed without clothes.
   b. Be sure that the scale is covered with a diaper or paper and is balanced before weighing.
   c. Many hospitals record the weight in both pounds/ounces and metric measurements.
   d This information is used to
      (1) Determine dosages of medications and anesthesia
      (2) Determine general condition and progress

3 Temperature
   a Electronic (rectal, axillary, oral, or ear) (see Fig. 25-2) thermometers are used depending on the policy of the hospital and patient care orders. The method may be altered, depending on the child's age, diagnosis, condition, and tolerance of the method.
   b Never leave a child alone with a thermometer in place (oral, rectal, or axillary). When rectal temperatures are secured, always have one hand on the thermometer and another on the child to ensure safety and accuracy.
   c. A glass thermometer should not be used for an oral temperature if the following occurs:
      (1) The child has seizures or poor muscular control. (There is danger that the child may bite the thermometer, causing self-injury.)
      (2) The child has difficulty keeping the mouth closed because of oral surgery, general condition, or breathing difficulties. (Mouth surgery itself may contraindicate oral temperatures.)
      (3) If the child is less than 5 years of age for safety reasons
   d. The following temperature elevations are defined as fever:
      (1) Oral and axillary temperatures above 100° F (37.8° C)
      (2) Rectal temperatures above 100.4° F (38° C)

   Temperature elevations should be reported promptly to the primary care nurse. Hypothermia is also significant; the infant is at greatest risk. Children with abnormal

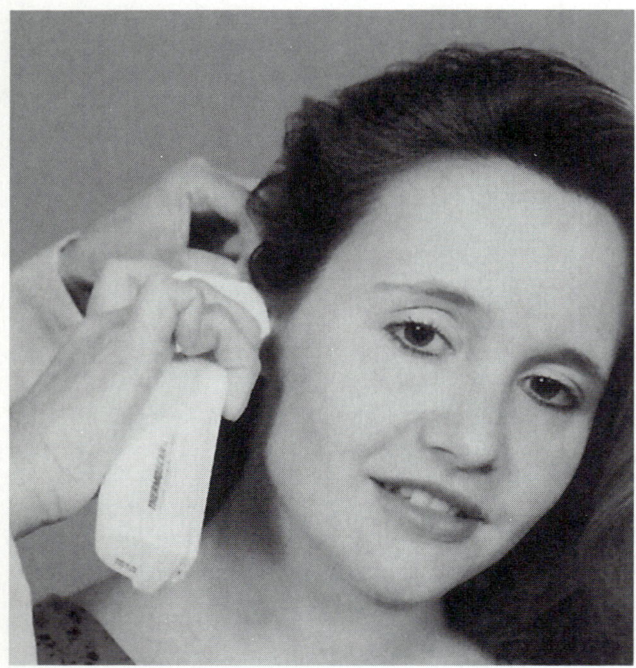

Fig. 25-2 Tympanic temperature measurement. (From Barkauska VH et al: *Health and physical assessment,* St Louis, 1994, Mosby.)

Nursing Alert

All children with diarrhea and vomiting or I&O problems are routinely weighed every morning before breakfast.

temperatures should have temperature checks more

e. Rectal temperatures are not generally recommended for children because of potential trauma and are contraindicated in young infants and persons with cancer, diarrhea, or rectal pathology.

Being consistent, minimizing trauma to the patient, and maximizing accuracy all should be considered when deciding on the best route for each patient.

4 Pulse
  a For infants the apical pulse rate is assessed by placing a stethoscope between the left nipple and sternum at the fourth intercostal space. It is too difficult to secure an accurate radial pulse rate using standard methods.
  b The radial pulse may be used with the older child.
  c Pulse determinations can be made by timing for 30 seconds and multiplying by 2, if the pulse is regular. In infants or if the pulse is irregular, the rate should be assessed for 1 full minute.

TABLE 25-1
Approximate Pulse and Respiration Rates at Rest Based on Age*

Age	Pulse	Respiration
Birth-1 mo	110-150	30-45
1 mo-1 yr	100-140	26-34
1-2 yr	90-120	20-30
2-6 yr	90-110	20-30
6-10 yr	80-100	18-26
Over 10 yr	76-90	16-24

*Pulse and respiration rates become slower with age.

  d Irregularity, quality, and rate should be noted.
  e The activity of the child should be taken into account. For example, it should be recorded if the child is sleeping.
  f For rate ranges see Table 25-1.

5 Respirations
  a The rate and character of respirations should be monitored for 1 full minute. The nurse should detect and describe wheezing and other respiratory abnormalities, such as sternal retractions.
  b For rate ranges see Table 25-1.

6 Blood pressure
  a The correct cuff size is very important. The cuff should cover two thirds of the upper arm measured from the shoulder to the elbow. The same cuff should be used consecutively if possible.
  b It is sometimes difficult to determine the blood pressure of an infant.
    (1) Infants should be supine.
    (2) The systolic pressure can be secured by palpation of the brachial pulse as the cuff is gradually deflated. This systolic reading is usually recorded over P (for example, 86/P).
    (3) A Doppler or arterial pressure transducer apparatus may be used. It provides both systolic and diastolic readings.
  c Any unusual activity of the child just before or during the blood pressure determination must be noted. Try to obtain a reading while the child is quiet.
  d The average blood pressure at birth is 80/46. For percentile readings for boys and girls ages 2 to 18 years of age, see Fig. 25-3.

Most children's blood pressures vary considerably. Charts may be used to compare the blood pressure readings with norms and

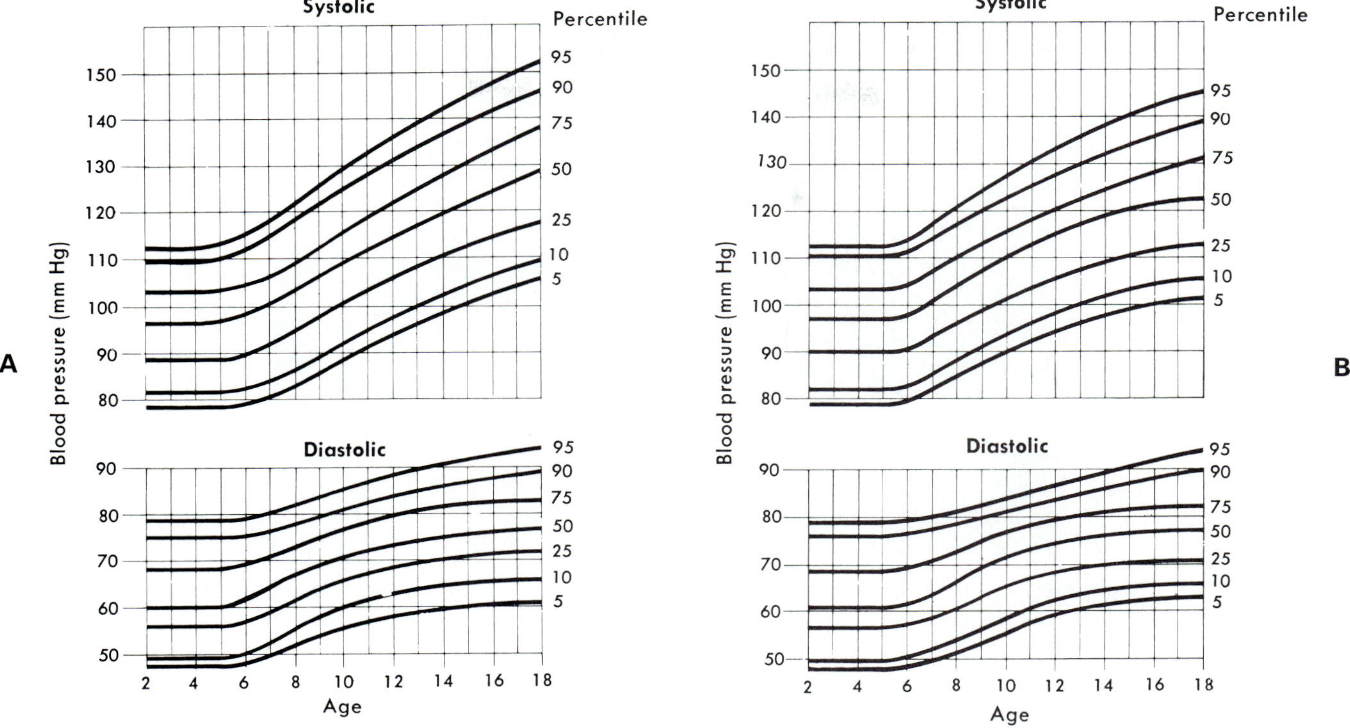

Fig. 25-3 **A,** Percentiles of blood pressure measurement in boys (right arm, seated). **B,** Percentiles of blood pressure measurement in girls (right arm, seated).

as a device for plotting blood pressure over time. Blood pressure measurements should be obtained and plotted at least once a year after the age of 3 years.

7 General appearance and behavior as evaluated through observation

- a Overall clinical appearance
  - (1) In no acute distress
  - (2) Mildly ill
  - (3) Severely ill
- b Growth and development
  - (1) Appropriate for age and gender of child
  - (2) Special physical considerations, such as orthopedic problems, vision or hearing loss, speech or language delay, malnutrition, obesity, cosmetic defects, prostheses (artificial eyes, limbs), surgically created stomas, history of seizures, dentures, glasses, contact lenses, hearing aids, and general health.
  - (3) Cultural, intellectual, and emotional considerations, such as cultural heritage (for example, Hispanic-American), gifted or delayed, parent-child-nurse interaction, temperament, and initial response to hospitalization
- c Skin manifestations
  - (1) Unusual color—flushed, pale cyanotic, or jaundiced
  - (2) Unusual birthmarks or scars
  - (3) Rashes, bruises, pustules, blisters, or possible infestations (body or head lice or scabies)
  - (4) Personal hygiene
- d Neurological system manifestations
  - (1) Level of consciousness
  - (2) Abnormally or unequally dilated pupils. Note PERRLA, the acronym for pupils equal round, reactive to light and accommodation
  - (3) Tremor, twitching, or periods of blank staring
  - (4) Bulging or sunken fontanels
  - (5) Limp, flaccid extremities
  - (6) Lower extremity weakness or paralysis, asymmetrical strength and tone
- e Other signs and symptoms important to note on admission
  - (1) Diarrhea, nausea, vomiting, or abdominal distention (type of stool or emesis)
  - (2) Nasal drainage or coughing
  - (3) Difficulty voiding, weak stream

The assessment phase of the admission process should be completed as soon as the child arrives on the pediatric unit. The specific reason for hospital admis-

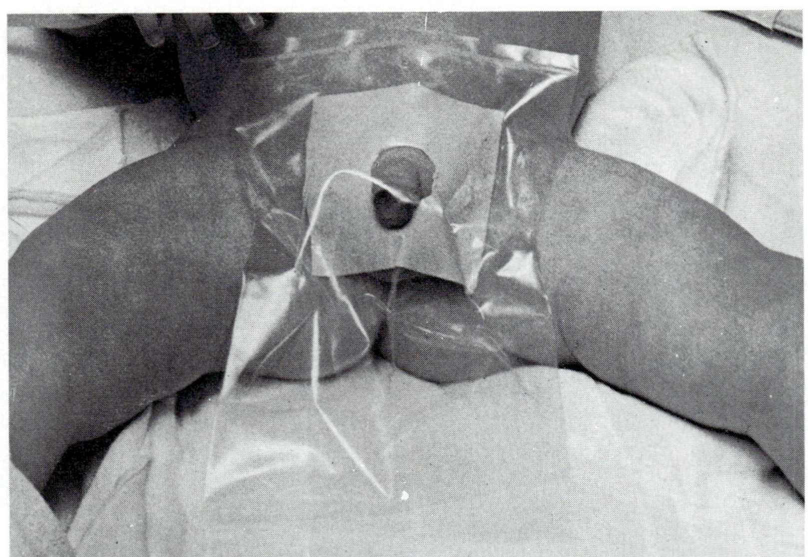

Fig. 25-4 Application of one type of adhesive-backed plastic bag for collection of urine specimen.

> **Nursing Alert**
>
> Signs of respiratory tract infection noted in a child scheduled for surgery should be reported immediately, since the surgery may be rescheduled.

sion should be determined and the assessment should be modified to gain additional data regarding the involved system or systems.

Collection of Specimens

In addition to the nursing assessment, the patient is routinely scheduled for urinalysis and a complete blood count. Special laboratory studies may also be ordered.

Urine specimens

The collection of a urine specimen in a toilet-trained child is seldom difficult. The collection of a specimen from an infant or young toddler may be more difficult. Various methods have been recommended. Most pediatric nurses, after careful cleansing of the perineal area, position small sterile adhesive-backed plastic bags over the urethra, which adhere to the perineal region or base of the penis (Fig. 25-4). These bags are usually satisfactory except when the child has a rash or perineal excoriations. The bag must be checked frequently to prevent losing the urine collection. When a prolonged urine collection is needed, a 24-hour pediatric urine specimen bag with an attached drainage tube may be used, or a small feeding tube may be inserted into the top of the routine collection bag and the bag periodically emptied with a syringe.

Blood samples

The nurse may help restrain the child as the physician or laboratory technician obtains a blood specimen. It may be obtained from a toe, heel, ear, finger prick, an arterial puncture of the arm, or a venous puncture of the arm or neck. If children must be restrained and if they are old enough to understand, they should be told that the restraint devices are used to help them hold still so that the doctors and nurses can help them get well. They should not think of the restraints as a means of punishment. Various types of restraints are used during a child's hospitalization (see Chapter 23). Common procedures or diagnostic tests that may be ordered at the time of admission are discussed in Chapter 24.

Diet and Fluid Orders

The diet of a newly admitted child depends on the reason for the hospitalization and the child's developmental age, food allergies, and general condition. Patients scheduled for pending surgery might not be allowed to eat or drink anything or may have orders for a certain amount of fluid until a designated time before surgery later in the day. Appropriate signs should be posted on the child's bed, and parents must be aware of restrictions.

Nursing Alert

Many children have allergies, not only to medicines, pollens, animal dander, fibers, and dust, but also to common foods. Chocolate, milk, wheat products, tomatoes, oranges, strawberries, nuts, and shellfish are common offenders.

Nurses should obtain a careful history regarding the allergens that have affected the child in the past. The nature of the reaction and the treatment should be recorded. Cultural patterns and preferences related to food should also be recorded. Larger hospitals attempt to develop culturally sensitive choices for various ethnic groups.

Admission Responsibility

The member of the nursing team who has the responsibility of admitting a patient depends on the condition and needs of the child. In certain situations the admission may be made in its entirety by a registered nurse. At other times it may be a joint or delegated responsibility carried out by both the registered nurse and the licensed vocational nurse. As a result of the nursing assessment, a plan for nursing care should be formulated based on the needs of the child and family.

DISCHARGE PLANNING

The discharge day is usually extremely busy for the child and parents. Arrangements must be made for transportation. For example, a child in a hip spica cast will not fit into most compact cars. The child's father or mother may have to take time off from work to provide transportation. Special child care arrangements may need to be made. The child usually must be dismissed in the morning to avoid a hospital charge for an additional day. The nurse should write out specific instructions for home care concerning prescribed medications and procedures, follow-up appointments, and important phone numbers to primary care providers and specialty clinics. Verbal instructions are insufficient.

Preparation for Home Care

When home care after discharge involves special skills, continued procedures, or particular stress, preparations for discharge needs to begin as soon as the child is stabilized to avoid a last minute rush. Preparation begins days before the actual departure of the child. Most hospitals employ a discharge, continuity care, or home-health nurse to assist parents or other care givers in planning for continued home care, teaching them necessary skills while the child is still hospitalized (e.g., instructions on gavage, dressing changes, stoma care, or intravenous observation). Ideally, more than one member of the family and the patient should be taught the skills that will be necessary for optimal care. At the time of discharge, every attempt should be made to send all of the child's belongings home with the parent. Return trips to the hospital to pick up articles left behind are annoying. Bedside stands, closets, cupboards, bedclothes, and flooring must be checked.

Before actually leaving the hospital premises, the parent or legal guardian must sign a form indicating who is taking the child. At this time a final check is made regarding any medications to be taken home or special instructions to be given. If possible the child should be taken to the car in a wheelchair, an isolette, or on a gurney. The child must always be accompanied by a nurse or hospital employee, and the nurse should make sure that the child is appropriately restrained in a child safety seat or a seat belt.

The discharge nurse may visit the home to assess needs and check patient progress. It may be necessary to change the location of the child's sleeping quarters to save steps and provide greater opportunity for observation. Special equipment or supplies may need to be improvised, borrowed, rented, or purchased. The services of a home health care nurse may be required. Patients are being discharged earlier from hospital settings and they frequently need special support.

Possible behavioral changes

Parents should be cautioned that hospitalization affects children differently. Occasionally, children experience a period of difficulty readjusting to life at home. They may regress developmentally, and activities that they had already mastered before their illness may not be attempted. Irritability and bedwetting by a previously toilet-trained child are common regressive behaviors.

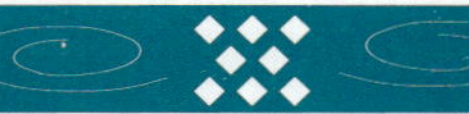

KEY CONCEPTS

1 Assets of a competent pediatric nurse include caring concern for children and families; effective communication skills; knowledge of the nursing process, child growth and development, common pediatric diagnoses, standards of care, hospital policies, and available resources; and a basic understanding of common legal and ethical issues affecting child health care.

2 The amount of parental participation in the care of the hospitalized child depends on the condition of the child and the motivation and desires of the parents. Parents should not be totally excluded from providing care; nor should they be given excessive responsibility.

3 During the admission assessment, the following information becomes part of the database: patient's history; height, weight, and age; temperature; pulse; respirations; blood pressure; and general appearance and behavior.

4 The patient is routinely scheduled for urinalysis and blood examinations. The nurse is usually responsible for obtaining the urine specimen and assisting the physician or laboratory technician in obtaining a blood specimen.

5 The diet of a newly admitted child depends on the reason for hospitalization and the child's age, food allergies, and general condition.

6 Discharge preparation should include written instructions for home care and arrangements for follow-up visits to the primary health care provider and specialty clinics. Because of early discharge, parents need specific instructions on how to care for their child in the home environment.

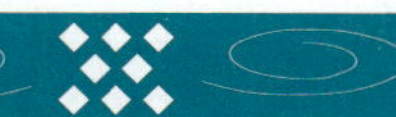

CRITICAL THOUGHT QUESTIONS

1 Pediatrics is viewed as a specialized area of nursing. Discuss the special skills and attitudes required of a nurse working in pediatrics. Are all well-educated nurses capable of being pediatric nurses?

2 How can the pediatric nurse best establish a trusting relationship with the child? With the parents? What can the nurse do to maintain this trust?

3 How does assessing vital signs (temperature, pulse, respirations, blood pressure) of a child differ from adult assessment? What particular safety precautions should be taken? Compare and contrast the methods used for an infant and a school-aged child.

4 Subjective data can be obtained from both parents and child. How would you attempt to get this type of information from the child? How would you vary your history taking technique based on the developmental age of the child?

5 What modifications and special nursing techniques are used when attempting to collect blood and urine specimens from a young child?

BIBLIOGRAPHY

Barkauskas VH et al: *Health and physical assessment,* St Louis, 1994, Mosby.

Callery P and Smith L: A study of role negotiation between nurses and the parents of hospitalized children, *J Adv Nurs* 16(7):772-781, 1991.

Dixon S and Stein M: *Encounters with children: pediatric behavior and development,* St Louis, 1992, Mosby.

Gottlieb SE: Documenting the efficacy of psychosocial care in the hospital setting, *J Dev Behav Pediatr* 11:6, 328-329, 1990.

Hester NO et al: Excerpts from the management of pain in infants, children, and adolescents undergoing operative and medical procedures, *MCN Am J Matern Child Nurs* 17:146-152, 1992.

Holt L and Maxwell B: Pediatric orientation programs: hospital tours allay children's fears, *AORN J* 54:3, 530-536, 1991.

Jarvis C: *Health and physical assessment.* Philadelphia, 1992, WB Saunders.

Whaley L and Wong D: *Nursing care of infants and children,* St Louis, 1992, Mosby.

Wong DL: *Essentials of pediatric nursing,* St Louis, 1993, Mosby.

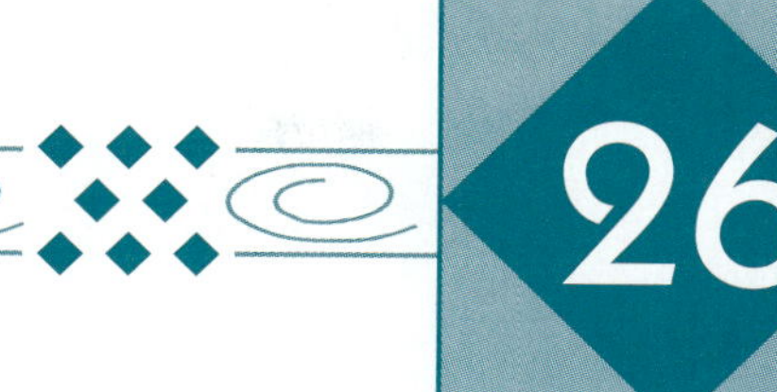
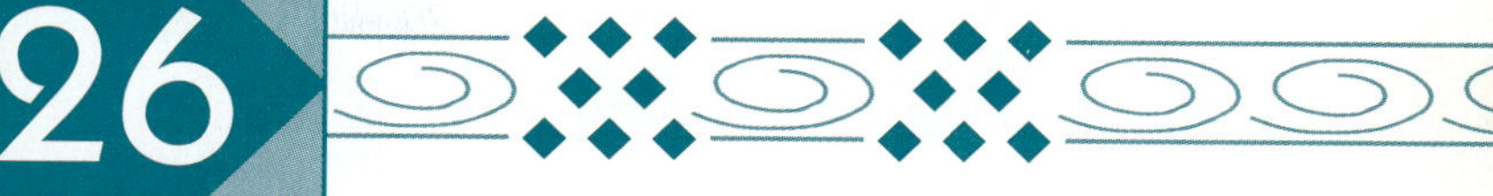

26

Health Maintenance of the Hospitalized Child

CHAPTER OBJECTIVES

After studying this chapter, the student should be able to:

1 Discuss patient safety in a pediatric nursing unit including why safety is more of an issue here than in other areas of the hospital.
2 Explain why restraints may be both a safety measure and a danger for patients.
3 Discuss ways in which one may successfully encourage a 3 year old to drink fluids.
4 Describe the three fluid compartments of the body and the movement of water from one area of the body to another.
5 Define *electrolyte, ion, pH, acid, base, acidosis,* and *alkalosis.*
6 List four main electrolytes in the body and the signs and symptoms of depletion of each.
7 Identify the formula for determining a child's maintenance fluid requirements based on weight and caloric expenditure.
8 Explain four reasons why an infant is more vulnerable than an adult to dehydration.
9 Describe five signs of dehydration in an infant.
10 Discuss three important principles to be considered when selecting toys.
11 Write three formulas used to determine pediatric dosage of medications.
12 State the five rights of medication administration.
13 Explain three ways that liquid medications may be given to an infant.
14 Describe the sites that may be correctly used for intramuscular injections in a 12-month-old girl.
15 Discuss how and why nose drops are given to infants.
16 Indicate the difference in the direction of pull on the earlobe when administering ear drops to a child older than and younger than 3 years.
17 Compare differences in the specialties of physical therapy and occupational therapy.

Basic patient needs and daily planning are affected by the trend toward early discharge and home health care. Thus parents and other family members must be taught procedures previously completed during inpatient hospitalization. Computerization at the bedside and the need for careful, concise documentation further affect the planning, implementation, and evaluation of nursing care.

BASIC PATIENT NEEDS

The nursing staff is responsible for the following:

1 Maintaining a safe environment
2 Assessment of the child and family
3 Planning and implementation of supportive care
  a Aiding respiration and oxygenation
  b Maintaining normal body temperature

- c Proper positioning and appropriate play activities
- d Adequate nourishment and hydration
- e Hygiene
- f Providing a restful environment
- g Promoting self-expression and coping mechanisms

4 Diagnostic procedures
5 Medications and special treatments
6 Rehabilitation
7 Documentation and evaluation

Safety

Maintaining a safe environment is a priority of nursing care. In a pediatric setting, safety is a constant concern. The environment must be continually evaluated to prevent injuries because patients are too young to regulate their own surroundings, and they lack the judgment to evaluate their own environments properly. Unrestrained or unattended children in high beds or cribs should always have the bed or crib sides securely raised. No nurse should turn away from an unrestrained child in a crib with the side lowered. Young children who are climbing should be placed in special protective beds unless supervision is constant (Fig. 26-1). Wall electricity, suction, and oxygen outlets should be out of the reach of young children. No antiseptics or other supplies, which may be ingested by a young child, should be left at the bedside. Toys should be checked for sharp edges, small parts, or other potential dangers. Plastic bags should not be used near young children. Known allergies should be clearly posted at the bedside and on the front of health records. All equipment should be in good working order and used properly. Special precautions should be observed when administering oxygen. When a child is transported in a wheelchair, a waist or jacket restraint may be used to prevent the child's tipping forward or sliding down. Unnecessary traffic and congestion in the halls should be avoided.

An important component of safety is clear, consistent discipline. A simple explanation of the rules to the child and family is essential. Discipline also means realistic expectations and prompt follow-through by the nurse responsible for caring for the child. Nurses must not give choices when alternatives are not possible. When possible, allowing the child to choose from several safe alternatives gives the child a sense of self-control. Promises kept, clear and consistent messages, and caring concern promote the child's sense of security and cooperation.

For protection, children may be restrained during treatments. Restraint should never be presented as a punishment but as one way to help children hold still.

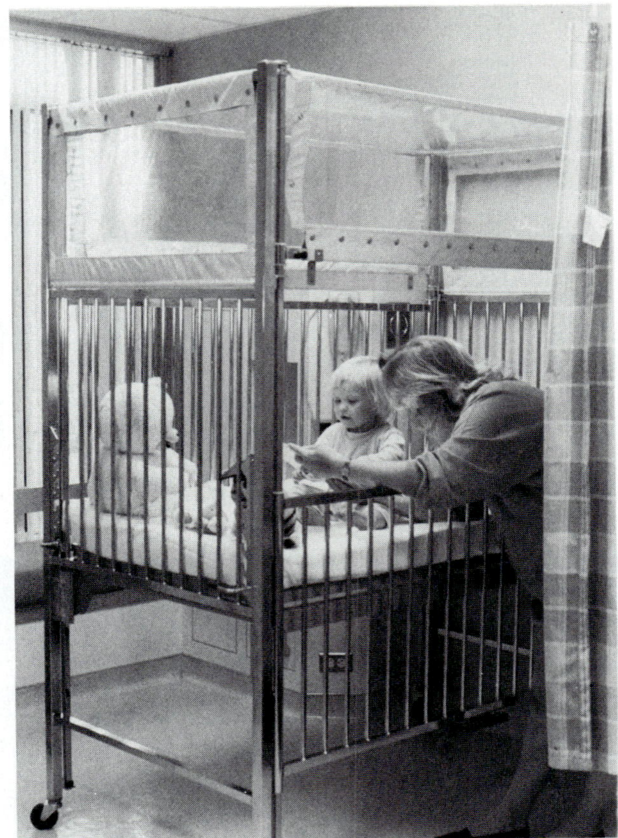

Fig. 26-1 High top cribs are designed to protect climbing toddlers. (Courtesy Children's Hospital and Health Center, San Diego, Calif.)

An example of such a restraint is the "mummy wrap" (Fig. 26-2). A commercial mummy restraint used in many emergency rooms is the Olympic papoose board shown in Fig. 26-3. Another type of control used to prevent children from touching their faces or pulling on gavage tubes is elbow restraints, which are usually fastened to the hospital gown (Fig. 26-4, *A*). Elbow restraints are not effective if the child can reach his or her face with a toy or an implement without bending the arms. To control leg and arm motion, specially constructed ankle and wrist restraints (Fig. 26-4, *B*) or the clove-hitch tie (Fig. 26-5) may be used. A pediatric Posey belt is used to allow some movement in bed while preventing the patient from rising. A jacket restraint is pictured in Fig. 26-6. Most restraints are removed at least every 2 hours to check circulation and exercise the body part involved. Restraints should be constructed so that they do not become tighter with increased tension, impairing circulation or endangering the child's respiration. Choking caused by restraint devices is a constant concern. Restraints must never be attached to bedrails.

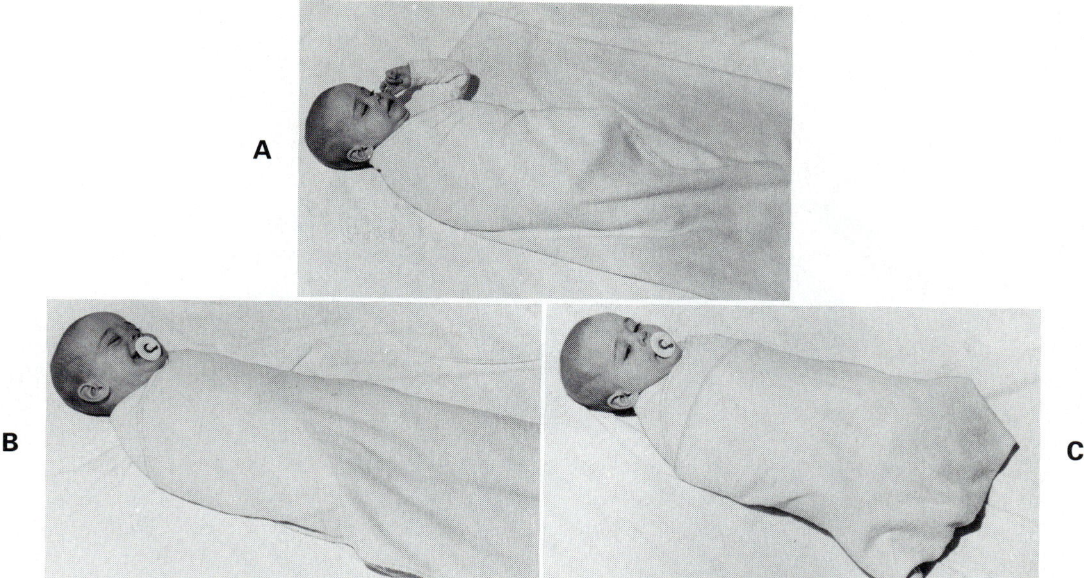

Fig. 26-2 Covered chest mummy wrap. **A,** Center infant's head at edge of "short side" of open baby blanket or sheet. Place one arm at infant's side and pull blanket snugly over infant's shoulder, arm, and chest and tuck the blanket under the infant. **B,** Position opposite arm similarly and pull opposite corner over and around infant. **C,** Open out loose end of blanket and bring it up and snugly around infant.

Assessment and Observation

A careful nursing assessment is the first step of the nursing process. The plan of care is based on a systematic assessment. Observation and inspection of the child are always important; however, when caring for the preverbal child it is of paramount importance. The child's unique temperament, stage of growth and development, family constellation, and cultural differences make this step complex. Observation of the patient should be made, especially in light of the patient's medical and nursing diagnosis. For example, if the medical diagnosis is pneumonia, the fact that the child is pale and has a frequent, loose cough producing thick, white mucus is significant. Negative observations are also important for baseline information and complete documentation. For example it is important to record that a child admitted because of convulsions has had no seizures for a certain period. The observation that a child hospitalized for vomiting and diarrhea retained a feeding and had no stools for a specific interval may be significant. When observing the whole patient and recording appearance, activity, and treatment, refer to the diagnosis. What is especially important for the primary nurse or physician to know? Moving the child closer to the nursing station is sometimes needed for closer observation.

Diagnostic Procedures

The diagnostic procedures ordered must be clearly understood to provide adequate preparation, execution, and follow-up. It is impossible to describe within this brief text all the diagnostic procedures encountered in a pediatric setting. For some of the more common tests and a description of specimen collection, consult Chapter 23 and the hospital procedure manual. It should be remembered that most diagnostic studies require the parent's or guardian's informed written consent.

In the morning the nurse must be careful to determine whether patients should not receive anything to eat or drink and whether they are listed as nothing by mouth (NPO). Many laboratory tests do not limit water intake. After the completion of a test for which a patient has been fasting, the nurse must be sure to inquire whether the patient may resume a regular diet. If so, the prescribed foods or liquids should be ordered.

Supportive Procedures

Various types of supportive procedures and techniques are used to promote the physical and emotional resources of the patient. These procedures may include

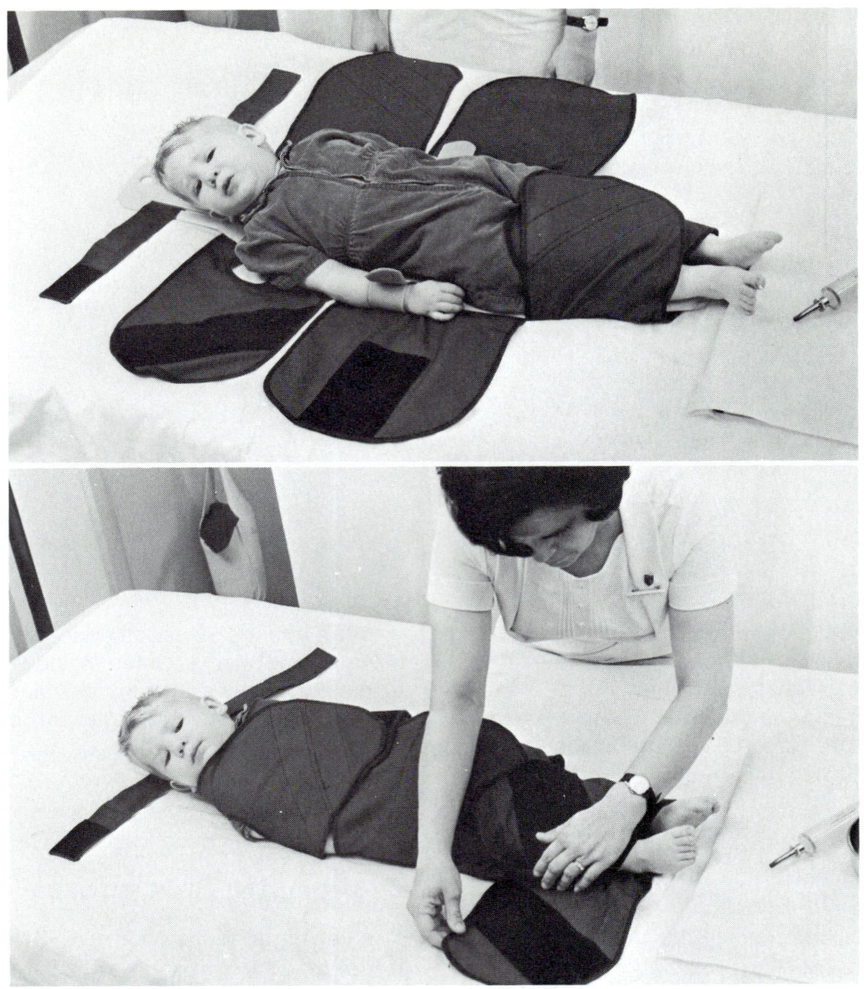

Fig. 26-3 Preparing to restrain child for gastric lavage using Olympic papoose board. Various wraps are possible with Velcro-lined restraining folds. (Courtesy Olympic-Surgical, Seattle, Wash.)

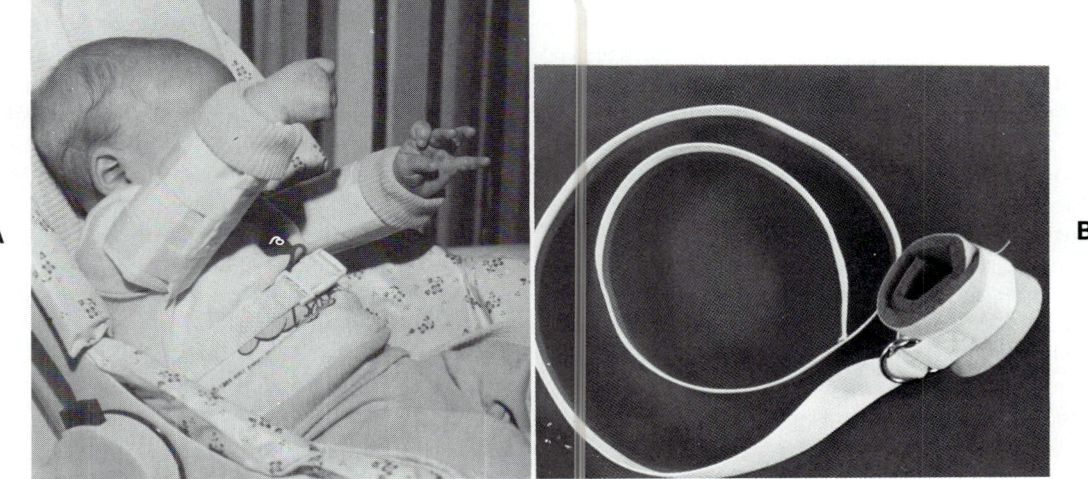

Fig. 26-4 **A,** Infant cannot touch cleft lip repair but can move arms, an advantage of elbow restraints. **B,** Extremity restraint incorporating Velcro fastener.

special provisions for aiding respiration or oxygenation, regulating body temperature, positioning, mobility, play, maintaining fluid balance or nutrition, pain control, or improving function. They also include the caring concern of parents, family, friends, and nurses; build or maintain the child's sense of trust; and buffer the stress of hospitalization. The use of oxygen and humidification equipment is discussed in a separate chapter, as are the methods of regulating body temperature. Positioning of the child in bed is described in the following sections.

Preventing complications of immobility

Children who are immobilized for long periods must maintain good body alignment, functional positions, range of motion, and tissue health. (Refer to section on skin care and positioning, Chapter 37.) Barring special treatments involving traction, casting, or specifically ordered body placement, the child in bed, whether supine (on back) or prone (on abdomen), must maintain a posture that would be considered well aligned if the child were standing. This is particularly critical for those who are not able to change their position easily. Included in this section are illustrations of examples of proper positioning. If patients remain in bed for extended periods without adequate foot support or with tight covers pressing down on their feet, they will develop tightening of the Achilles tendon, or heel cord, causing *footdrop,* which makes walking difficult. One leg may fall laterally *(external rotation)* causing deformity, or it may remain in a flexed position, which if not changed often, can result in fixation and *contracture* in a relatively short time. Arms positioned on top of the chest and a partially flexed head position decrease respiratory capacity. Persistently flexed arm and hand positions (typical of the arthritic patient) cause flexion contractures of the shoulder and elbow and *wristdrop,* with loss of function in the hand.

Fig. 26-7 illustrates how good alignment may be achieved with a footboard, pillows, and hand rolls. It should be noted whether a type of foot support is being used. Partially paralyzed patients who exhibit considerable muscle spasticity may be unable to tolerate a hard footboard without developing tissue damage. They may need a soft boot type of support. The knees are straight up, without rotation. Correct positioning is maintained by a rectangularly folded blanket that has been placed under the patients' buttocks. The long protruding end is then rolled under tightly toward the thigh to stabilize the leg in a neutral position. This is a *trochanter roll.* Some patients appreciate a small pillow placed in the small of the back. The arms are alternately rotated for comfort. Soft hand rolls help maintain functional finger-thumb position.

When the patient is in the prone or abdominal position (Fig. 26-8), the toes should be either over the end of the mattress pointing down between the foot of the bed and the mattress or over the edge of a pillow. A thin pillow support under the abdomen takes pressure off the chest and reduces the lumbar curve. The arms are usually comfortable if abducted and flexed. A small pillow may be positioned under the head. Excessive flexion of the neck must be avoided.

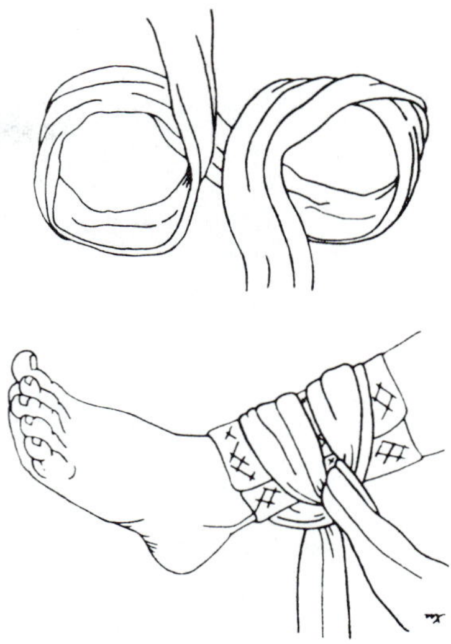

Fig. 26-5 Application of clove-hitch restraint. Formed loops are placed one on top of another and body part put through opening. Body part should always be padded.

The side-lying position is often preferred. The main problem with this position is the strain placed on the hip joint and lower back by the upper leg if it is allowed to fall forward. For a patient who has no back or hip problems and is able to move freely, this is not a problem. If these problems exist, however, the side-lying position should be properly maintained by adding one or two pillows to support the upper leg (Fig. 26-9). A pillow tucked lengthwise against the back is also comforting. A support for the upper hand and arm relieves the chest.

Good positioning and frequent turning at least every 2 hours prevent respiratory, circulatory, urinary, and musculoskeletal complications and speeds rehabilitation. Immobilized infants and toddlers need to be frequently turned and repositioned. Young infants should not be left unattended in the supine position if they have a history of vomiting or respiratory problems because of the danger of aspiration. A rolled blanket should be placed at the infant's back to maintain a side-lying position.

Nourishment and fluid balance

It is nursing's responsibility to keep an accurate intake and output (I & O) record on patients who are

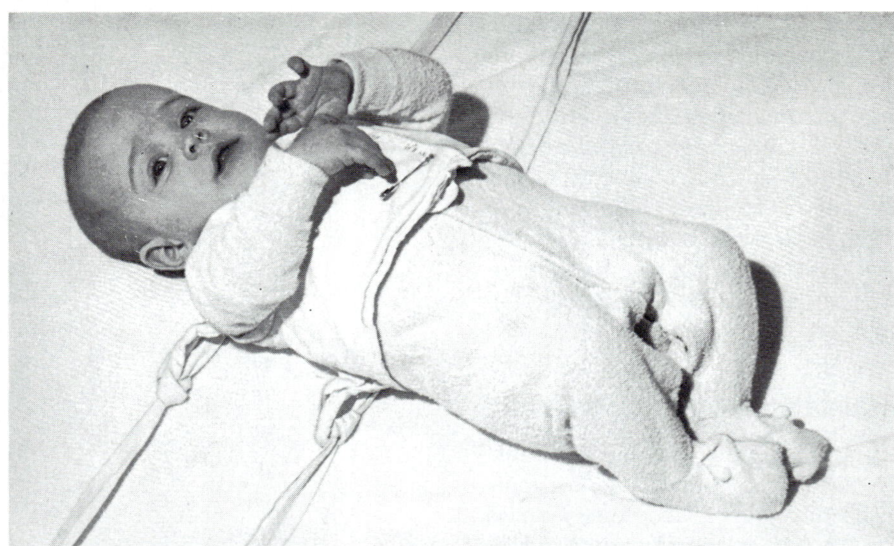

Fig. 26-6 Restraining jacket. Ties are fastened to bedspring frame, and pins are placed in front, on top, or underneath, depending on child's age. It is best, if possible, to elevate head of bed to avoid problems with aspiration. Ties may be modified to allow toddlers to sit up in bed. It may also be used as wheelchair restraint for small children.

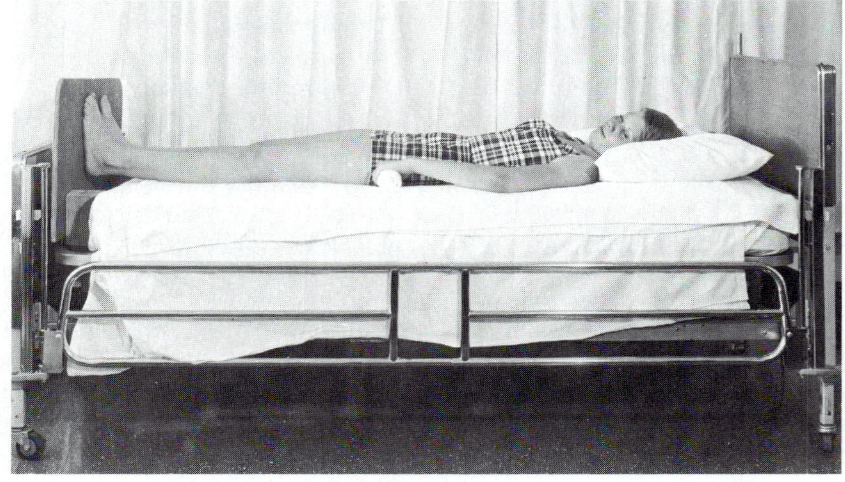

Fig. 26-7 Good body alignment in supine position. (Courtesy Children's Hospital and Health Center, San Diego, Calif.)

younger than 2 years and have experienced dehydration; major surgery; central nervous system disorders including meningitis; thermal burns, or injuries; intravenous, corticosteroid, or diuretic therapy; congestive heart failure; renal disease; diabetes mellitus; or oliguria. When I & O is ordered, it is important to record it from all sources.

The diet ordered by the health care provider and sent by the dietary department may be nutritious, but it is of no value if the child refuses to eat it. Before a tray is served to a patient, it should be checked carefully to see that it is developmentally appropriate and compatible with the diet order, food allergies, cultural preferences, and religious background. Nuts, raw carrots, and celery should not be served to toddlers who may aspirate these foods. Common diets served in the pediatric area are clear liquid, full liquid, soft, high protein, high carbohydrate, low residue, diabetic, and salt- or sodium-restricted. Nursing students should review these diets in a nutrition text or dietary department manual.

Infants and toddlers require assistance at mealtime.

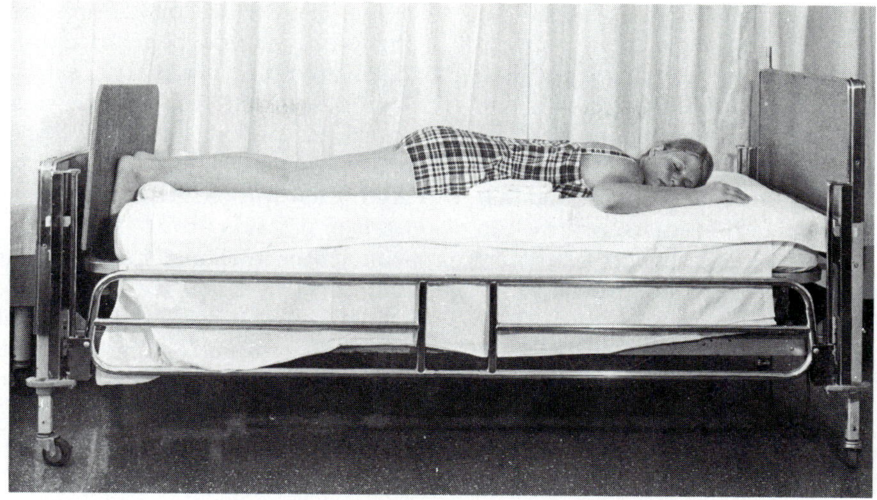

Fig. 26-8 Good body alignment in prone position. (Courtesy Children's Hospital and Health Center, San Diego, Calif.)

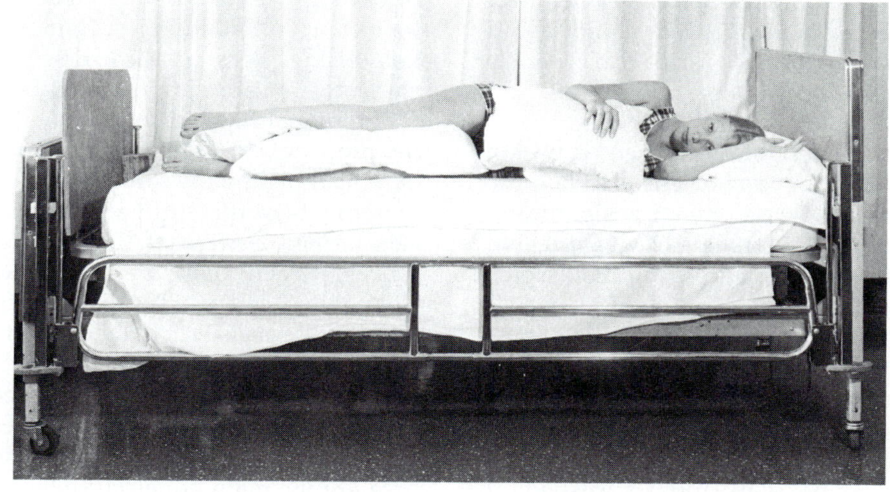

Fig. 26-9 Good body alignment in side-lying position. (Courtesy Children's Hospital and Health Center, San Diego, Calif.)

Some assistance must also be provided for older children. The utensils should be appropriate and the food must be easy to consume and attractive. Some young children prefer trying to feed themselves, but very young children enjoy being held during meals. Bibs and nurse's feeding gowns are helpful. Parents should be encouraged to assist with feeding as a comfort measure and to increase intake.

Infants often drink better if they have a break between their meal and their formula. Children who need to increase their fluid intake may be offered fluids before solid foods, when they are hungrier. Plastic bottles should be used with older infants who enjoy holding their own bottle.

The specificity of recording regarding intake depends on the diagnosis and the child's condition. A child with diabetes requires close observation and recording of food intake. The diet of a child with metabolic, growth and development, digestive, or feeding problems should be carefully recorded at the bedside and in the nurse's notes.

The intake of patients with stabilized conditions may be described as "ate well," "ate fairly well," or "ate poorly." *All* pediatric patients are routinely on a regimen of measured fluid intake, expressed in cubic centimeters (cc) or milliliters (ml). Output may also be recorded depending on the diagnosis.

Hydration. Fluid intake is of greater immediate importance than the feeding of solids. The hydration of a child is extremely important. A young child may become dehydrated more rapidly than an adult. An infant is especially vulnerable, having a greater surface area and higher metabolic rate per unit of weight than an adult. Maintaining an adequate fluid intake is one of the important responsibilities of the nurse. The amount of fluid that is urged depends on the child's size and condition. Nursing students are reminded that patients who are immobilized in casts or traction apparatus and all those with indwelling urinary catheters must have special attention to ensure adequate fluid intake.

Encouragement. Ensuring oral intake calls for a nurse's patience and persistence. Small amounts taken frequently are tolerated better by the ill child than copious amounts taken rapidly. Fluids taken rapidly are often not retained by children who are ill, upset, or excited.

The kinds of fluids offered to children depend on their diet orders and history of allergies. Clear fluids include any liquid through which one can see the bottom of the container—water, bouillon, strained fruit juices, popsicles, gelatin, and soft drinks. A full liquid diet includes unstrained fruit juices and milk products such as yogurt, ice cream, sherbet, milkshakes, and creamed soups.

Learning which fluids the child has accepted well in the past saves time. Offering a choice is also helpful. The manner in which fluids are offered is significant. Some older infants are in the process of weaning and drink well from a cup. Others regress and take fluids only from a bottle with a certain nipple. Propping a bottle is not a safe practice in any setting. Some children are accustomed to warm milk; others like it cold. Older children often reject milk unless it is ice cold. A nurse who sits down with the child and offers fluids in a relaxed manner is more likely to be successful than the nurse who appears rushed or verbalizes frustration. The use of straws (if gas is not a problem), doll tea-party dishes, colored ice cubes, or a paper star on the fluid intake record may help. Most children enjoy popsicles. Water should also be encouraged. With older children, the factual knowledge that intravenous feedings will be necessary to ensure hydration if oral fluid intake is inadequate may encourage them to try harder. A carton of milk and a glass of fruit juice at breakfast, a glass of some other fluid or dish of ice cream or gelatin equaling approximately 200 ml during midmorning, soup and beverage at lunch, and a midafternoon juice or milk serving provide an adequate fluid intake during the day.

Restriction. Children with renal disease, central nervous system disease, including meningitis, or heart disease may require restricted fluid intake. Patients scheduled for operative procedures are usually not allowed any oral intake for several hours before their surgeries. After the procedures the amount and type of fluids offered may be restricted. For instance, in some cases after heart surgery, oral liquid intake may be limited and offered only in small quantities for an extended period. Some postoperative patients are allowed nothing by mouth for a considerable period after their procedures, receiving intravenous fluids until oral fluids are ordered. The child who has had stomach or intestinal surgery is initially offered small amounts (1 to 2 tsp) at a time to ascertain tolerance and to decrease stress on the surgical site. Infants with severe diarrhea and vomiting are usually not allowed anything by mouth or are placed on intravenous fluids to rest the gastrointestinal tract.

Fluid and electrolyte balance. The content and volume of the body fluid are key considerations in the maintenance of cellular health and therefore the health of the whole patient. The body organs and systems function to maintain the proper internal and external cellular environment. The nurse's understanding of the physiology of fluid and electrolyte balance is an important foundation on which to build nursing knowledge. A simplified discussion of fluid and electrolyte balance is presented below.

The body functions in sensitive equilibrium. One of the most delicate balances maintained by the body is demonstrated by the composition of body fluid. Major ingredients of this fluid are water and certain chemicals termed *electrolytes.* Electrolytes develop electric charges when they are dissolved in water. Some electrolytes carry a positive charge and are called *cations.* Negatively charged electrolytes are called *anions.* In either case the electrolytes are referred to as *ions.* A small number of chemical compounds that do not ionize or carry electrical charges are also found in body fluid. Organic compounds such as glucose and urea are the main nonelectrolytes of body fluid (Table 26-1).

Body fluid occupies three permeable compartments (Fig. 26-10): blood vessels, tissue spaces (interstitial areas outside of tissue cells), and the areas inside the cells. *Extracellular fluid* (ECF) is located within the blood vessels and between the tissue cells, and *intracellular fluid* (ICF) lies inside the tissue cells.

Every tissue cell is surrounded by a semipermeable membrane that permits selective passage of certain substances and free passage of water molecules in both directions. Water passes from the side containing the least amount of electrolytes and other dissolved compounds to the side that contains more dissolved compounds. This water movement is called *osmosis.* In health a dynamic equilibrium of electrolytes and water is maintained between the two areas. Therefore although each of the fluid compartments of the body contains electrolytes, the concentration and composi-

◆ **TABLE 26-1**
Major Electrolytes and Imbalances

Electrolyte	Deficit	Excess
Sodium (Na^+)—normal value 136-143 mEq/L*	*Hyponatremia* Associated with dehydration; sodium losses from the body in excess of water losses; Na^+ below 130 mEq/L Muscular weakness; abdominal cramps; clammy skin; weak, rapid pulse; hypotension; drowsiness; confusion; coma Predisposing factors—excessive sweating and water intake; gastrointestinal suction and excessive oral water intake; glucose water infusion without sodium; diarrhea; renal disease; cystic fibrosis; central nervous system disease	*Hypernatremia* Associated with dehydration; water losses from the body in excess of sodium losses; Na^+ above 150 mEq/L Thirst; dry skin; loss of skin elasticity ("doughy" tissue turgor); fever; weight loss; scanty urine formation; confusion; stupor, seizures; circulatory embarrassment Predisposing factors—sodium chloride infusion; inadequate water intake; water diarrhea; renal concentrating disease; anorexia; nausea; vomiting; high fever Additional feeding factors—infant feedings of undiluted cow's milk; boiled skim milk; powdered electrolyte mixtures: salt and sugar mixtures; bouillon soup, and so forth
Potassium (K^+)—normal value 4.1-5.6 mEq/L	*Hypokalemia*† K^+ below 3.5 mEq/L Weak pulse; hypotension; muscular weakness; diminished reflexes; loss of peristalsis, cardiac arrest Predisposing factors—diuretics; diarrhea; vomiting; gastric suctioning	*Hyperkalemia* K^+ above 5.7 mEq/L Nausea; apprehension; muscular weakness; confusion; hypotension; cardiac arrest Predisposing factors—burns, excessive tissue damage; excessive infusion of potassium; kidney disease; severe dehydration with scanty urine formation; adrenal insufficiency
Calcium (Ca^{++})—normal value 10-12 mg/100 ml (5-6 mEq/L)	*Hypocalcemia* Ca^{++} below 9 mg/100 ml Tetany; tingling around mouth and fingers; muscular cramps; convulsions Predisposing factors—hypoactive parathyroid; malabsorption syndromes; chronic renal disease; distressed newborns	*Hypercalcemia (rare)* Ca^{++} above 12 mg/100 ml Vomiting; constipation; polyuria; abdominal pains; headache Predisposing factors—prolonged bed rest; overactive parathyroid; overdose of vitamin D

Continued.

tion of electrolytes in the water of each compartment vary. The electrolytes found in the fluid inside the cells differ greatly in amount from those found in the fluid outside the cells. Interstitial fluid in the tissue spaces is similar to plasma (the fluid portion of the blood), except that it contains little protein. In interstitial fluid the principal cation is sodium, and the main anions are chlorides and bicarbonates. Intracellular cations are mostly potassium and magnesium, whereas the anions are chiefly phosphates and bicarbonates. Thus chemical differences exist between the extracellular and the intracellular fluids.

Water equalizes quickly in all body compartments. Therefore rapid water intake does not result in edema

◆ TABLE 26-1
Major Electrolytes and Imbalances—cont'd.

Electrolyte	Deficit	Excess
Bicarbonate $(HCO_3)^-$ normal value 19-26 mEq/L	*Metabolic acidosis* HCO_3 below 12 mEq/L Apathy, drowsiness or lethargy; deep rapid breathing (Kussmaul type) disorientation; stupor; weakness; coma Predisposing factors—diabetes mellitus; starvation; kidney insufficiency; excessive parenteral NaCl; severe diarrhea; salicylate intoxication; respiratory alkalosis	*Metabolic alkalosis* HCO_3^- above 30 mEq/L Depressed, shallow respirations; hypertonic muscles; tetany; disorientation Predisposing factors—vomiting (pyloric stenosis); ingestion of alkali; chloride-deficiency diets or formulas; gastric suction; diuretics; respiratory insufficiency

*Milliequivalents per liter (mEq/L).
†Potassium may be given intravenously only after urinary output is well established.

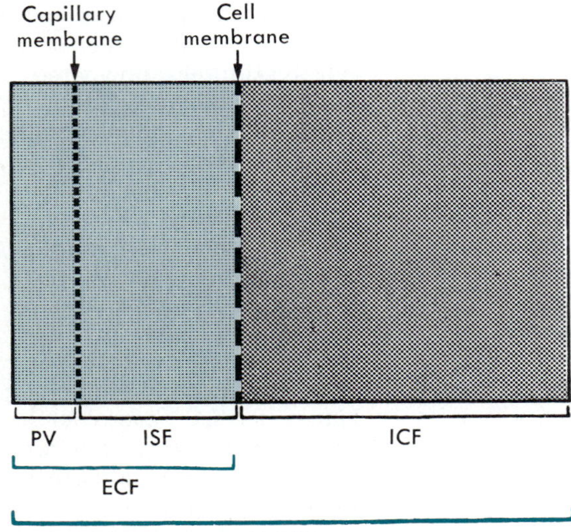

Fig. 26-10 Body fluid compartments. *PV,* Plasma volume; *ISF,* interstitial fluid; *ECF,* extracellular fluid; *ICF,* intracellular fluid.

but causes swelling of the body's cells and expands and dilutes both the intracellular and extracellular compartments. Salt- and protein-containing solutions remain primarily in the extracellular compartments. Excessive salt intake may lead to edema.

Acid-base balance. The acidity or alkalinity of a solution depends on the concentration of hydrogen or the H ions present. An acid may be simply defined as a compound that has enough H ions to give some away. A base or alkali is a compound possessing few H ions. An increase in H ions makes a solution more acid, and a decrease makes a solution more alkaline. The concentration of hydrogen ions is expressed by pH. A neutral fluid has a pH of 7 (a lower pH means higher hydrogen ion concentration). An acid solution has a pH value below 7; an alkaline solution has a pH value above 7. The acid-base balance of the blood is maintained in an extremely narrow pH range, normally 7.35 to 7.45. Any slight deviation from this range causes pronounced changes in the cellular functions, which in turn may threaten life. Blood is normally slightly alkaline (pH 7.4). The acid-base balance is maintained by the action of the lungs, kidneys, and buffer systems. The lungs assist in maintaining this equilibrium by varying the rate at which carbon dioxide is blown off, retaining it in acidic form when blood plasma is getting too alkaline or increasing the respiratory rate when the plasma is becoming too acid.

When disturbances in blood pH are primarily the result of disease or abnormalities of the respiratory system, the problems resulting are termed either *respiratory alkalosis* or *respiratory acidosis.* The kidneys assist in maintaining the normal pH of blood by regulating the rates of excretion of acids and bases in the urine. Excessive retention of base or loss of acids through diseases of body systems other than the respiratory apparatus results in *metabolic alkalosis;* likewise, excessive retention of acids or loss of base produces *metabolic acidosis.*

Chemical buffer systems protect the acid-base balance of solution by rapidly offsetting changes in its ionized pH concentration. Buffer systems maintain the pH of body fluids by protecting against added acid or base.

Fluid volume. The volume of blood plasma, interstitial fluid, and intracellular fluid normally remain relatively constant. Any blood plasma changes that

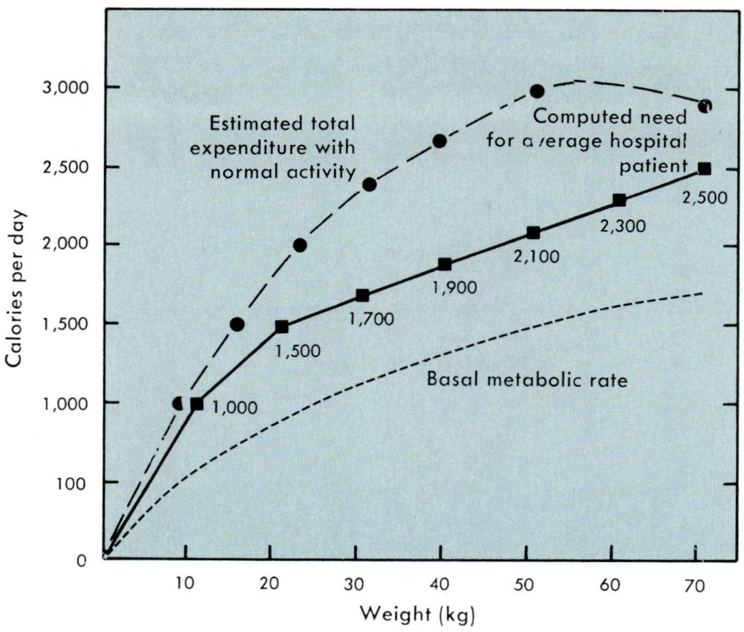

Fig. 26-11 Comparison of energy expenditure in basal and ideal state.

take place during illness usually reflect changes in all body fluids. Because plasma is relatively easy to obtain from the body and the other fluids are not, it is the chosen fluid for analysis.

Maintenance therapy. Fluid therapy aimed at replacing the patient's daily loss of water, electrolytes, and calories is termed *maintenance therapy.* The purpose of maintenance fluid is to keep the body in neutral balance for water, sodium, potassium, and chloride. Water and electrolyte requirements for normal maintenance depend on the child's metabolic rate (calories metabolized), which changes with maturation (Fig. 26-11). Pediatric caloric expenditure can be calculated using the formula with the infant's weight and the calories per ounce.

The store of fluid in the body comes from ingested liquid and food. A cardinal principle of fluid balance is that fluid intake must equal fluid output. Under normal conditions the requirement for water is usually derived from the need to replace water lost across the skin and lungs (insensible water losses), which maintain body temperature and dissipate the body's metabolic heat and water lost through urine and stool.

Fluid requirements may be greater in children with increased insensible losses associated with fever, burns, hyperthyroidism, increased respirations, or increased urine production (diabetes insipidus). Less fluid is required when insensible losses are reduced (e.g., when children are in croup tents, are on respirators with increased humidity, or have abnormal decreased urine output as in renal failure). Any condition that interferes with an adequate intake of fluid or produces excessive fluid loss threatens the life of the young child.

When fluids are administered parenterally, maintenance of electrolytes is necessary to replace urinary, stool, and skin losses of sodium, chloride, and potassium. A child usually requires 3 mEq of sodium, 2 mEq of chloride, and 2 mEq of potassium per 100 kcal expended to meet maintenance requirements. These electrolyte requirements usually do not need to be altered when maintenance water requirements are varied. It is important to note, however, that sodium is not given to patients in heart or renal failure. Potassium is excreted almost exclusively by the kidneys; therefore replacement of potassium is withheld until the child has demonstrated adequate renal function. Potassium is omitted if the child is oliguric.

To prevent acidosis and ketosis, reduce protein breakdown, and provide calories, glucose must also be added to most parenteral fluids. Although full caloric replacement is difficult to accomplish, about 5 gm/100 kcal/24 hr of glucose should be given. Fluid maintenance and electrolyte requirements should be administered over the greater part of the 24-hour period for which they were intended.

Fluid compartments. Fig. 26-12 illustrates that plasma is the only portion of body water in contact with the external environment. It is the first fluid storage supply to be tapped in gastrointestinal disturbances (vomiting or diarrhea), rapid respirations, or deficient fluid intake. Interstitial fluid is the reservoir

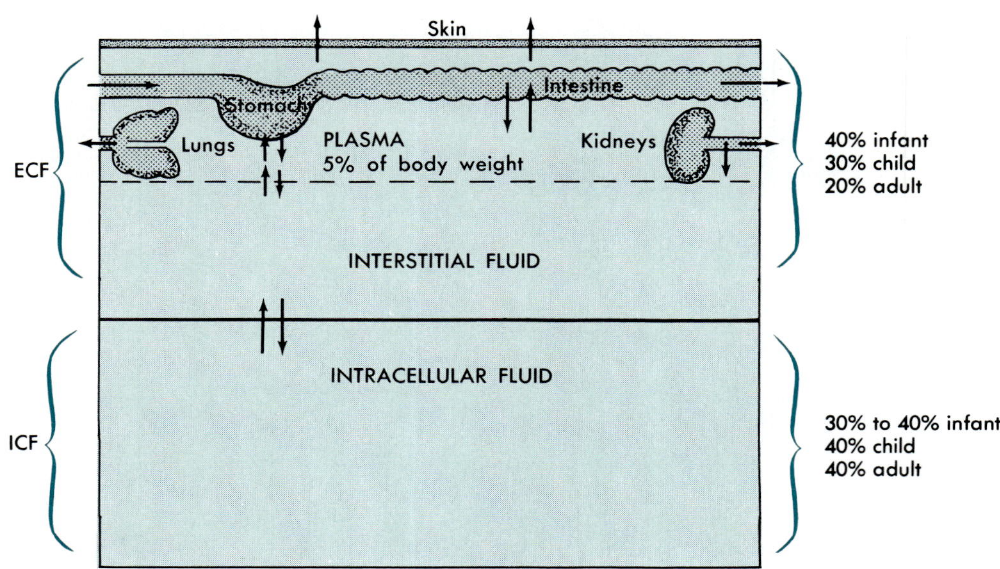

Fig. 26-12 Relative fluid balance in children and adults expressed in percentage of total body weight.

that responds most easily to the shifting fluid conditions present in disease (e.g., overhydration may cause edema, and dehydration causes the skin to lose its turgor and become wrinkled). The intracellular compartment represents the largest reservoir and is the least accessible. Here water is lost or gained over days. Without water a well infant in a temperate environment can live 3 days or more, and an adult can survive about 10 days. Several differences between body fluid compartments in the infant and older child must be considered.

A newborn infant's weight is approximately 80% water, the older child's is 70% water, and the adult's is 60% water. This percentage varies with the amount of fat. Because fat is essentially water-free, a lean individual has a greater proportion of water to total body weight. The proportion of intracellular fluid to body weight remains comparatively constant at all ages. Extracellular fluid constitutes about 40% of the infant's weight as compared with 20% of the adult's body weight. An infant, then, may approach a fluid loss of 10% of body weight before a severe fluid deficit occurs, whereas a weight loss of 5% represents a severe fluid volume deficit in the adult.

Although the infant's body has a greater fluid content per pound, an infant is *more vulnerable* to fluid volume deficit than the adult. Infants lose a proportionately larger volume of water daily for several reasons. The infant's body surface in relation to body weight is three times that of the older child. Therefore infants lose a relatively greater amount of fluid through the skin and gastrointestinal tract. Their high metabolic rate produces more waste products, which must be diluted for excretion. Their immature kidneys are less able to concentrate urine, thus adding to the volume of urine. Accumulation of acidic wastes (because of the high metabolic rate and immature kidneys) stimulates respiration, causing greater evaporation through the lungs. Infants may react to infections with higher temperatures, which also result in a higher water loss from evaporation. By reviewing these facts about the infant's body fluid balance, the nurse can more readily understand why the infant, at one-twentieth the adult's weight, requires one third as much water.

Dehydration. Inadequate fluid intake or excessive fluid loss causes dehydration. It is almost always associated with fever, burns, vomiting, diarrhea, hyperventilation, or hemorrhage. Dehydration seldom denotes water loss alone but rather loss of fluid volume, electrolytes, and water. During periods of dehydration, plasma volume is usually maintained at the expense of interstitial volume.

Clinically, dehydration is described as the percentage of body weight that has been lost as water. The most accurate method to assess the child's degree of dehydration is by noting changes in body weight.

Mild	5%
Moderate	7% to 10%
Severe	10% to 15%

Because accurate recorded weight before the episode of dehydration may not be available for comparison, the diagnosis is based on clinical signs. Early signs of dehydration in a patient are dry lips and mucous membranes, diminished urinary output, reduced weight,

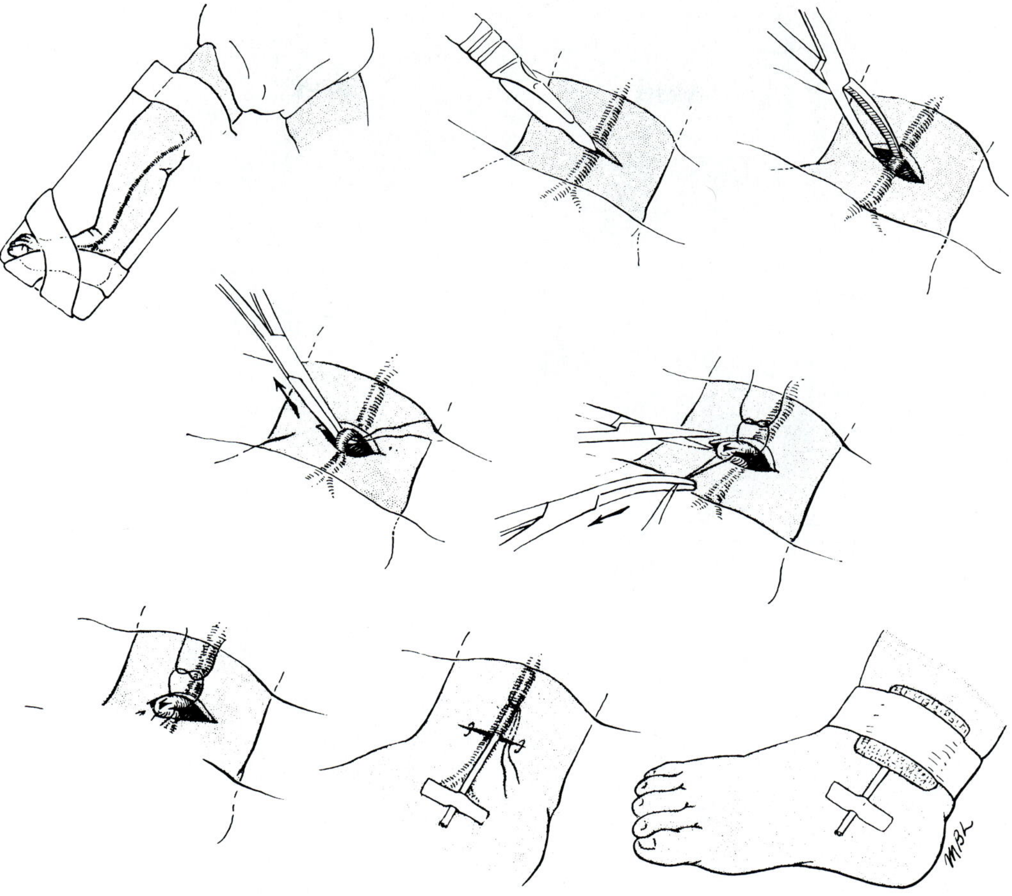

Fig. 26-13 Cutdown procedure. Great care is necessary in immobilizing leg to prevent impairment of circulation and pressure areas. Cutdown may be used for several days to help maintain fluid balance or administer medication. It is used when vein access is difficult.

and lethargy. Moderate dehydration is further characterized by depressed fontanels, sunken eyeballs, loss of skin turgor, and oliguria. As dehydration increases, the child becomes acutely ill, and the circulation may fail. The skin is grayish; the pulse is rapid and weak. Temperature elevation and low blood pressure are characteristic. Recorded output is scant, and weight loss is obvious—10% or higher. Apathy, restlessness, and even convulsions may occur. An infant's condition may require the use of preweighed diapers to determine output. Each gram increase in the weight of a wet diaper is counted as 1 ml of output. Obviously, diapers must be changed and weighed promptly. The blanket under the infant may need to be preweighed as well. It should be next to a waterproof pad. Excessively absorbent diapers interfere with the accuracy of measurement.

Intravenous therapy. Because it is often difficult to perform and maintain a conventional intravenous infusion for prolonged periods in the small child, a *cutdown* may be performed (Fig. 26-13). This minor surgical procedure is usually completed in the treatment room. The physician "cuts down" to a vein, directly exposing it. Small plastic tubing is inserted into a nick in the vein and sutured in place. This tubing is then joined to the intravenous tubing. The increased use of small angiocatheters, which are threaded through a needle puncture into a vein, has reduced the need for cutdowns.

Whether fluids are administered through a cutdown or a needle puncture through the skin into a vein of the scalp or extremity, it is important that the amount of fluid given to the child is monitored carefully to prevent overloading the circulatory system. The rate of flow must be marked on the bottle and meticulously observed. Special pediatric intravenous counting chambers simplify calculation. The typical drop size is 1/60 ml or 60 drops/ml. Although a number of semiautomatic infusion sets have added a special margin of safety to administering fluids, the nurse must continue to keep a close watch on the flow rate,

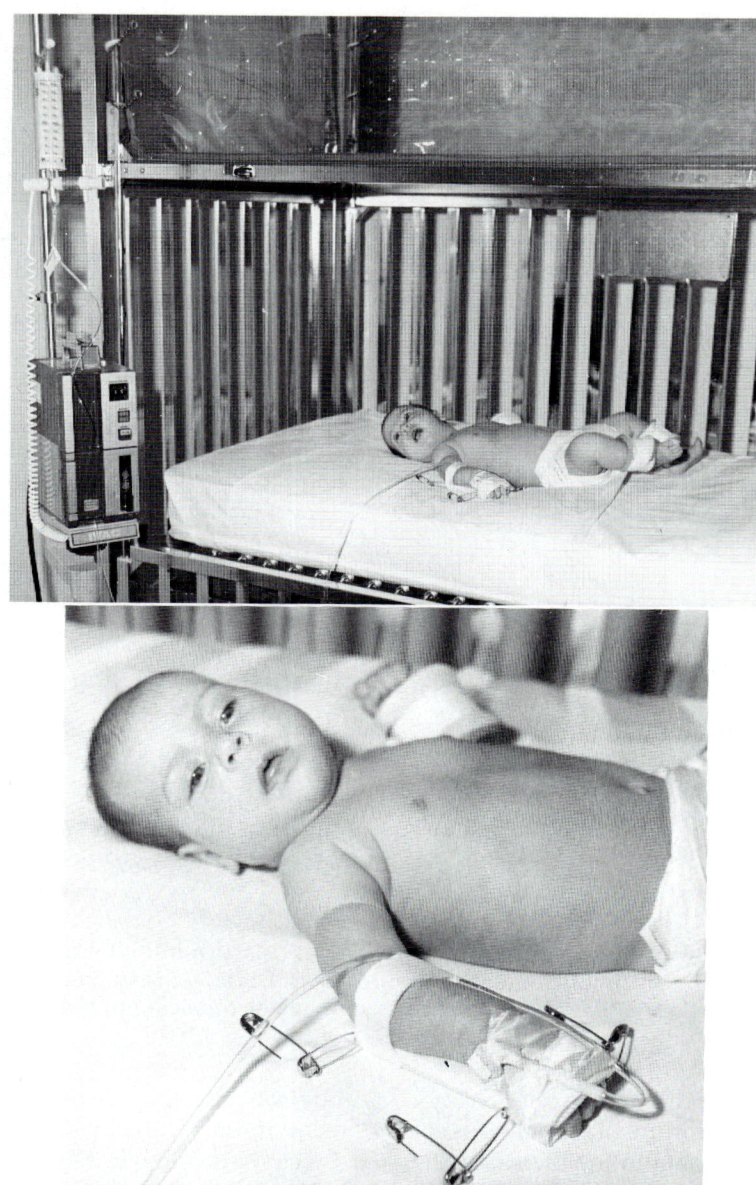

Fig. 26-14 Intravenous fluid with IVAC gravity flow infusion controller can be set for specific amount of fluid delivery and is able to detect infiltration. Siderail is down for the illustration only. Arm board is pinned to bedding. Close-up shows arm immobilization. (Courtesy Naval Hospital, San Diego, Calif.)

the infusion site, and the child's response to the fluid therapy. The infant and small child must be safely restrained to prevent dislodging the infusion. The nurse should be aware that changes in the child's position may slow or speed the infusion, and the nurse should frequently observe the rate of flow in the drip chamber (Fig. 26-14).

Extreme care should be exercised in moving the patient. The nurse shares responsibility for observation of the intravenous apparatus with the supervising primary nurse. If the nurse observes an infusion running more rapidly than ordered, it should be slowed to the correct rate. The physician's orders should be checked immediately for confirmation of the desired drip rate. The area surrounding the intravenous needle must be checked frequently to detect infiltration or inflammation. Pain and swelling are signs of possible dislocation of the needle. The responsibility for observation is critical if the child is receiving blood, since there is more danger of circulatory overload, tissue damage, and untoward reactions. Patients receiving blood should be carefully watched and, when

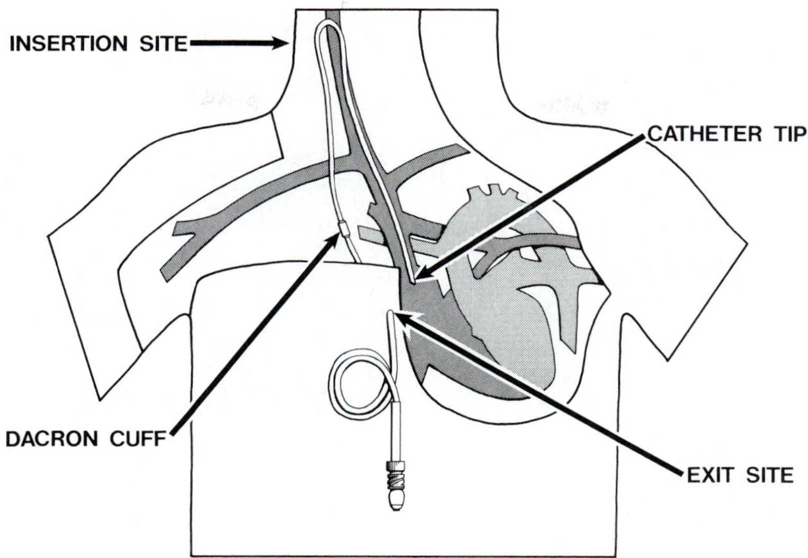

Fig. 26-15 The Hickman indwelling right atrial catheter provides long-term venous access for drawing blood and for giving TPN, medications, and blood products. (Courtesy Virginia Shumate, BSN, Children's Hospital and Health Center, San Diego, Calif.)

> **Nursing Alert**
>
> Stopcock ports are a source of contamination for peripheral and central vascular lines. When they are not being accessed, they should be covered at all times with a sterile cap or syringe. The sterile cap or syringe is changed if contaminated during access for blood collection or administration of medications.

necessary and possible, questioned regarding back or chest pain or chills. The temperature, pulse, and respiratory rate should be frequently determined and the skin observed for urticaria (hives) to detect blood incompatibility.

Parenteral hyperalimentation. Children who cannot tolerate oral or nasogastric feedings are fed by intravenous alimentation. Total parenteral nutrition (TPN) provides glucose, proteins, fats (lipids), minerals, vitamins, and fluids necessary for normal growth and weight gain. Two intravenous methods for TPN are currently used: (1) a central venous line may be established by threading a Silastic catheter through an incision on the side of the neck into a jugular vein to the superior vena cava, or (2) a multipurpose Hickman or Broviac catheter may be installed by way of the jugular vein into the right atrium, exiting via a subcutaneous tunnel on the right thorax or sternum (Fig. 26-15). Other long-term venous access devices include the Groshong catheter, which does not require heparin flushes, and the implanted ports, which have a reduced risk of infection because they are placed completely under the skin (Fig. 26-16).

Peripheral or surface veins may be used as a temporary method for more diluted nutritional supplement, that is, peripheral hyperalimentation. The first two approaches may be preferable, because a concentrated life-sustaining solution can be given at a uniform rate into large veins where it will dilute rapidly and thereby prevent thrombosis and phlebitis. Meticulous sterile technique is required to prevent infection. Hyperalimentation using peripheral veins runs the risk of severe tissue damage if infiltration occurs.

For short-term venous access, the heparin lock is used for patients receiving intermittent medicines. It allows more mobility without the need for continuous intravenous fluids or frequent venipunctures. The heparin lock (Fig. 26-17) consists of a short flexible catheter or scalp vein needle attached to plastic tubing sealed by a rubber insert that is maintained in a manner ensuring patency and sterility. The procedure on p. 539 is included to increase the nurse's understanding of the heparin lock technique.

Personal hygiene

Caring for the child's personal hygiene needs is the responsibility of the nursing staff in collaboration with

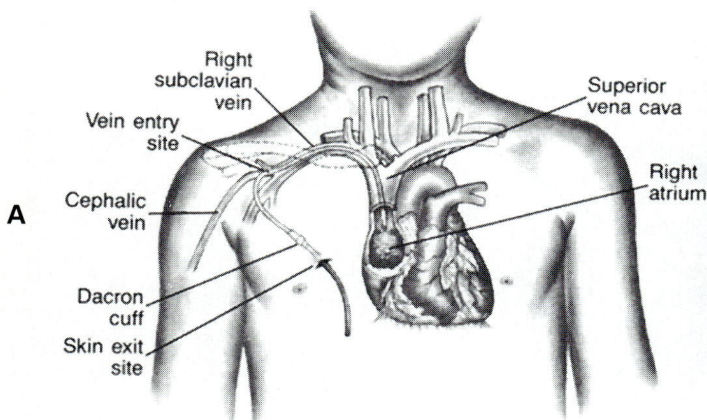

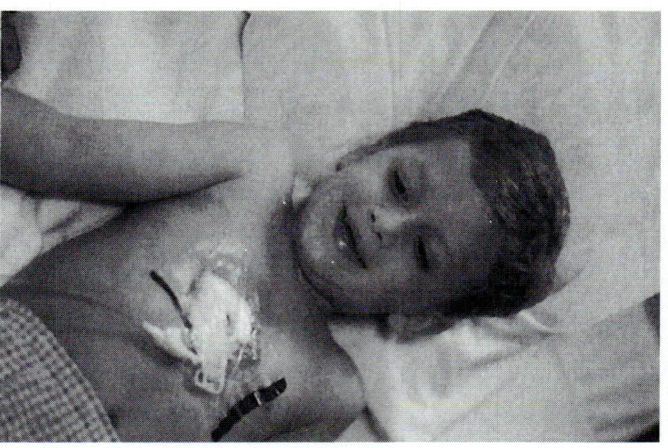

Fig. 26-16 Venous access devices. **A,** Central venous catheter insertion and exit site. **B,** Child receiving medication by way of implantable port. Note needle and extension tubing inserted into port and secured with gauze dressings and a transparent dressing. (From Wong D: *Essentials of pediatric nursing,* ed 4, St Louis, 1993, Mosby.)

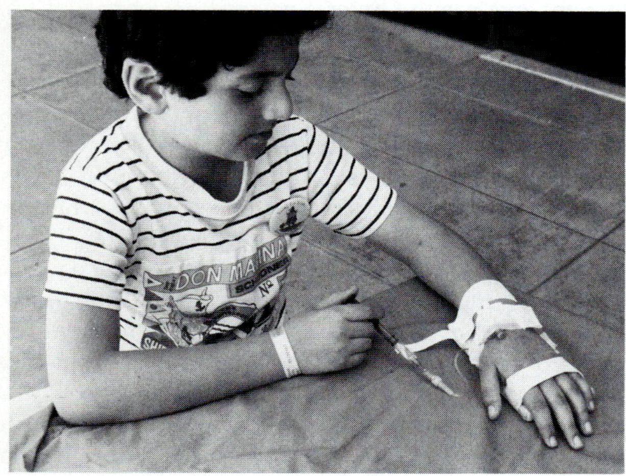

Fig. 26-17 Young boy with hemophilia injecting heparin flush into his heparin lock.

the child and parent. Methods of care depend on the child's developmental age, ability and desire for self-care, level of parental involvement, condition of the patient, and the facilities of the pediatric unit.

Nails. Cleansing and trimming the nails of young children are important components of personal hygiene. The nails may be cut straight across or filed. If the patient is diabetic or has peripheral circulatory, sensory, or bleeding disorders, a specific order must be written to trim the child's nails.

Oral hygiene. Oral hygiene should be carried out routinely. A child with a recent cleft lip, cleft palate, or dental repair is not allowed to have a brush or anything hard in his mouth. For infants with few teeth, oral hygiene may be a drink of water, and wiping the teeth with gauze. For older children, brushing several times a day and daily flossing are essential. A small toothbrush that can easily fit into the mouth is necessary. Massage of the gums and correct brushing and flossing techniques are important health habits. Cracked or dry lips may be lubricated with petrolatum.

Patients confined to a bed are usually dressed in pajamas, gowns, or sweatshirts and sweatpants. When children are convalescing, favorite playclothes may be a morale boost.

Care of the child's environment. Part of patient care is the care of the environment. The bath is not complete until the environment is clean and orderly. Whether a complete linen change is necessary depends on its condition. Most children's beds need frequent changes, but linen should not be used needlessly. The patient's bedside stand should be neat (inside and out). The goal is to provide a pleasant, orderly, well-ventilated, warm, safe environment that promotes health and healing. Children need their toys and freedom to play safely in their bed and surrounding area. In some hospitals, special bags are available for toy storage. Most children enjoy posters or pictures from home.

Bed bath. A bath is usually administered each day to prevent skin irritation and provide refreshment, stimulation, and comfort. It is also an excellent period for patient assessment, planning, and evaluation. Bed baths are given routinely to patients who are quite ill, are especially susceptible to chilling and respiratory tract infections, have dressings or incisions that require protection, or are in traction or casts. Most children with elevated temperatures have bed baths, although occasionally a tepid tub bath may be ordered to reduce fever. Tepid baths consist of placing the child in a warm

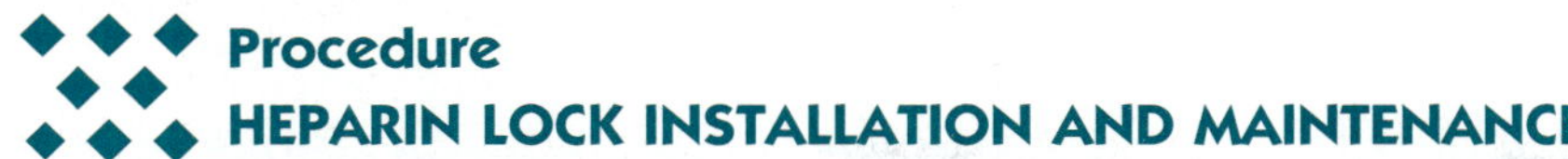

Procedure
HEPARIN LOCK INSTALLATION AND MAINTENANCE

MATERIALS/SUPPLIES

- Tourniquet
- Povidone-iodine solution sponges
- Adhesive tape
- 2 × 2 inch sterile gauze pads
- A special 22- or 24-gauge intravascular catheter (Quick-cath), or No. 23- or 25-gauge butterfly scalp vein needle
- Heparin lock injection adaptor
- Heparin lock flush (10 to 100 units/ml heparinized solution)
- 3-ml syringe for heparin lock flush
- 25-guage ⅝-inch needle for subsequent clearing of tubing, Quick-cath, or needle with saline and/or heparin lock flush
- Alcohol sponges
- 3-ml syringe for normal saline

Protocols vary in different agencies, and modifications may occur according to type of patient, equipment used, and medication administered. Refer to agency procedure.

STEPS

1. Skin is cleansed; intravascular catheter or needle is inserted into arm vein and taped in position.
2. Heparin lock injection adaptor is attached.
3. Injection port is cleansed with alcohol before any injection or infusion is performed. Small needles (23- to 25-gauge) must be used to prevent large puncture holes in the injection port.
   a. Saline can be used to clear tubing of any blood, or tubing can be flushed before a change in tubing solutions.
   b. Heparin lock flush is instilled last to maintain the patency of the line.
   c. A heparin lock should be checked for patency and flushed at least once per shift with saline or heparin lock flush 0.5 to 1.0 ml.
   d. Careful instructions and return demonstrations must accompany the outpatient use of this device.

bath and slowly adding some cool water, avoiding a dramatic temperature change. Bed baths are carried out in essentially the same manner for children as for adults. A bath blanket or towel should be used for a covering, and except in the case of an infant, the area should be curtained or screened. Unless contraindicated, a good light should be available for the bath area to aid in the detection of any special changes in skin color, rashes, or other abnormalities.

Perineal care. Children should be helped with the care of their genitalia if they are too young to cleanse the area properly. Any irritation of the penis or labia should be reported. If a little boy is uncircumcised, the foreskin should be retracted gently. Observation of the area for cleanliness and possible inflammation should be made. Occasionally, perineal care using an irrigation technique is desirable in the case of pubertal girls who are having their menses.

Tub bath. When tub baths are allowed, the amount of supervision required depends on the child's developmental age and condition. Young children should never be left alone because of the danger of burning from the hot water faucet, drowning, or falling while trying to climb out. Unless a prolonged tub bath is ordered for treatment purposes, the bath should not be too extended because the chance for chilling , increases, and others may be waiting in line. Prolonged bathing and the use of bubble bath and shampoo in bath water cause urinary tract irritation in many children, particularly little girls. The tub should be cleaned well after each use. Teenagers are modest and need only a minimum of supervision while bathing. Most school-aged children and teens prefer showering if they are physically able.

A prolonged tub bath lasts at least 20 minutes. It may be ordered to relax the muscles before physical therapy, to help remove dressings or crusts, or to apply a certain soothing medication to the skin, such as oatmeal or Alpha Keri. To help the patient relax in the bath and get the whole body in contact with the water, a pillow may be constructed from a rolled bath blanket to raise the head out of the water while the child lies flat in the tub. If a rubber headrest is available, it may be used for this purpose. If a child has a tendency toward urinary tract infections, a prolonged tub bath may be contraindicated.

Infant tub bath. The infant receiving a tub bath is placed in a small basin for greater security and easier handling. The following procedure can be used for a newborn infant whose umbilicus has healed or, with modification, for an older infant. It can be carried out at the bedside, at a special table or counter, or at home in a clean sink. Wherever the bath is given, the principles are the same, although the organization and

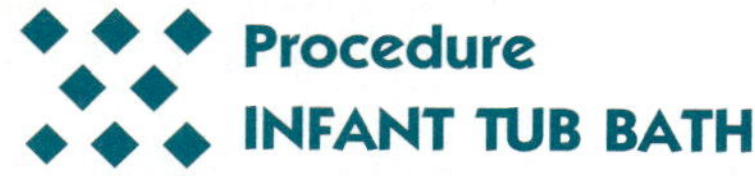

Procedure
INFANT TUB BATH

EQUIPMENT/SUPPLIES:

- Infant bathtub, large basin, or bathinette
- Suggested supplies on tray:
  a. Mild soap e.g., Dove, Johnson's Baby Soap, or Neutrogena
  b. Jar of cotton balls
  c. Jar of safety pins
  d. Bottle of sterile water
  e. Box of tissues
- Large towel or mat to dry area
- Bag or hamper for discard of dirty clothes
- Wastebasket to receive trash
- One soft towel for drying
- Two soft washcloths or paper mesh squares
- Clean baby clothes stacked in order of use:
  a. Diaper
  b. Shirt
  c. Kimono
  d. Receiving blanket

STEPS

1. Maintain infant warmth.
2. Bathe proceeding from clean to dirty areas. Refrain from referring to the genitalia or buttocks as "dirty" areas.
3. Support the infant appropriately, maintaining control of the head and guarding safety (Fig. 26-18).
4. Use bath time for careful assessment and stimulation.
5. Check the temperature of the room (should be 72° to 75° F [22° to 24° C] and free from drafts).
6. Wash hands thoroughly; put on apron.
7. Assemble equipment.
8. *Never leave baby alone in tub,* e.g., to obtain supplies or answer the phone.
9. Fill tub one third full of water at a temperature comfortable to your elbow.
10. Place the infant, still dressed to preserve body heat, on the towel or bath mat.
    a. Inspect eyes; wash lids proceeding from the inner corner of the eye outward. A fresh washcloth surface or cotton dipped in clear water is appropriate.
    b. Inspect the ears; wash outer folds. Do not probe canals.
    c. Wash the face with the washcloth and clear water from the tub. Dry.
    d. Soap the scalp; support infant, using the football hold. The infant's head is held over the tub; the ears are covered by the nurse's fingers. Rinse the scalp carefully. Dry. Check for "cradle cap."
11. Remove shirt and diaper. If the buttocks are soiled with stool, discard the washcloth used for the cleanup or use tissues. Use another washcloth to continue the bath.
12. The infant's body may be soaped either before being placed in the tub for rinsing or during the time the infant is in the tub, whichever way the nurse feels more secure.
13. Lift the child carefully into the tub, feet first, using appropriate positioning.
14. After a brief period, lift the infant out of the tub and place on a towel on the mat; pat infant dry.
15. Inspect and clean female genitalia with damp cotton balls or tissues as needed, wiping from front to back. Retraction of the foreskin on male infants should not be forced. Many infants have adhesions in the area. Gently cleanse the glans.
16. Dry the infant carefully; dress in clean clothes and a receiving blanket.
17. Offer drinking water and inspect the mouth.

Nursing Alert

The use of powder is not recommended and has been associated with aspiration pneumonia or pneumonitis. Baby oil should also be discouraged as it occludes pores and encourages infection.

details of equipment may be different. The nurse may wish to place the tub on a bedside table and use the bed for drying and dressing the infant. The older infant who enjoys the bath and is able to sit steadily may be allowed more freedom in the tub. This procedure should be a pleasant experience for the infant and the nurse. The child should never be left unattended.

Shampoo. The patient's general health, the length of the hair, and the condition of the scalp determine the frequency of shampooing. Hospital policy will determine whether an order is necessary. If their condition allows, older children may shampoo their hair in the shower. If assistance is needed a child can easily have his or her hair shampooed by lying on a gurney with the head extended over the end next to a sink or tub. A trough to guide the water may be constructed of plastic or rubber sheeting. If a wall spray hose is used, great care should be taken in regulating the temperature of the water before it touches the child.

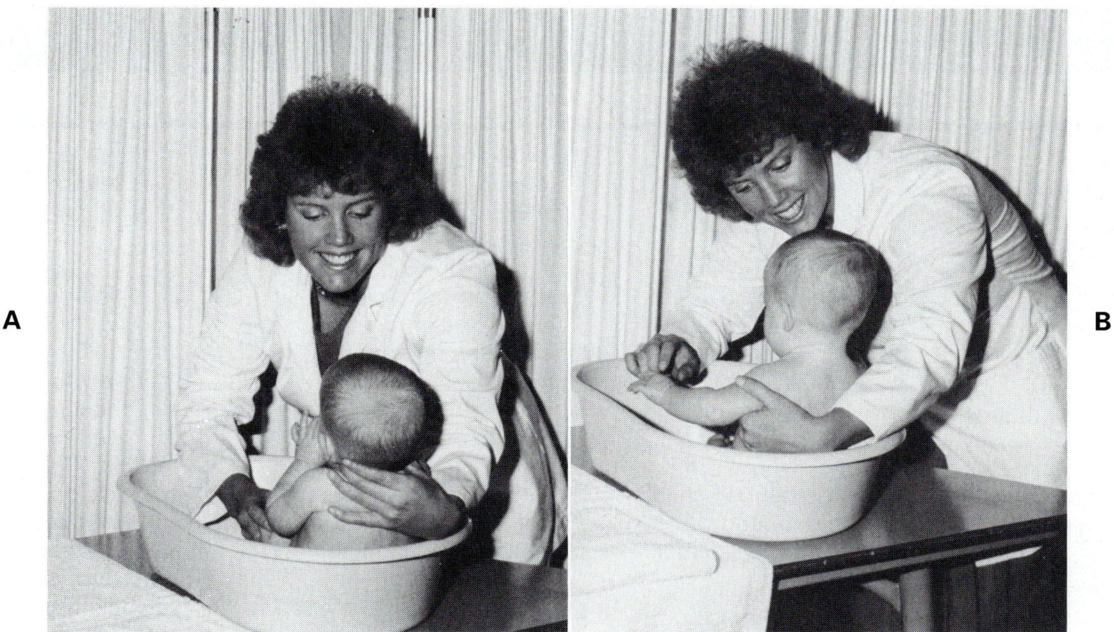

Fig. 26-18 **A** and **B,** Two methods of supporting infant during tub bath.

If the child is immobilized, a simple head basin and trough can be constructed from two bath blankets rolled together lengthwise and curved into a horseshoe shape, with the open end pointing toward the side of the bed. This form is draped by a plastic sheeting to make a waterproof basin that leads off the side of the bed into a large bath basin or infant tub. Some hospitals use inflated Kelly pads. Many units have bed shampoo basins, similar to those found in beauty salons. The hair must be rinsed well. Hair should be dried quickly and thoroughly to prevent chilling.

Rest

Adequate rest is critical to optimum child health promotion. Infants and toddlers may need two naps each day, whereas older children do well with a rest period after lunch, lasting at least 1 hour. Other nap times should be encouraged, depending on the child's needs. Shades should be drawn, the television turned off, and a warm, well-ventilated environment maintained. A reminder of something pleasant that will happen after a rest is often helpful. Some children respond well to soft music or relaxation tapes.

Diversion, self-expression, coping mechanisms (Table 26-2)

A convalescing child should not be expected to sit or lie quietly all day long without diversion and opportunities for self-expression. Although rest is important, a child may rest better when allowed moderate activity during the day. The nurse can help by supplying appropriate toys, books, and creative materials; providing suitable television programs or videos; setting up controlled group play for patients in the same room when possible; playing with the child; or enlisting the help of the child-life specialist. Occupational or recreational therapists and the hospital library are good resources.

Play is a learning activity that promotes physical, mental, emotional, and social growth. In play, children develop new abilities; acquire knowledge about themselves; and explore the feel, look, and taste of the world around them. They use play to express what they are thinking and feeling and to relate and interact with others. Dramatic play is recognized as a form of emotional release. The nurse can help children choose play materials that will be fun and satisfying. The following principles should be kept in mind when choosing toys: (1) developmental age, (2) safety, and (3) durability. Choosing the right play materials at the right time is not an easy task. Every child needs a well-balanced toy selection for overall development. The choice should be planned to stimulate (1) social play, (2) dramatic play, (3) creative play, (4) manipulation and constructive play, and (5) active physical play. Play activity is as vital to growth as nutrients, rest, nursing care, and medical treatment.

Administration of Medication

The administration of medication to young children entails special skills and knowledge. It is an enormous responsibility because dosages vary so greatly from

◆ TABLE 26-2
Play-and-Get-Well Chart

Age	Interest	Toys	Books
Infant (Birth to 1 yr)	Toys that attract the eye, make little sounds, and tempt grasping hands	Bright hanging objects; large plastic rings; string of bright-colored rings; rubber toys that squeak; tinkling bells	*Pat the Bunny,* Dr. Seuss Loves being read to if started early
Toddler (1 to 3 yr)	Toys that enable parallel play, provide security and attention, and help development of muscle coordination	Nest of blocks; mallet and wooden pegs; trucks and cars; cuddly toy animals; large dolls; rocking horse; toy telephone; musical toys; kiddie car	Large linen picture books; nursery rhymes; ABC books; farm and zoo animal stories Likes the same story over and over again
Preschooler (3 to 6 yr)	Toys that stimulate child's imagination and develop creative abilities	Nurse and doctor sets; trains and trucks; Tinker Toys; cabin logs; magnets; action figures; record player, hand puppets; crayons and color books; dolls and clothes; simple puzzles; modeling clay; scrapbooks; cuddly toy animals	Dr. Seuss books; Golden Books; once-upon-a-time-stories Enjoys stories about airplanes, trains, and police and fire stations Likes to look at pictures while being read to
Early school age (6 to 10 yr)	Application of mental and physical skills Interest and enjoyment in playing with children of same gender Realistic toys that bring child into contact with world outside hospital	Craft sets; models; picture painting; stamp collection; string marionettes; spool knitting; beadwork Games such as Monopoly, checkers, and Clue Paper and pencil games; jigsaw puzzles; paper dolls; video games	Comic books; riddle books; crossword puzzles; fairy tales; adventure stories; simple science books; how and why books; who-when-where books; *Highlights*
Middle school age (10 to 12 yr)	Adaptable to group activities Combine companionship and challenge and coordinate work and play in teams	Card games; photoelectric football; science toys; chess; checkers Skill crafts, such as sculpting and wood carving Walkie-talkie; telescope; transistor radio; camera; television; picture viewer	Comic books; school textbooks; biographies; adventure stories Junior classics such as *Heidi, Little Women, Treasure Island, Robin Hood, Alice in Wonderland, Andersen's Fairy Tales; Aesop's Tales*

child to child, as the result of weight, body area, and metabolic differences.

General principles

Pediatric dosages may be calculated in different ways. Age is used occasionally as a basis for determination.

Young's rule:

$$\textbf{Child's dose} = \frac{\text{Age of child in years}}{\text{Age of child in years} + 12} \times \text{Average adult dose}$$

Because the sizes of children who are the same age may differ, Clark's rule, which is based on weight, is the safer way to calculate dosage:

Clark's rule:

$$\textbf{Child's dose} = \frac{\text{weight of child in pounds}}{150} \times \text{Average adult dose}$$

Another concept used in computing pediatric dosage is based on the surface area of a child. With this method one must know the metric weight and height of the child to calculate the surface area in square meters. The average surface area of an adult is calculated to be 1.7 m^2.

The final formula used is:

$$\frac{\text{Surface are of child } (m^2)}{1.7} \times \text{Average adult dose}$$

A West nomogram may also be used for estimation of surface area.

Giving medication is sometimes difficult because the child may not recognize the need for the medicine and may resist its administration. Although the licensed vocational nurse may not be given major responsibility in the administration of medicines in the pediatric area, knowledge of the principles of administration, patient assessment, and evaluation of effectiveness are essential. The following information must be included:

1 The right patient (check ID bracelet)
2 The right medication in the right form
3 The right dosage
4 The right method of administration
5 The right time of administration

Before any medication is given, it should be identified on a medicine card or on the medication Kardex. In most hospitals, orders for certain medications must be renewed after a certain time. Common medications that are often automatically stopped unless reordered are broad-spectrum antibiotics and narcotics. Medications that are ordered on an as necessary or prn basis must be checked to see when they were last given to prevent too-frequent administration. The need for the medication also must be determined. The nurse should look up any unfamiliar medication before assuming responsibility for its administration. Knowledge of common usages, contraindications, side effects, common dosages, and optimum methods of administration is essential.

Common measurements

Before giving medications, the nurse should review the common measurements used in the metric and apothecary systems and frequently used conversions. An easily read table should be available for reference. Some of the most common conversions follow:

1 dram (L, dr) = 4 ml
1 teaspoon (tsp) = 5 ml
1 tablespoon (tbsp) = 15 ml
1 ounce (K, oz) = 30 ml
16 minims (Nxv or Nxvi) = 1 ml
15 grains (gr xv) = 1 gm
1 grain (gr i) = 0.06 gm or 60 to 65 mg

Oral medication

Preparation. If possible, medications for children are prepared as solutions for greater ease in administration. Suspensions must always be shaken well before being poured. Most may be diluted, although it is not wise to dilute medicines more than a few milliliters to wash out the measuring container. Children might not take the increased volume easily. Placing medication in an infant formula is not recommended. If the infant refuses to take all the formula, it is impossible to determine what amount of medication has been ingested.

Administration. Before giving any type of medication, the nurse must check the patient's identification. Always place a bib on a small child before administering oral medications. Such a simple maneuver saves extra clothing changes and nursing time. If a child is given fluids with a medication it must be recorded on the I & O record.

Liquid medications may be given easily to infants when placed in a nipple, a syringe, medication spoon, or rubber-tipped medication dropper. The infant will suck the medication while the nurse supports the head to prevent aspiration. Small medication cups are also used. Medicine is poured slowly with the infant in a sitting position or with the head elevated. Pills and capsules usually must be crushed or opened for children under 5 years of age; however, enteric coated medications may not be crushed. Giving nonliquid medication to younger children may also increase the danger of aspiration. The medication may be placed in applesauce or jelly and given from a spoon. Medications may taste bitter; thus a disguise is helpful. However, children must never be told that they are receiving candy when they are being medicated.

The child who takes medicine well should be praised. If children find it difficult to take medicine, they should be made to feel that the nurse understands their distaste and fear and wants to help. The nurse may find it necessary to hold the child on the nurse's lap with one of the child's hands wedged behind her and the other controlled by an encircling arm and hand (Fig. 26-19). Pouring medication down the throat of a struggling, crying youngster is an invitation to aspiration, emesis of the medication, and subsequent trying periods when medicine time comes again. At times children respond much better if allowed to hold the cup and drink at their own rate. Many of the small, disposable medicine cups are safe play objects for children, who in turn pretend to medicate their dolls and stuffed toys.

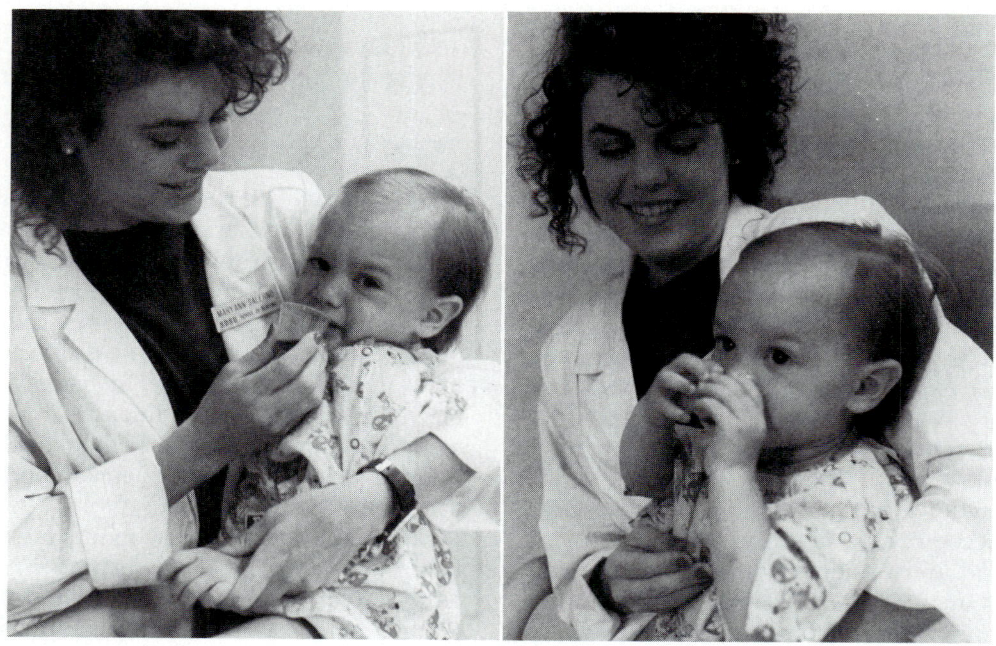

Fig. 26-19 **A,** Administration of medication. The nurse encircles child with arm and holds child's hand. Child's other arm is tucked behind nurse's back. The child will take the medicine in this position but much prefers **B,** to hold the cup and take the medicine.

Intramuscular injections

Intramuscular injections are a traumatic experience for most children; consequently injections are given only when the medication can be given by no other route (Wong, 1993). Small infants receive their immunizations in the vastus lateralis and offer minimum resistance. The larger infant can be restrained between the nurse's elbow and body (Fig. 26-20). When the nurse must give an intramuscular injection to a crying toddler or fearful older child, a second person may be needed to help support, distract, restrain, or comfort the child. If the child is old enough to understand, the nurse should explain the procedure just before administering the injection. Resistant, tearful children might be told that the medicine will help them get better so that they can go home sooner. The infant or younger child needs to be restrained adequately to ensure safe and correct administration. To lessen a child's fear and to maintain a sense of trust, the nurse should always comfort the child by holding afterward and should never administer an injection to a sleeping child. Role-play with a doll or stuffed animal may assist some children in coping more effectively with the stress of an injection.

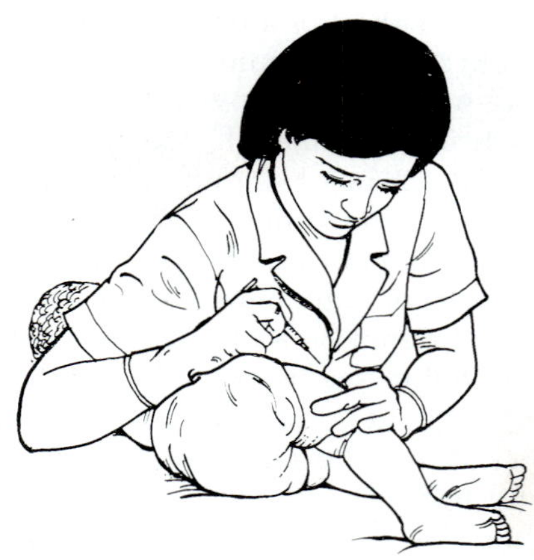

Fig. 26-20 Restraining small child for intramuscular injection. (From Perry AG and Potter PA: *Clinical nursing skills and techniques,* ed 3, St Louis, 1994, Mosby.)

Older children seem to be helped if they are distracted with conversation, or if they are given something on which to concentrate such as music, squeezing a bedrail, singing, or counting. The child may wish to hold the Band-Aid and place it on the puncture site after the injection. Using colorful Band-Aids or placing stickers on the Band-Aid may be helpful. The child should be comforted by the nurse administering the injection.

Suppositories

The rectal route is less reliable; however, it is used when the oral route is contraindicated. Acetamin-

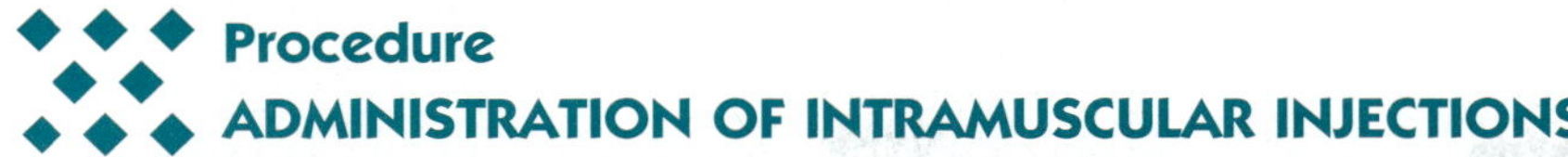

Procedure
ADMINISTRATION OF INTRAMUSCULAR INJECTIONS

EQUIPMENT/SUPPLIES
- Gloves
- Damp antiseptic sponge
- 1- or 3-ml syringe
- 22-gauge, 1-inch needle for infants and children
- 23-gauge, ⅝- to ¾-inch needle for infants less than 4 months old
- Band-Aid

Because the gluteal muscle is not well developed in the infant or young child, and permanent sciatic nerve damage is possible, the buttocks are never used for an intramuscular injection. The most desirable sites for pediatric injections are the lateral and anterior aspects of the thighs, the deltoid areas, and the soft tissue inferior to the iliac crests (ventrogluteal site) (Fig. 26-21). The medicine and syringe should be completely prepared and ready for use before the nurse enters the child's room.

STEPS
1. Place an ice cube or a cold compress on the site about a minute before the injection.
2. The site is cleansed with the antiseptic damp sponge, using a circular motion. The skin is pulled taut.
3. In young children who have minimal muscle, the needle is inserted at a slightly oblique angle with a dartlike motion; if the child is large and well developed, the needle is inserted perpendicularly.
4. The plunger is pulled back to ensure that the needle is not in a blood vessel, and the medicine is injected slowly.
5. The sponge is placed over the needle, the needle is quickly withdrawn, and the area is gently wiped with the sponge.
6. A bandage is usually placed over the site.

ophen, sedative drugs, and bowel stimulants may be given to children in the form of rectal suppositories. Most of these suppositories can be lubricated with a jellylike material before insertion. Because the suppositories are often refrigerated to preserve their shape, warming them, unwrapped, in a clean hand for about a minute may be helpful. A gloved finger is used to quickly but gently insert the suppository into the rectum 1 to 2 inches beyond the rectal sphincter. The child should be asked to take a deep breath. After insertion, pressure should be exerted on the buttocks, holding them or taping them together for 5 to 10 minutes to relieve pressure on the anal sphincter.

Nose drops

Nasal drops are ordered fairly often for infants and children. They are primarily used for nasal congestion and to make breathing, eating, and drinking easier. In the case of an infant, nose drops may be ordered 20 minutes before meals to improve sucking and breast milk or formula intake. If the nose is very congested, gentle suctioning of the nasal passageway may be indicated before the drops are administered. Young children do not understand the reason for nose drops and may need to be gently restrained by a second person or by a modified mummy restraint. The child should be lying down with the head tilted back over a folded towel or small pillow. The dropper should be pointed slightly toward the top of the nasal cavity. The child should maintain this position for several seconds after the instillation. Oily nose drops should be avoided because of the possibility of aspiration and lipoid pneumonia.

Ear drops

Ear drops are used in the pediatric area for external ear infections and to soothe the pain of middle ear infections. They should be close to body temperature because cold ear drops are painful. The child's head should be resting comfortably on the bed, turned with the ear to be treated exposed. When ear drops are given to children less than 3 years of age, the earlobe should be gently pulled down and back to straighten the canal. Older children and adults should have their earlobes pulled up and back for the same reason. After instillation, cotton should not be routinely inserted because it may interfere with drainage of discharge to the exterior or soak up the recently instilled medication.

Eye drops and ointments

Eye drops and ointments should be instilled in the lower conjunctival sac while the child, lying flat, looks up (Fig. 26-22). After instillation, the eyes should be closed but not squeezed shut, because the latter may force out the medication.

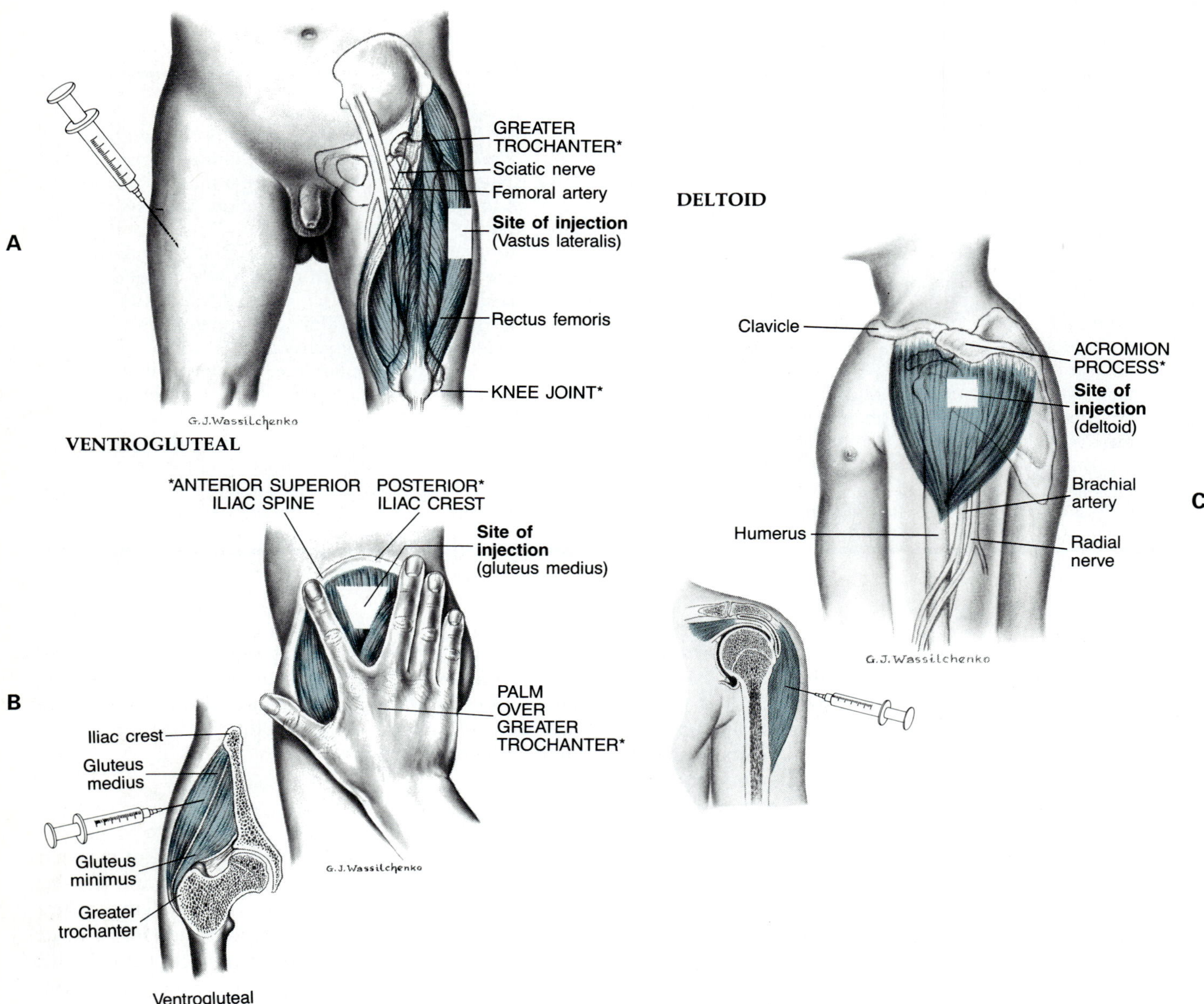

Fig. 26-21 Site of injection chart. Most desirable sites for pediatric intramuscular injections are **A,** rectus femoris muscle, **B,** vastus lateralis muscle, and **C,** deltoid muscle. (From Whaley L and Wong D: *Nursing care of infants and children,* ed 4, St Louis, 1991, Mosby.)

It is a good practice with some toxic medications, such as atropine, to put a little pressure at the inner angle of the eye after the drop has been placed to prevent drainage into the nose through the tear duct.

Topical medication

Ointments or creams may be applied to the skin with a finger cot or applied to gauze with a sterile tongue blade if the area is to be covered with a sterile compress. Lotions are applied with clean or gloved hands or cotton balls, depending on their contents and the condition of the area to be treated.

Special Treatments

Special treatments related to the particular physical problem that the child may be facing are discussed in separate chapters describing procedures involving the various body functions, systems, or diseases.

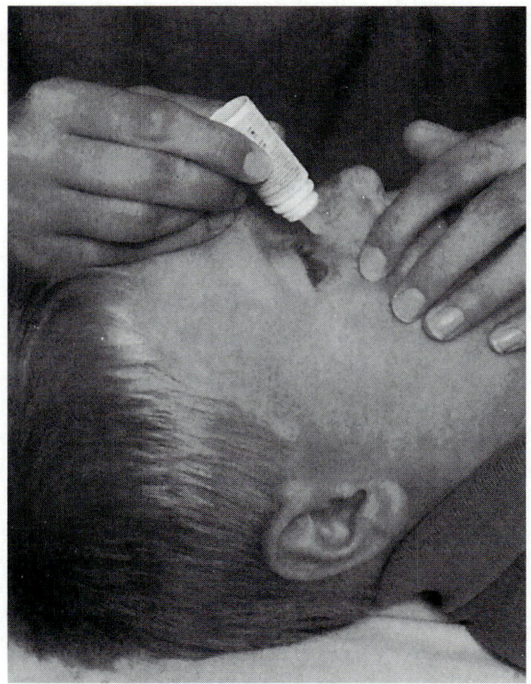

Fig. 26-22 Administering eye drops. (From Wong D: *Essentials of pediatric nursing,* ed 4, St Louis, 1993, Mosby.)

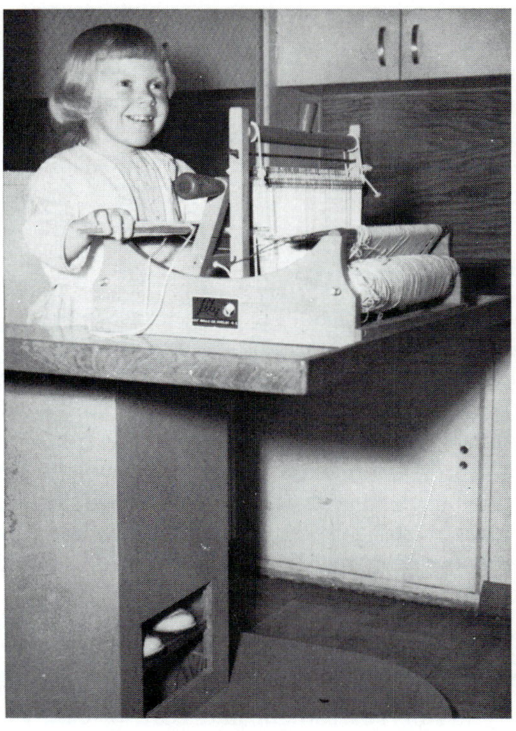

Fig. 26-23 The patient enjoys weaving in occupational therapy. Stand-up table with little gate at back helps maintain balance. Finger exercise encourages joint movement that is so necessary for rheumatoid arthritis patients. (Courtesy Children's Hospital and Health Center, San Diego, Calif.)

Provisions for Rehabilitation

As convalescence progresses, plans for rehabilitation are initiated. Rehabilitation usually begins during hospitalization and continues after discharge. In some cases the problem involved is not rehabilitation but *habilitation,* or the development of skills not previously mastered, particularly for patients suffering from neuromusculoskeletal problems. Emphasis is placed on the development of function with the least cosmetic defect and maximum appearance of normalcy. Priority is placed on skills needed for daily living and optimum health maintenance. Many hospitals have a special rehabilitation unit, or they collaborate with another community or state facility (see Chapter 37).

Physical therapy

Those engaged in the specialty of physical therapy concern themselves primarily with the treatment of disease and injury by using physical agents such as heat, cold, electricity, and water. The most common techniques used involve therapeutic exercises in and out of water. These specially prescribed exercises are fundamental to the treatment of delayed motor development and respiratory, orthopedic, and neuromuscular disease. They are designed to prevent and correct deformities, increase muscle strength and function, and establish normal postural reflexes. The physical therapist institutes normal patterns of motion and teaches coordination, balance, walking, and stair climbing (with and without orthopedic appliances), as well as other activities of daily living (ADL). Thus through the careful selection of techniques, the physical therapist prevents deformity, relieves pain, and promotes functional capacity.

Occupational therapy

Occupational therapy is more often concerned with the maintenance or stimulation of small muscle control necessary for the accomplishment of more refined but equally important skills involving finger and wrist manipulation (Fig. 26-23). Occupational therapy uses many crafts to motivate and involve the patient in activities that strengthen muscles or are psychologically stimulating. Weaving, ceramics, jewelry-making, woodworking, and painting are activities that may also improve patient function. The occupational therapy department can locate or design equipment to assist the patient in carrying out necessary ADLs: Appliances that help the hands to hold combs and toothbrushes, special cups, plate guards, angled spoons and forks to help with eating, and elastic shoelaces and long-handled gadget sticks to aid in dressing are just a few of many possibilities (see Chapter 32.)

Other specialties

Speech pathologists and audiologists (hearing specialists) are important members of the health care team. They assess the child's communication skills; decide whether assistive devices are necessary; and work with parents, teachers, and members of the team to plan for the optimum speech and language development and educational needs of the child. A bedside teacher provided by the public school system may make the return transition from hospital to regular school less difficult.

Documentation (Recording)

The nursing assessment and plan of care must be documented in a clear, concise, and appropriate format. Nursing notes are a permanent record of the patient's treatments, medications, and changing health status. Documentation is especially important because of dynamic changes of the developing child and inability of the preverbal child to communicate needs.

The nursing notes should be handwritten in ink. Errors in charting should never be erased. Instead, a line should be drawn neatly through the error, so that the entry can still be read, and the portion should be labeled "error." All notes should be signed with the first initial, last name, and title of the person making them. The reason for the child's hospitalization; known allergies; significant signs and symptoms; medical and nursing diagnosis; change in condition; I & O record; patterns of elimination including amount, consistency, and color; treatments, medications, and reactions; and parental presence and role in the care of the child are recorded. Special teaching including educational materials provided; demonstrations of procedures to patients or parents; and visits of health care providers, parents, and relatives should also be noted concisely and accurately. Excellent documentation develops as a result of concentrated effort and experience. Computerized documentation at the bedside is being used increasingly.

> **Nursing Alert**
>
> The nurse's notes influence interventions and treatment by the entire health care team, influence research questions, and may become of specific legal importance. The legal ramifications of complete or incomplete record-keeping are enormous.

DAILY PLANNING FOR PATIENT CARE

After a basic needs assessment, planning and implementation of nursing care is initiated. The student requires guidance in executing nursing care so that priorities are recognized and work progresses safely and efficiently, benefitting patients, families, and staff. When given the morning assignment and report, a student must plan individualized care to accomplish patient care goals according to established priorities. To achieve this goal, the student must be aware of the organization of the nursing unit and the staff utilization pattern. The charge nurse, primary nurse, team leader, or student instructor will assist and advise in planning. A quick tour of all assigned patients to check on any immediate needs is helpful. The following can be accomplished:

1 Introduce the child and family.
2 Check the general safety of the patient's environment.
   a Restraints and siderails, crib nets
   b Intravenous lines for rate of flow and possible infiltration and type of solution
   c Humidification devices
   d Oxygen equipment
   e Toy safety
3 Help set up and supervise breakfast, when appropriate, checking diet for accuracy. Note whether any patients need to be weighed before eating.
4 Evaluate the need for supplies.
   a Linen
   b Clothing, hospital gowns, or pajamas
   c Procedural supplies
      (1) Dressing supplies
      (2) Solutions, i.e., irrigating sets

In planning the daily schedule the following must be considered:

1 Any prior appointments that have been scheduled for patients.
   a Radiographic examination or therapy
   b Physical therapy
   c Speech and hearing services
   d Bedside tutoring
   e Scheduled dressing changes.
2 General condition of the patient
   a As a general rule, the patient who is least comfortable has the priority.
   b Presurgical patients who have had a preoperative medication are usually not disturbed.

c Patients who are sleeping and need the rest may, at the discretion of the supervising nurse, be left temporarily undisturbed.

3 Types of treatment that are ordered and when they are to be given

a Enemas are given before the bath and bed change.

b Shampoos are ordinarily given after the bath but before the bed change.

c A patient's care is preferably completed before a blood transfusion or other infusions are started.

4 Hospital routine

a Taking the vital signs, temperature, pulse, respiration, and blood pressure is routine for most patients; the time at which it is done depends on the hospital policy and the type of nursing organization pattern followed.

b Meal schedules: children usually need more supervision and aid than adults; infants are usually fed their ordered solids, bathed, and then given their fluids.

Policies and routines vary from one hospital to another; however, the underlying scientific principles and steps of the nursing process remain the same. Health care reform, computerization, shortened hospital stays, an emphasis on cost-containment, the growth of home health care, and expanded nursing roles will create dramatic change over the next decade.

KEY CONCEPTS

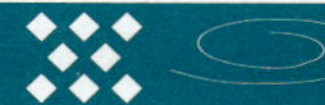

1 The nursing staff is responsible for helping to provide the following: safety, observation and assessment, supportive procedures, medications and special treatments, rehabilitation, and clear and concise documentation.

2 The pediatric hospital environment must be continually evaluated to prevent injuries.

3 Sometimes children must be restrained during treatment to protect themselves. Restraints should be constructed so that they do not become tighter with increased tension, impairing circulation or endangering respiration.

4 Observation and assessment of the pediatric patient are particularly important and complex because small children may be unable to express themselves and because many variables are associated with different stages of growth and development.

5 Diagnostic procedures must be understood so that assessment, planning, implementation, and evaluation can be provided.

6 Various types of supportive procedures and techniques are used to maintain or improve the physical and emotional resources of the patient. These include supervision of position and activity, nourishment and fluid balance, cleanliness, rest and diversion, self-expression, and coping mechanisms.

7 Children confined to bed for long periods must maintain good alignment, functional positions, range of motion, and tissue health.

8 All pediatric patients are routinely on a regimen of measured fluid intake; most are on a measured fluid output regimen as well.

9 Hydration is extremely important because a young child may become dehydrated more rapidly than an adult. The recommended amount of fluid depends on the child's size and condition. Ensuring adequate oral intake requires patience and persistence.

10 One of the most delicate balances maintained by the body is demonstrated by the composition of body fluid. Major components are water and electrolytes.

11 Body fluid occupies three permeable compartments: blood vessels, tissue spaces, and the areas inside the cells. Extracellular fluid is located within the blood vessels and between the tissue cells; intracellular fluid lies inside the tissue cells. Chemical differences exist between extracellular and intracellular fluids.

12 The four main electrolytes in the body are sodium, potassium, calcium, and bicarbonate. Deficits or excesses are called electrolyte imbalances and may require intervention.

13 Acid-base balance is maintained by the action of the lungs, kidneys, and buffer systems. Any slight deviation from the normal range causes pronounced changes in the cellular functions that may threaten life.

14 Fluid therapy aimed at replacing the patient's daily loss of water, electrolytes, and calories is termed *maintenance therapy.* The purpose of maintenance fluid is to keep the body in neutral balance for water, sodium, potassium, and chloride.

15 Infants are more vulnerable to fluid volume deficits than adults for the following reasons: (1) because their body surface in relation to body weight is greater, they lose a relatively greater amount of fluid through the skin and gastrointestinal tract; their high metabolic rate produces more waste products, which must be diluted for excretion;

their immature kidneys are less able to concentrate urine, resulting in greater urine volume; and accumulation of acidic wastes stimulates respiration, causing greater evaporation through the lungs.

16 Early signs of dehydration are dry lips and mucous membranes, diminished urinary output, weight loss, and lethargy.

17 It is important that the amount of fluid administered intravenously to a child be monitored carefully to prevent overloading the circulatory system. The nurse must keep a close watch on the flow rate, the infusion site, and the child's response to therapy.

18 Some children who cannot tolerate oral or nasogastric feedings can survive by intravenous alimentation. Total parenteral hyperalimentation provides glucose, proteins, fats, minerals, vitamins, and fluid necessary for normal growth and weight gain.

19 The heparin lock is used for patients receiving intermittent medication and allows more mobility without the need for continuous intravenous fluids or frequent venipunctures.

20 Bed baths, tub baths, shampooing, and other hygienic measures are the responsibility of the nursing staff.

21 Play is a learning activity that promotes physical, mental, emotional, and social growth. The following principles should be kept in mind when selecting toys for children: developmental appropriateness, safety, and durability.

22 The following factors must be identified before administering medication: the right patient, the right medication in the right form, the right dosage, the right method of administration, and the right time for administration.

23 Fluid medications may be easily given to infants by placing the medication in a nipple, a small medicine cup, a syringe, or a rubber-tipped medicine dropper.

24 The buttocks are never used for an intramuscular injection for an infant or young child. The most desirable injection sites are the lateral and anterior aspects of the thighs, the deltoid areas, and the soft tissue inferior to the iliac crests (ventrogluteal site).

25 Nasal drops are ordered frequently for infants and children, primarily to combat nasal congestion and make breathing, eating, and drinking easier.

26 As convalescence progresses, provisions for rehabilitation may be necessary, including physical and occupational therapy. Physical therapy is designed to prevent deformity, relieve pain, and promote functional capacity. Occupational therapy is more often concerned with the maintenance or stimulation of small muscle control necessary for the skills involving finger and wrist manipulation.

27 Nursing notes are a permanent record of the patient's treatments, medications, and changing health status. The nurse's notes may help influence therapy, research questions, or may become of specific legal importance.

CRITICAL THOUGHT QUESTIONS

1 Starting at birth, identify the developmental activities that increase the safety risks for children. Compare and contrast safety issues in the hospital and the home environment. Each student may select a different age and present pertinent material.

2 Discuss the reasons why careful monitoring and maintenance of fluids are of particular importance in children. How is fluid balance assessed? What special techniques are used for oral and intravenous intake? What special techniques may be used to measure output?

3 When injections are given to infants and children, how do the sites and equipment differ from those used for adults?

4 Play is often called the work of childhood. How do departments such as occupational therapy and physical therapy incorporate play activities into the plan of care? How might the nurse work in collaboration with these specialists in identifying developmentally appropriate toys?

REFERENCES

Daneck GD and Noris EM: Pediatric IV catheters: efficacy of saline flush, *Pediatr Nurs* 18(2):111-113, 1992.

Gablehouse BL and Gitterman BA: Maternal understanding of commonly used medical terms in the pediatric setting, *Am J Dis Child* 144:419, 1990.

Heiney SP: Helping children through painful procedures, *Am J Nurs* 20-24, 1991.

Whaley L and Wong D: Nursing care of infants and children, ed 4, St Louis, 1991, Mosby.

Wong D: *Essentials of pediatric nursing,* ed 4 , St Louis, 1993, Mosby.

27

The Child Experiencing Surgery

CHAPTER OBJECTIVES

After studying this chapter, the student should be able to:

1. Discuss ways infants and young children differ from adults regarding:
   a. Metabolic rate
   b. Reserve physical resources
   c. Healing ability
   d. Time orientation
2. Identify five factors that influence how a child is prepared for the experience of surgery.
3. Discuss five teaching methods that prepare a pediatric patient for a surgical procedure.
4. Identify four behaviors a preverbal child may exhibit when experiencing pain.
5. Describe three types of pediatric pain scales.
6. Discuss factors that influence perception and reaction to pain.
7. Indicate six nonpharmacological methods of pain control.
8. Describe the pediatric modifications for the following common hospital procedures:
   a. Skin preparation for surgery
   b. Cleansing enema
   c. Sterile dressing change
   d. Gavage feeding
   e. Gastrostomy feeding
   f. Nasogastric or intestinal tube irrigation

Anatomical relationships, physiological activity, and psychological responses are greatly influenced by the phenomena of child growth and development. This chapter highlights the differences that distinguish the child from the adult. This knowledge will assist the nurse in completing a comprehensive assessment and plan of care that reflects the unique needs and variability of children facing surgery.

CHILD-ADULT DISTINCTIONS

1. The metabolic rate of infants and young children is much greater proportionately than that of adults. Children need to be fed more frequently and cannot go as long preoperatively without some form of fluid intake.
2. Abnormal fluid loss is more serious in the infant and young child than in the adult. Fluid I & O must be calculated carefully, including fluid loss from diaphoresis or wound drainage. A 7-pound (3.2 kg) infant who sustains a blood loss of 1 oz (30 ml) is comparable to a 150-pound (68 kg) man who has lost 20 ozs (600 ml) of blood.
3. The child lacks the physical reserves that are available to the adult. The child's general condition may change rapidly, almost without warning.
4. The body tissues of the child heal quickly because of the rapid rate of metabolism and growth.
5. Young children are more oriented to the present than to the future.

PREPARATION FOR SURGERY

When uncomplicated surgery is planned, the trend is toward same-day surgery. Many youngsters, however, are still formally admitted to a hospital, even for minor surgery. Preparing a child for the experience of surgery must be based on the following factors: developmental age, the child's perception of hospitalization and the upcoming surgery, the surgical procedure to be performed, postoperative care, previous hospitalization experience, expected length of hospitalization, and parental attitudes.

Emotional Care

The method of preparation must be geared to the actual developmental level of the child or the regressed level, not merely to chronological age. Many nurses use role-play, imagery, puppets, dolls, drawings, films, and selected visitation to special areas of the hospital in conjunction with group and individual discussions as methods of preoperative preparation. Research has demonstrated that children who receive systematic psychological preparation and continued supportive care demonstrate less disturbed behavior, more cooperation in the postoperative period, and faster recovery time. Parents are also less anxious and more satisfied with the information and care received. The nurse should remember that in all contacts with patients, regardless of age, explanations and emotional support should be adapted to the individual's ability to understand and to personal needs. As parents are reassured and provided informational support, the confidence they gain helps them provide emotional support for their child. The presence of parents at the bedside immediately before and after surgical and diagnostic procedures is usually beneficial. Some hospitals admit parents to the post-anesthesia care unit (PACU).

Physical Preparation

Patients admitted for surgery should be assessed for the presence of respiratory infection and signs of malnutrition. Occasionally, surgery may be delayed until the child's general condition improves. Basic evaluative blood and urine tests are performed usually within 24 hours of the surgery. Other diagnostic studies may have been previously performed.

Except in emergency situations and same-day surgical centers, preparation for surgery usually begins the night before the procedure. Some children may be admitted to the hospital early in the morning of the day of minor surgery; many come into the hospital the previous afternoon.

If orthopedic surgery is planned, the child is usually given a povidone-iodine (Betadine) bath in the evening as ordered. Ask about allergies before using an iodine solution. The surgical site is carefully washed and inspected. The fingernails or toenails of any extremity involved are cleansed and trimmed. Frequently, any ordered shave of the operative area is delayed until the morning of surgery. If a shave preparation is requested, it often is done in the operating room suite just before the procedure to reduce the possibility of infection. For some types of surgery, preparatory enemas may be ordered. Food, fluids, and oral medications are withheld as ordered. This is dependent on the type of surgery planned, the age of the child, and the time of the procedure. The fact that the child must not receive anything by mouth should be posted at the bedside. This protocol should be explained to children so that they do not think that they have been forgotten when the breakfast trays are passed. Any loose or missing teeth should be noted and recorded on the chart.

Preoperative sedatives and analgesics may be ordered before certain procedures to control pain, to supplement and reduce anesthetic requirements, to lessen anxiety and body movement, to facilitate the induction of anesthesia, and to decrease airway secretions. There has been a trend, however, to reduce the use of preoperative medication because of possible complications and patient distress at the time of administration when weighed against the benefits obtained.

Each child is assessed individually. If such medication is given, every effort should be made to see that the young child is allowed to rest, whether in the parent's arms or in the crib with the siderails secure until surgery. More prospective controlled studies of sedation and analgesia in infants and children are necessary to discover the optimum preoperative medication for various situations.

Children may be taken to surgery in their cribs or on carts, or they may walk or have to be carried. Many take a well-labeled security item such as a stuffed animal or special blanket. Eyeglasses and hearing aids are important for communication and must be considered for this trip as well. Unless scheduled to go to an intensive care unit, the child's environment is prepared for his or her return. The bed, if present, is made up according to the child's postoperative needs, and any special equipment is placed conveniently. An orthopedic patient may need a special mattress, overbed frame and trapeze, and extra-firm pillows. Additional equipment that may be required, depending on the individual, includes a suction unit, intravenous standard, oxygen apparatus, properly sized restraints, emesis basin, and warm blanket.

POSTOPERATIVE CARE

Assessment

When patients return to the nursing unit from the PACU, their general condition must be noted. Vital signs, temperature, pulse, respirations, and blood pressure are assessed and recorded. Until patients are responsive and alert, they should be kept in a side-lying position unless the surgery performed contraindicates these positions. The nurse should note the condition and placement of any dressing and describe any apparent drainage. The presence of a plaster cast or mold should be recorded. Arms or legs in casts should be elevated, and frequent checks for circulatory disturbances should be made. Intravenous infusions should be checked for possible infiltration and correct rate of flow. Needleless systems may be preferable. Children should be protected from harming themselves (pulling out needles or tubes or tampering with suture lines) by the use of appropriate restraints, as necessary. If a child is immobilized with restraints for an extended time, it is imperative that appropriate range of motion be included in the plan of care and that explanation be given to the child and family. Urinary catheters should be connected to dependent drainage and stabilized properly. The type and amount of urinary drainage should be observed. The patient's skin color and temperature are checked. The nurse must always watch for and quickly report signs of shock: low blood pressure; cold, moist, pale, or cyanotic skin; rapid pulse; dilated pupils; and restlessness.

Diet

Whether oral fluids are allowed after the child is responsive depends on the surgeon's orders and the child's general condition. Sometimes surgical patients are not allowed oral fluids for a considerable time; instead, they are fed intravenously. When oral feedings are introduced, they are begun gradually, and the patient's tolerance is observed. The routine postsurgical diet follows this sequence with modifications for different age groups—clear liquid, full liquid, soft foods and regular foods. Rich, spicy, highly seasoned, or gas-forming foods and red gelatin products should be avoided (red gelatin may discolor the stools).

Ambulation

For the general surgery patient, early progressive ambulation is expected. In only a few situations does the surgeon delay ambulation beyond the first postoperative day. The general surgery patient usually has orders to stand at the bedside and take a few steps the evening of the surgery. The nurse should be sure to follow these orders because ambulation increases patient stamina, aids in the restoration of gastrointestinal function, and helps prevent complications such as pneumonia, the formation of blood clots, and pressure areas.

When the patient's condition makes it impossible or inadvisable to get out of bed, the nurse must be sure that the child is turned frequently, receives good skin care, and breathes deeply at regular intervals. The surgeon may order the use of incentive spirometers or intermittent positive-pressure treatments to aid lung expansion. After surgery, toddlers and preschoolers usually move about spontaneously in their cribs or beds; ambulation presents few problems for them. Older children, however, may express the same timidity and fear of pain that many adult patients exhibit when asked to move or get up and may need a great deal of initial support and encouragement from their parents and the nursing staff. Usually these same children soon are enjoying the freedom of the playroom. Most recover quickly and are discharged in 1 to several days.

Methods of Preventing Pain and Promoting Comfort

Although the following discussion of pain prevention has been placed in the context of the child surgical patient, it is readily understood that pain is experienced in many settings. The following considerations should benefit surgical, medical, emergency, and long-term patients of all ages in numerous places.

One of the major goals in patient care is to prevent pain and maintain optimal comfort. The assessment and management of pain in children, therefore, is of critical importance. Eland (1985) initially drew attention to the fact that undertreatment of pain in children was widespread. Many research studies have been directed toward pain management in children. Much has been learned and our ability to detect and manage pain in children continues to improve.

The physiology of how pain occurs requires an understanding of many different apsects of both the central and peripheral nervous systems. Emotional and psychological components also contribute significantly to the individual's response to pain. Pain is extremely complex and difficult to assess objectively and reliably. It is difficult to determine the best treatment, especially in the young child whose verbal skills and level of understanding are limited. The importance and challenge of accurate pain assessment cannot be overestimated.

Assessment of pain in children must include their physiological and behavioral responses and shared perceptions. Although the infant and toddler are too young to reveal much about their perception of the pain they are experiencing, consultation with their parents may offer some of this missing data. Physiologically, the body responds to a painful stimulus by activating the autonomic nervous system. This response causes an increase in the heart rate, pulse, blood pressure, sweating, muscle tension, and gastrointestinal motility. Although these signs and symptoms can be due to other causes as well, they should always be assessed when determining whether pain exists. Behavioral clues are especially important when assessing the infant and toddler because these children are unable to use verbal means of describing their pain.

Four multidimensional behaviors have been researched and suggested as useful in improving the nurse's assessment of the infant believed to be experiencing pain: vocalization or cry, facial expression or grimacing, body movements involving all four extremities, and the autonomic nervous system responses just described. The assessment process is greatly enhanced by using an organized and consistent approach. The toddler often responds to pain through aggressive behavior such as biting, hitting, temper tantrums, and even verbal hostility. The toddler may also exhibit ritualistic behaviors, such as thumbsucking, rocking, and teeth clenching, or be silent and regressive.

The preschool child can verbalize fears and discomfort better than the toddler, but may distort reality significantly because of his or her self-centered perspective (egocentricity) and magical thinking. Preschoolers cannot clearly separate themselves from the cause of illness or pain and have a very limited understanding of body intactness, which can greatly enhance fears in the hospital situation, and thus also increase pain.

School-aged children can usually describe the type, quality, and quantity of pain, especially if given some preparation beforehand. They are able to respond to scales or questionnaires developed specifically to assist with a more accurate and reliable measurement of pain in both children and adults.

From preschool age on, it is possible and highly desirable to elicit the child's own perception of pain experience. One of the most widely used definitions of pain is that of McCaffery (1989)—that pain is whatever the person experiencing it says it is. A variety of scales are available for use, and a few are applicable to children as young as age 3. The "faces" scale, in the form of drawn faces with progressive gradations of unhappy expressions (Table 27-1), and the Oucher scale, which shows photographs of a child in various stages of pain, are both applicable to the preschool child. The poker chips scale uses five white plastic chips to depict "pieces of hurt" and is recommended for use starting at age 4. The validity and reliability of all scales increase with age. It is important to remember that some preparation of the child before the painful event greatly enhances any scale's usefulness. Additional scales are the thermometer, the color scale, and the visual analog scale (a horizontal line depicting pain intensity from 0 to 10), as well as a variety of questionnaires and body diagrams that encourage more specific description and localization of the pain. It is most important to select a scale and/or questionnaire that is appropriate to the patient's age, to introduce it at a nonthreatening and pain-free time, and then to use that same scale in a consistent manner at regular intervals as long as pain remains a problem. It is only with this three-dimensional measurement of pain—physiological, behavioral, and perceptual information—that the nurse can reliably decide first how to manage the child's pain and then determine the effectiveness of that management.

While attempting an accurate assessment of the patient's pain, the nurse must also be aware of the multitude of influential factors at work in determining reactions to painful experiences. Age, gender, culture, previous experience with pain, fear, the presence of parents, the amount of preparation, and the child's individual temperament and personality all play a role in determining how each child responds to a given situation. A clear understanding of these factors is necessary to help the patient manage pain.

After an accurate pain assessment is achieved, the goal of pain management must be threefold: (1) to eliminate suffering to the greatest degree possible, (2) to enhance each child's ability to cope, and (3) to respond when possible to the underlying reason for the pain. For instance, if the pain is caused by swelling and the edematous extremity is below the level of the heart, elevation of the affected extremity should be the immediate initial intervention.

When everything has been tried to treat the cause of the pain, the possible use of medication becomes of primary consideration. Parenteral narcotics are usually the best means of relieving severe pain. However, they should never be used alone, without consideration of additional pain relief measures. An awareness of the respiratory depression and other side effects that may occur with their use. Parenteral narcotics not only reduce the pain and stress of hospitalization but also maximize the effectiveness of additional nursing

◆ **TABLE 27-1**
Pain Rating Scales for Children

Pain Scale/Description	Instructions	Recommended Age
Faces Scale* (Wong and Baker, 1988): Consists of six cartoon faces ranging from smiling face for "no pain" to tearful face for "worst pain"	Explain to child that each face is for a person who feels happy because there is no pain (hurt) or sad because there is some or a lot of pain. Face 0 is very happy because there is no hurt. Face 1 hurts just a little bit. Face 2 hurts a little more. Face 3 hurts even more. Face 4 hurts a whole lot, but Face 5 hurts as much as you can imagine, although you don't have to be crying to feel this bad. Ask child to choose face that best describes own pain.	Children as young as 3 years
 0 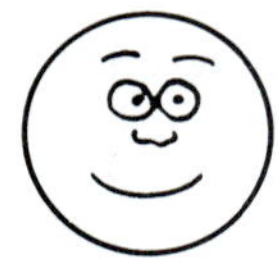 1 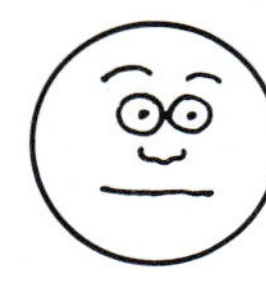 2 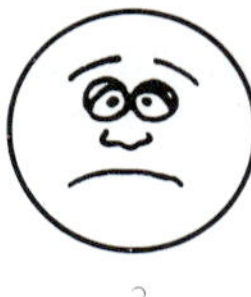 3 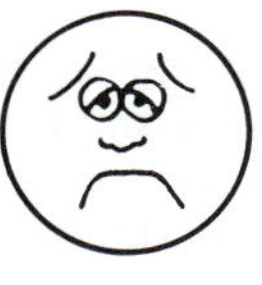 4 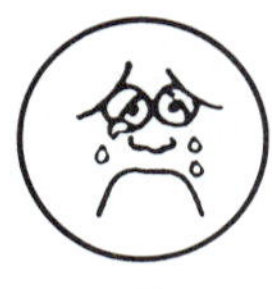 5		
Oucher† (Beyer, 1987): Consists of six photographs of child's face representing "no hurt" to "biggest hurt you could ever have"; also includes a vertical scale with numbers from 0 to 100	*Photographs*: Explain to child that face at bottom has "no hurt, no hurt at all"; second picture, "just a little bit of hurt"; third picture, a "little bit more"; fourth picture, "even more hurt"; fifth picture, "*pretty* much hurt"; and last picture, "biggest hurt you could ever have." Ask child to choose face that best describes own pain. *Numbers*: Explain to child that 0 means you have "no hurt"; 0 to 29, "little hurts"; 30 to 69, "middle hurts"; 70 to 99, "big hurts"; and 100, "biggest hurt you could ever have." Ask child to choose any number between 0 and 100, not just numbers pictured on Oucher, that best describes own pain.	Children as young as 3 years; use numeric scale if child can count to 100; otherwise use photographic scale; scales for African-American and Hispanic children have been developed (Villarruel and Denyes, 1991)
Numeric Scale: Uses straight line with end points identified as "no pain" and "worst pain"; divisions along line are marked in units from 0 to 10 (high number may vary)	Explain to child that at one end of the line is a 0, which means that a person feels no pain (hurt). At the other end is a 10, which means the person feels the worst pain imaginable. The numbers 1 to 9 are for a very little pain to a whole lot of pain. Ask child to choose number that best describes own pain.	Children as young as 5 years, provided they can count and have some concept of numbers
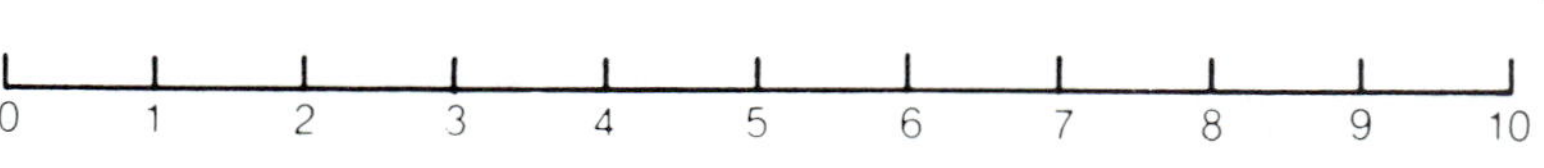		

Continued.

pain relief measures. They also can help in preventing postoperative complications. A young child cannot breathe deeply and will refuse to ambulate or even move at all if in a moderate to severe amount of pain.

Other types of medications such as nonsteroidal antiinflammatory drugs, muscle relaxants, and antiemetics are often ordered on an as-needed basis at the same time. These drugs can provide additional relief for specific complaints that may be contributing to the overall discomfort of the patient. The nurse must consider safety and comfort together when making the all-important determination of the right medication for the individual patient. A sound knowledge of pharmacology will direct appropriate use of narcotics for severe pain and a liberal use of nonnarcotic analgesics as the pain is lessening. Conscientious follow-up

◆ TABLE 27-1
Pain Rating Scales for Children—cont'd.

Pain Scale/Description	Instructions	Recommended Age
Poker Chip (Hester, Foster, and Kristensen, 1990): Uses plastic (poker) chips; several variations in color and number of chips have been described; original used four white chips	Explain to child that these are "pieces of hurt." One piece is a "little bit of hurt," and four pieces is the "most hurt." Ask child to choose number of pieces that describes own pain. If child replies "no pain," record a 0.	Children as young as 4 to 4½ years, provided they can count and have some concept of numbers
Color Tool (Eland, 1985): Uses crayons or markers for child to construct own scale	Ask child to identify things that have hurt in the past and what has hurt the worst. Give child eight crayons or markers (yellow, orange, red, green, blue, purple, brown, and black) in a random order. Ask child which color is like the worst pain experienced. Place that crayon or marker aside and ask child to identify crayon that is like a hurt not quite as bad as the worst hurt. Place that crayon aside and ask which other crayon is like something that hurts just a little. Place that crayon with the others and ask child which crayon is like no hurt at all. Show four crayon choices to child in order from worst-hurt color to no-hurt color. Ask child to show on body outline where it hurts using crayon of color that is most nearly like own pain. When colors are ranked, assign them a numeric value of 0 to 3.	Children as young as 4 years, provided they know their colors, are not color blind, and are able to construct the scale if in pain

*Several variations of faces scales exist. Wong/Baker Faces Scale is available from Purdue Frederick Co., 100 Connecticut Ave., Norwalk, CT 06856; (203) 853-0123, ext. 4010.
†Oucher is available for a fee from Judith E. Beyer, Ph.D., R.N., Associate Professor, University of Colorado Health Sciences Center, School of Nursing, Campus Box C288, 4200 E. Ninth Ave., Denver, CO 80262; (303) 270-4317.
From Wong D: *Whaley and Wong's essentials of pediatric nursing*, ed 4, 1993, St. Louis, Mosby.

assessment to detect side effects and determine ongoing pain management is necessary.

In addition to medication, the nurse has available a multitude of comfort-enhancing interventions. Probably the most important among these is a positive attitude toward the benefit of each pain-relieving measure proposed and the development of trust between the nurse and the patient. Trust enables the patient to relax and relate more honestly and openly. Including the parents whenever possible is also crucial because their anxiety clearly contributes to the child's pain. Their assistance, when they are supported and informed enough to give it, can help immeasurably in alleviating the child's discomfort.

There are cognitive, behavioral, and physical ways in which to offer pain relief. Cognitive measures include a careful, age-appropriate, and well-timed preparation for hospitalization, surgery, and painful procedures. This is essential to allaying anxiety and fear of the unknown. The child's level of understanding and concept of time help determine how much preparation should be given and when it should occur. For the younger child, the simpler, more concrete, visual explanation is the most desirable, and the closer its timing to the actual event, the better. Behavioral methods of assisting with pain relief include a variety of relaxation techniques such as rhythmical breathing, massage, rocking, therapeutic touch, and the soothing voice of a parent, close friend, or concerned nurse. Guided imagery and hypnosis can be effective, particularly with specially trained personnel. The concept of distraction can be effective when assisted by the right person in the right way. Play therapy, music, story telling, videos, reading, and various types of games all can be used for distraction. These tools may help the child gain a degree of mastery and control over the environment. In most children, this greater sense of control helps to decrease pain intensity. Physical measures of pain control consist of transcutaneous electrical nerve stimulation (TENS), rest, repositioning, application of heat or cold, and elevation of the injured body part, any or all of which may be appropriate depending on the circumstances.

The nurse's judgment often determines what methods of pain control will be used. This responsibility is challenging, exciting, and sobering all at once. In accepting the responsibility, the nurse needs to maintain a current knowledge base, understand the degree to which personal experience and values influence decision making, and communicate readily with other members of the health team. The nurse must realize that it is only with multidisciplinary collaboration that the goal of optimum pain relief will be accomplished.

When working with a patient with chronic, persistent, or unresolved pain, the use of a pain flow sheet can be invaluable. It necessitates frequent documentation of pain assessment parameters, the patient's rating of the pain, methods used to relieve the pain, and both beneficial and adverse effects of those relief measures. Whether or not a pain flow sheet is used, however, the nurse must conscientiously document in the patient's record the reason for, use of, and effects from each pain-relieving measure administered. By following this routine and by constantly reassessing the patient's condition, the nurse can make reliable judgments for ongoing pain management and help co-workers accomplish the same.

Many promising prospects for improved pain man-

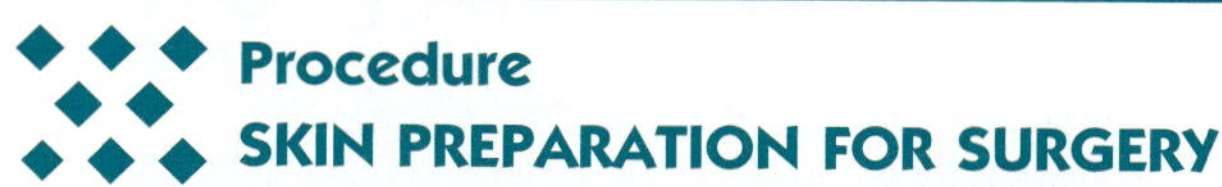

Procedure
SKIN PREPARATION FOR SURGERY

SKIN PREPARATION FOR SURGERY

PURPOSES:

To cleanse the area to help prevent infection, to provide a clearly visible operative field, and to carefully inspect the skin for possible pustules, lesions, or signs of poor circulation. Skin preparations are now frequently performed in the operating room just before surgery. Many surgeons are omitting a shave-preparation of the operative site. Clipping rather than shaving is current practice in many institutions.

EQUIPMENT/SUPPLIES:

1 Gloves
2 Sharp, sterile razor (if shave-prep is ordered)
3 Clean bowl for warm water
4 Prescribed soap or antibacterial solution
5 Waterproof pad or sheeting
6 Towels (2)
7 Washcloth or gauze sponge
8 Clean cotton applicators, if the areas to prepare involve the umbilicus or toes
9 Nail clippers, if extremities are involved
10 Bath blanket or drawsheet
11 Gooseneck lamp or other good light

STEPS:

1 Check the order, the operative permit, and the time preoperative medications will be given.
2 Identify the patient.
3 Explain the procedure to patients according to their level of understanding. Small children usually respond to the explanation, "We're going to wash your tummy to make it very clean." Continue to provide explanations.
4 Position the lamp and raise the bed to a convenient working level.
5 Wash your hands. Apply gloves.
6 Place the waterproof pad and towel under the patient to protect the bed.
7 Prepare and place the warm water and any ordered antibacterial agent conveniently.
8 Apply tension to the skin with a washcloth or gauze sponge if you shave. If the feet or fingernails are very dirty, they may be soaking in a basin of warm water while the adjacent areas are being shaved.
9 Get at eye level frequently to look *across* the surface of the skin to check for remaining hair.
10 Retain your "prep setup" until the skin preparation has been checked by the primary nurse or instructor.
11 Record the procedure. Any skin lesions (for example, pustules) must be reported. Pustules are *not* to be opened. Razor nicks should be treated with direct pressure with a sterile sponge and should be reported. Great care must be used in shaving, especially in areas of old scars, insect bites, or bony prominences, where nicking may easily occur. Due to the potential for injury, clipping is a preferred alternative.
12 In some cases a povidone-iodine (Betadine) scrub of 10 minutes may be ordered after the shave is complete. The surgeon may order the prepared area wrapped in sterile towels until surgery.

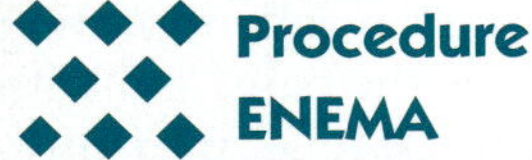

Procedure ENEMA

ENEMA (FIG. 27-1)

In contrast to the adult, an enema for an infant or child differs in the amount and type of fluid administered (see box on p. 559).

PURPOSE:

To cleanse the lower bowel before surgery or for diagnostic procedures, to relieve constipation or flatulence, and to aid in the expulsion of parasites.

EQUIPMENT/SUPPLIES:

1 Appropriately sized rectal catheter and clamps,
   a. For infants, size 12 to 16 French
   b. For young child, size 12 to 20 French
   c. For older child, size 16 to 22 French
2 Container of ordered solution—An infant or young child should not be expected to retain a cleansing enema until the total amount of fluid is given. Small amounts should be instilled and then allowed to return around the catheter. The output should be measured if possible.
3 Lubricant and wipes
4 Asepto syringe barrel or enema bag, depending on the amount of fluid to be given and the size of the child

   Disposable enema setups may be used depending on amount of solution needed. At times commercially prepared enemas may be ordered for children older than 2 years, simplifying the procedure (e.g., Fleet phosphate-type ready-to-use enema, as ordered by the surgeon).

STEPS:

1 Check the order.
2 Identify the patient.
3 Explain to the child what will be done as you do it according to the level of understanding. In the case of the very young child, understanding will not be complete, of course, but the tone of voice and the socialization such explanation offers can be helpful. Telling a child that you are "going to put a little water in to help you go to the bathroom" sometimes helps.
4 Provide privacy and position the child. A number of positions are advocated when giving an infant or toddler an enema.
   a. For most children the side position with the upper leg flexed seems to be the most comfortable. The left side is preferred because this placement puts the descending colon lowest; however, a left-sided position is not mandatory. Infants and small toddlers often do well if placed on a firm pillow, which has been draped with a lightweight plastic sheet and covered with an absorbent towel, with the hips pulled to the edge. The plastic extends over the side of the pillow into or beside a curved basin or small bedpan, which is placed snugly against the buttocks just below the rectum (Fig. 27-1). For warmth, the child is covered by a bath blanket or towel.
   b. Older children with sphincter control are usually positioned on their sides and given enemas in basically the same way as an adult.
5 Place the ordered amount and type of solution in an Asepto barrel attached to a clatal tube. Expel the air from the tube and lubricate the tip. Do not occlude the eyes of the catheter.
6 Gently insert the tubing. Hold the container of solution no higher than 12 to 18 inches (30 to 46 cm) above the patient's hips.
7 Observe the patient closely during the procedure for an increase in respiratory and pulse rates and exhaustion.
8 As needed, put the child on a bedpan or potty chair, or allow the child to go to the bathroom.
9 Remove equipment from the area.
10 Record the procedure, the solution used, and the results obtained.

   Rather than an enema, a preoperative bowel preparation solution given orally or through a nasogastric tube may be preferable. The electrolyte lavage solution mechanically flushes the bowel without significant absorption (Konings, 1989).

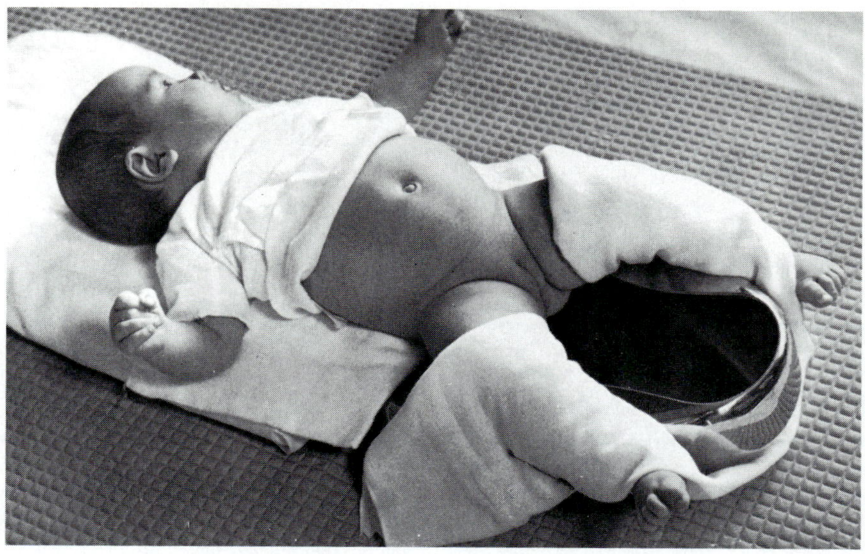

Fig. 27-1 Example of infant positioning for enema.

PROPER ADMINISTRATION OF ENEMAS TO CHILDREN

AGE	AMOUNT (ML)	INSERTION DISTANCE (CM/INCHES)
Infant	120-240	2.5 (1 inch)
2-4 years	240-360	5.0 (2 inches)
4-10 years	360-480	7.5 (3 inches)
11 years	480-720	10.0 (4 inches)

From Wong D: *Whaley and Wong's essentials of pediatric nursing,* ed 4, St Louis, 1993, Mosby.

Nursing Alert

To prevent rectal damage and perforation, proper insertion of the enema catheter tip is critical.

agement are being carefully researched and more frequently used in pediatrics. One example is patient-controlled analgesia (PCA).

The total amount of pain medication allowed with PCA is kept within safe limits. Children as young as 9 years of age have learned to use this system successfully. It is extremely encouraging to see the increased attention and research now being directed toward pain relief in children. It is hoped that this research will stimulate all nurses to use the knowledge at their disposal and the concern for the child's well-being to meet the challenge of safe and effective pain management for children of all ages.

Nursing Alert

PCA allows the child to determine when pain medication is needed and to administer that medication by pushing a button that sends the narcotic into the bloodstream through an existing intravenous line.

COMMON PROCEDURES

A few of the common procedures encountered when caring for pediatric surgical patients are described in the following sections. Some of these treatments may also involve medical patients. At times parents may be instructed regarding these techniques as they assume nursing responsibilities for their child at home. They include skin preparation for surgery, cleansing enema, dressing change, gavage feeding, gastrostomy feeding, and irrigation of nasogastric or intestinal tubes.

One of the most satisfying aspects of the role of the pediatric nurse is watching children master their fears and anxieties about impending surgical procedures. The nurse assists the child and family to cope effectively with a potentially traumatic situation.

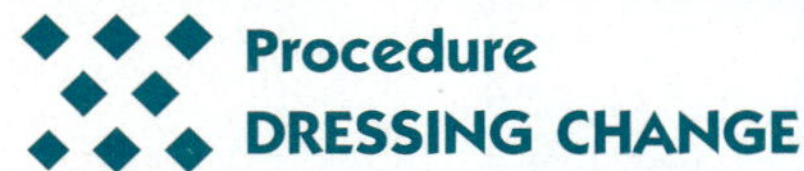

Procedure
DRESSING CHANGE

DRESSING CHANGE
PURPOSE:

To protect the incision or wound from contamination by replacing soiled or wet dressings, to allow direct observation of the incision or wound to evaluate the healing process or measure wound drainage, to increase the cleanliness and comfort of the patient, and, in some instances, to apply local medications, carry out irrigations or debridement procedures (wet to dry dressings).

EQUIPMENT/SUPPLIES:

Materials vary according to the area to be dressed and whether sutures are to be removed or local debridement attempted, and according to physician's instructions. The following supplies may be needed, although not all the supplies listed are needed every time. Simple dressings may require only sterile compresses, handling forceps, adhesive tape, and a biohazard bag.

1. Dressing tray containing the following:
   a. Basic instrument kit with sterile instruments
      (1) Suture-remover scissors
      (2) Clip removers
      (3) Sharp-pointed suture scissors
      (4) Tissue forceps
      (5) Smooth forceps
      (6) Small hemostat
      (7) Probe
   b. Wrapped, sterile cotton applicators
   c. Wrapped, sterile dressings of various thicknesses and sizes
      (1) Thick, absorbent pads (ABD or composite pads)
      (2) 4×4-inch and 2×2-inch gauze squares (flats)
      (3) Nonadherent dressings (Telfa)
      (4) Soft gauze dressings that have been fluffed out (fluffs)
   d. Various sizes of gauze roller bandage, Kerlix, or Ace tensor bandage
   e. Various sizes and kinds of adhesive tape or Montgomery straps
2. Sterile gloves
3. Biohazard bag to receive old dressings utilizing universal precautions
4. Clean kidney basin for antiseptic pour-off overflow
5. Bandage scissors
6. Appropriate antiseptic, irrigating solution, or medication; sterile syringe and basin
7. Clean paper towels

STEPS:

1. Check the order.
2. Select a time when there is little bedmaking or housekeeping activity in the area. These activities increase the bacteria count in the air.
3. Identify and screen the patient and explain the purpose of the dressing change according to the level of understanding. At times positioning assistance may be needed.

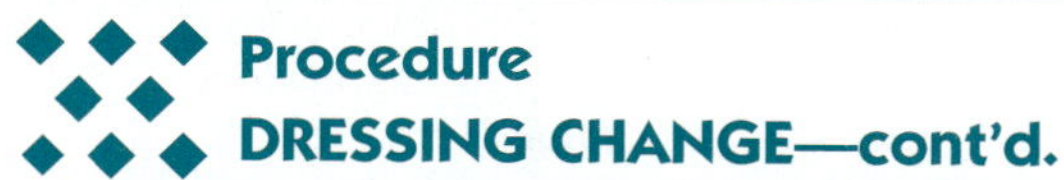

Procedure
DRESSING CHANGE—cont'd.

4 Drape the patient appropriately.
5 Adjust the lamp, if needed; position and open discard bag and kidney basin, if needed.
6 Good handwashing.
7 Open only those supplies needed.
8 Place sterile handling forceps on the edge of a sterile wrapper—points on the sterile surface, handles over the edge.
9 Remove bandages or adhesive tape. (Always pull tape toward the incision or wound to prevent undue strain or pain.)
10 Lift off the top dressing, with clean gloves. Touch only the side of the dressing that was exposed to the exterior. Drop dressing and gloves into a biohazard bag.
11 Lift off any remaining inner dressing with the sterile handling forceps or use sterile gloves. Be careful not to pull drains, if present. Dressings that stick to the skin usually may be moistened with a small amount of sterile saline solution to facilitate their removal. Always note the presence of a drain when recording the dressing change.
12 Wash hands after removing contaminated dressings and gloves. Then apply sterile gloves.
13 Cleanse the area gently of any old drainage present with mild antiseptic or solution as ordered, using sterile gauze sponges mounted on handling forceps with sterile gloves. Pour the solution onto the sponge over the discard kidney basin or use a sterile basin. Dry the area with a sterile compress.
14 Place the new sterile dressing, appropriate for size of the incision and amount of drainage present, using handling forceps or sterile gloves. Remove gloves, if used, before handling tape.
15 Secure with adhesive tape, Elastoplast, or Montgomery tapes prelabeled with date, time, and initials. If using adhesive tape, turn back the ends slightly "sticky side against sticky side" to make the tape easier to remove.
16 Discard used dressings in biohazard bag, wash your hands, and tidy up the area.
17 Record the procedure and the condition of the wound or incision. Describe the type and amount of any drainage present and report any unusual odor. Note any skin irritation caused by adhesive. Note any drains present.
18 If the patient is having the sterile dressings weighed to calculate the amount of wound drainage, you may:
  a. Weigh the total amount of dressings to be used in their sterile wrappers using a gram scale and mark their weight on the outside.
  b. Apply the dressings and save the wrappers carefully after marking the time and date of the dressing change next to the weight previously indicated.
  c. At the time of the next dressing change, discard the old dressings on the saved wrappers and weigh them again. The difference in weight expressed in grams will equal the milliliters of drainage present. A biohazard bag and universal precautions must be utilized.

Procedure
GAVAGE FEEDING USING AN INDWELLING NASOGASTRIC TUBE OR ORAL FEEDING TUBE

GAVAGE FEEDING USING AN INDWELLING NASOGASTRIC TUBE OR ORAL FEEDING TUBE

PURPOSE:

To avoid mouth and lip motion when it may endanger surgical repair, to nourish a child who is too weak to be fed orally in the normal fashion, and to supplement oral feeding when nutritional buildup is imperative and sufficient intake by oral route is impossible.

When needed, feeding tubes for premature infants are inserted orally before each feeding. Such an approach keeps the nose unobstructed and untraumatized, helps maintain a sucking reflex, and reduces incidence of bradycardia during insertion.

EQUIPMENT/SUPPLIES:

1. Sterile Asepto or piston type of syringe (If the child is receiving sterilized formula, a sterile syringe will be secured for each feeding. If the child is not receiving sterilized formula, the nurse may wash and store the syringe in a clean manner for use next time.) Equipment is changed every 24 hours. The time and date are labeled on the equipment.
2. Container of formula (Infants who receive sterilized formula will have the feeding tube sterilized.)
3. Glass of water (bottle of sterile water for infants)
4. Towel or napkin
5. Possibly a bib and infant seat
6. Appropriate tube and tape as needed
7. Stethoscope

STEPS:

1. Check the order.
2. Identify the patient and explain the procedure according to the patient's needs and level of understanding.
3. Briefly warm the formula, if necessary, so that it will be tepid at the time of the feeding. Feeding cold formula, if not given by pump or slow drip, can be upsetting to the patient and may initiate vomiting. Evaluate the consistency of the feeding: Is it too thick? Will it clog the tube? Many times you cannot dilute a feeding and administer the entire amount to maintain the caloric count ordered without overloading the stomach.
4. Unless contraindicated, raise the backrest of a child's bed or place a baby on his side, head elevated. An elevated position lets gravity aid the flow of the formula. Restrain as necessary.
5. Protect the area next to the tube opening with a towel.
6. If insertion of an oral tube is indicated:
   a. Measure the tube for insertion from the tip of the nose, to the lobe of the ear, to ½ inch below the xiphoid process; mark with tape.
   b. Gently pull down on the chin and advance the tube over the tongue to the tape marker.
   c. Observe the infant continually for color change, gagging, coughing, or respiratory distress. Withdraw the tube if any occurs.
   d. Secure the tube to the face with the tape or hold it in place with one hand.
7. Test the position of the end of the tube by each of the following methods:
   a. Observe the length of the tube exposed.
   b. Inject approximately 1 to 5 ml of air (depending on patient) into the tube. Listen with a stethoscope just below the sternum for sound of air passage. Withdraw the air and suction further for evidence of stomach contents, or, if ordered, measure entire aspirate to help determine digestion of previous feedings and current stomach capacity. Measured aspirate is usually returned to the stomach and the amount of the ordered feeding reduced by the amount of the aspirate.
   c. Ask the patient to hum, if possible. If the tube is in the trachea, the patient cannot hum.
8. Continue with the administration of the formula. In most instances allow the formula to flow by gravity. Exerting additional pressure may be dangerous. If the flow is sluggish, raise the barrel. If it is too fast, lower the barrel or pinch the tube. If the flow has stopped, change position of the patient slightly. If the flow still does not continue, *gentle* pressure with a syringe bulb or piston may *start* the flow. If no response is forthcoming, the tube must be removed and another inserted. If the infant is crying, flow will be slower than when the child is quiet.
9. Add more formula before the barrel is empty to avoid introducing additional air into the stomach. If the tube is to be left in place, when the formula is finished (just before the last few drops leave the barrel) add 5 to 15 ml of water to rinse the tube. (Failure to include this step will cause a clogged tube.) If the tube is to be removed, pinch it tightly before and during its quick removal to prevent drops of formula from entering the airway.
10. An infant must be burped after gavage just as after routine oral feeding. Position with head elevated 30 degrees for 30 to 60 minutes to prevent aspiration.
11. Record any aspirate obtained, the amount and type of feeding, and the tolerance of the patient.

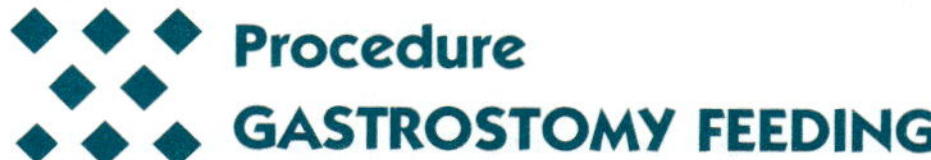

Procedure GASTROSTOMY FEEDING

GASTROSTOMY FEEDING (FIG. 27-2)
PURPOSE:

To provide nourishment by way of a tube that has been surgically inserted through the abdominal wall into the stomach because of obstruction or surgical repair of the child's oroesophageal tract or to avoid the constant irritation of a nasogastric tube when oral feedings are not possible.

EQUIPMENT/SUPPLIES:

1 Tray containing the following:
   a. Syringe barrel (sterile for small infants receiving sterilized formula)
   b. Container of formula (sterile for small infants)
   c. Container of water (sterile for small infants)
2 Towel or napkin

STEPS:

1 Check the order.
2 Identify patient and explain the procedure according to the patient needs and level of understanding.
3 Evaluate the formula as for a gavage feeding. Position the child either flat with the head raised or elevated in a semisitting position.
4 Attach the syringe barrel to the tube and fill with formula before unclamping the tube. There may be orders to aspirate the contents of the stomach into the barrel. The amount aspirated is noted and is allowed to return to the stomach. The feeding to be given is decreased accordingly to prevent overloading.
5 Unclamp the tube and allow the fluid to flow slowly by gravity. Never use pressure of any kind to start the flow of formula into the gastrostomy tube. This may cause unwanted backflow into the esophagus.
6 Continue to add formula to the barrel before it completely empties to avoid introducing air into the stomach.
7 Finish the feeding by adding 15 to 30 ml of water to rinse the tube. Clamp off the tube before all the water leaves the barrel to avoid introducing air into the stomach. In some cases involving infants, the physician may order the tube not to be clamped but left opened with the barrel attached and elevated above the infant's body. The formula is allowed to return to the barrel as the child cries or changes position.
8 Record the amount and type of feeding and the tolerance of the patient. Position with head elevated 30 degrees for 30 to 60 minutes to prevent aspiration.

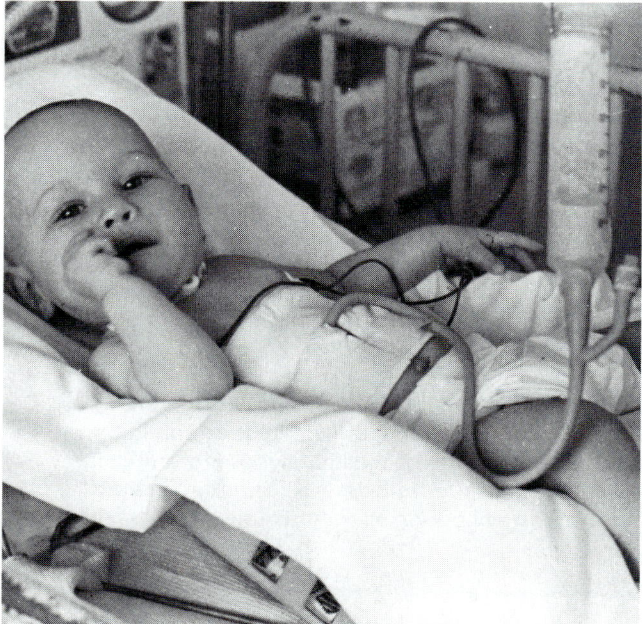

Fig. 27-2 Gastrostomy feeding. Syringe barrel suspended to allow thick formula to enter stomach by gravity. Note child sucking thumb for oral gratification. (From Whaley L and Wong DL: *Nursing care of infants and children,* ed 4, St Louis, 1991, Mosby.)

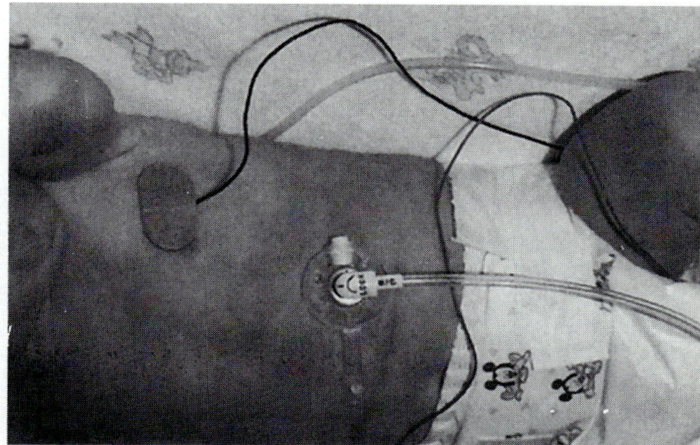

Fig. 27-3 Child with skin level gastrostomy device (MIC-KEY), which provides for secure attachment of extension tubing to gastrostomy opening. (From Wong DL: *Essentials of pediatric nursing,* ed 4, St Louis, 1993, Mosby.)

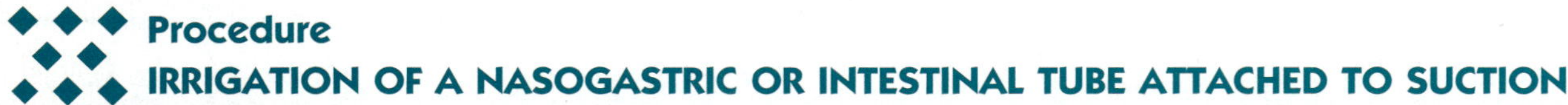

Procedure
IRRIGATION OF A NASOGASTRIC OR INTESTINAL TUBE ATTACHED TO SUCTION

IRRIGATION OF A NASOGASTRIC OR INTESTINAL TUBE ATTACHED TO SUCTION

PURPOSES:

To prevent clogging and ensure the patency of an indwelling nasogastric or intestinal tube. The tube may have been inserted (1) to prevent vomiting or (2) to relieve postoperative abdominal distention, discomfort, and pressure on surgical repairs.

When the tube has been inserted it is attached to some type of suction or drainage device. Usually the suction ordered is intermittent; occasionally it may be continuous. High or low negative pressure may be prescribed. Sometimes only gravity drainage is ordered. Most children are placed on low intermittent suction. Irrigation is carried out only on instructions of the physician. Double-lumen or sump-type nasogastric tubes are frequently used. A small tube, or sump, which serves as an "airway," is incorporated into the larger suction tube. As the suction pulls out gastric contents, it also pulls in air via the airway; this helps prevent the end of the suction tube from "grabbing" the stomach mucosa and causing tissue damage.

EQUIPMENT/SUPPLIES:

Unless the type of surgery makes it necessary to use sterile technique, the materials used to irrigate a tube must be kept meticulously clean but need not be sterile. Universal cautions are maintained. The type and amount of irrigating fluid to be used are ordered by the physician.

1 Syringe (10 to 30 ml, depending on amount to be used)
2 Basin or solution reservoir
3 Clamp
4 Towel and emesis basin
5 Ordered solution
6 Gown
7 Goggles
8 Mask

STEPS:

1 Identify the patient.
2 Explain the procedure to the child according to the level of understanding. For young children it is usually sufficient to say that you are putting a little "water" in the tube.
3 Draw up the amount and kind of solution ordered in the syringe.
4 Place a folded towel and emesis basin under the junction of the tube leading to the suction apparatus or gravity drainage.
5 Turn off any mechanical suction device.
6 Clamp the tubing that leads to the suction or drainage bag and disconnect the two parts of the tubing; wrap the end of the tubing that leads to the suction machine in a towel, cover it with a cap, and hang it from a support on the machine or hold it between your last two fingers. Goggles, gown, and gloves must be utilized when disconnecting.
7 Fit the syringe of irrigating fluid into the patient's tube and gently instill the ordered amount. Whether the nurse will be allowed to withdraw any of the irrigating solution with the attached syringe will depend on the preferences of the physician. If a sump type of tube is being irrigated, the saline may be instilled in either the end of the sump or "airway" or the end of the suction tube. Regardless of the route used for irrigation after the instillation, approximately 10 cc of air should be injected into the sump to clear the tube. The sump tube outlet should never be clamped while the suction is in operation.
8 Detach the syringe and reconnect the tube either to the suction machine (removing the clamp and restarting the suction) or to the gravity drainage. (Recheck any suction setting.)
9 Remember, this patient is usually not allowed oral fluids except perhaps *small* amounts of ice chips. However, lubrication of the nares, renewal of the tape maintaining the tube's position, and oral hygiene are fairly common patient needs.
10 Record in the patient's output record the amount of irrigating fluid used. (NOTE: If a tube is not draining and resistance is encountered during an attempted ordered irrigation, the nurse should notify the supervisor immediately.)

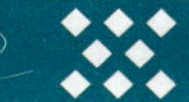

KEY CONCEPTS

1 Child-adult distinctions that may help the nurse evaluate the needs of children include the following: (1) the metabolic rate of infants and young children is much greater than that of adults, (2) fluid loss is more serious in the infant and the young child than in the adult, (3) the child lacks the physical reserves available to the adult, and (4) the body tissues of the child heal more quickly.
2 Preparing a child for surgery is based on the following factors: developmental age; the child's perception of hospitalization and the upcoming surgery; the surgical procedure to be performed; postoperative care; previous hospital experience; expected length of hospitalization; and parental attitudes.
3 Psychological preparation must be geared to the child's developmental level, not merely to chronological age. Emotional and informational support must be provided to parents.
4 Vital signs, temperature, pulse, respirations, and blood pressure are assessed and recorded in the postoperative period. The nurse must assess and immediately report signs of shock.
5 The assessment and management of pain in children are of critical importance. The level of pain experienced is influenced by both physiological and emotional factors. It is difficult to assess pain objectively and reliably; thus pain assessment scales are helpful.
6 Physical signs of pain include increased heart rate, pulse, blood pressure, perspiration, muscle tension, and gastrointestinal motility.
7 In addition to the physical signs of pain, the nurse should assess an infant for vocalization or cry, facial expression or grimacing, and body movement.
8 The toddler often responds to pain through aggressive or ritualistic behavior.
9 The preschool child can verbalize fears and discomfort better than the toddler but may significantly distort reality.
10 School-aged children can usually describe the type, quality, and quantity of pain.
11 A variety of scales and questionnaires have been developed to assist with the measurement of pain. The validity and reliability of these tools increase with the child's age. Some preparation regarding these tools should be provided for the child before the painful experience.
12 The goal of pain management must be threefold: (1) to eliminate suffering to the greatest degree possible, (2) to enhance each child's ability to cope, and (3) to treat the underlying cause of the pain when possible.
13 Narcotic and nonnarcotic medications may be used to relieve pain. Side effects and other pain relief measures must also be considered when determining the most appropriate medication for each patient.
14 Nonpharmacological methods of pain management are important nursing interventions.
15 Early progressive ambulation is ordered for the general surgery patient. When the child's condition makes it impossible or inadvisable to get out of bed, the nurse must be sure that the child is turned frequently, receives good skin care, and breathes deeply at intervals.
16 Common procedures experienced by pediatric surgery patients include skin preparation for surgery, cleansing enema or electrolyte lavage, dressing change, gavage feeding, gastrostomy feeding, and irrigation of nasogastric or intestinal tubes. Parents are instructed regarding these techniques if they are to care for their child at home.

CRITICAL THOUGHT QUESTIONS

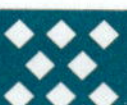

1 What critical factors must be considered when preparing a child for surgery? Give some examples of child's age and developmental level.
2 Minor surgical procedures are being performed on a "day surgery" basis. How can proper preparation be done if the patient does not arrive until 1 or 2 hours before surgery?
3 With the trend toward early discharge, parents are becoming increasingly responsible for the nursing care of children having recently undergone surgical procedures. What would you explain to the parents regarding diet, activity, good handwashing, care of the incision, and specific observations?
4 Identify the specific safety precautions that may be required to prevent injury postoperatively. Why is it essential for the nurse to observe a child more often than an adult?
5 Do you think that children experience as much postoperative pain as adults? Why? How would you assess a child for signs of pain or discomfort?

REFERENCES

Eland JM: The child who is hurting, *Semin Oncol Nurs* 1(2):116-122, 1985.

Konings K: *Preop use of Golytely in pediatrics,* Pediatric Nursing 15(5):473-474, 1989.

McCaffery M and Bube A: *Pain: clinical manual for nursing practice,* St Louis, 1989, Mosby.

Villarruel AM and Denyes MJ: Pain assessment in children: theoretical and empirical validity, *Adv Nurs Sci* 14(2):32-41, 1991.

Wong D: *Whaley and Wong's essentials of pediatric nursing,* ed 4, St Louis, 1993, Mosby.

BIBLIOGRAPHY

Avigne G and Phillips TL: Pediatric preoperative tours, *AORN J* 53(6):1458-1465, 1991.

Craft M and Denehy J: *Nursing Interventions with infants and children,* Philadelphia, 1991, WB Saunders.

Noonan AT et al: Family-centered nursing in the post-anesthesia care unit, *J Post Anesth Nurs* 6(1)13-16, 1991.

Ogilvie L: Hospitalization of children for surgery: the parent's view, *Child Health Care* 19(1):49-56, 1990.

Principles of analgesic use in the treatment of acute pain and chronic cancer pain. Skokie, IL, 1992, American Pain Society.

Rivera WB: Practical points in the assessment and management of postoperative pediatric pain, *J Post Anesth Nurs* 6(1):40-42, 1991.

Vessey J, Caserza L, Bogetz M: Parental participation in anesthetic induction, *Child Health Care* 19(2):116-118, 1990.

Visintainer MA and Wolfer JA: Psychological preparation for surgical pediatric patients: the effect of children's and parent's stress responses and adjustment, *Pediatrics* 56(2):187-202, 1975. (Classic)

Whaley L and Wong D: *Nursing care of infants and children,* ed 4, St Louis, 1991, Mosby.

Wong D: *Whaley and Wong's essentials of pediatric nursing,* ed 4, St Louis, 1993, Mosby.

28

Maintaining Oxygenation

CHAPTER OBJECTIVES

After studying this chapter, the student should be able to:

1. Define respiration, Pa_{O_2}, Sa_{O_2}, and hypoxemia.
2. List six signs of respiratory difficulty.
3. Give the normal values for arterial blood gases in children.
4. State the purpose of chest physiotherapy and identify four of its components.
5. Explain the purpose of the cuff on an endotracheal or tracheostomy tube.
6. Name three possible complications of suctioning endotracheal and tracheostomy tubes.
7. Discuss four safety considerations associated with the administration of oxygen.
8. Explain three reasons for placing patients on mechanical ventilation.

The process of respiration refers to gas exchange or the movement of oxygen from the atmosphere into the bloodstream and the movement of carbon dioxide from the bloodstream into the atmosphere. In some diseases, ventilation of air into and out of the lungs, transfer of gases across the alveolar-capillary membrane, or blood flow is inhibited, thereby decreasing the amount of oxygen available for cellular function. To remedy this problem, various procedures, apparatuses, and medications have been developed. Clearing the airway, enriching the oxygen content of inspired air, stimulating or maintaining adequate ventilatory effort, or achieving adequate circulation of blood are treatment goals.

Nurses can do a great deal to maintain oxygenation and improve the respiratory function of their patients. They need to work closely with respiratory therapists to sustain optimal breathing and prevent respiratory dysfunction. In many hospitals the responsibilities of respiratory therapists include supervision of gaseous and ventilator therapy, and performance of chest physiotherapy and resuscitation measures.

BARRIERS TO OXYGENATION

To understand more clearly the types of problems encountered and the rationale of many of the treatments ordered, the student should review the structure and function of the respiratory system (Figs. 28-1 and 28-2). The passageways from the exterior of the body to the microscopic air sacs (alveoli), which make up the functional tissue of the lungs, must remain open to ensure proper oxygenation. Any obstruction, whether caused by the position of the tongue, aspiration of a foreign body, edema, a tumor, the presence of tenacious secretions in the laryngotracheobronchial "tree," or spasm of the bronchioles, will lead to respiratory difficulty. Conditions such as atelectasis, pneumonia, pulmonary edema, tuberculosis, and malignancy that cause an inability of the lung tissue to receive air and transfer oxygen and carbon dioxide may cause respiratory distress. Common pulmonary disorders in infants and children are respiratory distress syndrome (RDS), aspiration, pneumonia, bronchiolitis, croup, and asthma. Less common but most challenging is cystic fibrosis.

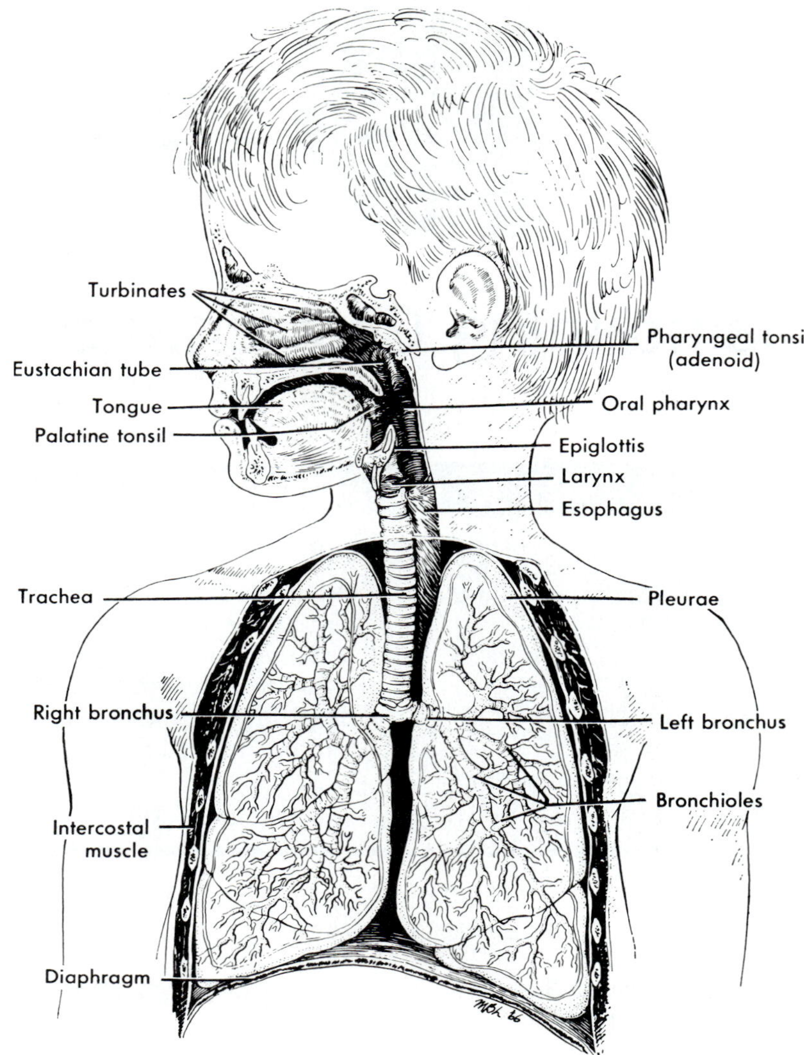

Fig. 28-1 Normal respiratory tract.

Any interruption in the mechanisms of breathing also affects respiration and therefore oxygenation. The circulatory system must also be adequate to deliver oxygen to each body cell.

CLINICAL SIGNS AND SYMPTOMS OF RESPIRATORY DIFFICULTY

Signs of respiratory difficulty include the following:

1 Depressed or elevated respiratory or cardiac rates at rest for the age of the child considered
2 Any chest retractions, note kinds (Figs. 28-3 and 28-4 show types of retractions in infants)
3 Noisy, labored breathing, grunting, wheezing
4 Flaring nostrils and the use of facial and neck muscles in attempts to aid respirations
5 Pallor, cyanosis (gray to purple skin coloring), which may be localized or generalized
6 Restlessness, apprehension, and disorientation
7 Inflamed respiratory tract with or without thick nasal discharge and blockage of the nasal passageways
8 Frequent productive or nonproductive coughing (however, the absence of coughing is not necessarily a sign of respiratory improvement)

The observation of any of the preceding signs and symptoms deserves prompt report and evaluation. If a child becomes cyanotic and a bedside oxygen unit is available, it should first be determined that the child's airway is open. Then the oxygen should be started and

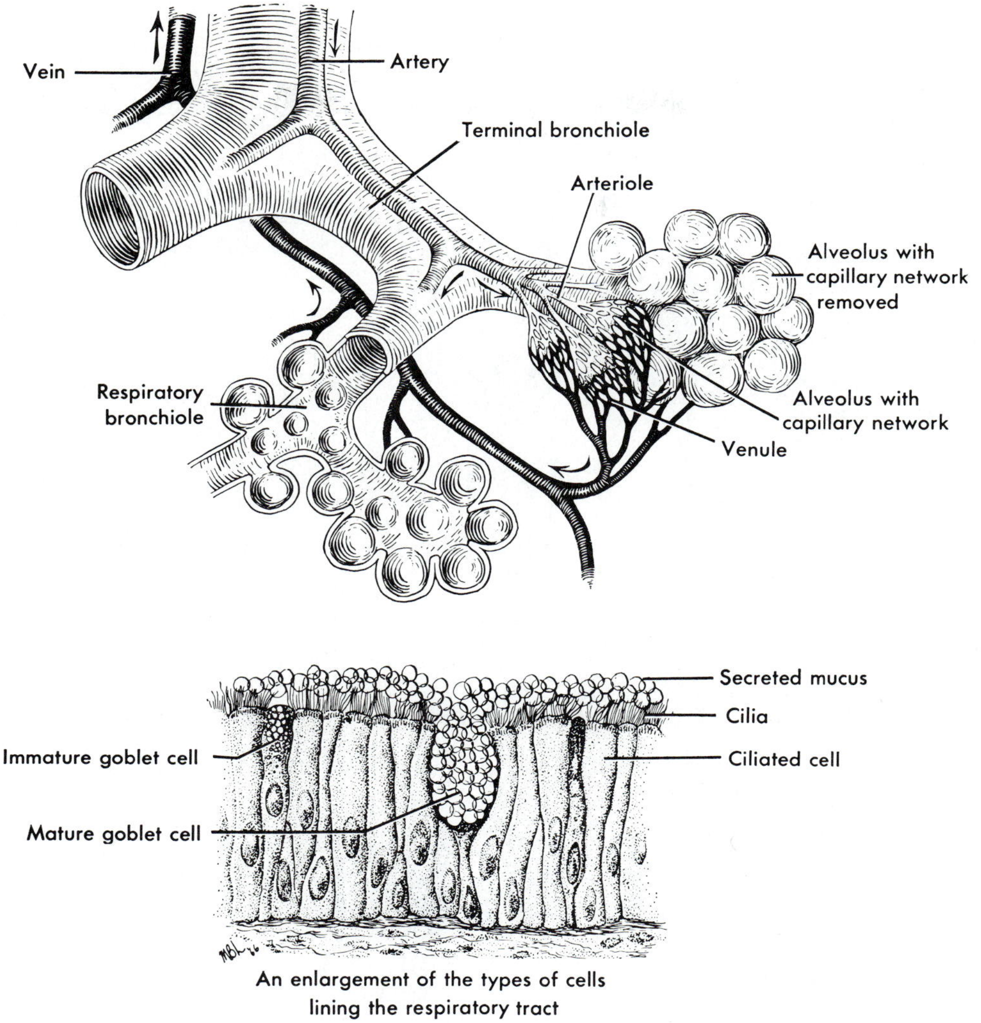

Fig. 28-2 Microscopic anatomy of lower respiratory tract.

assistance sought for further evaluation of the patient. The pulse rate and respirations should be counted. Many children with circulatory and respiratory problems in which fluid tends to collect in the chest or abdomen breathe more easily when propped in a semi-Fowler's position or supported in an infant seat. The most accurate way to determine the extent of oxygenation of a patient's blood is by a chemical analysis of the oxygen and carbon dioxide levels in arterial blood. This is called an arterial blood gas sample.

LABORATORY EVALUATION OF OXYGENATION

The term *hypoxemia* describes the presence of subnormal amounts of oxygen dissolved in arterial blood plasma. Tissue hypoxia occurs when a subnormal amount of oxygen is delivered to the body cells.

Clinical signs of tissue hypoxia may be identified. Tachycardia and tachypnea are common mechanisms triggered to correct the hypoxia. Other signs are hypertension, polycythemia, dysrhythmias, and low urine output. When more than one third of the body's hemoglobin is not oxygen-saturated, cyanosis may be present. A myriad of neurological symptoms, such as headache, anxiety, agitation, confusion, weakness, double vision, and drowsiness, may be experienced. Eventually, coma may develop.

Although the clinical signs and symptoms of hypoxia are important manifestations, they are nonspecific and can relate to other organ dysfunction. Because tissue hypoxia cannot be directly measured, the most accurate way to determine the extent of

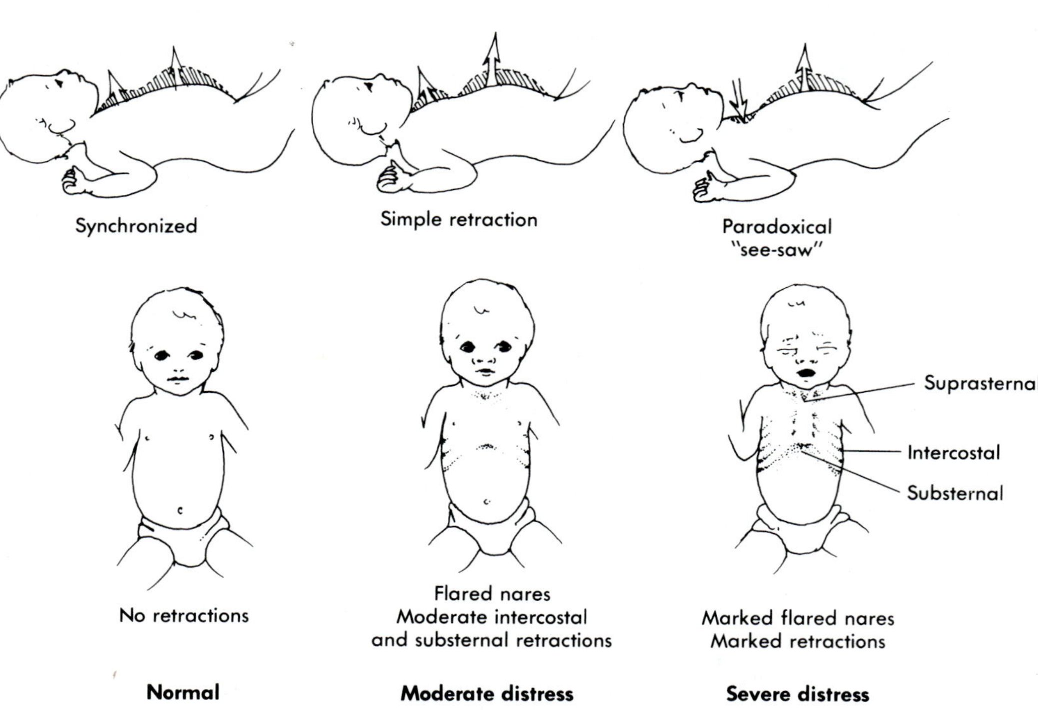

Fig. 28-3 Types of respiration—visible signs of respiratory distress.

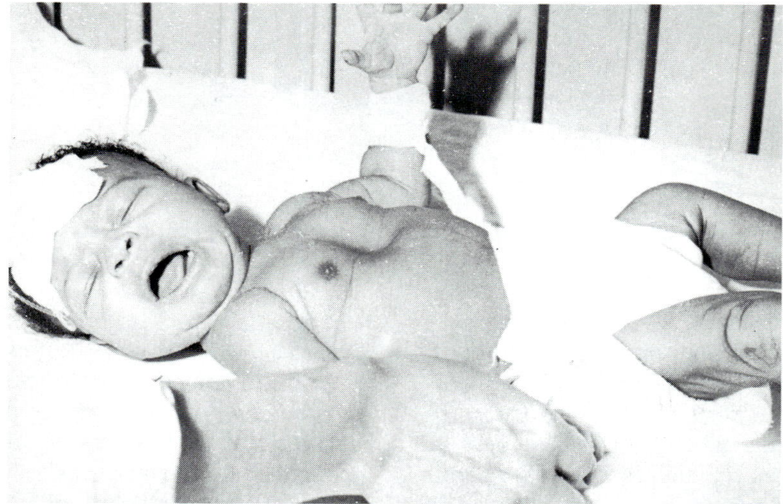

Fig. 28-4 Deep substernal retractions caused by pneumonia. (Note hollow in chest area.) The retractions lessened when the infant was placed upright in an infant chair. (Courtesy Naval Hospital, San Diego, Calif.)

oxygenation is through the measurement of the oxygen ($Pa{O_2}/P{O_2}$) and carbon dioxide ($Pa{CO_2}/P{CO_2}$) levels in an arterial blood sample. Indwelling arterial lines are often established when frequent arterial samples are needed. Pulse oximeters are also used clinically to measure oxygen saturation after comparison with arterial blood gases. Pulse oximeters measure the percentage of hemoglobin saturated with oxygen and have the advantage of being noninvasive. A direct relationship exists between the percentage of hemoglobin saturated by oxygen in an arterial blood sample ($Sa{O_2}$) and the partial pressure of oxygen in an arterial blood sample ($Pa{O_2}/P{O_2}$) (see Tables 28-1 and 28-2).

◆ TABLE 28-1
Normal Ranges for Arterial Blood Gases (ABGs) for Infants and Children Beyond Newborn Period*

ABGs	Range
pH	7.35-7.45
$Paco_2/Pco_2$	35-45 mmHg
Pao_2/Po_2	83-108 mmHg (Adult value 80-100 mmHg)

*Measurements at sea level—21% O_2.

◆ TABLE 28-2
Approximate Relationships Between Pao_2 and Sao_2 Values*

Partial Pressure of Oxygen in Arterial Blood (Pao_2)	Percentage of Hemoglobin Saturated by Oxygen in Arterial Blood (Sao_2)
100 mmHg	98%
60 mmHg	90%
45 mmHg	80%
30 mmHg	60%

*An Sao_2 of 90% or less signifies hypoxemia.

SECURING AND MAINTAINING AN AIRWAY

Position

The first concern in maintaining oxygenation always involves the airway. Occasionally, it may be obstructed because of the position of the tongue, especially in the unconscious patient. The tongue is not actually swallowed, but falls backward and obstructs the pharynx. An open airway may be obtained by placing the patient on the back with the head in "sniffing" position and the lower jaw held up. This returns the tongue to normal position. At times the insertion of a plastic oropharyngeal airway is needed.

If the airway is obstructed by a foreign body or secretions, the emergency relief usually attempted *first* involves gravity drainage. In cases of choking, in which the patient is unable to speak or cough, several repeated, controlled, upward thrusts of the thumb-side of a fist just below the patient's rib cage are used (Heimlich maneuver) (see Fig. 28-12J). This causes the diaphragm to suddenly force air out through the airway, which may dislodge a foreign body. Further references and detailed instruction should be sought. Occasionally, the bronchi may need to be visualized for removal of a foreign body. A relatively small, flexible, fiberoptic bronchoscope is then used.

To prevent aspiration, a child in danger of vomiting or regurgitating should be maintained on his side or abdomen. If this is impossible because of other more important considerations (such as the type of surgery or administration of an anesthetic), the head should be lowered and turned to the side during episodes of nausea and vomiting. Infants are sometimes placed upright in infant seats to help prevent vomiting.

Nasopharyngeal Suction

Suction of the nasooropharyngeal passages may be necessary to clear the airway. Suction is accomplished by using a bulb syringe or a catheter setup attached to wall or portable suction (see Fig. 17-1). The following procedure points should be remembered when a catheter is used:

1. Catheter sizes vary with the size of the patient, usually as follows:
   a. Infants, size 5 to 8 French
   b. Children, size 8 to 10 French
   c. Youths and adults, size 12 to 14 French
2. An individual suction apparatus is used for each patient and is kept free from contamination. Although in some instances clean rather than sterile techniques would be acceptable for suctioning limited to the nose, mouth, and throat, trauma and hazards of infection are still possible. Therefore sterile precautions are used, especially when dealing with infants, young children, and patients who are particularly vulnerable to injury or sepsis. A two-glove technique (one sterile, one clean) is consistent with universal precautions.
3. At the outset, the drainage bottle should contain about 1 inch of disinfectant solution to make cleaning it easier and to reduce the number of organisms in the bottle.
4. Catheters should be lubricated with saline or water-soluble gel to ensure greater ease of insertion. Suctioning saline through the catheter before use will also verify that the suction is functioning properly.
5. During catheter insertion suction should be temporarily discontinued by pinching the catheter or uncovering the Y-tube. To suction the nose, the catheter should be guided along the floor of the nasal cavity, parallel with the roof of the mouth.

SUGGESTED SUCTION RANGES

Neonate	60-80 mmHg
Child	80-100 mmHg
Teenager	100-120 mmHg

6 The lowest amount of suction necessary should be intermittently applied as the catheter is being rotated and withdrawn (see box above). Suction should not be prolonged (no more than 10 seconds). If administered too frequently, suction may aggravate rather than relieve congestion.

7 The catheter and connection tubing should be rinsed during and after use to prevent clogging.

8 The child usually needs to be restrained during the procedure.

9 The catheter should be discarded after each suctioning procedure.

10 The type and amount of suctioned material obtained and the patient's tolerance of the procedure should be recorded.

ENDOTRACHEAL AND TRACHEOSTOMY TUBE PLACEMENT AND SUCTION

Endotracheal Intubation

When the patient's airway and oxygenation cannot be maintained using the previously mentioned treatments, an artificial airway or endotracheal tube must be inserted. The patient often needs to be supported on a mechanical ventilator at this time.

The indications for endotracheal intubation are generally of an emergency nature, such as need for airway maintenance, removal of secretions, prevention of aspiration in a compromised patient, respiratory insufficiency or failure, and/or the need to enhance oxygenation. An endotracheal tube is the most common artificial airway for short-term airway management, although it may be used for several weeks when prolonged ventilation is required.

Immediately after intubation, the adequacy of tube placement should be determined by observing symmetrical chest movement, auscultating bilaterally equal breath sounds, and absent breath sounds over the stomach. A radiograph should be taken to confirm its position. Occasionally, an endotracheal tube can slip into the right mainstem bronchus, which is more nearly vertical to the trachea than the left. A reference mark should be made at the point of insertion into the mouth or nose to detect subsequent tube movement. After intubation, the tube should be secured to the patient's face with a velcro strap chin guard or tape.

Tracheostomy

When it is anticipated that a child will need ventilatory support or airway maintenance for more than a few weeks, a tracheostomy is performed. A tracheostomy is an artificial surgical opening into the trachea, usually at the second through fourth tracheal rings, performed electively in the operating room. Today an emergency tracheostomy is almost nonexistent. A tracheostomy provides the best route for long-term airway maintenance because of easier secretion removal, increased patient acceptance and comfort, and the ability to eat and sometimes talk with the tube in place.

Types of Artificial Airways

Most tubes are made of plastic material and have an inflatable cuff attached (usually if the child is older than 8 years old). This cuff or balloon is built into the end portion of an endotracheal or tracheostomy tube. When inflated, it creates a seal between the tube and the patient's trachea to prevent air leakage and provide a closed system, thereby enabling the patient to be adequately ventilated. The cuff should be of the low pressure and high volume type and should be inflated with an intentional minimum air leak to prevent tracheal wall damage.

Tracheostomy tubes may be single or double lumen. Single-lumen tubes consist of the tube and the cuff and an obturator, which is necessary during insertion. In addition, double-lumen tubes have an inner cannula that can be removed for cleaning. The obturator of the patient's indwelling (in situ) tube and another tube of the same size must be at the bedside in case of accidental removal.

Suctioning (Endotracheal and Tracheostomy Tubes)

When the upper respiratory tract is bypassed, the defense system becomes impaired, and warming and humidification of gases must be accomplished externally. Studies show contamination of the lower airways 24 hours after endotracheal intubation.

The cough reflex is also compromised and tracheal suctioning must be performed through the artificial airway. The technique must be sterile to prevent infection. Universal precautions, including goggles and a mask, are recommended.

Complications of tracheal suctioning via endotracheal tube or tracheostomy include hypoxemia and

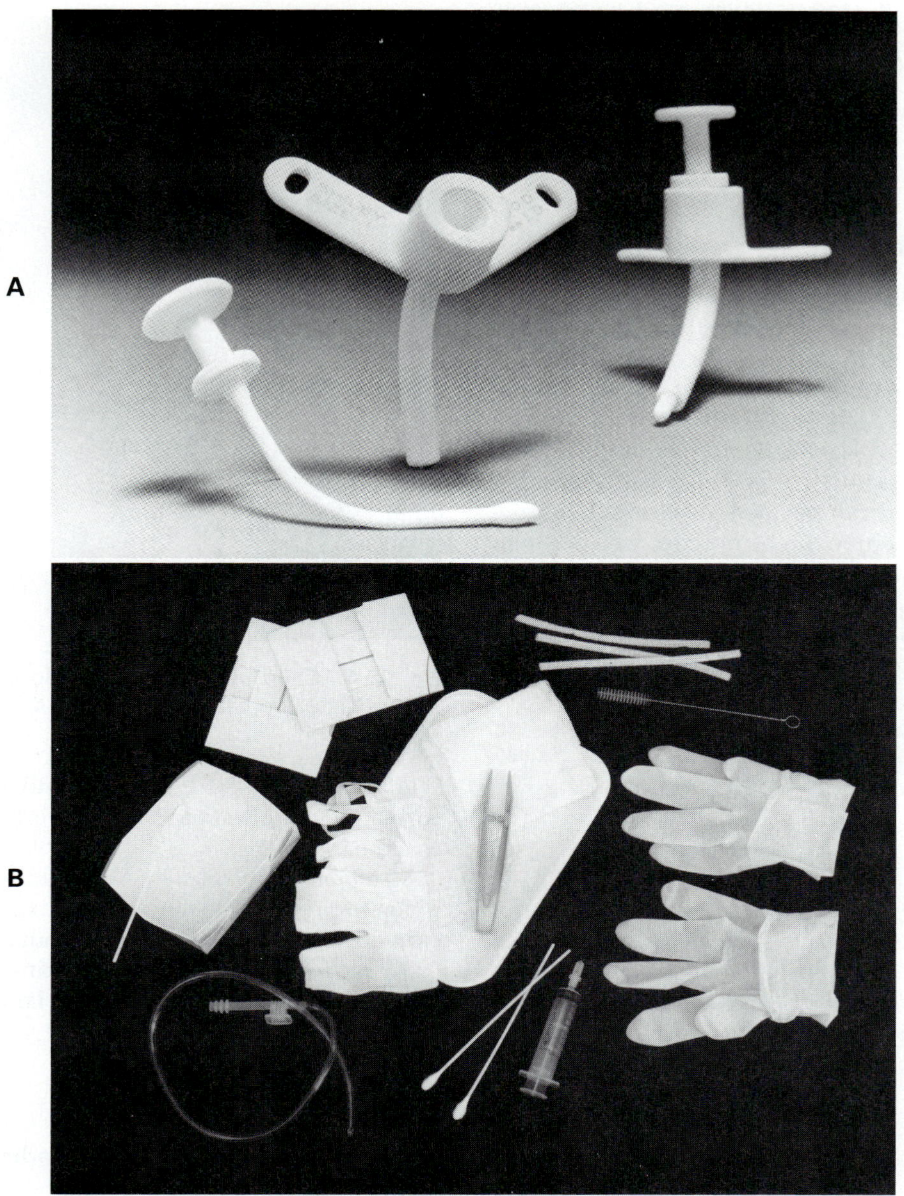

Fig. 28-5 **A,** *Left to right,* Shiley pediatric tracheostomy tube obturator, pediatric tube, Shiley neonatal tracheostomy tube with obturator in place. **B,** Contents of tracheostomy suctioning and cleaning tray (Pharmaseal). (*A,* Courtesy Shiley, Inc.)

resulting cardiac arrhythmias and bronchospasm, airway irritation and possible infection caused by catheter, and atelectasis from applying too much suction. Suctioning should be performed only when necessary, that is, when secretions are audibly or visibly obstructing the artificial airway. Basically, the technique for endotracheal suctioning is as follows:

1 Oxygenate the patient. The patient should be given oxygen for several minutes before, during, and immediately after suctioning. (The concentration of O_2 used is usually 100% except in the case of newborns for whom lower oxygen concentrations are typically used.)
2 Use a sterile disposable suction tray equipped with gloves, catheter, and saline solution. Rinse catheter in saline and test suction (Fig. 28-5, *A* and *B*).
3 Install 0.5 to 2 ml of sterile saline in trachea to help thin secretions during inspiration (an optional procedure; may initiate productive cough).
4 Insert the catheter without applying suction (finger off vent) during inspiration when the airways are open wider. The alert patient can be

instructed to take a breath as the catheter is inserted.
5 Apply suction intermittently during expiration while rotating catheter in a circular motion.
6 Limit total time in which catheter is in trachea to 10 seconds.

Communication

Patients cannot talk with a patent endotracheal tube or a tracheostomy tube; therefore, they must rely on the health care team to provide a means of communication. A young child who cannot yet write but cries for attention may be especially frightened. Signal cords or handbells should always be available. Communication devices like magic slates, cards, talkboards, and a simple pen and pencil can be used for older children. When a tracheostomy tube can be plugged or a talking trach inserted, a patient with a tracheostomy is able to talk. Body language usually can be easily interpreted. A nurse with a calm, reassuring manner is most helpful.

MEDICATIONS

Medications are frequently ordered to aid in clearing the airway.

Nasal Drops

Nasal drops or nasal sprays such as phenylephrine hydrochloride (Neo-Synephrine) may be ordered to shrink mucous membranes and ease nasal congestion. Excessive use of these products may cause a rebound worsening of congestion. Saline nose drops are a safer alternative.

Expectorants

Oral expectorants, which increase the bronchial secretions and may help thin mucus, are occasionally ordered. Common expectorants are potassium iodide and guaifenesin syrup.

Aerosols

Acetylcysteine (Mucomyst) reduces the thickness and tenacity of mucus and is used primarily for patients with cystic fibrosis. It is, however, administered *with caution* because it has been known to cause bronchospasm and/or bleeding. Cephalosporin antibiotics are now being aerosolized to provide direct bactericidal effects in cystic fibrosis patients.

Cromolyn sodium (Intal) must be taken daily as prescribed for prophylaxis to prevent both allergy and exercise-induced asthma.

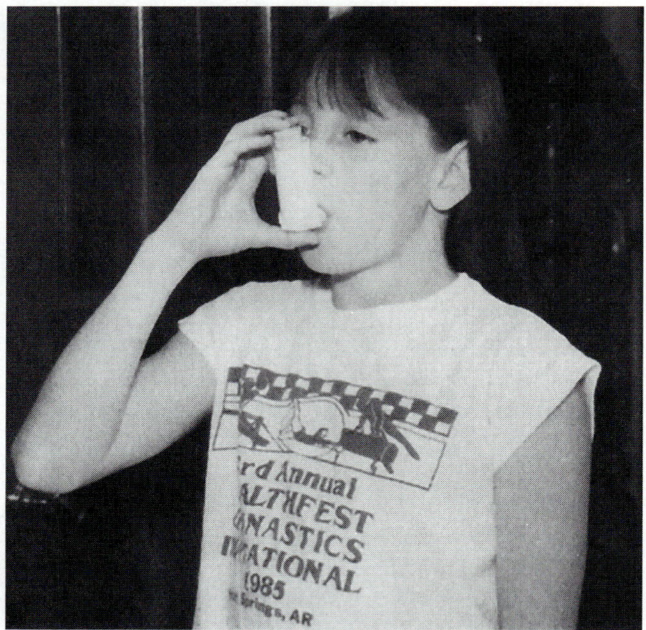

Fig. 28-6 Child using a metered-dose inhaler (Wong D: *Essentials of pediatric nursing,* ed 4, St Louis, 1993, Mosby).

Albuterol (Proventil, Ventolin) and terbutaline sulfate (Brethine) are often used to relieve bronchospasm and dyspnea.

Metaproterenol sulfate (Alupent, Metaprel) is also given to provide bronchodilation but has more cardiac side effects than albuterol or terbutaline.

Racemic epinephrine (Vaponefrin) has been used successfully to treat symptoms of laryngotracheobronchitis, also known as *croup.*

Inhalers

The most effective method of administering rapid-acting bronchodilators is with metered-dose inhalers (Fig. 28-6). Children older than 4 years become quite adept with this method. For young children a spacer device, which does not require the coordination of the delivery of medication with inspiration, may be used. Spacer devices aid in getting the medication beyond the oral cavity.

Injections

Epinephrine hydrochloride (Adrenalin) is indicated for the emergency treatment of anaphylactic allergic reactions to insect bites, foods, drugs, and other allergens, as well as exercise-induced anaphylaxis. It can be given subcutaneously or intramuscularly. It is rapid-acting and may produce cardiac and/or neurological side effects, such as tachycardia, palpitations, hypertension, headache, and nervousness.

Aminophylline or *theophylline ethylenediamine* (Aminophyllin) may be given intravenously for acute bronchospasm associated with status asthmaticus. It may produce numerous side effects or adverse reactions (usually because of overdose), such as tachycardia, palpitations, flushing, hypotension, and tachypnea, as well as epigastric pain, nausea, vomiting, headache, and irritability. Generalized convulsions may also occur.

Oral Medication

Theophylline (Theo-Dur, Slo-bid, Slo-Phylline) is also available in various oral forms, which have multiple side effects. Some types are immediate release; others are time-released to produce prolonged bronchodilation for preventing and treating asthma attacks. The use of the metered-dose inhaler often prevents the need for oral forms of theophylline.

CHEST PHYSIOTHERAPY

Some respiratory diseases (e.g., cystic fibrosis and bronchitis) produce such exaggerated amounts of tenacious secretions deep in the lungs that it may be difficult for the patient to expel them even with the aid of medications, humidification, and suction techniques. These secretions interfere with proper pulmonary ventilation and set the stage for frequent respiratory tract infections that further endanger the patient.

Chest physiotherapy is a therapeutic modality designed to improve pulmonary hygiene in patients with acute or chronic sputum production. It incorporates the use of breathing exercises, gravity-assisted positioning, percussion and vibration of the chest wall, followed by purposeful coughing and possible suctioning. When respiratory therapists are available, they usually perform these maneuvers and instruct the family if continued treatment is necessary at home. If respiratory therapists are not available, nurses may be asked to learn the techniques. Anyone responsible for performing them should receive special instruction and be initially supervised in their use. The following brief explanation is not intended to take the place of such instruction.

The treatment is most effective when preceded by aerosol therapy and is enhanced by diaphragmatic breathing. It may be prescribed as a prophylactic and therapeutic measure.

Various postures assumed by the patient help to drain different parts of the lungs. Therefore the position or positions in which the patient is placed depend on the site of the congestion and the general aims of the therapeutic program. The placement of the patient enlists the forces of gravity and the sweeping action of the respiratory cilia in clearing the lungs. In infants the right upper lobe is frequently infected. In children, bronchial secretions tend to collect in the lower lobes of the lung by gravity. Positions that drain the lower lobes use the Trendelenburg position. Any constrictive clothing should be removed. The patient's knees and hips should be flexed in various positions to promote relaxation and exert less strain will be on abdominal muscles when coughing is encouraged. When a patient's chest must be lowered, all that is needed for an infant or young child is a well-positioned, firm pillow (Fig. 28-7). Premature infants should *not* be placed in head-down positions because of the increased danger of intracranial hemorrhage. An infant or toddler may respond best when positioned on the nurse's or therapist's lap. An older child may assume a modified jack-knife position, lying over an elevated knee-gatch. The bed may be placed in the Trendelenburg position for teenagers.

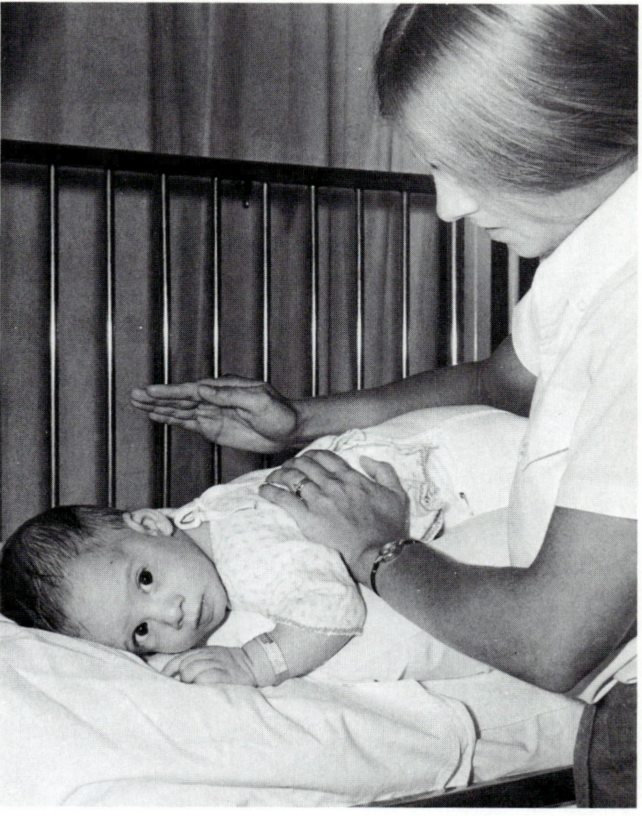

Fig. 28-7 Respiratory therapist is performing early morning, before breakfast ritual on small patient with congenital structural weakness of bronchi. Scheduled percussion and vibrating have proved particularly helpful. (Courtesy Children's Hospital and Health Center, San Diego, Calif.)

These assisted postural drainage techniques should be performed before meals or at least 1 hour after

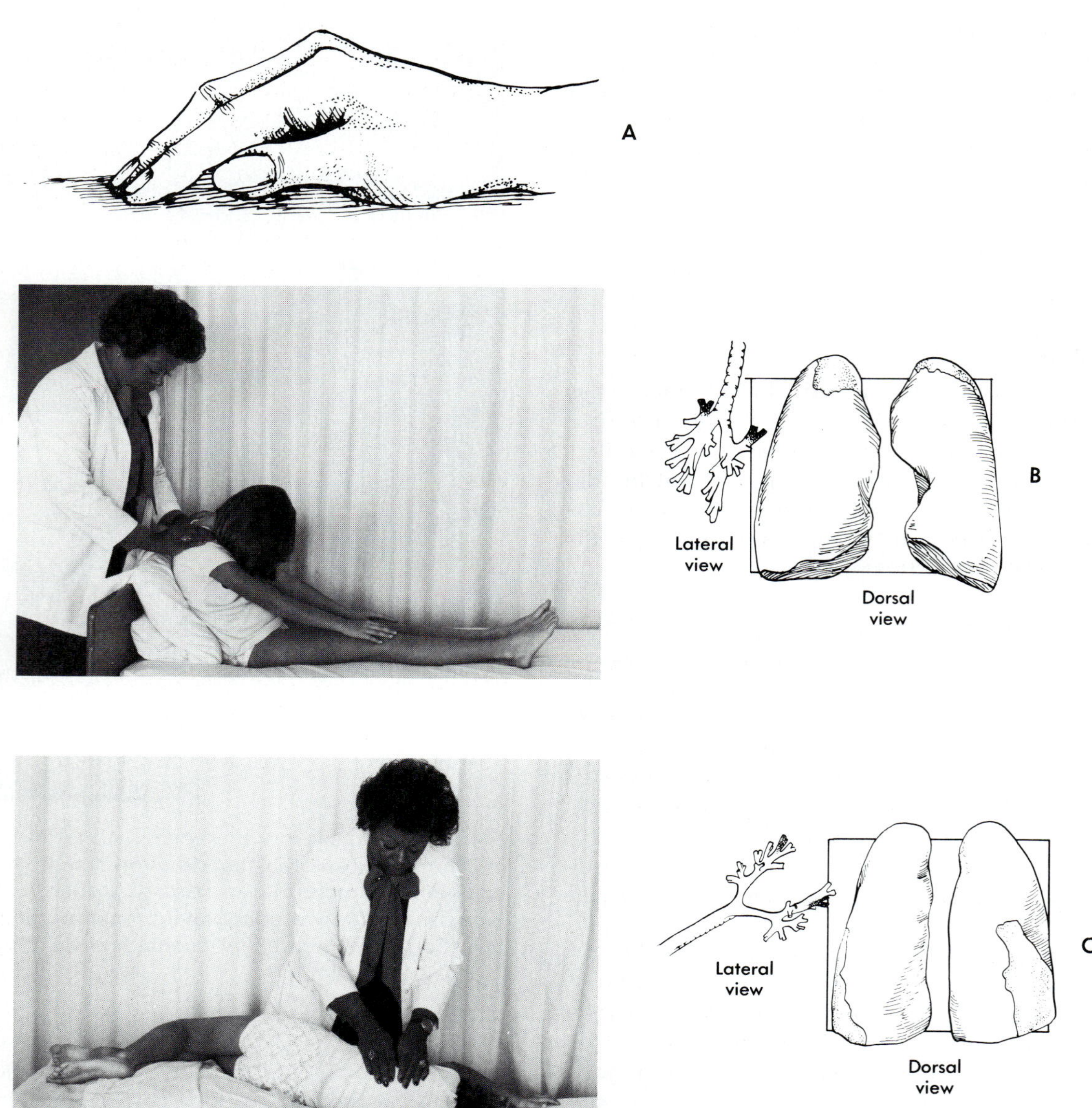

Fig. 28-8 Chest physiotherapy usually includes breathing exercises, positioning (postural drainage), percussion, vibration, and effective coughing or suctioning to clear congested areas of the lung. Vibration is more difficult to perform but is considered more effective than percussion. The entire range of possible positions is not illustrated. **A,** Percussion is accomplished by striking the cupped hand rhythmically against the chest wall, creating an air pocket between the therapist's hand and the chest wall. **B,** Position for drainage from upper lobes, apical segment. **C,** Position for drainage from lower lobes, lateral basal segments.

eating. They are never initiated if the patient is hemorrhaging or in pain. Two basic maneuvers are used: (1) percussion, also known as cupping or clapping, and (2) vibrating. The first is performed with the palm of the hand raised, the fingers and thumb forming the sides of a firm cup (Fig. 28-8, *A*). When the cupped hands are gently but abruptly applied to the patient's chest wall, the wrist is alternately flexed and extended. A characteristic hollow sound is produced. The technique is continued for about 1 minute over the affected area while the patient inhales and exhales. It is then followed by the vibrating motion, only while the patient is exhaling. This second maneuver is accomplished by tensing the hands, arms, and shoulders and producing fine, gentle vibratory movements on the chest wall for five or six exhalations. The two maneuvers are then repeated several times, depending on patient tolerance.

Soft percussion aids made from nipples or small face masks may also be used with infants and small children. Mechanical vibrators are very effective and less tiring than manual vibration. Electric toothbrushes may be used on infants and a G-5 apparatus on larger children. Vibration is thought to be more effective than percussion. Percussion techniques are performed over a light shirt or diaper. Neither maneuver should be performed directly over the spine, kidney area, abdomen, sternum, or developed breast tissue. Coughing should be encouraged after each postural drainage position. If the patient is unable to cough productively, suctioning should be used. The effectiveness of the treatment should be evaluated by chest auscultation before and after the procedure.

Incentive spirometers, devices that indicate the approximate volume of inspiratory intake of patients during breathing exercises, are found at the hospital bedsides of persons of all ages. They help to encourage deep breathing for postoperative or relatively inactive patients to avoid the onset of respiratory complications such as pneumonia. The patient is encouraged to practice voluntary sustained inspiration. Deep breaths should be held for at least 2 seconds.

ADMINISTRATION OF OXYGEN

Safety Factors

Various methods and devices are used to make inspired air richer in oxygen. The oxygen content of air in a well-ventilated room is about 21%. Therefore any device used to increase the oxygen content must be capable of administering oxygen of a higher percentage. Preterm infants may suffer eye damage and loss of sight as a result of retrolental fibroplasia caused by oxygen excesses in the blood. Inspired air must contain more than 40% oxygen to meet the needs of some infants. The most accurate way of assessing the actual oxygen needs of preterm infants is by periodic blood gas determinations. The results of these tests are compared with the oxygen concentrations monitored by oxygen analyzers delivered in the hood or incubator.

When oxygen is being used, other safety factors involved must be clearly understood to avoid fire. Oxygen readily supports combustion, and all sources of possible ignition of flammable materials should be removed from the environment. If oxygen cylinders are used, they must be safely stored and maintained to avoid fire and explosion hazards.

Rules for oxygen administration

The following rules should be observed during oxygen administration:

1 No open flames, cigarettes, cigars, matches, cigarette lighters, or candles should be allowed in a room in which oxygen is being used. Signs should be clearly posted.
2 Electrical appliances are not used unless they have been safety-checked. A device capable of producing a spark should not be operated in the oxygen-enriched environment. Any electrical equipment used must be specially grounded to be safe.
3 All enclosed oxygen units (e.g., incubators or tents) should be "flushed" with oxygen before the patient is enclosed within them.
4 Because of the potential danger of excess carbon dioxide accumulation, all tents or enclosures should provide some method of ventilation or chemical control that will prevent this problem.

Methods of Oxygen Enrichment Specifically for Infants

Incubators

An incubator with increased oxygen and/or mist may be used to provide both increased oxygen and humidity to the infant, as well as a controlled environmental temperature. Incubator temperatures and oxygen concentrations (whenever supplementary oxygen is being used) should be recorded at least every 2 hours. Some incubators have oxygen delivery controls that limit the percentage to 40% and below unless an adjustment is made. This system was devised to prevent permanent blindness from oxygen toxicity in premature infants; however, some infants need to have concentrations above 40% to survive.

Hoods

Oxygen hoods are often used for ill neonates receiving care under a warmer in intensive care units. Occasionally, they are placed within incubators to avoid wide variations in oxygen concentration, which may occur when the incubator is entered. The oxygen should be warmed and humidified. (Cold air blowing on an infant's face increases O_2 consumption and dries the mucus membrane.) Hourly oxygen concentration and temperature checks are recommended (Fig. 28-9).

Oxygen and/or Mist Tents

A large oxygen tent may be ordered for an older child. Such a tent is usually a plastic canopy suspended

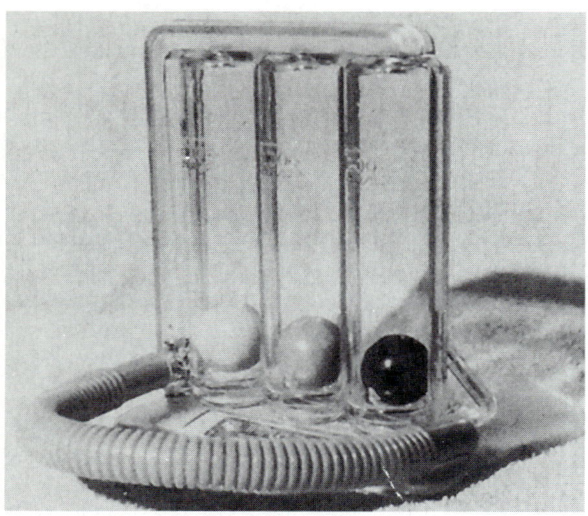

Fig. 28-9 Triflo incentive spirometer; patient inhales and raises the balls. (Photo by Bob Burgin, courtesy Children's Hospital and Health Center, San Diego, Calif.)

from an overhead rod and attached to a cabinet containing a machine that, when properly adjusted, regulates the tent's ventilation and temperature and may also provide a control for increased humidity along with an opening for the appropriate oxygen flow (Fig. 28-10). A tent may be set up in the following manner:

1 Place a bath blanket between the bed mattress and the bedspring to prevent snagging the plastic canopy, which can be easily torn.
2 Set the air circulation or ventilation control halfway between low and high. Set the temperature control at 70° F (21° C). In extremely hot weather the temperature setting should not be more than 10° to 15° F (5.5° to 8.3° C) below the room temperature to maintain the working efficiency of the tent. Arrange the ventilation deflectors so that the cool air entering the tent does not blow directly on the patient. Turn motor on, if so equipped.
3 Connect the oxygen inlet tube to the wall flow meter or oxygen cylinder regulator and start the flow at 15 L/min. Maintain this rate for 30 minutes and then analyze the oxygen concentration. The same concentration can be achieved by holding a flush valve open for at least 2 minutes after the tent has been placed around the patient. Always start oxygen or compressed air before closing a tent.
4 Many tents of this type seem drafty to patients. The amount of clothing necessary to protect the child from cold depends on the patient's own body temperature.
5 Mold the tent canopy around the child's body to prevent oxygen loss. If the tent is not tucked in properly, leakage will occur.
6 Plan nursing care so that the tent is opened as little as possible and many of the patient's needs are met during one interval.

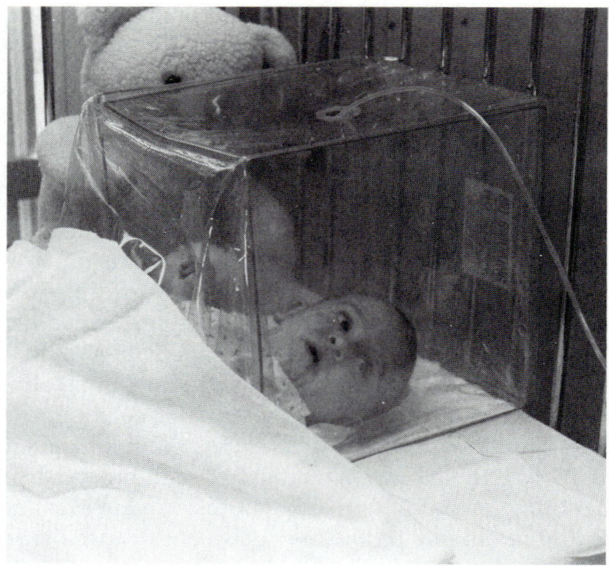

Fig. 28-10 A 12- × 12-inch pediatric oxygen tent or "Care-Cube." (Courtesy Children's Hospital and Health Center, San Diego, Calif.)

Respiratory secretions may be so thick that they are difficult to drain by gravity or remove by suction. Various procedures may be used to help thin out the mucus, such as simply increasing fluid intake, breathing cool moistened air provided by a convenient bedside humidifier, and, in the hospital setting, using a tent and humidification device to help relieve congestion. (Warm mist or steam tents are no longer used because of the danger of burns.) High humidity concentrations may be achieved with the addition of jet nebulizers to many types of tents. Sterile distilled water alone or additional ordered medications may be used. Tents may often use compressed air rather than oxygen to achieve desired mist (Fig. 28-11). Patients placed in the cool, high-humidity environments produced in such tents must be checked frequently to see whether their hair and clothing are damp. If a patient does not have a fever, undershirts may be worn under cotton gowns. Infants seem to do best when dressed in long-sleeved, footed sleepers.

Nasal Cannula

A common mode of delivering low concentrations of oxygen is by nasal cannula (Fig. 28-12). Between 1 and 6 L/min will provide a fraction of inspired oxygen (FiO_2) concentration of 24% to 44%. The cannula is a lightweight, disposable soft plastic tube with two

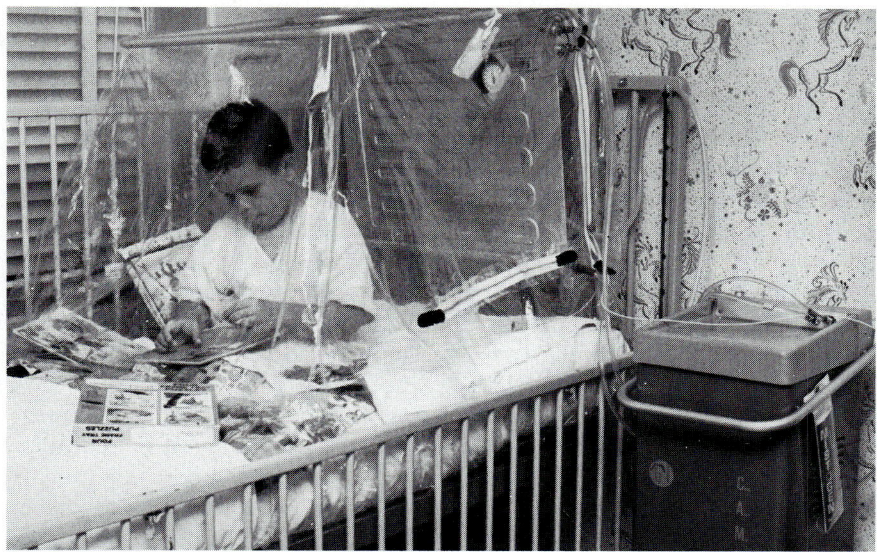

Fig. 28-11 CAM tent, used for oxygen or mist therapy, is cooled and ventilated electrically. Working apparatus is not near patient, and more room is available for activity. Siderail down for picture only. (Courtesy Children's Hospital and Health Center, San Diego, Calif.)

prongs that insert shallowly into each nostril. The prongs should not obstruct the nares, and the patient (if old enough) should be instructed to breathe through the nose. Oxygen administered by cannula should be passed through a humidifier to prevent uncomfortable drying of the mucous membranes.

Oxygen Masks

Oxygen by mask is usually administered through a tube leading from the oxygen supply to a light, disposable, plastic face mask. Masks are capable of providing high oxygen concentrations quickly and are ideal for emergency use.

The simple mask is commonly used. It is an open-face mask that covers the nose and mouth, has vents for exhaled air, and can deliver oxygen concentrations of up to 60%. Oxygen flow rates of 5 to 6 L/min should be used to wash out the exhaled carbon dioxide that accumulates within the mask. One of the main uses of the simple mask is to deliver humidity or aerosol therapy.

A nonrebreathing mask is a mask with a reservoir bag system designed to deliver 90% to 100% oxygen when there is a tight seal over the face. Exhaled air is diverted to the atmosphere so that carbon dioxide cannot be rebreathed.

Masks can be uncomfortable because they need to fit tightly on the face and because of the headstrap used to hold them in place. They must also be removed for the patient to eat or cough. Nurses should be well acquainted with the particular oxygen equipment used in their setting. Pressure points on the cheek bones, behind the ears, and on the nostrils should be assessed for skin irritation.

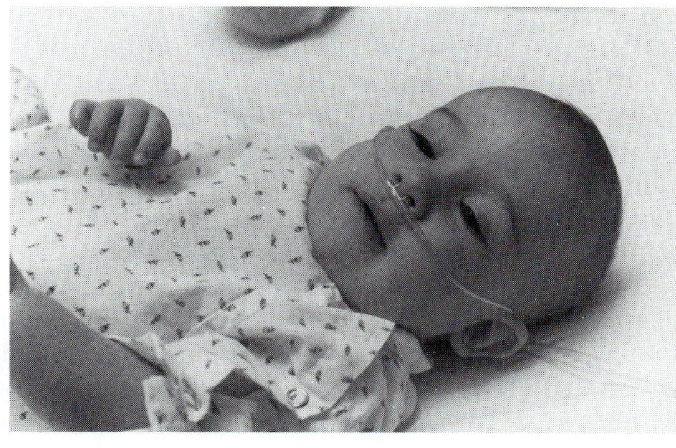

Fig. 28-12 Infant receiving oxygen by nasal cannula. (Courtesy Children's Hospital and Health Center, San Diego, Calif.)

STIMULATION AND MAINTENANCE OF RESPIRATORY EFFORT

If respiratory effort is decreased, various methods may be used to stimulate or maintain respiration. They all presuppose an *adequate airway.*

In the delivery room or nursery, if a newborn is not breathing regularly, the nurse often stimulates more effective respirations by gently rubbing the infant's back, flicking the soles of the feet, or jarring the bed or incubator.

Mouth-to-mouth Resuscitation

If respiration has actually ceased, mouth-to-mouth resuscitation is a practical, prompt source of aid because it requires no additional equipment. To prevent exposure to infection during mouth-to-mouth ventilation, however, and for consistency with universal precautions, nurses must carry airways or specially designed disposable patient "masks" wrapped and ready for use during emergency resuscitations. The following is a description of mouth-to-mouth resuscitation, which can be used alone if cardiac function is adequate or with cardiac compression in the absence of heartbeat. (Fig. 28-13, *A-K*). Often children respond to mouth-to-mouth resuscitation alone.

If the child is found face down at the scene of a possible accident, the child must be rolled over in a manner that avoids twisting the neck or back and must be placed supine on a firm surface. If head or neck injury is suspected, the head tilt/chin lift maneuver is not used to open the airway. Instead, the jaw thrust maneuver is substituted. The care giver is positioned behind the patient's head with the elbows on the supporting surface and reaches on each side of the child's head. The nurse then places the middle and index fingers of each hand under the child's jaw while resting the thumbs near the corners of the child's mouth and lifts the jaw.

If head or spinal injury is not considered to be a problem, the standard head tilt/chin lift procedure is followed. The child's head is tipped slightly more than in the neutral position used with infants. Only slight hyperextension is used with infants to avoid the possibility of collapsing the infant's trachea. The rescuer places his or her hand closest to the victim's head on the victim's forehead. Gently, the rescuer tilts the victim's head backward while using the other hand to raise the child's chin by placing his or her fingers against the bony jaw and lifting it upward. The head tilt/chin lift method clears the tongue and epiglottis from the airway and allows greater air exchange.

Obvious foreign material in the mouth should be removed. However, finger sweeps should be used only if you can visualize the object.

Two breaths of 1 to 1.5 seconds are performed (mouth-to-mouth with a child or youth, with the nose pinched; mouth-to-nose-and-mouth with an infant). Controlled breaths of air from the cheeks should be used with an infant, and gentle breaths just large enough to make the chest rise and fall with a child.

In children and adults, continued foreign body airway obstruction may be relieved by the Heimlich maneuver. In the case of infants, abdominal thrusts (Heimlich maneuver) are not recommended because of possible injury to the abdominal organs, chiefly the liver. Instead a combination of four back blows and four chest thrusts is delivered. Chest thrusts in the infant are a succession of four external chest compressions similar to those performed during cardiac pulmonary resuscitation (CPR).

After a clear airway is established, the circulatory status of the victim is evaluated. In infants it is advised to feel for the brachial pulse instead of the apical pulse, because some infants may have good cardiac function but a heartbeat that is difficult to palpate. Although less accessible in infants, the carotid pulse is sought in young children, as it is in adults.

If the pulse is present, rescue breathing is continued at a rate of 20 ventilations per minute for infants, 15 ventilations per minute for a child, and 12 to 15 ventilations per minute for children older than 8 years of age and for adults. Resuscitation is continued until the victim responds spontaneously or is pronounced dead or until the rescuer is physically unable to continue.

Cardiopulmonary Resuscitation

1. See basic procedure in Fig. 28-13 and in the following text.
2. Chest compressions are not without danger. However, the danger of injury (broken ribs, traumatized liver) is less than the danger of circulatory collapse.
3. A precordial thump or blow on the chest is not recommended for children. It is used only on adults who display an arrest on a cardiac monitor, and the practice is controversial.
4. CPR is usually not attempted in cases in which such dramatic efforts would delay a death that will take place in minutes or hours after the treatment is terminated (e.g., in a child dying of a malignancy).

A nurse must update CPR certification annually and should review resuscitation measures during nonemergency situations. It is imperative to know where emergency resuscitation and oxygenation equipment is stored including knowledge of the location of the following items:

1. Resuscitation apparatus
2. Suction setup
3. Oxygen mask and cylinder
4. Emergency drug supply

Manual Resuscitators

The use of manually controlled bag-valve-mask ventilation devices can be of great assistance in emergencies and for relatively short-term respiratory

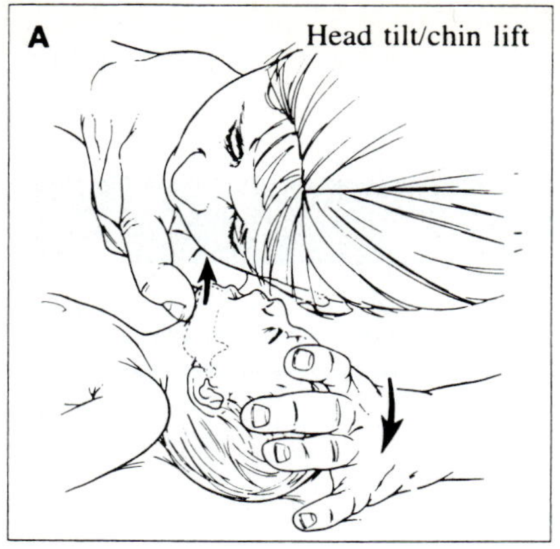

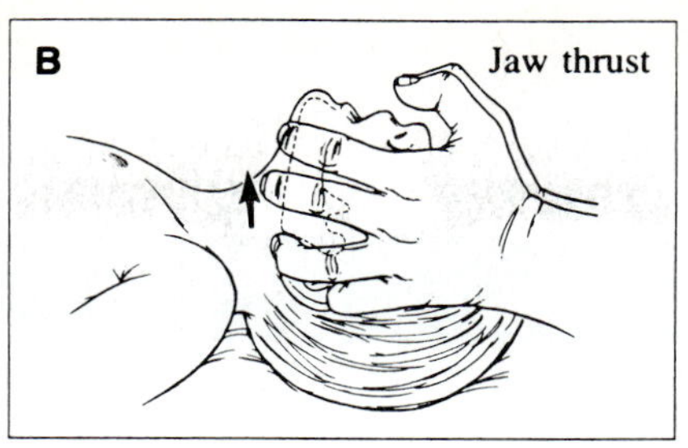

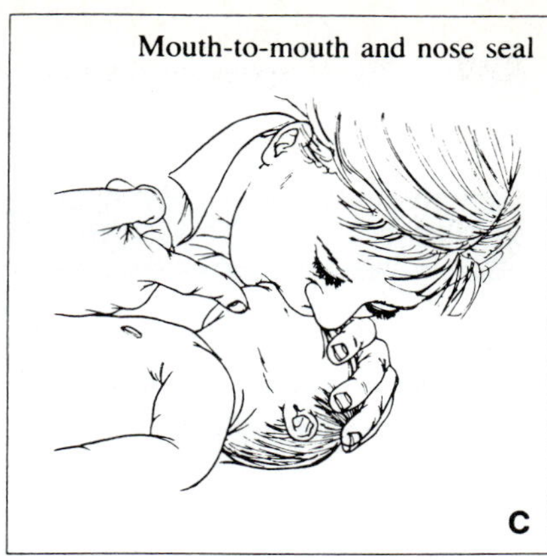

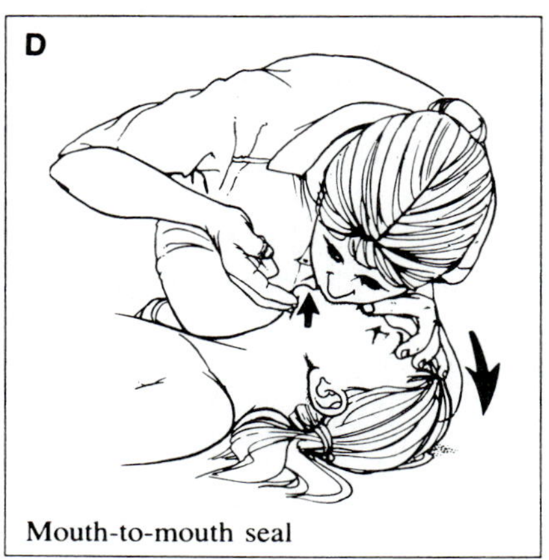

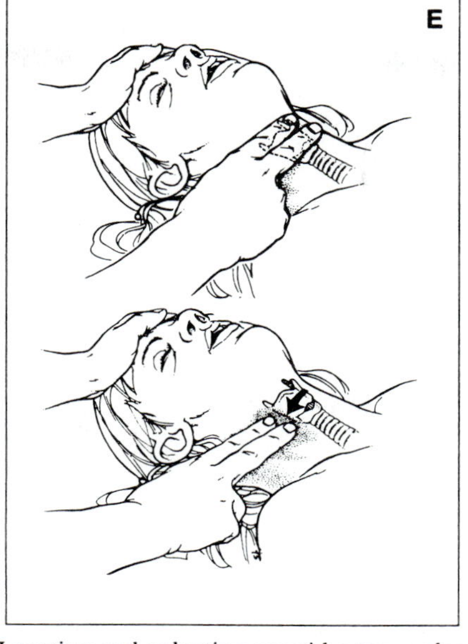

Locating and palpating carotid artery pulse

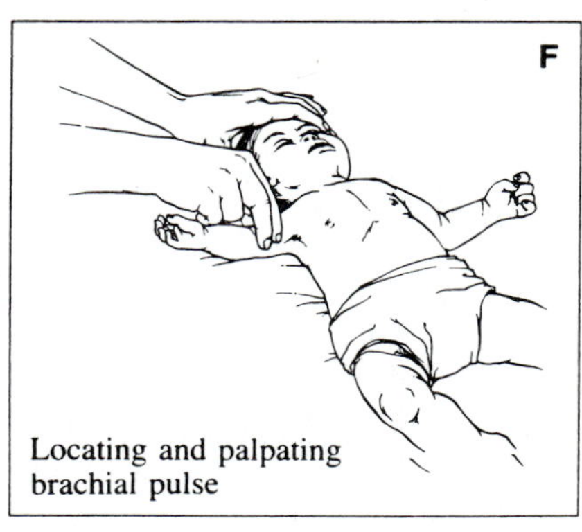

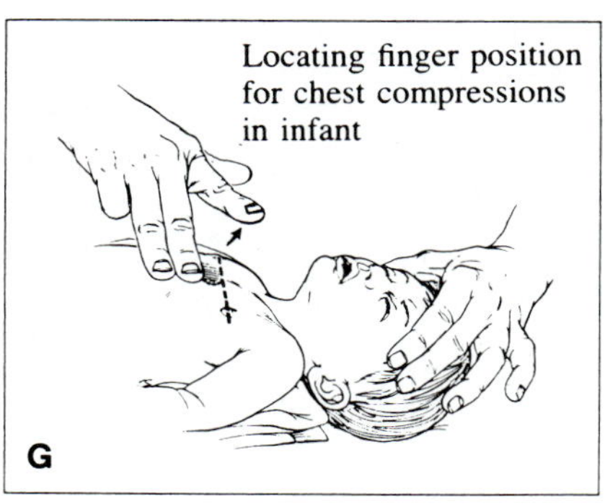

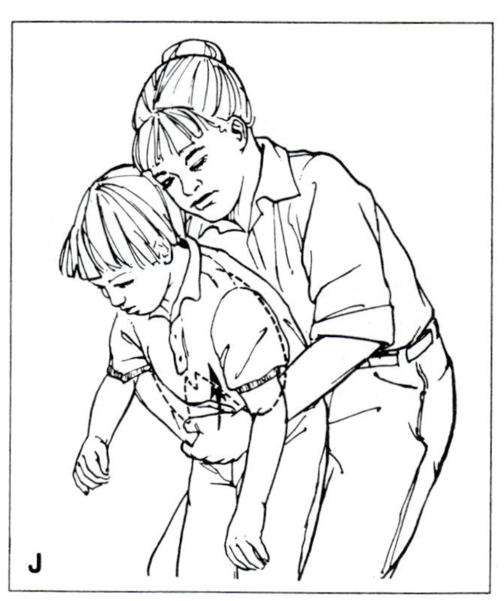

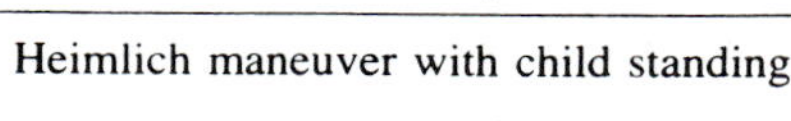

Heimlich maneuver with child standing

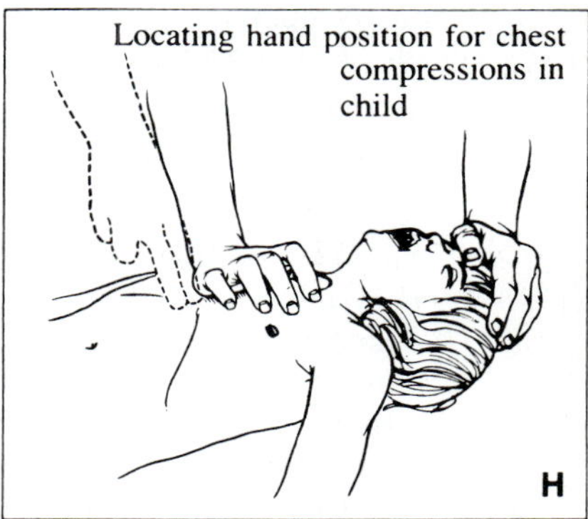

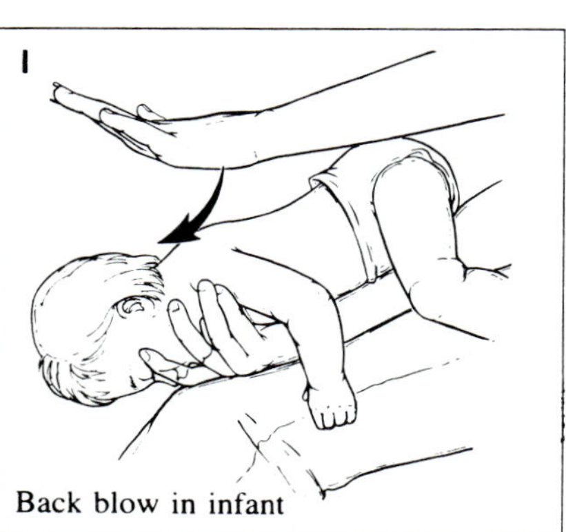

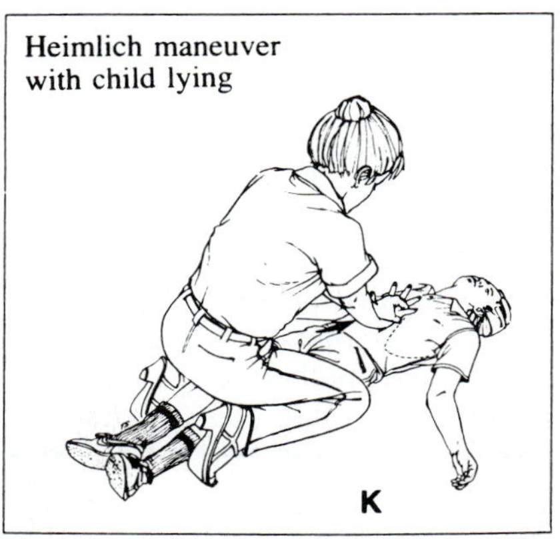

Fig. 28-13 Procedures for cardiopulmonary resuscitation, *A* to *H,* and airway obstruction, *I* to *K.* (Modified from Emergency Cardiac Care Committee and Subcommittees, American Heart Association: Guidelines for cardiopulmonary resuscitation and emergency cardiac care. V. Pediatric basic life support, *JAMA* 268(16):2251-2261, 1992. From Wong DL: *Essentials of pediatric nursing,* ed 4, St Louis, Mosby.)

◆ **TABLE 28-3**
Emergency Cardiopulmonary (CPR) Reminders*

	Infants (Less than 1 Year)	Children (1 Year through 8 Years)	Older Children and Adults
CPR basic sequence 1. Identify problem a. Gasping or struggling for breath b. Lack of respiratory effort c. Cyanosis d. Limp extremities 2. Stimulate a. Shout, gently shake b. If unable to arouse, call out for help (if child unconscious and rescuer alone, perform CPR 1 minute before calling out for help) 3. Open airway (*A*) a. Head tilt/chin lift (if no neck injury suspected) b. Jaw thrust (without head tilt; safest when neck injury suspected) c. If airway remains obstructed, use Heimlich maneuver (abdominal thrusts) on children or adults d. Back blows, chest thrusts used for obstructed airway in infants (less than 1 year)	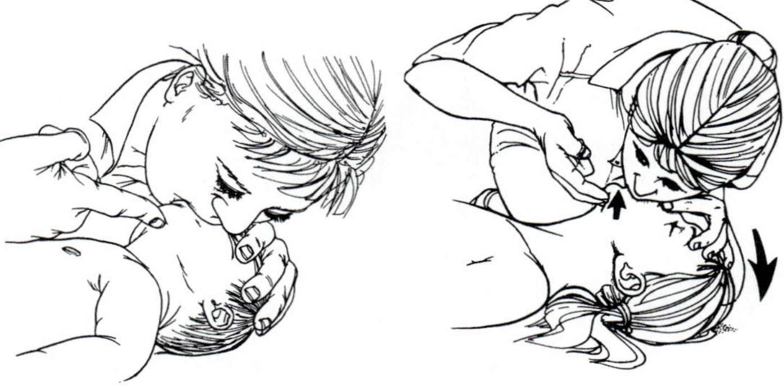		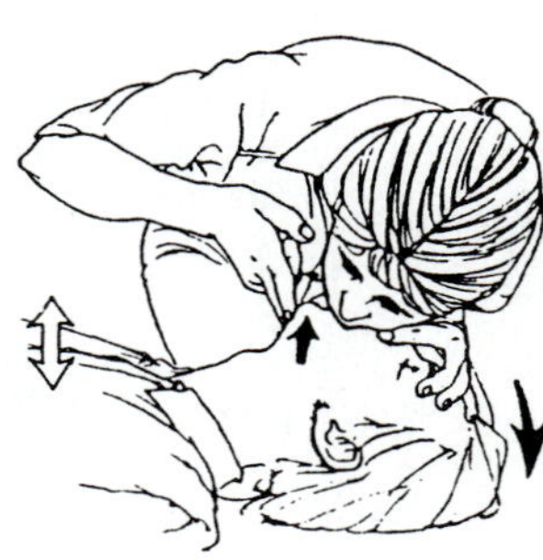

Continued.

◆ **TABLE 28-3**
Emergency Cardiopulmonary (CPR) Reminders*—cont'd.

	Infants (Less than 1 Year)	Children (1 Year through 8 Years)	Older Children and Adults
4. Evaluate breathing (*B*) Look, listen, feel 5. Give two initial breaths a. 1 to 1.5 second each b. Only enough volume to make chest rise and fall 6. Evaluate circulation (*C*) a. Palpate for carotid pulse in children and adults b. Palpate infant's brachial/femoral pulse 7. Use rescue breathing or CPR as needed	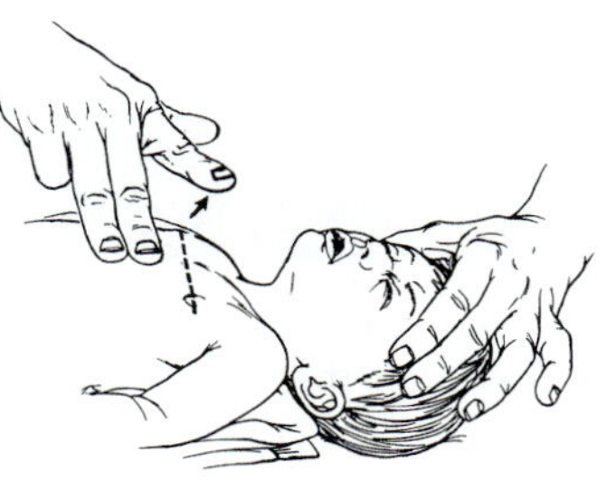	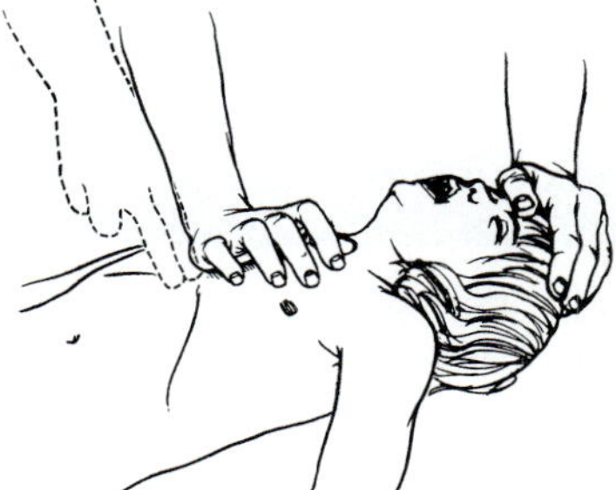	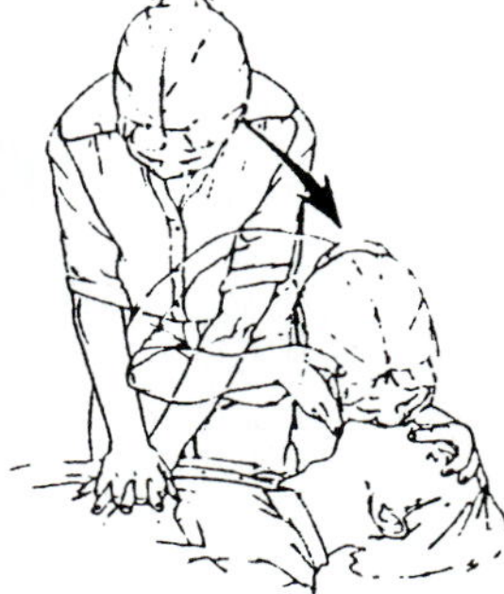
Consideration			
Pressure point	Midsternum—one finger breadth below the nipple line	Lower third of sternum	Lower half of sternum (Locate the xiphoid process and measure up about two finger widths.)
Hands	Tips of two fingers	Heel of one hand	Both
Compression distance	½ to 1 inch (1.3 to 2.5 cm)	1 to 1½ inches (2.5 to 3.8 cm)	1½ to 2 inches (4 to 5 cm)
Compression/ventilation (C/V)	5/1 (3-second cycle)	5/1 (4-second cycle)	Alone—15C/2V Two rescuers—5/1 (V = 1.5 seconds each)
C/V ratio	100C/20V/minute	80-100C/15V/minute	80-100C/12-15V/minute

*Victims should be supported on firm surface for best results. Breathing techniques now recommended make gastric distention and aspiration less likely. Effective CPR is accompanied by improvement in skin color and pupillary constriction. Check briefly for pulse after approximately 10 cycles or 1 minute of compression/ventilation and periodically thereafter. Each compression/relaxation phase should be equal duration and performed in a smooth fashion.
(Illustrations reproduced with permission. *Instructor's manual for basic life support*, 1992, American Heart Association.)

support (Fig. 28-14). Use of such devices is much less fatiguing for the care giver than mouth-to-mouth or mouth-to-airway resuscitation and also helps avoid the problem of possible disease transmission.

To be successful, one must be able to maintain an adequate airway using the typical techniques of head tilt/chin lift and/or oropharyngeal airway placement while also providing adequate support for the mask over the nose and mouth. The person providing ventilation may stand or sit behind the supine patient's head with the top of the patient's head stabilized against the body of the person providing ventilation. With one hand this person holds the mask firmly against the patient's nose and mouth while maintaining the airway. With the other hand, the person squeezes the air bag at a rate and depth compatible with the size and needs of the patient. Usually, only enough bag pressure to achieve a rise and fall of the chest is recommended.

The typical rates are the same as those used for

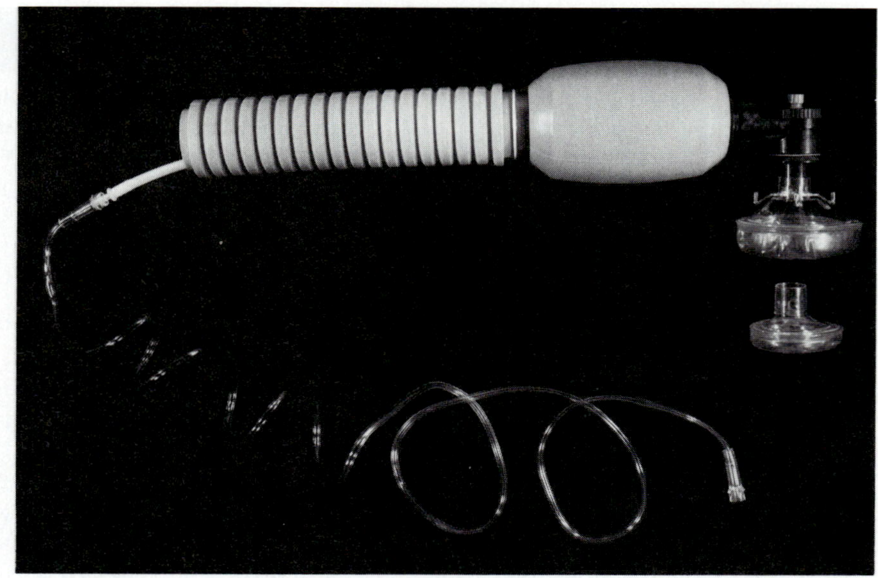

Fig. 28-14 Puritan Bennett PMR II. A manual resuscitator that administers 40% oxygen unless equipped with an oxygen reservoir that provides a 100% oxygen concentration capability.

mouth-to-mouth resuscitation: infants, every 3 seconds; children 1 through 8 years (or size), every 4 seconds; and older children, every 4 to 5 seconds. Too rapid, excited compression of the bag will cause greater respiratory distress. Time must be allowed for the patient to exhale adequately. When the patient makes an effort to breathe spontaneously, the treatment may be discontinued while the patient's respiratory attempts are evaluated.

There are two basic types of bag-valve-mask devices. The most commonly used are self-inflating or automatic recoil bags (Ambu, Hope, Laerdal, and Penlon). Adult and pediatric size bags, masks, and oropharyngeal airways should be available. Concentrations of oxygen up to 40% may be obtained by attaching the green tubing from a standard cylinder wall source to the port at the base of the bag. However, a reservoir tubing can be adapted to most bag-breathing apparatuses to provide as much as 100% oxygen concentration. Some, but not all, self-inflating bags have pressure relief safety valves set at 35 to 40 cm H_2O, or they incorporate an intentional fixed leak to guard against the application of too much pressure and the danger of pneumothorax.

The second type of bag-valve-mask device is the thin rubber flow-inflating bag used commonly by anesthesiologists. During use they are constantly connected to a flow of gas, usually an oxygen-air mixture, but 100% oxygen concentrations can also be achieved. A manometer should be attached to the system to provide a visual indication of the applied pressure. Nurses should be knowledgeable about the equipment available.

Mechanical Ventilators

If breathing needs to be supported for a prolonged time, mechanical ventilators are used. The most common indication for mechanical ventilation is impending or actual respiratory failure. Patients are placed on mechanical ventilators to treat hypoxemia and tissue hypoxia, to provide adequate ventilation for the patient who no longer can breathe on his or her own, to maintain positive pressure in the airways throughout the respiratory cycle, and to reduce the work of breathing.

Mechanical ventilators deliver air into the lungs through masks or endotracheal or tracheostomy tubes and administer any desired amount of oxygen from 21% to 100%. Positive pressure ventilators (PPV) are the most commonly used. They accomplish lung inflation by applying intermittent positive pressure ventilation (IPPV) or continuous positive pressure ventilation (CPPV) to the airway. Three different types of positive pressure ventilators are volume-cycled, pressure-cycled, and time-cycled. Volume-cycled ventilators deliver a preset volume, pressure-cycled ventilators deliver gas until a preset pressure is achieved, and time-cycled ventilators deliver gas during a preset time interval.

High-frequency ventilation is a type of PPV that delivers small tidal volumes at a high ventilatory rate in an effort to reduce barotrauma and cardiac complications associated with normal frequency mechanical ventilation.

Positive end-expiratory pressure (PEEP) is used to maintain an airway pressure greater than atmospheric pressure at the end of exhalation. Alveolar volume is thereby increased, in the hopes of decreasing hypoxemia and reducing the Fio_2 to less toxic levels. PEEP is often used in infant respiratory distress syndrome (IRDS). For a discussion of ECMO and CPAP see Chapter 34.

KEY CONCEPTS

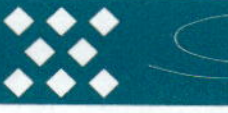

1 Signs of respiratory difficulty include the following: altered resting respiratory or cardiac rates, chest retractions, labored breathing, flaring nostrils, pallor, cyanosis, restlessness, disorientation, inflamed respiratory tract, and frequent coughing.

2 Because the clinical signs and symptoms of hypoxia are nonspecific, laboratory evaluation of arterial blood is performed to determine the extent of oxygenation. Pulse oximeters are also used clinically to measure oxygen saturation.

3 Methods for securing and maintaining an open airway include positioning, nasopharyngeal suctioning, endotracheal or tracheostomy tube placement and suctioning, medications, and chest physiotherapy.

4 An open airway may be maintained or established by positioning the patient so that obstructions are cleared and aspiration is prevented.

5 Suction of the nasooropharyngeal passages is accomplished by using a bulb syringe or a catheter setup attached to mechanical suction.

6 When positioning and nasopharyngeal suctioning are insufficient to maintain the patient's airway and oxygenation, an artificial airway must be inserted. An endotracheal tube is most commonly used for short-term airway management; a tracheostomy provides the best route for long-term maintenance. Gentle tracheal suctioning should be performed only when necessary.

7 Medications to aid in clearing the airway are nasal drops or sprays, expectorants, aerosols, inhalers, injections, and oral forms of medication.

8 Chest physiotherapy is designed to improve pulmonary hygiene in patients with acute or chronic sputum production. It incorporates breathing exercises, gravity-assisted positioning, percussion and vibration of the chest wall, followed by purposeful coughing and possible suctioning.

9 Rules for oxygen administration must be understood and carefully followed to avoid fire.

10 Methods of oxygen enrichment include incubators, hoods, oxygen and mist tents, nasal cannulas, and oxygen masks.

11 In the presence of an adequate airway, the following methods may be used to stimulate or maintain respiration: mouth-to-mouth resuscitation, cardiopulmonary resuscitation, manual resuscitators, and mechanical ventilators.

12 If respiration has ceased, mouth-to-mouth resuscitation is a practical, prompt source of aid.

13 The use of manually controlled bag-valve-mask ventilation devices is consistent with universal precautions.

14 Patients are placed on mechanical ventilators to treat hypoxemia and tissue hypoxia, to provide adequate ventilation when the patient cannot do so, to maintain positive pressure in the airways throughout the respiratory cycle, and to reduce the work of breathing.

CRITICAL THOUGHT QUESTIONS

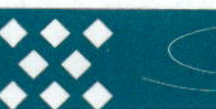

1 Identify various conditions that can result in airway obstruction. Which of these are most commonly seen in children?

2 What methods are used to relieve or reduce airway obstruction?

3 A variety of medications are used to improve respiratory function. Identify the most common medications. Compare and contrast the therapeutic effects and side effects of these medications.

4 What techniques are used to facilitate drainage of fluids from the lungs? Why are many different positions necessary? What precautions should the nurse take when performing chest therapy?

5 What mechanical equipment is used to assist ventilation?

6 When maintaining oxygenation, what universal precautions must be considered?

7 Compare and contrast CPR for the infant and for a five-year-old child.

BIBLIOGRAPHY

Comer DM: Pulse oximetry: implications for practice, *JOGN Nurs* 21(1):35-41, 1992.

Hodge D: Endotracheal suctioning and the infant: a nursing care protocol to decrease complications, *Neonatal Netw* 9(5):7-15, 1991.

Runton N: Suctioning artificial airways in children: appropriate technique, *Pediatr Nurs* 18(2):115-118, 1992.

Tolles CL and Stone KS: National survey of neonatal suctioning practices, *Neonatal Netw* 9(2):7-14, 1990.

Whaley L and Wong D: *Nursing care of infants and children,* ed 4, St Louis, 1991, Mosby.

Wong D: *Essentials of pediatric nursing,* ed 4, St Louis, 1993, Mosby.

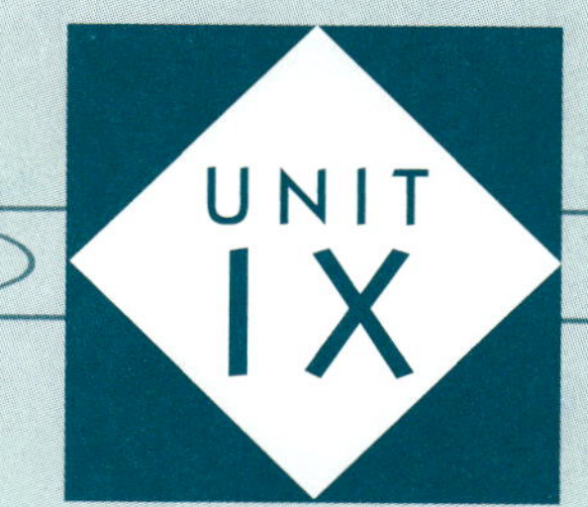

CHILD HEALTH PROBLEMS

29

Alterations in Body Temperature

CHAPTER OBJECTIVES

After studying this chapter, the student should be able to:

1 Identify the criteria used by parents and professionals to assess an elevated temperature in infants and children.
2 State the definition of fever taken by the oral, rectal, axillary, and tympanic membrane routes.
3 List four mechanisms by which the body produces heat and regulates its own temperature.
4 Describe six methods that help a person maintain or increase body temperature.
5 Discuss disorders associated with an elevation in the body's temperature set point, and what method of temperature control is commonly used for each disorder.
6 Identify six methods that help a person lower body temperature.
7 Define the terms *evaporation, radiation, conduction,* and *convection* as they relate to the regulation of body heat; cite an example of each.
8 Define *neutral thermal environment* as it relates to the body temperature maintenance of an infant.
9 Identify characteristics of a febrile seizure, including prevention, treatment, and instructions for parents.
10 Convert the following into thermometer reading ranges: neutral or warm, hot, and very hot.
11 Discuss possible dangers involved in the local surface application of heat or cold.
12 Explain what is meant by reflex vasoconstriction or vasodilatation.
13 Describe an acceptable method of administering a tepid water sponge bath.

One of the most common reasons for pediatric office visits, emergency room visits, or telephone calls from anxious parents is a child's elevated temperature. If a fever persists for more than 3 to 5 days for no apparent reason the diagnosis of fever of unknown origin (FUO) is made and the child may be hospitalized for a diagnostic work-up. In either setting the nurse plays an important role in assessment, planning, treatment, and education related to alterations in body temperature.

The regulation of body heat and the effects of localized temperature change on body parts are significant considerations in the nursing care of children. Although the goals and methods of temperature control are not without controversy, the perceptive regulation of body temperature through the use of selective therapies not only may bring greater comfort to the patient but also may prevent complications that occur in the presence of high temperature or abnormal loss of body heat. Appropriate temperature maintenance is particularly critical for infants due to their immature thermoregulation system.

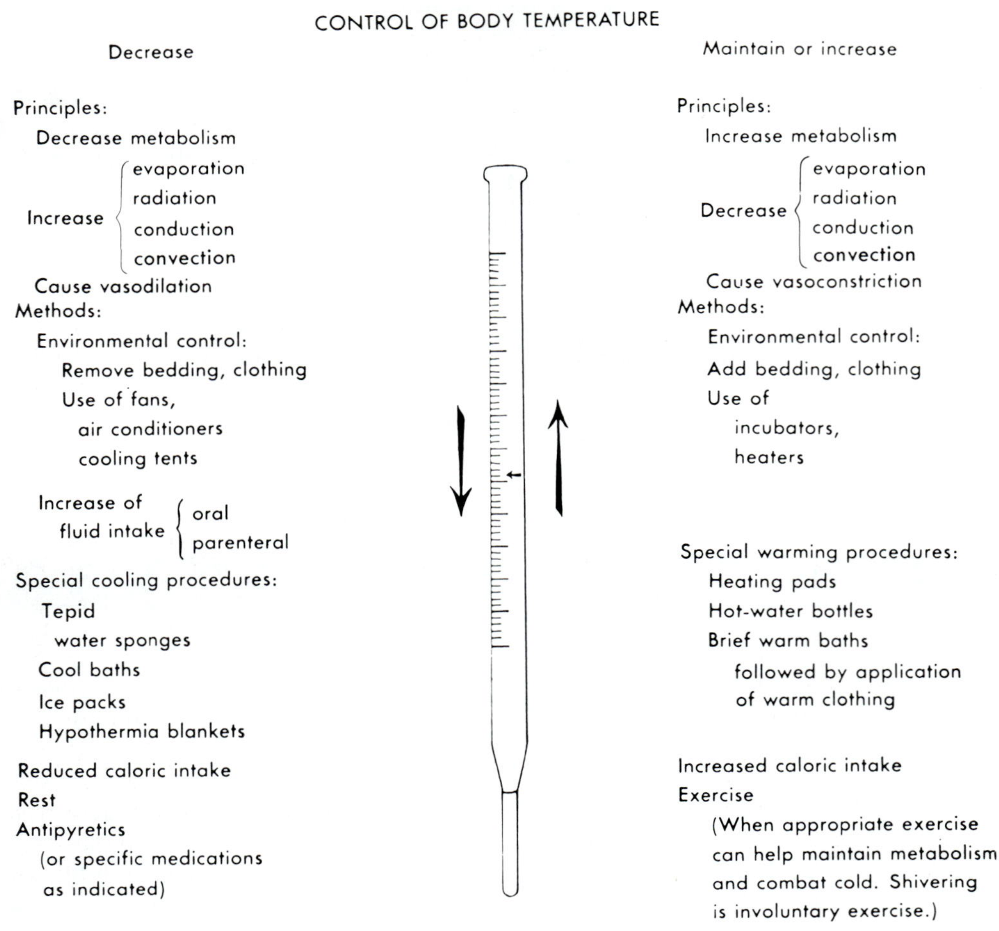

Fig. 29-1 In health the body keeps its temperature within safe ranges. However, during unusual conditions or illness, normal temperature controls may be disturbed, and special regulating measures may be needed.

BODY TEMPERATURE

Regulation (Fig. 29-1)

Although the normal oral temperature is often cited as 98.6° F (37° C) (see Table 29-1), these figures indicate an average normal oral temperature. However, even the normal *range* of oral temperature is variously defined. Oral temperatures ranging from 97.6° to 99° F (36.4° to 37.2° C) are not considered abnormal. A number of authors consider an oral or axillary reading greater than 100° F (37.8° C) to be fever. Rectal temperatures higher than 100.4° F (38° C) indicate fever.

Most texts report that rectal temperatures are about 1° F higher than those taken orally and that axillary temperatures usually register about 1° F lower. This relationship has not been supported by careful investigation. Axillary temperatures are increasingly favored for infants and young children. They are accurate and less invasive than other routes.

Infants and young children have relatively high metabolic rates and higher normal temperatures than older people. During a 24-hour period, people typically demonstrate a predictable change in body temperature. Readings taken between 4 and 8 PM usually are higher, whereas those taken during the usual sleep interval are characteristically lower. Environmental conditions, type of dress, and activities all influence a person's body temperature.

Normal body temperature in a human being represents a balance between heat production and heat loss in the body. Most body heat is inadvertently created in the process of normal body functions. Production of body heat is the result of the activity of all cells and made possible by the oxidation or burning of foodstuffs within those cells. Blood, flowing through the various parts of the body helps distribute heat. When measured by different methods (oral, rectal, axillary, tympanic membrane, or skin probe), these measurements do not differ greatly. Temperatures measured

◆ TABLE 29-1
Approximate Celsius/Fahrenheit Temperature Conversions

	Celsius	Fahrenheit
Boiling point	100°	212°
	41.7	107.0
	41.6	106.8
	41.4	106.5
	41.2	106.2
Harmful fever*	41.1	106.0
	41.0	105.8
	40.8	105.4
	40.6	105.1
	40.5	105.0
	40.4	104.7
	40.2	104.4
	40.0	104.0
	39.8	103.6
	39.6	103.3
	39.4	103.0
	39.2	102.6
	39.0	102.2
	38.9	102.0
	38.8	101.8
	38.6	101.5
	38.4	101.1
	38.3	101.0
	38.2	100.8
	38.0	100.4
	37.8	100.0
	37.6	99.7
	37.4	99.3
	37.2	99.0
Average oral temperature	37.0	98.6
	36.8	98.2
	36.7	98.0
	36.6	97.9
	36.4	97.5
	36.2	97.2
	36.0	96.8
	35.8	96.4
Freezing point	0.0	32.0

*Note: Generally the appearance and behavior of a person is more significant than the degree of temperature recorded. The rapidity of the rise of a fever is also important. A rapid rise in temperature is often associated with seizures. Controversy continues regarding the definition of harmful fever 106° vs. 107° F (Schmitt BD: Pediatrics 74(5):929, 1984 Reeves-Swift R: MCN 15(2):82, 1990).
Temperature measured orally
Conversion Formulas: °C × 9/5 + 32 = °F
°F − 32 × 5/9 = °C

near arteries are often called *core temperatures.* Examples are oral, rectal, tympanic membrane, and axillary readings in contrast to those measured by a skin probe.

Body heat is conserved by the involuntary constriction of the blood vessels of the skin, forcing more blood into the warm interior of the body and cutting it off from cooler areas near the skin's surface. Body heat is also conserved by the automatic reduction of perspiration. The maintenance of body heat is also aided by the voluntary activity of the person. Adding a sweater or coat to provide better insulation or exercising to increase metabolism and circulation increases tolerance to cold. Much heat is produced through the activity of the skeletal muscles. When additional warmth is necessary, these muscles may even contract involuntarily to produce heat, a process called *shivering.* Conversely, removing insulation, increasing surface evaporation, and reducing muscular activity decrease body heat.

Body heat is lost primarily through the dilatation of the capillaries in the skin, the *evaporation* of increased perspiration on the skin's surface, and the process of warming inspired air, which is subsequently exhaled. Heat naturally moves from a warmer to a cooler area or surface. Heat transfer occurs even when objects of different temperatures do not touch. This heat loss, called *radiation,* is more rapid if a significant difference in the temperatures of neighboring objects exists. Placing a body part directly in contact with a surface cooler than itself causes heat loss by *conduction.* Some surfaces remove body heat much more rapidly than others. They are called *good conductors of heat.* Cooler air flowing on the body, particularly the face, can be the source of considerable heat loss by *convection* (conduction to air). All of these mechanisms of heat transfer or loss may become operative, and the nurse trying to conserve a patient's body heat must understand them. For example, the newborn has an immature thermoregulation system; thus the health status of the newborn or young infant is at greater risk if exposed to environmental cold stress.

The area of the body that ultimately controls the unconscious processes necessary for the regulation of heat production, heat maintenance, and heat loss is thought to be located deep in the brain. The part of the brain considered most responsible for heat regulation is the hypothalamus, the "thermostat" of the body responsible for setting the systemic temperature. Through the action of the autonomic nervous system, the hypothalamus controls the processes of vasoconstriction and vasodilatation, the associated activity of the sweat glands, and the involuntary skeletal muscle motion. The hypothalamus influences various aspects of body temperature through hormonal stimulation and control.

In infants and young children, temperature regulation is not perfected, and rather wide swings in body temperature occur readily. During the first days of life an infant is more likely to be influenced by the temperature of the environment; hence, the frequent use of incubators. Toddlers and young school-age children may react to the common infectious diseases of childhood by running temperatures of 104° F (40° C) or more. A child may initiate a temperature elevation during a prolonged episode of crying.

Causes and Effects of Elevated Body Temperature

Elevated body temperature may be caused by three basic processes:

1. Elevation of the body's temperature set point or control located in the hypothalamus—associated with infection, allergy, malignancy, radiation, and central nervous system disorders
2. Excessive heat production by the body not involving an elevation in temperature set point—associated with aspirin overdose, hyperthyroidism, and "malignant hyperthermia" (a serious condition involving an inherited muscle disorder and the administration of anesthesia and neuromuscular blocking agents)
3. Defective heat loss mechanism preventing the body from dissipating excess heat not involving an elevation in temperature set point—associated with heat stroke, burns

Most episodes of body temperature elevation involve the resetting of the body's thermostat or set point. An elevated systemic temperature, whether initiated by infectious processes, dehydration (inadequate intake, vomiting, or diarrhea), overdressing, or other mechanisms, causes considerable discomfort and distress for pediatric patients and their parents. Young children may experience a rather rapid rise in temperature, especially in response to viral infections. In general the rapidity of a rise in body temperature is more significant than the fact that a moderately high fever exists. However, patients may be ill without a fever.

Studies suggest that fever is a therapeutic response by the body that helps support the immune system and fight infection. This research has changed the management of low-grade fevers, under 102 degrees F. For example, routine orders such as "acetaminophen (Tylenol) to reduce fever of 101° F" are less common than a decade ago. Efforts are concentrated on finding the cause of the fever and prescribing appropriate therapy to eliminate its initial cause. If acetaminophen is given when a child has a low-grade fever, it is administered primarily for its analgesic effect.

To evaluate fever it is necessary to assess the patient's total condition and behavior and to monitor the temperature consistently. A rapid rise in temperature (especially spiking fevers) even in the "lower readings" can cause a seizure. A high fever of 105° F or more may *depress* the immune system. Some patients may have underlying cardiorespiratory problems that may cause the elevated metabolism and accompanying rising pulse and respiratory rates associated with fever to be detrimental to their conditions. Other problems, such as neurological disease, may cause special concern.

Simple febrile seizures

About 2% to 5% of children with a fever may exhibit convulsions or seizures. Two thirds of these children will experience only one seizure. These *simple febrile seizures* may occur at temperatures that are not extremely elevated. Febrile seizures usually occur early in an illness, with the initial temperature spike or rapid rise. Whether the temperature or some other factor causes the seizures is not clear. Although a seizure is frightening and parents are especially fearful regarding the possibility of brain damage, studies indicates that such damage does not occur from fever in itself until levels of 106° to 107° F (41.1° to 41.7° C) are reached or unless there is an underlying neurological disorder or infection.

Simple febrile seizures occur more often in boys, last several minutes, and have a positive family history. The initial first seizure usually occurs before the age of 3 years with the peak age range being 6 to 18 months.

Prevention of simple febrile convulsions is best accomplished by keeping the child healthy, well-nourished, and well-rested. Febrile convulsions most often accompany respiratory infections. These are prevented by good handwashing and optimal health

Nursing Alert

Treatment with anticonvulsant medication for 1 year is recommended if the seizures occur before 1 year of age, are focal or localized, last longer than 15 minutes, if the child has an underlying neurological disorder, or if the EEG is abnormal 3 weeks after the seizure (Leung and Robson, 1991). These variations suggest that the child is not having a simple febrile seizure. Complex seizures, epilepsy, and infection must always be considered.

maintenance. Parents should be given a brief explanation of fever, its risks and benefits, how to take a temperature, home management, and when to seek advice from the health care provider. Explaining to parents that although simple febrile seizures are frightening, they are benign, that two thirds of children who have them experience only one, and that their incidence decreases dramatically after the age of 3 years.

Causes and Effects of Depressed Body Temperature

A depressed body temperature may simply reflect inactivity. The early morning temperature reading may be low only because body processes are at a naturally low ebb. However, an abnormally low systemic temperature may also indicate circulatory collapse or the tiring of basic body processes before death.

For children undergoing cardiac and thoracic surgery, it may be desirable to slow down metabolism during surgery and postoperative care by cooling the body to extremely low temperatures to rest the heart and respiratory system. The narrowing of the blood vessels in the skin that results from surface cooling, forces the blood into the interior of the body, increases viscosity (thickens the blood), slows the blood flow, and necessitates less oxygen intake. Uncompensated by muscle activity, the drop in temperature is of therapeutic importance. However, such a severe reduction in metabolism requires special equipment and personnel and cannot be safely maintained indefinitely. A less dramatic reduction in body temperature may increase metabolism because of the body's continuing compensatory efforts to maintain a normal temperature. Such efforts may decrease blood glucose used for fuel and consume more oxygen. This is particularly important to remember when caring for the neonate. At-risk infants subjected to this type of continued cold stress rapidly become hypoglycemic and, in addition, are unable to increase their oxygen intake sufficiently to meet their metabolic needs.

Cellular metabolism in the absence of adequate oxygen produces lactic acid, and acidosis results. Such a sequence of events is avoided by maintaining a neutral thermal environment in which an infant is able to maintain body temperature with the least expenditure of energy as measured by oxygen consumption. Adequate weight gain and proper acid-base balance is enhanced. A neutral thermal environment for an infant is usually when the abdominal skin temperature registers between 97.7° F (36.5° C) and 98.6° F (37° C) (AAP, 1992).

Maintaining or elevating body temperature

The nurse maintains or in some cases raises body temperature to provide comfort, regulate metabolism, or treat exposure. This may be accomplished by increasing room temperatures, applying more blankets, adding clothing, and offering warm fluids.

In the postnatal period a newborn's optimal temperature may be maintained effectively when placed in skin-to-skin contact on the mother's abdomen. An infant can also be easily warmed by a radiant warmer or in an incubator.

Infant incubator

Incubators are often used to maintain or gradually increase the body temperature of newborn infants. They allow close observation of a nude or partially clad infant without jeopardizing body temperature. Incubators are plastic enclosures that also may provide additional humidity and oxygen for the infant. Three basic designs are available: (1) those with hinged lids that are lifted up to expose the infant; (2) those that, in addition to hinged lids, provide special portholes or panels for access to the infant (Fig. 29-2); and (3) those that lift up from the side, creating an open, horizontal slitlike access to the infant (Fig. 29-3). Before opening any part of an incubator, the nurse should read the temperature of the air inside and record any oxygen concentration percentage. The infant's body temperature should be recorded with that of the ambient air temperature on the infant's graphic chart. How warm an incubator is kept to conserve the infant's energy depends on the infant's gestational age at birth, chronological age, weight, and condition.

In some incubator models the temperature of the artificial environment may be automatically controlled by the infant's own skin temperature through the use of a heat-sensitive probe taped to the infant. This may be advantageous in maintaining body temperature. Such incubator controls are to achieve a neutral thermal environment. However, an early abnormal rise in an infant's temperature may be masked unless the simultaneous records of the temperature of the incubator and the skin of the infant are compared. This is because, as the infant's temperature rises, the heat source will not be activated and the incubator temperature will decrease. Conversely, if the probe becomes detached from the infant undetected, the unit may overheat. The temperature setting of incubators may also be adjusted manually, depending on the results of intermittent temperature readings.

The application of local heat is helpful in raising total body temperature. The use of hot-water bottles,

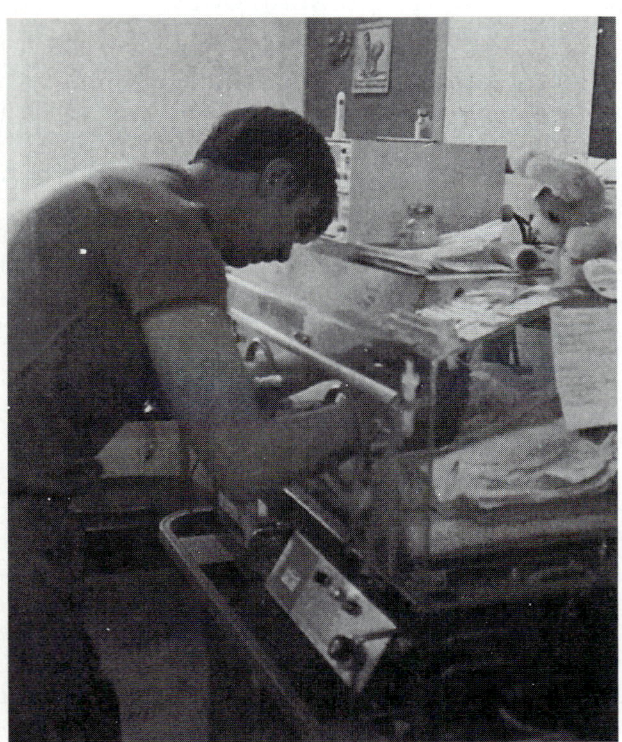

Fig. 29-2 Nurse caring for infant in incubator. (Courtesy Wong D: *Essentials of pediatric nursing,* ed 4, St. Louis, 1993, Mosby.)

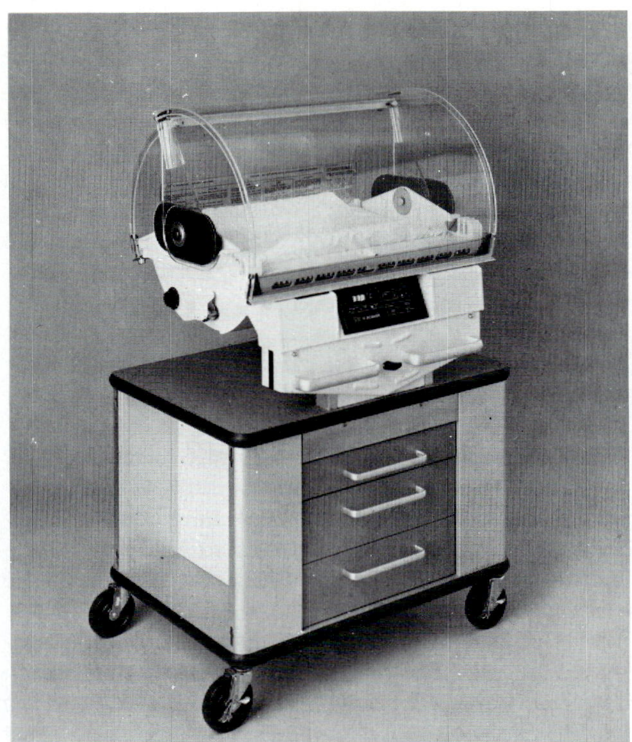

Fig. 29-3 Intensive care incubator. (Courtesy Ohio Medical Products, Madison, Wis.)

heating pads, and hypothermia blankets, which may be regulated to function like heating blankets, is discussed later in the chapter.

Reducing Body Temperature

Six methods of lowering body temperature are fluid intake, environmental control, medication, tepid tub bath, tepid sponge bath, and hypothermia blankets.

Fluid intake. Dehydration is a common cause of fever. Maintaining and encouraging fluid intake is an important nursing intervention. If oral fluid intake cannot be maintained due to the child's condition, fluids must be administered intravenously.

Environmental control. Body temperature may be lowered and the patient made more comfortable by altering the immediate environment. The removal of extra blankets and heavy clothing (unless the patient is complaining of chills and shivering) is often helpful. A well-ventilated, draft-free room is important to optimal health promotion. In warm weather, well-placed fans that circulate the air without directly blowing on the patient may be used.

Medication. Antipyretics may be ordered to help reduce fever. The most frequently prescribed medication for fever reduction and analgesia is the nonsalicylate acetaminophen (Tylenol or Tempra). Acetaminophen helps to reduce the elevated set point of the hypothalamus. Ibuprofen, a nonsteroidal antiinflammatory and antipyretic, may be prescribed for older children.

Antipyretics are not ordered for low-grade fever, usually considered to be less than 102° F (38.8° C), because of the role that fever plays in boosting the immune system. There is also a concern that a fever (a possible sign of a disease process) may be masked by their use, obscuring one indication of diagnosis or progress in treatment.

Tepid tub or sponge baths. Cooling by means of a tepid water tub bath or sponging techniques in the crib or bed have long been used in pediatrics in an effort to control elevated temperatures and relieve discomfort. However, this method is controversial because too rapid cooling may cause shivering, a rebound effect,

> **Nursing Alert**
>
> Aspirin, acetylsalicylic acid, is not recommended for use as an antipyretic in children because of its relationship to Reye Syndrome.

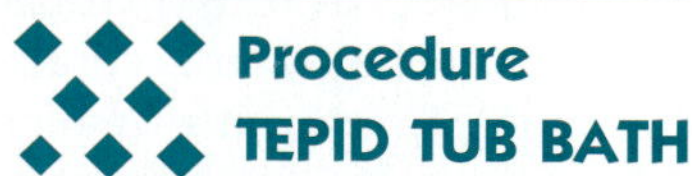

Procedure
TEPID TUB BATH

EQUIPMENT/SUPPLIES NEEDED:

1. Wash cloths, towels
2. Convenient baby tub or standard bath tub
3. Floating toys, plastic headrest
4. Light gown or pajamas
5. Appropriate water supplies

STEPS:

1. Explain procedure according to child's understanding.
2. Place warm water about 98° F (36.6° C) in tub, only enough for a shallow bath.
3. Support child as necessary in tub—supine if possible. Never leave child alone.
4. Place a moist washcloth on child's forehead, if appropriate.
5. Pour warm water over child's body.
6. Gradually reduce temperature of bath water by adding cooler water if tolerated.
7. Observe carefully for onset of chilling or shivering. Discontinue if chilling is observed.
8. Continue bath for about 20 to 25 minutes.
9. Pat dry and dress in lightweight clothing.

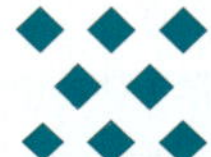

Procedure
TEPID SPONGE BATH: BEST FOR MOST TODDLERS

EQUIPMENT/SUPPLIES:

1. Waterproof sheet
2. Absorbent bath blanket or towels, depending on the size of the child
3. Light bath blanket to place over child
4. Basin of tepid water at about 85° to 90° F (29.4° to 32.2° C)
5. Four washcloths

STEPS:

1. Explain the procedure to the child in simple terms.
2. Place the child on top of waterproof sheeting and absorbent blanket (unless this is already part of the base of the bed) fairly close to the side of the bed so that it may be easily reached. Remove pillows.
3. Undress the child and cover with the light bath blanket.
4. Rub the skin of the anterior trunk and extremities briefly with a dry washcloth to bring the blood to the surface to decrease the sensation of chilling and aid in heat reduction when the tepid moist washcloths are applied.
5. Place moist, not dripping, folded washcloths on the axilla and groin on the side of the child you will sponge last.
6. Wash the child's face and neck; place a wet washcloth on its forehead.
7. Expose only the area being sponged. Use firm, long strokes in sponging the upper extremity, thorax, abdomen, and lower extremity on the side farthest away. Place the washcloths on the groin and axilla of the opposite side. Continue sponging the patient—first the upper extremity, then the thorax, abdomen, and lower extremity.
8. Evaluate periodically the child's reaction, skin pulse, and respirations. (If the child seems to be chilled or shivering or becomes agitated, discontinue the bath, lightly cover it, and report to the supervising nurse.)
9. Turn the child on its side. Rub and sponge the back firmly.
10. Gently pat the skin dry at the end of the sponge bath with a towel, and dress the child in a light gown. The procedure should take about 20 to 25 minutes.
11. Cover the child with a light sheet or blanket. Remove the bed protectors and encourage rest.

NOTE: An alternative to the tepid water sponge bath described above is wrapping with moist tepid towels instead of sponging with washcloths. These towels must be changed as soon as they become warm.

shock, and convulsions. Thus a tepid bath should be a warm bath with cool water added gradually. Tepid tub or sponge baths are said to be most effective for the treatment of temperature elevations *not* caused by a rise in set point. PREPARATION: The procedure selected and the materials needed depend on the age, condition, and reaction of the individual child.

About 30 minutes after completing the procedure:

1 Check the child's temperature, pulse, and respiration.
2 Report to the supervising nurse.
3 Record the procedure, child's reaction, and results.

Hypothermia blankets

Children with temperature elevations that are exaggerated or fail to respond to other methods of treatment may be placed on hypothermia blankets. Several types of hypothermia blankets are manufactured. Although the operating instructions on each may differ, the principles involved are similar. Cold, distilled water, or alcohol and distilled water (depending on the model), are circulated through tubes embedded in a plastic mat or mats. The water is cooled and circulated by a refrigeration pump unit to which the pads are attached. With some units, adjustment of the pad temperature is accomplished manually by the nurse, depending on the child's temperature. With others, a rectal probe is inserted, facilitating continuous monitoring of the infant's temperature. The temperature of the child, registered by the probe, may regulate the temperature of the pads automatically, according to predetermined temperature settings. Several pads of various sizes may be used both under and over the child, according to need. A light bath blanket or sheet is always placed between the child and the plastic pad. The pad should not be folded or creased, and no pins should be used to secure it. The temperature desired and the duration of time the pad is to be used should be ordered by the attending physician.

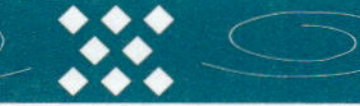

KEY CONCEPTS

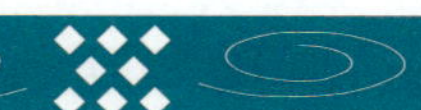

1 Fever is usually indicated with oral temperatures of more than 100° F (37.8° C), rectal temperatures over 100.4° F (38° C), and axillary readings over 100° F (37.8° C).
2 Normal body temperature represents a balance between heat production and heat loss. Most body heat is created in the process of normal body functions. Heat loss or conservation is controlled by vasoconstriction and vasodilatation, activity of the sweat glands, and involuntary skeletal muscle motion.
3 Elevated body temperature may be caused by three basic processes: (1) elevation of the body's temperature set point, (2) excessive heat production not involving an elevation in set point, or (3) defective heat loss mechanism.
4 Simple febrile convulsions occur more often in boys, last less than 15 minutes, have a positive family history, are not focal, result in a normal EEG, and have a peak incidence in children aged 6 to 18 months.
5 It may be desirable to cool the body to an extremely low temperature to slow down metabolism for children undergoing cardiac and thoracic surgery. A less dramatic reduction in body temperature may increase metabolism and is an important factor to remember when caring for the neonate.
6 Body temperature may need to be maintained or raised to provide comfort, regulate metabolism, or treat exposure. This may be accomplished by various methods, including increasing room temperature, adding clothing or blankets, offering warm drinks, placing an infant in an incubator, or applying local heat.
7 There are six basic methods of reducing body temperature: increased fluid intake, reduced environmental temperature, administration of antipyretics, tepid tub bath, tepid sponge baths, and hypothermia blankets.

CRITICAL THOUGHT QUESTIONS

1 Why do infants and children experience wide swings in body temperature? What internal and external factors can contribute to elevated body temperature? To decreased body temperature?
2 Discuss the nursing measures that help to prevent rapid change in body temperature in infants and young children.
3 What nursing measures are used to reduce elevated body temperature? What nursing measures are used to raise lowered body temperature?
4 Describe the characteristics of simple febrile seizures, their prevention, treatment, and parent counseling.

REFERENCES

American Academy of Pediatrics and American College of Obstetricians and Gynecologists: *Guidelines for perinatal care,* ed 2, Elk Grove Village, Ill, 1992.

Davis K: The accuracy of tympanic membrane measurement in children. *Pediatr Nurs* 19(3):267-272, 1993.

Leung AK, Robson WL: Febrile convulsions, how dangerous are they? *Postgraduate Medicine,* 89(5), 217-224, 1991.

Moss JR: The ups and downs of fever management, *Small Talk* 5(1), 1-8, 1993.

Newbold J: Evaluation of new infrared tympanic thermometer: a comparison of three brands. *J Pediatr Nurs* 6(4):281-283, 1991.

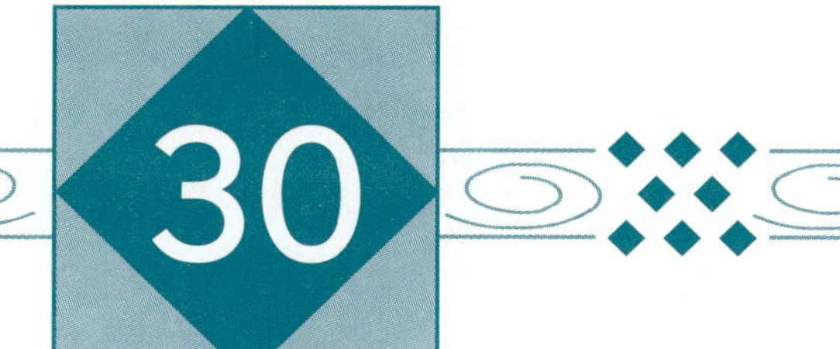

Skin Problems

CHAPTER OBJECTIVES

After studying this chapter, the student should be able to:

1 Discuss three ways in which the appearance and condition of the skin may reveal significant information regarding a person's physical and emotional status.
2 Define these terms often used to describe skin conditions: macule, papule, vesicle, pustule, petechiae, contusion, excoriation, laceration, fissure, and ulcer.
3 Differentiate primary and secondary skin lesions.
4 Identify seven descriptive characteristics of a skin lesion.
5 Discuss the etiology, prevention, signs and symptoms, treatment, and nursing implications of these common infant skin problems: miliaria rubra (prickly heat), seborrheic dermatitis (cradle cap), and diaper rash.
6 Describe the typical appearance of infantile eczema, frequent factors associated with its onset, and four objectives that must be considered as treatment is begun.
7 Explain the use of wet compresses in the treatment of weeping, crusted lesions of eczema and how the compresses should be applied.
8 Describe impetigo and indicate why systemic antibiotics are often prescribed as part of its treatment.
9 Compare tinea capitis, tinea corporis, and tinea pedis, as to location, description, treatment, and nursing care.
10 Discuss the identification, incidence, treatment, and nursing implications of infestations of pediculosis capitis (head lice) and the itch mite (scabies) in the young school-age population.
11 Identify the etiology, treatment plan, and typical duration of acne vulgaris.
12 Explain why the "rule of nines" used in the evaluation of the extent of a burn injury cannot be used without modification in evaluating an infant or young child.
13 Describe minor, moderate, and major burn injuries and indicate the first-aid care of burn victims.
14 Identify five goals of burn therapy.
15 Define these terms associated with burn injury and therapy: eschar, debridement, granulation tissue, isografts (autografts), allografts (homografts), Curling's ulcer, and flexion contractures.
16 Discuss how the nursing staff may provide emotional support to the burn patient and family.

The integumentary system consists of the skin, hair, nails, sweat and oil glands, and superficial sensory nerve endings. These organs form the first line of defense against bodily injury. The integumentary system prevents both excessive loss of fluid from the body and the entry of certain poisons and microbes into the body. It is of special importance in the regulation of body temperature, principally through capillary dilatation and constriction and the formation of cooling perspiration. The skin can be an important avenue of fluid loss. However, it has only limited powers of absorption. It is of considerable aid in the evaluation of environmental conditions and therefore in the determination of individual safety. Embedded within the tissues of the integumentary system are nerve endings that relay sensations of pressure, touch, hot, cold, and pain to the brain.

The health of the skin is a reflection of the health of the individual. Skin color, hydration, surface irregularities, and disturbances in sensation reveal significant information about an individual's health habits and status. The skin also reveals a patient's emotional reactions.

KEY VOCABULARY

Specific terms describe the condition of the skin and are used routinely in nursing assessment. These terms are used to describe primary, secondary, and special skin lesions:

abrasion (adj., abraded) Loss of superficial tissue by friction (chafing).

ecchymosis (adj., ecchymotic) Bruise; a black-and-blue irregularly formed hemorrhagic area.

erythema (adj., erythematous) Reddened areas of the skin.

jaundice or **icterus** (adj., jaundiced or icteric) Yellow tinge to the skin or sclerae.

laceration (adj., lacerated) Jagged cut or tear.

lesion Any change or irregularity in tissue caused by disease or injury.

pruritus (adj., pruritic) Itching.

Primary or Initial Lesions:

bleb or **bullae** (adj., bullous) Blister.

macule (adj., macular) Flat spot or stain; freckle.

papule (adj., papular) Small, solid elevation on the skin; the typical early stage of a pimple is papular.

pustule (adj., pustular) Pus-filled vesicle; a superficial cutaneous abscess.

urticaria (wheals and hives) (adj., urticarial) Large, slightly raised, reddened or blanched areas, usually accompanied by intense itching.

vesicle (adj., vesicular) Small elevation of the skin obviously containing fluid, such as a blister.

Secondary Lesions or the result of changes in Primary Lesions:

crust (adj., crusted) Temporary covering of a lesion formed primarily by dried blood or serum (scab).

erosion (adj., eroded) Moist, circumscribed, often depressed lesion.

excoriation (adj., excoriated) Self-inflicted abrasion; a scratch.

fissure Ulcer or crack-like sore

ulcer (adj., ulcerated) open sore, often depressed or forming a cavity, caused by loss of normal tissue.

Special Lesions:

petechiae (adj., petechial) Small bluish purple dot caused by capillary hemorrhage.

LAYERS OF THE SKIN (FIG. 30-1)

The epidermis is paper thin and consists of several microscopic layers. The uppermost layer consists of dead cells ready to be shed from the body's surface. They are constantly being replaced by new cells, which are formed in the lower layers. The lower layers of the epidermis secure their nourishment from the dermis, or true skin, over which they lie.

The dermis, also called the *corium,* is a dense layer of connective tissue well supplied with blood vessels and nerves. It also contains sweat and oil glands and hair follicles, some of which may extend into the deeper subcutaneous tissue. Small muscle fibers may be attached to the hair follicles.

The subcutaneous layer is chiefly fatty tissue in a framework of elastic and fibrous tissue. It serves multiple functions, including those of lipid storage and insulation.

Assessment of the skin is a critical component of the overall nursing assessment. Skin problems may be of secondary importance in the diagnostic picture. However, the condition of the skin is significant as the nurse assesses the whole child.

A skin lesion should be described so that the following information is included:

1. Size (e.g., 1 cm in diameter)
2. Elevation (e.g., raised, flat, depressed)
3. Quality (e.g., smooth, rough, scaly, moist)
4. Color
5. Distribution (e.g., localized, scattered, generalized)
6. Associated sensory disturbances (numbness, itching, pain, burning)
7. Type of drainage or exudate noted

COMMON SKIN PROBLEMS

Infant and Toddler

Miliaria rubra (prickly heat or heat rash) Miliaria rubra is a common problem caused by blockage of the

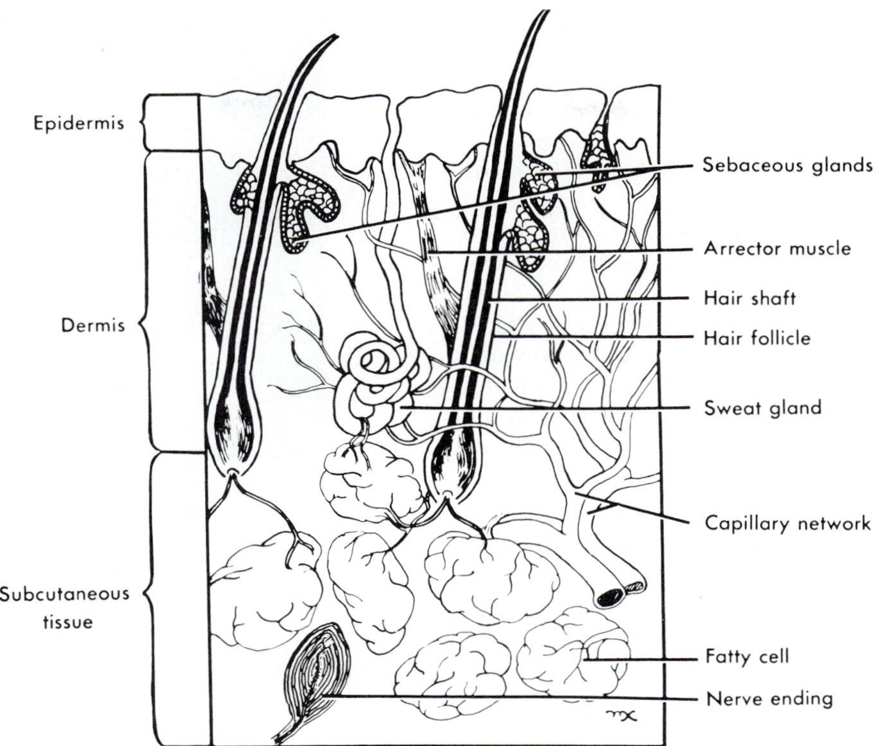

Fig. 30-1 Schematic drawing of skin layers.

sweat glands. The exits of the sweat ducts are plugged, causing sweat to seep into the dermis or epidermis. This produces a red, pinhead-sized vesicular-papular rash that is associated with underlying erythema, especially in areas where perspiration or friction is common. It may be accompanied by pruritis (itching). The rash may include pustular lesions. Prevention is easier than treatment. Overdressing children should be avoided. A 1% hydrocortisone cream may be recommended for persistent cases. In the event of secondary infection an antibiotic may be prescribed.

Intertrigo

Intertrigo *(chafing)* is found in the folds of the skin where friction occurs and hygiene is inadequate. Examples of problem areas include the creases in the neck and the folds of the groin and gluteal muscles where the skin may become inflamed. As in miliaria rubra, prevention is simpler than a cure. Good hygiene and keeping the area dry are of great importance.

Seborrheic dermatitis (cradle cap) (Fig. 30-2)

Seborrheic dermatitis is a common dermatitis of infancy. It is caused by a lipophilic, skin surface-dwelling yeast. The organism thrives in the oily

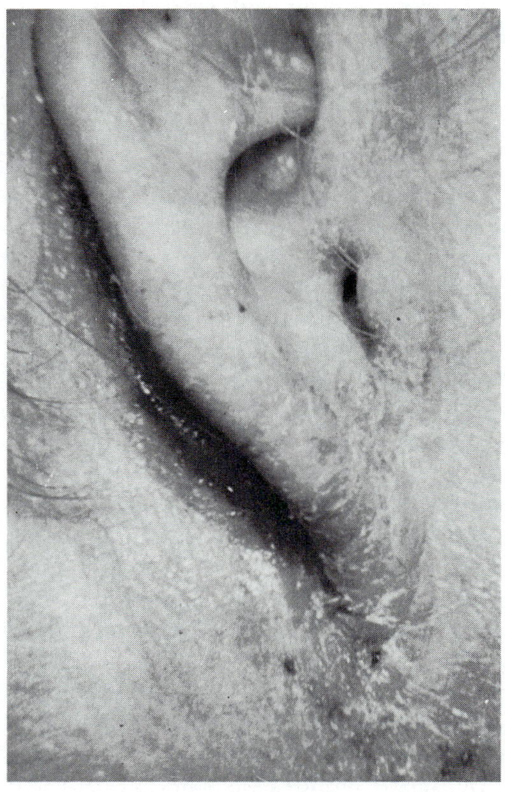

Fig. 30-2 Seborrheic dermatitis. (Courtesy WW Duemling, San Diego, Calif.)

environment induced by maternal transplacental hormone stimulation of the oil glands. The condition is usually benign and self-limiting, but it can be chronic and is often confused with atopic dermatitis.

Clinical manifestations. Seborrheic dermatitis or cradle cap is characterized by a dry or greasy scaly eruption on an inflammatory base. It chiefly affects the scalp, eyebrows, eyelids, and pubic regions. Seborrheic dermatitis is comprised of yellowish, slightly adherent large scales found principally on the top of the head. It sometimes is related to a parent's reluctance to wash the soft spot on the infant's scalp for fear of causing injury. It also develops in the groin and may become secondarily infected with yeast (*Candida* or *Monilia*) or bacteria.

Treatment. Frequent shampooing and the use of mild medications containing sulfur, salicylic acid, or hydrocortisone are often prescribed for seborrheic dermatitis. In adolescents it is often associated with acne. When the condition involves the scalp, the common name is *dandruff*. Some children are affected by another form called *intertriginous seborrhea*, which is usually moist and involves areas behind the ears and the axillary and inguinal regions. Moderate to severe cases may be managed with a topical agent, ketoconazole cream 2% (Nizoral), which kills the lipophilic yeast organism.

Diaper rash

The most common cause of diaper rash is irritant dermatitis. Moniliasis (yeast-like fungi), seborrheic dermatitis, and eczema are also common causes. The rash may take multiple forms, from simple erythema to blisters and ulceration, depending on the causes. As a group, children with irritation of the diaper area may have a hereditary predisposition and sensitive skin. Unfavorable conditions quickly trigger an unfavorable response. Contributing factors are poorly washed and rinsed diapers, infrequent diaper changes aggravated by prolonged use of plastic diaper covers, and incomplete or infrequent washing and drying of the diaper area. Careful attention to cleanliness is necessary; however, overzealous cleansing with harsh soaps can also cause problems.

Prevention. To reduce the formation of irritating ammonia produced by the action of bacteria on urine, every effort is made to cut down the bacterial population on the diaper area. The use of gentle antiseptic final rinse, such as methylbenzethonium chloride sometimes may be recommended. The use of antiseptic rinses by diaper laundries is standard practice.

Exposing the diaper area to the air is extremely helpful. Sunshine may be used for 10 minute periods several times a day; however, the infant must be carefully observed to prevent overexposure.

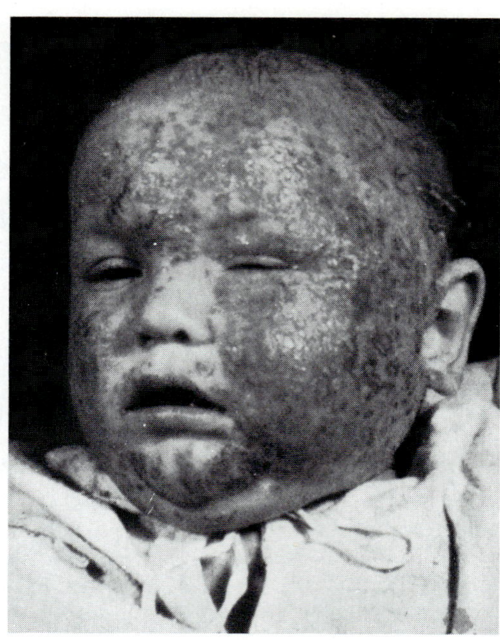

Fig. 30-3 Infant with severe eczema. (Courtesy RB Pappenfort, San Diego, Calif.)

Treatment. In the hospital setting the cautious application of dry heat to diaper rash may produce good results; however, safety remains a critical factor. A heat lamp must be out of the child's reach and away from bed linens. The bulb should be at least 12 inches (20.3 cm) from the child's buttocks. During heat treatments the diaper area should be free from medications.

Desitin or hydrocortisone may be used for irritant rashes, whereas lotrimin or nystatin cream may be ordered for fungal rashes. Because of the occlusive effect of ointments, cream preparations are preferred. Rarely, diaper rashes become secondarily infected with bacteria. Thus topical or systemic antibiotics will be ordered.

Infantile eczema (atopic dermatitis) (Fig. 30-3)

Infantile eczema appears after the second month of life and usually subsides after the second year. Infantile eczema is an allergic or atopic response. It is a symptom of a disorder rather than a disorder itself. Infantile eczema is the most common manifestation of allergic disease in infancy. It is not always clear what agents, or allergens, cause the dermatitis. Exposure to allergens may occur in any of the following ways:

1 By ingestion (common foods causing difficulties in infancy are cow's milk, egg whites, wheat products, and citrus juices)

2 By inhalation (dust, pollen, and animal dander)
3 By skin contact with some medications and materials (rubber, plastic, and wool).

There is often a family history of allergy manifested by eczema, asthma, or hay fever. Eczema usually improves during the summer months and worsens during the winter. To identify substances that may initiate the dermatitis, a careful history is taken.

Clinical manifestations. Eczema is characterized by skin lesions, which first appear as localized, scaling, red areas, usually on the head, neck, wrists, flexor surfaces of the elbows and knees, although involvement may become more extensive. Small vesicles that break and weep serum (a yellow, sticky fluid) develop rapidly in these areas. The fluid dries, forming crusts on the skin. Lesions on various parts of the body may be in different stages of development—some moist, others dried and scaling. The skin may become thickened and fissured. Since itching is intense, the child scratches the lesions, thus secondary infection is common.

Treatment. Many factors must be considered in the treatment of eczema. If possible, the offending allergens should be identified and eliminated from the infant's environment. Discomfort (pruritus or itching) and secondary infection should be treated. The goals of treatment include: clear the scaling, minimize discomfort, and improve appearance. Informational and emotional supportive for the child and the family is essential.

For the infant or toddler an elimination diet is often prescribed in which the foods that are allowed are listed in detail. If the baby is not breast fed, soy milk may be prescribed. The importance of rigidly following the diet must be impressed on the parents. As time goes on, more foods are added, one by one, to the diet. The child is carefully observed for changes in skin condition and general health after each addition.

The home environment of the infant must be carefully controlled also. Since many children with allergic symptoms of the respiratory tract show sensitivity to dust, their nurseries are stripped of all drapes, rugs, stuffed toys, and books. The crib mattress is encased in a nonallergic cover, and wool blankets or clothing are eliminated. The presence of a dog or cat in the household may cause significant problems, and pets must sometimes find new homes. Approximately 20% of the general population is allergic to cats, and 5% are allergic to dogs. The house should be vacuumed weekly with special attention to the child's bedroom. Skin testing with special patch and scratch techniques in an effort to determine allergens is usually reserved for children over the age of 3 years.

The child with eczema should avoid people who have known staphylococcal, streptococcal, or viral infections, such as herpes simplex (which is the cause of the common fever blister). Good handwashing is critical.

To help reduce scratching, which increases the possibility of secondary infection, various methods are used. Efforts are made to decrease the itching by using a minimum of clothing, all softly textured. Diapers are changed frequently. Fingernails and toenails are trimmed short. Restraints are no longer recommended unless all other methods of control fail.

A variety of medications may be used. Systemic antihistamines may ease itching. Sedation allows the infant to sleep. Topical or systemic antibiotics may be used to treat secondary infections. Topical creams containing hydrocortisone are used to reduce inflammatory response if infection is not present.

If coal tar preparations are used, care should be taken not to expose the areas to sunshine, which causes a chemical reaction that in itself is irritating to the skin. Jars containing coal tar preparations should be tightly closed to prevent deterioration. Coal tar ointment should be removed in special baths or with liquid petrolatum before a new application is made.

Medications are applied with clean hands or a finger cot or glove. They are generally used on a small area on a trial basis to test skin reaction. Many of these medications are expensive and should not be wasted.

Special baths or soaks are prescribed for the infant to remove crusts and reduce pruritus and weeping. Common ingredients added to the bath water are cornstarch, oatmeal preparations (such as Aveeno), or bicarbonate of soda solutions. The water should be tepid, about 95° F (35° C). If possible, a small baby bathtub should be used. Sometimes the skin of the infant is so dry that bathing is restricted. In routine bathing a soap substitute is regularly used. Continual, tepid, wet medicated compresses are sometimes employed to dry weeping crusted lesions. Therapeutic compresses must be kept wet to accomplish the goals of treatment. This type of compress or gauze bandage is not covered by waterproof material but is left exposed to cool the area by evaporation.

Older children may undergo desensitization procedures. Through the injection of small but gradually increasing amounts of allergen, the body is sometimes eventually able to tolerate the allergen without reaction. The course of infantile eczema is usually not steady improvement. The child improves, has a re-

Nursing Alert

Excessive bathing should be avoided because of the excessive dryness that it causes. Lotions or medications should be applied immediately after the bath to seal in moisture.

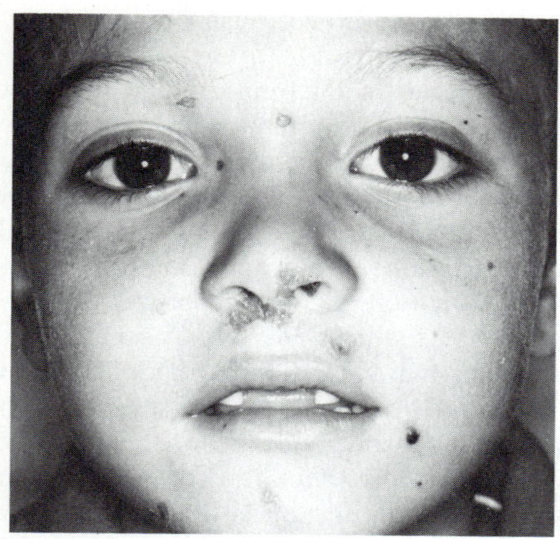

Fig. 30-4 Impetigo. (Courtesy David Allen, San Diego, Calif.)

lapse, and improves again. The parents should be told to prepare themselves for a rather long siege. However, the child over 2 years can usually expect a respite. Unfortunately, as eczema disappears other types of allergy manifestations, such as asthma or hay fever, may develop.

Preschoolers and School-age Children

Impetigo (Fig. 30-4)

Impetigo is a skin infection caused by either coagulase-positive staphylococci or group-A beta-hemolytic streptococci. It is highly contagious and serious in newborns. Impetigo is contagious but less serious among children and adults. It is often associated with poor hygiene.

Clinical manifestations. Inflammation begins with the appearance of erythematous lesions on the skin, which develop into small blisters. The blisters become pustules and break, causing thick yellow-red crusts on older children but few crusts on infants. When the crusts are removed, small superficial erosions are seen. The face and hands are most frequently affected, but other areas may become involved. In the hospital, contact precautions are used.

Treatment. Treatment of impetigo includes careful cleansing and removal of the crusts with compresses. A small amount of the topical antibiotic, mupirocin ointment 2% (Bactroban), is applied to the affected area three times daily until clear. Bactroban is highly effective but expensive. A course of penicillin or erythromycin administered systemically may be recommended because of the demonstrated association of certain strains of group-A beta-hemolytic streptococci and nephritis. Also, more rapid erradication of lesions is seen when systemic therapy is used. The nurse should be especially cautious in the care of the lesions and disposal of infected material because the infection spreads easily. The child's fingernails should be clipped short. Good handwashing for the child, family members, and other care providers is essential.

Furuncles and carbuncles

Furuncles and carbuncles are deep infections of the hair follicles. They may occur singly or in groups. If the furuncles run together, forming one sore with several draining points, the resulting lesion is called a *carbuncle.* Carbuncles are uncommon in small children but seen with greater frequency among adolescent boys.

Clinical manifestations. A furuncle begins as a single papule associated with a hair. The papule becomes a pustule, which enlarges and forms a head.

Treatment. Mupirocin ointment 2% (Bactroban) may stop progression of the lesion and preclude the need for systemic antibiotics or incision and drainage by the health care provider. If multiple furuncles are present, systemic antibiotic therapy will be prescribed.

Sty (Hordeolum)

A sty is an infection involving an eyelash follicle and may clear spontaneously. However, warm compresses several times a day and erythromycin ophthalmic ointment will speed resolution.

Ringworm of the scalp, skin, and feet (Fig. 30-5)

Ringworm of the scalp, or *tinea capitis,* is common among school-aged children and is more prevalent in urban areas when crowded living conditions exist. It can be caused by several kinds of fungi. Some types of fungi are contracted from human beings, whereas others are contracted from animals.

Clinical manifestations. The fungus attacks hairs at their bases, causing them to break off close to the skin and leave circular balding areas. The scalp in the area of the hair loss may become red and scaly. Mild itching may be present. Diagnosis is usually made on the basis of the clinical history, observation with an ultraviolet light called *Wood's lamp,* or a microscopic examination of the affected hairs. Fungi that cause ringworm of the scalp fluoresce brightly when exposed to the rays of Wood's lamp.

Treatment. The oral administration of griseofulvin has been successful. The medicine does not kill the fungus but prevents its spread into uninfected cells. As

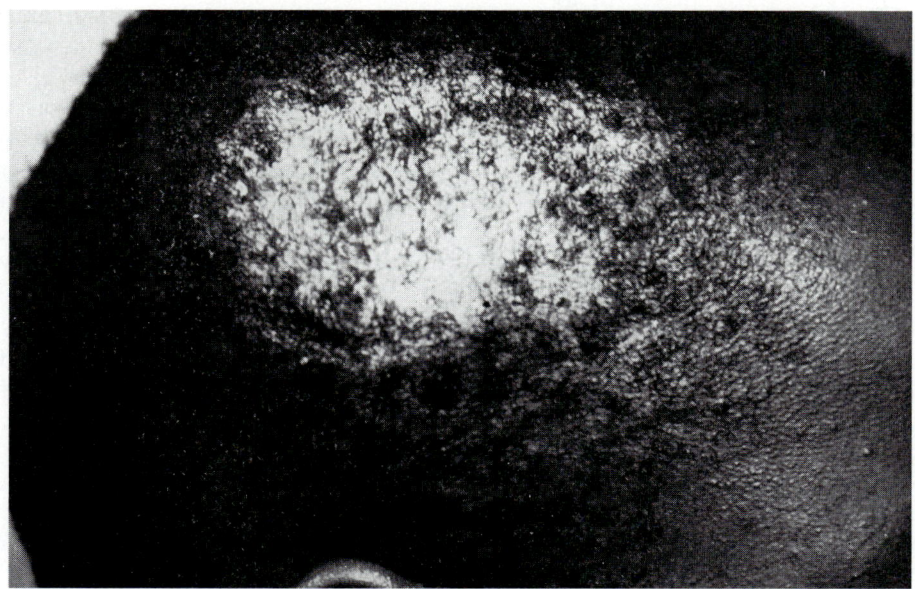

Fig. 30-5 Tinea capitis (ringworm of scalp). (Courtesy WW Duemling, San Diego, Calif.)

the infected cells are shed or removed, they are replaced by healthy cells. Clipping of the affected hair after a few weeks of treatment is also desirable. In addition, a local antifungal ointment may be ordered.

Clinical manifestations. Ringworm of the skin, *tinea corporis,* may involve various areas, including the face, neck, arms, and hands. Although there are exceptions, the classic lesion of ringworm of the skin is rounded or circular with a gradually extending, small, raised vesicular border and with central healing. The lesion may vary considerably in size, but it is usually about the size of a quarter.

Treatment. Treatment consists of prevention of scratching and topical application of the following: clotrimazole (Lotrimin), tolnaftate 1% (tinactin), haloprogin (Halotex), or Monistat-Derm. Local treatment is combined with systemic use of griseofulvin in severe cases.

Ringworm of the feet, *tinea pedis,* or so-called athlete's foot, is common in school-age children and adolescents. Younger children with scaling of the feet may have some form of eczema.

Clinical manifestations. Ringworm of the feet is most often characterized by itching or burning of the feet, blisters, and painful cracks between the toes. At times it may extend to involve other areas and become serious if secondarily infected. It is caused by several kinds of fungi.

Treatment. Treatment consists of the use of topical Nizoral or griseofulvin. Over the counter anti-fungal preparations such as Desenex or Whitfield's ointment may be effective in mild cases. Better ventilation and the reduction of moisture are helpful. Frequent changing of socks is a necessity. If the infection has been intense and tends to recur, the advisability of discarding shoes worn during the infection should be considered. The feet should be carefully dried. A prophylactic antifungal dusting powder is often advised for susceptible persons. Clean municipal showers are essential to the prevention of spreading the infection.

Pediculosis or lice infestations

Although there are three types of lice—head lice, body lice, and pubic lice—only one type is of significance to children, *pediculosis capitis,* or infestation of head hair by lice. This condition is seen in all socioeconomic groups. Children often contract the infestation in the school setting.

Clinical manifestations. The parasitic head louse causes itching as it travels on the scalp. Small, grayish, oval eggs called *nits* are laid and attached to the base of the hair shafts with a type of mucus that is produced by the louse (Fig. 30-6). As the hair grows, the nits become more visible; they resemble tiny flakes of dandruff except that they do not brush out. New lice hatch within 1 week, and the cycle repeats. Pediculosis is often accompanied by excoriation and secondary infection caused by scratching.

Treatment. Treatment is comprised of lindane (Kwell) or crotamiton (Eurex) shampoos. Because of the potential systemic absorption of lindane and potential nervous system toxicity causing seizures if

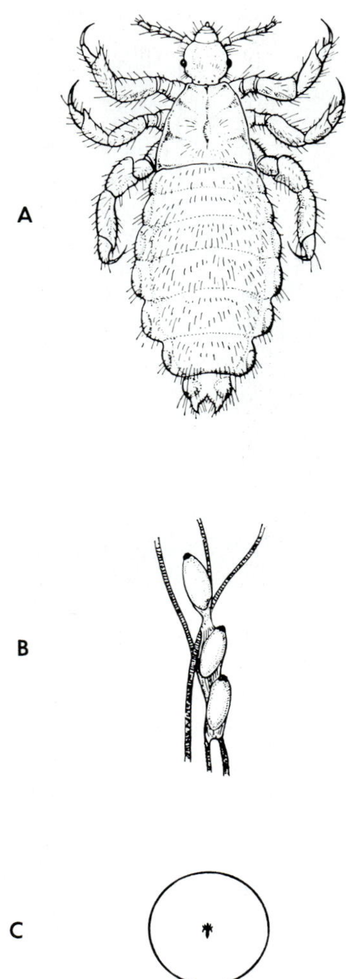

Fig. 30-6 **A,** The female head louse (enlarged). **B,** Enlargement of nits on hair shafts. **C,** Life-sized louse.

product directions are not observed, some clinicians are prescribing crotamiton for children under 50 pounds. At the end of the treatment, the hair should be combed with a fine-tooth comb to remove the devitalized nits. Warm vinegar solution also aids in the mechanical detachment of nits. The entire family of an affected person should be treated. Bed linens, hats, and headbands should be washed in hot water.

Scabies

Scabies is a superficial infestation by the itch mite (*Acarus scabiei*, or *Sarcoptes scabiei*).

Clinical manifestations. The female mite burrows under the skin, making a tunnel about ½ inch (1.2 cm) long, which is visible as an elevated line from the skin's surface. The insect is so small that it is rarely visible to the naked eye. Scabies usually involves those body areas where the skin is moist and thin—between the fingers and toes, in the axillae, and on the groin and abdominal areas. The itch mite causes itching, as the name indicates.

Treatment. Various treatments are available. Lindane (Kwell) may be applied in cream form to cool, dry skin. The use of Kwell, however, is not recommended in infants because of questionable neurotoxicity. The pyrethrin-containing pediculicides and scabicides have a much greater margin of safety and their efficacy is well established. Instructions for application and removal of nits should be carefully followed. The entire family of an affected person should receive therapy. Bed linens should be washed in hot water.

Adolescence

Acne vulgaris

Vulgar means "common," and acne vulgaris is a skin disease that is exceedingly common among teens. It may exist in a very mild form, or it may be extremely severe. There are several causes that, appearing together, produce the problem. Acne first appears at the onset of puberty. Hormone levels are believed to play a role. Parents of the affected child may have experienced similar difficulty; therefore, hereditary factors are not ignored.

Clinical manifestations. The production of sebum, or fatty secretion of the oil glands, is stimulated by certain hormones during adolescence, and several types of skin microorganisms utilize sebum as a food source and change it into fatty acids that cause acne. The pores clog, and blackheads (plugs of keratin, sebum, and microorganisms, also called *comedones,* the primary lesions of acne) form. The pores may also be clogged with dirt; however, blackheads are not commonly caused by dirt particles but rather oxidation of the top of the plug, a process that may occur no matter how carefully the adolescent bathes. Plugging of the oil ducts may lead to papules, pustules, and, at times, cyst formation and permanent scarring.

Since acne most often occurs on the face, shoulders, and back, it is of cosmetic and psychological concern. The teen should be given professional help during this distressing period so that the interval is as short and free from complications as possible. Acne may cause low self-esteem at an already challenging stage of development.

Treatment. Treatment is based on reinforcing self-care. General health habits are reviewed. A well-balanced diet is emphasized (see Food Guide Pyramid, Chapter 22). The avoidance of carbohydrates and fatty foods, such as chocolate, nuts, and peanut butter is not necessary as long as they are consumed in moderation. Six to eight hours of sleep each night, eight glasses of water each day, stress management, and aerobic exercise at least three times a week contribute to overall health status.

Cleansing several times a day is encouraged. Mild cases are treated topically with antibacterial soaps or skin cleansers (Fostex or Acne-Aid), lotions or pads containing *keratolytic* compounds (salicylic acid, resorcin) or other agents (benzoyl peroxide, tretinoin [Retin-A]). Girls are advised to avoid oily makeup and moisturizers. Tinted antibacterial creams or lotions are available that help heal and mask the lesions. Flare-ups may occur premenstrually.

Frequent shampooing is helpful. Picking and squeezing lesions should be discouraged because this may break down tissue walls and spread infection. The health care provider may remove comedones in the office with a special extractor or give careful instructions to the patient's family regarding the removal of comedones. The treatment of choice in severe cases includes either tetracycline or erythromycin to kill the bacteria. Minocycline hydrochloride (Minocin) or isotretenoin (Accutane) may be necessary if these measures fail.

Acne is usually self-limited and subsides in 3 to 4 years. However, severe cases may persist into middle age. The partial removal of scarred tissue may be accomplished, in selected cases, by superficial abrasion, a technique called *dermabrasion.* X-ray treatment is no longer recommended by dermatologists because of the possibility of causing skin changes later in life and the availability of effective alternatives.

Herpes Simplex (Type 1)

Herpes simplex type 1, a viral infection, usually causes an irregular vesicular lesion on the margin of the lip (fever blister) or gums. The blister breaks, and a crust develops and eventually clears. These lesions have a tendency to recur in the same area, causing considerable annoyance, discomfort, and cosmetic concern. Occasionally herpes simplex takes on a more important aspect. It is serious when a newborn infant or very young child is involved because the lesions have a tendency to multiply, and when the eye is involved impairment of vision may result.

Treatment. Acyclovir, an antiviral agent, is effective in the management of herpes simplex.

Dermatitis venenata

Dermatitis venenata may be seen at any age. It is an inflammatory skin response to external contact with some irritating substance, such as fibers, plants, synthetics, or adhesive tape. However, it is most often observed in those groups who hike in the midst of poison oak or poison ivy.

Clinical manifestations. Signs of skin irritation usually occur several hours after exposure and consist of redness, swelling, and small blisters at the point of contact. Itching is intense.

Treatment. If children know that they have been exposed, the best immediate treatment before the appearance of symptoms is washing the area well. The best course of action is an initial proper identification and avoidance of the offending plants. After the blisters have developed, the urge to scratch must be resisted to prevent spreading. Calamine lotion and cortisone preparations applied locally helps to relieve itching.

BURNS

Burns may be caused by exposure to hot liquids, strong chemicals, direct flame, radiation, sunlight, or electric current. Toddlers and young children are most often scalded by hot coffee, grease from frying pans, or hot water from unguarded bathroom faucets. Older children are frequently burned when their clothes catch fire while they are playing with matches, using kerosene, or standing too close to household heaters. In the United States approximately 500 children are hospitalized each day because of burns, and about 1500 die each year.

Classification

Burns are classified into four categories, depending on the depth of penetration of the body's surface.

A *first-degree* (partial-thickness) burn involves only the epidermis. It is very superficial; a tender, slightly swollen redness results. A common example of a first-degree burn is sunburn. A *second-degree* (partial-thickness) burn involves the epidermis and dermis. This category is further divided into superficial and deep dermal burns. Some epidermal appendages must be intact for these burns to heal spontaneously. Deep dermal burns may change from partial-thickness to full-thickness wounds by infection, trauma, or obstruction of the blood supply to the affected part. A second-degree burn is characterized by blister formation or a reddened, discolored region with a moist, weeping surface. A *third-degree* (full-thickness) burn involves the entire dermis and portions of the subcutaneous tissue. The region affected has a brown, leathery appearance with little surface moisture. A *fourth-degree* (full-thickness) burn involves subcutaneous tissue, fascia, muscle, and perhaps bone. The tissue appears blackened and contracted. Partial-thickness burns can heal without grafting. Full-thickness burns must be grafted for healing to occur. Evaluation of the depth of a burn is not always easy immediately after the injury.

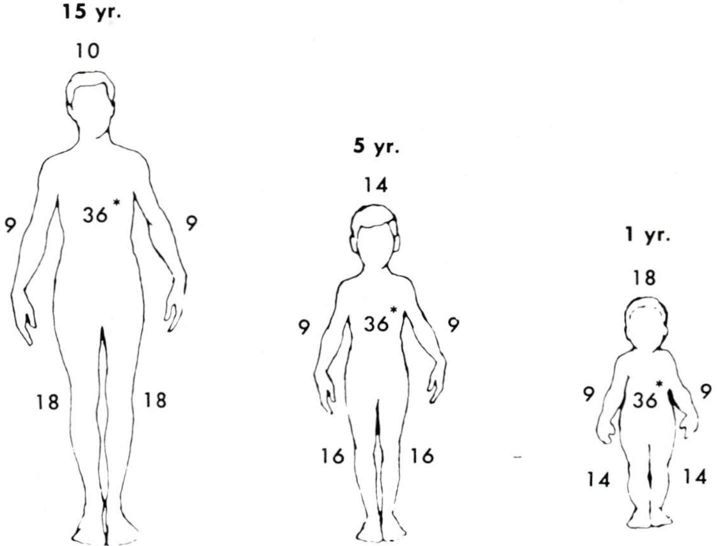

Fig. 30-7 Modification of "rule of nines." (Courtesy Burn Institute, Galveston Unit, Shriners Hospital for Crippled Children, Galveston, Tex.)

It is not only the degree of burn that is significant but also the amount of body surface affected. A person can tolerate a deep burn only if a small area is involved. In evaluating the extent of a burn on an adult, the so-called rule of nines can be applied; it gives a certain percentage value to each part of the body—a percentage that is almost always nine or a multiple of nine. This method of calculation, unless modified, is not helpful when working with children because of the relatively large size of a child's head and the reduced length of the legs. (One example of modification based on size differences is illustrated in Fig. 30-7.)

The area, extent, and depth of a burn determine its severity, and treatment is planned according to severity.

Minor burns are described as partial-thickness first- or second-degree burns covering less than 15% of the body surface and not involving strategic areas such as the face, hands, feet, or genitalia. Minor burns are treated on an outpatient basis. *Moderate burns* are described as partial-thickness, second-degree burns covering over 15% but less than 30% of body surface or as full-thickness burns involving less than 10% of body surface. Moderate burns usually require hospitalization. *Major burns* are described as partial-thickness, second-degree burns covering at least 30% of the body surface or as full-thickness, third-degree burns involving more than 10% of the body surface. Most burns—either partial- or full-thickness—that involve a large part of the face, hands, feet, or genitalia are considered major burns. Children with major burns always require hospitalization, and children with critical burns are transferred to a major burn center if possible.

Therapeutic Management and Nursing Responsibility

Initial considerations

The Burn Institute recommends that children and adults be taught to Stop! Drop! and Roll! should they be directly exposed to fire. If an abundant source of water from a hose or bucket is available it should be used; if not, blankets or throw rugs may be used to smother the flames, since fire cannot continue in the absence of oxygen. If neither water nor blankets are available, the victim should be rolled on the ground or floor to smother the flames. When the fire has been extinguished, the burned area should be rinsed with cold water. The victim should be taken immediately to a hospital for evaluation and care. The victim should be transported wrapped in a clean sheet and blanket. No medication of any type should be administered.

When a burned child is admitted to an emergency room or other hospital receiving area, the child's clothes should be removed gently, cutting along the seams of the garments if necessary. The child should be placed on and covered by sterile sheets in a room with good lighting. All those in attendance should wear face masks and should be provided with sterile gowns and gloves. The severity of the burn is estimated by the attending physician, and the need for hospitalization is determined.

Minor burns. Initial treatment includes immersing the area in cold water to reduce pain and edema. Care of minor burns usually consists of cleansing the area with mild soap and water. Iodophor soaps are currently used for their antibacterial effect. The area may be covered with a fine-mesh gauze, lightly lubricated with water-soluble antimicrobial cream (for example, nitrofurazone, neomycin, or bacitracin) and wrapped with a bulky, protective dressing. Depending on the condition of the dressing, the condition of the patient, and the health care provider's preference, this dressing may be left in place for 4 or 5 days. The child's tetanus immunization should be validated and, if not documented as up to date, should be given. Acetaminophen (Tylenol) may be prescribed for pain, and the patient should return to be seen by the health care provider in 48 hours.

Moderate or major burns. The first phase of therapy when moderate or major burns are present includes maintenance of an airway and prevention of shock. The airway is not a problem in all cases, but occasionally, because of the location of the external burn, the inhalation of fumes, or internal burning of the respiratory tract, it is of great importance. Blood gas analysis is mandatory. A complete blood count, electrolyte determination, and blood typing provide a baseline that is vital for evaluating the child's state of health on admission. An endotracheal tube may be needed. Humidified oxygen should be administered and the airway suctioned as necessary.

A nasogastric tube (double-lumen sump) may be inserted to prevent paralytic ileus or tachypnea, associated with acute gastric dilatation and vomiting. Intravenous fluid therapy is the most important aspect of the early care of the burn patient. Loss of plasma into the burn area and evaporation of water from the burn results in a rapid decrease in plasma volume, a concentration of red blood cells, and ultimately an increase in hematocrit. Fluid replacement must be initiated immediately and continued at a high rate for about 24 hours, after which a plasma shift occurs. Fluid that has leaked into the burn area returns to the vascular area. In young children a peripheral cutdown is performed, or a central venous line is inserted.

An indwelling urinary catheter is usually necessary. The amount and type of urine formation is observed and recorded hourly to determine the rate of intravenous therapy and to provide an index of the patient's general condition. An initial specimen should be sent to the laboratory for a baseline urinalysis, specific gravity and electrolyte studies. A dwindling urinary output may serve as a warning of developing hypovolemia and possible circulatory collapse. A urinary output of 1.0 to 2.0 ml/kg/hr for a child is desirable (approximately 10 to 30 ml/hr). Signs of overhydration revealed by excessive output require a reduction in fluids given intravenously. Electrolyte, specific gravity, and BUN/creatinine levels are followed regularly and frequently. It is extremely important to report irregularities in the urinary output, loss of a urine specimen, or an error in the measurement of a urine specimen because of the danger of miscalculating the rate and amount of intravenous fluids needed.

Careful assessment is necessary to prevent overloading the circulatory system—an important concern requiring close monitoring. The patient is weighed to provide a baseline for subsequent weight loss or gain. Vital signs are checked frequently, although meaningful blood pressure readings may be difficult to secure because of the age of the child and the location of the burn area. Some children need central venous pressure determinations.

Hospitalized children with serious burns are usually treated with intravenous antibiotics to prevent infection by the staphylococci and streptococci present on the skin. Prophylactic antibiotics are given as indicated by the child's clinical course and specific cultures of the wound. Many hospitals routinely isolate their burn patients in an effort to prevent or reduce infection.

Pain medication is administered intravenously. The child should be made comfortable but should not be oversedated. More pain accompanies a partial-thickness burn than a full-thickness burn because in the partial-thickness burn, nerve endings are still intact. (Refer to Chapter 27 for a discussion of pain management and control.)

The shock phase of the body's response to extensive burns usually lasts from 48 to 72 hours. After 48 hours, the initial ileus that may be seen with major burns has passed, and either oral or nasogastric feedings should be initiated. Hypermetabolism is seen in all patients with extensive burns and continues until the wound is covered. Calorie and protein intake must be increased to facilitate wound epithelialization and graft acceptance. Increased nutritional requirements often necessitate tube feedings to supplement oral feedings. An antacid is given either orally or through the tube to prevent Curling's ulcer, a stress ulcer associated with serious burns. Frequent milk feedings, which children usually take well, provide greatly needed calories and fluid. Children usually require about 80 calories per kg of body weight and 3 gm of protein per kg of body weight daily. Adequate nutrition maintains basal weight and enhances wound healing, helping to prevent infection. The vocational nurse and registered nurse will work as care partners with severely burned children during this critical period.

Wound Care

After the child is initially stabilized, the burn wound is treated. Hair adjacent to the burn wound should be shaved carefully and the burned area cleansed with water and small amounts of iodophor soap or saline solution. Cleansing is performed preferably in a hydrotherapy tub. At the time of admission the loose skin and blisters of partial-thickness burns are surgically removed in a procedure called *debridement*. Gradually a thick black crust (eschar) composed of the drying wound secretions and nonviable tissue forms. An escharotomy may be necessary to relieve compression from circumferential burns. For the little girl in Fig. 30-8, an incision through the eschar was required to release pressure and to permit adequate respirations.

A modified exposure treatment is used for the immediate care of moderate and major burns. Partial-thickness burns are prepared for spontaneous healing by covering the area with fine-mesh gauze that is impregnated with antibacterial ointment or cream. The gauze is held in place by elastic netting or a Surgifix dressing. A sterile blanket may be applied to prevent chilling, and burned extremities should be elevated to minimize edema.

The surface of the burn wound must be kept clean by vigorous daily cleansing in the form of povidone-iodine (Betadine) tub baths, whirlpool treatment, or local soaks. All dressing materials should be ready to reapply in a sterile manner after the soak. Soaking in the hydrotherapy tub facilitates removal of loose, sloughing tissue, exudate, and the topical medication.

Days later, as the eschar begins to separate, the physician cuts away portions of the dried crust, revealing new granulation tissue. When the granulation tissue is exposed (by removal of the eschar), antibiotic gauze is laid over the open granulation areas. Through soaks and redressings or intermittent surgical debridements, the burned areas are cleaned and the developing granulation tissue is prepared for elective grafting, which saves time and gives a better end result. Granulation tissue is a deep-pink, fragile tissue that bleeds easily. When the tissue is sufficiently prepared, the child undergoes grafting. Donor sites are selected on the patient's body. The donor site is usually covered with fine gauze and a pressure dressing. Later, when bleeding has been controlled, the outer pressure dressing may be removed. Donor sites heal in about 2 weeks. The newly grafted area is kept covered. The dressing should be observed for amount and type of drainage and odor. Exposed adjacent areas are observed for edema and circulatory problems. Grafts are usually firmly attached by the twelfth day after the grafting procedure.

Full-thickness major burn wounds are treated soon after admission by primary (tangential) excision. In the operating room under hypotensive anesthesia, which minimizes bleeding, devitalized burned tissue is cut down to the live tissue, and skin grafts are immediately applied. The primary objective of wound care is to reduce the size of the wound as rapidly as possible, thereby increasing the patient's chance for survival. When the wound is reduced to less than 20% of the body surface area, the chance for survival approaches 100%. Full-thickness major burns are, preferably, covered with the patient's own skin. These *autografts* from undamaged parts of the patient's own body provide permanent coverage (see box above). Unfortunately, often too little skin remains, and homografts, heterografts, and synthetic grafts are used as temporary surface coverings. These biological dressings are used to cover the wound and prevent infection in preparation for skin autografts or donor grafts.

TYPES OF SKIN GRAFTS

PERMANENT	
Isografts (autografts)	Undamaged tissue from the patient's own skin (may also be from patient's identical twin)
TEMPORARY	
Allografts (homografts)	Tissue taken from a member or cadaver of the same species
Xenografts (heterografts)	Tissue taken from another species, for example, pig skin (porcine xenograft)
Synthetic grafts (Epigard)	Man-made grafts

Immediate coverage of the burn wound with grafts or medication after debridement or primary excision is very important to the child's recovery. Such treatment reduces pain, fluid loss, and infection and provides the best environment for wound healing.

After surgery the child is placed in protective isolation. Round the clock primary nursing care is essential, with particular attention given to respiratory therapy, nutrition, the newly grafted area, and prevention of complications. The use of biological dressings in the treatment of deep dermal and full-thickness burns has revolutionized the treatment and rehabilitation of burn patients.

Topical medications

Systemic antibiotics cannot reach the damaged area because of thrombosed or burned vessels; thus topical

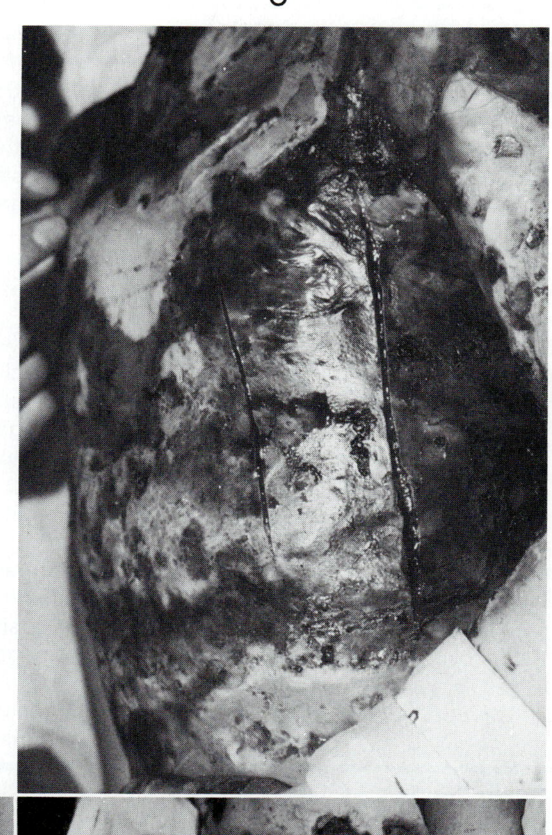

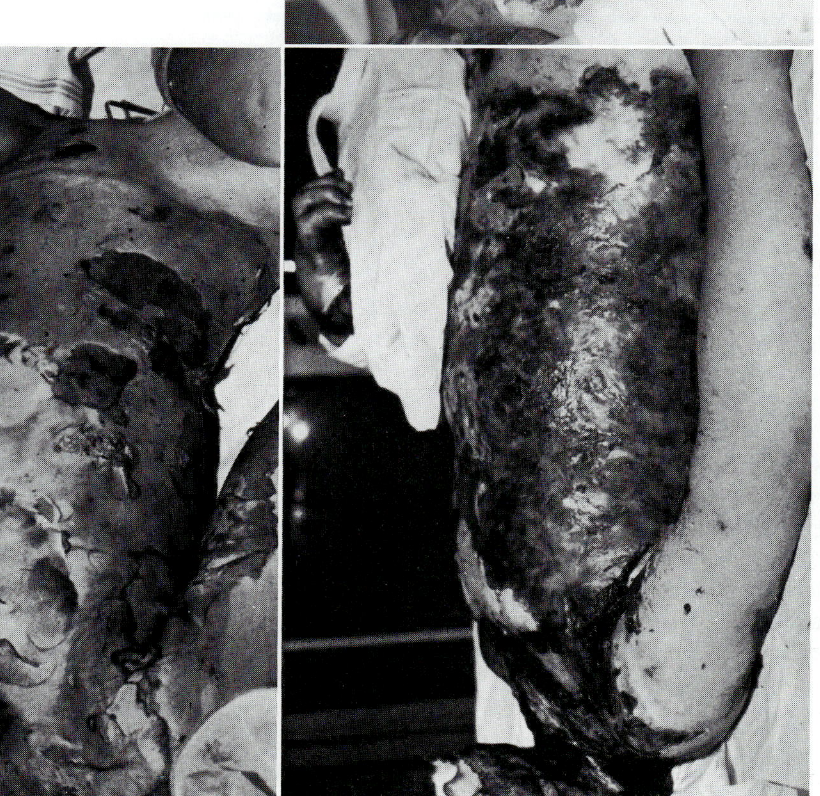

Fig. 30-8 **A,** This 6-year-old child has just been admitted to emergency room because of second- and third-degree burns. She is receiving oxygen by nasal cannula. **B,** Heavy eschar formed over trunk. **C,** Escharotomy incisions performed to permit deeper respirations. (Courtesy Matthew Gleason, San Diego, Calif.)

◆ TABLE 30-1
Comparison of Three Common Topical Antimicrobials

Agent	Cost	Advantages	Disadvantages
Mafenide cream 10% (Sulfamylon)	Least expensive	Penetrates eschar Easy application Effective against all gram-positive and gram-negative organisms	Tendency to cake; should be removed by tub bathing Burning pain on application May cause metabolical acidosis Requires a minimum of two applications daily Patient may develop sensitivity rash
Povidone-iodine (Betadine) ointment 10%; also available in foam preparation (Helafoam)	More expensive	Very wide spectrum Effective against gram-positive and gram-negative organisms, fungi, yeasts, protozoa, and viruses Sensitivity is infrequent	Ointment becomes liquid and runs off surface, staining linen Mild burning on application Foam dries out rapidly to a thick powder Inactivated by wound exudate
Silver sulfadiazine cream 1% (Silvadene)	Most expensive	Painless Effective against gram-positive and gram-negative organisms and *Candida albicans* Sensitivity is infrequent No discoloration	Poor penetration Supplemental systemic therapy usually needed

medication is an essential method of therapy. A thin layer of medication may be applied directly to the injured area with a sterile glove or tongue blade, or the medication may be embedded in sterile gauze strips that are positioned as needed. A spray form may also be available (Table 30-1).

Mortality caused by infection has declined as a result of the effectiveness of new and improved topical antimicrobial agents. The most desirable topical agent should be inexpensive, painless, nonallergenic, easy to apply, and effective against all microbial contaminants. It should also penetrate the wound without causing systemic effects or harm to viable tissue. Unfortunately, although several topical agents have led to excellent results, no single agent offers all these characteristics.

Mafenide hydrochloride (sulfamylon cream), povidone-iodine (Betadine) ointment, and silver sulfadiazine cream are useful for exposure treatment, combined with frequent hydrotherapy and reapplication of the agent.

Treatment goals

No matter which burn therapy methods are selected, all treatment is intended to accomplish the following goals:

1. Preserve life
2. Promote healing
3. Prevent infection
4. Control pain
5. Prevent deformity
6. Provide emotional and physical rehabilitation.

Maintaining good nutrition is essential for the survival and satisfactory healing of extensively burned children. An important aspect of the nurse's responsibility is the provision of optimal nutrition. Initially the child with extensive burns is maintained on tube feedings, followed by oral feedings with or without a nasogastric tube, depending on the child's progress. It is very important for the nurse to keep an accurate record of all nourishment and fluids taken. A detailed daily intake record must be kept for analysis by the dietitian for caloric and foodstuff (protein, fat, carbohydrate, vitamin, and mineral) content. Protein consumption is particularly important. Supplemental vitamins including C and E, iron, and zinc are ordered.

Frequent milk feedings and the prophylactic administration of antacids may prevent a Curling's ulcer, but the nurses should be alert for any signs of blood in the stool or nasogastric tube. The child's appetite should not be discouraged with servings that are too large. Feedings should be judiciously planned. The child

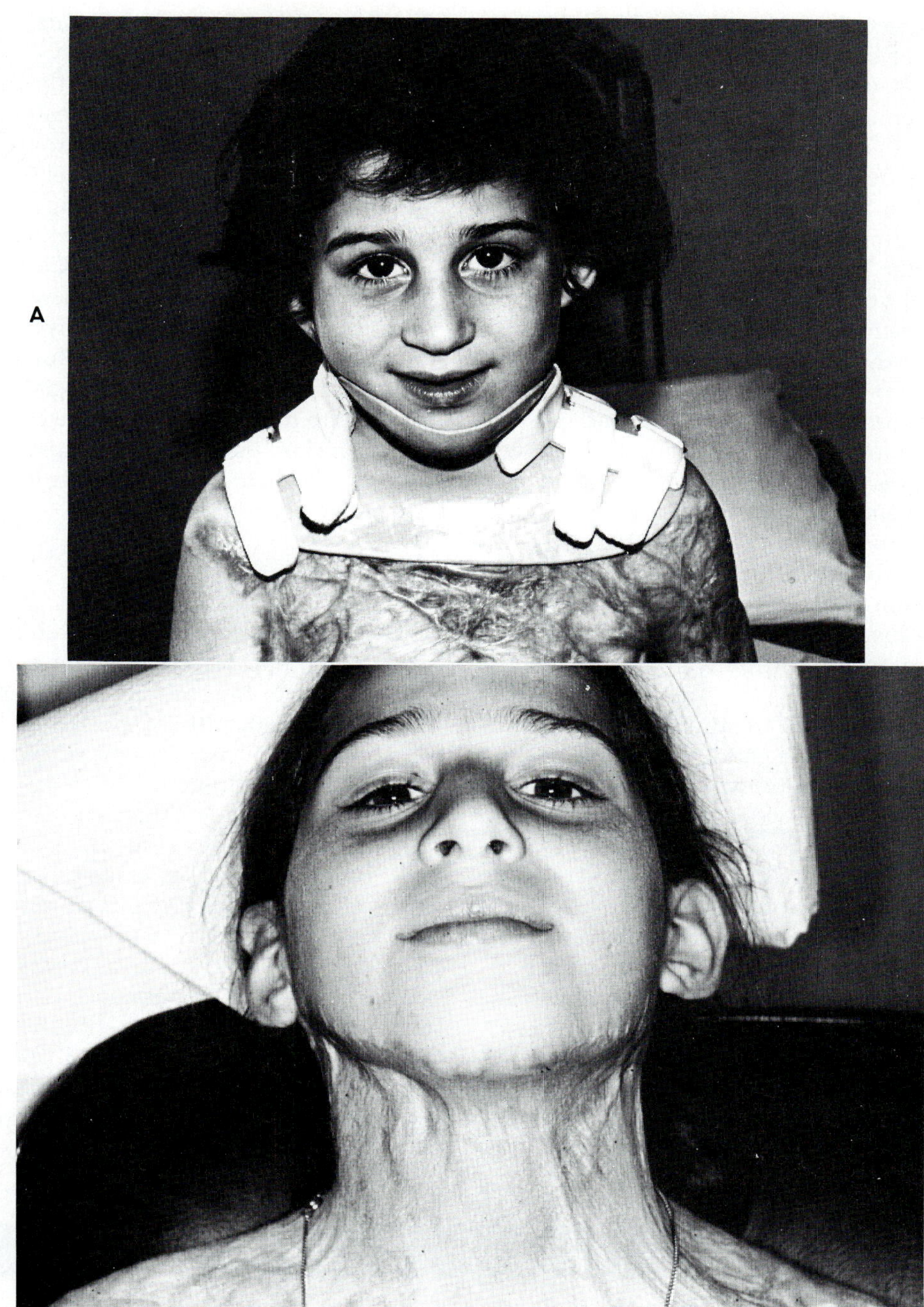

Fig. 30-9 **A,** Same patient as in Fig. 30-8; splint to prevent neck contractures. **B,** Same child 5 years later; Treatment included skin grafting and splinting. (Courtesy Matthew Gleason, San Diego, Calif.)

should not be expected to eat directly after an exhausting dressing change. A different schedule for the kitchen on some days or better planning of procedures on other days may be necessary, but children should receive their meals when they can *best* eat. Preferences should be noted. The foods selected should be high in calories and protein. Sometimes permission to bring food from home brings forth happy cooperation by both parents and children. Children must be weighed periodically to determine their nutritional status.

The immediate and long-term positioning of a seriously burned child is critical in preventing extensive deformity. Although the position of flexion may be the position of greatest comfort to the child, it also may become the cause of crippling contractures. The posture of extension is uncomfortable, but in the final analysis such placement of the head and extremities may save the burn victim weeks, if not months, of needless hospitalization and additional pain. Patient-controlled anesthesia is recommended for school-age and adolescent children during therapy. The pain scale discussed in Chapter 27 is helpful in determining the anesthesia needs of younger children.

The neck splint pictured in Fig. 30-9, *A* is made of a type of plastic, "Orthoplast" Isoprene, which, when molded and fitted to the individual child, has been successful in preventing deformities that had previously been difficult to prevent (Fig. 30-9, *B*). If active and passive exercises of the affected body parts are neglected convalescence may be retarded significantly. It is the responsibility of the nurse and the physical therapy staff to see that these important movements, which the child often resists, are carried out. Appropriate exercises plus good positioning to prevent flexion contractures can contribute greatly to early rehabilitation.

During the entire period of treatment and observation of the extensively burned child, the morale of the parents and their child is of tremendous importance. Often the parents feel guilty concerning their child's injury. They may be appalled at its condition and appearance. Some will be overly protective; others may hardly be able to make themselves approach the child. All will be extremely upset, whether they appear so or not. Children may feel extreme guilt if they consider themselves responsible for the injury. Children who have extensive burns characteristically regress in their behavior. Frequent and consistent parental visits are extremely important. Some children who have had a history of emotional disturbance before their accident develop extreme hostility toward their parents and others involved in their care.

Good communication among the health care providers, the family, and the child is essential. Parents need to be informed of the child's progress and helped in their efforts to cope with their feelings while providing support to the child. A feeling of acceptance and freedom to talk without being criticized are important for both the child and family. Clear, simple explanations of the plan of care are essential.

Play therapy, availability of toys and television, and an empathic approach to painful procedures are all helpful. Often additional specialized assistance is required to meet the needs of the child and family. The social worker, psychologist, or psychiatrist should be called on to help maintain a healthy support system whenever necessary.

Rehabilitation

The rehabilitation of a burned child may be long and exhausting, but despite the pain and fatigue, the end result is worth the continued effort. Fortunately, with the greater availability of specialized burn care units or centers and the use of new surgical techniques, the time needed for rehabilitation promises to be much shorter. Splinting, traction, and frequent visits to the physical therapy department's pool or exercise room may be necessary. Plastic surgery is needed in some cases to relieve contractures or remove keloid formation (exaggerated scar tissue). Special tutoring may be required to prevent educational delay, and social contacts must be maintained, particularly for older children. A positive, constructive attitude toward therapy should be encouraged. The care of children who have been seriously burned is among the nurse's most challenging and rewarding experiences.

KEY CONCEPTS

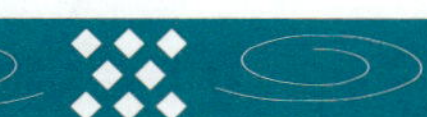

1 Skin color, hydration, surface irregularities, and disturbances in sensation may reveal significant information about a person's health habits and status.
2 The description of a skin lesion should include the following information: size, elevation, quality, color, distribution, associated sensory disturbances, and type of any existent drainage or exudate.
3 Common skin problems in infants and toddlers include miliaria rubra, intertrigo, seborrheic dermatitis, diaper rash, and infantile eczema.
4 Infantile eczema is considered to be essentially an allergic response. Care should include identifying the allergens, eliminating them from the infant's environment, treating secondary infections, preventing scratching and exposure to known infections, treating the lesions, and providing emotional and informational support to the child and parents.
5 Common skin problems in preschool- and young school-age children include impetigo, furuncles and carbuncles, sty, ringworm, pediculosis, and scabies.
6 Impetigo is a skin infection often associated with poor hygiene. Treatment includes careful cleans-

ing, removal of crusts, and application of Bactroban, a topical antibiotic ointment. Bactroban or systemic antibiotics are necessary for complete resolution.

7 Ringworm may be found in the scalp *(tinea capitas)*, skin *(tinea corporis)*, or feet *(tinea pedis)*.

8 Treatment of pediculosis (head lice) includes shampoos of pyrethrin, lindane or crotamitron and manual removal of devitalized nits with a fine-tooth comb.

9 Common skin problems in adolescents include acne vulgaris, herpes simplex type 1, and dermatitis venenata.

10 Acne first appears at puberty, is usually self-limiting, and subsides in 3 to 4 years. Treatment includes components of self-care, ensuring a well-balanced diet and adequate rest, thorough cleansing, application of medicated lotions, and antibiotic therapy.

11 Burns are classified into four categories, depending on the depth of penetration of the body's surface: first-degree, second-degree, third-degree, and fourth-degree. The area, extent, and depth of a burn determine its severity and treatment.

12 Initial burn therapy includes the following: maintenance of an airway, prevention of shock, replacement of fluids, insertion of a nasogastric tube, monitoring vital signs and laboratory values, pain control, and providing adequate nutrition.

13 Care of a burn wound includes cleansing, debridement, and application of dressings and topical medications. Treatment may also include skin grafts.

14 The goals of burn therapy are to preserve life, promote healing, prevent infection, prevent deformity, and provide informational and emotional support and physical rehabilitation.

15 Rehabilitation of a burned child may include splinting, traction, physical therapy, plastic surgery, and special tutoring.

CRITICAL THOUGHT QUESTIONS

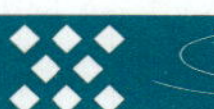

1 Which skin problems would you expect to see in infants and toddlers? Develop a chart that lists the problem, etiology, and nursing care. Which skin problems are seen most often in preschool- and early school-age children? Expand the chart as described above.

2 Why are preschool- and young school-age children at increased risk for skin diseases of a contagious nature? What are the implications for the nurse working in a school setting? How might preventive measures be initiated?

3 Why is a condition such as acne vulgaris a major problem and concern in adolescence? What nursing interventions help to promote self-care among adolescents?

4 Identify the major causes of burns in the various age groups. How can the nurse help in the prevention of burns? How are the extent and severity of burns measured?

5 How does medical and nursing treatment differ in relation to minor and major burns? What nursing measures, both physiological and psychosocial, are most significant in the treatment of burn victims?

REFERENCES

Adler R: Burns are different: the child psychiatrist on the pediatric burn ward, *J Burn Care Rehab* 13(1):28-32, 1992.

Atchison NE: Pain during burn dressing change in children: relationship to burn area, depth, and analgesia regimens, *Pain* 47:41-45, 1991.

Brimhall CL, Esterly NB: Uninvited guests: skin manifestations of childhood, *Contemp Pediatr* 7(1):18-57, 1990.

Dershewitz RA: *Ambulatory pediatric care,* ed 2, Philadelphia, 1993, JB Lippincott.

Honig PJ: The dermatology masquerade: don't be fooled twice, *Contemp Pediatr* 8(9):15-28, 1991.

Hunt TK: Basic principles of wound healing, *J Trauma* 30(12):S122-S128, 1990.

Krusinski P, Flowers F: *Handbook of pediatric dermatology,* St. Louis, 1990, Mosby.

Martinez S: Ambulatory management of burns in children, *J Pediatr Health Care* 6(1):32-37, 1992.

Philips T, Dover J: Recent advances in dermatology, *N Engl J Med,* 326(3):167-178, 1992.

Ratner MH: A short course in wound care for children, *Contemp Pediatr* 8(8):22-38, 1991.

Truhan AP: Sun protection in childhood, *Clin Pediatr,* 30(7):412-421, 1991.

Wong DL: Diapering choices: a critical review of the issues, *Pediatr Nurs* 18(1):41-54, 1992.

Wong D: *Essentials of pediatric nursing,* ed 4, St. Louis, 1993, Mosby.

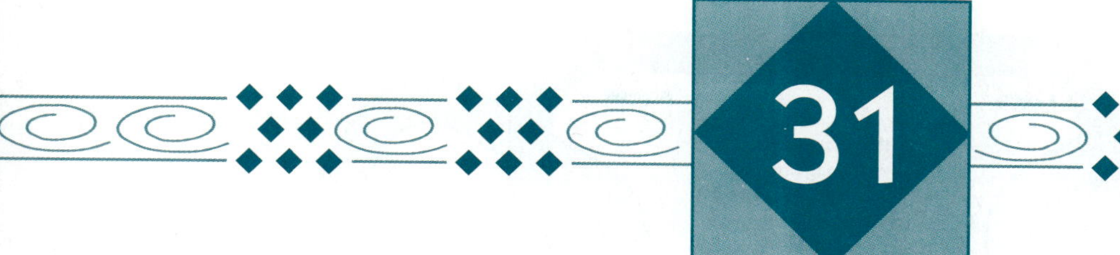

Infectious Disorders

CHAPTER OBJECTIVES

After studying this chapter, the student should be able to:

1 Define the key terms.
2 Describe the so-called chain of infection.
3 Explain how to break the chain of infection, listing six methods that could be used.
4 State how gowns, gloves, masks and eye protection can be used effectively as barriers during nursing care.
5 Contrast the three systems of isolation precautions recommended by the CDC: category-specific, disease-specific, or "design your own."
6 Describe the CDC's "universal precautions" to reduce the risks of transmission of bloodborne infectious agents.
7 Describe and demonstrate proper handwashing technique.
8 Discuss how the nurse can reduce the anxiety level of the isolated child and family.
9 Using the headings provided in Table 31-1, describe the following contagious childhood diseases: chickenpox (varicella); 2-week measles (rubeola); German measles (rubella); infectious parotitis (mumps), and whooping cough (pertussis).
10 Indicate three infectious agents mentioned in Table 31-1 for which, as of yet, there is no active immunization.
11 Discuss the transmission of and detection guidelines for mycobacterium tuberculosis.

Infection precautions in the hospital are necessary for the safety of patients, visitors, students, and staff. The rationale for using certain barriers or techniques should be based on knowledge of how a contagious disease is transmitted—the chain of infection (Fig. 31-1). If the chain is broken, no new incidence of disease develops as a result of an infectious person's presence. Breaking the chain of infection is a critical responsibility for all health care providers.

It is also important that barrier techniques be as physically and psychosocially nontraumatizing as possible for all concerned. The ill pediatric patient is undergoing considerable stress. The burden of hospitalization and isolation techniques is particularly heavy for small children and their families.

With greater knowledge of the transmission modes of most infectious diseases and of methods for stopping contagion, many old concepts involving communicable disease control are changing. As this knowledge influences the activities and attitudes of health care personnel, it benefits the nursing care of all patients. Hospital policies and procedures related to infection prevention and control are under continual scrutiny. Recommendations from the Centers for Disease Control and Prevention (CDC) affect ongoing change.

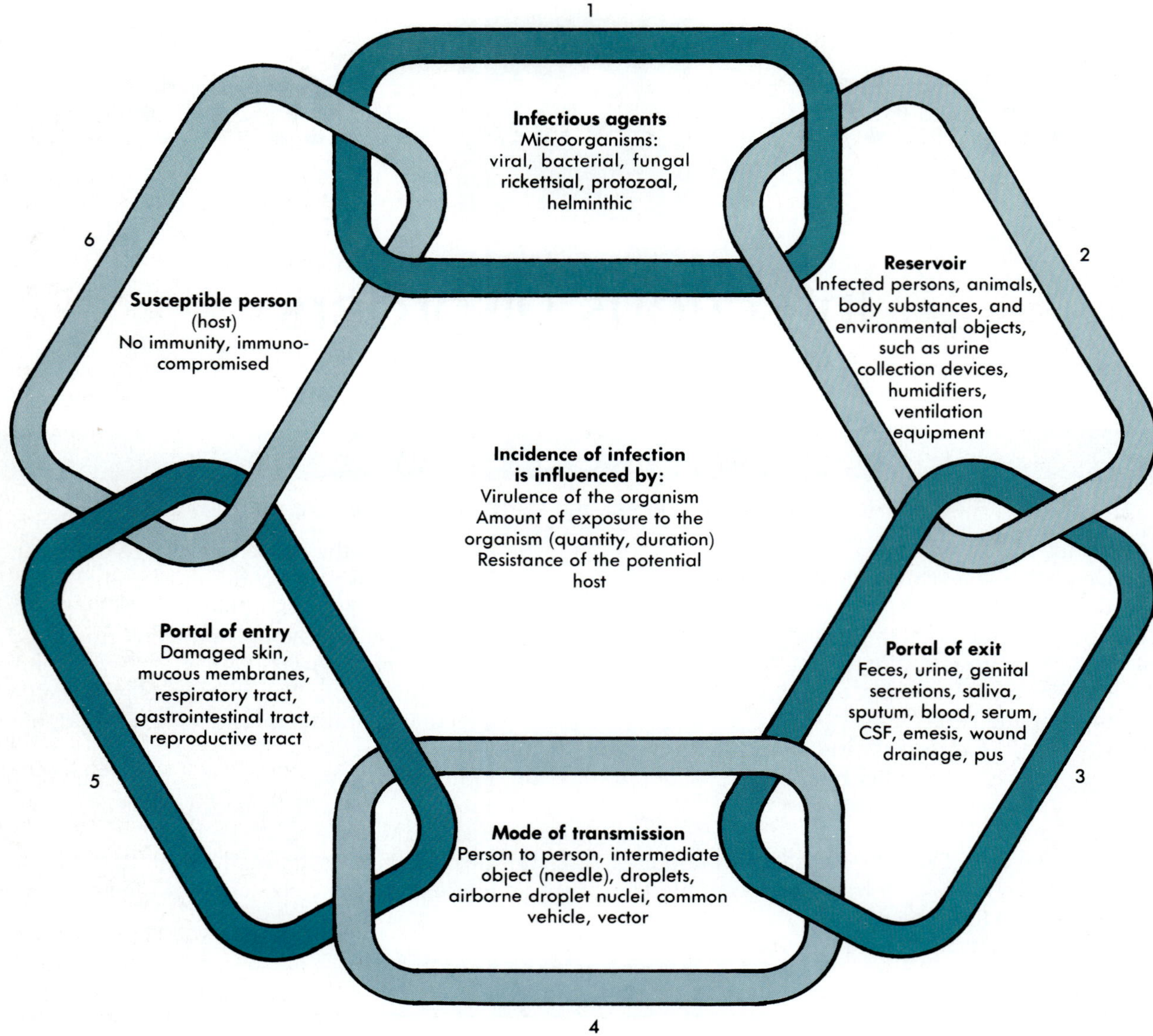

Fig. 31-1 The Chain of Infection.

In many ways the newer recommended CDC Guidelines for bloodborne pathogens and tuberculosis are less rigid and less ritualistic, encouraging nurses and other health care providers to use independent judgment. In fact, the CDC is currently revising all of the Guidelines for Isolation Precautions to reflect current knowledge and practice and to incorporate changes made during the past decade. New guidelines will be published in 1995.

The facility's infection control practitioner will have access to the latest information and can be a valuable resource. Change simply for its own sake should not be endorsed. For example, the issue of what type of mask should be used depends on what is the purpose of the mask. It would be unwise to fail to change when sound study and research indicate that certain patterns of care are unsafe, are wasteful of financial resources or personal energies, or cause needless patient distress.

In this regard the expanded role of the infection control practitioner (ICP) in the hospital setting is important. This professional, usually a nurse with specialized training and certification, collects and analyzes data about infection in both patients and health care providers. The ICP uses this information to influence change in patient care practices associated with infection risk. The ICP initiates review and evaluation of appropriate interventions to reduce infection risk, using both facility-specific data and appropriate research data. The ICP helps interpret and prepare protocols for hospital procedures, including infection precautions, and provides valuable consultation and educational resources for the entire multidisciplinary health care team.

KEY VOCABULARY

During clinical assignments the student encounters certain terminology associated with infection risk or isolation precautions that need to be reviewed. The following key terms are designed to help in that review.

body substances A general term used to describe body products that are characteristically moist and that support the growth of organisms. Examples are feces, urine, emesis, wound drainage, pus, saliva, sputum, genital secretions, blood, serum, and cerebral spinal fluid.

carrier A person or animal capable of transmitting a disease without having any signs or symptoms of the disease.

colonization The presence and multiplication of organisms in body substances or on the body that do not cause tissue invasion or damage.

contagious (communicable or transmissible) disease Illness caused by living microorganisms or their toxins, which may be transmitted to susceptible persons by contact with persons carrying the organisms, their infected body substances, or other reservoirs. Transmission may occur by direct, indirect, or droplet contact or by airborne route. (See box on p. 620.)

contamination The presence of disease-producing agents on a person or in or on inanimate objects (e.g., clothing, water, food, or medical supplies).

epidemiology The study of the occurrence, distribution, and causes of disease and other conditions.

hyperimmune globulin Human immune globulin that contains a high titer of antibodies designed to prevent or lessen the impact of specific contagious disease (e.g., rubeola or hepatitus B).

immunity The ability to protect oneself against development of a contagious disease by the action of antibodies. Immunity may be active or passive. (See box on p. 620.)

incubation period Time that must elapse between the infection of a person at a time of exposure and the appearance of signs or symptoms of the disease. The incubation period of most infectious diseases have two phases: (1) the period between initial contact with an infectious agent and communicability of the agent to others and (2) the period of communicability before the appearance of clinical signs and symptoms in the infected person. This second phase is often called the *prodrome* of the infection, and during this phase the patient is usually most infectious to others. This phenomenon explains why childhood diseases such as varicella (chickenpox) spread so efficiently—the infected person passes the infection to others during his prodromal period. By the time the child becomes ill, others are already infected.

infection The presence and multiplication of microorganisms in the body that cause tissue invasion and damage. Mild or low-grade infections are not always recognized. Any microorganism has the potential for producing disease, but many are prevented from causing illness by the person's own body defenses: the health condition of the body tissues may stop the entry or significant multiplication of an organism, or the activity of the immune system may form protective antibodies.

infectious disease A clinically manifest disease of human or animal resulting from an infection. Those illnesses caused by microorganisms.

isolation precautions Observance of barrier techniques that are designed to interrupt transmission of infectious agents from a reservoir (usually an infected patient) to a susceptible host (either the caregiver or another patient). Which barriers are employed depends on the portal of exit, modes of transmission, and portal of entry characteristic of the infection. Thorough handwashing is always used. Gloves, gowns, masks, goggles, or special room assignments may also be used.

nosocomial infection (NI) An infection associated with hospitalization. Over half of these infections are not considered to be preventable because of the poor condition of the patient's body defenses. As a result, usually benign microorganisms normally present in a patient's body may become pathogenic. Potentially preventable NIs are usually associated with invasive devices or procedures, many of which are performed by nurses, for example, intravenous placement and maintenance, urinary catheterization, and wound care.

portal of entry The way in which microorganisms gain entrance into a person's body, for example, broken skin or mucous membranes in the nose, mouth, and urethra.

portal of exit The way in which microorganisms leave the body, for example, feces, emesis, urine, semen, water, and blood.

reservoir of infectious agents Place where microorganisms live and multiply, for example, in people, animals, plants, and soils.

toxoid A preparation containing a toxin or poison produced by a pathogenic organism capable of providing active immunity against a disease but too weak to cause the disease itself.

vaccine A preparation containing killed or weakened (attenuated) living organisms that, when introduced into the body, causes the formation of antibodies against that type of organism.

ISOLATION PRECAUTIONS: HISTORICAL BACKGROUND

In 1983 the Centers for Disease Control (CDC) published *Guideline for Isolation Precautions in Hospitals.* Additional recommendations for the prevention of transmission of bloodborne diseases were issued in 1987 and 1988 and recommendations for preventing

METHODS OF TRANSMISSION

I. Contact transmission
   A. Direct (person to person)
   B. Indirect (requires intermediate object, such as hands of nurse or needle, as in needlestick injuries)
   C. Droplet (droplets usually do not travel more than 3 feet; droplets rapidly settle on horizontal surfaces)
II. Airborne transmission (from residue of evaporated droplets [droplet nuclei] that can remain suspended in air for long periods or from dust particles in the air that contain infectious agents; pulmonary tuberculosis is a major disease transmitted by droplet nuclei)
III. Common vehicle transmission (such as food poisoning of many people who consumed the same batch of contaminated potato salad at a picnic)
IV. Vector-borne transmission (such as mosquito-transmitted malaria)

ACTIVE AND PASSIVE IMMUNITY

I. Active immunity is relatively long-lasting but takes longer to achieve than does passive immunity. It is attained when a person's own body produces protective antibodies in response to an infective organism, its toxin, or its vaccine. This occurs under the following conditions:
   A. By having had the disease
   B. By receiving specially prepared materials (toxins or vaccines) that stimulate the immune system to produce antibodies (in these instances, the body *actively* protects itself)
II. Passive immunity is comparatively short-lived but may be achieved relatively quickly. It is attained under the following conditions:
   A. By receiving a prepared injection of antibodies (antitoxin), which are manufactured in the body of another person or, rarely, by an animal
   B. By an unborn baby receiving antibodies from his mother across the placenta
   C. By a breastfeeding baby receiving antibodies from his mother's breast milk (in these instances, the body *passively* receives the protection)

transmission of tuberculosis were updated in 1990. In the earlier guidelines the CDC offered the possibility of choosing one of three alternative isolation systems. The first is based on a modification of the previously used *category-specific isolation precautions,* which are primarily influenced by the mode and ease of transmission of an illness. The second is a system that describes *disease-specific isolation precautions.* Institutions were invited to study and select one of the two systems described or choose the third alternative by designing their own system for consistent use within their own setting.

The isolation system based on categorization of diseases is more likely to overisolate and to use supplies unnecessarily. However, it is thought to be easier to administer and to teach personnel. The disease-specific system requires more understanding of each illness and requires increased independent decision-making. It also allows more individualized care and conserves resources by using fewer supplies.

The possibilities presented by the third alternative have stimulated a thoughtful, fundamental critique of the problems associated with diagnosis-driven isolation practices as described in the first two systems and an emphasis on the danger of unidentified, undiagnosed infectious contacts. Indeed, it is the unknown contagious person who is potentially the most dangerous to his caregivers and other patients.†

Category-specific Isolation Precautions (system A)

A category included in former CDC recommendations and conspicuous by its absence in the 1983 guidelines is that of protective or reverse isolation. The absence of this category does not mean that hospitals should never employ special protective techniques, particularly for the care of patients who, for a predictable, temporary period, are very vulnerable to infection (for example, those receiving total body irradiation some types of bone marrow transplants or those with severe burns or dermatitis). However, it has been recognized that protective isolation, as it was previously outlined and practiced, may fail to reduce the risk of infections. Many persons at risk (immunocompromised patients) are infected by their own (endogenous) microorganisms or flora, or they are colonized or infected by microorganisms transmitted by the inadequately washed hands of personnel or nonsterile items used routinely within the former protective isolation protocol. Gowns, gloves, and masks are usually not the most effective protective devices for this patient's safety. Private rooms, conscientious handwashing, and careful instruction of all personnel and visitors seem to be more appropriate, except in special periods of high risk for specific patients where additional measures such as special ventilation may be indicated.

Disease-specific Isolation Precautions (system B)

The disease-specific isolation precautions are based on the mode of transmission of the individual disease. The CDC guidelines indicate suggested precautions, which material is considered infective, and how long isolation precautions are appropriate. A black-and-white instruction card should be completed (front and back) and displayed near the patient, indicating what precautions should be observed (Fig. 31-2).

Universal precautions

In 1987, Category VII in system A, entitled Blood/Body Fluid Precautions, was extended to include *all* patients (not merely those diagnosed or suspected of having bloodborne disease). This extension was primarily developed to reduce the risks of transmission of the HIV virus, which causes AIDS, and the hepatitis B virus (HBV); however it would reduce the spread of all bloodborne disease. The term *universal precautions,* as employed by the CDC, refers to the application of certain limited precautions to all caregiver/patient contacts within the health care setting.

"Universal precautions" may require the use of barrier equipment, such as gloves, plastic aprons, gowns, eyeglasses, goggles, face shields, masks, and leak-resistant bags. Such precautions also mandate careful handwashing and thoughtful patient room assignment. They are always to be implemented when there is a risk of contact with blood, specific body tissues, or fluids or other body products containing visible blood.

Application of these precautions has significantly changed methods of performance. For example, maternity nurses wear eye protection and glasses to protect themselves from splashing blood-contaminated fluid during patient care at the time of labor and delivery. Some also wear plastic aprons or gowns. Gloves are worn by those caring for the newborn after birth. The principle behind universal precautions is the realization that all blood is potentially infectious and that the caregiver cannot know whose blood is or is not infected (Jackson, 1990).

The universal precautions principle has been more broadly applied to all body fluids, excretions, and secretions in the "body substance isolation" (BSI) system, an alternative to the category-specific and disease-specific systems for isolation precautions. The

(Front of Card)

Visitors—Report to Nurses' Station Before Entering Room

1. **Private room indicated?** ________ No
   ________ Yes
2. **Masks indicated?** ________ No
   ________ Yes for those close to patient
   ________ Yes for all persons entering room
3. **Gowns indicated?** ________ No
   ________ Yes if soiling is likely
   ________ Yes for all persons entering room
4. **Gloves indicated?** ________ No
   ________ Yes for touching infective material
   ________ Yes for all persons entering room
5. Special precautions indicated for handling blood? ________ No
   ________ Yes
6. **Hands must be washed after touching the patient or potentially contaminated articles and before taking care of another patient.**
7. Articles contaminated with ________________________ should be
   infective material(s)
   discarded or bagged and labeled before being sent for decontamination and reprocessing.

(Back of Card)

Instructions

1. On Table B, Disease-Specific Precautions, locate the disease for which isolation precautions are indicated.
2. Write disease in blank space here: ________________________
3. Determine if a private room is indicated. In general, patients infected with the same organism may share a room. For some diseases or conditions, a private room is indicated if patient hygiene is poor. A patient with poor hygiene does not wash hands after touching infective material (feces, purulent drainage, or secretions), contaminates the environment with infective material, or shares contaminated articles with other patients.
4. Place a check mark beside the indicated precautions on front of card.
5. Cross through precautions that are *not* indicated.
6. Write infective material in blank space in item 7 on front of card.

Fig. 31-2 Instruction Card.

BSI system is conceptually simple because the nurse plans the use of barriers based on the interaction with *every patient's body substances* rather than on the patient's diagnosis. The BSI perspective stresses the critical nature of handwashing and involves increased use of gloves in patient care. It minimizes the possibility of disease transmission from dry surfaces while emphasizing the precautions needed in caring for body substances that are moist or wet. BSI has been evaluated clinically (Lynch, 1990; Jackson, 1989).

BARRIER PROCEDURES AND CONCEPTS

Isolation procedures may differ in various settings; the hospital infection prevention manual and patient care nursing manual (PCN) should be consulted. Before specific barrier techniques are described, one should also consider the concepts discussed here.

Essential Characteristics of the Caregiver

The nurse working with any patient should be:

A. Free from communicable infections (of importance when caring for *any* patient).
B. Knowledgeable regarding possible special need to reevaluate assignment.
   1. Pregnancy—fetus especially vulnerable in early trimester to teratogens: rubella, cytomegalovirus (CMV), and others
   2. Open wounds—may become infected
   3. Increased susceptibility
      a. Type of medications taken
      b. No record of varicella (chickenpox) infection. Many hospitals now require a varicella titer (blood test) to determine if the individual has developed antibody to the disease.
      c. Appropriate immunization not current
C. Cognizant of the need to maintain good general health. Essential health habits include:
   1. Proper nutrition
   2. Adequate rest
   3. Good personal hygiene
   4. Use of stress reduction techniques
D. Knowledgeable and dependable regarding infection precautions needed.

Routine handwashing

The most important procedure for preventing the transmission of infectious agents is appropriate handwashing. Handwashing has been defined as a vigorous, systematic, brief rubbing together of *all* surfaces of lathered hands, followed by rinsing under a stream of water. When washing, the hands should be kept lower than the elbows so that contaminated water does not soil the arms. Faucets are closed with a paper towel after handwashing is completed. The ideal duration of handwashing is not specific, but for most activities (excluding special, longer presurgical, predelivery, or nursery hand scrubs), a vigorous wash of about 10 seconds is needed. If hands are visibly soiled, more time is required. Many transient microbes representing recent contaminants and about 80% of resident microbes are effectively removed with plain soaps or detergents and running water. Resident microorganisms in the deep skin layers usually can be killed or inhibited by handwashing with products containing antimicrobial agents. Transient microorganisms, especially in hospital settings, may be pathogenic and cause nosocomial infections. Resident flora are more likely to cause infections when a patient is severely immunocompromised.

The fingernails of all health care personnel should be short and clean because body secretions and stool may collect under nails and be difficult to remove. The indications for handwashing depend on the type, intensity, duration, sequence, and area of activity. Except for emergencies, hands should always be washed in the following situations:

Before:

A. Initiating individual patient nursing care
B. Performing any sterile or invasive procedures or touching a wound
C. Pouring medications or touching food

After:

A. Completing individual patient nursing care
B. Touching wounds, mucous membranes, or body substances
C. Using the bathroom
D. Touching inanimate objects that are likely to be contaminated, such as used urine-measuring devices and catheters
E. Removing sterile or clean gloves

   If health care personnel question if their hands need to be washed, they need to be washed.

Gloves

Disposable, single-use gloves, clean or sterile, depending on the patient's needs, are recommended to protect patients from microorganisms from personnel and to protect personnel from patient's microorganisms. Unless a careful "no touch" technique is employed, gloves are recommended when contact with body substances (excretions, secretions, blood, and body fluids) is possible.

Isolation gowns

The use of isolation gowns formerly was combined with considerably detailed protocol. This is chiefly because the definition of contamination often was "touching anything in the room of a patient with a contagious disease" and because of the now obsolete practice of reusing gowns for the same patient unless they became visibly soiled or damp. Currently, gowns are less frequently used and seldom reused. Gowns or aprons are used primarily to protect against splashing body fluids. They are stored in a clean area and put on with clean hands. After use, gowns are carefully removed. If they are intended to be laundered and used again, they are placed in a laundry bag. If they are made of paper or other disposable material, they are discarded in the trash. The nurse should practice thorough handwashing after gown disposal.

Masks

There is no proof that even high-efficiency disposable masks protect the caregiver from airborne droplet nuclei as air travels the path of least resistance and may get behind a mask through gaps between the face and the mask at the sides. However, masks, like gowns, may help prevent splashes from reaching skin, mouth, or nose. A mask also may be of some value in preventing disease because it keeps the wearer from touching his own nose or mouth. Masks should be replaced when moist and never reused. It is important to use masks in combination with eye protection. Special masks are also available that reduce the risk to the caregiver of inhaling droplet nuclei from the air if the patient is diagnosed or suspected of having pulmonary or laryngeal tuberculosis.

Eye protection

Protective eyewear (glasses, face shields, and goggles) should reduce the risk of contamination of the mucous membranes of the eyes. However, sometimes they are a nuisance and may fog over, impairing vision.

Needle safety

Needles and sharps (knife blades, razors) should be deposited immediately after use in rigid puncture-resistant receptacles. Syringe needles should not be separated from disposable syringes nor should they be recapped, unless a proper receptacle is not readily available. In that case a one-handed recapping technique may be used by placing the correctly sized cap on a flat surface and with one hand sliding the needle into it. The other hand should be kept behind the back. The cap should not be placed over the needle with the free hand. The cap should be secured by covering the needle by using pressure on both sides.

Bagging of articles

Articles that are possibly contaminated should be enclosed in sturdy bags impervious to moisture. If there is a possibility that the outer surface of the bag is also contaminated the CDC recommends double-bagging. Most trash from a hospital room may be single-bagged for routine disposal. However, there are many different kinds of trash. It is important to consult the hospital regulations regarding disposal of different types of waste.

Food service

The use of paper plates for certain isolation patients is thought to be unnecessary. Emphasis should be placed on patient handwashing before eating and after use of the bedpan or toilet.

Discharge housekeeping

Methods of cleaning a patient's room should be standardized and the same methods used for all hospital rooms. The use of fogging devices is not recommended.

ADMISSION OF A PEDIATRIC PATIENT NEEDING ISOLATION PRECAUTIONS

Parental Needs and Fears

Almost without exception, admission to the hospital is a stressful period for parents and child. The anxiety and feeling of helplessness often experienced by parents are increased considerably when the admission necessitates the use of certain barrier techniques and entry into a special room labeled "Isolation." The sight of health care providers wearing gowns or gloves and perhaps masks and the sound of alarming terms such as *contaminated* and *contagious* do not reassure parents. Many parents worry, "If Johnny has to be here, he must be terribly ill. I wonder what the other children here have. Couldn't Johnny catch something else from them?" Parents need emotional and informational support and instruction at such a time. The assistance of the infection control practitioner is especially useful. Fortunately, isolation in a single room, complete with a nurse in gown and mask is not encountered often in pediatrics today. For example, if strict isolation is needed, it is typically limited to the first 24- to 48-hour period until antibiotics are able to render the patient noncontagious.

Unit Preparation

Sometimes the admission of a new patient is anticipated, and an individual isolation unit can be set up before the child's arrival. Pediatric patients are not usually placed together in a room unless it is confirmed that their diagnoses are the same and the attending physicians grant permission. However, patients with diarrheal diseases or respiratory infections that appear to be caused by the same organism may sometimes share a room, having the same type of isolation while maintaining separate bed units. The room should be comfortably warm and well-ventilated. In addition to a correctly sized bed or crib, a bedside stand, and the overbed table found in all standard patient units, the room should include the following:

1. Access to a sink, running water, and toilet
2. A box of gloves
3. A "hand-washing agent" in a dispenser that works for hand and arm care of personnel
4. Paper towels in a dispenser
5. Laundry hamper support and laundry bags
6. Plastic bags for collection of trash for discard
7. Other barriers, such as gowns, masks and eye protection, if care activities warrant their use; some facilities put these items in a cart outside the door of the patient's room
8. All other articles needed for admission and daily care

Routine stocking of supplies is essential because much time is wasted if the nurse must leave the patient to obtain equipment.

Admission modifications

Currently, in-room visitation by family members of isolated patients is much more liberal than in the past. Just who is allowed to enter depends on the type of infection and the visitor and patient being considered.

At admission, the child's clothes are usually placed in a clean bag and returned to the parents. Parents often ask, "What do we do with Johnny's clothes when we get them home?" and "What about all the things that Johnny used at home while he was sick?" Usually it is sufficient to suggest that the parents wash the child's clothes, using a hot water setting on an automatic washer and regular laundry detergent, and dry them in a dryer.

Parents should be encouraged and welcomed at the bedside. They should be shown where the supply of clean gowns is kept and taught to remove the gowns and place them in the laundry hamper and to wash their hands just before leaving.

Urine and stool specimens are collected in the usual way, and the outside of the container used to send them to the laboratory should be clean. Containers may be placed in plastic bags.

Psychosocial Implications

Much has been written about the impact of hospitalization on the child and his family. (See Chapter 24.) Less has been published regarding the additional stress experienced from various isolation precautions. One study examined school-aged children's perceptions of isolation.

The first research question sought to discover whether the children understood the reasons for their hospitalizations. The 9 year olds correctly expressed the reason for isolation, but the 6- and 7-year-old children did not. One of these children poignantly stated, "Because I was bad and got sick, I was supposed to stay in my room." Clearly, when possible, there needs to be exploration of the child's concept of the reason for his isolation and some of the procedures it involves. If children understand that punishment is not a part of the reason for isolation, more of their energy can be directed toward becoming well more quickly.

If the nurse must wear a mask, letting the child visualize the face before coming into the room may dispel some fears. A nurse's isolation regalia may be frightening. One of the children in the study explained that the nurse's gown was used "so she can operate on you." A number of children probably received the impression that the presence of people in gowns indicated impending unpleasant procedures because their nurses, trying to economize on time, always included a procedure when they came to see their patients. Perhaps nurses should consider the many different kinds of treatments that help children get better—playing games, talking, cuddling, and making friends or family members welcome in the hospital setting.

SIGNIFICANT COMMUNICABLE DISEASES OF CHILDHOOD AND THEIR NURSING CARE

Descriptions of some of the communicable diseases seen or mentioned most often in pediatrics are included in Table 31-1. Also summarized are nursing points to remember in each case. Fortunately, not all the diseases described are encountered by nurses today. However, all those described pose a potential threat to communities (Figs. 31-3 to 31-5). Diseases such as diphtheria, typhoid, and polio, for which prevention exists, could again ravage the population if public health standards decline and public education and support for immunization programs are not constantly maintained.

◆ TABLE 31-1
Communicable Childhood Diseases

Disease	Infectious Agent and General Description	Importance	Mode of Transmission	Communicable Period
Acquired immunodeficiency syndrome (AIDS) and human immunodeficiency virus (HIV) infections (Figs. 31-3 to 31-5)	Human immunodeficiency virus (HIV-1)—a human retrovirus. Diagnosis of AIDS is based on clinical, immunological serological, and virological findings and exclusion of primary or secondary immunodeficiency states	Relentlessly progressive, devastating disorder of extraordinary morbidity and mortality	Blood and certain other body fluids are epidemiologically associated with transmission; urine, feces, saliva (unless visibly bloody), and vomitus are not associated with transmission of HIV. At risk persons include men who have sex with men, intravenous drug users, infants born to infected mothers, sexual partners of persons with AIDS or HIV infection. Health care workers are at risk from percutaneous injuries (e.g., needlesticks) and blood splashes to mucous membranes and nonintact skin.	Potentially infectious for indeterminant period before symptoms and during duration of disease

Special precautions are sometimes necessary in a hospital setting to prevent the transmission of certain infections. A resource for current information is the facilities' infection control practitioner.
*Centers for Disease Control: Recommendations for prevention of HIV transmission in health care settings, MMWR 36(25); 1, 1987; Centers for Disease Control: Update: Universal Precautions for the prevention of transmission of HIV, HBV and other blood born pathogens in health care settings, MMWR 37(24):377,1988.
†New Universal Precautions.
‡Centers of Disease Control: Protection against viral hepatitis, MMWR 39(RR2):1, 1990.
Centers for Disease Control: Initial therapy for tuberculosis in the era of multidrug resistance, MMWR 42(RR-7):3, 1993.
§American Academy of Pediatrics: Report of the Committee on Infectious Diseases. In the Red Book, ed 22, Elk Grove Village, Ill, 1994.

Incubation Period	Symptoms	Treatment and Nursing Care	Prevention
Interval between exposure and infection is short and measurable with the HIV-antibody test within 3 to 6 months after exposure; interval between infection and illness is highly variable and can be up to several years. Infants born to infected mothers will have maternal antibody measureable for up to 15 months; some infants with true HIV infection will show signs and symptoms within a short time after birth; others will have no signs or symptoms for several years; HIV-antibody testing of children born to infected mothers should be repeated periodically to determine whether or not the infant is truly infected.	Opportunistic infections or unusual forms of malignancy Early signs and symptoms; recurrent otitis media, sinusitis or pneumonia, failure to thrive, persistent thrush, fever of unknown origin, chronic unexplained diarrhea, hepatomegaly, generalized lymphadenopathy, and developmental delay	Antiretroviral therapy is available to treat cell-mediated immunodeficiency that results in infections with opportunistic agents Antimicrobial, antitumor therapy and nutritional support have prolonged lives	Exclusion of blood donors with a positive antibody test for HIV Transfusions and plasma infusions should be avoided whenever possible. The use of clotting factor concentrate should be restricted to hemophiliacs with essential clinical indications Deglycerolized RBCs for other blood product recipients. Use of autogenous transfusions. Abstaining from high-risk sexual practices and from intravenous drug use

Continued.

◆ **TABLE 31-1**
Communicable Childhood Diseases—cont'd.

Disease	Infectious Agent and General Description	Importance	Mode of Transmission	Communicable Period
Bacillary dysentery (shigellosis)	*Shigella sonnei* (most common), *S. flexneri*, and *S. dysenteriae* Acute inflammation of colon	Extremely widespread in areas with poor sanitary facilities and hygiene practices Disease often severe in infancy but mild after 3 years of age	Direct or indirect contact with feces of infected patients or carriers Contaminated food, water, and flies play important role	As long as patients or carriers harbor organisms (until three consecutive stool or rectal swab cultures are negative) Healthy carriers uncommon
Chickenpox; see varicella Chlaymdia infection, see p. 250 Cytomegalovirus (CMV) infection, see p. 97				
Diphtheria	*Corynebacterium diphtheriae* (Klebs-Löffler bacillus) Severe, acute infectious disease of upper respiratory tract and perhaps skin Toxins produced may affect nervous system and heart	Rarely seen because of routine childhood immunization, more comprehensive public health regulations, and enforcement of milk standards and carrier control 5% to 10% mortality Serious complications include neuritis, paralysis, and myocarditis	Direct or indirect contact with secretions from respiratory tract or skin lesions of patient	Variable: 2 to 4 weeks in untreated persons, or 1 to 2 days after antibiotic therapy initiated Isolation until two negative cultures 24 hours apart, from both nose and throat or skin lesions, obtained after end of antimicrobial therapy; contacts may be isolated
German measles (rubella, 3-day measles)	Rubella virus Acute infectious disease characterized chiefly by rose-colored macular rash and lymph node enlargement	Very common, frequently occurring in epidemic form Complications rare for victim but may cause deformities of fetus if contracted by pregnant woman during first trimester—nonimmune persons should avoid persons known to have this disease	Usually direct contact with secretions from mouth and nose May be acquired in utero	From 1 week before rash appears until approximately 7 days after its onset For discussion of congenital rubella syndrome see p. 97; affected infants may be infectious up to 1 year of age unless nose, pharynx, and urine cultures are negative 3 months after birth

Incubation Period	Symptoms	Treatment and Nursing Care	Prevention
1 to 7 days (usually 2 to 4 days)	Mild to severe diarrhea; in severe cases blood, mucus, and dehydration Abdominal pain, fever, and prostration may be present	Treatment depends on severity of infection Trimethoprim, sulfamethoxazole (Septra) drug of choice Keep patient warm; oral fluids may be restricted; intravenous therapy may be necessary to prevent dehydration	Attack appears to confer limited immunity No preventive known other than improved individual and community hygiene
2 to 5 days (occasionally longer)	Depends on type and part of upper respiratory area inflamed Formation of fibrinous false membrane, which may or may not be visible in throat or nose Nausea, possible muscle paralysis, and heart complications	Administration of antitoxin, analgesics, erythromycin, or penicillin Prednisone lessens incidence of myocarditis in severe disease Absolute bed rest; gentle throat irrigations; bland, soft diet; humidification Possible need for tracheostomy Watch for muscle weakness	Immunity after one attack, but person may be immune without history of disease Immunity determined by Schick test Routine primary schedule—Td (tetanus-diphtheria toxoids) booster injection recommended at 10-year intervals
14 to 21 days (usually 18 days)	Rose-colored macular rash occurring first on face, then on all body parts; enlargement and tenderness of lymph nodes; mild fever	Supportive nursing care with good personal hygiene	Rubella vaccine Immune after one attack

Continued.

◆ **TABLE 31-1**
Communicable Childhood Diseases—cont'd.

Disease	Infectious Agent and General Description	Importance	Mode of Transmission	Communicable Period
Gonorrhea (pp. 249-250)				
Hepatitis, viral; several types identified: Hepatitis A (HAV), hepatitis B (HBV) hepatitis C (HCV)	All types manifest similarities and differences; may vary with age and general condition of person infected	Hepatitis of all types represented third most commonly reported communicable disease in 1994		
(1) Type A (infectious) (HAV)	Hepatitis A virus (HAV): usually abrupt onset	HAV: Highest incidence in civilian populations in persons under 15 years, typically subclinical in children (very common in mentally retarded children)	Person-to-person; generally through fecal-oral route Transmission is facilitated by poor sanitation and close contact; ingestion of fecally contaminated food and water (e.g., shellfish, milk) Many outbreaks are traced to infected food handlers.	Uncertain; probably infectious 2 weeks before onset of jaundice; minimal risk of 1 week after onset of jaundice
(2) Type B (serum) (HBV)	Hepatitis B virus (HBV): characterized usually by insidious onset	HBV common in adolescents and young adults; more often complicated by relapse and prolonged liver dysfunction; long-term consequences (i.e., chronic liver disease and carcinoma of liver); typically more severe in infants and debilitated patients.	HBV reported more frequently; transmitted through sexual contact, also transmitted from infected mother to infant during perinatal period; contaminated blood products, occupational risks from needlesticks and other blood exposures	Infectious for indeterminate period before and 4 to 6 months after acute illness; persists for the lifetime of chronic carriers. Neonates acquire illness from infected mother and have high risk of developing chronic active hepatitis

Incubation Period	Symptoms	Treatment and Nursing Care	Prevention
	Jaundice for three types may be inapparent, fleeting, or persistent with or without itching	No specific therapy available; supportive care, rest, and high-calorie diet	
15 to 50 days; average 28 days	Fever, malaise, anorexia, nausea, enlarged liver, abdominal discomfort, dark urine, weight loss, jaundice Children usually have less-severe clinical manifestations, and illness may not be accompanied by jaundice	Supportive care	HAV attack confers immunity for HAV IG recommended for HAV contact; IG is protective if given before exposure or during incubation period; best if given within 72 hours after exposure IG for travelers into areas where HAV is common. Handwashing before food preparation, proper personal hygiene. IG immune globulin (formerly called "immune serum globulin," ISG, or "gammaglobulin")‡
45 to 180 days; average 60 to 90 days	Urticaria and arthralgia more characteristic of HBV Various combinations of anorexia, malaise, nausea, vomiting, abdominal pain, and jaundice Occasionally a rapid, severe (fulminating) type characterized by mental confusion, emotional instability, restlessness, coma, and internal bleeding; usually progresses to a fatal outcome within 10 days	Bed rest for symptomatic patients; well-balanced diet as desired; supplements of all vitamins, especially B complex Infants born to infected mothers should be given HBIG (within 12 hours of birth) and the first dose of hepatitis B vaccine as soon as possible (may be given at same time as HBIG, or within 7 days)	HBV attack confers immunity for HBV; Hepatitis B vaccine confers immunity after three doses; second injection 1 month after first, third 6 months after first‡; hepatitis B—immune globulin (HBIG) primarily for those exposed to HBV-contaminated blood (i.e., by needle stick); optimal effect if given within 48 hours after exposure HBV vaccine for all infants, health care workers and others at risk. Condom use. Effective screening of blood donors; absolute sterilization of equipment used for drawing blood, or use of disposable equipment

Continued.

◆ TABLE 31-1
Communicable Childhood Diseases—cont'd.

Disease	Infectious Agent and General Description	Importance	Mode of Transmission	Communicable Period
(3) Type C non-A, non-B viral hepatitis	Causative agent or agents have not been identified Clinical features resemble HBV, insidious onset	Acute hepatitis, neither HAV or HBV, affects all age groups; common among low socioeconomic groups, such as commercial blood donors; most common type of hepatitis associated with blood transfusion (70% to 80%)	Blood to blood contact*	Potentially infectious for indeterminate period before and after active symptoms; carrier state possible
Herpes simplex infections, see pp. 250-251				
Measles (rubeola, or 2-week or red measles)	Measles virus Acute infection characterized by moderately high temperature, inflammation of mucous membranes of respiratory tract, and macular rash	Very common, highly infectious disease frequently occurring in epidemic form Possible serious complications include pneumonia, otitis media, conjunctivitis, and encephalitis	Direct contact with secretions from nose and throat, airborne*	From time of "cold symptoms" (about 4 days before rash) until about 4 days after rash appears
Meningitis (*Haemophilus influenzae* and *Escherichia coli* see pp. 665-668)				
Meningococcal meningitis (cerebrospinal fever)	*Neisseria meningitidis (N. intracellularis)* Meningococcus Serious, acute disease caused by bacteria that invade bloodstream and eventually meninges, causing fever and central nervous system inflammation	Occurs fairly often where concentrations of people are found (army bases, schools) because of healthy carriers Very severe or relatively mild Mortality depends on early diagnosis and treatment Complications include hydrocephalus, arthritis, blindness, deafness, impairment of intellect, and cerebral palsy	Direct contact with patient or carrier by droplet spread*	As long as meningococci are found in nose and mouth Usually not infectious after 24 hours of antibiotic therapy

Incubation Period	Symptoms	Treatment and Nursing Care	Prevention
Mean range 2 to 12 weeks	Sama as HBV; sypmtoms may not be as severe	Same as HBV	Screening donated blood; avoidance of blood-to-blood exposure for at-risk health care providers
8 to 12 days from exposure to onset of symptoms	Catarrhal symptoms like a common cold; conjunctivitis; photophobia Fever followed by maculopapular rash, which starts behind ears and at the hairline and forehead, and moves progressively down the body, becoming more confluent over the face. Koplik's spots (eruption on mucous membrane of mouth) diagnostic, best seen before the rash	Antibiotics (for treatment of secondary bacterial infections) Acetaminophen (Tylenol) and tepid sponge baths for severe cases; various soothing lotions Boric acid eye irrigations; protection from bright lights—eyeshade Observation for onset of pneumonia or ear infection	Live measles vaccine; IG immune globulin will prevent or modify disease if given within 6 days of exposure. Usually immune after first attack
1 to 10 days (usually 4 days)	Sudden onset of fever, chills, headache, and vomiting (convulsions fairly common in children) Cutaneous petechial hemorrhages, stiffness of neck, opisthotonos; joint pain, possibly delirium, convulsions	Spinal tap and culture needed to confirm diagnosis Temperature control; penicillin G, cefuroxime or ampicillin, analgesics, and sedatives Watch for clinical signs of increasing intracranial pressure or meningeal irritation and eye and ear involvement Maintain dim, quiet atmosphere; turn gently; watch for constipation and urinary retention; attention to fluid balance	Meningococcal polysaccharide vaccines for group A and C meningococcal infections Extent of immunity after attack unknown Rifampin should be given to any person having intimate contact with secretions

Continued.

◆ **TABLE 31-1**
Communicable Childhood Diseases—cont'd.

Disease	Infectious Agent and General Description	Importance	Mode of Transmission	Communicable Period
Mononucleosis, infectious (glandular fever)	Epstein-Barr (EB) virus Mildly contagious disease characterized by increase in monocyte-type white cell in blood, splenomegaly, lymph node enlargement, fever, and fatigue Heterophil agglutinin studies positive fairly late in course of disease	Typically, disease of teenagers or young adults Trauma rarely may cause ruptured spleen; hepatitis in 8% to 10% of cases May involve prolonged convalescence	Probably droplets from nose and throat, saliva, or intimate contact*	Not known Probably only during acute stage
Mumps (infectious parotitis)	Virus Acute infectious disease causing inflammation of salivary glands and, at times, testes and ovaries	Possible serious consequences for male after puberty when an attack is more severe; sterility can be complication Meningitis or encephalitis occurs infrequently Mild pancreatitis may be encountered	Direct or indirect contact with patient by droplet spread*	From 1 to 7 days before parotid swelling until up to 9 days after onset
Rabies (hydrophobia)	Virus Only two nonfatal cases reported, acute infectious encephalitis, causing convulsions and muscle paralysis	Exceedingly dangerous Household pets may acquire rabies through bite of rabid wild animals All dogs should be immunized periodically; cats may also be carriers, but impractical to insist on immunization	Bite of rabid animals or entry of infected saliva through previous break in skin or mucous membrane*	Throughout clinical course of disease plus 3 to 5 days before appearance of symptoms (as demonstrated in dogs and cats)

Incubation Period	Symptoms	Treatment and Nursing Care	Prevention
Unknown (probably 4 to 7 weeks)	Sore throat, malaise, depression, enlarged spleen, liver, and lymph nodes Possible jaundice with liver damage	Symptomatic, no specific therapy known Bed rest, high carbohydrate and protein intake Possible use of corticosteroids with severe throat involvement and airway obstruction	No immunization available
14 to 21 days (usually 18 days)	Tender swelling chiefly of parotid glands in front of and below ear Headache; moderate fever; pain on swallowing	Bed rest; bland, soft diet; analgesics; warm or cold applications to swollen glands Watch for tenderness of testes—scrotal support may be necessary	Mumps vaccine Usually immune after first attack
Usually 2 to 6 weeks	Mental depression, headaches, restlessness, and fever Progresses to painful spasms of throat muscles, especially when attempting to drink Delirium, convulsions, and coma	No effective treatment known Supportive nursing care to help prevent convulsions; analgesics Death usually occurs in about 7 days	Vaccination of dogs; 10-day confinement of any dog who has bitten human Laboratory investigation of brain of dog that dies during this period; if rabies is diagnosed, person bitten must receive rabies vaccine; consult AAP Red Book for specific treatments§

Continued.

◆ **TABLE 31-1**
Communicable Childhood Diseases—cont'd.

Disease	Infectious Agent and General Description	Importance	Mode of Transmission	Communicable Period
Staphylococcal infections	Coagulase-positive staphylococci (*Staphylococcus aureus*); coagulase-negative (*S. epidermidis*); pus-producing coccus Descriptions variable	Found almost everywhere; causes many hospital infections; does not respond well to usual antibiotic therapy; extremely difficult to control; anyone may be carrier at intervals Complications include skin lesions, pneumonia, wound infections, arthritis, osteomyelitis, meningitis, and food poisoning	Depends on body area infected Via hands of hospital personnel Asymptomatic nasal carriers common Open suppurative lesions May be airborne Direct or indirect contact with infected secretions (Type of isolation depends on area infected—Contact)*	As long as lesions drain or carrier state persists
Group A streptococcal infections (GAS)	Strains of group A beta-hemolytic streptococci Diseases include septic sore throat, scarlet fever (scarlatina), erysipelas, impetigo, puerperal fever	Interrelated group of infections; septic sore throat probably most common Early complications include otitis media May cause serious complications not contagious in themselves—nephritis and rheumatic fever, with possible arthritis and carditis	In septic sore throat and scarlet fever, direct or indirect contact with nasopharyngeal secretions from infected patient; probably airborne In erysipelas, impetigo, and puerperal fever, direct or indirect contact with discharges from skin or reproductive tract*	Variable
Group B streptococcal infections (see p. 370)				
Syphilis (see pp. 248-249)				
Tetanus (lockjaw)	*Bacillus clostridium tetani* Acute infectious disease chiefly attacking nervous system Wounds deprived of good oxygen supply especially vulnerable	Always considered in event of burns, automobile accidents, or puncture wounds Mortality of about 35%	Entrance of spores into wounds through contaminated soil Direct or indirect contamination of wounds	None

Incubation Period	Symptoms	Treatment and Nursing Care	Prevention
Variable; 1 to 10 days to several weeks	Depend on area infected Fever and characteristic signs of inflammation typical	Antibiotics according to drug sensitivity pattern of organisms; methicillin, oxacillin, cephalosporins, vancomycin Topical antibiotics: bacitracin, neomycin, polymyxin, mupirocin	Good hygiene and aseptic technique best preventive
2 to 5 days pharyngitis 7 to 10 days impetigo	Depends on manifestations Septic sore throat, severe pharyngitis, and fever Scarlet fever, pharyngitis, fever, fine reddish rash, and strawberry tongue Erysipelas, tender, red skin lesions, and fever often recurrent Impetigo, refer to p. 604 Puerperal fever, refer to p. 271	Depends on manifestation Penicillin for at least 10 days to prevent rheumatic fever (erythromycin for persons allergic to penicillin)	No artificial immunization available Penicillin prophylaxis may be used with special groups Good asepsis important
3 to 21 days (usually 8 days)	Irritability, rigidity, painful muscle spasms, and inability to open mouth Exhaustion and respiratory difficulty	Specific—tetanus immune globulin Parenteral Pen G is effective in reducing the number of vegetative forms of the organism Sedation plus muscle relaxant Quiet, dim room Possible suction and tracheotomy Observation of fluid balance; watch for constipation and respiratory distress; protect from self-injury during convulsions	Routine primary immunization; DPT booster at school age and Td every 10 years (see pp. 454-455)

Continued.

♦ **TABLE 31-1**
Communicable Childhood Diseases—cont'd.

Disease	Infectious Agent and General Description	Importance	Mode of Transmission	Communicable Period
Tuberculosis (TB) (see pp. 247-248)	*Mycobacterium tuberculosis* (tubercle bacillus) Typically chronic infection that may affect many body organs Human type most often causes pulmonary infection Bovine type causes much of tuberculosis affecting areas outside lungs	Serious world health problem, particularly in economically deprived areas Infants and young children highly susceptible Pulmonary complications, hemoptysis, spontaneous pneumothorax, or spread to other organs with varied symptoms; possible orthopedic problems	Pulmonary TB: Mycobacterium tuberculosis is transmitted by airborne route (e.g., coughing). A person with active pulmonary or laryngeal TB expels organisms into the air where they are rapidly transformed into tiny droplet nuclei that can remain suspended in the air to be inhaled into respiratory tract of a susceptible person. Transmission from persons with extrapulmonary disease is very rare but can occur under circumstances where organisms are aerosolized (e.g., from a lesion irrigated with a high pressure device). Bovine type may result from drinking milk from infected cows (now rare in United States)*	Children with uncomplicated primary TB are usually noninfectious because of minimal pulmonary lesions. Communicable as long as organism is discharged in sputum or other body excretions Communicability may be reduced by anti-TB therapy Body often walls off a primary infection, controlling spread and preventing active disease
Typhoid fever (enteric fever)	*Salmonella typhosa*, bacillus (one of many types have been identified) Relatively severe febrile systemic infection (sepsis) with symptoms involving lymphoid tissues, intestine, and spleen; may be accompanied by complete prostration and delirium Condition has prolonged course and convalescence	Always of potential public health importance when community hygiene breaks down Carrier states may persist Complications include intestinal hemorrhage and perforation, thrombosis, cardiac failure, and cholecystitis	Direct or indirect contact with urine and feces of infected patients and carriers Food and water supplies may be infected by contaminated flies or unsuspected carriers; community sewage facilities should be evaluated; excreta has to be disinfected before being added to local system*	As long as typhoid organism appears in feces or urine, 2% to 5% of those affected become permanent carriers

Incubation Period	Symptoms	Treatment and Nursing Care	Prevention
From exposure to infection (measured by a positive PPD skin test) is about 10 to 12 weeks; from infection to active disease highly variable; over 90% of infected people never develop active tuberculosis	Active pulmonary tuberculosis: anorexia, weight loss, night sweats, afternoon fever, cough and dyspnea, fatigue, and hemoptysis; in children, dyspnea and cough often absent Diagnosis based on symptoms and microscopic studies of sputum, gastric washings, CSF, tissue; bronchoscopy; PPD skin test; chest x-ray examination	Specific—Isoniazid (INH), Rifampin (RIF), Pyrazinamide (PZA), and Ethambutol+ (EMB), or Streptomycin (SM) Nursing care includes provision for mental and physical rest; nutritious diet; observation for toxic drug reactions and increasing respiratory distress; provision for and instructions in personal hygiene	Early detection and control of known cases through annual skin test, and close medical supervision INH prophylaxis for neonate exposed to infected mother; separation from mother depends on mother's status Skin testing family members and case contact studies are paramount
1 to 3 weeks (usually 2 weeks)	In children, symptoms may be atypical, may at first resemble upper respiratory tract infection; intestinal tract becomes inflamed and even ulcerated; spleen enlarges; fever mounts; pulse relatively slow; rash, or "rose spots," may be present	Ampicillin or chloramphenicol for typhoid fever Supportive nursing care; liquid to bland, soft diet as tolerated; bed rest Watch for abdominal distention and hemorrhage; small enemas may be ordered; observation of fluid balance	Immunity usually acquired after one attack Vaccine available

Continued.

◆ **TABLE 31-1**
Communicable Childhood Diseases—cont'd.

Disease	Infectious Agent and General Description	Importance	Mode of Transmission	Communicable Period
Varicella-zoster infections	Virus capable of causing varicella (chickenpox), or zoster (shingles)		Direct or indirect contact with respiratory secretions or moist skin lesions of varicella or zoster Special ventilation in room for outbreak control*	Approximately 1 to 2 days before rash appears until 6 days after its onset; dried crusts not contagious
Varicella (chickenpox)	Response to primary infection Mild, chiefly cutaneous infectious disease	Very common, highly contagious, usually mild disease Complications other than secondary infection from scratching rare; however, encephalitis possible	See precautions above	
Zoster (shingles)	Reactivation in debilitated persons or in persons receiving immunosuppressive therapy	Overwhelming severe infection seen in children receiving immunosuppressive therapy	Zoster less contagious, but susceptible children exposed to zoster lesions may develop chickenpox	
Whooping cough (pertussis)	*Bordetella pertussis* (pertussis bacillus) Acute infection of respiratory tract characterized by paroxysmal cough ending in "whoop," often accompanied by vomiting	Severe disease in infants, may terminate fatally Complications include bronchopneumonia and convulsions, widespread hemorrhages, hernia, and possible activation of pulmonary tuberculosis	Direct or indirect contact with nasopharyngeal secretions of infected patients (droplet infection)*	From 7 days after exposure to 3 weeks after onset of typical cough Greatest in catarrhal stage before onset of paroxysms

Incubation Period	Symptoms	Treatment and Nursing Care	Prevention
10 to 21 days (usually 14 days)	Zoster lesions confined to skin over sensory nerves preceded by local pain, itching, and burning	Keep fingernails short and clean to minimize secondary infections caused by scratching Calamine lotion, oral antihistaminics reduce pruritis	None; immune after one attack, Vaccine for high-risk patients Passive immunization of susceptible immunodeficient patients exposed to either varicella or zoster virus may be obtained with varicella-zoster immune globulin (VZIG) given within 96 hours of exposure; distributed by the American Red Cross Blood Services Regional Centers
	Slight fever; malaise; rapidly progressing papulovesiculopustular skin eruption in all stages of development, first appearing on trunk and scalp	Children with varicella should not be given salicylates because of potential development of Reye syndrome	None; immune after one attack, OKA vaccine for high-risk patients
7 to 10 days (rarely more than 2 weeks)	Early symptoms resemble typical common cold Cough worsens and may become violent and paroxysmal Vomiting may be caused by coughing or nervous system irritation; cough may linger after convalescence	Diagnosis confirmed with bacterial studies of mucus from the nasopharynx; immunofluorescent antibody technique will identify organism after it has been isolated Erythromycin antibiotic of choice; provision for rest and quiet; sedatives Light nutritious diet; judicious fluid intake to prevent dehydration; weight determinations Observed for onset of respiratory distress or other complications	Immunity usually produced after one attack Routine primary schedule plus boosters until 7th birthday Erythromycin therapy shortens the period of communicability to 5 days or less

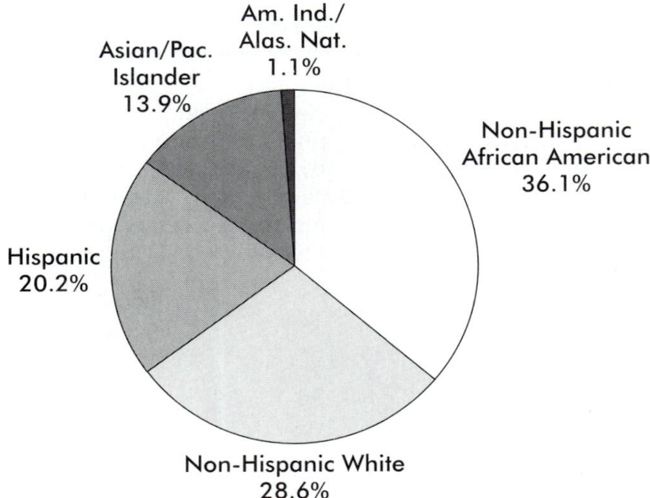

Fig. 31-3 Tuberculosis: percentage of cases, by race and ethnicity, United States, 1992. Excludes 32 cases (0.1%) with race and ethnicity unknown. (From Centers for Disease Control: Summary of notifiable diseases, United States 1992, *MMWR* 41(55):60, 1993.)

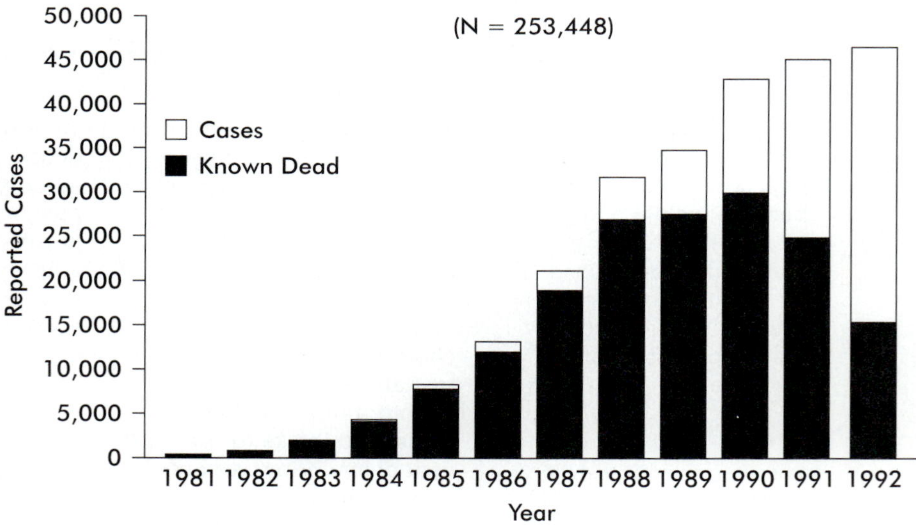

Fig. 31-4 Acquired Immunodeficiency Syndrome (AIDS): deported cases and known deaths, by year, United States, 1981-1982. Includes Guam, Puerto Rico, the US Pacific Islands, and the US Virgin Islands. (From Centers for Disease Control: Summary of notifiable diseases, United States, 1992, *MMWR* 41(55):15, 1993.)

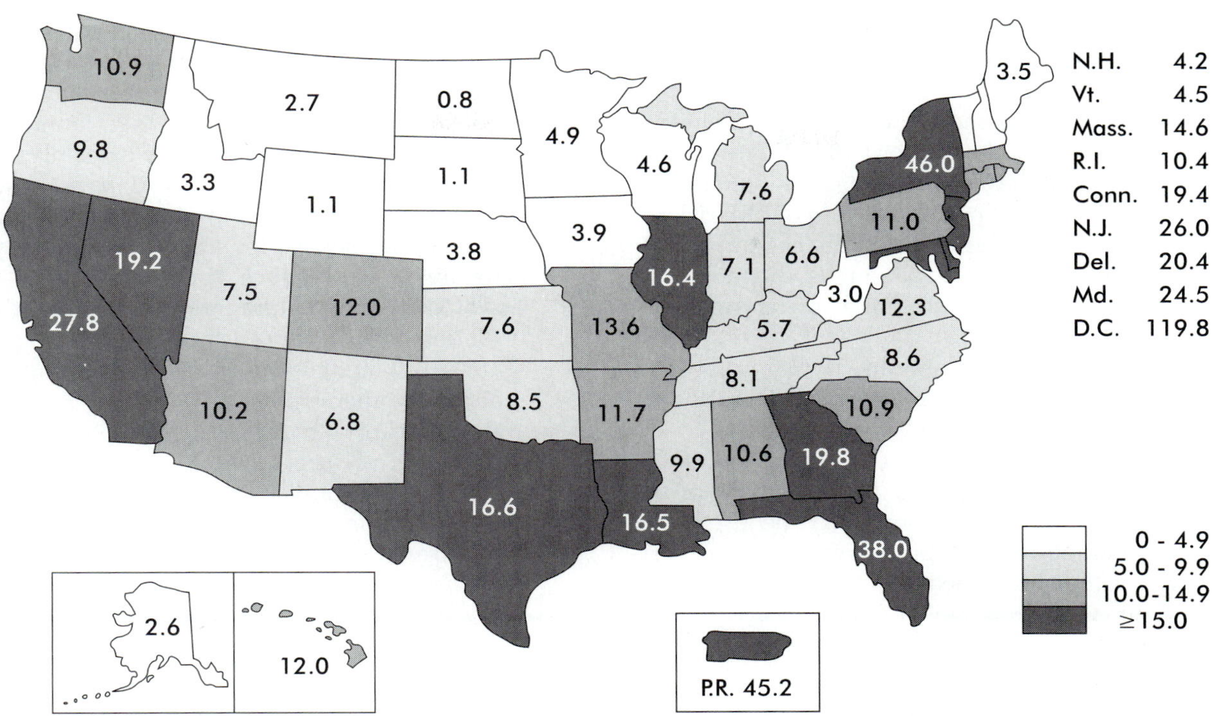

Fig. 31-5 Acquired Immunodeficiency Syndrome (AIDS): Reported cases, per 100,000 population, United States and Puerto Rico, 1992. Denominators for computing rates are based on extrapolations from US Bureau of the Census population data from the 1980 and 1990 censuses. (From Center for Disease Control: Summary of notifiable diseases, United States, 1992, *MMWR* 41(55):17, 1993.)

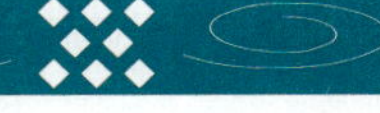

KEY CONCEPTS

1 Centers for Disease Control and Prevention (CDC) guidelines offered the possibility of choosing one of three alternative isolation systems: category-specific, disease-specific, or a system designed for use within the particular institution. These guidelines are currently under revision.

2 Disease-specific isolation precautions are based on the mode of transmission of the individual disease.

3 In 1987 the CDC extended Category VII, blood/body fluid precautions, to include all patients. The term *universal precautions* refers to the application of certain limited precautions to all caregiver/patient contacts within the health care setting.

4 The Body Substance Isolation (BSI) system is an alternative to the category-specific and disease-specific systems. With the BSI system the nurse plans the use of barriers based on the interaction with every patient's body substances, including body fluids, excretions, and secretions.

5 To minimize the transmission of infectious agents the care giver should be free of communicable infections, knowledgeable regarding the need to reevaluate patient assignment, knowledgeable about the need to maintain good general health habits, and knowledgeable and dependable regarding isolation precautions needed.

6 The most important procedure for preventing the transmission of infectious agents is appropriate handwashing. Except in emergencies, hands should always be washed in the following situations: before initiating individual patient care, performing any sterile or invasive procedure and touching a wound, pouring medications and touching food; and after completing individual patient care, touching wounds, mucous membranes, or body substances, using the bathroom, touching inanimate objects that are likely to be contaminated, and removing gloves.

7 Disposable, single-use gloves, clean or sterile, are recommended to protect patients and personnel from microorganisms.

8 Gowns or aprons are primarily used to protect against splashing body fluids.

9 Although masks may not protect the caregiver

from airborne droplet nuclei, they may help prevent splashes from reaching the skin, mouth, or nose.

10 Protective eyewear should reduce the incidence of contamination of the mucous membranes of the eyes. Masks should be worn in combination with eye protection and special masks to reduce risks to caregivers of inhaling droplet nuclei from the air should be worn if the patient is diagnosed or suspected of having pulmonary or laryngeal tuberculosis.

11 Needles and sharps should be carefully and properly disposed of to prevent accidental puncture.

12 The parents of an isolated child need emotional and informational support. The assistance of the infection control practitioner may be especially useful. Parents should be encouraged and welcomed at the child's bedside.

13 The room of an isolated pediatric patient should include the following: access to a sink, running water, and toilet; a box of gloves; a handwashing agent; paper towels in a dispenser; laundry hamper support and plastic laundry bags; plastic bags for collection of trash for discard; barriers such as gowns and/or masks and eye protection; and all other articles needed for admission and daily care.

14 The nurse can reduce the anxiety level of an isolated child by helping him understand that the isolation is not a punishment, and by playing games, talking, cuddling, and welcoming friends and family members.

15 When caring for children with communicable diseases, the nurse should be knowledgeable about the infectious agent, mode of transmission, communicable period, incubation period, symptoms, treatment and nursing care, and prevention.

CRITICAL THOUGHT QUESTIONS

1 Identify the links in the chain of infection. Which nursing measures are able to "break" each link of the chain?

2 In addition to isolation technique, health care institutions today use universal precautions. How are isolation technique and universal precautions used in a pediatric setting? What modifications are necessary because of the age and developmental stage of the child?

3 Why do reported cases of varicella (chickenpox) exceed all other common communicable diseases of childhood? Why does chickenpox spread rapidly? Is there any risk to the parents of children with chickenpox?

4 It has been observed that some of the early measles vaccines did not give lifelong immunity. What problems and nursing concerns does this raise?

5 What implications does the growing number of AIDS cases and persons who are HIV positive have for the pediatric nurse? What are the most common ways in which infants and children acquire HIV?

REFERENCES

Centers for Disease Control: Summary of notifiable diseases, United States 1992, *MMWR* 41(55):15, 17, 60, 1993.

Jackson MM: Implementing universal body substance precautions, *State Art Rev Occup Med* 4:39 (special issue) 39, 1989.

Jackson MM and Luncy P: In search of a national approach. *Am J Nurs* 90(10):65, 1990.

Jackson MM et al: Why not treat all body substances as infectious? *Am J Nurs* 87(9):1137, 1987.

Keen TP: Nursing care of the pediatric multitrauma patient, *Nurs Clin North Am* 25(1):131, 1990.

Lynch P et al: Implementing and evaluating a system of generic infection precautions: body substance isolation, *Am J Infect Control* 18(1):1, 1990.

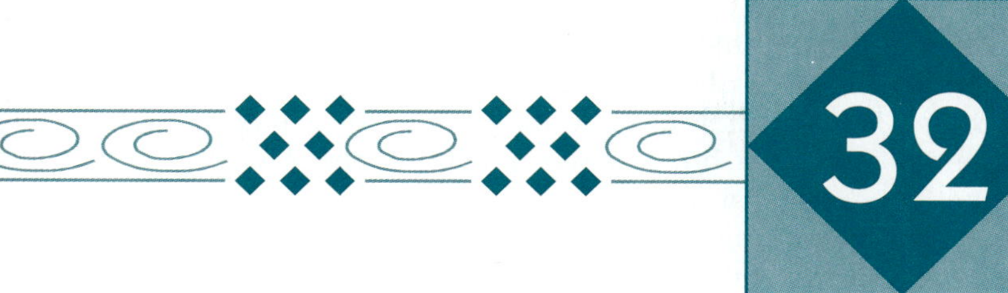

32

Conditions Involving the Neuromuscular and Skeletal Systems

CHAPTER OBJECTIVES

After studying this chapter, the student should be able to:

1 Discuss fractures: the most characteristic type of childhood fracture, signs and symptoms, first aid measures, and early medical care.

2 Describe Bryant's or vertical traction, when it is used, and two potential problems of which the nurse should be aware.

3 Define the following orthopedic procedural terms: *closed* and *open reductions*, *arthrodesis*, *osteotomy*, *bone block*, *arthroplasty*, and *epiphyseal arrest*.

4 Discuss how the nurse can lessen the following problems facing the child with rheumatoid arthritis: joint pain, decrease in activity, potential deformity, and other signs and symptoms not directly related to orthopedics.

5 Describe the problem of scoliosis, what population it most frequently affects, signs of its development, screening programs, and why early identification of affected children is so important.

6 Describe briefly the basic physical and psychosocial problems children with the following medical diagnoses may encounter: torticollis, Duchenne's muscular dystrophy, osteomyelitis, and Legg-Calvé-Perthes disease.

7 Discuss why early intensive evaluation and treatment of the child with suspected meningitis is crucial.

8 Describe four key components of the nursing care of the child with meningitis.

9 Indicate the proper immediate care of a 3 year old who suddenly has a generalized seizure and discuss what the nurse should observe.

10 List four possible causes of cerebral palsy and the types of problems that a moderately to severely affected child may demonstrate.

11 Demonstrate how to proceed with a neurological check of a school-age child.

12 Review six signs and symptoms of increasing intracranial pressure in a preschool-age child.

13 Discuss the frequency of head injuries in children and the reported incidence of skull fracture and intracranial bleeding; differentiate the terms *concussion*, *cerebral contusion*, and *laceration*.

14 Indicate possible signs of a basilar skull fracture that may develop in the hours following the admission of a head-injured child.

15 Identify three types of pediatric visual difficulties that should be referred to an ophthalmologist and describe how they reveal themselves.

16 Explain the relationship between strabismus, notable inequality in right or left eye visual acuity, and the development of amblyopia.

17 Discuss six behavioral clues a child may demonstrate indicating a poor ability to hear.

All the systems of the body are interrelated. If dysfunction in one part of the body is severe or prolonged, many body systems—in fact, the whole person—will be affected. The interdependence of the neuromuscular, skeletal, and sensory systems is especially noteworthy; thus these systems are presented together.

Traumatic, infectious, or toxic injury to the nerve centers or nerve fibers that control the skeletal muscles often leads to wasting of those muscles and an inability to control or perhaps even initiate motion in related parts of the body. Poorly developed, abnormal, or damaged muscles may cause orthopedic deformities. Broken bones frequently cause muscle spasm and pain.

Some of the more common neuromuscular and skeletal problems found in children, the methods of treatment, and the nursing care involved are discussed in this chapter. The first section presents fractures, joint and extremity problems, and other conditions involving the bones and muscles, followed by a discussion of nervous system diseases that affect the bones and muscles; and finally sensory assessment of vision, hearing, and related disorders.

A number of problems affecting these interrelated systems are present at birth or are congenital in nature. The more common congenital defects are discussed in the chapter treating abnormalities of the newborn infant. For a brief description of hydrocephalus, cranial stenosis (craniosynostosis), microcephaly, spina bifida, clubfoot, congenital dislocated hip, syndactyly, and polydactylism, refer to Chapter 18.

FRACTURES, JOINT AND EXTREMITY PROBLEMS

Fractures

A common problem in childhood is a broken bone or fracture. Team sports, roller blades, skateboards, bicycles, and the active lives of youngsters contribute to the high incidence of fractures. More broken bones would occur in childhood if it were not for the relatively plastic condition of the child's skeletal system. Children's bones tend to bend rather than break. Frequently, if a bone does break, it is not completely severed; a portion of the bone remains intact. This type of fracture is called an *incomplete* or *greenstick fracture* (Fig. 32-1).

Classifications

Other common types of fractures described according to the course of the break sustained include *transverse, spiral,* and *oblique*. A *comminuted fracture* is especially difficult to repair because the bone is broken into more than two pieces. A *depressed fracture* is particularly important when the fractured bony area is the skull and abnormal pressure is exerted on sensitive brain tissue. Fractures can result from excessive or sudden direct pressure, exaggerated muscular contractions, or an unsound bony structure. If an unsound bony structure is the case, the fracture is termed *pathological*. Some of the causes of pathological fractures are osteomyelitis (infection of the bone marrow and surrounding bone cells), primary bone tumors (or metastases), and osteogenesis imperfecta congenita (congenital brittle bones). Osteogenesis imperfecta is a disease of unknown origin in which bones may fracture even before birth, causing characteristic skeletal malformations occasionally accompanied by deafness. If a child has an underlying bone disease, great care and gentleness must be practiced in turning and positioning him or her (Fig. 32-2).

Careful assessment and documentation must be made of the general condition of a child who enters the hospital with a fracture of unknown origin, multiple fractures, repeated fractures, bruising, or malnutrition. These children may be victims of abuse. Parents, who are unable to meet the daily frustrations of parenthood in a mature manner or who have deep-seated psychological problems may abuse their children. Other adults and older children have also been the perpetrators of child maltreatment (Fig. 32-3).

Every fracture, regardless of the course or extent of the break or its basic cause, may be placed in one or two main categories. If a bone is broken, but the skin overlying the fracture has not been pierced by the end of the broken bone and no opening in the skin has occurred, the result is called a *closed fracture*. Some closed fractures may be emergencies depending on their location. If, however, the skin has been broken, exposing the bone to infection, the resulting trauma is called an *open* or *compound fracture*. Open fractures are surgical emergencies because of the increased danger of infection and extensive soft tissue damage usually involved.

First-aid considerations

A nurse encountering an accident victim with unknown injuries should take the following action:

1. Evaluate the safety of the immediate environment (for example, turn off ignition of car, set out warning flares if on highway). Send someone for help, if possible. Use universal precautions.
2. Establish an airway if respirations are not present.
3. Control hemorrhage if present.

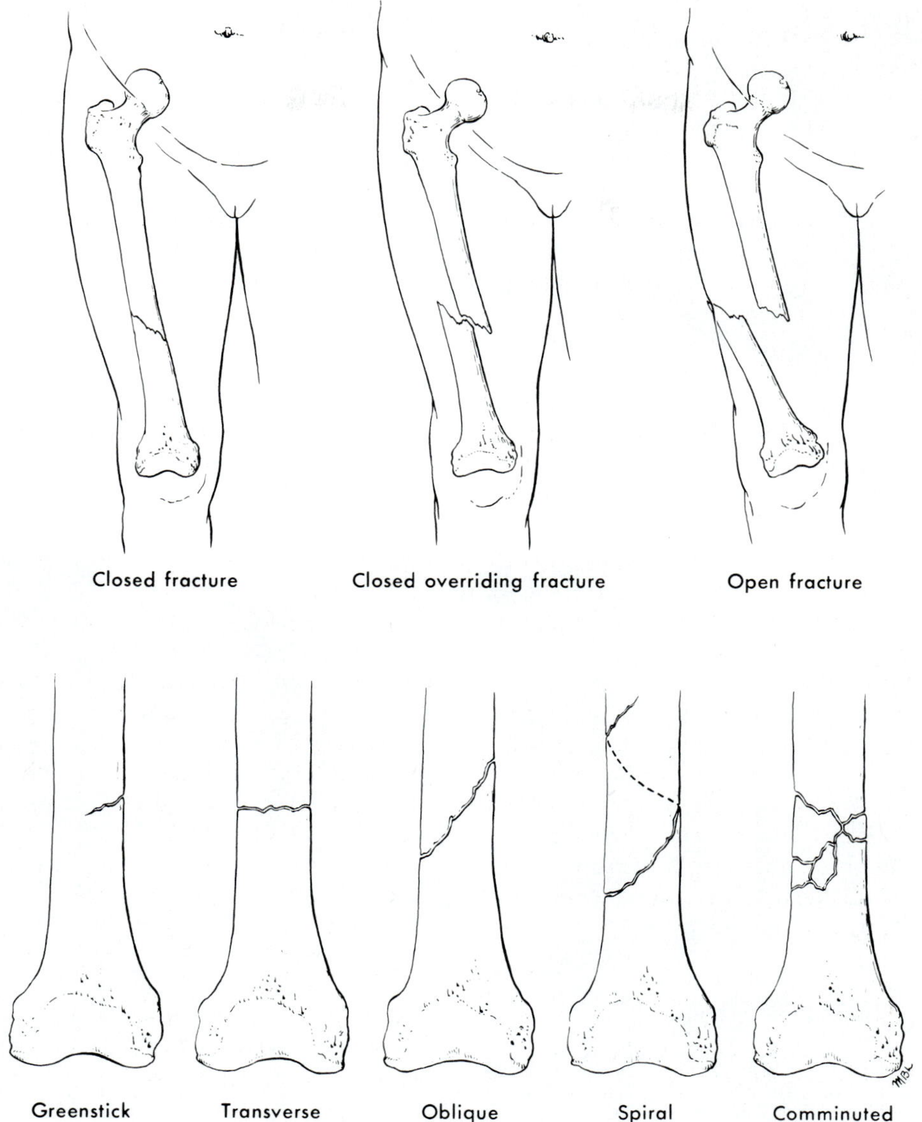

Fig. 32-1 Types of fractures.

4 Restore and maintain respiratory status.
5 Restore and maintain pulse (CPR) if necessary.
6 Evaluate for spinal injury and fracture. Do not move victim until proper help is available.
7 Keep the patient flat, warm, and quiet to prevent and treat shock.

If a victim with spinal injury is moved improperly, the injury may be increased and permanent paralysis or even death may occur. If the victim is conscious but cannot move any extremity, the nurse must consider the possibility of a cervical fracture or a fracture of the thoracic spine. A child with a possible broken neck should be moved by a team so that no twisting or injurious movement of the spine takes place. The individual should be securely positioned with sandbags and transported on a rigid support while supine with the chin up. Persons with suspected spinal injuries should be moved as little as possible. They should be frequently observed to detect the onset of respiratory difficulty and abdominal distention. The higher the injury on the spinal cord, the more body functions affected. Nonspinal fractures are less serious but still necessitate careful attention and first aid.

Clinical manifestations

A fracture of an extremity is considered in the presence of the following:

1 Deformity in alignment and swelling

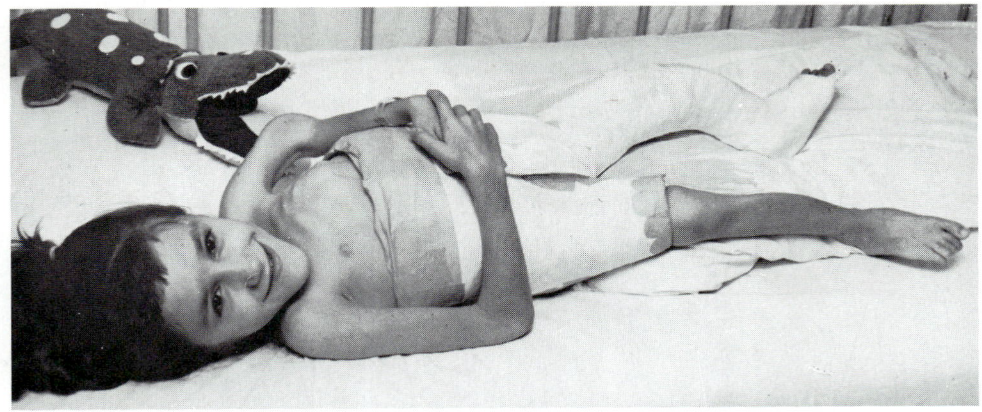

Fig. 32-2 This child is a victim of osteogenesis imperfecta congenita. She was hospitalized for corrective surgery involving previous fractures. (Courtesy Children's Hospital and Health Center, San Diego, Calif.)

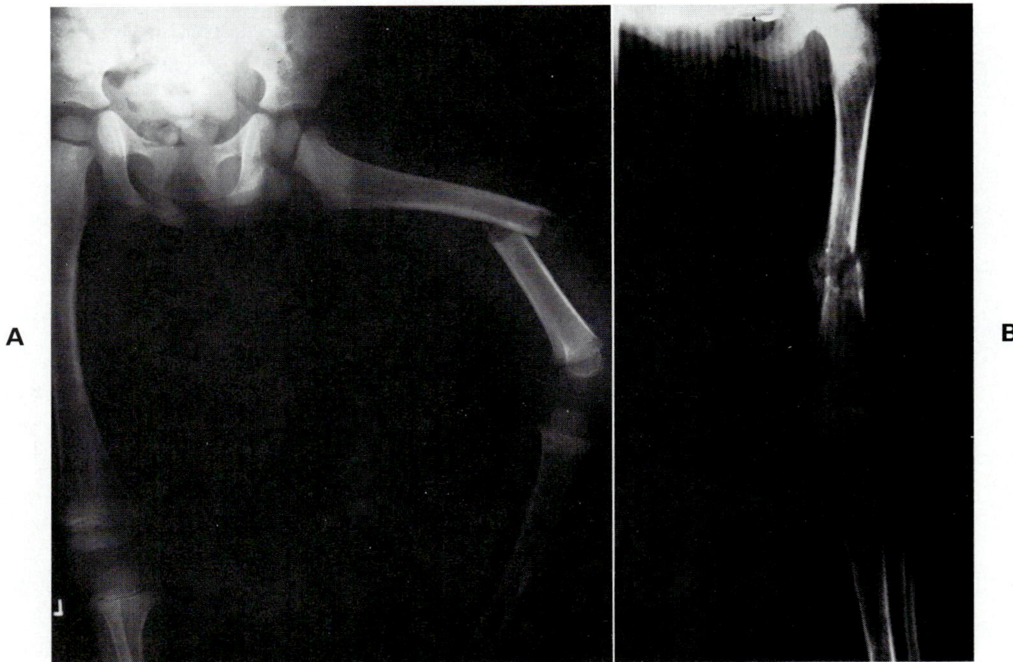

Fig. 32-3 ***A,*** X-ray of left femur of 19-lb, 2 ½-year-old child who entered hospital with multiple body bruises. Provisional diagnosis: "nonaccidental injury." ***B,*** X-ray showing same leg after reduction of fractured femur. Shadowy outline around break is callus. (Courtesy Naval Hospital, San Diego, Calif.)

2 Pain or tenderness at the fracture site
3 Loss of function or abnormal mobility of the part
4 A "grating sensation" heard or felt at the suspected point of fracture (crepitus)
5 Black-and-blue areas caused by subcutaneous hemorrhage (ecchymosis)

Confirmation of the presence of fracture is obtained by x-ray. Sometimes clinical symptoms are virtually lacking or inconclusive, but the x-ray film reveals a

Nursing Alert

The acronyms RICE (REST, ICE, COMPRESSION, ELEVATION) and ICES (ICE, COMPRESSION, ELEVATION, SUPPORT) should be kept in mind and initiated when caring for a child or adult with a suspected fracture or soft tissue injury.

break. Every suspected skeletal injury should be treated as a fracture until proved otherwise.

Use of splints

First-aid treatment of a possible fracture includes limiting the movement of the injured part by stabilizing the part and the joint above and below the break to relieve muscle spasm and pain and to prevent further injury. A rolled newspaper, a cardboard box, or a magazine can be used for a splint. The splint should be applied in a position comfortable for the child. The arm or leg should be splinted without an attempt to correct any deformity. No attempt should be made to straighten it because this may cause further damage. No attempt should be made to push back a broken bone protruding from the skin in the case of an open fracture. The area should simply be covered.

If bleeding is present, direct manual pressure to obtain control should be used. A tourniquet should not be used because prolonged application can cause gangrene and loss of a limb. Rings and bracelets on a fractured upper extremity should be removed in the event of swelling. The application of icebags may decrease the possibility of swelling. Heat should not be applied. For bleeding from an arm or leg, the part should be elevated if possible.

When a fracture occurs involving the bones of an extremity, the involved muscles usually contract as a result of loss of proper skeletal support. The muscles go into spasm in an effort to splint the injured part. If this spasm is exaggerated, the severed ends of the broken bone can be pulled farther out of alignment or can override, causing abnormal shortening of the limb.

Care of the Hospitalized Child

Observation

When children with possible fractures are admitted to the hospital, their general condition is evaluated in detail. Neurovascular checks and vital signs (temperature, pulse, respiration, and blood pressure recordings) are obtained. Elevated blood pressure is important to report because of the possibility of skull fracture. Low blood pressure is equally important because of the possibility of shock. The level of consciousness should be evaluated and the pupils of the eyes checked for abnormal pupil dilation or inequality of pupil size (other signs of possible skull fracture and brain injury). Depending on the child's condition, intravenous solutions or blood may be given, but no food or fluid should be given by mouth because corrective surgery may be indicated. An x-ray of possible fracture sites should be made.

Reduction and casting

If overriding or angulation of a fractured bone has occurred, the displaced bone is pulled into alignment through some form of traction until the broken fragments are in proper position. The process of bringing the fragments into proper relationship is termed *reducing* or *setting* the fracture. If the fractured bone can be set without performing a surgical operation that actually exposes the involved bone, the procedure is called a *closed reduction.* If it is necessary to expose the site of the fracture to direct view to secure proper alignment and optimum healing or to use some method of internal immobilization, such as the installation of a nail, pin, or screws, the procedure is called an *open reduction.* Most children's fractures can be treated by closed reduction.

At times the x-rays will reveal a break, but the alignment is not disturbed because the bony segments are still in proper relationship. If this is the case, no mechanical traction apparatus is needed. A plaster cast or protective splint is applied to maintain correct positioning to ensure proper healing. Occasionally only a relatively minor disturbance in alignment has occurred that can be reduced easily at the time the child is first seen or may not even require reduction. In children a fracture often stimulates the formation of bone, and at times the physician may desire a certain amount of overriding to prevent excessive growth of the fractured extremity.

If satisfactory alignment is difficult or impossible to achieve and maintain, some form of constant pull, or traction, must be exerted to reduce the fracture and bring the ends of the broken bone into proper alignment. The position of the bone and the progress of healing are intermittently checked by x-ray studies. When a sufficient amount of new bone (callus) is formed at the fracture site to help hold the bone segment in position, traction is discontinued and a protective cast is applied, allowing the child more mobility. For a discussion of the basic nursing care involved in the hospitalization of a child in traction or a cast, refer to Chapter 33.

The healing of a broken bone, or *union* of a fracture, is accomplished through the deposit of new bone cells. In children, union is usually achieved in a relatively short time. Healing is seldom delayed, and it is rare to see a case in which union never takes place.

Rehabilitation

After the bone has united, the weakened muscles attached to the bone may require gradual strengthening through a program of exercise as prescribed by the physician. This part of therapy is less necessary with young children because they start using the part

COMMON ORTHOPEDIC PROCEDURES

1. *Arthrodesis* is the fusion of a joint to gain stability for weight bearing. It can be accomplished by removing the cartilage from the opposing ends of the bones that form a joint or by grafting bone into the area and then immobilizing it in a cast for a prolonged period to promote fusion. A *triple arthrodesis* is occasionally performed on a foot; as the name implies, it involves fusion of three joints. It prohibits some lateral movements of the foot itself but preserves ankle motion. Considerable bleeding can be expected after this type of surgery, and considerable pain may be involved. Weight bearing by the newly fused part is delayed until fusion is secure, in about 2 to 3 months.
2. *Arthroplasty* is the reconstruction of a joint to provide greater movement. The joints usually involved in the procedure are the hip and knee. Other procedures that involve total replacement of those joints have largely supplanted arthroplasty.
3. *Arthroscopy* is the visualization of a joint, most often the knee, by means of an arthroscope, which can be inserted via a trochar through a tiny skin incision. Magnification allows diagnosis and some treatment procedures such as partial removal or repair of meniscal injuries.
4. *Osteotomy* is an opening into or a controlled fracture of a bone to correct a congenital or acquired skeletal deformity. In a *rotational osteotomy* the distal fragment of the bone is rotated to secure the desired correction.
5. *Tendon transplant* is a procedure in which a tendon from one part of the body is transplanted to another. It is performed for various reasons: to substitute the action of neighboring strong muscles for paralyzed or weak muscles, to replace badly damaged tendons, or to decrease a deformity caused by exaggerated muscle pull.
6. *Epiphyseal arrest* may be performed to slow the growth of one extremity that is unequal in length. A partial arrest can also aid in the correction of deformities such as knock-knees or bowlegs. It is accomplished by a bone block or by the placement of stainless-steel staples into the epiphyseal area, where bone growth takes place. This procedure stops normal growth. The staples are removed when the desired results are obtained.
7. *Leg lengthening* is a difficult but possible alternative procedure for leg-length inequality. An osteotomy is performed followed by separation of the bone, bone grafting if necessary, and external fixation that allows gradual stretching over a period of several weeks.
8. *Open reduction and internal fixation* (ORIF) is the operative procedure used when a fracture requires open visualization to reduce it and stabilization by means of metal fixation. In children, fractures often heal as well and as quickly without this surgical procedure.

immediately and usually do not need the encouragement required by many adults. The resources of the physical therapy department may be used on either an inpatient or an outpatient basis. The aims of treatment are return to function, freedom from pain, and normal appearance.

JOINT AND EXTREMITY PROBLEMS

The skeletal system can become distorted for reasons other than fracture. Some congenital deformities and intervening paralytic or inflammatory diseases of the skeletal system can cause muscular weakness or bone destruction, producing joint instability that prevents normal weight bearing. Some disorders reduce joint mobility so that the usefulness of a body part is greatly reduced. Other conditions affect the growth patterns of individual extremities. Various surgical procedures have been devised to increase the effectiveness of various body joints, either by increasing their ability to bear weight (increasing joint stability) or by permitting greater motion. If a choice between motion and stability in the lower extremity must be made, the decision is made in favor of stability. The box above describes common procedures used to treat a wide variety of orthopedic problems.

CONDITIONS INVOLVING THE BONES AND MUSCLES

Because many pediatric nursing courses are organized according to developmental sequence the following conditions are presented according to the age group primarily affected. Such an approach is not without inconsistencies. Some conditions extend to children of all ages; moreover, many problems are present in infancy but are not diagnosed until later in childhood. See Chapter 18 for conditions commonly diagnosed in the neonatal period.

Infant

Torticollis

Torticollis, or wryneck, is a congenital muscular abnormality often associated with birth trauma. (Fig. 32-4) Although the defect is minimal at birth, within 2 weeks a palpable fibrous tumor appears in the sternocleidomastoid muscle. The cause of these tumors is unknown. Within a few months the fibrous tumor gradually disappears, leaving behind a contracture (shortening) of the muscle. The head of the infant is tilted toward the side of the affected muscle, and the chin is rotated to the opposite side. When the condition is recognized early, treatment consists of passive stretching of the involved muscle. Parents are instructed as to positioning and specific maneuvers to be performed four or five times daily. Physical therapy may be recommended. The reward for faithful treatment is complete and permanent correction in at least 90% of the cases. When torticollis does not respond to conservative measures or when treatment is not consistent, surgery is indicated. The affected muscle is divided or partially excised. The head is immobilized in the correct position for a period of time. If surgery is delayed until the child is older, postoperative exercises are necessary to prevent a recurrence.

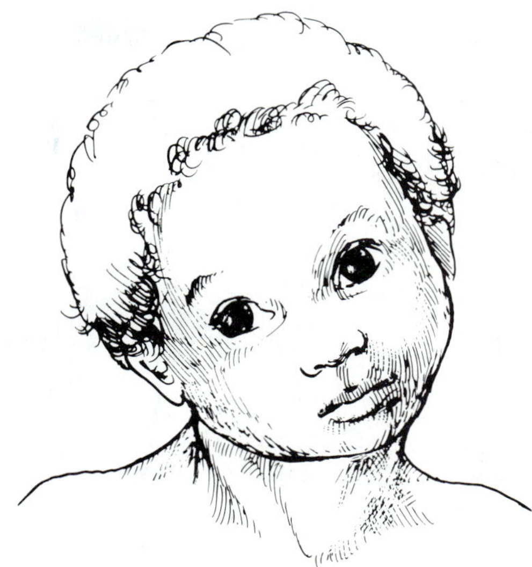

Fig. 32-4 Torticollis or wryneck: in this case, shortening of right sternocleidomastoid muscle.

Childhood rickets

One disease resulting from nutritional disturbance is common childhood rickets. The name is misleading because now a classic example of this disease is sometimes difficult to find in the United States. Rickets is always a potential health hazard in communities where there is little sunshine or little exposure of children to the outdoors and a diet deficient in vitamin D, calcium, or phosphorus. Vitamin D is crucial because it regulates the absorption and deposit of calcium and phosphorus. Most formulas are specially irradiated or fortified to provide adequate levels of vitamin D to infants and children. Other rich sources are the fish-liver oils. Sunshine, if it is not screened by window glass and clothing or rendered unavailable by air pollution, is the most inexpensive source of vitamin D. Of course, vitamin preparations can be purchased. Cases of rickets can be mild and pass undetected or very severe and remarkable. Classic manifestations are knock-knees or bowlegs, kyphosis (humpback) or scoliosis (an abnormal lateral spinal curvature), delayed closure of fontanels and protruding forehead (bossing), thickened wrists and ankles, enlargement of the cartilaginous area of attachment of the ribs to the sternum *(rachitic rosary)*, pigeon breast, and contracture of the pelvis. Treatment consists in greater intake of vitamin D, calcium, and phosphorus. It is possible but not likely for a person to have an excessive vitamin D intake. Discretion should be used in the selection and dosage of therapeutic vitamins.

Toddler

Duchenne's muscular dystrophy

A number of conditions are characterized by a progressive weakening of the musculoskeletal system and eventual wasting of muscle tissue. They differ in the main muscles affected, the course of the disability, and the typical age of onset. Duchenne's or (pseudohypertrophic) progressive muscular dystrophy is the most common form of the progressive types of muscle weakness. The onset of this disease usually occurs between the third and sixth years. It is a hereditary, sex-linked, recessive condition that affects males almost exclusively. Recently the gene that causes the disease was discovered. This genetic breakthrough allows for accurate carrier detection, prenatal diagnosis and, it is hoped, a successful treatment.

In this type of dystrophy a fatty infiltration of the muscle cells may produce a deceptively large muscle lacking strength, hence its title *pseudohypertrophic* muscular dystrophy. This condition is seen most often in the calf muscles. Intramuscular enzymes, creatine phosphokinase (CPK), and serum aldolase, leak into the blood serum as muscle tissue breaks down. Serum values of these enzymes are high in the early stages of

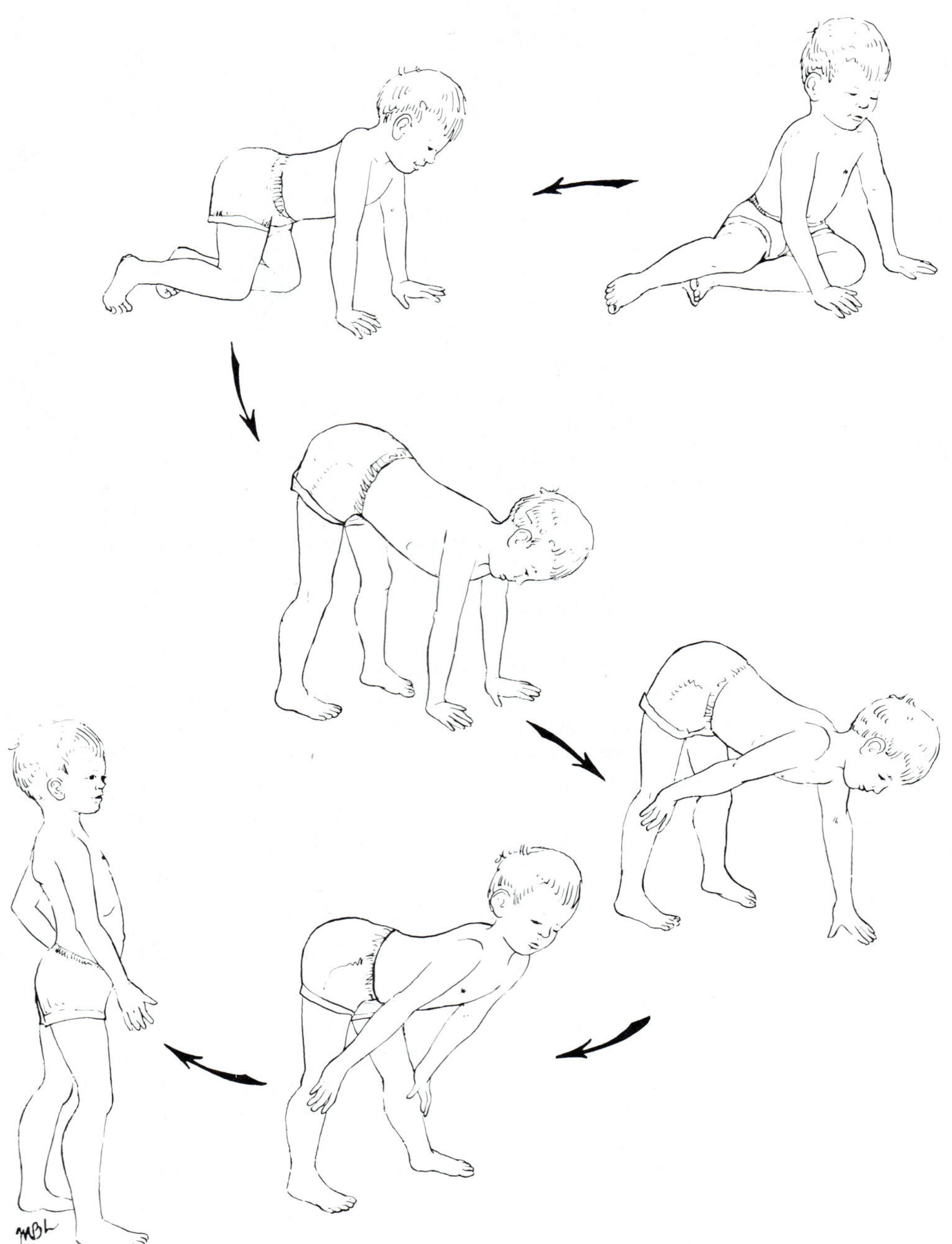

Fig. 32-5 Gower's sign, "self-climbing procedure," characteristic of pseudohypertrophic muscular dystrophy.

the disease but decline as the disease progresses, and in the final stages they are only slightly above normal (apparently because so little muscle tissue is left).

The affected young child has difficulty in walking and falls easily as the muscular weakness attacks, in sequence, the muscles of the legs, pelvis, and abdomen. A pronounced lordosis develops as the youngster struggles to remain upright. These children display a characteristic method of supporting themselves when attempting to rise to their feet from a seated posture on the floor. They rise to their knees, extend their legs and arms, grasp the lower part of their legs with their hands, and gradually push themselves upward in a self-climbing procedure. This maneuver is referred to as *Gower's sign* and is one of the most characteristic signs of muscular dystrophy (Fig. 32-5). The genetic background of the family, the history and examination of the child revealing the progressive nature of the

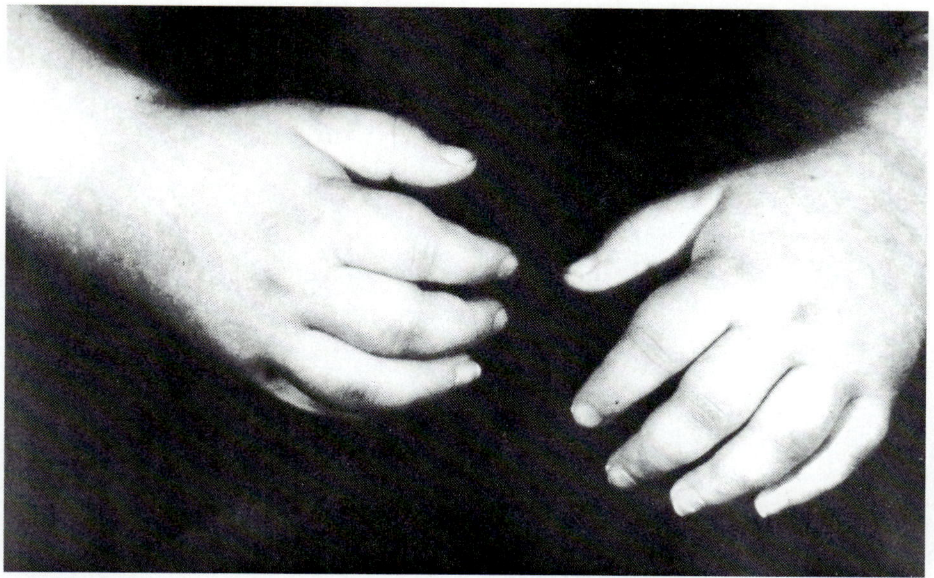

Fig. 32-6 Juvenile rheumatoid arthritis. Spindle-shaped fingers in 2½-year-old boy. (Courtesy Naval Hospital, San Diego, Calif.)

disease, serum enzyme tests, electromyogram, and muscle biopsy confirm the diagnosis. Muscle biopsy is especially valuable in determining the exact type of muscular problem. It is currently possible to diagnose preclinical cases through determination of serum enzyme levels. Counseling of affected families and potential carriers is an important preventive measure.

A diagnosis of muscular dystrophy (no matter what type) is difficult for parents to accept. The term alone produces anxiety and fear in parents, so it must be emphasized that nonprogressive and indeed treatable muscle disorders may mimic Duchenne's. Only with confirmation by available techniques should parents be informed of this diagnosis. Duchenne's muscular dystrophy is a tragic model of neuromuscular disease. Life expectancy is late adolescence to young adulthood. Death often results from respiratory weakness and intervening infection. The course of the disease is downhill, and it is particularly disheartening for parents to see their child confined to a wheelchair or immobilized in bed. Much can be gained if parents can meet together to share their common stressors and to learn from one another how certain problems can be met. The Muscular Dystrophy Association sponsors numerous clinics for these children.

The nurse sees the child with muscular dystrophy in the hospital setting chiefly at the time of diagnosis. He or she may also see the child when orthopedic appliances, such as braces and splints, are being evaluated or when the child is admitted for other health problems that make home nursing difficult.

Juvenile rheumatoid arthritis

The most common form of chronic arthritis encountered in pediatrics is juvenile rheumatoid arthritis (JRA). This disease is grouped with the collagen vascular diseases and affects the child's overall health pattern. The three major types of JRA are (1) a systemic form, characterized by fever, rash, internal organ involvement, and arthritis; (2) a polyarticular form (arthritis in numerous large and small joints); and (3) a pauciarticular form (arthritis in only a few joints). The arthritis manifests itself with joints that become swollen, stiff, painful with movement, and occasionally warm. The arthritis may involve the knee or ankle or nearly all joints. The fingers often assume a spindle shape, as a result of edema of the middle joint (Fig. 32-6).

Signs and symptoms of JRA other than arthritis can occur, particularly in the systemic form, and may include enlargement of the liver, spleen, and lymph nodes, anemia, anorexia, pallor, and a salmon-colored, blotchy rash. Pericarditis and myocarditis are seen occasionally. Fever may be a significant manifestation of the disease. The child's temperature may swing daily, reaching as high as 105° F (40.5° C) in the evening and return to normal by morning. The pattern on the temperature chart is usually characteristic and of great value in diagnosing systemic JRA.

Uveitis is a complication of juvenile rheumatoid arthritis in about 5% of patients. Inflammation in the anterior chamber of the eye can occur with no symptoms; therefore children with JRA need to be

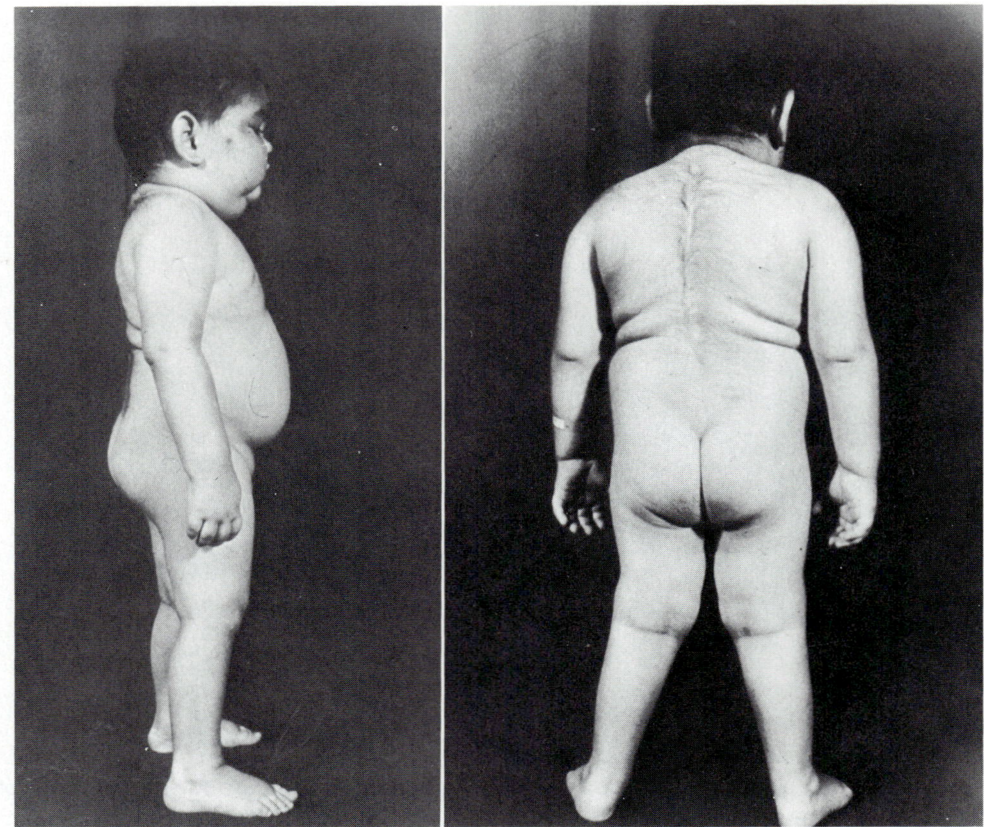

Fig. 32-7 Hypercortisonism in 2½-year-old boy as result of intensive steroid therapy. Note moon facies, excessive growth of hair (hirsutism), prominent fat pads, buffalo hump, and marked weight gain. (Courtesy Naval Hospital, San Diego, Calif.)

followed on a regular basis by an ophthalmologist. Uveitis can be so severe that blindness can result.

Antiinflammatory medications, physical and occupational therapy, kind and understanding parental support, and promotion of general health all are important aspects of therapy. Nonsteroidal antiinflammatory drugs (NSAIDs) are the drugs of choice to relieve pain, reduce swelling, and increase range of motion. When aspirin is used, it is prescribed four times daily at high doses. Blood salicylate levels are evaluated to ensure that proper doses are given. Children are carefully monitored and the parents cautioned about early signs of toxicity (p. 405). NSAIDs other than aspirin, such as ibuprofen, tolmetin, and naproxen, are beginning to be used more often because of their lower toxicity and less frequent dose requirements as compared with aspirin. These drugs can be just as effective as aspirin when used in significant doses and do not require blood level monitoring. They do require instruction regarding possible side effects.

A second drug for treatment of patients with JRA is gold salts. This medication, often given in addition to an NSAID, can slowly relieve joint symptoms in difficult cases. It is given weekly usually by injection, although it is now available in oral form. Renal and hematological complications can occur with gold therapy, so a complete blood cell count and urinalysis are performed before each dose of gold.

In rare instances, prednisone or other corticosteroids may also be used for the treatment of JRA, particularly in systemic disease, refractory polyarticular disease, and uveitis. Steroids can greatly alleviate the symptoms of arthritis but do not affect the basic disease process. The usefulness of steroids is limited by their toxicity. Unwanted manifestations of such hormone therapy include decalcification of the skeleton, altered tissue response to infections and other injuries, personality changes, moon face, obesity, and excessive body hair (Fig. 32-7). The JRA patient is likely to assume positions of comfort, which, if maintained for prolonged periods, can cause deformities that interfere with motions necessary for meeting the needs of daily living. Mobility should be encouraged as much as can be tolerated even during periods of active disease and inflammation. When pain and inflammation are suppressed by NSAIDs, children are then encouraged to ambulate and resume as close to normal activities as possible.

The most effective, continuous therapeutic exercise program is provided through the child's own play activities. Play activities should be directed to provide the maximum exercise for the joints most involved. The physical therapist can teach children and their parents exercises designed to give improved range of motion in each joint. Play activity and formal exercises help prevent the stiffness and deformity that result from inactivity. JRA often gradually improves over a period of years, and usually subsides in the teen years. In rare cases, it may persist actively into adulthood. Even though JRA often "burns out" eventually, children can be left with difficult, lifelong joint deformities as a result of their years of active disease.

Orthopedic complications of hemophilia

The subject of damaged joints should not be completely closed without at least mentioning another interesting cause of joint difficulty. The child with hemophilia, the classic bleeder, may sustain considerable joint destruction because of "insignificant injuries" followed by hemorrhages into the joints of the knees and elbows. At times these children must be placed in traction and protective casts to treat this problem.

Preschool Child

Legg-Calvé-Perthes disease (coxa plana)

Legg-Calvé-Perthes disease is a self-limited disease of the hip produced by lack of circulation to the femoral head. The initial degeneration of the femoral head is followed by absorption and regeneration of bone. The entire process takes an average of 4 years.

This developmental disease of the hip is commonly seen in children between 4 and 8 years of age and has a much higher incidence in boys. Usually the initial complaint is a limp of several months' duration. Some children have a limp with pain (referred to the knee) that is aggravated by activity and relieved by rest. The primary cause of Legg-Calvé-Perthes disease is unknown. Trauma and synovitis of the hip have preceded some cases. A great variety of treatments has been used in the past, including 4 years of bed rest. Modern successful treatment of the disease centers around two basic principles: (1) maintaining full range of motion and (2) keeping the femoral head deep in the socket during its period of healing. In this way the physician seeks to obtain a femoral head that fits well and to prevent the development of degenerative arthritis in the later years.

Treatment consists of traction until symptoms are resolved, followed by hip bracing in an abducted and slightly internally rotated position to maintain properly the femoral head in the acetabulum. Such bracing removes pressure from the avascular head of the femur. It helps to keep the child ambulatory with the least discomfort and limitation of activity during the years of necessary management. Surgery on the pelvis or femur may be indicated in the more severe cases of Legg-Calvé-Perthes disease. In general the younger child at the time of diagnosis has a more favorable prognosis for development of a normal hip.

Osteomyelitis

Inflammatory bone conditions caused by disease-producing organisms were more common in the past. With the increased availability of different types of antibiotics, osteomyelitis (inflammation of the bone resulting from infectious agents) has decreased remarkably. Osteomyelitis can result from various types of infection, but *Staphylococcus aureus* is the most common invading organism. Less common causes are *H. influenzae,* group A *beta-hemolytic streptococcus,* and *Mycobacterium tuberculosis.*

Osteomyelitis is sometimes preceded by some type of local injury to the bone that either introduces the organism directly or weakens the bone so that it is more susceptible to any offending organisms brought to the area by the bloodstream from some distant source of infection. Blood-borne infections are most common. Boys are more frequently affected than girls. Fever and pain near the end of a long bone are clinically associated with osteomyelitis. The characteristic pain is initially very severe and unremitting because pressure is building up in a closed space. Pseudoparalysis is a common presenting symptom in the young child who refuses to move the affected area because of pain. When purulent drainage begins to track out under the periosteum, the area is extremely tender, more so than a fracture. Treatment is started on the basis of the clinical examination alone. The child is placed on a regimen of bed rest, and the affected limb is immobilized. Analgesics are given to lessen the pain. Although blood cultures are positive in only 50% of patients with osteomyelitis, they are taken immediately and during the first few days after examination in the hope of identifying the causative organism. Aspiration and culture of fluid at the suspected site of infection, and radionuclide bone scans may also aid in the specific diagnosis.

Initially large doses of broad-spectrum intravenous antibiotics are given. X-ray evidence of osteomyelitis is not seen for 10 days after the onset of symptoms. Surgery is considered necessary if improvement is not seen within 36 to 48 hours after antibiotic therapy is instituted. The area of maximum tenderness is drilled to decompress the bone and to allow the purulent drainage to drain. The organism responsible for the infection is identified, and a cast may be applied to the affected limb. Intravenous antibiotic therapy is continued for another 1 to 6 weeks. A central venous catheter may be inserted to enable antibiotic therapy at home. During this time progress of the infection may be monitored by frequent sedimentation rates. When the results of this test are nearly normal, antibiotics can be stopped, with the hope that the risk of chronic osteomyelitis and extensive bone damage has been minimized.

School-age Child

Bone tumors

Some of the symptoms of infectious osteomyelitis are duplicated when the cause is not pathogenic organisms but the development of abnormal cells producing a tumor within the bone. Some of these masses of abnormal tissue are *benign* and of purely local importance. They may cause pain, at times accompanied by fever and deformity. These tumors may weaken the structure of the bone, but they do not spread (metastasize) to distant parts of the body. Other types of bone tumors grow rapidly and metastasize early through the bloodstream. These tumors are *malignant*. An osteosarcoma originates in connective tissue (of which bone is one example) and is the most common primary malignant tumor of bone. School-age boys are affected almost twice as often as girls.

The most common sites are characterized by active epiphyseal growth (for example, the distal end of the femur and the proximal ends of the tibia and humerus). Initially the child complains of mild pain in the affected part, but in a matter of days to weeks, the pain is constant and severe. As the condition progresses, the tumor mass becomes obvious. Limitation of adjacent joint motion is common. Early diagnosis and immediate treatment are crucial.

X-rays are characteristic, but the diagnosis of bone tumor is made only after biopsy and pathological studies of the tissue. Occasionally tumors of the bone in children may be secondary to tumors located elsewhere. When a tissue of bony origin is malignant, aggressive anticancer chemotherapy and radical methods of treatment, including amputation, must be endorsed in an effort to save the child. The prognosis has been vastly improved with recent advances in surgical treatment combined with multiple drug chemotherapy. Various limb salvage procedures have been developed to allow removal of bone tumors with maintenance of good form and function. The most recent development involves the use of an expandable internal prosthesis that can be lengthened as the child grows.

Spinal curvature

Scoliosis (S-shaped lateral curvature), kyphosis (exaggerated thoracic curvature), and lordosis (exaggerated lumbar curvature) are abnormal types of spinal curvature.

Scoliosis. Of the three kinds of abnormal spinal curvatures, scoliosis (lateral curvature) is probably the most common spinal deformity encountered in childhood. Lateral curvature of the spine can be divided into two major groups: nonstructural (functional) and structural. The patient can voluntarily correct a nonstructural curve by altering position. In functional scoliosis, a condition outside the spine (such as poor posture, pain or muscle spasm, or short leg) can cause a temporary misalignment of the vertebrae. A structural scoliosis is an irreversible lateral curvature that leads to permanent anatomical changes unless early preventive measures are taken.

Three basic types of structural scoliosis are seen: congenital, paralytic, and idiopathic. Congenital scoliosis results when one side of the vertebral column grows faster than the other. Surgical correction at 1 or 2 years of age may be indicated to prevent greater asymmetrical growth. Paralytic scoliosis may result from poliomyelitis, Duchenne's type of muscular dystrophy, myelomeningocele, or other neuromuscular disorders.

To prevent respiratory complications, some type of stabilization of the spine must be considered either through external support or surgery. Idiopathic scoliosis is the most common type, accounting for 80% of the cases classified as structural. It is called idiopathic because the cause is unknown. However, there seems to be a definite familial tendency that suggests a dominant inheritance pattern. The condition is more common in girls and is most apparent during adolescence, although it usually begins much earlier. The level of the curve may be cervical, thoracic, lumbar, or a combination of these. The most important aspect of the deformity is its progression with skeletal growth. As the lateral curvature and rotation of the spine increases, permanent secondary changes develop in the vertebrae and ribs. Misalignment of the spinal joints worsens and eventually leads to painful degenerative spinal joint disease in adulthood. In addition to a "crooked back" with a high shoulder and prominent hip, the deformity of the spine may compromise cardiopulmonary function and shorten the patient's life expectancy. The progression of the curvature is slow and steady, seldom arousing the concern of the

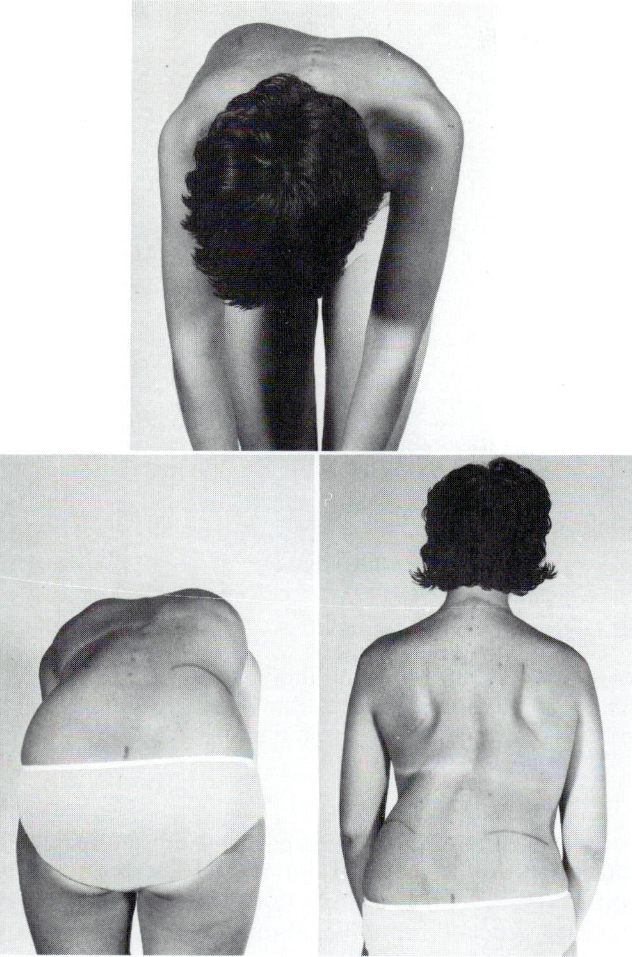

Fig. 32-8 Idiopathic scoliosis in 14-year-old girl seen in first visit to orthopedist. Screening positions: standing and forward bend. Observe for (1) general posture and alignment of spine: (a) lateral angulation and (b) balance of head, neck, and shoulders over pelvis; and (2) asymmetry: (a) exaggerated flank crease—more prominent on opposite side, (b) high shoulder, (c) position of scapulae, (d) convexity on side of major curve (caused by protruding ribs), (e) prominent hip, and (f) one arm longer than other when hanging free in forward bend position. (Courtesy Naval Hospital, San Diego, Calif.)

parent or child. Poor posture, an uneven hemline, and inability to get a proper fit in clothing are common complaints that cause the parents to bring the child in for evaluation.

Because pain is not associated with the progressive curve, the deformity often reaches 30 degrees before it is detected. The deformity can be clinically evaluated in three positions (Fig. 32-8). Radiological studies confirm the extent of the deformity. The primary (major) curve is greatest in angulation and is the least flexible.

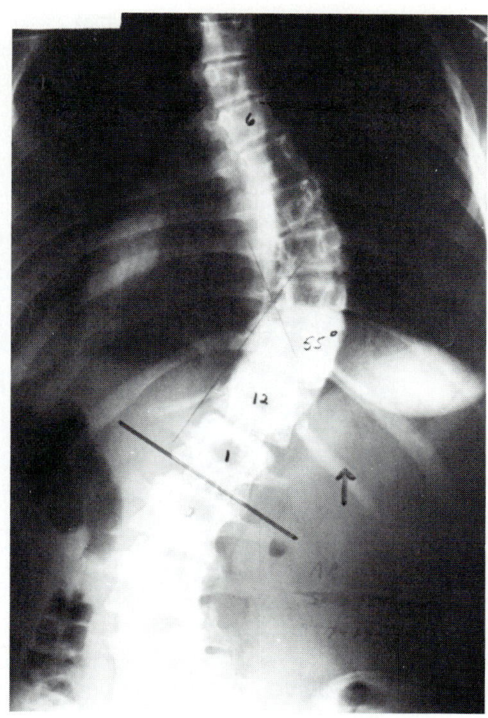

Fig. 32-9 Radiograph of 14-year-old girl (same as in Fig. 32-8) shows 55-degree right thoracic curve of spine. (Courtesy Naval Hospital, San Diego, Calif.)

Nursing Alert

Scoliosis screening programs should begin before 10 years of age and include boys as well as preadolescent girls. It is most important to detect the curve before puberty and its associated period of rapid skeletal growth. School nurses play a major role in scoliosis screening.

It is always more marked than would be expected from the physical appearance (Fig. 32-9).

Screening. The only sure way of preventing the severe curvatures of idiopathic scoliosis, which usually involve major surgical procedures and their inherent risk, is early recognition. The presence of a mild deformity allows the use of reliable, safe, effective nonsurgical treatment. Most children who demonstrate a curve at 11 or 12 years of age have almost always had it for a number of years.

Treatment. An orthopedist should determine the need for correction and examine the child with scoliosis at regular intervals to detect any progression of the curve. Curves up to 20 degrees can probably be left alone and watched. Curves between 20 and 40 degrees and progressing are stabilized with a brace.

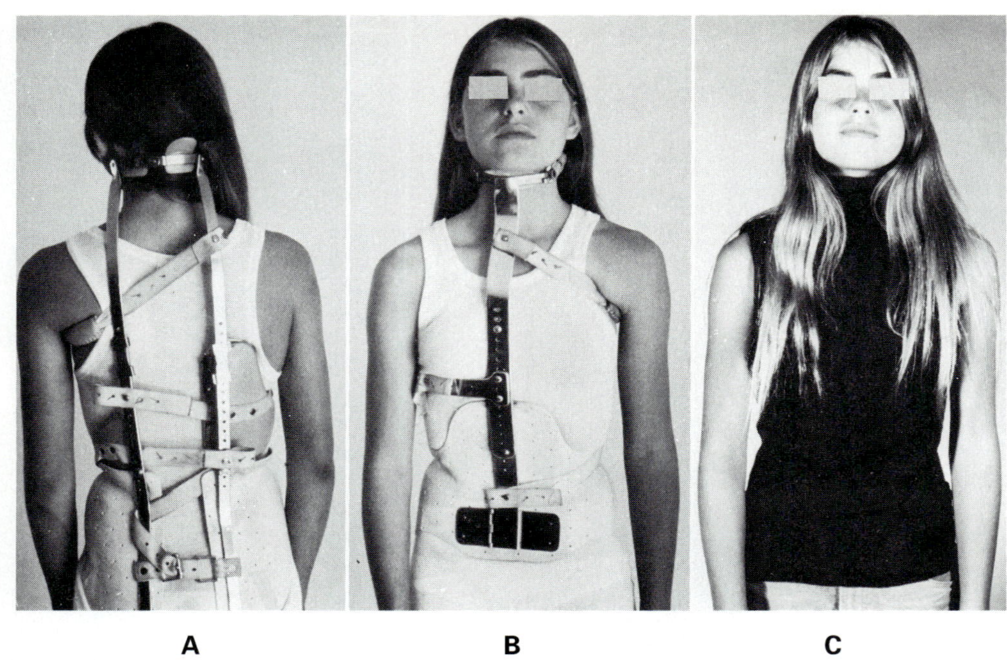

Fig. 32-10 ***A,*** Thirteen-year-old girl wearing Milwaukee brace with right thoracic pad, left axillary sling, and left lumbar pad. Overall alignment is good. ***B,*** Same child, front view. Brace is contoured closely to body. ***C,*** Brace can be worn under clothing without being noticed.

Milwaukee braces. The *Milwaukee brace* (Fig. 32-10) is a device used in the nonoperative treatment of high spinal curvatures. It is designed to provide dynamic correction that incorporates a vertical pushing force between the head and pelvis through adjustable, rigid uprights, as well as a lateral corrective force directed toward the convex side of the major curve. The brace is well contoured and cosmetically acceptable.

To prevent worsening of the scoliosis, it is necessary to wear the brace full time for several years until complete maturation of the spine has occurred. Prevention of progression of the curve is likely when treatment is begun at an early age. Normal activities (such as bike riding and skating) are encouraged while wearing the brace. In fact, an active exercise program is required to maintain good muscle tone. Most children learn to accept and live with the brace and have good results. Underarm braces are used with lower spinal curves as an alternative to the Milwaukee brace. Brace removal for personal hygiene measures is acceptable.

Surgical correction is usually considered for curves that are over 40 degrees. Surgery offers the best outcome for (1) curves that are cosmetically objectionable (over 60 degrees) in the preadolescent or postadolescent child, (2) for maximal respiratory function, and (3) a growing child in whom conservative measures have failed. The operation consists of a spinal fusion supplemented by the insertion and spinal attachment of an internal apparatus. The Harrington rod serves to obtain correction and to provide an internal type of immobilization (Fig. 32-11). Recent advances in surgical technique involve more flexible rods and several points of attachment. This technique allows earlier stabilization and recuperation and a more normal body contour. After spinal fusion the patient may be placed in a corset, body cast, or brace postoperatively; then progressive ambulation is encouraged (Fig. 32-12). Complete union and maturation at the fusion site may take up to 1 year.

Spinal fusion. Casts, which may be worn for an extended period after a spinal fusion, make turning the child much simpler and safer. However, if a cast is not applied after a spinal fusion, care must be exercised so that the spinal column is not twisted during changes in position. The child's bed should be kept flat unless specific permission has been granted to allow the child to be on a slight incline while in *supine* position (on the back). A noncasted child who is allowed to be turned should be gently log-rolled from back to side with the use of a turning sheet and at least two health care providers. Such a child, casted or not, who is turned from the back to a side-lying position, should have a pillow between the thighs to prevent the adduction of the top leg and pull on the small of the back. Just how much motion is allowed depends on the patient's

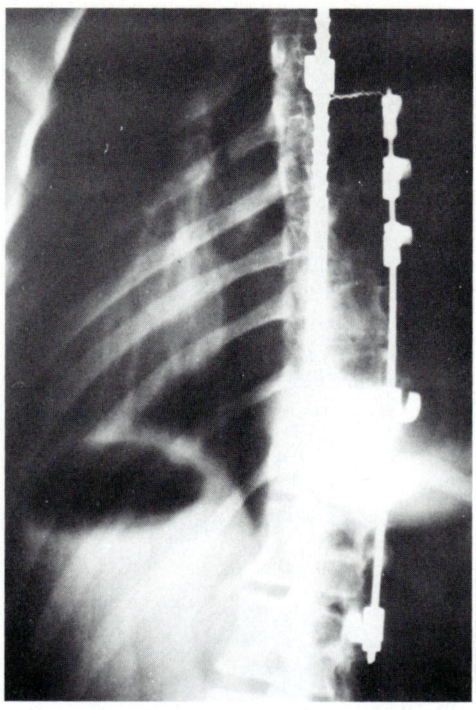

Fig. 32-11 Radiograph of back of patient in Fig. 32-8, 6 months after spinal fusion and Harrington instrumentation. (Courtesy Naval Hospital, San Diego, Calif.)

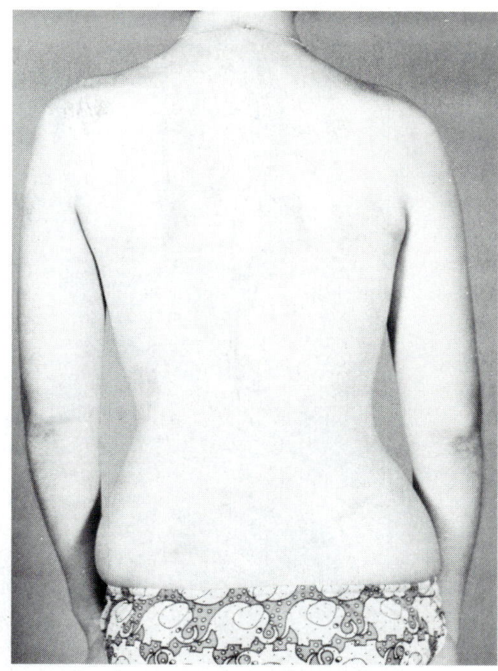

Fig. 32-12 Postoperative standing position shows spine reasonably well compensated (same child Fig. 32-8). (Courtesy Naval Hospital, San Diego, Calif.)

orders. Assessment for nerve damage from the surgery is important to consider, especially in the early postoperative period.

Children who have had a spinal fusion need the same basic preoperative and postoperative care required for all surgical patients. In addition, they need the special attention necessary for all casted patients (Chapter 33). Constipation is a particular problem; therefore the type of diet, fluid intake, and usual time of elimination should be assessed.

Therapy for severe scoliosis is usually long-term. It characteristically involves innumerable visits to the physician for evaluation, hospitalization at intervals for cast changes, brace adjustments or surgical interventions, and physical therapy. The parents and child (young woman or man) must be constantly encouraged to continue treatment faithfully until optimum, lasting results are achieved.

NERVOUS SYSTEM DISEASES AFFECTING BONES AND MUSCLES

Infant

Seizure disorders

The term *convulsive seizure* denotes an excessive and disorderly impulse discharge from nervous tissue, resulting in involuntary muscular activity or lapses in consciousness. It is really not a diagnosis but simply a description of a transient disturbance of the central nervous system (Fig. 32-13). As noted, seizures are caused by a number of conditions. Significant fever may be the precipitating cause, especially in children aged 6 to 36 months. Seizures also originate from congenital brain deformities or increased intracranial pressure caused by tumors, abscess formation, or edema of the brain. Cerebral irritation resulting from toxic or infectious agents may be implicated.

A chronic or recurrent convulsive disorder may also be called *epilepsy*. Some writers reserve the term *epilepsy* for recurrent convulsions of the idiopathic variety (cases of unknown cause). Opinions differ regarding the role of heredity in idiopathic seizures. Some authorities believe that heredity may be a significant cause. Because some states and communities have laws limiting the activities of those persons who have been diagnosed as epileptic and because the public does not always understand what the word means in a specific case, health care providers hesitate to use this term when describing the child's problem. It is estimated that approximately 1% of the population has some type of epileptic disorder. An additional 2% have had febrile seizures.

The two main types of seizures are partial and generalized (Table 32-1). Children with partial seizures

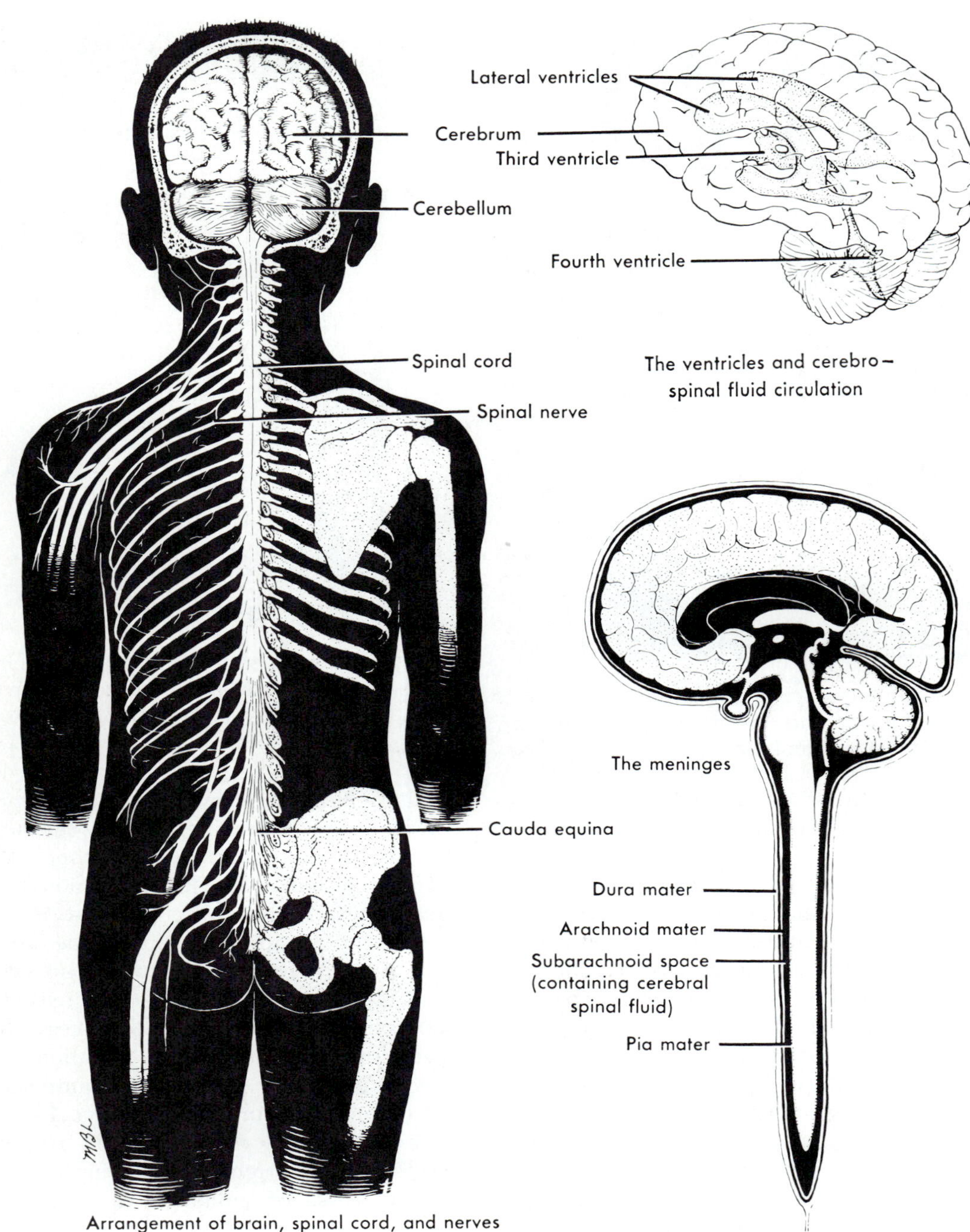

Fig. 32-13 Simplified central nervous system anatomy and peripheral nerve relationships.

experience focal symptoms such as motor, sensory, or experiential phenomena. Partial seizures are called *simple partial* if there is no loss of consciousness and *partial complex* if consciousness is impaired. Seizures are classified according to specific signs and/or symptoms (see Table 32-1). The generalized, tonic-clonic type represents one half of all seizure disorders, and the absence type, also known as petit mal, represents about 10% of all seizure disorders.

About 20% of epileptics have mixed seizure disorders, which manifest characteristics of more than one type. Generalized or tonic-clonic seizures affect the large muscle groups of the body. Usually the entire body becomes involved in dramatic, involuntary muscular contractions of considerable force. Absence seizures, on the other hand, are characterized by brief losses of consciousness revealed perhaps only by a prolonged blank stare or by minor tremors or the

◆ TABLE 32-1
Classification of Seizures

Type of Seizure	Clinical Manifestation
Partial	Begins locally
1 Simple	Without loss of consciousness
a With motor symptoms	Focal motor (Jacksonian seizure)
b With somatosensory or special sensory	Abdominal disturbances or visual, auditory, and olfactory symptoms and/or dizziness
2 Complex	With impairment of consciousness (temporal lobe or psychomotor)
Generalized	Bilateral, symmetrical onset
1 Absence	Brief loss of awareness (petit mal)
2 Tonic-clonic	Major tonic-clonic motor activity (grand mal)
3 Infantile spasms	Myoclonic (brief symmetrical flexion of head or trunk with mild clonus of arms and legs)
4 Atonic	Sudden loss of postural tonic and consciousness

dropping of an object held in the hand. The frequency of either type of seizure can be variable. A child may experience a seizure rarely or many times during a 24-hour period. Diagnosis is aided by a study of the child's brain waves, or an electroencephalogram (EEG). Children who have tonic-clonic seizures may experience a subjective warning of an impending episode. Such a warning is called an *aura.* It usually occurs a few minutes before the attack. It may come in the form of a vague feeling of uneasiness or as some type of sensory cue. For example, the child may hear, see, or smell things in a particular manner. Such auras are useful because the child can seek out places of safety and privacy if they are forewarned of an attack. In small children the presence of an aura may only be detected through the awareness of a child's repetitive actions, such as climbing into mother's lap, preceding a seizure.

The tonic-clonic seizure usually begins with a period of rigidity and temporary respiratory arrest. The first sign of an attack may be involuntary movements of the eyeball (eyes rolling upward or to the side) and a stiffening of body parts. The child temporarily suspends respirations and may become cyanotic. Saliva is not swallowed, and the child may drool and may utter a high-pitched cry. This first period, called the *tonic phase,* is usually followed by intermittent contractions of the muscles. This secondary period is the so-called *clonic phase.* During this time the tongue and lips may be bitten, and saliva, as a result, may be blood-tinged.

Nursing care. The nursing care of a child having a convulsion emphasizes the need to protect him or her from accidental injury and the importance of close observation and documentation. If possible, the child should be placed on the side or lie with face turned to one side to prevent aspiration. He or she should be placed in an area where the possibility of personal injury because of uncontrolled muscular contractions is at a minimum: on the floor on a rug, if possible, or in bed. The beds or cribs should be equipped with side rails padded with folded blankets or pillows. Most hospitals have discontinued use of a tongue blade unless ordered by a physician, and the Epilepsy Society does not advise placing anything into the person's mouth.

After first securing a safe position for the convulsing child, the nurse should focus the assessment on describing the preceding circumstances and the seizure itself. The following should be recorded:

1 The time the seizure began and what type of activity immediately preceded its occurrence;
2 What part of the body was first affected, the position of the eyes, and how the seizure progressed;
3 How long the seizure lasted and whether fever preceded or followed the attack;
4 Whether the child was incontinent;
5 Whether prolonged cyanosis or profuse saliva appeared (may signal the need for the use of oxygen or possible suctioning); and
6 What was the child's behavior and level of consciousness after the seizure?

In the majority of cases the seizure (ictus) subsides, and the child falls into a deep sleep called the *postictal state.* When awake again, the child may not remember the seizure but may feel tired and sore. Children should be reassured regarding the episode and be gently questioned to determine whether they had any warning, or aura, of the attack.

Almost all children who suffer from idiopathic epilepsy and many with organically initiated seizures receive some type of anticonvulsant therapy. A number of medications are available, prescribed according to

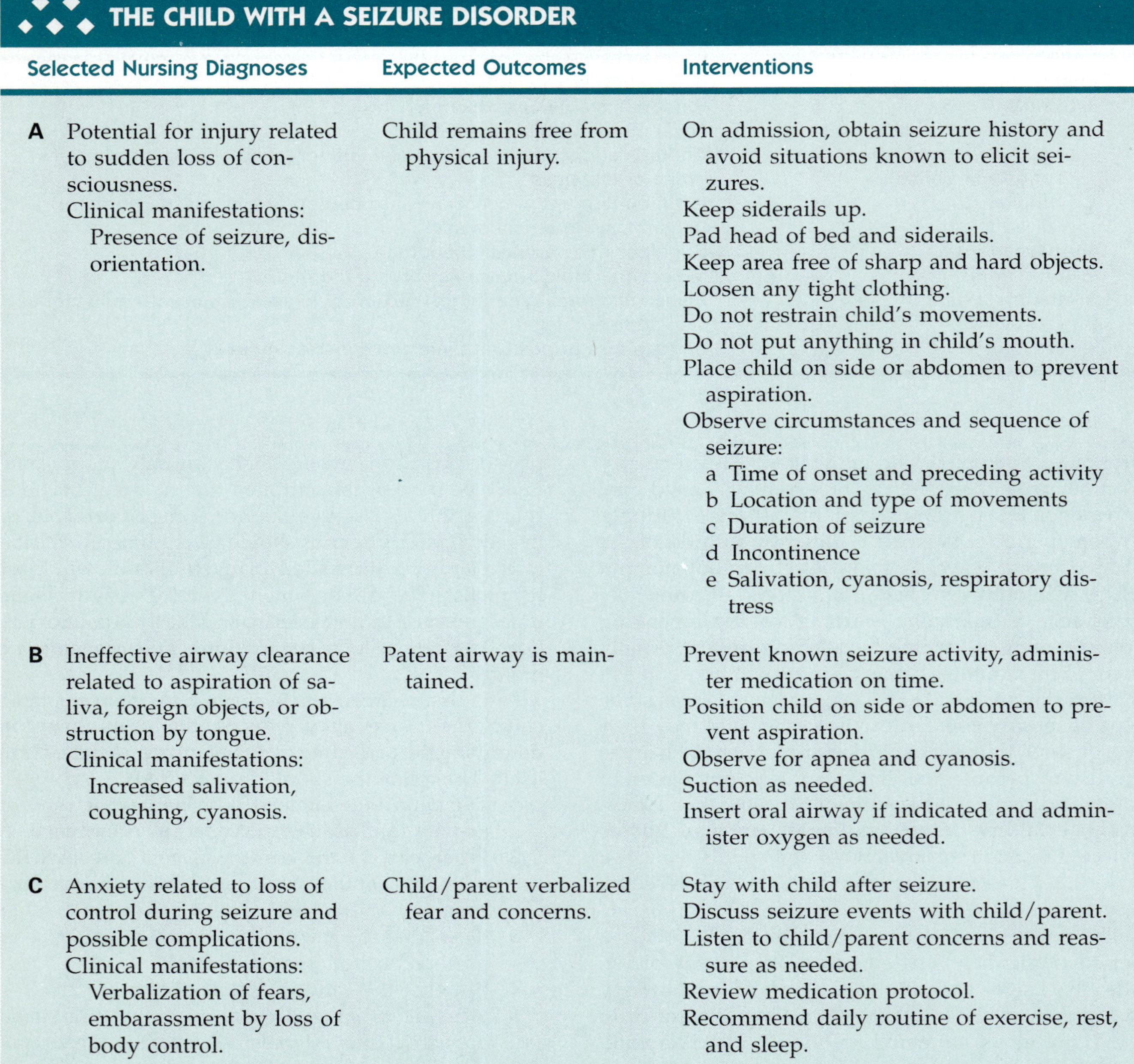

Nursing Care Plan
THE CHILD WITH A SEIZURE DISORDER

	Selected Nursing Diagnoses	Expected Outcomes	Interventions
A	Potential for injury related to sudden loss of consciousness. Clinical manifestations: Presence of seizure, disorientation.	Child remains free from physical injury.	On admission, obtain seizure history and avoid situations known to elicit seizures. Keep siderails up. Pad head of bed and siderails. Keep area free of sharp and hard objects. Loosen any tight clothing. Do not restrain child's movements. Do not put anything in child's mouth. Place child on side or abdomen to prevent aspiration. Observe circumstances and sequence of seizure: a Time of onset and preceding activity b Location and type of movements c Duration of seizure d Incontinence e Salivation, cyanosis, respiratory distress
B	Ineffective airway clearance related to aspiration of saliva, foreign objects, or obstruction by tongue. Clinical manifestations: Increased salivation, coughing, cyanosis.	Patent airway is maintained.	Prevent known seizure activity, administer medication on time. Position child on side or abdomen to prevent aspiration. Observe for apnea and cyanosis. Suction as needed. Insert oral airway if indicated and administer oxygen as needed.
C	Anxiety related to loss of control during seizure and possible complications. Clinical manifestations: Verbalization of fears, embarassment by loss of body control.	Child/parent verbalized fear and concerns.	Stay with child after seizure. Discuss seizure events with child/parent. Listen to child/parent concerns and reassure as needed. Review medication protocol. Recommend daily routine of exercise, rest, and sleep.

individual needs of the child. Some commonly used drugs to stop or control seizures are listed in Table 32-2. The time schedule established for taking anticonvulsants should be faithfully followed to prevent any interruption in treatment and the possible appearance of a seizure. Other methods to prevent seizures stress a high-fat–low-carbohydrate (ketogenic) diet.

Complete or almost complete control can be obtained in approximately one half of cases. The condition of many children can be well regulated with medical therapy, and these persons are able to live normal lives. A few types of epilepsy (for example absence seizures) may disappear after puberty; some change their form; others, unfortunately, persist throughout the person's life. The nurse should realize that tension, fatigue, illness, excitement, hyperventilation, blinking lights, and especially failure to take anticonvulsants or a change in anticonvulsant therapy may bring on certain seizures.

The child and family need ongoing emotional and

◆ TABLE 32-2
Anticonvulsant Guide

Medication and Therapeutic Blood Level	Indication for Use
Phenobarbital (15-40 μg/ml)	Tonic-clonic seizures Simple and complex partial seizures
Phenytoin (Dilantin) (10-20 μg/ml)	Tonic-clonic seizures Simple and complex partial seizures
Carbamazepine (Tegretol) (4-12 μg/ml)	Complex partial seizures Tonic-clonic seizures Simple partial seizures
Valproate (Depakene) (50-100 μg/ml)	Absence seizures Myoclonic seizures
Ethosuximide (Zarontin) (40-100 μg/ml)	Absence seizures
Clonazepam (Clonopin)	Absence seizures Myoclonic seizures (anticonvulsant not usually used)
Primidone (Mysoline) (4-12 μg/ml)	Complex partial seizures Tonic-clonic seizures
Clorazepate (Tranxene)	Partial and generalized seizures refractory to other medicines

informational support. The normal aspects of the child's life should be emphasized. The range of cognitive abilities of children with epilepsy is reflective of the general population. The epilepsy societies have provided considerable public education regarding seizure disorders, attempting to remove false ideas and any legislation that unjustly limits the activities of affected individuals.

Meningitis

Meningitis is inflammation of the meninges. Not all types of meningitis are infectious, but the infectious types are far more common.

Etiology

The *Haemophilus influenza* bacillus, meningococcus, and pneumococcus are common etiological agents responsible for acute bacterial meningitis in children past 1 month of age. Meningitis usually affects children under 2 years of age, and *H. influenza* is the most common causative agent. New research shows the *H. influenza* vaccine is reducing the incidence.

Assessment

Whatever the cause of or age at onset, the treatment of meningitis is always considered a medical emergency. Early recognition and prompt treatment are essential for a favorable recovery. A long and severe infection may result in permanent neurological damage or death (Fig. 32-14).

Typically the child is irritable and restless or drowsy. Previous upper respiratory tract infections and ear infections are frequently associated with *H. influenzae* meningitis. For this reason the nurse should impress on parents the importance of continuing medications (for otitis media or other infections) and all antibiotics prescribed for as long as ordered. *H. influenzae* meningitis was far more common before the initiation of the vaccine in infancy. Fever, vomiting, chills, headache, rigidity of the neck and back, and convulsions are common. In more severe cases the child may be in shock or may exhibit an involuntary arching of the back known as *opisthotonos*. A high-pitched cry is characteristic. Meningococcal meningitis is usually accompanied by petechiae, a hemorrhagic skin rash caused by meningococcal invasion of the bloodstream. However, meningococcemia may occur without central nervous system involvement.

Diagnosis

A lumbar puncture is performed at the slightest suspicion of meningitis. Both parents and children fear a lumbar puncture. Parents should be reassured of the importance, relative safety, and necessity of this procedure. Children, if conscious and old enough to understand, should be mentally prepared just before the procedure. They should be told what is going to happen and that they are likely to feel discomfort. Reminding them that it is important to lie still during the procedure can provide a sense of control and thereby reduce feelings of helplessness. During the procedure, the child should be told that it is okay to cry but that lying still is the best help. The assisting nurse must understand the importance of maintaining the position of the

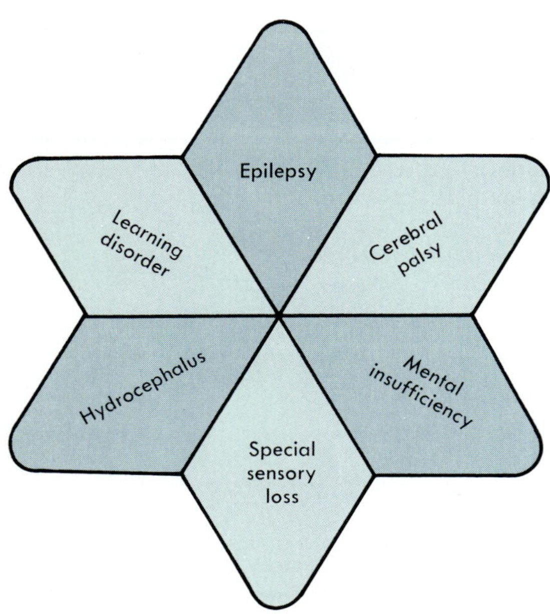

Fig. 32-14 Residual complications of meningitis may include any one or all of these conditions.

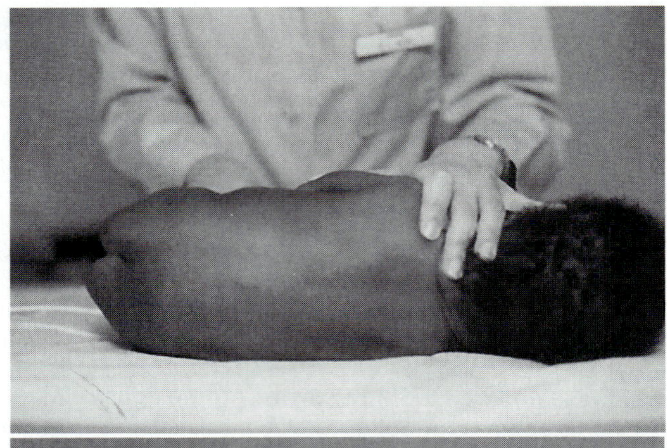

A

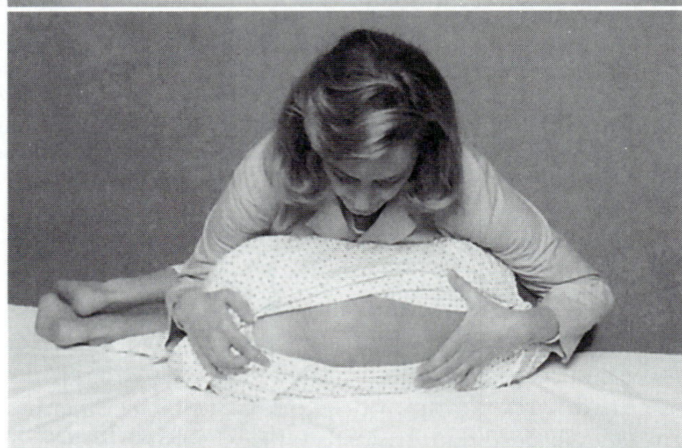

B

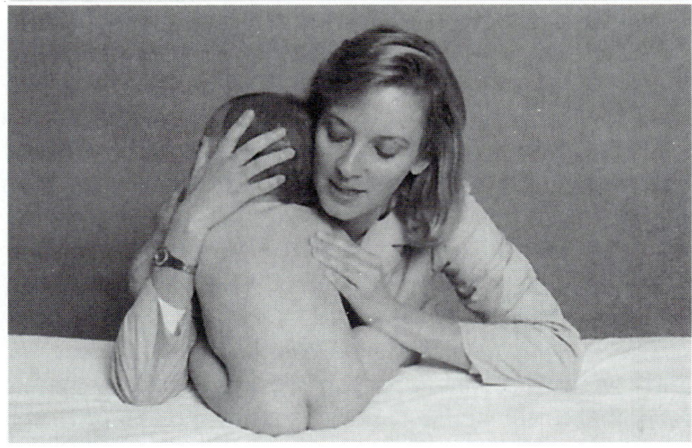

C

Fig. 32-15 Positioning for lumbar puncture. Adhere to universal precautions. (From Wong D: *Essentials of pediatric nursing,* ed 4, St. Louis, 1993, Mosby.)

child. Several holds are possible, depending on the size of the child; however, positioning the child on the side (lateral decubitus) is usually preferred (Fig. 32-15). The back of the patient is arched to provide greater room for the insertion of the needle between the vertebrae at the level of the iliac crest. The skin is prepared with an antiseptic by the gloved physician. At the time of the lumbar puncture the pressure of the fluid within the meninges can be measured by attaching a measuring tube or manometer to the spinal needle.

Three specimens of spinal fluid are collected consecutively in specially numbered sterile specimen containers using universal precautions. All three containers are sent to the laboratory where they should be immediately examined for cellular and chemical content. From the contents of the first tube, a Gram's stain and cultures are done to identify any organisms that may be present. Gram's stain may identify the structure of an organism at once, before the culture report. Countercurrent immunoelectrophoresis may often identify an organism within a few hours. Culture results usually take 24 to 48 hours. The second tube is examined for chemical content, usually glucose and protein. The third tube is examined for blood cell content. The selection of the third tube for this procedure reduces the possibility that minor bleeding from insertion of the needle will alter the cell count. At the conclusion of the puncture procedure, care should be taken to remove iodine-containing preparations that were used to prepare the skin. This prevents the occurrence of serious contact rashes. A bandage is placed over the site of the needle insertion.

Nursing care

The child is placed in respiratory isolation for 24 hours after the start of antibiotic therapy. The purpose of isolation and why the nurse wears a gown and mask should be explained to the parents.

Intravenous fluids are started as soon as the lumbar puncture is completed. Fourth generation cepha-

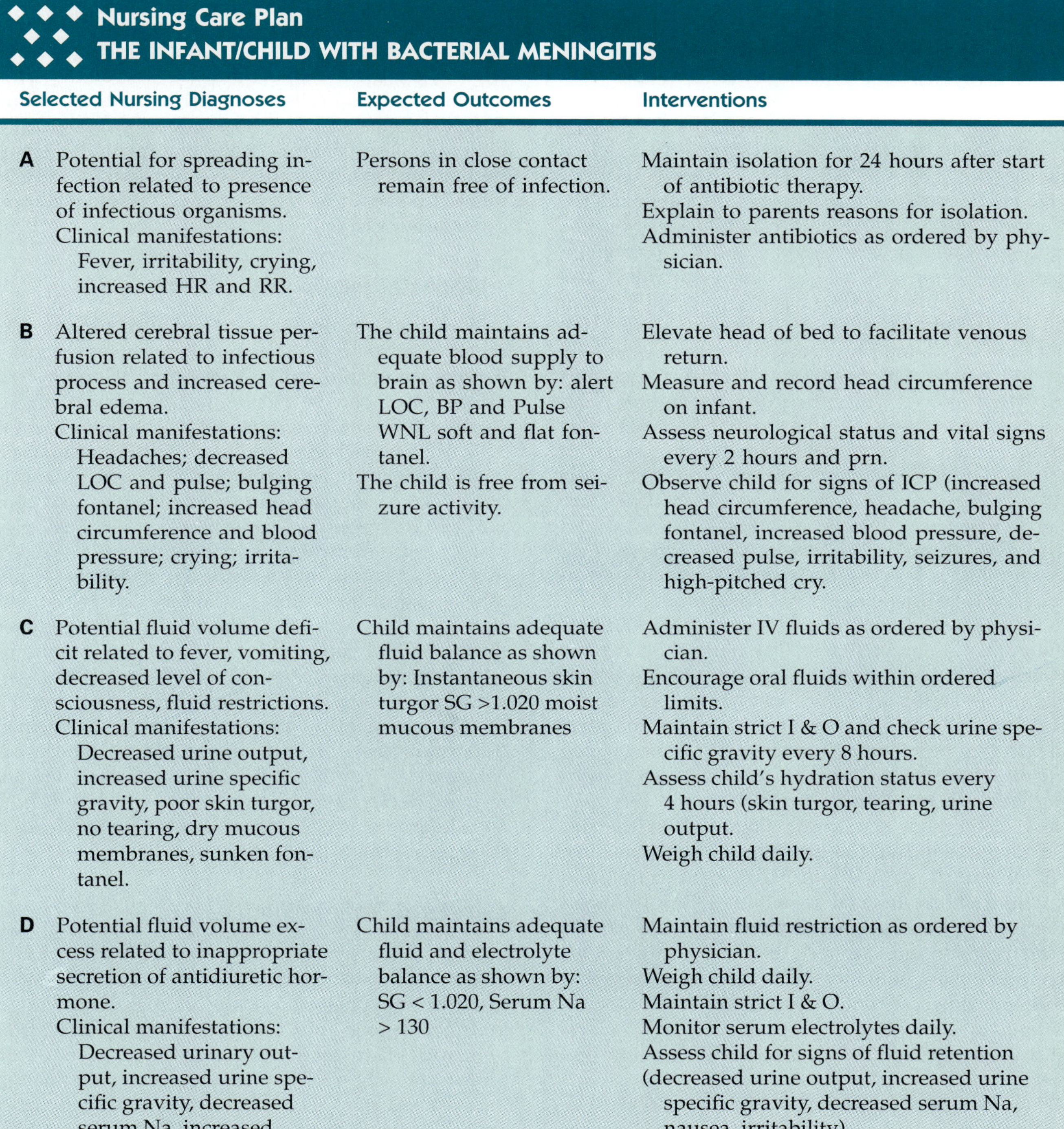

Nursing Care Plan
THE INFANT/CHILD WITH BACTERIAL MENINGITIS

	Selected Nursing Diagnoses	Expected Outcomes	Interventions
A	Potential for spreading infection related to presence of infectious organisms. Clinical manifestations: Fever, irritability, crying, increased HR and RR.	Persons in close contact remain free of infection.	Maintain isolation for 24 hours after start of antibiotic therapy. Explain to parents reasons for isolation. Administer antibiotics as ordered by physician.
B	Altered cerebral tissue perfusion related to infectious process and increased cerebral edema. Clinical manifestations: Headaches; decreased LOC and pulse; bulging fontanel; increased head circumference and blood pressure; crying; irritability.	The child maintains adequate blood supply to brain as shown by: alert LOC, BP and Pulse WNL soft and flat fontanel. The child is free from seizure activity.	Elevate head of bed to facilitate venous return. Measure and record head circumference on infant. Assess neurological status and vital signs every 2 hours and prn. Observe child for signs of ICP (increased head circumference, headache, bulging fontanel, increased blood pressure, decreased pulse, irritability, seizures, and high-pitched cry.
C	Potential fluid volume deficit related to fever, vomiting, decreased level of consciousness, fluid restrictions. Clinical manifestations: Decreased urine output, increased urine specific gravity, poor skin turgor, no tearing, dry mucous membranes, sunken fontanel.	Child maintains adequate fluid balance as shown by: Instantaneous skin turgor SG >1.020 moist mucous membranes	Administer IV fluids as ordered by physician. Encourage oral fluids within ordered limits. Maintain strict I & O and check urine specific gravity every 8 hours. Assess child's hydration status every 4 hours (skin turgor, tearing, urine output. Weigh child daily.
D	Potential fluid volume excess related to inappropriate secretion of antidiuretic hormone. Clinical manifestations: Decreased urinary output, increased urine specific gravity, decreased serum Na, increased weight, nausea, irritability.	Child maintains adequate fluid and electrolyte balance as shown by: SG < 1.020, Serum Na > 130	Maintain fluid restriction as ordered by physician. Weigh child daily. Maintain strict I & O. Monitor serum electrolytes daily. Assess child for signs of fluid retention (decreased urine output, increased urine specific gravity, decreased serum Na, nausea, irritability).

losporins are routinely started for broad-spectrum antibiotic coverage. When these are not available due to cost, ampicillin and gentamicin are the treatment of choice for meningitis and should be started immediately. A reduction in the incidence of hearing loss has been demonstrated by the use of steroids introduced early in the management of some form s of bacterial meningitis. Good supportive care requires that dehydration be avoided, but fluids may be limited to decrease the possibility of cerebral edema.

Effective restraints may be used to safeguard the infusion. The nurse should carefully position the restrained child in a side-lying position during intravenous therapy in case he or she convulses and aspirates vomitus. Constant nursing care and frequent observation of the child are necessary during the acute phase. Monitoring the vital signs is especially important when increased intracranial pressure is suspected. Slowed pulse, irregular respirations, and elevated blood pressure, which may be accompanied by an altered level of consciousness, are signs of increased intracranial pressure and should be called to the physician's attention at once. Cerebral pressure may be reduced by hyperventilating with a mask and bag, which decreases P_{CO_2}, by infusion of drugs, such as mannitol, or by surgical intervention. Such methods are often lifesaving.

The infant may be placed in an oxygen-enriched environment in an incubator. The older child may be placed on oxygen by nasal canula. Other nursing responsibilities include control of body temperature by sponging and maintenance of a quiet environment. Tylenol can be of great benefit to these very often irritable children, as long as care is taken not to interfere with monitoring the temperature response, which determines the length of antibiotic therapy. Accurately recording the intravenous intake and the urinary output is important. (Urinary retention and fecal impactions are real possibilities.) As the child progresses, the nurse may safely encourage the parents to hold their infant or toddler during intravenous therapy, allowing for body contact and love, as well as position change. Granting as much freedom from restraint and providing for psychological comforts (such as a pacifier) is consistent with therapy and safety.

The convalescent period should be long enough to permit the child to regain the previous physical status. Young children should be carefully reevaluated at intervals during the convalescence. Residual complications may include epilepsy, hydrocephalus, cerebral palsy (incoordination or weakness), mental insufficiency, special sensory loss, such as hearing and vision, and behavior or learning disorders.

Aseptic meningitis syndrome

The term *aseptic meningitis syndrome* includes a number of viral disorders that have an acute onset and usually a self-limited course with varying meningeal manifestations. Meningismus, meningeal irritation resulting in complications such as nuchal (neck) or spinal rigidity, is present. Lumbar puncture reveals abnormal numbers of blood cells and a sterile bacterial culture. To rule out other diseases, hospitalization for at least 48 hours for observation is necessary. Treatment is supportive and symptomatic. Like bacterial meningitis, follow-up should be provided, since residual complications can occur.

Neonatal meningitis

Newborns are frequent victims of meningitis. The organisms most often affecting these babies are group B streptococci followed by *Escherichia coli* and *Listeria*. Mixed infections in meningitis are almost always confined to the neonatal age group. About one in every 1000 to 2000 newborns is affected. These infections are often associated with low birth weight. Maternal infection, premature rupture of membranes, and complicated deliveries are often part of the obstetrical history. Signs of meningeal irritation are minimal. The infant characteristically is lethargic and irritable and refuses to suck. Vomiting, respiratory distress, convulsions, and temperature instability, including hyperthermia and hypothermia, are common symptoms. Fourth generation cephalosporins, ampicillin, gentamicin, and other medications are given intravenously. Intensive supportive nursing care is essential. Because of the difficulty in recognizing the disease early and the inability of the debilitated small infant to respond to treatment, survival may be as low as 60%, and children who do survive have a high incidence of residual complications.

Cerebral Palsy (Fig. 32-16)

Cerebral palsy is a nonprogressive disorder of motion and posture resulting from brain injury or insult during a period of early brain growth. It is not in itself a disease but a condition that may result from numerous diseases that damage those parts of the brain responsible for voluntary muscular coordination. Such causes may include pressure on the brain or oxygen deprivation to the brain before or during birth (cerebral anoxia), direct injury, embolus or hemorrhage, arrested hydrocephalus, and infection or toxicity occurring any time after birth. Cerebral palsy is usually diagnosed in infancy, since it is commonly caused by events associated with the prenatal or perinatal period. Treatment is directed toward limiting

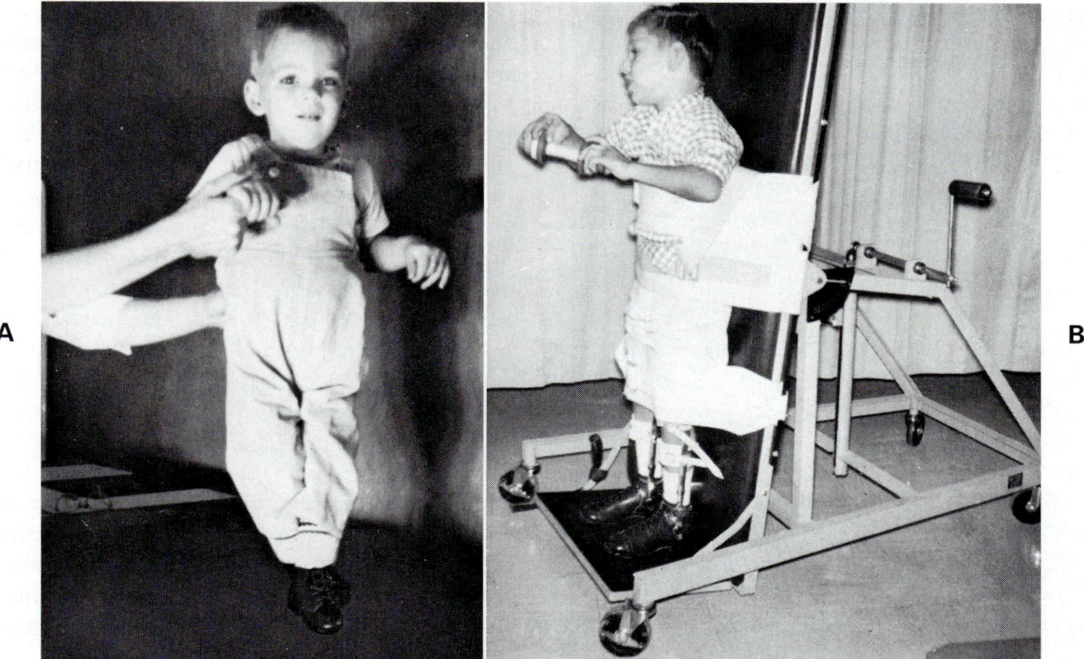

Fig. 32-16 This preschooler cannot walk without support. **A,** With support, scissors gait is present (one foot crossing the other caused by adductor spasticity). **B,** Many hours on tilt table, consistent therapy with a multidisciplinary health care team and parents have greatly strengthened this child's legs. (Courtesy Crippled Children Services, Department of Public Health, San Diego, Calif.)

the disability and may continue throughout the affected person's life. The disorder may be limited and mild or severe and far-reaching, involving many body functions. There are approximately 1.3 cases of cerebral palsy per 1000 persons in the general population.

The child with the disorder of movement called *cerebral palsy* may have injuries to the brain involving other functions. Some patients with cerebral palsy have associated seizures, mental insufficiency, behavior problems, special sensory difficulties, especially related to vision or hearing, and learning disturbances. The muscles of the mouth, tongue, and throat may be affected, influencing the ability to receive, chew, and swallow food, as well as speech and language.

Types of cerebral palsy (CP)

The box on p. 670 describes the types of cerebral palsy.

Nursing considerations

The care of children with cerebral palsy and their families requires a multidisciplinary team approach including: the nurses in the hospital, home, and primary care settings, the pediatrician, orthopedist, physical therapist, occupational therapist, speech pathologist, audiologist, psychologist, medical-social worker, public health workers, nurses, and educators.

These children and their families often have considerable emotional problems, which may be expressed in the way the parents treat the child and in their aspirations for the child's future. Parents may be overprotective and do too much for their child, making it difficult for him to master the skills of which they are capable. On the other hand, they may expect too much and cause painful frustrations. Parents may need help in establishing realistic goals and in providing an environment conducive to positive mental and physical health. That the problem is not inherited should be clarified early to decrease parental feelings of guilt.

Informational and emotional support provided by other parents and health care providers is invaluable. A hopeful aspect of cerebral palsy is that the initiating cause is not progressive in character, and so the neuromuscular involvement, with treatment, does not worsen. Cerebral palsy is not a degenerative disease like muscular dystrophies, and considerable improvement can usually be gained. Through physical and occupational therapy, surgical techniques, and medication, children with cerebral palsy are able to meet

TYPES OF CEREBRAL PALSY

1 The spastic type, the most common form, affecting 65% of the patients, is characterized by increased muscle stiffness or tone, exaggerated contraction of affected muscle groups when stimulated (stretch reflex), jerky motions, and a tendency to have contractures. The lower extremities are most often involved. A scissors gait is common.

Patterns of Spasticity

The following body patterns of spastic cerebral palsy are:

- **a.** *Hemiplegia,* involving two limbs (an arm and a leg) on the same side;
- **b.** *Double hemiplegia,* involving arms and legs on both sides, with one side more severely involved;
- **c.** *Quadriplegia,* involving all four limbs, with the legs slightly more affected;
- **d.** *Diplegia,* involving all four limbs, with the legs affected to a significantly greater degree.

2 Extrapyramidal (nonspastic) types, comprising about 15% of cases, are characterized by a variety of emotional, postural, and sleep states. This type includes the following:

- **a.** *Athetoid,* characterized by involuntary, uncoordinated, purposeless movements involving joint motion rather than single muscle action (The upper extremities are more often involved.);
- **b.** *Ataxic,* characterized by loss of a sense of balance and problems in evaluating spatial relationships and the relative positions of body parts;

3 Mixed type of cerebral palsy combines features of types 1 and 2 and represents about 20% of affected patients.

their daily personal needs and, in some cases, to prepare for self-supporting occupations. Special public school programs geared to meet the needs of disabled children are available in most communities. Children may attend regular public school classes as well as special sessions designed to meet their individual needs during the school day. The school nurse places an important role in coordinating their care.

When children with cerebral palsy are hospitalized, it is very important that the hospital staff know their capabilities as individuals. Information regarding successful feeding and dressing techniques, toileting practices, communication aids, and special challenges saves hours of frustration and distress. The care of children whose total neuromuscular involvement is slight requires little modification. The care of others requires considerable study and adjustment. Children with a history of seizures or upper extremity or head involvement should not have their temperatures taken orally until the safety of the procedure is evaluated.

Each child's diet must be evaluated to ensure that it is appropriate for his or her age, nutritional needs, and ability to handle and swallow. Although self-feeding may take considerable time and cause some disorder, these children should feed themselves as much as possible, using techniques they have been taught. Aids, such as swivel spoons, plate guards, training cups, and rocker knives, are invaluable (Fig. 32-17). Special weights can be attached to the child's arms to help control involuntary motion. Children may need patient, caring assistance with feeding. Since severely affected children may require the occasional use of suction, an apparatus should be available. During feedings, the nurse should hold the child in such a way that the child's arm closest extends behind him or her. This often causes the child's head to rotate comfortably to the same side (tonic neck reflex). Gentle support of the chin or stroking the neck on either side of the esophagus may help lip closure and swallowing. Some children who have difficulty swallowing find carbonated drinks a problem. Stirring until the carbonation is minimal or serving other types of liquid is helpful.

Excessive stimulation, sudden jarring movements, and the pressure of "having to hurry" induces greater tenseness and makes performance of relatively simple tasks arduous. These children find it very difficult to relax, and they become fatigued easily. The simplest kind of controlled movement may require a tremendous amount of concentration and energy.

When possible, the child with cerebral palsy should have contact with other children and should not be socially deprived. Contact with other youngsters is frequently limited. However, even those who have moderately severe muscular involvement often enjoy working with modeling clay, finger paints, large blocks, and hand puppets. Many enjoy music, television, and reading. An occupational therapist can work with the children to improve skills needed to meet everyday needs. These are presented to the young child in the form of games or special projects. Progress, though at times seemingly small, should be recognized and praised. The child usually responds to this recognition and continues efforts to improve.

Although it may seem to some critics that a tremendous amount of time, effort, and financial expense is expended in community programs to help youngsters with CP, such programs are rewarding. It is less expensive to educate individuals to

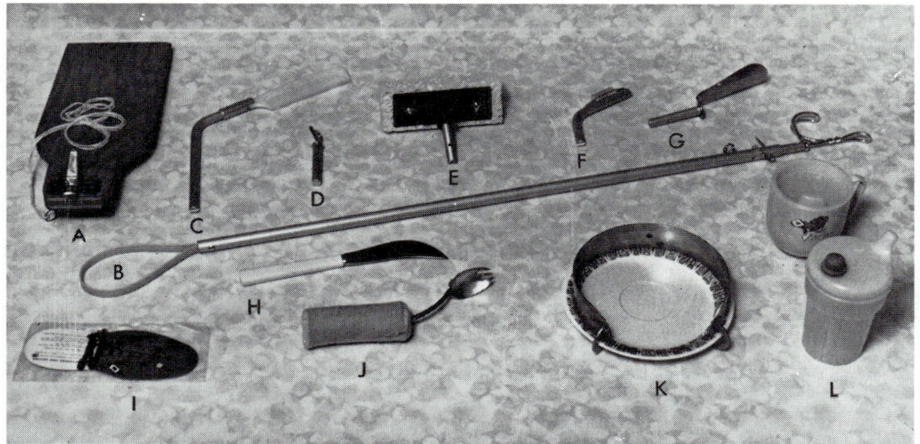

Fig. 32-17 Various aids for everyday activities for handicapped. ***A,*** Nail clippers on wooden base, operated by string and foot action; ***B,*** gadget stick with hook attachment; ***C,*** comb attachment; ***D,*** clip attachment; ***E,*** mop or sponge attachment; ***F,*** magnet attachment; ***G,*** shoehorn attachment; ***H,*** rocker knife; ***I,*** elastic shoelaces; ***J,*** built-up handle on swivel fork (Spork); ***K,*** plate and plate guard; ***L,*** two types of weighted "trainer cups." (Courtesy Children's Hospital and Health Center, San Diego, Calif.)

achieve their potential than to provide the type of state-supported custodial care offered in the past. Programs are designed to promote self-care and self-esteem and to provide emotional and informational support to children and families.

TODDLER

Encephalitis

Encephalitis is an inflammation of the brain (encephalon). When the inflammation involves both the meninges and the brain tissue, the condition is referred to as *encephalomyelitis.*

Encephalitis is characterized by personality change, headache, drowsiness, fever, and often convulsions. Cranial nerves may become paralyzed, affecting speech, swallowing, and protective airway reflexes. Double vision may also be reported. Encephalitis may produce the same complications as does meningitis.

Encephalitis is caused by infectious agents, most often viral. Probably the most common epidemic viral encephalitis is due to enteroviruses and the most common sporadically occurring viral encephalitis is due to herpes simplex. Some types of encephalitis are caused by viruses spread by vectors, such as mosquitoes, ticks, or mites. Encephalitis following rubeola (2-week measles) was relatively common before immunization programs were available, occurring once in every 600 to 1000 cases of measles.

Nursing care

Nursing care of a child with encephalitis is much like that of a child with meningitis. Lumbar punctures may be performed to relieve intracranial pressure, and pressure intracranial monitoring is frequently used. The difference between encephalitis and meningitis may not always be clinically demonstrated by symptoms. Differentiation is then made on the basis of laboratory examinations.

Lead Poisoning

Symptoms of encephalitis caused by toxic exposure are more properly referred to as *encephalopathy.* Lead exposure from ingestion or inhalation is significant in the United States. Lead poisoning (plumbism) is prevalent and preventable. All furniture and toys used by young children should be protected by nontoxic, lead-free paint. Although life-threatening encephalopathy is rare, many asymptomatic children have significant elevation of lead levels which can lead to neurological and intellectual damage. For the classification of risk and treatment for lead poisoning refer to Table 32-3.

PRESCHOOLER

Brain Tumors (Fig. 32-18)

Although brain tumors are not found as frequently in children as in adults, nervous system tumors are the second most common malignancy in children. Pediat-

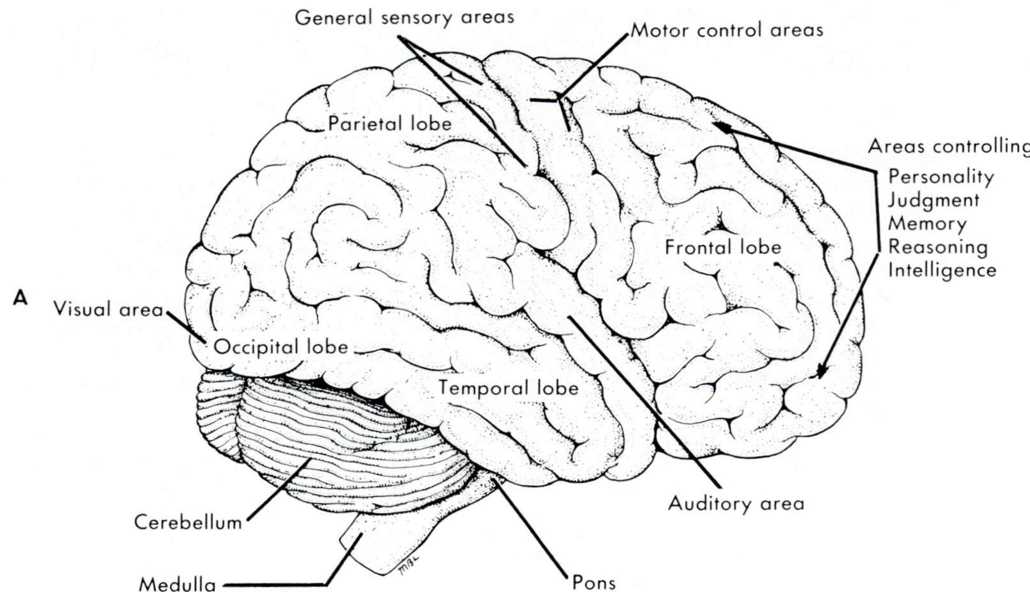

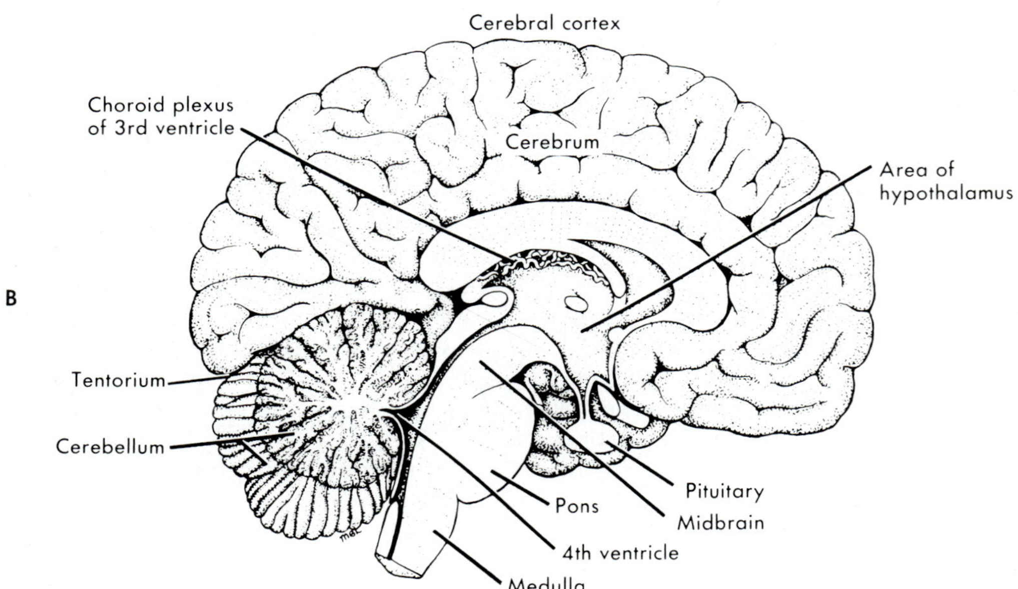

Fig. 32-18 ***A,*** Surfaces of brain showing cerebrum, cerebellum, pons, and medulla with identification of specialized areas of cerebral function. ***B,*** Simplified sagittal section of brain showing internal relationships. Brain tumors in children often involve the cerebellum.

ric brain tumors are situated rather deeply within the brain structure, making it difficult to ensure complete removal of the abnormal cells. About three fourths of brain tumors occurring in childhood involve the supportive connective tissue of the brain, called *glial cells.* The two most common gliomas are astrocytomas and medulloblastomas. Total resection of an infiltrating cerebral astrocytoma is seldom possible, but a cystic cerebellar astrocytoma is relatively slow-growing, usually encapsulated, and easier to remove.

Assessment

Early symptoms of a developing brain tumor may appear gradually in the case of a slowly progressing lesion. However, some tumors (for example, medullo-

◆ **TABLE 32-3**
Classification of Risk and Treatment for Lead Poisoning

Blood Lead Concentration (μg/dl)	Intervention
≤9	Child is not considered to be lead poisoned.
10-14	Many children with blood lead levels in this range should trigger community-wide childhood lead poisoning prevention activities. Children may need to be rescreened more frequently.
15-19	Child should receive nutritional and educational interventions and more frequent screening. If blood lead level persists in this range, environmental investigation and intervention should be done.
20-44	Child should receive environmental evaluation and remediation and a medical evaluation; may need pharmacological treatment of lead poisoning.
45-69	Child will need both medical and environmental interventions, including chelation therapy.
≥70	Child is a medical emergency; medical and environmental management must begin immediately.

Modified from Centers for Disease Control and Prevention: *Preventing lead poisoning in young children*, Atlanta, Ga., 1993.

blastomas) grow rapidly and cause remarkable signs and symptoms rather soon. The signs and symptoms are caused by increased intracranial pressure. They include headache, dizziness, lethargy, indifference, and irritability. Emesis occurs typically in the morning. This is the result of fluid and pressure shifts as the child moves from a recumbent to a standing position. After vomiting the child can eat a normal breakfast because there is no nausea. Double or blurred vision and speech problems are reported fairly often. The pupils may be abnormally or unequally dilated or slow to react to changes in light intensity. Balance and gait may be affected because 60% of childhood brain tumors are infratentorial and often involve the cerebellum, a part of the brain that plays a significant role in the maintenance of equilibrium (Fig. 32-18, *B*). Rigidity, tremors, or convulsions occasionally occur. Local muscle weakness may be present. Periodic testing of the handgrip is sometimes ordered.

In children younger than 2 years of age, when the cranial suture lines are not completely knit, there may be considerable enlargement of the head and fontanel because of the enlarging tumor or its obstruction of cerebrospinal fluid drainage. The blood pressure may be elevated, and the pulse may be slowed when compared with the normal values for the child's age group. Respirations may be of the Cheyne-Stokes variety. Fever or wide swings in temperature occasionally occur.

Diagnosis

Diagnosis is confirmed through various procedures: magnetic resonance imaging (MRI), skull radiographs (x-ray films), brain scans, electroencephalograms (EEGs), ventriculograms, and arteriograms, as well as clinical observation. Some of these procedures, though often necessary, are uncomfortable. Computed tomography (CT) and magnetic resonance imaging (MRI), cause the patient much less discomfort and risk.

If a nurse is responsible for the care of a child with a possible brain tumor, he or she must carefully assess the child's capabilities before attempting to ambulate the child. The nurse should ensure that he or she has sufficient assistance to prevent falls because some of these children have poor balance. The child should be observed for any of the signs and symptoms previously described. Observation of vital signs including blood pressure and eye reactions should always be part of the nursing care.

Treatment

Surgery, radiation, and chemotherapy are the treatments currently available. A craniotomy (the surgical opening of the skull) is preferred. The complete removal of a well-confined tumor almost always produces a more optimistic prognosis. When only incomplete removal is possible, radiation and chemotherapy are used to retard tumor progression.

Nursing care

Nursing care of the craniotomy patient is complex. The vocational nurse and registered nurse work as care partners because the child's condition may be unstable. The child must be turned slowly and gently to prevent dizziness, nausea, vomiting, and a rise in blood pressure. Because crying elevates the blood pressure, all measures designed to prevent fear or distress are especially important. The head dressings may become damp from cerebrospinal fluid drainage and require reinforcing until they can be changed by the physician. The face, especially the eyes, may be bruised and swollen. Special eye irrigations may be necessary to prevent infection or ulceration resulting from disturbances in tear formation and drainage because of trauma. Suctioning may be necessary, although it is avoided if possible since this procedure can elevate intracranial pressure. The child may appear unconscious but may be able to hear well; so conversations at the bedside should be prudent.

As children with brain tumors improve, efforts toward rehabilitation should be made. They may live relatively satisfying lives for months or years. Children and their families need informational and emotional support to make the most of this time.

Neuroblastoma

A neuroblastoma is an undifferentiated malignant tumor arising during embryonic development from the adrenal medulla or from any of the nervous system's sympathetic ganglia located in the head, neck, chest, abdomen, or pelvis. It is the most common of all solid cancers of children. Both genders are equally affected, and although the tumor may be diagnosed at any age, a preponderance is diagnosed during the first 4 to 5 years of life.

Assessment

Four common clinical manifestations of the neuroblastoma are (1) a mass usually involving the abdomen or lymph nodes; (2) neurological signs, such as weakness in an extremity or paraplegia; (3) pain, usually in the bone or joints; and (4) orbital signs, such as local ecchymosis or proptosis (protruding eye). In addition, children with neuroblastoma often come to the hospital with varied constitutional symptoms, including weight loss, fever, anorexia, and anemia.

Diagnosis

When a neuroblastoma is suspected, a number of diagnostic studies must be performed at once because the neuroblastoma is a highly malignant tumor with tendencies to produce widespread metastases. The sequence of studies includes a complete blood cell count; electrolyte, glucose, and other blood chemistry determinations; a urinary assay for catecholamines; intravenous pyelogram; radioactive bone scan; chest x-ray examination; computed tomography (CT); and bone marrow aspiration. In seven out of ten cases the tumor secretes excess quantities of catecholamines or metabolites or both into the blood. Urine measurements of their metabolic end products, vanillylmandelic acid (VMA) and homovanillic acid (HVA), make the 24-hour VMA and HVA urine determinations a valuable diagnostic test. A good prognosis is associated with diagnosis in children under 1 year of age with localized tumor. Staging of this tumor is important for planning treatment and estimating prognosis. See box above.

The cure rate decreases as the extent of disease increases. Unfortunately, more than 50% of cases have metastasized at the time of initial diagnosis.

STAGING OF NEUROBLASTOMA

Stage I Localized tumor, well encapsulated
Stage II Tumor extended to regional lymph nodes
Stage III Extensive tumor spread across the midline
Stage IV Tumor with distant metastases and bone involvement
Stage IVS (S for *special*). Small primary tumor with metastases to the liver, skin, or bone marrow with no bone involvement

Treatment

An aggressive therapeutic approach, combining surgical excision, irradiation, and chemotherapy is used in an attempt to save these children. Surgery alone is probably acceptable in Stages I, II, and IVS. Spontaneous resolution of residual tumor in stages II and IVS is a common event with high cure rates (75% to 90%) in these children.

Because neuroblastoma is radiosensitive, x-ray therapy to the tumor site and to any areas of local extension may be an indicated addition. Palliative x-ray therapy is used for metastatic lesions in bones, lungs, liver, and brain. Chemotherapy has improved survival and is useful in shrinking previously unresectable tumors. It is especially indicated in children with bone involvement, when the urinary catecholamines remain elevated after all identifiable tumor has been removed, or when recurrence or late metastases are detected.

Currently, multidrug chemotherapy is employed, using vincristine (Oncovin), cyclophosphamide (Cytoxan), doxorubicin (Adriamycin), cisplatin (Platinol), and VM-26, in addition to surgery and radiation therapy. No single chemotherapeutic agent or combination of drugs has been uniformly effective. When chemotherapy is given, control of anemia, specific antibiotic therapy for infections, and prevention of high blood levels of uric acid are necessary. Liberal fluids and allopurinol (Zyloprim) should be given to prevent uric acid kidney damage.

After surgery, children with neuroblastomas should be reevaluated often because, in spite of the use of chemotherapy and radiotherapy, results to date have been poor. Although an increasing number of long-term survivors are receiving chemotherapy, this tumor often has a rapid downhill course despite all the therapy that is currently available. The value of bone marrow transplantation for children with disseminated disease and in first remission is being assessed.

SCHOOL-AGE CHILD

Head Injuries

Approximately 200,000 children are hospitalized annually with head injuries. Although most of these children have simple, closed head injuries, about 17% have skull fractures. One out of ten has active intracranial bleeding, and two out of ten have other body injuries associated with head injury. Identifying children with active intracranial bleeding and those with other injuries is a significant role of the nurse. The patients are typically boys between the ages of 4 and 9 years. Child auto restraint and bike helmet laws are critical factors in the prevention of head injury in children.

Concussion

The term *concussion* implies a loss of consciousness with a temporary neuronal dysfunction caused by jarring but with no pathological evidence of damage to the underlying brain. The period of unconsciousness is usually brief and is measured in terms of minutes to hours. The period of memory loss that surrounds a concussion is termed *posttraumatic amnesia* (PTA). It is important to be aware of the PTA phenomenon because it explains why the patient often cannot provide information about the injury. Usually the longer the PTA period, the greater the likelihood of brain injury rather than simple concussion.

PTA is divided into retrograde amnesia, loss of memory for the period of time after the actual injury, and anterograde amnesia, the loss of memory for the period of time preceding the injury. Most children display some persistent residual loss of memory surrounding the period of injury. A long retrograde amnesia is particularly significant in evaluating the extent of a head injury. Any head-injured child who shows a neurological deficit should be admitted to the hospital for observation. Sports injuries and motor vehicle accidents are major contributors to the incidence of concussion in children.

Contusion and laceration

A contusion is an actual bruising of the brain. A laceration involves tearing of cerebral tissue. This bruising or tearing of cerebral tissue is frequently accompanied by hemorrhages or bleeding into the brain substance. Contusions and lacerations, in contrast to concussion, are characterized by specific (focal) findings. Changes in motor function, speech, and vision are important clues for determining the area of damage; for example, the left side of the brain controls the arms and legs on the right side of the body, speech is most often generated by the left side of the brain, and a visual center is located at the back of the brain. When disruption of brain tissue is associated with bleeding, intracranial pressure may begin to rise.

Since the cranium containing the brain, cerebral blood vessels, and cerebrospinal fluid is rigid, any enlargement of one of these three components results in compression of the others. The brain substance is more vulnerable to compression than are blood and cerebrospinal fluid, and when no further compensation is possible, intracranial pressure begins to rise.

Like other tissues, when the brain is subjected to injury, it becomes edematous. This swelling also causes increased intracranial pressure. Increasing intracranial pressure (ICP) is manifested by a change in orientation and loss of consciousness, changes in the child's baseline blood pressure and pulse rate, and irregularity of breathing. These are the classic neurological signs indicating that the head-injured child is deteriorating.

A basic neurological check (see the box on p. 676) is used for observing a child who is beginning to manifest subtle signs of increasing intracranial pressure or who is admitted to the hospital for observation after a head injury. Consciousness is a bihemispheric and brainstem function. Nerve centers in the brainstem also control vital functions, such as respiration, heart rate, and blood pressure. The brainstem may be directly injured, or it may be compromised by potentially reversible lesions that cause compression, such as increasing intracranial pressure and brain shifts or lesions that cause cerebral oxygen deprivation (ischemia).

The brainstem centers that control vital functions are anatomically close to those that regulate pupil responses. Observations of changes in pupil size, therefore, aid in detecting damage to the brainstem.

NEUROLOGIC CHECK

ASSESSMENT	TECHNIQUE OR OBSERVATION USED
I Level of consciousness	
A Alert, oriented, responsive to	Ask the following questions:
1 Person	1 "What is your name?"
2 Time	2 "What is your favorite TV show? What day is today?"
3 Place	3 "Where are you? Where do you go to school?"
B Lethargic—drowsy	Patient responses are delayed.
C Disoriented—confused	Patient gives inappropriate responses.
D Responsive to verbal stimuli	Patient answers simple commands, e.g., "Open your eyes."
E Responsive only to painful stimuli	Pinch patient's upper arm.
1 Purposeful	Patient withdraws from stimulus—pushes it away.
2 Nonpurposeful	Patient may only grimace.
a Flexor response	
b Extensor response	
F Coma	Patient gives no response of any kind.
II Pupil response	
A Appearance	Observe both pupils simultaneously; pupils should be round (constricted in bright room and dilated in dark room) and equal in size.
1 Shape	
2 Size	
3 Equality	
B Reaction to light	
1 Direct light reflex	Shine light directly into one eye; pupils should constrict briskly.
2 Consensual light reflex	Shine light into one eye note alternate pupil constriction.
C Extraocular movements	Ask patient to follow your finger from side to side and up and down with eyes to detect limitation in movement.
III Motor function	
A Facial symmetry	Ask patient to show teeth—to make a "funny face."
B Movement	
1 Upper extremities	Ask patient to raise arms and extend both arms forward.
2 Lower extremities	Ask patient to move each leg individually upward and laterally.
C Strength	
1 Upper extremities	Ask patient to squeeze examiner's hand or two fingers and to pull against resistance of examiner.
2 Lower extremities	
D Babinski reflex	Stroke outside sole of each foot with tongue blade. Normally toes, especially big toe, turn down. Reflex is present when big toe rises (dorsiflexion) and other toes fan out. Reflex is normally present up to about 18 months of age.
IV Vital signs	Elevation is usually associated with infection elsewhere unless hypothalamus (temperature-regulating center) has been damaged.
A Temperature	
B Pulse	Slowed pulse and irregular respirations associated with rising systolic pressure indicate increased intracranial pressure.
C Respiration	
D Blood pressure	

It is important to note the degree of alertness when the child is admitted to the emergency department or pediatric unit and to note the vital signs exactly. Changes in these important parameters as indicated above are classic signs that the patient is in need of prompt medical assistance. The physician should be notified at once.

This, however, is a late sign of increased intracranial pressure.

Intracranial hematoma

Intracranial hematomas are space-occupying lesions that produce signs of intracranial pressure. They should be suspected in every case of head injury with coma or one-sided weakness. Short-term increased intracranial pressure may occur because of an expanding hematoma, or long-term pressure may occur because of cerebral edema caused by the injury. Unless the intracranial pressure is reduced, neurologic deterioration follows, which can prove to be fatal.

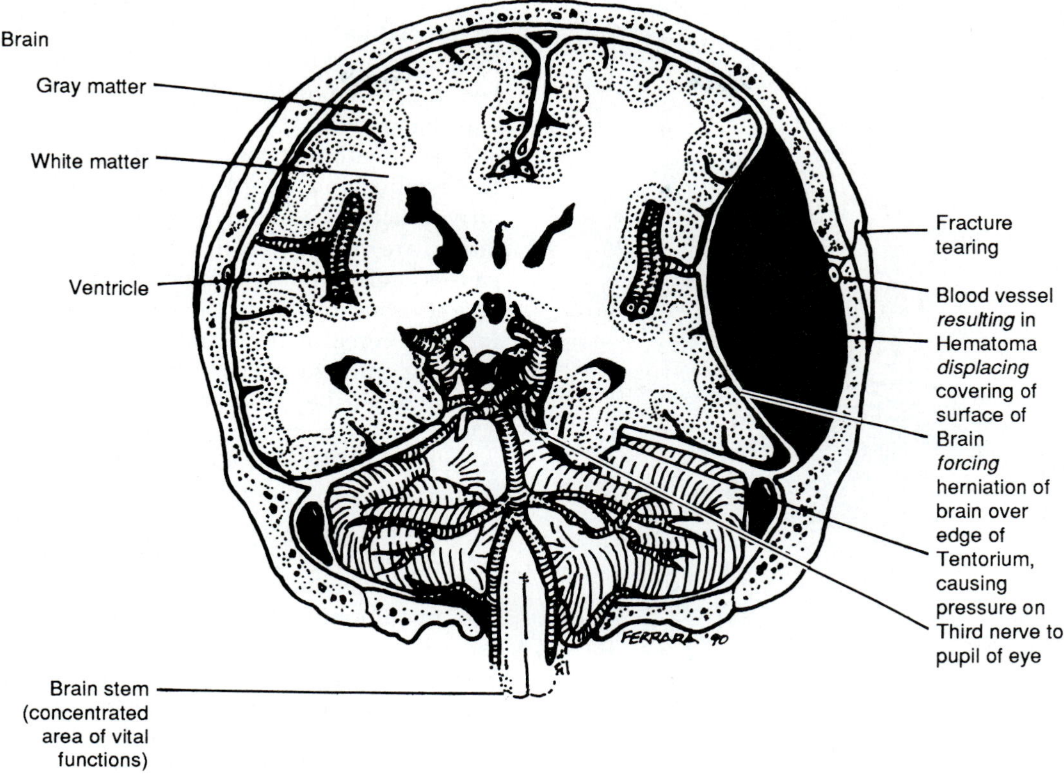

Fig. 32-19 Epidural hematoma located between skull and outer covering of brain.

Epidural hematoma

About 75% of epidural hematomas are associated with a skull fracture (Fig. 32-19). This lesion, located between the skull and the outer covering of the brain (dura), results from a torn high-pressure arterial system. It characteristically demonstrates a relatively rapid downhill course unless identified and treated. Since the expanding hemorrhage cannot get through the bone, the hematoma presses down on the substance of the brain. Usually a brief period of unconsciousness is followed by a lucid interval of variable duration, after which the child is progressively confused, lethargic, difficult to arouse, and finally, comatose.

Pulse and respirations become slow, and blood pressure rises. A dilated pupil and hemiparesis of the opposite side of the body, accompanied by a deterioration in state of consciousness and vital signs, indicate a prompt need for surgical intervention. The high mortality from this kind of injury usually results from a failure in recognition and a delay in operation.

Subdural hematoma

Subdural hematomas are usually caused by rupture of low-pressure bridging veins in the space under the dura and may be associated with severe brain injury. Subdural hematomas are divided into three categories, depending on the time interval from onset of the injury to the course of symptoms. *Acute subdural hematomas* usually cause immediate unconsciousness with a rapid, downhill, progressive deterioration, resulting from massive bleeding and fatal brain compression. *Subacute subdural hematomas* develop slowly because bleeding is less profuse. Clinical manifestations usually appear between 2 and 14 days after injury. *Chronic subdural hematomas* manifest themselves weeks or months after the injury (Fig. 32-20). This condition occurs most frequently in infancy. A vascular membrane forms around the blood as the mass slowly enlarges because of leakage of plasma protein from the capillaries. Intracranial pressure mounts over a period of weeks to months and is manifested by vomiting (especially projectile type), a tense fontanel, and separation of the cranial sutures. Because chronic subdural hematomas are usually bilateral, the skull may become deformed and broad with a high forehead. The infant becomes irritable and is often underweight and anemic. Bilateral subdural taps confirm the diagnosis, and the fluid is removed. If the fluid is removed in time, repeated subdural taps can provide a complete cure; otherwise, a shunting procedure is necessary for the more persistent hematomas.

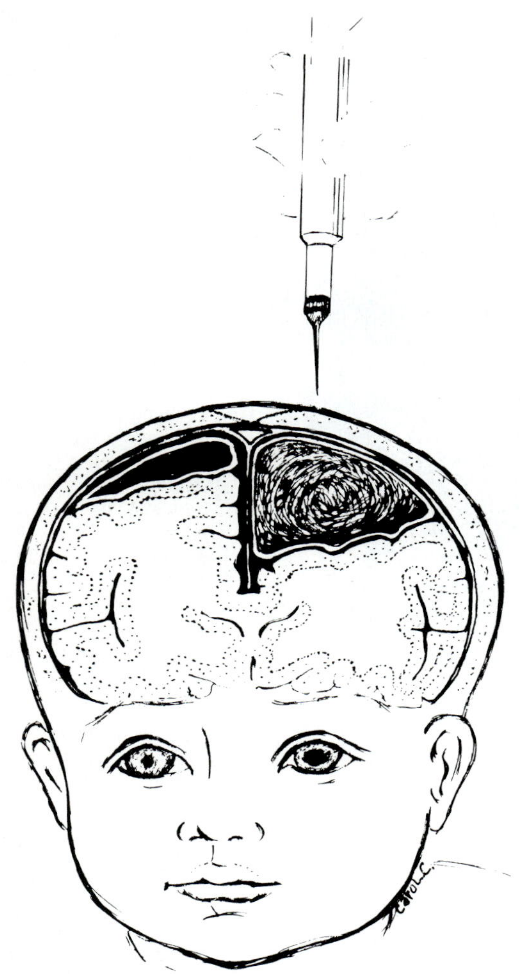

Fig. 32-20 Bilateral, chronic subdural hematomas. Subdural taps are performed on infants by insertion of special subdural needle through lateral suture line.

Skull fracture

Skull fracture is often associated with brain injury. A *linear skull fracture* (lengthwise) may often cause an underlying hematoma. This is particularly true if the fracture line crosses the normal distribution of blood vessels. In children, 50% of skull fractures are in the parietal bone, and these usually are evident on x-ray examination. A *depressed skull fracture* occurs when the bone is displaced or is pressing on the brain tissue. Debridement and surgical restoration of normal contour are required. Basal skull fractures are not always seen on x-ray examination. However, the nurse may suspect the presence of a basilar skull fracture by a special finding not always initially present when the child is admitted. On the second day the nurse may notice black-and-blue marks around the eyes (raccoon sign) or behind the ear (battle sign). A third finding is watery fluid that runs out of the ear (cerebrospinal fluid otorrhea) or a watery discharge from the nose (cerebrospinal fluid rhinorrhea). Cerebrospinal fluid leaking from the ear or nose causes increased concern because of the danger of infection and meningitis.

Nursing care. *Cerebral anoxia* is the most frequent cause of death in a child with skull fracture. Therefore the establishment and maintenance of an adequate airway, accompanied by proper ventilation and circulation, are critical. Obstruction of the airway not only causes atelectasis and infection but also produces a serious abnormality in the gaseous exchange that can increase cerebral flow and cerebral edema, thus increasing intracranial pressure. When possible, blood gases should be periodically checked to validate the adequacy of ventilation. Tracheal suction may be essential to clear secretions, and a tracheostomy may be necessary to maintain a patent airway.

Because vomiting frequently accompanies increased intracranial pressure, insertion of a nasogastric tube and removal of stomach contents may prevent aspiration pneumonitis. These children should be kept in a lateral, slightly elevated position, unless contraindicated, because of the potential for aspiration. They should be turned hourly.

Hypotensive shock is seldom caused by head injury unless hemorrhage from a severe scalp wound occurs or the brain injury itself is so severe that the vital centers are failing and death is imminent. The presence of clinical shock should alert the nurse to notify the physician and to search elsewhere in the body for hemorrhage. Careful examination of the abdomen and extremities is necessary to detect the possibility of a ruptured spleen or fractured long bone. Blood should be obtained for grouping and cross-matching because replacement of lost fluid volume by intravenous route may be lifesaving.

The presence of shock usually means injuries involving other organs. With the exception of a life-threatening lesion, such as hematoma, neurosurgical management should be postponed until other injuries are investigated and treated.

Disturbance in cerebral function

A detailed neurological examination is included with the initial medical examination of the head-injured child. This not only allows for a more accurate diagnosis of the extent of the injury, but observations made during the examination form the baseline from which subsequent progress can be judged. The general state of the child, level of consciousness, heart rate, blood pressure, and breathing should be evaluated immediately with primary attention to vital circulatory and ventilatory functions on which life depends. Headache, vertigo, vomiting, increasing irritability, and restlessness often characterize the response of young children to head injury. These factors may or may not be evidence of intracranial pressure. Restlessness can be caused by cerebral hypoxia or by an overdistended bladder, which may be relieved by an indwelling catheter. Other causes of restlessness include extensive soft tissue injuries, fracture, and improperly applied cast or dressing. Seizures also frequently accompany head injuries in small children.

Careful systematic serial observations and recordings of changing factors and physical signs are constantly compared with the baseline. In addition to the nurse's responsibility for the care of the child, the nurse must report at once any significant change in the child's condition. Problems associated with raised intracranial pressure demand solution before irreparable brain damage is inflicted. A *neurological check,* which includes evaluation of level of consciousness, pupillary signs, extremity movement, strength, and sensation, as well as vital signs, should be done every 15 to 30 minutes as necessary. Careful observation of the child, especially the level of consciousness, yields by far the most important information for further management (See the box on p. 679).

A child who is alert or is improving does not require any therapeutic measures. However, when serial examinations suggest that intracranial pressure is increasing significantly, various measures are employed to minimize this complication. Administration of dehydrating agents, such as mannitol, can be given over a 4- to 6-hour period every 12 hours to control cerebral edema. Dexamethasone (Decadron) and methylprednisolone sodium succinate (Solu-Medrol) are two glucocorticoids commonly used to prevent cellular decompensation and increasing cerebral edema. Anticonvulsant drugs may be necessary to control seizures. Normal daily maintenance fluids should be given at a uniform rate over a 24-hour period. An accurate record of fluid intake and output is essential and should be followed closely, because lethargy, confusion, and convulsion can result from electrolyte imbalance and not an intracranial hematoma.

Hematomas can be differentiated from cerebral edema by computed transaxial tomography (CT scan). This technique permits identification of hemorrhage and cerebral edema and clearly outlines ventricular cavities. The CT scan is the safest, fastest, and best initial study for the child who exhibits further neurological deterioration or who is comatose. If scanning is not available, cerebral angiography is used to diagnose intracranial hematomas that may need to be evacuated by craniotomy.

Coma. Coma is defined as the inability to open the eyes, obey commands, or speak. Various degrees of impaired consciousness occur with head trauma.

GLASGOW COMA SCALE

RESPONSE	SCORE*
Eye opening	4 Spontaneous
	3 To speech
	2 To pain
	1 None
Best verbal	5 Oriented
	4 Confused
	3 Inappropriate
	2 Incomprehensible
	1 None
Best motor	6 Obeys commands
	5 Localizes pain
	4 Withdraws
	3 Flexion to pain
	2 Extension to pain
	1 None

*Eye + Motor + Verbal = 3 to 15. Any combination equal to 7 or less defines coma.

Recognition of the depth of responsiveness is essential in determining the initial severity of the patient's brain insult. The Glasgow Coma Scale (GCS) is a reliable instrument designed to define the degree of responsiveness. Scoring of responsiveness depends on the ability to open one's eyes, obey commands, and speak in response to verbal or tactile stimuli. The worst score obtainable is 3; the best is 15. Patients who do not spontaneously open their eyes within 24 hours of head trauma have the poorest prognosis. (See box above.)

In summary, the nurse must remember that intracranial monitoring remains the single most important aid in determining when the previously mentioned therapeutic measures should be initiated. Although children have a remarkable capacity to survive even the most severe type of head trauma, the management of each child remains a challenge.

SENSORINEURAL DEFICIT

Vision

Approximately 20 to 35 per 1000 children are considered vision impaired. One per 1000 is considered legally blind; that is, visually unable to distinguish light from darkness. The majority of children who are blind have significant visual impairment, but retain some measurable or functional vision. The nurse's primary role is detection of vision impairment, referral to an opthalmologist, and rehabilitation in specialized settings. The basic anatomy of the eye is presented in Fig. 32-21.

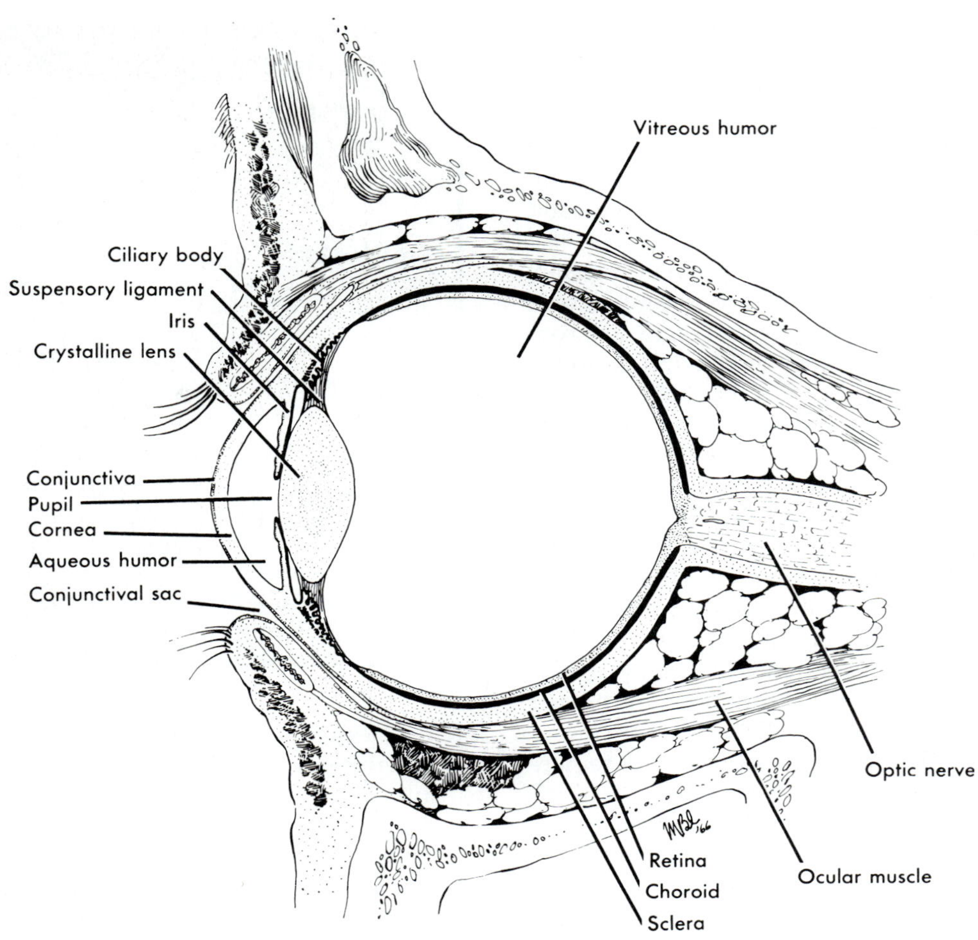

Fig. 32-21 Basic anatomy of eye.

> **Nursing Alert**
>
> If an infant fails to react to light or if parents express concern regarding vision impairment, blindness should be suspected.

Common causes of visual impairment in infancy and childhood are (1) trauma, (2) strabismus (malalignment of the eyes), and (3) refractive error (image not clearly focused on the retina). A decreased incidence in severe visual disorders is due to:

1. Recognition of the cause of retrolental fibroplasia
2. Prevention and control of rubella
3. Early diagnosis and treatment of developmental eye problems
4. Technological advances in eye examination and surgery

Pediatric eye examination

The gift of sight is indeed precious. Eye care should be taught to parents and growing children. Prevention of eye disease is the ideal, but early recognition of eye disorders with proper definitive treatment is the ultimate goal. Children should be observed for signs and symptoms of the following possible visual difficulties:

1. Poor vision: inability to follow objects visually or visual inattentiveness to the environment in infants and preschoolers; difficulty with near or distant reading in school-age children;
2. Strabismus: intermittent or persistent crossing of the eyes; squinting, blinking, or closing one eye in bright light or during visual tasks; head turning or tilting;
3. Uncorrected refractive error: irritability with near or distant visual tasks or avoidance of these tasks; tearing, rubbing, or squinting of the eyes; recurrent eyelid inflammations.

Nursing Alert

Children with the following findings should be referred to an opthalmologist immediately: strabismus, inability to fixate and follow in the young infant; a visual acuity difference between eyes of two lines or more on the eye chart or vision in either eye of 20/40 or less (in preschoolers or school-age children); evidence of structural deformity of the eye; or a family history of retinoblastoma, congenital cataracts, or genetic or metabolic eye diseases.

4 To identify and treat visual problems as early as possible, a professional eye examination should be performed for every child immediately after birth, at 6 months, and once in the preschool years between ages 3 and 5. Annual follow-up visual screening by the school nurse is optimal.

The examination should include measurement of visual acuity, estimation of ocular alignment by corneal light reflexes or alternate cover testing, and examination of ocular structures for pathological findings.

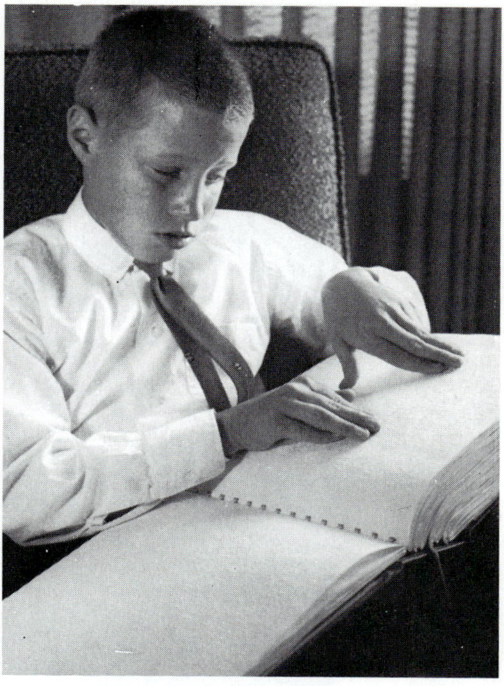

Fig. 32-22 This industrious boy, reading from his Braille Bible, is blind as result of retrolental fibroplasia.

Retinopathy of Prematurity (Retrolental Fibroplasia)

Administration of oxygen, which saves the lives of premature low-birth-weight infants, also causes the development of abnormal retinal vascularization. Ultimately a contraction of this retinal scar tissue can result in a detachment of the retina and the appearance of a white fibrous sheath on the posterior surface of the lens. The incidence of retinopathy of prematurity (ROP) has decreased, but it is reemerging as the use of oxygen therapy rises in the high-risk infant population (Fig. 32-22).

Amblyopia and strabismus

Strabismus (malalignment of the eyes) affects about 4% of the population (Fig. 32-23). This imbalance of the extraocular muscles can lead to amblyopia (decreased vision in one eye resulting from disuse), poor binocular vision (decreased depth perception), and an unacceptable appearance ("cross-eyed," "wall-eyed"). Although strabismus is the most common cause of amblyopia, the next leading cause is a notable difference in refractive error (the eye most out of focus "turns off"). Specific treatment of amblyopia may include glasses or occlusive (patching) therapy. Patching the nonamblyopic eye stimulates the increased visual maturation of the amblyopic eye. Specific treatment of strabismus depends on the cause and may include glasses, occlusive therapy, orthoptics (visual exercises), or surgery. Surgical treatment of a congenital strabismus in the first year of life significantly improves changes for binocular vision and an acceptable appearance.

Strabismus surgery involves either shortening or repositioning the extraocular muscles controlling the position of the eyeball. Postoperative care is usually dictated by physician preference and the child's needs. Although restraints have been used frequently in the past, there is no substitute for an attentive parent or nurse. Parents have usually been instructed by the surgeon to expect that the child will have red eyes. The child may become needlessly frightened by occlusive eye dressings or the inability to open the eyes because of crusted secretions on opposing lid margins. Proper postoperative care can prevent both these situations.

Refractive Errors

Poor visual acuity in one or both eyes may be the result of myopia (nearsightedness), hyperopia (farsightedness), or astigmatism (Table 32-4). Astigmatism is an irregularity in the curvature of the cornea or lens

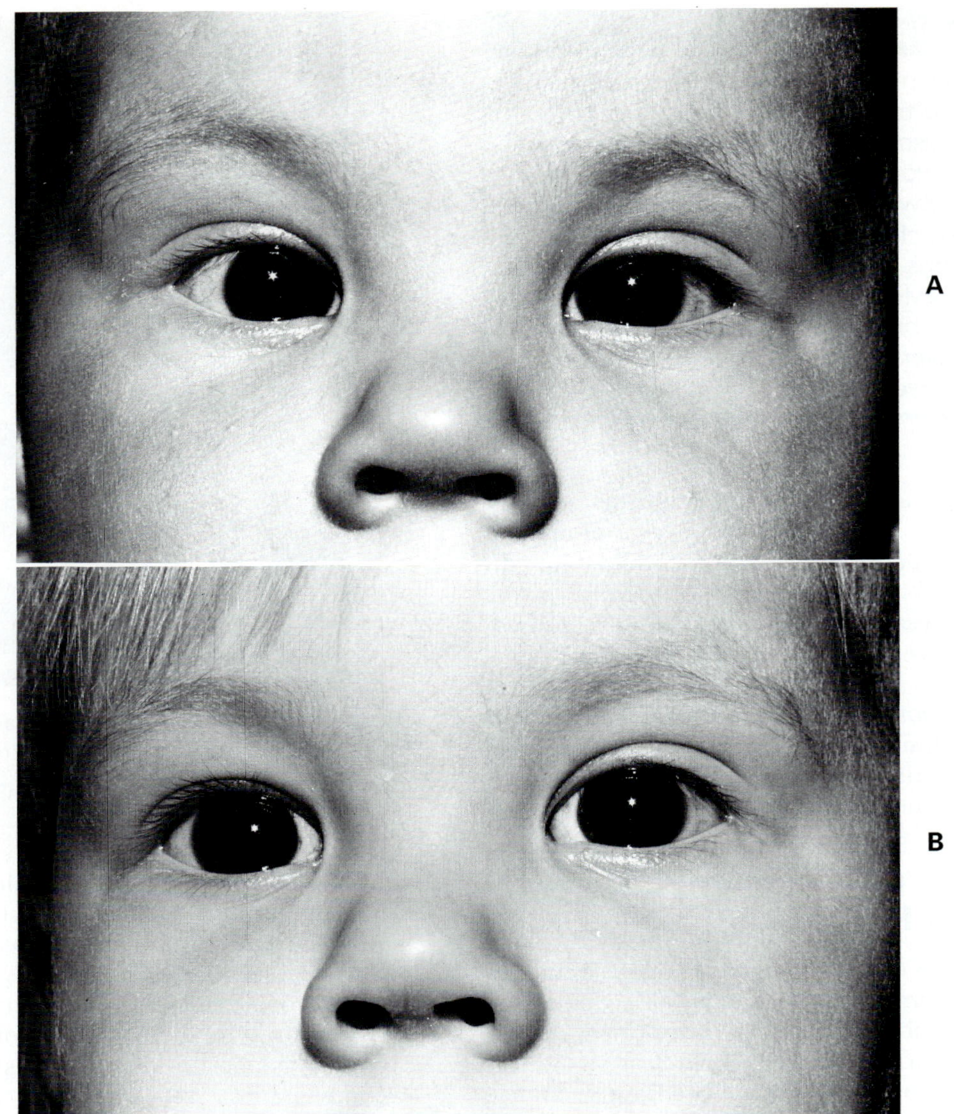

Fig. 32-23 Infantile esotropia. ***A,*** Age 7 months—preoperative; ***B,*** age 12 months—postoperative (strabismus surgery at age 11 months). Note that although postoperative alignment is straight (i.e., true strabismus has been eliminated), there are still typical facial characteristics for pseudostrabismus (flat nasal bridge, wide epicanthal skin folds, narrow interpupillary distance, and greater nasal than temporal scleral visibility). (Courtesy David G. Martin, San Diego, Calif.)

that blurs focal points; it may be associated with either myopia or hyperopia. When there is a significant difference in the ability of the eyes to focus—in their refractive powers—the condition is known as *anisometropia.* Refractive errors usually do not cause difficulties until the child reaches school age. Vision usually can be corrected to a normal level in both eyes with proper glasses. Only if amblyopia is present do uncorrected or poorly corrected refractive errors cause permanent loss of vision.

Children who wear glasses must be taught to keep their glasses in a case when they are not being worn. Proper methods of handling and cleaning the lenses should also be demonstrated. When a young child wearing glasses or contact lenses is admitted to the hospital, a note concerning them should be included in the child's admission record.

Cataracts

Congenital and early developmental cataracts constitute one of the most important causes of visual impairment in children. A cataract is an abnormal opacity of the crystalline lens, located just in back of the pupil. By obstructing the pathway of light to the retina, cataracts can cause partial or total blindness. Cataracts may be congenital, such as those caused by maternal rubella. Some cataracts are hereditary—most commonly autosomal dominant. Nonhereditary cataracts may develop as a result of trauma, infection, retrolental fibroplasia, retinitis pigmentosa, or prolonged administration of corticosteroids. Surgical removal of the cataract lens is the only effective method of treatment available for all but a few infants and children. The postoperative period is usually short. It usually requires a sterile eye pad and protective shield and occasionally involves some limitation of activity. Every effort should be made to reduce crying and prevent vomiting, because that increases intraocular pressure, strain on the sutures, and possible bleeding. Occasionally the child's eyes are bandaged. Before touching a child who cannot see, the nurse should speak so that he or she is not startled. A radio is a comfort when vision is limited by bandages and movement is restricted. Again, orientation to the hospital setting, preparation for the postoperative period, and parental support are extremely important.

Retinoblastoma

Retinoblastoma is a malignant tumor arising from retinal tissue. The tumor may be familial or sporadic and may be identified by a thorough eye examination at birth. Frequently the diagnosis is made because of the presence of a white reflex from the pupil (leukokoria), strabismus, or ocular inflammation. Retinoblastoma is the most frequent ocular malignancy of childhood. Early recognition and immediate treatment are essential to prevent the rapid metastasis of this tumor.

Trauma

Serious injury may be associated with a decrease in vision. Nearly one third of monocular blindness follows trauma in childhood years. Arrows and other pointed objects are the chief instruments of blinding injuries in children under 15 years of age.

Of all possible injuries to the eye, traumatic *hyphema* (hemorrhage within the anterior chamber of the eye) is probably the most common ocular injury necessitating hospitalization. Bleeding usually arises from a tear or laceration in the anterior ciliary body rather than in the iris itself.

Prognosis for normal vision decreases as the amount of bleeding in the anterior chamber increases. This is the primary reason for the classic preventive regimen of bed rest with the head of the bed elevated 30 to 45 degrees, bilateral eye patches, and sedation. Patients should *not* be placed on the affected side. Long-term evaluation should include careful examination of the peripheral retina for tears and periodic evaluation for development of glaucoma. *Glaucoma,* a condition that results from high intraocular pressure, ultimately can lead to loss of optic nerve function and blindness.

Children with a visual loss are confronted with complex, interrelated problems throughout their childhood years. These problems are by no means exclusively personal. The burden is far-reaching, presenting major challenges to parents, teachers, and physicians and to nurses caring for such children in the hospital setting. Those who share this responsibility should be committed to assisting these children in achieving both physical and psychosocial well-being so that they can develop the skills necessary to live safely and happily.

Specific Language Disability (Developmental Dyslexia)

Developmental dyslexia can occur in children in the presence or absence of visual deficit, and in children of normal intelligence. A multidisciplinary team comprised of speech pathologists, educators, psychologists, school nurses, and developmentalists is best qualified to deal with learning disorders and language delay. A thorough ophthalmological and audiological examination and general health assessment should precede the individualized learning evaluation.

HEARING

The auditory system is the primary channel through which children learn speech and language, develop educationally, and dynamically adjust to the challenges of their environment. The importance of the integrity of the auditory system is both simple and complex. The degree of auditory dysfunction (hearing impairment), the developmental time at which hearing impairment occurs, and the duration of the impairment all determine to what extent the child develops normal speech, language, and educational and psychosocial skills. Because hearing impairment itself is generally physically invisible and manifests itself in problems of communication, learning, and psychological and social behavior, it is sometimes misdiagnosed and subsequently managed as childhood autism, emotional disturbance, and mental retardation. As a result of such errors in diagnosis and treatment, hearing-impaired children can be denied the opportunity to realize their potential and take their places as contributing members of society. For children

◆ **TABLE 32-4**
Refraction: Three Common Defects in Children

Normal Refraction	Normal Eye
Emmetropia (no refractive error) Light is focused on retina	Emmetropic eye 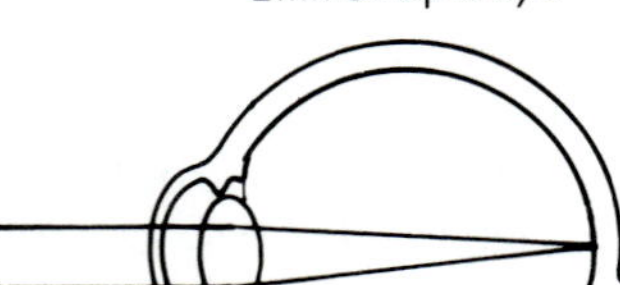

Abnormal Refraction	Cause	Optical Defect	Corrected with Lens
Myopia (near-sightedness) Sees near objects more clearly than distant objects	Elongated eyeball Parallel rays are focused anterior to the retina	Myopic eye 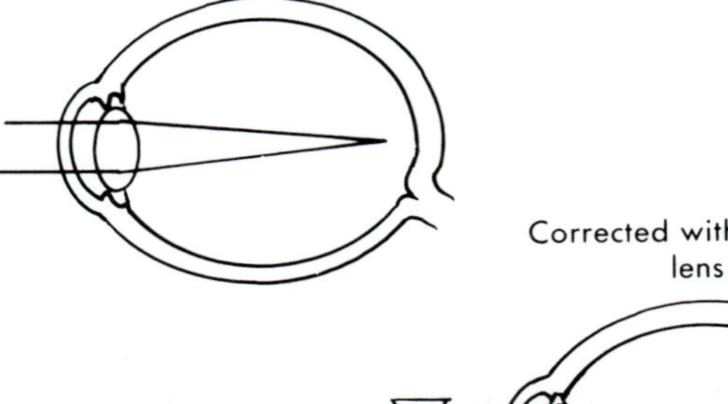	Corrected with concave lens 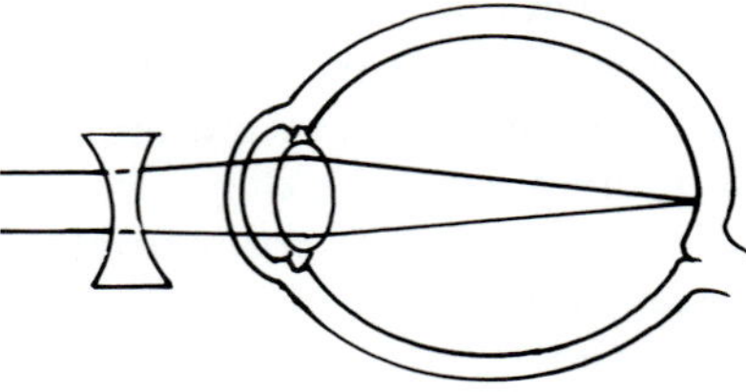
Hyperopia (far-sightedness) Sees objects more clearly at a distance	Shortened eyeball Parallel rays are focused posterior to the retina	Hyperopic eye 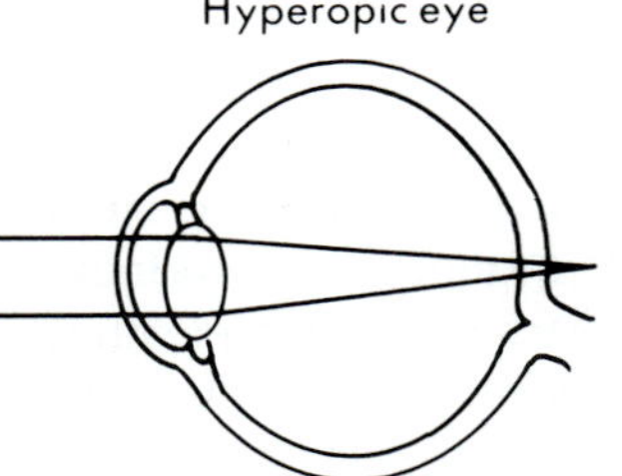	Corrected with convex lens 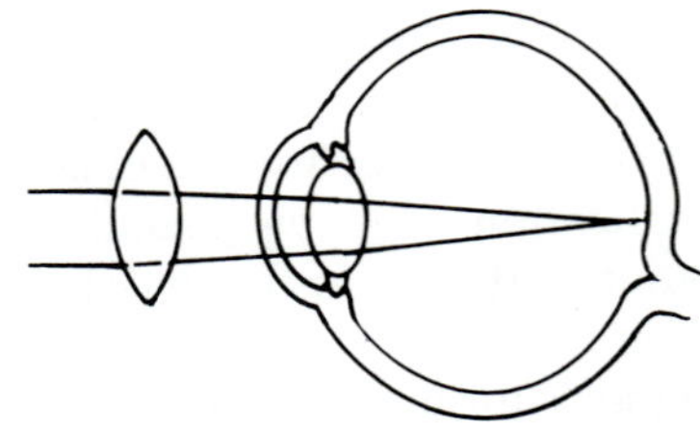

◆ TABLE 32-4
Refraction: Three Common Defects in Children—cont'd.

Abnormal Refraction	Cause	Optical Defect	Corrected with Lens
Astigmatism (may be associated with myopia or hyperopia) Sees distorted image	Irregular corneal curvature Rays entering eye are not refracted uniformly in all meridians	Myopic astigmatism	Corrected with myopic cylinder Axis 90°

with congenital hearing loss, it is important to identify the loss and initiate intervention within the first 6 months of life to minimize the effect of the hearing loss on their communication and psychosocial development.

Types of Loss

It is important to remember that the auditory system is divided primarily into two parts: the peripheral auditory system and the central auditory system.

The peripheral auditory system is composed of the outer, middle, and inner ears. The central auditory system is composed of afferent and efferent neurons connecting the sensory end organs of the inner ear to the brainstem and cortical structures.

The three main categories of hearing disorders are as follows: (1) *peripheral impairments,* resulting from lesions to the outer, middle, and inner ears and eighth cranial nerve; (2) *central impairments,* resulting from lesions to the brainstem and auditory cortex; and (3) *functional impairments* nonorganic, which are psychological with no physiological basis. There may, of course, be combinations of any or all of these in a given individual.

Disorders of both the peripheral and central auditory systems can be either congenital or acquired. Congenital and acquired losses can be *conductive* (caused by medically treatable pathological conditions of the outer or middle ears); *sensory* (caused by permanent damage to the cochlea); *neural* (caused by damage to the eighth nerve); *mixed* (combination of conductive and sensori-neural); or *central* (caused by neural disease in the central auditory nervous system). Since the cochlea is composed of both sensory and neural structures, hearing loss secondary to cochlear damage is frequently referred to as *sensori-neural hearing loss.*

Incidence of Hearing Loss

Total deafness is relatively rare, but partial hearing impairment is not uncommon. The incidence of significant hearing impairment is 1 in 50 in neonates discharged from intensive care nurseries, and about 1 in 1000 in well neonates. Most of these losses occur within the cochlea—that is, sensorineural hearing losses.

Common Causes of Hearing Impairment and Deafness

Hearing loss can occur during the prenatal, perinatal, or postnatal stages of a child's development. The most common prenatal factors associated with hearing loss are of genetic origin or occur as a result of maternal rubella in the first trimester.

The most common perinatal factors include prematurity, low birth weight (less than 1500 gm), hyperbilirubinemia (indirect bilirubin of 15 mg or greater), anoxia, and infection; for example, **TORCHES** disorders.

The most frequent postnatal factors are otitis media, meningitis, and other types of bacteriological and viral infections (for example, scarlet fever, measles, mumps, and meningitis), and head injury.

An increasingly common cause of sensorineural hearing loss in the adolescent is exposure to excessively loud noise or music. In preschool, kindergarten, and elementary school children, otitis media is by far the most common cause of hearing loss. Although otitis media is a disease of the middle ear that can result in conductive loss of fluctuating severity, it appears from more recent research that the reoccurrence of otitis media in young children can have an irreversible effect on the development of the entire auditory system. Children with significant hearing loss associated with persistent or episodic otitis media before age 2 may have impairment in cognitive, language, and emotional development.

The following criteria are suggested as indications of significant hearing loss in young children (see box at right).

1 Hearing levels of 15 dB HL or greater for one or more of the speech frequencies (500, 1K, 2K, 4K Hertz)
2 Indications of otitis media during more than half the time for a period of 6 months in a child under 18 months
3 Fluctuating hearing levels from less than 15 dB HL to over 15 dB HL 6 months or more during the first year of life

Early detection of hearing loss

Early detection and treatment of hearing loss are the key to reducing its damaging effects. All newborns meeting one or more of the *high-risk criteria* listed in the box at the left on p. 687 should be tested and followed up for the presence of hearing loss.

An infant meeting any of these criteria should be referred for an in-depth audiological evaluation within the first 2 months of life. Even if hearing seems normal at that time, the child should receive subsequent regularly scheduled hearing evaluations. Regular evaluations are important because many genetically related hearing impairments and hearing losses resulting from ototoxic drug therapy do not appear until some time after birth. Currently audiometric evaluation can begin in the neonatal nursery. Audiometric procedures that allow for the testing of very young children and children previously thought untestable include: (1) the brainstem auditory evoked response (BAER) test, which objectively measures brainstem neural responses to auditory stimulation in relaxed or sleeping subjects (cortical-evoked responses to auditory stimulation can also be recorded; however, this must be done with an awake and cooperative subject); (2) the crib-o-gram, which is a completely automated crib assembly designed for auditory signal presentation and recording of infant response; and (3) the impedance test battery. This test objectively measures tympanic membrane mobility, middle ear pressure, eustachian tube patency, and the presence of a functioning acoustic reflex (seventh to eighth cranial nerve reflex arc); this test is most reliable for children who are 7 months of age or older; (4) screening for the presence (normal) versus absence (abnormal) of evoked cochlear emissions.

Also included in the test battery are the more traditional behavioral tests of sensitivity to pure tones (see the Box at right on p. 687), calibrated noises, and speech. Reflex responses to sound and classic condi-

PARAMETERS OF STIMULI USED TO TEST HEARING

INTENSITY LEVELS—"LOUDNESS"

Hearing levels (HL) * for pure-tone hearing testing are measured in *decibels* (dB). Zero dB HL is the threshold at which sounds are normally first detected. The levels used to measure human hearing thresholds range from 0 dB to 110 dB HL. Normal hearing levels for children for all frequencies tested are considered to be 0 to 15 dB.

PURE-TONE FREQUENCIES—"PITCH"

Pure-tone frequencies are measured in cycles per second, or *hertz* (Hz). Hertz refers to the number of vibrations per second that a sound source makes to produce each pure tone. The fewer the vibrations per second, the lower the frequency—"pitch"; the greater the number of vibrations, the higher the frequency. The human ear (fully intact) can usually hear frequencies from 20 Hz (very low) to 20,000 Hz (very high), but hearing tests usually monitor frequencies of 250, 500, 1000, 2000, 4000, and 8000 Hz (frequencies most important for hearing speech and most environmental sounds).

* From American National Standards Institute (ANSI): Specifications for audiometers, New York, 1970, American National Standards Institute.

HIGH-RISK CRITERIA FOR HEARING LOSS

1 History of hereditary childhood hearing impairment
2 Rubella or other intrauterine infections (TORCHES)
3 Defects of ear, nose, throat, or larynx (malformed, low-set, or absent pinnae, cleft lip or palate, including submucous clefts, preauricular tags or pits)
4 Birth weight of less than 1500 gm
5 High serum bilirubin concentrations associated with jaundice that appear in the first 24 hours after birth.

tioning methods are used to obtain this information from young children.

With previously undiagnosed or newly developing hearing impairment, certain behaviors may alert the observant nurse to the presence of peripheral or central hearing dysfunction in a child. Examples of these are discussed in the Box above right.

Peripheral hearing loss is commonly measured using pure tones. Each pure tone has a single frequency of vibration that is perceived as a particular pitch and can be presented to the listener at a variety of levels of intensity or loudness. Presentation of pure tones at different intensity levels to a listener's ears is called the *pure-tone hearing test.* The purpose of this test is to find the intensity level for each frequency at which the listener can "just barely" detect that the tone is present. This hearing level for each pure-tone frequency is called the listener's *threshold* for that tone.

For young children, mild hearing loss is considered to be hearing threshold levels of 15 dB or greater for *any one* or all the frequencies considered important for the ability to detect and understand speech (500 Hz, 1000 Hz, 2000 Hz, 4000 Hz). Thresholds of 40 dB to 65 dB HL are moderate losses; 70 dB to 85 dB HL are severe losses; and 90+ dB HL are profound losses. An individual with thresholds of greater than or equal to 90 dB HL for a particular frequency is generally classified as being "deaf" for that frequency.

Conventional hearing aids should be considered at the first detection of sensorineural hearing impairment for all children with mild to profound degrees of hearing loss. The earlier that hearing aids are applied, the better is the prognosis for development of speech and language skills. For a congenital sensorineural hearing loss, hearing aids ideally should be in place by 6 months of age. A referral to an otolaryngologist and an audiologist should be made. Cochlear implants are currently being developed to help children and adults who cannot use more traditional hearing aids or who have essentially no cochlear function with intact central auditory systems. These "hearing aids" are surgically implanted electric devices that run on batteries; they stimulate eighth nerve fibers directly rather than cochlear sensory cells, as do traditional hearing aids. The nurse should consult an audiologist or otolaryngologist for further information and referral.

BEHAVIORAL CUES FOR HEARING LOSS

1 Better responses in quiet than in noisy environments
2 Hyperactivity
3 Disinterest in or lack of attention to sounds in the environment
4 Absence of a startle reflex in neonates and infants in the first 6 months of life
5 Difficulty following verbal instructions unless accompanied by visual demonstrations
6 Inadequate vocabulary
7 Defective sentence structure
8 Problems maintaining concentration
9 Social isolation
10 Inadequate reading or spelling
11 Poor reading comprehension
12 Discrepancy between achievement level and potential for learning
13 Significant discrepancy between verbal and performance IQ scores

Nursing considerations

Before speaking to hearing-impaired children, one should face them directly and obtain their visual attention. This allows them to supplement their limited sound perception with visual cues from your lips and face. Parents and nurses should take every opportunity to expose these young children to meaningful auditory stimulation to help improve use of their residual hearing. With abundant and early exposure to meaningful speech and environmental sound, hearing-impaired children have a much better prognosis for maximum utilization of their auditory systems.

The fact that a child has a hearing defect or wears a hearing aid on admission to the hospital is an important nursing observation. If the child is scheduled for surgery, permission should be sought to allow the child to wear the aid until he is anesthetized in the operating room. The aid should be reapplied as soon as the child has awakened from surgery. Such permission reduces the fear of the young patient and facilitates the entire procedure.

It is important for the nurse to remember that he or she may well be the first health care professional to suspect the presence of a hearing loss in a child. Sensitivity to the potential of hearing loss and swift and appropriate referral and follow-up can be critical factors in the child's attainment of his or her full potential.

KEY CONCEPTS

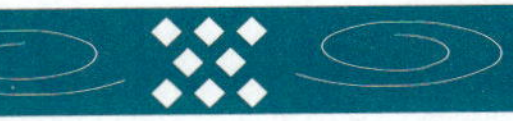

1 Types of fractures are greenstick, transverse, spiral, oblique, comminuted, and depressed. Every fracture may be placed in one of two main categories: closed fracture, in which no opening in the skin has resulted; and open fracture, in which the skin has been broken, exposing the bone to infection.
2 The fracture of an extremity may be indicated by the presence of deformity in alignment and swelling, pain or tenderness at the fracture site, loss of function or abnormal mobility of the part, a "grating sensation" heard or felt at the suspected point of fracture, and black-and-blue areas caused by subcutaneous hemorrhage.
3 First-aid treatment of a possible fracture includes limiting the movement of the injured part by stabilizing the part and the joint above and below the break to relieve muscle spasm and pain and to prevent further injury.
4 The process of bringing the fragments of a broken bone into proper relationship is termed *reducing* or *setting the fracture.* Alignment may be restored surgically or through the application of traction. Casting or splinting is done to maintain correct positioning to ensure proper healing.
5 Various surgical procedures have been devised to increase the effectiveness of various body joints either by increasing their ability to bear weight or by permitting greater motion. Some of the more common procedures are arthrodesis, arthroscopy, osteotomy, tendon transplant, epiphyseal arrest, leg lengthening, and open reduction and internal fixation.
6 Torticollis, or wryneck, is a congenital muscular abnormality often associated with birth trauma.
7 Childhood rickets is caused by minimal sun exposure and a diet deficient in vitamin D, calcium, or phosphorus.
8 Duchenne's muscular dystrophy is the most common form of progressive type muscle weakness. Onset usually occurs between 3 and 6 years of age; life expectancy is usually limited to the teenage period.
9 The most common form of chronic arthritis encountered in pediatrics is juvenile rheumatoid arthritis (JRA). There are three major types: (1) systemic, characterized by fever, rash, internal organ involvement, and often arthritis; (2) polyarticular, characterized by arthritis in numerous large and small joints; and (3) pauciarticular, in which arthritis affects only a few joints.
10 Therapy for JRA includes antiinflammatory medications, physical and occupational therapy, kind and understanding parental support, and promotion of general health. Mobility should be encouraged as much as can be tolerated to avoid lifelong joint deformities.
11 Legg-Calvé-Perthes disease is a self-limiting disease of the hip produced by lack of circulation to the femoral head. Treatment consists of traction until symptoms are resolved, followed by hip bracing to properly maintain the femoral head in the acetabulum.
12 Osteomyelitis, or inflammation of the bone resulting from infectious agents, has decreased remarkably with the increased availability of antibiotics. Treatment includes bed rest, immobilization of the affected limb, analgesics, and broad-spectrum antibiotics.
13 An osteosarcoma originates in the connective tissue and is the most common primary malignant tumor of bone. Early diagnosis and immediate treatment are crucial. When a tissue of bony origin is malignant, aggressive anticancer chemotherapy and radical methods of treatment, including amputation, must be endorsed to save the child.
14 Abnormal types of spinal curvature are scoliosis, kyphosis, and lordosis. Scoliosis, S-shaped lateral curvature, is the most common spinal deformity encountered in childhood. Idiopathic scoliosis is the most common type.
15 Screening is the only sure way of preventing the severe curvatures of idiopathic scoliosis. Screening programs should begin before 10 years of age and should include both boys and girls.
16 Treatment for scoliosis depends on the stage in which scoliosis is diagnosed and the severity of the curvature. Curves up to 20 degrees are usually left

alone and watched. Curves between 20 and 40 degrees and progressing are stabilized with a brace. Surgical correction is usually considered for curves that are over 40 degrees.

17 When maximum correction of the spinal curve has been achieved, a spinal fusion is usually performed. Patients who have had a spinal fusion need the same basic pre- and postoperative care required for all surgical patients. In addition, they need the special attention necessary for all casted children.

18 The two main types of seizures are partial and generalized. The nursing care of a child having a convulsion emphasizes the need to protect the child from accidental injury and the importance of close observation and thorough reporting.

19 Meningitis is always considered a medical emergency; early recognition and prompt treatment are essential for a favorable recovery. Diagnosis is confirmed by the results of a lumbar puncture. The nurse assisting with this procedure must understand the importance of maintaining the position of the child.

20 Nursing care of the child in the acute phase of meningitis includes correction of dehydration, restraints to safeguard intravenous infusion, frequent monitoring of vital signs, control of temperature, and recording of intake and output.

21 Cerebral palsy is a nonprogressive disorder of motion and posture resulting from brain injury or insult during a period of early brain growth. Treatment is directed toward limiting a disability and may continue throughout the affected person's life.

22 The three main types of cerebral palsy are spastic type, extrapyramidal (nonspastic) type, and mixed cerebral palsy, which combines the spastic and extrapyramidal types.

23 A team approach is necessary for the care of a child with cerebral palsy and his family. Through physical and occupational therapy, surgical techniques, and medication, youngsters with cerebral palsy are able to meet their daily personal needs and, in some cases, to prepare for self-supporting occupations.

24 Encephalitis is an inflammation of the brain caused by infectious agents. The nursing care of a child with encephalitis is much like that of a child with meningitis.

25 Signs and symptoms of brain tumors are headache, dizziness, lethargy, indifference, irritability, morning vomiting, double or blurred vision, speech, balance, and gait problems, and local muscle weakness. Care of the child with a possible brain tumor includes observation for any of these signs and symptoms in addition to assessment of vital signs and precautions to prevent falls during ambulation.

26 Four common clinical manifestations of neuroblastoma are (1) a mass usually involving the abdomen or lymph nodes, (2) neurological signs, (3) pain, usually in the bone or joints, and (4) orbital signs. Because the neuroblastoma is a highly malignant tumor with tendencies to produce widespread metastases, aggressive therapy usually includes surgical excision, irradiation, and chemotherapy.

27 The term *concussion* implies a loss of consciousness with a temporary neuronal dysfunction caused by jarring with no pathological evidence of damage to the underlying brain. The period of memory loss that surrounds a concussion is called post-traumatic amnesia (PTA).

28 Contusions and lacerations are characterized by specific findings, and are frequently accompanied by hemorrhages or bleeding into the brain substance. A basic neurologic check includes assessment of level of consciousness, pupil response, motor function, and vital signs.

29 Intracranial hematomas should be suspected in every case of head injury with coma or one-sided weakness. Unless the intracranial pressure is reduced, neurological deterioration follows and can prove to be fatal.

30 Epidural hematomas result from a torn high-pressure arterial system and characteristically demonstrate a relatively rapid downhill course unless identified and treated.

31 Subdural hematomas may be associated with severe brain injury and are divided into three categories (acute, subacute, and chronic), depending on the time interval from injury to onset of symptoms.

32 Skull fractures are either linear or depressed. Symptoms that may alert the nurse to a skull fracture after the child's hospital admission include black-and-blue marks around the eyes or ears on the second day and watery fluid or discharge from the ear or nose.

33 Nursing care of children with skull fractures includes establishment and maintenance of an adequate airway and proper ventilation and circulation. Children should be kept in a lateral, slightly elevated position and should be turned hourly.

34 Initial examination of the head-injured child consists of a detailed neurological examination to

facilitate a more accurate diagnosis of the extent of injury and to form the baseline from which subsequent progress can be judged. The nurse is responsible for careful systematic serial observations and recording of changing factors and physical signs.

35 Recognition of the depth of responsiveness is essential in determining the initial severity of the comatose child's brain insult. The Glasgow Coma Scale (GCS) is a reliable instrument designed to define the degree of responsiveness.

36 Common causes of visual impairment in infancy and childhood are trauma, strabismus, and refractive error.

37 A professional eye examination should be performed on every child immediately after birth, at 6 months, and once between ages 3 and 5. Annual follow-up screening in the schools is recommended.

38 Children with the following findings should be referred to an ophthalmologist: possible strabismus; poor visual fixation preference or a visual acuity difference between the two eyes of two lines or more on the eye chart; vision in either eye of 20/40 or less; evidence of structural deformity of the eye; and family history of retinoblastoma, congenital cataracts, or genetic or metabolic eye diseases.

39 The incidence of retinopathy of prematurity (ROP) has decreased but is reemerging as the use of oxygen therapy rises in the salvage of high-risk infants.

40 Developmental dyslexia can occur in children in the presence or absence of visual deficit. A multidisciplinary team is best qualified to deal with such learning disorders.

41 The imbalance of the extraocular muscles in strabismus can lead to poor alignment, amblyopia, and poor binocular vision. Specific treatment of strabismus depends on the cause and may include glasses, occlusive therapy, orthoptics, or surgery. Specific treatment of amblyopia may include glasses or occlusive therapy.

42 Refractive errors are myopia, hyperopia, and astigmatism, and usually do not cause difficulties until the child reaches school age. Vision usually can be corrected to a normal level with proper glasses.

43 Surgical removal of cataracts is the only effective method of treatment for all but a few infants and children. The postoperative period is usually short and requires a sterile eye pad, protective shield, and some limitation of activity. Every effort should be made to reduce crying and prevent vomiting.

44 Retinoblastoma is the most common ocular malignancy of childhood. Early recognition and treatment are essential to prevent rapid metastasis.

45 Traumatic hyphema (hemorrhage within the anterior chamber of the eye) is probably the most common ocular injury necessitating hospitalization. Treatment includes bed rest, bilateral eye patches, and sedation. Children should not be placed on the affected side.

46 The degree of auditory dysfunction, the developmental time at which hearing impairment occurs, and the duration of the impairment all determine to what extent the child develops normal speech, language, and educational and psychosocial skills.

47 The three main categories of hearing disorders are (1) peripheral impairments, (2) central impairments, and (3) functional impairments.

48 Hearing loss can occur during the prenatal, perinatal, or postnatal stages of a child's development. The following criteria may indicate significant hearing loss in young children: hearing levels of 15 dB HL or greater, indications of otitis media during more than half the time for a period of 6 months in a child under 18 months, and fluctuating hearing levels from less than 15 dB HL to over 15 dB HL 6 months or more during the first year of life.

49 All newborns meeting one or more of the following criteria should be tested and followed up for the presence of hearing loss: history of hereditary childhood hearing impairment; rubella or other intrauterine infections; defects of ear, nose, throat, or larnyx, birth weight of less than 1500 g; and high serum bilirubin concentrations associated with jaundice that appear in the first 24 hours.

50 Behaviors that may alert the nurse to the presence of peripheral or central hearing dysfunction in a child include the following: better response in quiet than noisy environments, hyperactivity, disinterest in or lack of attention to sounds in the environment, difficulty following verbal instructions unless accompanied by visual demonstrations, inadequate vocabulary, problems maintaining concentration, and social isolation.

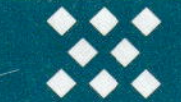

CRITICAL THOUGHT QUESTIONS

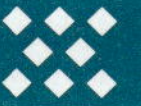

1 In contrast to the adult, why are fractures a common problem in childhood and adolescence? How does this correlate to the developmental stages? Identify the types of fractures and their medical treatment, and review the nursing implications for care of the child with a cast or in traction.

2 Discuss how chronic musculoskeletal problems, such as rheumatoid arthritis, scoliosis, Duchenne's muscular dystrophy, cerebral palsy, and osteomyelitis, can make an impact on a child's growth and development. What is the role of the nurse in caring for children with these conditions?

3 What are the major causes of head injuries in infants and children? How are head injuries classified? How are cranial checks performed on a child? What signs indicate increased intracranial pressure?

4 Seizure disorders are frequently diagnosed during childhood. Identify the major seizure disorders. What should the nurse record regarding seizure activity? What safety precautions should be taken if a major seizure is witnessed? What is involved in the treatment of seizure disorders?

5 List two of the most common vision problems that occur in childhood. How can these be detected? What is their medical treatment? What are the nursing considerations?

6 What are the most common causes of hearing loss in infants and children? What can the nurse do to aid in the detection and prevention of hearing loss?

REFERENCES

American Academy of Otolaryngology-Head and Neck Surgery Subcommittee on Cochlear Implants. In Kveton J, Balkany TJ: Status of cochlear implantation in children, *J Pediatr* 118(25): 1-7, 1991.

Apt L: The eye. In Burg FD, Ingelfinger JR, and Wald ER, editors: *Gellis and Kagan's current pediatric therapy*, Philadelphia, WB Saunders, 1993.

Brosnan H: Nursing management of the adolescent with idiopathic scoliosis, *Nurs Clin North Am* 26(1): 17-31, 1991.

Campbell LS, Campbell JD: Musculo-skeletal trauma in children, *Crit Care Nurs Clin North Am* 3(3):445-456, 1991.

Carrol NC: Treatment of Bone Tumors and Limb Salvage. In Burg FD, Ingelfinger JR, and Wald ER, editors: *Gellis and Kagan's current pediatric therapy*, Philadelphia, WB Saunders, 1993.

Consensus Conference: Noise and hearing loss, *JAMA*, 263(23): 3185-3190, 1990.

Cotton LA: Unit rod segmental spinal instrumentation for the treatment of neuromuscular scoliosis, *Orthop Nurs* 10(5): 17-23, 1991.

Davidson PW: Visual impairment and blindness. In Levine MD, Cary WB, and Crocker AC, editors: *Developmental-behavioral pediatrics*, ed 2, Philadelphia, WB Saunders, 1992.

Friedman EM: Foreign bodies in the external ear. In Burg FD, Ingelfinger JR, and Wald ER, editors: *Gellis and Kagan's current pediatric therapy*, Philadelphia, WB Saunders, 1993.

Friedman EM: Injuries to the middle ear. In Burg FD, Ingelfinger JR, and Wald ER, editors: *Gellis and Kagan's current pediatric therapy*, Philadelphia, WB Saunders, 1993.

Gagliardi BA: The impact of Duchenne muscular dystrophy on families, *Orthop Nurs* 10(5): 41-49, 1991.

Gregg JR and Ergin TM: Orthopedic trauma. In Burg FD, Ingelfinger JR, and Wald ER, editors: *Gellis and Kagan's current pediatric therapy*, Philadelphia, WB Saunders, 1993.

Hall DE: Head injuries. In Hoekelman RA et al, editors: *Primary pediatric care*, ed 2, St. Louis, Mosby, 1992.

Harrison LL: Minimizing barriers when teaching hearing impaired clients, *MCN* 15(2): 113, 1990.

Healy GB: Hearing loss. In Burg FD, Ingelfinger JR, and Wald ER, editors: *Gellis and Kagan's current pediatric therapy*, Philadelphia, WB Saunders, 1993.

Kaplan SL: Bacterial meningitis and septicemia beyond the neonatal period. In Burg FD, Ingelfinger JR, and Wald ER, editors: *Gellis and Kagan's current pediatric therapy*, Philadelphia, WB Saunders, 1993.

Kenna MA: Labyrinthitis. In Burg FD, Ingelfinger JR, and Wald ER, editors: *Gellis and Kagan's current pediatric therapy*, Philadelphia, WB Saunders, 1993.

Kotecki J et al: The miracle of little Carlos (pediatric head injury), *Nursing '90*, 20(5): 52, 1990.

Langman CB: Rickets. In Burg FD, Ingelfinger JR, and Wald ER, editors: *Gellis and Kagan's current pediatric therapy*, Philadelphia, WB Saunders, 1993.

Mason KJ: Congenital orthopedic anomalies and their impact on the family, *Nurs Clin North Am* 26:1-16, 1991.

McIlvain-Simpson G and Singsen B: Decreasing morning stiffness, *Small Talk* 3(6): 8, 1991.

Mier RJ: Torticollis. In Burg FD, Ingelfinger JR, and Wald ER, editors: *Gellis and Kagan's current pediatric therapy*, Philadelphia, WB Saunders, 1993.

Olson EV: The hazards of immobility, *Am J Nurs* 90:43-52, 1990.

O'Shea JS: Otitis media. In Burg FD, Ingelfinger JR, and Wald ER, editors: *Gellis and Kagan's current pediatric therapy*, Philadelphia, WB Saunders, 1993.

Park TS and Owen JH: Surgical management of aseptic diplegia in cerebral palsy, *N Engl J Med* 326(11): 745-749, 1992.

Pomeroy SL et al: Seizures and other neurologic sequelae of bacterial meningitis in children, *N Engl J Med* 323: 1651-1657, 1990.

Powell KR: Meningitis. In Hoekelman RA et al, editors: *Primary pediatric care*, ed 2, St. Louis, Mosby, 1992.

Roddy SM, McBride MC: Seizure disorders. In Hoekelman RA et al, editors: *Primary pediatric care,* ed 2, St. Louis, Mosby, 1992.

Roush J: Acoustic amplification for hearing-impaired infants and young children, *Inf Young Child* 2(4): 59-71, 1990.

Saez-Llorens X and Siegel JD: Neonatal septicemia, meningitis and pneumonia. In Burg FD, Ingelfinger JR, and Wald ER, editors: *Gellis and Kagan's current pediatric therapy,* Philadelphia, WB Saunders, 1993.

Siegel IM: Muscular dystrophy and related myopathies. In Burg FD, Ingelfinger JR, and Wald ER, editors: *Gellis and Kagan's current pediatric therapy,* Philadelphia, WB Saunders, 1993.

Servodio CA, Abramson DH, Romanella A: Retinoblastoma, *Cancer Nurs* 14(2), 117-123, 1991.

Sherman DW: Managing acute head injury, *Nursing '90* 20(4):47-51, 1990.

Southwood TR et al: Unconventional remedies used for patients with juvenile arthritis, *Pediatrics* 85 150-154, 1990.

Sussman MD: Disorders of the spine and shoulder girdle. In Burg FD, Ingelfinger JR, and Wald ER, editors: *Gellis and Kagan's current pediatric therapy,* Philadelphia, WB Saunders, 1993.

Szer HS: Juvenile rheumatoid arthritis. In Burg FD, Ingelfinger JR, and Wald ER, editors: *Gellis and Kagan's current pediatric therapy,* Philadelphia, WB Saunders, 1993.

Thabit G and Mitcheli LL: Orthopedic disorders of the extremities. In Burg FD, Ingelfinger JR, and Wald ER, editors: *Gellis and Kagan's current pediatric therapy,* Philadelphia, WB Saunders, 1993.

Thompson M and Thompson G: Early identification of hearing loss: listen to parents, *Clin Pediatr* 30(2): 77-80, 1991.

Torfs C et al: Prenatal and perinatal factors in the etiology of cerebral palsy, *J Pediatr* 116: 615-619, 1990.

Wallace CA and Levinson JR: Juvenile rheumatoid arthritis outcome and treatment for the 1990s, *Rheum Dis Clin North Am* 17: 891-905, 1991.

Watts HG: Bone and joint infections. In Burg FD, Ingelfinger JR, and Wald ER, editors: *Gellis and Kagan's current pediatric therapy,* Philadelphia, WB Saunders, 1993.

Yager JY and Vannucci RC: Brain tumors. In Hoekelman RA and others, editors: *Primary pediatric care,* ed 2, St. Louis, Mosby, 1992.

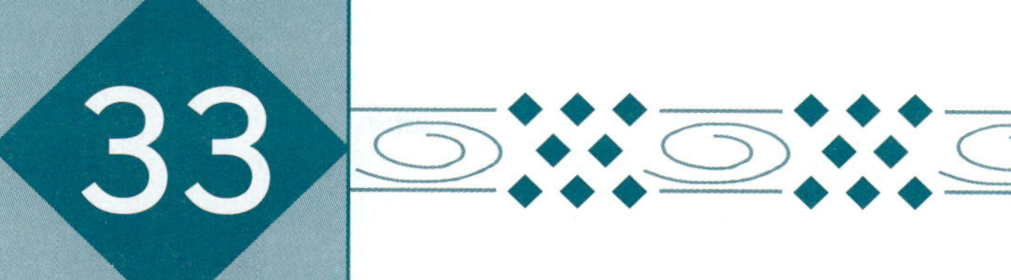

33

Orthopedic Technology: Traction, Casting, and Braces

CHAPTER OBJECTIVES

After studying this chapter, the student should be able to:

1. Define traction and enumerate four reasons for its use in orthopedics.
2. Compare and contrast skin and skeletal traction in three different ways.
3. Identify three ways in which countertraction may be created to prevent the loss of traction.
4. Discuss four ways to help prevent pressure areas.
5. Describe four different traction setups noted in the chapter and the conditions for which they are usually prescribed.
6. Explain why casts are often "petaled" or lined and edged with stockinette.
7. List eight signs of possible neurovascular complications involving a casted or wrapped extremity.
8. Explain one method of measuring a supine patient for crutches.

This chapter presents basic nursing procedures and responsibilities involved in the care of patients receiving therapy in traction, casts, or braces. These patients may be hospitalized for various reasons. Fractures, musculoskeletal diseases, and neurological disorders account for most diagnoses. For more information regarding specific illnesses in this grouping, the student is referred to Chapter 32, which discusses in greater detail some of these problems and the nursing care they require.

TRACTION

Traction, or methods of exerting pull, is discussed first because it often precedes casting. Traction is used primarily to decrease muscle spasm or tightening and may be applicable in any of the following situations:

1. To bring a broken bone back into alignment (reduce a fracture) and provide immobilization for correct union
2. To secure a corrected position to treat a congenital or acquired deformity not involving a fracture (reduce a dislocated hip)
3. To prevent or treat contracture deformities
4. To relieve the pain of muscle spasm.

Basic Types

Traction may be exerted manually or by means of certain appliances. There are two main types of traction—skin and skeletal.

Skin traction

Skin traction indirectly helps position the bone by pulling on the skin and muscles. It is relatively simple to apply, involves no surgical operation, and may be accomplished in a home setting. However, only a limited amount of weight may be added with this type of traction, and occasionally the maximum amount allowed is insufficient to produce the desired results. Also, the skin may show signs of irritation—allergic reactions, circulation difficulties, or friction—caused by the supportive wrapping. The weight is usually secured to the skin by running strips of adhesive material, cotton or perforated plastic-backed adhesive tape, or foam rubber up both sides of the extremity and securing the strips with a compression (Ace) bandage. The ends of the strips are then attached to a foot spreader, which in turn is connected to the desired weight.

Skeletal traction

Skeletal traction is secured by inserting a mechanical device directly into or through the bone and attaching the prescribed weight. The bone may be fixed with wires, pins, or tongs. Considerable weight may be attached to such devices, and no bulky or irritating skin wrappings are necessary. Nevertheless, skeletal traction, too, has its drawbacks. Since the bone is actually pierced, danger of infection is always present, and a surgical procedure is involved in the insertion of the mechanical attachment. The areas where the holding devices are inserted through the skin must be frequently inspected for signs of inflammation, infection, drainage, and odor. Special pin care may be ordered, usually involving the cleansing of the skin around the pin with half-strength hydrogen peroxide, followed by the application of a protective antimicrobial ointment.

Nursing Considerations

The first time a student cares for a patient in traction may be a challenge. There seems to be a surplus of weights, ropes, pulleys, and bars, which fit together to produce a desired result. The mechanical apparatus used may seem complex, but the basic principles of traction are simple and clear.

Maintenance of proper traction

The maintenance of proper traction depends on the correct direction and amount of pull exerted through the use of ropes, pulleys, and weights and on the correct positioning or alignment of the patient. Therefore it is important that the nurse understand the orders concerning the care of each individual patient in traction and maintain the correct relationship of the various parts of the traction apparatus to the patient. The following points should be noted:

1 Pulleys increase the amount and change the direction of pull on a body part by a weight. A rope should ride smoothly on a pulley to exert the ordered weight.
2 Weights should not be added or subtracted by the nurse. Too much weight may cause the nonunion of a break; too little weight may cause unwanted overriding and an extremity of unequal length. Weights should always hang freely. Weights should be frequently observed so that they do not come to rest on a rung of the bed, a poorly placed chair, or the floor, or become altered in any way by the curious hands of ambulatory children.
3 The amount of time that traction is applied should be clearly understood. Skin traction may occasionally be removed, but such removal always depends on the physician's order. Skeletal traction is continuous and should not be interrupted.
4 Ropes should be in good condition and frequently inspected for signs of wear. Knots should be taped for additional safety. Multiple weights attached to the same rope should be taped together so that they cannot easily fall or be removed.

Countertraction

Pull in one direction must be balanced by pull in the opposite direction for traction to remain effective. This opposing pull is called *countertraction,* not to be confused with *balanced traction.*

Countertraction may be exerted in various ways. If the weights used to create the initial pull are not extremely heavy, it may only be necessary to keep the patient in a certain place in bed, checking periodically to see that the patient has not slipped. The patient's body provides the countertraction.

If the pull is stronger, the end of the bed where the initial traction is applied may need to be elevated so that gravity increases the countertraction created by the patient's body weight. Elevation may be achieved through the use of grooved blocks under two legs of the bed, a mechanical bed lift, or special positioning of an electric bed.

If it is very difficult to maintain the child in the proper position in bed, sometimes a restraint may be used (a restraining jacket or waist restraint). However, such devices may cause pressure areas. The use of restraints must be carefully evaluated.

Sometimes the treated body part is placed in a frame or splint that is lifted off the surface of the bed. When this arrangement is used, a counterweight may often be connected to the frame, exerting force in the opposing direction. In review, countertraction is created in four basic ways:

1 Maintenance of body position in bed by constant observation and correction, if needed
2 Elevation of the part of the bed closest to the weights
3 Use of restraints
4 Application of a counterweight

The method employed depends on the desires of the physician and the responses of the patient. Failure to maintain correct placement in bed while the patient is in traction may (1) cause the weights to rest on the floor or some other surface and temporarily stop traction altogether, in some cases allowing possible displacement, or (2) change the angle of pull and distort the result desired. Both situations are potentially harmful. When a nurse is told, "Keep Susie's hips at the level of the tape markers on the bed," or "Be sure that Roger is kept pulled up in bed," it is to prevent these situations.

Activity and body position

The amount of movement and activity allowed for the patient in traction should be understood and promoted, and good body alignment and support should be maintained. Bedboards may be placed under the mattress to prevent sagging.

Some patients are allowed relatively little movement or position change because of their particular musculoskeletal problems or traction arrangements. If the nurse allows these patients to sit up or turn on their sides, the traction may be lost or altered so that treatment fails or complications may result. However, a patient who has a leg in a Thomas splint support, which is raised off the surface of the mattress, is allowed considerable movement. Such traction maintains proper alignment when the patient's trunk is raised. Even a slight amount of turning toward the splinted leg is usually possible. Such an arrangement is termed *balanced traction*. When balanced, traction is used in conjunction with an overhead bar and trapeze. The patient enjoys considerable activity, and nursing care is greatly simplified.

Although it is important that patients not be moved in a way that disrupts their traction, it is also important that they be moved to the extent permitted to encourage proper body function, elimination, respiration, and circulation and to avoid pressure areas. Exercise and correct positioning of the uninvolved extremities are necessary to prevent other problems (stiffness or deformity) from occurring in some patients. As in all cases of prolonged immobilization, a high fluid intake should be encouraged. A diet well supplied with roughage and natural laxatives, such as prunes, helps prevent constipation. Special attention should be given to the prevention of footdrop or undesired internal or external rotation of the lower extremities.

Circulation and skin condition

The circulation and skin condition of a patient in traction or other immobilization devices, such as casts, should be frequently evaluated.

The skin of any patient who is immobilized for long periods and is permitted only limited movement must be meticulously observed and protected. Pressure areas are most likely to develop over bony prominences, such as the hips, sacrum, ankles, elbows, scapulae, and shoulders. Areas exposed to continuous friction are also likely spots for skin breakdown. If a Thomas splint is used, the skin area under the padded ring must be frequently inspected. The heels of both the affected and nonaffected leg should be carefully observed. Often the foot that is not being treated may develop a sore heel because the patient moves up in bed by digging the heel into the mattress to obtain leverage. To prevent unnecessary pressure, the linen must be kept smooth and tight, and crumbs and other irritating small objects must be eliminated from the bed. Skin traction wrappings may cause circulation and nerve interference similar to that occasionally encountered with the casted patient. Inability to dorsiflex the exposed big toe of a wrapped affected lower extremity should be reported to the physician promptly.

Pressure areas are much easier to prevent than to treat. Frequent inspection and cleansing of susceptible areas; use of an egg crate mattress; maintenance of wrinkle-free linen; continual elevation of the bed's head to an angle of less than 30 degrees; and encouragement of as much movement as is allowed, consistent with the patient's well-being, greatly reduce, if not entirely eliminate, pressure areas. Every complaint of skin tenderness, burning sensation, or aching should be investigated. It does not take long for a small red area to become an enlarged, open sore, particularly in areas where circulation may already be impaired. All devices that lift a pressure area off a surface must be used with caution and frequently evaluated, since they may sometimes cause circulatory disturbances themselves. Patients who are paralyzed or suffer from sensory loss must receive special care and observation. A child in traction should routinely receive back and skin care during baths and at least twice more during the day. The use of an overhead bar and trapeze can greatly facilitate back and skin care when such aids are feasible. If no such arrangement is possible, a nurse may press down on the mattress with one hand to allow her other hand to massage, or two nurses may

◆ **TABLE 33-1**
Common Types of Traction

Name	Basic Type	Most Common Indications	Major Nursing Considerations
Bryant's	Skin—to lower extremities	Fractured femur in child under 30 lb	Report immediately any signs of neurovascular problems
Buck's	Skin—to lower extremities	Hip or knee contractures or immobilization	Avoid skin breakdown around ankles and heels
Russell's	Skin (may incorporate skeletal)—to lower extremities	Hip contractures or immobilization for fractured femur	Maintain proper alignment with patient flat
90°—90°	Skeletal	Fractured femur—preschool- and school-age child	Avoid any movement of bed or traction setup

work together to lift the child *slightly* to facilitate skin care, depending on the type of traction used.

Sometimes the use of imitation or genuine lamb's wool mats under the patient is helpful. Duoderm, opsite, and granulex spray are agents used to toughen areas of potential pressure. However, benzoin may stain the sheets.

Bed making

Some hospitals are supplied with special traction linen designed to fit under or around different traction appliances, such as the Thomas splint. A special "split" top sheet may be used on either side of the splint. More commonly a large sheet is simply pulled to one side over the uninvolved leg, and a light baby blanket is draped over the splinted leg at night. Another satisfactory and modest arrangement uses two blankets, each contained within a separate folded sheet. One such blanket-sheet combination is placed over the chest and abdomen of the patient, with open edges under the chin; the other is placed on top of the uninvolved leg and below the suspended leg, with open edges toward the foot of the bed where they are tucked in. The upper and lower blanket-sheet combinations are then pinned together around the thigh of the leg in traction. This makes a very neat bed. Traction patients may have special snap-on pajamas (tops and bottoms) to facilitate dressing, or perineal drapes or G-strings may be used.

Types of traction equipment

Traction equipment may vary depending on the individual needs of the patient (see Table 33-1).

External fixation

External fixation is a new adaptation of an older method of treating complicated fractures and may be used instead of traction, casting, or internal fixation (Fig. 33-1). The external fixation device consists of pins inserted through the fractured bone and attached to a metal frame, which provides reduction and stabilization. Possible indications for its use are open comminuted fractures, fractures that occur with multiple injuries, or infected bone that fails to heal properly. The advantages of external fixation are an immediate and rigid stabilization of the fracture, an early mobilization of adjacent joints, and a shorter bed confinement. At the same time, it allows for complete visualization and treatment of an open wound. The major disadvantages lie in the cumbersome nature of the device and the sometimes frightening appearance of the open wound. In addition, the multiple pin sites present the possibility of infection. It thus becomes extremely important for the nurse to prepare the child ahead of time, to explain carefully the reason for its use to the child and his parents, and to provide meticulous pin-site care to prevent infection of the pin tract. External fixation is less frequently seen in younger children because of their ability to heal rapidly, but it can offer earlier mobilization and rigid stabilization for the older child with a complicated fracture.

Bryant's traction

Bryant's traction is often used for the treatment of fractured femurs in young children or to lengthen the muscles adjacent to a dislocated hip (Fig. 33-2). Such patients must be carefully observed for developing circulation problems because the leg wrappings may interfere with the blood flow. Swollen, cool, or "blotchy" looking toes, slow blanching on pressure, or delayed return of skin color after pressure is released from a toenail bed all are signs that should be promptly reported. The pulse at the ankle may be checked to detect circulatory problems. Unexplained restlessness, crying, and complaints or indications of leg pain must be further evaluated immediately, and assessment for circulatory impairment must be carried out on both the

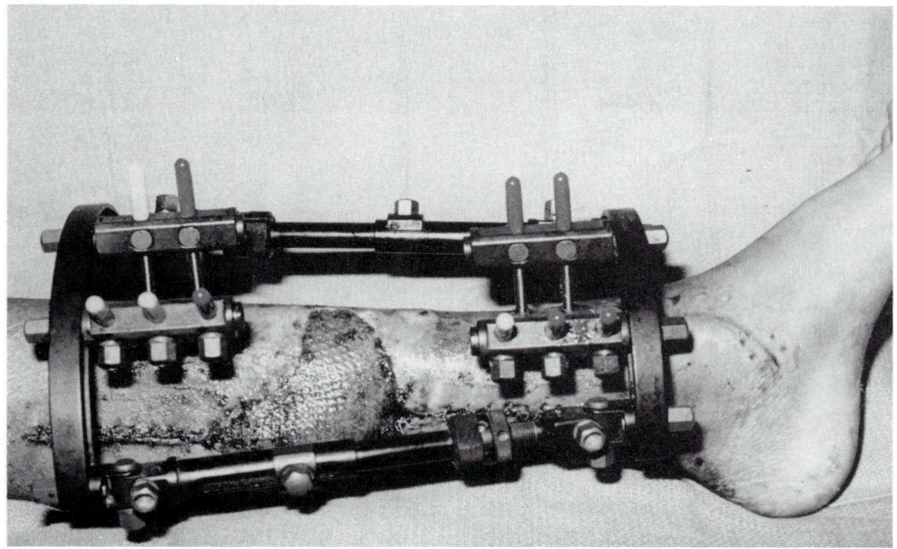

Fig. 33-1 External fixation. Severe open fracture of tibia has been stabilized with Ace-Fisher external fixator. Skin defect has been closed with soleus muscle flap and covered with split-thickness skin graft. (Courtesy F. Craig Swenson, MD, La Jolla, Calif.)

affected and unaffected extremity. This type of patient should be raised slightly during feedings to prevent aspiration. The jacket restraint can be loosened or removed if a responsible person is at the bedside but it should be in place when the child is alone. If the nurse is rewrapping the compression bandages, care must be taken to wrap them tightly enough to secure the traction but not so tightly as to impair circulation or prevent a slight degree of flexion in the knees. To make the bed, one nurse must lift the child's body just enough to allow another nurse to slide the bed sheets under the hips and back. The weights should not be removed. Frequent back care and diaper changes are a necessity.

Russell's traction

Russell's traction, a skin traction using a sling and single rope arrangement attached to one weight supported by multiple pulleys, is used to treat undisplaced fractures and provide postoperative hip and knee immobilization in older children (Fig. 33-3). If the traction pull of the sling is separate and in the opposite direction, it is called *split Russell traction.* Because the extremity is suspended, more patient movement is allowed, and nursing care is considerably easier.

90°-90° traction

90°-90° traction is commonly used to reduce a fractured femur (Fig. 33-4). Both the hip and knee are placed in 90-degree flexion. A pin is inserted through

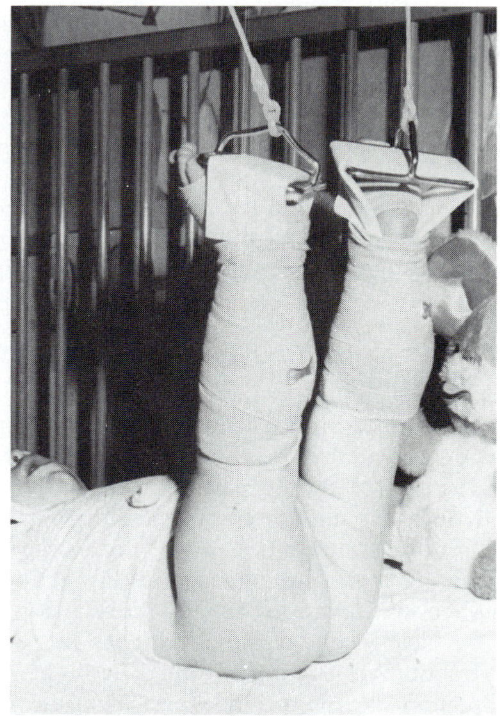

Fig. 33-2 Bryant's or vertical traction may be used for infants or young children weighing less than 30 pounds. Pelvis is no longer lifted above mattress by traction, since this has been associated with circulatory problems in legs. Knees should be slightly flexed. Both legs are placed in traction even though only one may be fractured. Better alignment is maintained. (Courtesy Children's Hospital and Health Center, San Diego, Calif.)

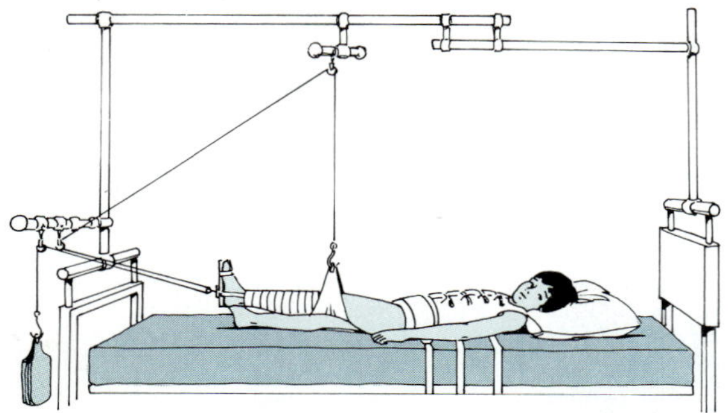

Fig. 33-3 Russell's traction can be used to treat fractures in older children and adults. (From Wong DL: *Essentials of pediatric nursing,* ed 4, St Louis, 1993, Mosby.)

the distal femur or proximal tibia, and traction is applied. A sling or cast on the lower leg is used for suspension.

Buck's extension

A rather simple, frequently used skin traction for treatment of hip synovitis or muscle spasm of the lower extremities or lower back is called *Buck's extension* (Fig. 33-5). Note the adhesive strips on the sides, the elastic bandage wrapping, the foot spreader (to prevent pressure of the adhesive strips against the ankle), the pulley, and the rope leading to the freely hanging weight. Some physicians order the placement of a small flattened pillow under the leg just above the Achilles tendon to protect the heel from pressure. In this figure the angle of the pull elevates the heel slightly off the bed.

Cervical traction

The patient in cervical traction may have a sling or halter arrangement around the chin and occiput (Fig. 33-6), or the patient may be placed in skeletal traction, which involves the placement of metal tongs into (but not through) the cranium (Fig. 33-7). Orders regarding the positioning of the patient, the movement allowed, and whether any elevation of the backrest is permitted should be clearly understood. Patients in skeletal-cervical traction are often positioned in slight hyperextension, and flexion of the cervical spine is not permitted. If cervical skin traction is used, foam rubber padding may be necessary in the chin area to prevent skin irritation. Gum chewing may relieve aching jaw joints.

Pelvic traction

Occasionally pelvic traction may be ordered to relieve lower back pain. Pelvic traction is created by a pelvic band or girdle attached to a weight or weights. Sometimes a thoracic belt may be used for countertraction. Such an arrangement is designed to relieve muscle spasm and lessen pressure on nerve roots. Pelvic traction may be ordered for continuous or intermittent application. Many patients are given bathroom privileges.

Balanced traction

Balanced traction, involving the suspension of the affected limb above the surface of the bed, provides the opportunity for more movement and activity by the patient. Patients may raise their hips, have their backrests elevated, or turn slightly toward the side of the splinted lower extremity. An overhead bar and trapeze greatly facilitate lifting. The suspension device takes up the slack created and maintains the line of traction. The nurse should remember that no matter how much these patients want to stay up they should intermittently rest flat, without the elevation of the backrest, to prevent hip contractures.

Although suspended traction gives greater liberty of movement and effectively relieves heel pressure, the area where the ring of the Thomas splint rests must be frequently inspected for the development of skin problems. Each day the skin may be gently pulled up or down from under the ring and washed, dried, and massaged. The ring, if leather, can be polished with saddle soap. Fig. 33-8 shows a Thomas splint with a complete ring and a Thomas half-ring splint with a Pearson attachment, which is used to support the extremity. Fig. 33-9 shows a young girl with a balanced skeletal traction, including an extra support to prevent foot drop and an additional weight to correct a tendency toward internal rotation of the leg. Not long after this photograph was taken the girl was sent home in a long-leg plaster cast.

Neufeld's traction

More mobility is possible with this recent type of balanced traction setup that incorporates a skeletal pin into a plaster of Paris cast, ensuring both secure immobilization and substantial traction at the same time. An overhead pulley system enables maximum mobility, even to the point of the patient's moving to a bedside chair. It is used to treat a fractured femur in the older school-age child or adolescent who may be facing a prolonged period of time in traction.

CASTS

Casts are often applied subsequent to treatment by traction, supplying a form of external immobilization

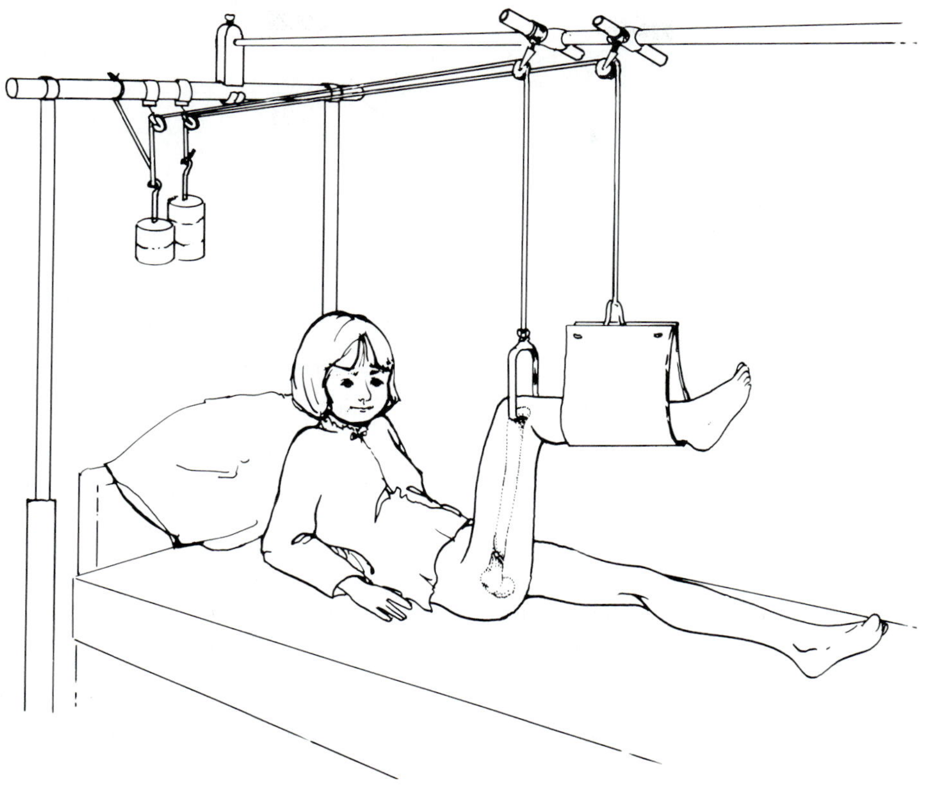

Fig. 33-4 90°-90° traction through distal femur, commonly used for preschool- or school-age child.

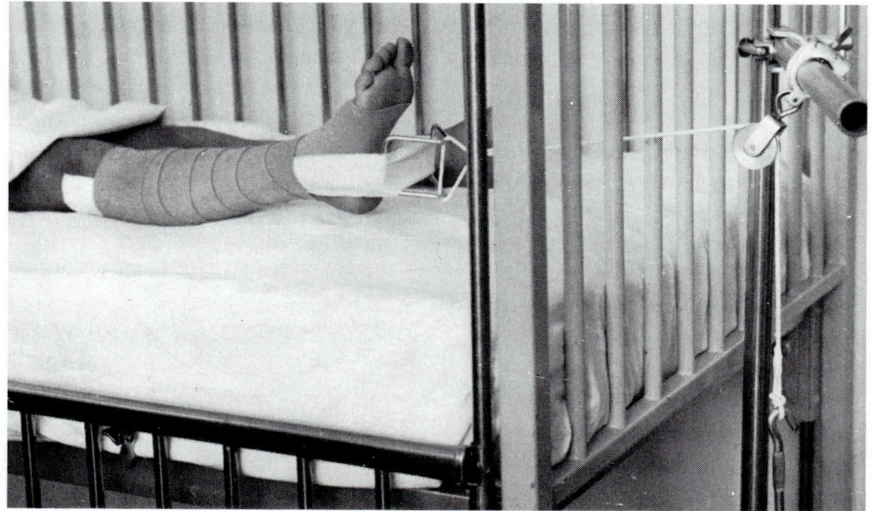

Fig. 33-5 Buck's extension. Note that heel clears mattress. Some physicians use small flat pillow under leg to provide clearance. (Courtesy Children's Hospital and Health Center, San Diego, Calif.)

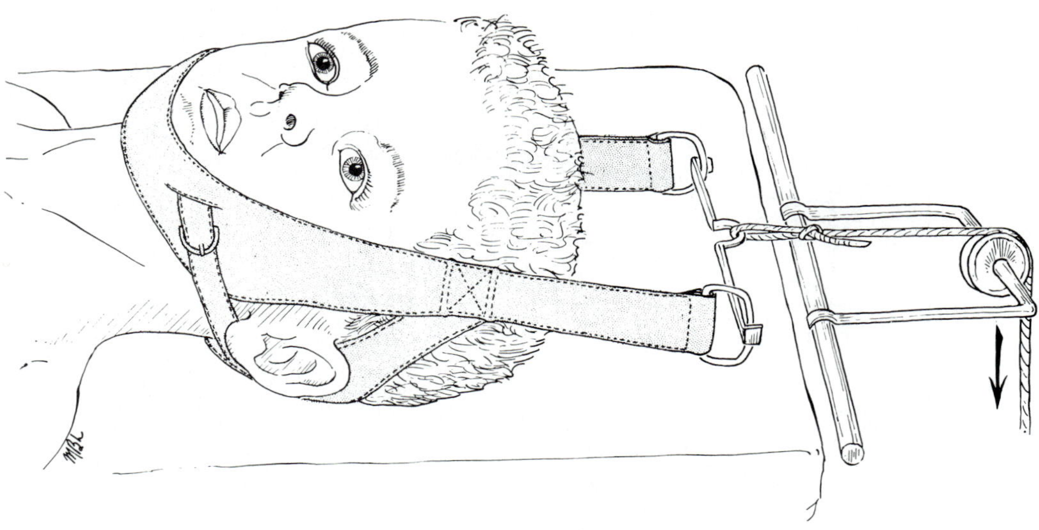

Fig. 33-6 Cervical skin traction with halter.

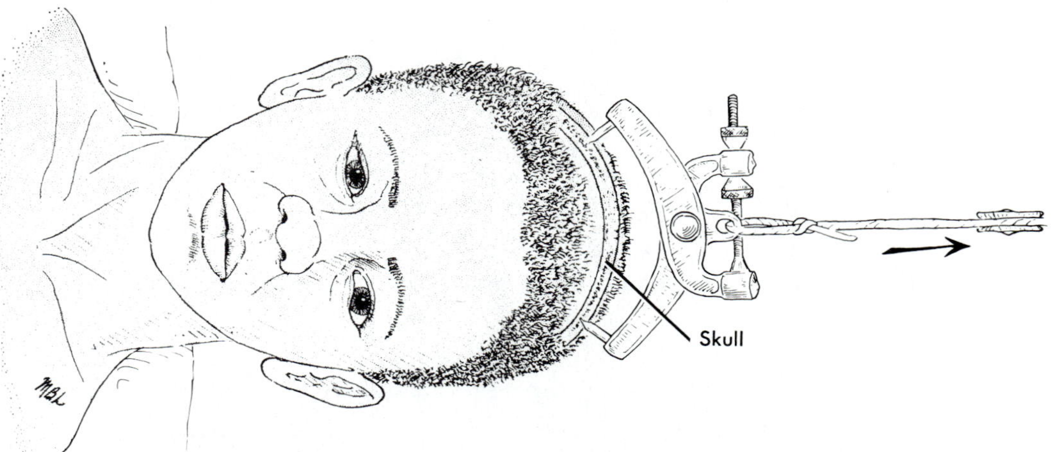

Fig. 33-7 Crutchfield tongs, cervical-skeletal traction.

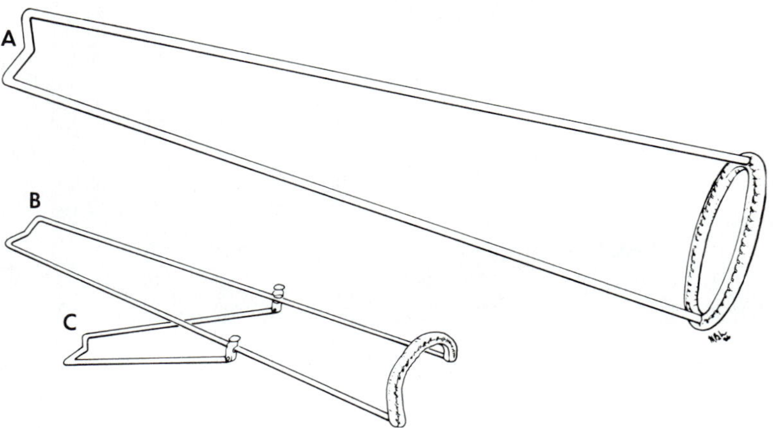

Fig. 33-8 **A,** Thomas splint with complete ring. **B,** Half-ring Thomas splint. **C,** Pearson attachment.

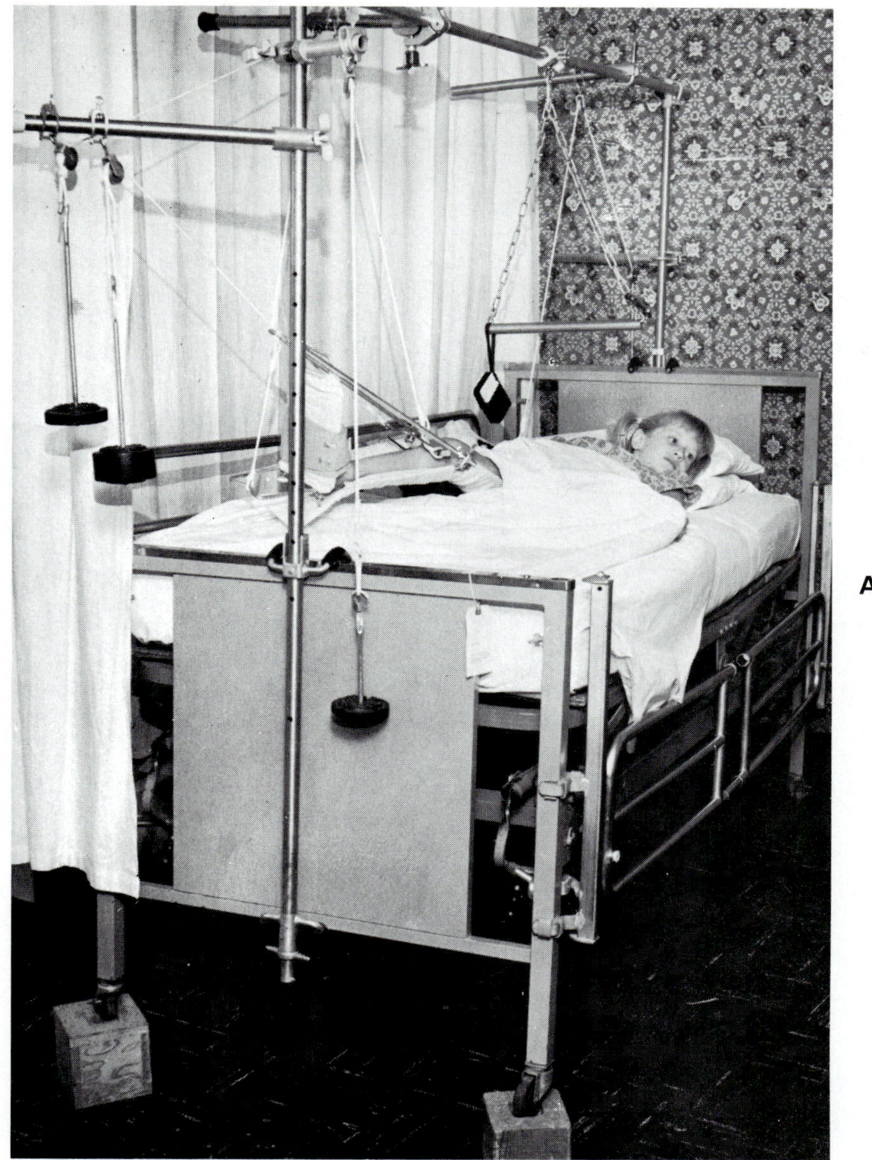

Fig. 33-9 **A,** Patient in balanced traction. (Courtesy Children's Hospital and Health Center, San Diego, Calif.)

Continued.

of a body part. Occasionally, a cast may be applied over a skeletal pin, thus continuing traction, as well as contributing to immobilization. Such a procedure is called *plaster traction.* The ends of the protruding pins should be covered with plaster or some sort of protective device to prevent the snagging of clothing or bed coverings or injury to others. Plaster traction allows greater mobility for the patient (when feasible). In addition to immobilization and possible traction, casts may also be a means of aiding proper positioning or resting a body part.

The most common kind of cast consists of plaster of Paris—impregnated crinoline bandages that have been applied and molded while moist over some type of soft, protective layer and allowed to dry to a hard, resistant shell. Dry plaster of Paris is a form of calcium sulfate; when mixed with water, it forms the substance known as *gypsum.*

Plaster is most often used in the casting of the hospitalized child, but despite their greater expense, synthetic materials (fiberglass and plastic) are increasingly being used to form casts for ambulatory patients. They set rapidly and, depending on the substances and techniques used, may be ready for weight bearing 3 to 30 minutes after application. They are less bulky, light weight, and porous. When applied over special non-

B

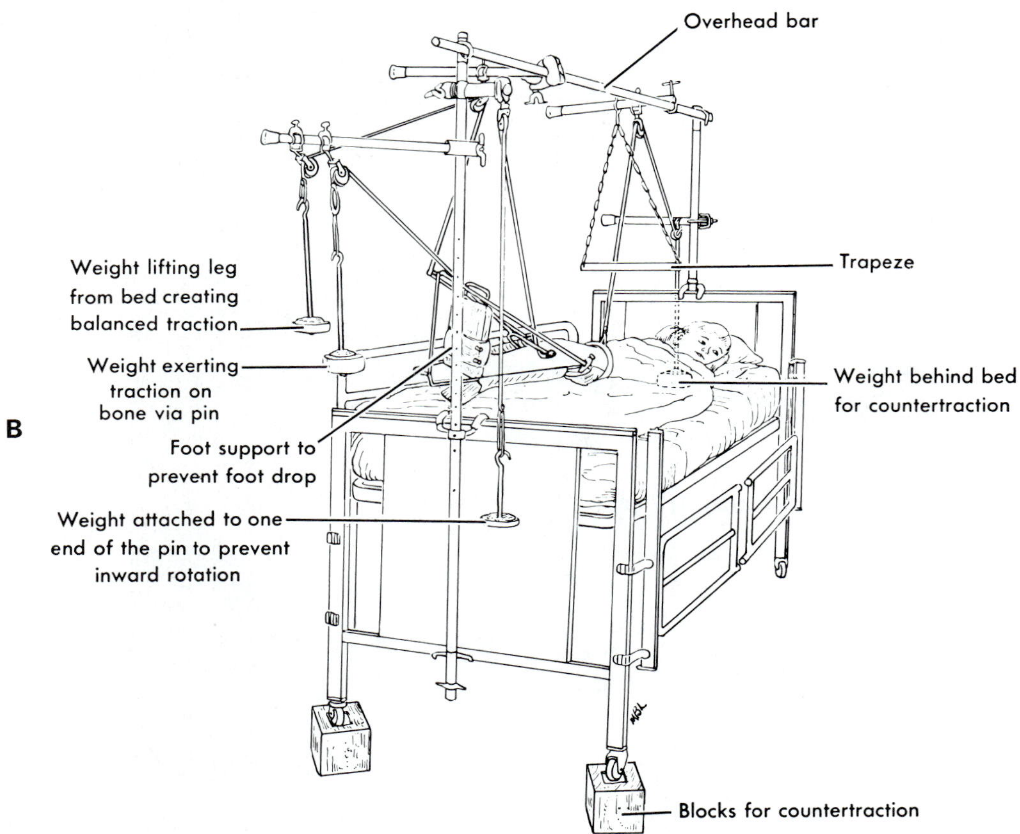

Fig. 33-9, cont'd. B, Explanatory drawing.

C

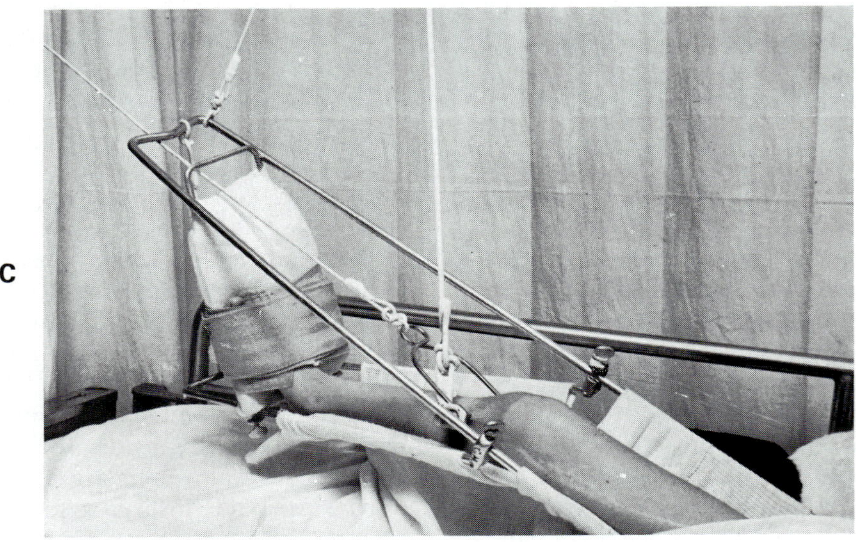

Fig. 33-9, cont'd. C, Close-up view of leg.

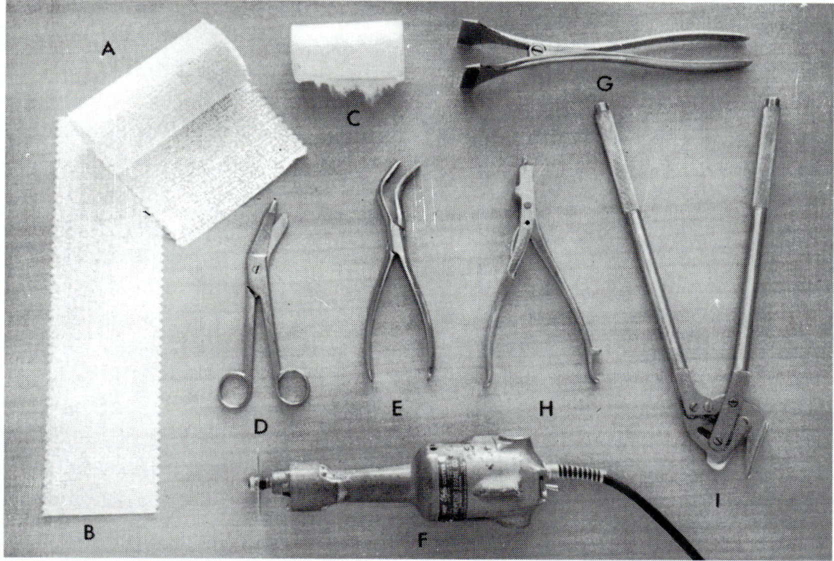

Fig. 33-10 Instruments and materials used in preparing or removing plaster casts. **A,** Plaster roll. **B,** Plaster strip or splint. **C,** Webril (sheet wadding). **D,** Plaster shears (large bandage scissors). **E,** Cast bender. **F,** Cast cutter or saw (electric). **G** and **H,** Cast spreaders. **I,** Cast cutter (manual). (Courtesy Children's Hospital and Health Center, San Diego, Calif.)

absorbent linings, they may be immersed in water if the physician permits. If they do get wet for any reason, they must be carefully dried, a process that takes about an hour. Manufacturer's instructions must be consulted for details of application and care. Because they are more difficult to mold than plaster, synthetics are usually considered less effective for immobilizing severely displaced bones or unstable fractures until initial swelling has subsided. Parents and patients need to be aware that vigorous activity can misalign a fracture or even break a synthetic cast. The exterior of the cast is often rough and can snag clothing or scratch furniture or skin unless precautions are taken.

Application of the Cast

Because of the "orderly disorder" that invariably accompanies plaster applications, it is preferable to schedule cast work in a room especially designed for such procedures—a room that is easily cleaned and contains all the equipment and supplies usually needed.

Commonly needed supplies are as follows:

1 Materials that protect the skin, to be wrapped around the body part before application of plaster or synthetics
   a Sheet wadding (Webril)
   b Tubular stockinette
2 Various widths of plaster of Paris bandages and strips (splints) or synthetic tapes
3 Materials to reinforce or protect areas of the cast or body that are under special pressure or strain
   a Felt
   b Yucca board
   c Wire netting
   d Rubber heels (for leg casts of ambulatory patients)
4 Special tools (Fig. 33-10)
   a Various types of cast knives
   b Plaster shears
   c Cast spreaders and cast benders
   d Manual and electric cast cutters
   e A bucket for water to moisten the cast materials (temperatures vary)
5 Other possible needs
   a Cover gowns
   b Gloves, caps, and masks
   c Special lamps to cure certain synthetic casting materials (Lightcast II)

The furnishings of a cast room need not be elaborate. Usually an examining table, some benches, good lighting, an x-ray film view box, and a sink are sufficient. A sink with a plaster trap is convenient because the water used to soak the plaster of Paris rolls may be discarded into the drain without much danger of plugging the plumbing. If large body casts or scoliosis jackets are applied, additional supportive frames, tables, or slings are needed. Newspapers placed on the floor under the working area aid cleanup.

Preparation of the patient

Some patients undergoing casting procedures are anesthetized to aid muscle relaxation, relieve pain, and facilitate the entire procedure. Of course, patients who have open reductions of fractures or have had other operative procedures just before casting are always anesthetized. Small children are frequently anesthetized for closed reduction procedures. Such patients are given nothing by mouth for several hours before the procedure and usually receive preoperative sedation.

The nurse must make certain that the child and the parents have been informed of this procedure beforehand and know what to expect after the cast has been applied. Sometimes meeting another youngster with a cast or seeing a doll with a casted arm or leg is a helpful preparation for the young child.

Nursing considerations

The nurse assigned to the cast room is responsible for making available all the necessary equipment and supplies. When plaster of Paris is used, the desired width of plaster bandage is removed from its waxed paper wrapper and immersed on end in tepid water. When air bubbles no longer rise from the roll, the bandage is lifted from the water. The sides of the closed bandage are gently squeezed to remove water while retaining the plaster. The loose end of the bandage is unrolled slightly, and the roll is handed to the physician nurse practitioner, or orthopedic technician for application. The bandage should not be dripping at the time of the transfer. The nurse may assist by holding the extremity being casted or support part of the newly formed cast. The palms of the hands should be used in rendering such support to prevent the formation of pressure areas.

Cast Changes and Removal

Sometimes a patient must have one cast removed and another applied (Fig. 33-10). The frequency with which a child must have a cast changed depends on the child's rate of growth, the condition of the cast, and the progress of the desired correction. The plaster cast may be cut manually with a cast knife shaped like a short kitchen paring knife and a hand cast cutter. The cut is made along a line dampened by vinegar solution, hydrogen peroxide, or water from a syringe. A metal strip may be inserted just below the cutting line to protect the body part. An electric vibrating-blade cast cutter may be used instead. The electric saw makes a great deal of noise, which sometimes frightens the patient. When the cast has been carefully cut, the sections are separated by a cast spreader, and the padding underneath is released with large bandage scissors. The body part that was casted must be gently supported and handled and not forced into new, unfamiliar positions. Sudden lack of support or movement often causes considerable stress.

Professional opinion differs regarding the skin care of a patient who has been in a cast for a considerable time and who will almost immediately be enclosed in a cast again. Some physicians want their patients to have baths; others believe that the least amount of handling as possible is best. All wish to prevent trauma to the skin, which leads to trouble during the subsequent period of casting. If the use of a cast is discontinued permanently or for a considerable time, the physician may order a combination of gentle baths and the application of baby oil to help loosen the crust of old skin and sebaceous material that has collected on the body part that was under the cast. With patience and time this crust can be removed with no injury to the underlying epidermis.

Care of the Newly Casted Patient

A newly casted patient may complain of the heat generated by the plaster as it undergoes physical reaction with the water. This heat of crystallization is transitory; however, in body casts it may cause considerable annoyance. Newly applied casts are soft, damp, and grayish white and have a slightly musty smell. They must be handled carefully.

Transfer of the patient

When transferring a newly casted patient, the nurse should lift the cast with the palms of the hands rather than grasp it by the fingers. Finger pressure may cause indentations, tissue injury, and disturbances in circulation. If the patient is in a body cast (hip spica) covering the trunk or hips and legs, many hands may be necessary to make an efficient, smooth transfer from cart to bed.

Preparation of the unit

The unit of a patient who is having a new body cast applied requires special preparation. Bed boards should be placed under the mattress to prevent sagging. Numerous firm pillows should be available to support the contours of the soft cast. If the child is old enough and able to benefit from them, an overhead bar and trapeze should be attached to the bed. The room should be well ventilated to assist in the drying of the cast. Occasionally, special cast driers are available, or an undraped heat cradle may be used to help speed drying. A new cast should be exposed to the air.

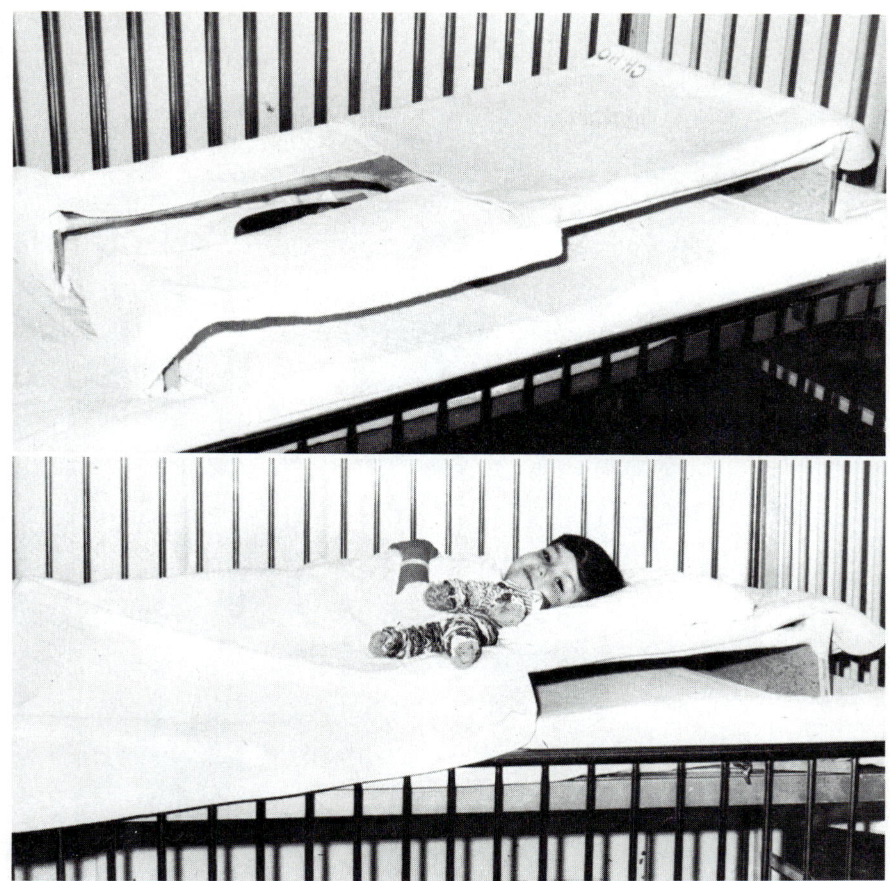

Fig. 33-11 Cast board premeasured for patient. Note incline and positioned bedpan. (Courtesy Children's Hospital and Health Center, San Diego, Calif.)

However, for modesty's sake a diaper may be positioned over the perineal area. A fracture pan should be available in the bedside stand. In many hospitals, infants and small children in body casts are measured for so-called cast boards or for a Bradford frame, which holds the child at a slight incline, elevated from the bed mattress (Fig. 33-11). A bedpan is kept positioned under the child at all times, and plastic strips, which are tucked into the perineal area of the cast, guide waste material into the pan below. Very young children who are incontinent can be "taped" with urine collection bags until the cast is dry enough to be protected against accidental soiling. If this is done before cast application, soiling can be more effectively prevented.

For patients with newly casted extremities, often all that is necessary for the nurse to have ready in the patient's unit is a supply of firm pillows to elevate the body part above the level of the heart to help prevent swelling. Sometimes elevation is best maintained through the use of a gatch bed, placement of pillows under the end of the mattress, or suspension of the affected part from an intravenous pole. The cast should be left exposed to the air to facilitate drying, and the patient should be turned frequently. Most casts dry in approximately 24 hours.

Care of the cast

When the cast is dry, as indicated by a chalky white finish and a hard nonmoist surface, it should be protected against accidental wetting in the perineal region. This may be done in several ways. Various types of plastic material can be cut to fit under the perineal edge of the cast and to protect the curved band of the adjacent plaster. It can be held in place by pieces of water-repellent adhesive tape. Plastic adhesive tape can be cut into wedge-shaped pieces and positioned around and under the perineal rim and on the outer surface. Regardless of the method selected to protect the cast, the waterproof material should not be applied until the cast is dry because the adhesive usually does not stick until then. When the cast is dry, all rough or potentially rough edges of the cast should be covered.

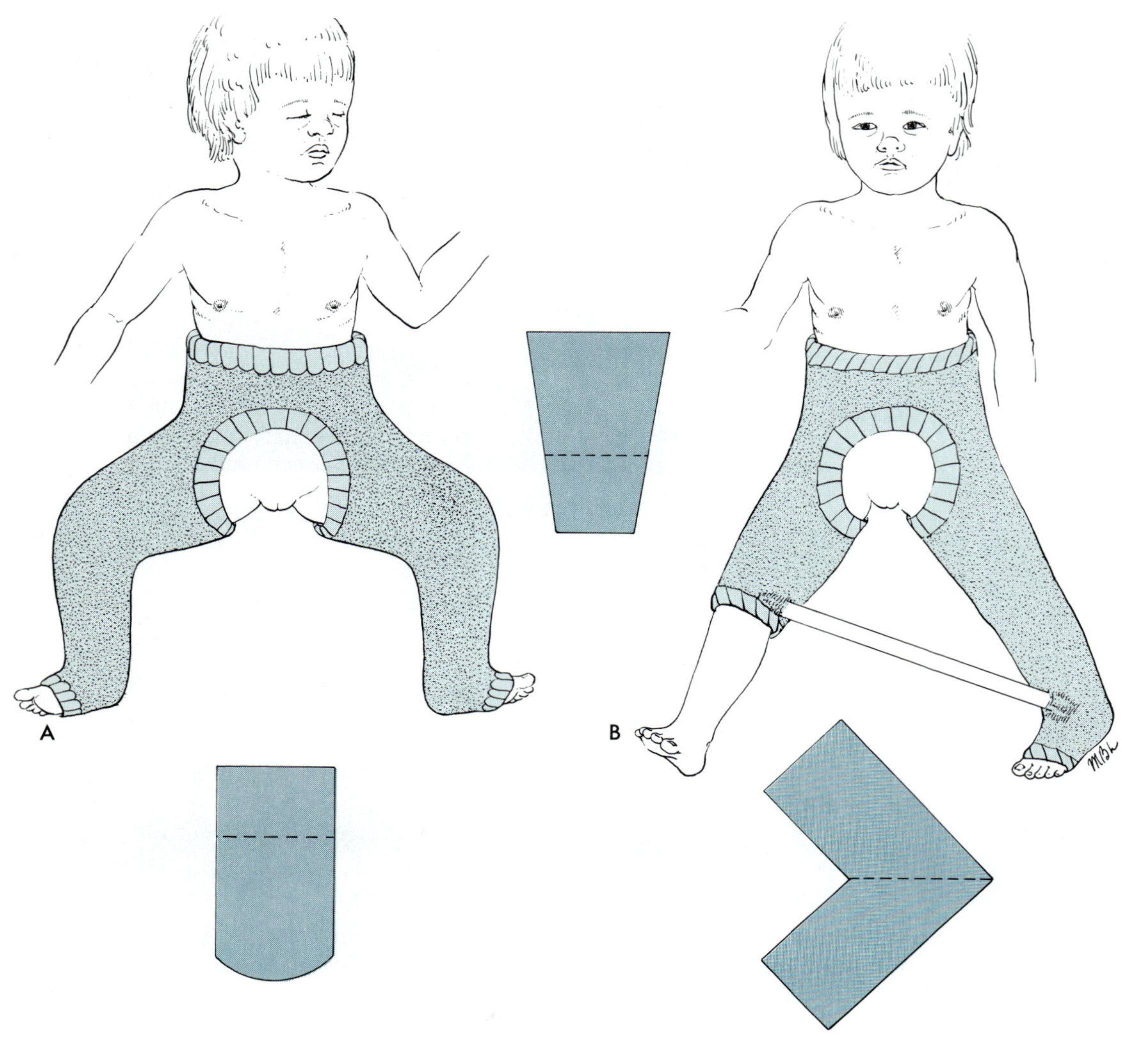

Fig. 33-12 Different types of petaling. **A,** Bilateral hip spica cast. **B,** Unilateral hip spica cast with abductor bar.

This process is termed *petaling* because the pieces of adhesive tape first used for this purpose were cut in the shape of flower petals. However, nurses currently use adhesive tape cut like chevrons, circles, or wedges, as well as the traditional petal, to protect cast edges (Fig. 33-12). Petaling keeps small bits of plaster from the cast edges from falling into the cast, helps prevent skin irritation around the cast, and may waterproof and improve the appearance of the cast. If tubular stockinette is applied before the plaster bandage during the construction of the cast, it can be neatly trimmed, brought up over the cast edge, and secured with adhesive or plaster strips to make a smooth, attractive edging when the cast is dry. (See Table 33-2.)

Various methods have been used to enhance the appearance of a cast and help protect it from damage and soil. A nonaerosol plastic spray may be applied to a dry cast to increase its longevity and help keep it clean. It is best not to get a cast dirty or stained in the first place, but if it does become soiled, the nurse may clean the area with a damp, not wet, cloth and a small amount of white cleanser or fast-drying white shoe polish. Some dry, dirty areas may be covered by adhesive tape or additional plaster of Paris strips. Children should be cautioned against getting their casts damp, thus swimming is prohibited.

Casts are a great help in correcting various musculoskeletal problems, but they may also cause or accentuate problems. The casted patient must be carefully observed to detect the development of any difficulties.

Observation for complications

A newly casted extremity may suffer impaired circulation. Sometimes circulatory problems compound themselves. Because of injury, operative proce-

◆ **TABLE 33-2**
Cast Care

Objective	Intervention
Detect circulatory impairment early	Assess and report unexplained pain, edema, cool temperature, poor capillary refill, or loss of pulse in affected extremity.
Ensure even drying	Turn at least every 2 hours Use palms and avoid pressure from fingers. Air dry as much as possible.
Prevent skin breakdown	Assess skin at cast edges every 4 hours Use padding or cut away sharp cast edges. Turn patient often and support comfortably with pillows. Avoid use of sharp objects for scratching underneath cast. Keep skin clean and dry, giving special attention to perineal area.
Maintain integrity of cast	Do not allow plaster of Paris cast to contact water. Do not use abduction bar to facilitate turning. Use of metal frame or cast board may facilitate toileting.
Promote maximum mobility	Facilitate optimal use of unaffected extremities. Change environment often. Place child near center of activity. Support upright position whenever possible. Use wagon or adapted "stroller."

dure, or a tight cast application, there may be swelling under the cast. The increasingly tighter cast impedes circulation further, and tissue damage may take place. Certain signs and symptoms that indicate abnormal pressure and swelling should be reported to avoid significant tissue damage. Patients should be assessed frequently after casting and periodically thereafter (see box on p. 708).

Excessive bleeding after surgery, as estimated by bloody drainage seeping through the cast layers, may be worrisome. The type of surgical procedure involved is a consideration. Physicians differ in opinion about marking the drainage stains and the time noted on a cast because it may alarm patients unduly.

When possible, the corresponding unaffected extremity should be compared with the casted arm or leg. Some people have cold hands most of the time, with or without casts. Any complaint of a burning sensation or pain should be promptly reported and investigated. Considerable damage can occur in a relatively short period. The body part may become numb and no additional complaints may be heard for some time, until tissue damage is significant.

The usual emergency procedure involves cutting the cast in half and forming upper and lower, or anterior and posterior, shells. The inner wrappings should also be cut, since they may cause considerable pressure. The extremity may be maintained in the shell with the halves held loosely together by elastic bandage. Such a cast is said to be *bivalved*. Physicians intentionally bivalve casts to provide support, allow some movement and exposure, and facilitate the skin care of an area. Bivalved casts are often used as splints in conjunction with elastic bandages with excellent results.

Even when the cast is dry and relatively old, the daily care of the patient in a body cast or a hip spica cast should continue to include observation for disturbances in circulation and possible areas of pressure, skin breakdown, and infection. A peculiar, sweet, musty odor may indicate the presence of pus. The skin next to the cast edges must be carefully inspected and massaged. The heel and heel cord and

Nursing Alert

A swelling casted extremity must be relieved promptly. Inability to move the exposed part, pallor, cyanosis, pain, lack of pulsation, or warmth requires immediate intervention. A nurse should not hesitate to call a physician if circulation is impaired even though the hour is inconvenient. In the unusual situation in which no physician can be contacted, the nurse should be prepared to cut the cast herself. Certainly such a situation is extraordinary, but if no help is available for a considerable period, it is better to have a damaged cast than a gangrenous extremity.

SIGNS OF NEUROVASCULAR COMPLICATIONS	
Pain	Patient feels discomfort or burning sensation, especially when toes or fingers are passively stretched. Very small children are unable to verbalize subjective symptoms; they should be watched for unexplained "fussiness."
Edema	Toes or fingers are swollen.
Pallor	Toes or fingers are cold (they should be pink and warm). The nurse should compare them with uninvolved extremity if possible.
Purple tint	Toes or fingers are cyanotic or mottled.
Pressure response delay	Blanching sign is absent or delayed. Pressure is made on the nail beds to blanch the area. When the pressure is removed, the normal nail color should return immediately. If the area does not blanch, this is also significant because it indicates local congestion and lack of good circulation.
Pulselessness	A pulse in an extremity cannot be found (when the area to be palpated is accessible).
Paralysis	Toes or fingers cannot be moved properly by the child.
Paresthesia	Patient feels numbness and tingling.

the perineum especially should be watched for signs of irritation.

Turning the patient

The patient in a dry body cast is routinely turned at least every 2 or 3 hours in an attempt to prevent pressure sores and promote respiration and elimination. The number of people needed to turn a patient in a body cast depends on the size and general condition of the patient and the age of the cast. Remember the following when turning a patient in a large body cast:

1. If there is a choice, plan to turn the patient toward the nonoperative side.
2. Before turning the patient, pull or lift the child to the side of the bed, placing the "turning side" toward the center of the bed. Have the patient lift the hands above the head or, if this is not feasible, have them held against the patient's sides with a towel or diaper placed between the hands and the cast just before turning to prevent injury. Do *not* use the abductor bar to turn the patient. It is held in place with only a few turns of plaster bandage. It helps support the cast, but it is not a handle.
3. If possible, place the protective pillows needed under the cast in the new position before the patient is turned.
   - a If the patient is placed *on his or her abdomen,* a flat pillow just below the chest area sometimes helps chest expansion and respiration. A small pillow for the patient's head increases comfort. Legs should be supported to prevent the toes from digging into the bedding and the problem of footdrop. Curved up-and-down contours of the cast also should be protected from strain. The abdominal position is preferred for older children at mealtime to aid in swallowing and self-feeding.
   - b If the patient is *supine,* place a small pillow under the head. Curved up-and-down contours of the cast should be protected from strain, and the heels should be lifted from the mattress.
   - c Ensure that the edges of the cast do not press against the patient's skin. The patient should be made as comfortable as possible.
   - d A young child who is incontinent and does not have a cast board may be placed on a horseshoe-shaped pillow arrangement, and a small bedpan or large kidney-shaped basin may be positioned under the patient with a plastic strip tucked under the cast leading to the pan or basin (Fig. 33-13). Such a pillow support should elevate the child on a slight incline to prevent urine backflow into the cast.

Safety factors

Children in casts of any type must be carefully observed and taught not to put anything into the cast. Small objects, such as crayons and bobby pins, can cause pressure areas, pain, and infection. The nurse must also be vigilant regarding the use of so-called scratchers, used to relieve itching. If scratchers are allowed at all, they must be relatively soft, such as a strip of gauze that has been strategically placed before the cast application is begun. Even pipe cleaners may cause excoriation and are not recommended for such purposes. Blowing air from a syringe or from a hair dryer set on *cool* air under the rim of the cast may be soothing. One must be sure that the child is not scratching a healing surgical incision.

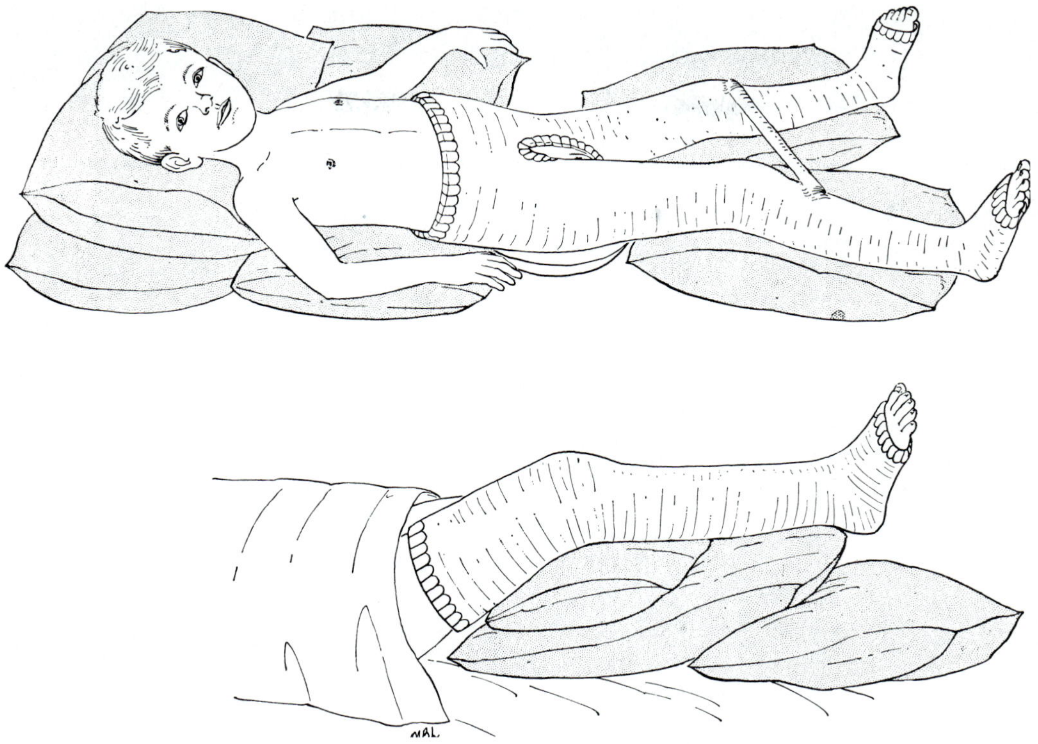

Fig. 33-13 Methods of using pillows to support cast. Child shown at top is on bedpan.

> **Nursing Alert**
>
> Hot fans or dryers may cause burns from heat conduction or cause the cast to dry on the outside while remaining wet on the inside.

Nursing considerations

Bathing. Parts of the body that might be overlooked during the daily bath are the fingers and the areas between the toes. Plaster crumbs may collect between the digits and cause pressure areas. Cotton-tipped applicators dipped in baby oil help clean these areas satisfactorily.

Diet and fluids. The child who is immobilized needs not only meticulous skin care but also special attention to diet and fluid intake to promote healing and prevent constipation and urinary stasis. A liberal fluid intake should be maintained, and a high-protein diet is often encouraged. At times prune juice or a mild laxative is indicated.

Support of a casted extremity. When a child with a casted extremity is allowed to be up in a chair, there is still a potential for edema, thus the cast should be elevated and not permitted to become dependent. The physician may order that a casted arm be supported in a sling. Several types of slings are available. The classic sling is formed from a triangular bandage. The fingers are exposed but the wrist is supported, and the hand is higher than the elbow. The knot should not rest over the cervical spine. This is uncomfortable and may cause a pressure area. Fig. 33-14 shows a commercially prepared hammock-type sling. It is available in several sizes.

When local swelling of an extremity is present or possible, some physicians order that the arm be elevated with pillows. If such elevation is to be effective, the child's wrist must be higher than the elbow, the elbow must be higher than the shoulder, and the entire extremity must be elevated above the level of the heart.

Diversion and intellectual stimulation. A person may be clean, free from pain, on the mend physically, but not particularly happy. The nurse should provide diversion, intellectual stimulation, and interpersonal contacts for patients. During confinement older children may develop constructive hobbies and lasting interests.

Discharge. Many casted patients do not remain in the hospital for very long. Often the cast is applied, dried, protected, and petaled, and the patient's discharge is written within 8 to 48 hours. The family

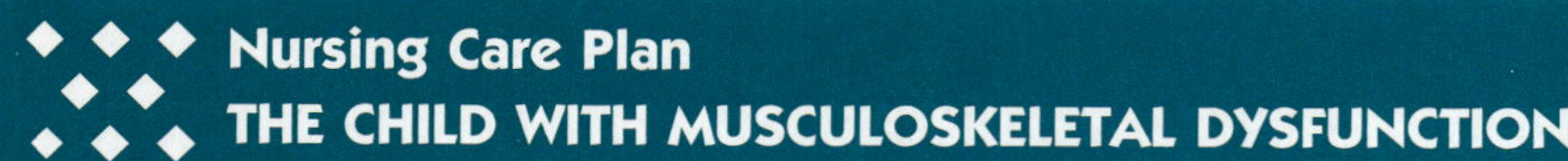

Nursing Care Plan
THE CHILD WITH MUSCULOSKELETAL DYSFUNCTION

Selected Nursing Diagnoses	Expected Outcomes	Interventions
A Altered peripheral tissue perfusion, related to bleeding, edema, and increased pressure. Clinical manifestations: Progressive pain, positive passive stretch, weak or absent peripheral pulse, slow capillary refill, weakness or tingling in affected extremity.	Child maintains adequate peripheral circulation to affected extremity, as seen by: absence of pain negative passive stretch strong peripheral pulse immediate capillary refill.	Assess for circulatory impairment every hour during first 24 hours following surgery or trauma, and every 4 hours thereafter. Notify physician if child has progressive pain in spite of analgesia and/or other signs of circulatory impairment. Compare affected extremity to unaffected, and note any changes from previous assessment. Elevate affected extremity at or above level of the heart. Ensure even drying of plaster of Paris cast by turning child frequently and avoiding pressure on any one area. If rewrapping Ace bandages, ensure secure but well-distributed tension. Teach child and/or parent signs and symptoms to report that indicate circulatory impairment.
B Impaired physical mobility related to cast or traction. Clinical manifestations: Mechanical restriction of normal movement, inability to move out of bed.	The child maintains maximum mobility within the limits of a cast or traction, and remains free of complications from decreased activity as seen by: frequent use of trapeze; change of position every 2-4 hours; resilient muscle tone—4-5 (0-5) strength in affected extremity; maintenance of skin integrity at cast edges and overall areas of pressure or friction; regular, soft bowel movements; voiding at least every 4 hours and absence of bladder distention; clear, symmetrical BRSs.	Explain limitations of movement necessitated by treatment plan, and rationale to child and/or parent. Discuss possible complications of restricted mobility and means of prevention. Encourage maximum movement possible while still maintaining optimal position of safety, function, and comfort. Assess joints, skin, abdomen, and lungs to ensure full function and absence of complications. Have child perform full ROM, active if possible, to all uninvolved extremities every shift. Help child minimize friction with movement and avoid prolonged pressure over bony prominences by changing position every 2 hours, use of trapeze, egg crate mattress, and back care every shift. Monitor frequency and character of bowel movements; encourage diet with high fluid and fiber content; and secure order for stool softeners if needed. Maintain accurate I & O; offer bedpan to empty bladder at least every 4 hours; cleanse perineum well during bath and after each bowel movement.

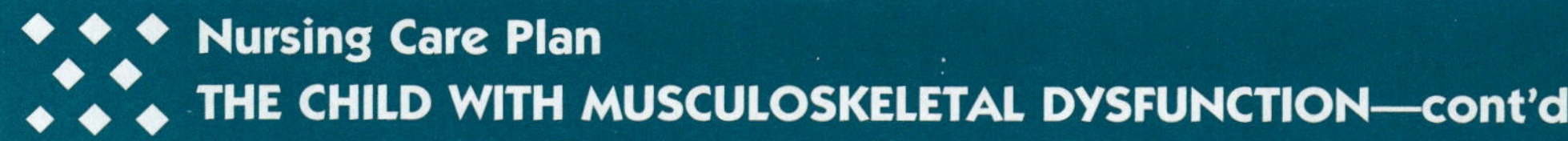

Nursing Care Plan
THE CHILD WITH MUSCULOSKELETAL DYSFUNCTION—cont'd

Selected Nursing Diagnoses	Expected Outcomes	Interventions
		Encourage semi-Fowler's position or higher while awake, deep breathing every 4 hours; and use of incentive spirometer if indicated by unwillingness to deep breathe.
C Diversional activity deficit related to restricted movement, unfamiliar surroundings, inability to participate in customary play activities. Clinical manifestations: Verbal and nonverbal expressions of boredom, disinterest in surroundings, flat emotional affect, restlessness.	Child participates actively in both structured and unstructured age appropriate play activities each day of hospitalization.	Learn of child's individual interests and favorite play things from child and parent. Schedule with child and parent each day to include times for both structured and unstructured play. Help decorate the bedside with objects of interest and reminders of home. Encourage frequent use of playroom and change child's environment often, if possible. Place child in room with peers, especially if school age or older, and foster interaction between roommates. Secure toys, games, and supplies for projects feasible for use in bed, and with consideration of child's individual age, interests, hobbies, and talents. Consider acquisition of tape recorder, video games, and/or radio. Encourage its use for music, sports, and storytelling. Secure reading books appropriate to child's age and interests, and make time/effort to foster their use via nurse, parent, or volunteer. Facilitate contact with school teacher from home and plan time for help with assignments. Encourage contact by phone, letters, or visits with siblings and friends in addition to parents. Refer to Child Life Director if indicated. Allow use of television and video movies occasionally but only after participation in more productive activities.

must be provided with detailed instructions regarding skin care, observation for circulatory problems, cast protection, and cleansing. The need for maximum mobility within the child's limitations should be emphasized to enhance normal growth and development. Using proper body mechanics and seeking assistance when necessary may prevent injury to both parent and child. Appropriate transportation must be arranged. Patients in long-leg casts or hip spica casts cannot be comfortably placed in all automobiles.

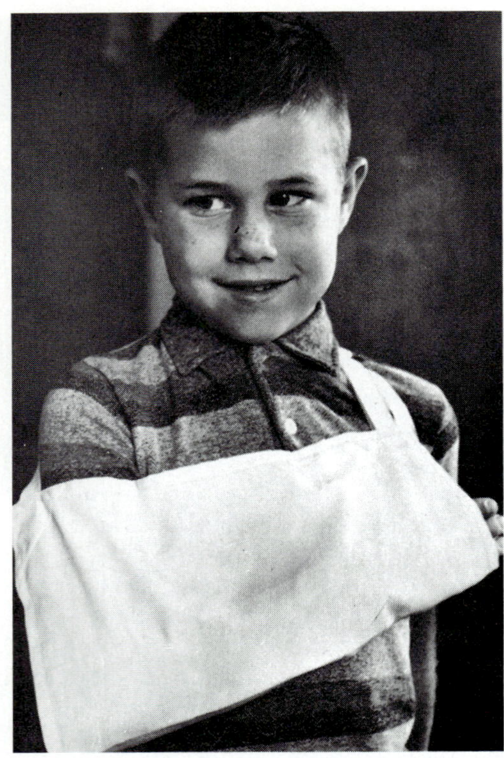

Fig. 33-14 Commercial hammock-type sling. Note that arm enters sling from top, not from side.

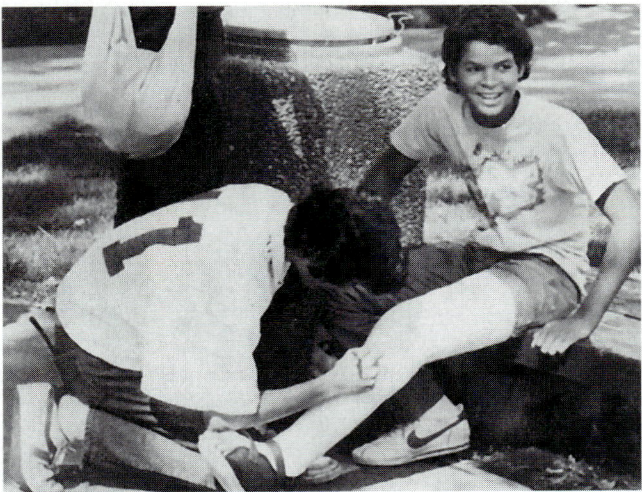

Fig. 33-15 A cast serves as an excellent medium for graffiti and autographs.

Discharging a patient with a cast should not be taken lightly, and sufficient time for teaching must be given to anticipate and answer the parents' questions. Videotapes and instruction handouts can be used to supplement direct teaching. Creativity regarding cast graffiti should be encouraged (Fig. 33-15).

BRACES

A removable, external support used to maintain position and to provide stability to a body part is called a *brace.* A brace may be made of numerous kinds of material but characteristically is constructed of metal, leather, felt, and lacings. Braces are expensive but helpful pieces of equipment. They are individually fitted and produced, and they demand the respect of both patient and nurse. Braces furnish support by exerting pressure on at least three points of the body. There are many different types of braces. The Milwaukee brace for the treatment of scoliosis is one example of a body brace (See Chapter 32). Short, below-the-knee braces for ankle or foot support or full-length leg braces for both knee and ankle stabilization are available. Some patients with cerebral palsy must have combined body and long-leg braces because of extensive muscle involvement. Many braces include movable joints that can be locked with various mechanisms to provide greater stability for weight bearing.

Maintenance of the Brace

The routine care of a brace includes protecting it from rust, carefully cleaning and oiling any hinges with a fine-grade oil, and removing any excess oil to prevent staining of leather supports or clothing. It also includes the care of any leather parts by the periodic application of saddle soap, followed by polishing. Nontoxic cleaning fluids may be used on felt pads. Laces should be maintained intact and free from pressure-causing knots. Shoes incorporated in any leg brace should be frequently inspected for abnormal wear. Any missing parts (such as felt kneepads or screws) should be promptly reported because the loss may seriously jeopardize the brace's function.

Nursing responsibilities

The nurse, the patient, and the patient's family should be familiar with the purpose of each brace, the way in which it should be applied and positioned, when it should be worn, the length of time it should be worn, and its mechanism and maintenance. Patients wearing braces should be frequently inspected for bruises and pressure areas. Bony prominences can be protected beforehand by rubbing tincture of benzoin or a wet tea bag over the skin area. Trial periods should be gradually lengthened. Those wearing leg braces should have well-fitted, "no-hole" stockings. A body brace is usually worn over a cotton shirt. It should be applied with the patient lying flat in bed. Back braces are buckled or laced from the bottom up, then adjusted as necessary with the patient in a standing position. A good orthotist (maker and fitter of braces) and a cooperative patient and family are essential to the successful use of a brace. In the event of the patient's persistent refusal to wear the brace, psychological counseling may be advisable. A power struggle between parent and child must be prevented at all costs.

CRUTCHES

Often a patient is required to use crutches, with or without braces, to be ambulatory. The physical therapist is usually responsible for teaching crutch walking and the particular gait best suited to the individual patient. However, the nurse may be asked to measure patients for crutches and assist them in developing good habits involving their use.

One method of measuring a patient in the supine position for the standard type of crutches is to measure the distance from the patient's axilla to a point 4 to 8 inches (10 to 20 cm) out from the patient's heel while the leg is extended and adducted. Ideally patients should wear the shoes that they will be using while walking. Another method involves subtracting 16 inches (41 cm) from the patient's height. Crutch length depends also on the condition of the patient and the gait selected.

The nurse should be sure that the rubber guards on the crutch ends are not worn smooth. The patient should not lean on the axillary (armpit) rests. The weight of the body should be borne by the hands. It is easier for a patient using crutches to rise from a firm rather than an overstuffed chair. When walking with a patient who is learning to use crutches, the nurse should walk behind the patient. In case of difficulty the nurse may grasp the patient by the belt, trousers, or waist.

Orthopedic nursing can be extremely satisfying. Straightening a back or correcting a foot deformity is a multidisciplinary effort requiring skill, determination, patience, time, and caring.

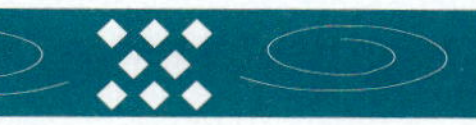

KEY CONCEPTS

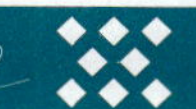

1 Traction is used for the following reasons: to bring a broken bone back into alignment and provide immobilization for correct union, to secure a corrected position, to treat a congenital or acquired deformity not involving a fracture, to prevent or treat contracture deformities, and to relieve muscle spasm and pain.

2 The two main types of traction are skin and skeletal. Skin traction indirectly helps position the bone by pulling on the skin and muscles. Skeletal traction is secured by inserting a mechanical device directly into or through the bone and attaching the prescribed weight.

3 The maintenance of proper traction depends on the correct direction and amount of pull exerted through the use of ropes, pulleys, and weights and on the correct positioning or alignment of the patient.

4 Countertraction is created in four basic ways: maintenance of body placement in bed, elevation of the part of the bed closest to the weights, use of restraints, and application of a counterweight.

5 Although it is important that patients not be moved in a way that disrupts traction, it is also important that they be moved to the extent permitted to avoid pressure areas and encourage proper body function, elimination, respiration, and circulation.

6 The skin of a patient in traction must be meticulously observed and protected. Pressure areas may be reduced or eliminated by frequent inspection and cleansing of susceptible areas, use of an egg crate mattress, maintenance of wrinkle-free linen, continual elevation of the head of the bed to an angle of less than 30 degrees, and encouragement of as much movement as is allowed.

7 Some hospitals are supplied with special traction linen designed to fit under or around different traction appliances.

8 Traction equipment varies depending on the patient's individual needs. Common types are Bryant's, Buck's, Russell's, and 90°-90°.

9 External fixation may be used instead of traction, casting, or internal fixation. It is less frequently used for the younger child, but it can offer earlier mobilization and rigid stabilization for the older child with a complicated fracture.

10 Bryant's traction is often used for the treatment of fractured femurs in young children. Such patients must be carefully observed for circulation problems because the traction may interfere with blood flow.

11 Russell's traction, a skin traction using a sling and single rope arrangement attached to one weight supported by multiple pulleys, is used to treat undisplaced fractures and provide postoperative hip and knee immobilization in older children.

12 In 90°-90° traction, both the hip and the knee are placed in 90-degree flexion. This type of traction is used to reduce a fractured femur.

13 Buck's extension is a rather simple, frequently used skin traction for treatment of the lower extremities or lower back.

14 Balanced traction, involving the suspension of the

affected limb above the surface of the bed, provides the opportunity for more movement and activity by the patient.

15 In addition to immobilization and traction, casts may also be a means of aiding proper positioning or resting a body part. The nurse assisting the physician in applying a cast is responsible for making available all equipment and supplies. The nurse may also be asked to hold the extremity being casted or to support part of the newly formed cast.

16 Objectives of cast care include early detection of circulatory impairment, ensuring even drying, prevention of skin breakdown, maintenance of cast integrity, and promotion of maximum mobility.

17 Sometimes a patient must have one cast removed and another applied. The frequency with which a child must have a cast changed depends on the rate of growth, the condition of the cast, and the progress of the desired correction.

18 The unit of a patient with a newly applied body cast requires special preparation, including placement of bedboards under the mattress, numerous pillows, and a fracture pan or bedpan. Patients with newly casted extremities usually require a supply of firm pillows to elevate the body part.

19 When the cast is dry, all rough or potentially rough edges are covered using a process called petaling. Petaling prevents small bits of plaster from the cast edges from falling into the cast, helps prevent skin irritation around the cast, and may waterproof and improve the appearance of the cast. Skin protection is also achieved by lining and edging the cast with a tubular stockinette.

20 Patients should be assessed frequently after casting and periodically thereafter. Signs of neurovascular complications are pain, puffiness, pallor, purple tint, pressure response delay, pulselessness, paralysis, and paresthesia.

21 The patient in a dry body cast is routinely turned at least every 2 to 3 hours to prevent pressure sores and promote respiration and elimination.

22 Nursing considerations for the casted patient include bathing, diet and fluids, support of the casted extremity, diversion and intellectual stimulation, and preparation for discharge.

23 Braces are individually fitted and produced, and various types are available. The nurse and patient should be familiar with the purpose of each brace, the way in which it should be applied and positioned, when and for how long it should be worn, and its mechanism and maintenance.

24 The nurse may be asked to measure patients for crutches and assist them in developing good habits involving their use. Crutch length can be measured in different ways and depends on the patient's condition and the gait selected.

CRITICAL THOUGHT QUESTIONS

1 How do traction, countertraction, and balanced traction differ?

2 Explain the two basic types of traction? Identify the specific forms of traction used for children?

3 Discuss the advantages of fiberglass casts.

4 What modifications are made regarding hygiene activities, bed making, and skin care when a pediatric patient is restricted by traction or a cast?

5 What special nursing precautions are taken when a cast is newly applied? What special nursing observations are required when a cast is applied? Because many patients are discharged soon after cast application, the parent needs to be aware of how to care for the child. What would you explain about bathing, diapering, foreign objects, and circulation checks?

REFERENCES

Jones-Walton P: Clinical standard in skeletal pin site care, *Orthop Nurs* 10(2):12-17, 1991.

National Association of Orthopedic Nurses: Cues for orthopedic patient care: common concerns, *Orthop Nurs* 19(5):73-74, 1991.

National Association of Orthopedic Nurses: *Guidelines for orthopedic nursing,* Pitman, NJ, 1992, Anthony J. Jannetti.

Salmond SW, Mooney NE, and Verdisco LA, eds: *National association of orthopedic nursing core curriculum for othopedic nursing,* Pitman, NJ, 1991, Anthony J. Jannetti.

Speers AT, Speers M: Care of the infant in a Pavlik harness, *Pediatr Nurs* 18(3):229-232, 1992.

Wong D: *Essentials of pediatric nursing,* ed 4, St Louis, 1993, Mosby.

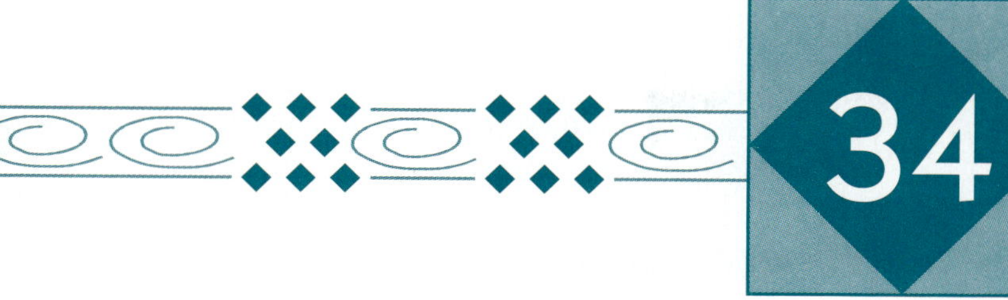

Respiratory and Cardiovascular Problems

CHAPTER OBJECTIVES

After studying this chapter, the student should be able to:

1. Define the terms listed in the key vocabulary.
2. Discuss pneumonia in the pediatric patient: types, etiological factors, general signs and symptoms, treatments, and nursing care.
3. Indicate the basic genetic hereditary pattern of cystic fibrosis, affected organs/systems, signs and symptoms, diagnostic tests used, nutrition, treatment, and nursing care.
4. Compare croup (LTB) and epiglottitis, considering typical patients, anatomy affected, symptoms, treatment, and nursing care.
5. Describe the first-aid treatment of epistaxis (nosebleeds).
6. Define the terms *otitis media* and *myringotomy*.
7. Discuss complications of otitis media.
8. List five nursing considerations to remember when caring for a 4-year-old child recently returned from the recovery room after a "T and A."
9. Explain why the identification of a strep throat is important in the prevention of disease.
10. Identify five nonimmunological factors that can trigger an attack of asthma in susceptible persons.
11. Outline the treatment of an 8-year-old child suffering from a severe asthmatic attack; include the definition of status asthmaticus and care in a hospital setting.
12. Discuss nursing care for a 2½-year-old child who has just undergone a cardiac catheterization.
13. Indicate five cardiac signs and symptoms demonstrated by infants with congenital heart disease.
14. Describe the following congenital heart defects: patent ductus arteriosus, atrial and ventricular septal defects, tetralogy of Fallot, complete transposition of the great vessels, and coarctation of the aorta.
15. Discuss six key components of the nursing assessment of the child with a moderately severe heart defect.

The respiratory and cardiovascular systems are closely interrelated; thus they will be discussed together in this chapter.

KEY VOCABULARY

apnea Absence of breathing.

atelectasis Airless segment of lung; collapse of lung.

bronchiectasis Abnormal dilation of the bronchi in response to inflammation, which, if prolonged, leads to associated structural changes and a chronic, productive cough.

Cheyne-Stokes respiration Irregular, cyclic breathing characterized by a period of increasing respiratory action followed by an interval of apnea.

dyspnea Difficult breathing.
edema Abnormal, excessive amount of fluid within the body tissues.
emphysema Abnormal dilation and loss of elasticity of the microscopic air sacs, or alveoli, of the lung.
empyema Collection of pus in a body cavity, especially the pleural cavity.
eupnea Normal breathing.
orthopnea Condition in which breathing is possible by the patient only when in a standing or sitting position.
pneumothorax Abnormal collection of air or gas in the pleural cavity.
stenosis Abnormal narrowing of a passage or opening.

THE RESPIRATORY SYSTEM

In conjunction with the study of disorders of the respiratory system, the student should review Chapter 28, which briefly outlines the basic anatomy and physiology of the respiratory system and discusses methods of maintaining oxygenation, Chapter 32 Infectious Diseases including tuberculosis.

Respiratory difficulties (such as respiratory distress syndrome, tracheoesophageal fistula, and diaphragmatic hernia) that are particularly associated with the newborn period are discussed in Chapters 18 and 19. This presentation of respiratory pathological findings begins with a brief anatomical review, followed by a consideration of those common problems affecting children in various stages of development.

ANATOMICAL REVIEW

Nose

The nasal structures prepare air for entry into the interior of the body. It filters, warms, and moistens the air. If humans breathe through their mouths, the air is not filtered, warmed, or humidified properly.

The nose is also involved in the identification of different odors because the olfactory nerve endings are located within the nasal cavity. Many of the finer perceptions of the palate are influenced by the sensitivity of these nerves. Consider how uninteresting food seems when one has a cold and the proper ventilation of the nose is disturbed. The nasal structures also contribute to normal vocal response.

Pharynx and Trachea

The pharynx is a passageway shared by both the respiratory and digestive systems. It extends from the back of the nasal cavity down past the posterior portion of the oral cavity to the level of the larynx and esophagus. Consequently the pharynx is divided descriptively into three parts: nasal, oral, and larynx and trachea extending from the hypopharynx complete the upper respiratory system.

Lower Respiratory Tract

The lower respiratory tract includes the bronchi, bronchioles, alveoli, which form the tissues of the lungs, and pleurae, or coverings of the lungs. Infectious conditions involving the lower respiratory system are usually more serious.

RESPIRATORY DISORDERS

Infant

Bronchiolitis

Bronchiolitis is a viral respiratory illness with clinical manifestations attributed to inflammatory narrowing of the small airways. The bronchioles are partially or completely obstructed as a result of mucosal swelling and exudate. The condition is more common in infants and toddlers. The causative organism is respiratory syncitial virus (RSV) for which a vaccine is being developed.

Bronchiolitis begins as an upper respiratory infection. After a few days the infant develops a low-grade fever, shallow, rapid respirations, a cough, and an expiratory wheeze. Air can usually enter the bronchioles, but expiratory narrowing causes it to be trapped distal to the obstruction. Suprasternal and subcostal retractions are noted on inspiration. The infant is fatigued, irritable, anxious, and unable to eat or sleep. In severe cases, some infants become cyanotic.

A trial of bronchodilator therapy is warranted in moderate to severe cases, but it may not be effective in young infants who do not have adequate smooth muscle development. Aerosol therapy with ribavirin, terbutaline or albuterol, intravenous aminophylline, or subcutaneous epinephrine may be used.

Acute bronchiolitis in infants presents a frightening picture. Parents feel helpless, anxious, and fearful that the life of their child is in jeopardy. Fortunately mortality is very low, and the most severe period lasts only a few days. Recovery is almost always complete within 2 weeks. The parent's questions should be answered clearly and simply, and they should be encouraged to stay with their child. Careful assessment of vital signs and skin color are essential as apneic episodes may occur in severe cases. Rest, oxygen, and hydration are most important. Fluids should be encouraged hourly and in small amounts (2 to 3 ounces). Nasal suctioning may be necessary before feeding. A

CAUSES OF PEDIATRIC PNEUMONIA

1 Primary pneumonias (no predisposing condition)
   a. Bacterial
      1 Pneumococcal
      2 Staphylococcal
      3 Streptococcal
      4 *Haemophilus influenzae*
   b. Nonbacterial
      1 Viral
      2 Mycoplasma
      3 Chlamydia
2 Secondary pneumonias (other predisposing conditions diagnosed)
   a. Hypostatic—caused by stasis of respiratory secretions resulting from lack of adequate inflation and drainage
   b. Asthmatic—caused by narrowed airways and increased mucus
   c. Associated with cystic fibrosis—caused by the presence of viscid respiratory secretions
   d. Aspiration pneumonias—involving accidental inhalation of
      1 Hydrocarbons—petroleum distillates, such as gasoline, kerosene, and furniture polish
      2 Foreign bodies—popcorn, peanuts, buttons, and other objects
      3 Gastric contents—associated with gastroesophageal reflux (GER) and other congenital anomalies of the esophagus or trachea and neuromuscular disorders

cool-mist humidifier may be helpful if the room air is dry. The child's head should be elevated via an infant seat.

Pneumonia

Pneumonia is an inflammation of the lung parenchyma. Multiple microorganisms, as well as certain noninfectious agents, environmental toxins, and chronic conditions, cause pneumonia. The anatomical and pathological changes may involve the lobar, lobular, interstitial, or bronchial areas. Pneumonia, most commonly seen in infants and young children, can be a serious condition, and one of the major causes of mortality in the age group of 1 to 14 years. Early recognition and prompt treatment will prevent hospitalization and reduce the incidence of complications. Causes of pneumonia in infants and children are presented in the box above.

Clinical manifestations. The onset and clinical manifestations of pneumonia vary with the age of the child and the etiological agent. The disease occurs most frequently in winter and spring. Bacterial pneumonias are often preceded by a viral upper respiratory tract infection, which alters the defense mechanisms of the lower respiratory tract. The classic signs and symptoms are fever, anorexia, listlessness, and cough. At first the cough is wet and loose, but soon it becomes dry and painful. The pain associated with lower lobe pneumonia is frequently referred to the abdomen. Therefore one should think of pneumonia when a child has abdominal pain and fever because the abdominal pain can be caused by a lower lobe pneumonia. In the young child the temperature mounts rapidly, and seizures may occur. Respirations become rapid and shallow and are accompanied by flaring of the nostrils, grunting, and retractions. The pulse rate is extremely rapid (it may be doubled). Meningeal irritation, such as stiff neck, is sometimes present with upper lobe pneumonia, and a spinal tap is necessary to rule out coexisting meningitis. Cyanosis coupled with a rapid, weak pulse is always a grave sign. Since proper therapy depends on knowledge of the causative agents, the common pneumonias are discussed according to their cause.

Types.

Bacterial primary pneumonias. *Pneumococcal (strep pneumoniae) pneumonia* is the most common type encountered in infants and young children. Typically, after symptoms of a mild cold, the infant refuses to eat and becomes listless. The temperature rises rapidly, and respiratory distress is soon apparent. Fortunately, the pneumococcus is responsive to antibiotic therapy. A good response to penicillin usually takes place within 24 to 48 hours in uncomplicated cases. Response to therapy is delayed in cases that are complicated by fluid in the pleural space (pleural effusion), empyema, otitis media, or meningitis.

Staphylococcal pneumonia is the most serious of the pneumonias in infancy. It may follow an upper respiratory tract infection, or it may spread to the lungs by way of the bloodstream from a staphylococcal infection elsewhere in the body. Unless recognized and treated early, the disease characteristically progresses rapidly, causing severe respiratory distress, and may be associated with the formation of abscesses and air cysts (pneumatoceles). Intravenous antibiotic therapy with nafcillin, oxacillin, or cephalosporin is initiated, followed by a course of oral antibiotics. Respiratory isolation technique is observed. Pneumothorax can occur, resulting in deterioration of respiratory status. A chest tube may be inserted. Mortality is high in untreated infants.

Streptococcal pneumonia is more common in young children than in infants. It is usually preceded by a viral infection, such as rubeola, rubella, or varicella.

The onset of chills and pleuritic pain may be sudden, or the pneumonia may start with a gradual rise in temperature, accompanied by cough. Streptococci cause an interstitial type of pneumonia, and occasionally abscesses and pneumatoceles can develop. Empyema usually requires chest tube insertion. Penicillin G is the antibiotic of choice and is highly effective.

Haemophilus influenzae type b pneumonia is a serious disease. The onset of illness is usually acute, and the clinical course cannot be distinguished from other bacterial pneumonias. Infants and children under 5 years of age are most often affected and seem susceptible to bacteremia and empyema. There is a high incidence of associated infections such as URI, otitis media, epiglottitis, and meningitis. Cephalosporins or sulfa derivatives are effective.

Nonbacterial primary pneumonia. Many viruses cause pneumonia. A low-grade fever and coryza (runny nose) precede the interstitial pneumonia, which appears suddenly with the onset of tachypnea and a nonproductive, tight cough. Treatment is symptomatic, since antibiotics are of no value unless secondary bacterial complications occur. One exception is respiratory syncytial viral pneumonia, which is treated with ribavirin aerosol.

Mycoplasmae pneumonia is an atypical pneumonia caused by a pathogenic "filterable" microorganism known as *Mycoplasmae pneumoniae* (Eaton agent). It is a tiny, free-living microorganism that has properties between those of bacteria and viruses. Infection usually results in a self-limited, interstitial pneumonia. Mycoplasmal pneumonia occurs most commonly in the school-age child and adolescent. The onset is abrupt, and symptoms include fever, headache, malaise, chills, and a characteristic dry, hacking cough. Later the cough becomes productive, sometimes producing blood-streaked mucus. Erythromycin is the antibiotic of choice in treating this type of pneumonia in children. Doxycycline may be used in adolescents.

Chlamydia pneumonia is transmitted to the infant in the birth canal. It may also cause conjunctivitis. The age of onset is 2 to 12 weeks, and onset is gradual. The infected infants may be afebrile. The most prominent symptom is staccato cough. It may be very severe and paroxysmal. Physical examination reveals rales and chest x-ray examination shows hyperexpansion with infiltrates. The antibiotic of choice is erythromycin.

Secondary aspiration pneumonias. Infants and children have been known to aspirate not only their formula but also all kinds of foods, poisons, and objects. The right upper lobe is frequently involved. Mucosal swelling and obstruction can occur. Symptoms vary depending on the child, the substance, and the amount aspirated. Treatment is supportive and aimed at preventing intercurrent infections. Of course, prevention of these incidents is the best therapy.

Aspiration of petroleum distillates, such as kerosene, gasoline, lighter fluid, and furniture polishes, causes a severe chemical pneumonitis, characterized by edema and inflammation. Some petroleum distillates are absorbed from the intestines and then excreted through the lungs. Treatment is symptomatic and may include steroids to reduce inflammatory changes or antibiotics to combat secondary infections.

Foreign bodies, including seeds, coins, jewelry, nuts, popcorn, hot dogs, safety pins, and bones, have been removed from the respiratory passages of young children. Foods that frequently cause choking should not be offered to children under the age of 5 years. Foreign bodies inhaled into the lungs occlude the bronchi, causing atelectasis or hyperinflation. The young child manifests dyspnea, cyanosis, and asymmetric respirations. Incomplete obstruction causes wheezing, and, if it is untreated, fever and cough-producing purulent sputum soon develop. Delay in removal of the foreign object by bronchoscopy seriously alters the prognosis. Usually the foreign body becomes embedded, injuring the tissues and causing infection. Larger foreign bodies can get lodged in and obstruct the larynx and trachea, causing acute suffocation.

Diagnosis. A high white blood cell count (WBC) of over 10,000 with increased polymorphonuclear cells and a shift to young forms (bands) is suggestive of bacterial infections. A low WBC (5000 or less) is more typical of viral infections in general; therefore a differential white blood cell count is routinely requested. Blood cultures obtained before antibiotic therapy is initiated are helpful in the identification of specific organisms if septicemia is present. Nasopharyngeal cultures are not of great value because pneumococci, streptococci, *H. influenzae,* and staphylococci organisms can be isolated from healthy children. Tracheal cultures obtained by suction techniques are more helpful in identification of organisms. X-ray films are a valuable diagnostic tool in evaluating the extent or type of the pneumonia.

Bronchoscopy, a visualization of the tracheobronchial tree, may be performed when other procedures have failed to make an adequate diagnosis. Fluid or tissue may be obtained for a culture or for cytological studies. Lung biopsy is sometimes necessary when protracted pulmonary disease cannot be diagnosed by other means and when the clinical situation is serious.

Treatment and supportive nursing care. Specific therapy is important in the treatment of pneumonia. Differentiating viral and bacterial infections initially is difficult. Antibiotic therapy is essential for the prevention of bacterial pneumonia.

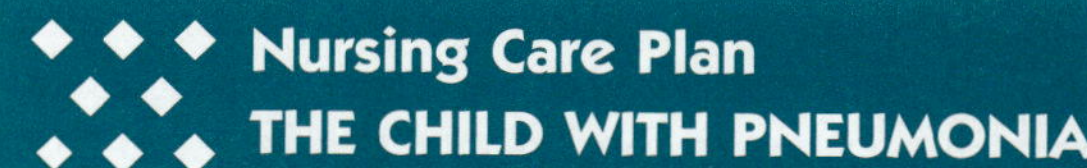

Nursing Care Plan
THE CHILD WITH PNEUMONIA

	Selected Nursing Diagnoses	Expected Outcomes	Interventions
A	Ineffective airway clearance related to inflammation and obstruction of the respiratory tract. Clinical manifestations: Increased respiration rate, dyspnea, cough, elevated temperature, retractions, nasal flaring, grunting, and cyanosis.	Child regains/maintains normal respiratory function.	Assess child's respiratory status (lung sounds, color, respirations, rate, presence of nasal flaring and retractions, use of accessory muscles) every 4 hours and prn. Monitor intravenous antibiotics as ordered. Encourage clear oral fluids/intravenous hydration as needed. Monitor intake and output. Assure respiratory treatments are given as ordered and assess child's response. Suction nares before feeding and prn. Elevate head of bed/place infant in infant seat to facilitate air exchange.
B	Fluid volume deficit related to decreased oral intake and fever. Clinical manifestations: Poor skin turgor, dry mucous membranes, no tears, decreased urinary output, increased urine specific gravity.	Child maintains adequate hydration.	Assess child's hydration status every shift (mucous membranes, skin turgor, tearing, urine output, urine specific gravity). Encourage clear oral fluids/intravenous hydration as needed. Maintain strict intake and output. Administer antibiotics and antipyretics as ordered.
C	Anxiety related to respiratory distress and unfamiliar environment. Clinical manifestations: Verbalizes fear/anxiety, crying, restlessness.	Child and parents cope effectively and decrease level of anxiety.	Provide a quiet, restful environment. Remain with child when he or she is in distress. Explain procedures and treatment to child (age-appropriate) and parents. Encourage parents to participate in care of child. Prevent recurrence of respiratory infection through thorough handwashing. See Nursing Care Plan for The Hospitalized Child.

Supportive care is also extremly important. Fluids are encouraged, and acetaminophen is given for fever. Rest in bed is recommended during the febrile stage. Humidification and increased amounts of fluid are necessary for liquefaction of bronchial secretions. Expectorants may help to loosen secretions and initiate a productive cough. In general, cough suppressants, such as codeine, are not recommended in pneumonia because coughing is a valuable defense mechanism used to help clear the bronchial tree. Respiratory therapy is important in the hospital setting. Bronchial drainage is carried out three or four times daily before meals and at bedtime. Viscid secretions do not drain from the bronchi by gravity alone, but deep breathing, reinforced coughing, and respiratory therapy techniques, such as chest percussion and vibration, assist in their removal. Oxygen administration is used for hypoxic children.

When the child's appetite improves, an appealing, nutritious diet should be ordered. Before feeding an infant, the nurse should remove nasal secretions. One or two drops of saline solution may be ordered, followed by gentle suctioning. A restless infant who cannot breathe does not eat.

A careful assessment of respiratory patterns, pulse, color, and the general condition of the patient is essential. Frequent position change is also critical. Patients breathe better when their upper body is elevated; infants are often placed in infant seats. Conversely, unresponsive or neurologically impaired patients should be positioned on their sides so that pharyngeal secretions can drain thus preventing aspiration.

Respiratory isolation techniques are observed, mainly for contagious conditions such as staphylococcal pneumonia. Convalescence should not be hurried. Adequate time for recuperation is important to allow the child to regain strength and weight and to prevent relapse or complications.

After the first 3 to 6 months of life, most children with pneumonia are treated at home or on an outpatient basis. The parents should be carefully instructed regarding therapeutic and nursing measures. They should understand that medicines must be taken on time and in the correct amount. In general, home care is best for young children. Nevertheless, hospitalization may be advisable during the first 2 or 3 days of illness to provide respiratory therapy and parenteral administration of drugs and fluid. Children are hospitalized when they become too sick to take fluids, when they require intensive supportive measures (such as intravenous or oxygen therapy or surgical drainage) because of their diagnosis or condition, or when the family cannot or does not adequately care for them. Pneumonia remains a potential threat to the future health of the child.

Cystic fibrosis (mucoviscidosis)

Cystic fibrosis (CF) is a hereditary, multisystem disorder in which generalized dysfunction of the exocrine glands occurs, especially involving the mucous and sweat glands. It is usually characterized by the triad of chronic, severe disease, pancreatic insufficiency, and abnormally high concentrations of electrolytes in the sweat.

Cystic fibrosis is transmitted as an autosomal-recessive trait. It is possible to identify carriers of the CF gene, located on the long arm of chromosome 7, within affected families. Analysis of blood samples and chorionic villi for the presence of specific DNA markers linked to the CF gene allow for prenatal diagnosis. The immunoreactive trypsin (IRT) test of blood spots indicates whether the unborn child has the disease.

If one child has CF, the risk for each subsequent pregnancy is one in four. Each conception has the same 25% chance of producing an affected child (see Chapter 20). The incidence of cystic fibrosis in the United States is 1 per 1600 to 2000 live births. Boys and girls appear to be equally affected. About 5% of the white population and less than 1% of the black population are estimated to be genetic carriers of this trait. Although the survival rate is steadily improving, cystic fibrosis remains a serious condition. Couples who have a child with cystic fibrosis should be made aware of the genetic implications of the disease and appropriate counseling should be provided.

Clinical manifestations. Clinical expression of the disease varies because of individual variation in age at onset and severity of involvement of the various organs and systems. However, the altered function of the exocrine glands leads to clinical manifestations, primarily in the respiratory and digestive systems (Fig. 34-1).

Patients with cystic fibrosis have varying degrees of chronic pulmonary disease. The degree of pulmonary involvement and rate of progression usually determine the prognosis. Involvement occurs through a progressive sequence of events that are experienced by all patients. Secretions of the mucus-producing glands become extremely thick and tenacious in the bronchi and bronchioles, causing coughing, wheezing, respiratory obstruction, emphysema, and frequent infection. As a result, the defense in the lungs against microbes is severely compromised. In severe cases the chronic respiratory disease causes a barrel-like chest deformity, cyanosis, and clubbing of the fingers and toes. As hypoxemia and secondary pulmonary arterial hypertension develop, dilation of the right side of the heart and thickening of the right ventricular wall occur. When untreated, this process can result in heart failure and death. Cardiac disease secondary to pulmonary disease is termed *cor pulmonale* (Fig. 34-2).

Approximately 85% of patients with cystic fibrosis have digestive system problems. Since the pancreatic digestive enzymes in these patients are reduced or absent, foodstuffs (fats and proteins especially) may be poorly digested and assimilated. As a result, the infant or child fails to thrive. Because much of the food eaten does not undergo the normal process of digestion and assimilation, the child will pass large amounts of feces and develop a protuberant abdomen. This bulky, foul-smelling stool has a greasy appearance and floats in the toilet bowl because of undigested fat.

In a small percentage of cases (about 10%) the disease is recognized in the newborn nursery because of the detection of meconium ileus. In this condition the meconium, or stool formed in utero by the newborn infant, is thicker and stickier than normal meconium because of the absence or reduction of normal pancreatic digestive enzymes. The abnormal stool sticks to the walls of the ileum like paste and obstructs the lower digestive tract. The obstructed intestine becomes distended, and abdominal distention, or bloating, is noted, and no passage of stool occurs. Vomiting and dehydration may ensue. Any newborn who does not

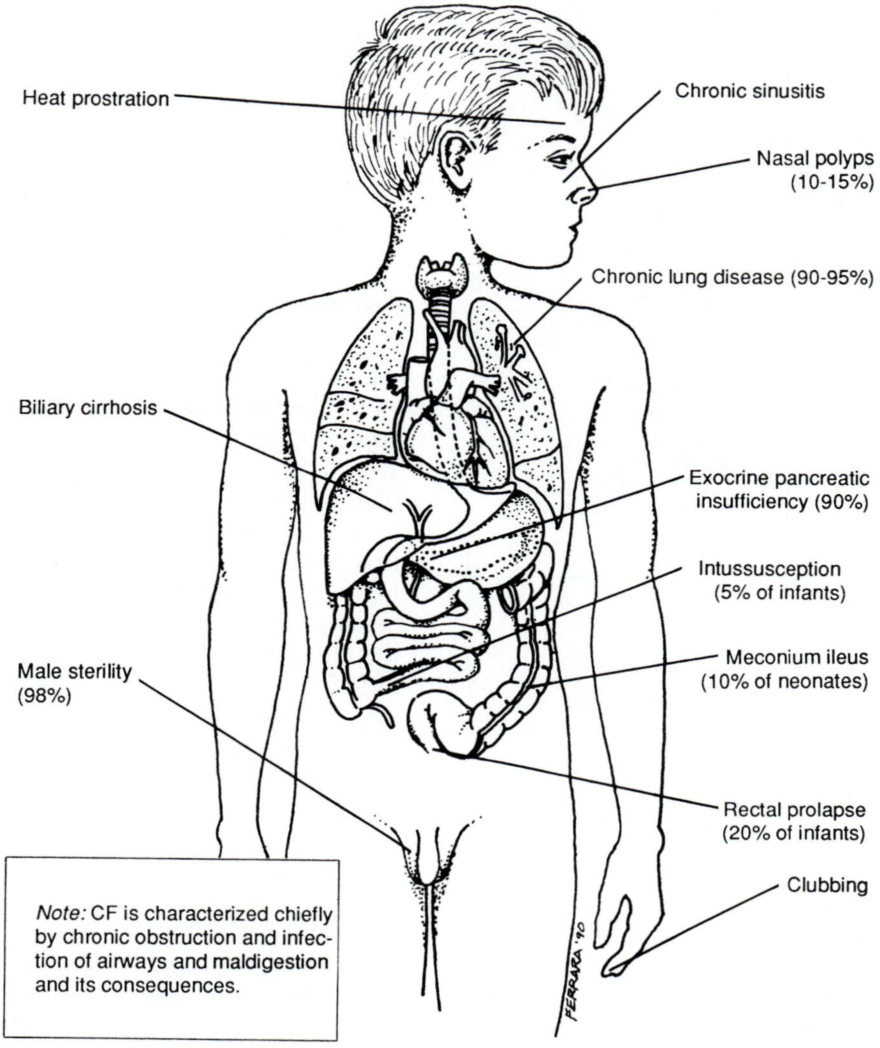

Fig. 34-1 Clinical manifestations of cystic fibrosis in a child.

pass stool within 24 hours after birth should be carefully evaluated and examined for possible obstruction. Other clinical conditions in infancy that indicate the possibility of cystic fibrosis include obstructive jaundice, hypoproteinemia, prolonged bronchiolitis, and rectal prolapse.

Diagnosis. A high degree of clinical suspicion is usually the first step in the diagnosis of cystic fibrosis. Infants and children who suffer from recurrent respiratory tract infections or fail to thrive should be evaluated. The diagnosis is confirmed by laboratory evidence of abnormally elevated sweat chloride levels. A positive reaction implies an elevation of the concentration of chloride above 60 mEq/L. This feature is so pronounced that parents report that their affected children have a "salty taste" when they are kissed.

The quantitative sweat test by pilocarpine iontophoresis is definitive for confirming the diagnosis of cystic fibrosis. Because of the seriousness of the disease and to ensure reliability, at least two positive tests are required before the final diagnosis is made.

When the diagnosis has been established, further tests may be performed to determine the extent of system involvement and to establish a baseline for

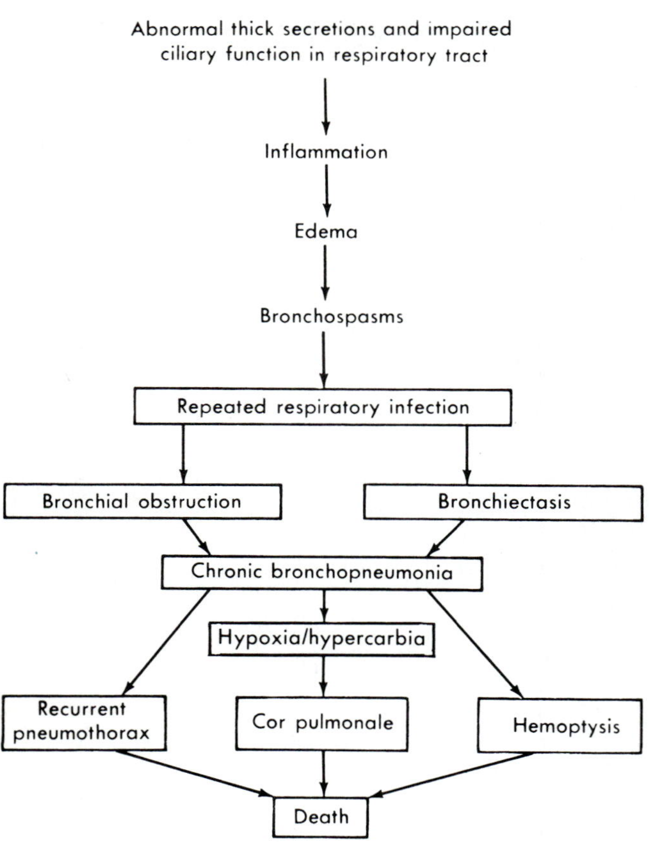

Fig. 34-2 Pathological sequence characteristic of cystic fibrosis.

◆ TABLE 34-1
Pulmonary Therapy

Treatment	Purpose
Intermittent aerosol therapy	To deliver medications and water to the lower respiratory tract
Antibiotic therapy	To treat infection and minimize progression of lung disease
Chest physical therapy	To facilitate the removal of secretions and prevent mucus accumulation
Breathing exercises	To establish and maintain a good breathing pattern

future assessment of treatment and disease progress. Chest x-ray examinations and pulmonary function tests are performed to assess respiratory involvement. Abdominal x-ray examinations, stool analysis, and pancreatic function tests are performed to assess gastrointestinal involvement.

Treatment. Treatment of patients with CF is directed toward the organs involved and designed to meet the needs of the individual patient. Since the chief cause of death in patients with cystic fibrosis is directly related to the degree of lung involvement, maximum therapeutic efforts are directed to the lungs (Table 34-1). Thick mucus obstructing the lungs leads to recurrent pulmonary infection and tissue damage. Early in the course of the disease, the accumulates in the bronchi and bronchioles is so viscid that the cilia are unable to expel it. As the mucus stagnates, it becomes contaminated, usually by *Staphylococcus aureus* and *Pseudomonas aeruginosa*. Resultant infection intensifies mucus production, and the accumulation leads to airway obstruction.

Control of pulmonary infection requires the use of appropriate antibiotics and adequate drainage of bronchial secretions by respiratory therapy. A fine-mist environment may be beneficial to some children; however, studies have not confirmed a positive effect. The use of a continuing home pulmonary care program that prevents progression and complications has improved the life expectancy of children with cystic fibrosis. Children with advanced and steadily increasing pulmonary disease or severe pulmonary infections usually must be hospitalized for intravenous antibiotic therapy. Intravenous administration of antibiotics to inpatients and outpatients with acute and chronic infection may be accomplished by use of the heparin lock. In fact, hospitalizations may be avoided by teaching children or parents this convenient method. The heparin lock IV consists of a venous catheter attached to a small plastic tube that is sealed by a plastic cap in such a way as to protect sterility and patency. It facilitates frequent high intravenous doses of antibiotics without limiting activity. The patient can move about freely with only the lock in place, and the other equipment needed for the intravenous administration of medications remains at the bedside until the next dose is due. Postural drainage and percussion treatments vital in combating these infections can also be performed. For details of heparin lock IV see Chapter 26.

An implantable intravenous access device, the medi-port, has been used in CF patients. This allows for the administration of intravenous medications without venipuncture. The medi-port has been valuable for children who require frequent and prolonged intravenous antibiotic therapy, as well as intravenous hyperalimentation. In severe cases, long-term intravenous antibiotics are used, and in selected cases, heart-lung or lung transplant has been done successfully.

Nutrition. Maintaining nutritional goals becomes increasingly difficult as CF progresses. Initially the aim is to encourage 100% of the recommended dietary

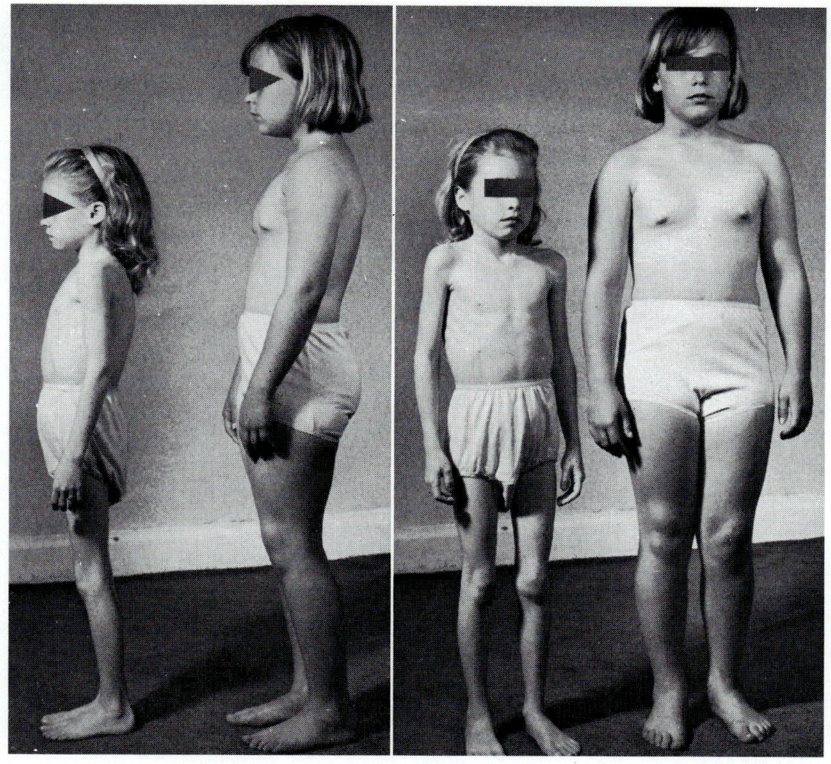

Fig. 34-3 Both of these girls are 10 years old. The child on the left demonstrates effects of severe cystic fibrosis.

allowance (for age) plus extra calories to make up for the calories lost because of malabsorption. Pancreatic insufficiency limits the patient's capacity for digesting fats and proteins. The child usually has good appetite; however, because of malabsorbtion and respiratory complications, failure to thrive and growth retardation are seen in untreated cases (Fig. 34-3). Fortunately the digestive problems usually improve with the addition of pharmaceutical preparations of pancreatic enzymes given with each meal. A major advance in this area is the enteric-coated enzyme, Pancrease, which allows for delivery of predictable levels of enzymes to the duodenum at the same time as food. Other products include Creon and Pancrease MT 16. The enzymes are taken by mouth with meals; the dosage varies, depending on the amount of food, the kind of food (particularly the fat content), and the degree of pancreatic insufficiency. The goal of pancreatic enzyme therapy is to increase intestinal absorption of foodstuffs and allow the patient as nearly normal a diet as possible while decreasing the number of bulky, foul-smelling stools. Fat restriction is generally unnecessary, with the exception of the fat load of whole milk and excessive grease in food. Children should be offered skim or 2% milk after the age of 2 years.

Studies demonstrate that better nutrition has a positive effect on the overall prognosis of the patient with CF. Nutritional supplements supplied by nasogastric tube, jejunostomy, and gastrostomy feedings, and by long-term intravenous hyperalimentation are advocated. Medium-chain triglycerides (MCTs) are more easily absorbed than other fats and provide an important source of calories. The MCT oil enables the preparation and digestion of fried foods, salad dressings, and mayonnaise. The diet should also be supplemented with twice the recommended daily dose of vitamins, prepared in such a way that they can be combined with water (water-miscible) because of malabsorption of the fat-soluble vitamins in cystic fibrosis. The water-miscible vitamins make supplementation of vitamins A, D, and K accessible to the patient. Supplementary vitamin K is recommended, especially for infants, to prevent blood clotting problems. In hot weather, extra salt intake is necessary because of the large amounts lost in the perspiration. The prescribed amount can be incorporated in the preparation of food and need not be given separately. Heat prostration caused by salt depletion is a real danger for these children, especially on hot summer days and during periods of exertion. If excessive sweating is anticipated, salt intake should be increased.

Cystic fibrosis centers. Because cystic fibrosis is

Nursing Care Plan
THE CHILD WITH CYSTIC FIBROSIS

	Selected Nursing Diagnoses	Expected Outcomes	Interventions
A	Ineffective airway clearance related to thick secretions, inflammation and infection of lung tissue. Clinical manifestations: Rales/rhonchi, increased cough, change in sputum characteristics, cyanosis, tachypnea, fever, decreased activity tolerance, retractions, and nasal flaring.	Child regains/maintains baseline respiratory function. Child is relatively free from respiratory infection.	Assess child's respiratory status (color, lung sounds, respiratory rate, use of accessory muscles) every 4 hours and prn. Administer intravenous antibiotics as ordered. Observe and document amount, color, and quality of sputum. Assure respiratory treatments (vigorous chest physiotherapy) are given as ordered and assess child's response. Administer oxygen prn. Encourage oral fluids/intravenous hydration as needed.
B	Altered nutrition: less than body requirements related to decreased respiratory function, inadequate enzyme secretion, and food digestion. Clinical manifestations: Poor weight gain and anorexia.	Child maintains adequate caloric intake to promote growth.	Give child small, frequent meals. Administer vitamins and enzymes with meals and snacks. Assist child/parent in selecting food choices. Supplement with high-caloric snacks (Sustacal Shakes). Assess need for and administer nasogastric tube/gastrostomy feedings, if ordered.
C	Activity intolerance related to increased respiratory effort, decreased caloric intake, and presence of infection. Clinical manifestations: Tires easily, frequent naps, unable to perform ADLs.	Child regains/maintains baseline activity level.	Provide adequate rest periods throughout the day. Allow child to participate in planning daily schedule (children with CF tend to have more energy in the afternoon.) Ensure adequate caloric intake for age and activity level. Administer respiratory treatment and antibiotics as ordered to facilitate return to baseline activity level.

chronic and many organs and systems are involved, care is complex and requires a team effort to coordinate the services of many specialists. Comprehensive, coordinated services are the key to good management, and all children with cystic fibrosis should be referred to a cystic fibrosis center, where a team of experts in all aspects of the disease can design an individualized treatment plan. In addition to a specific treatment plan that includes instructions on medication, diet, and exercise, the patient and family are trained in techniques of postural drainage. Cystic fibrosis centers can also provide initial and continuing psychological, psychosocial, genetic, and vocational counseling.

Nursing care. Nursing care entails a careful observation of the dietary intake and its effect on the child with CF and on elimination. Every effort should be made to offer a variety in meals within the limitations imposed and to make eating a pleasant experience.

Provision for frequent changes in position to prevent pneumonia and reduce skin problems is an important consideration in sick, malnourished patients with cystic fibrosis. Some of these children are emaciated,

◆ TABLE 34-2
Comparison of Croup Syndromes

	Acute Epiglottitis (Supraglottitis)	Acute Laryngotracheobronchitis	Acute Spasmodic Laryngitis (Spasmodic Croup)	Acute Tracheitis
Age-group affected	1-8 years	3 months-8 years	3 months-3 years	1 month-6 years
Etiological agent	Bacterial, usually *H. influenzae*	Viral	Viral with allergic component	Bacterial, usually *S. aureus*
Onset	Rapidly progressive	Slowly progressive	Sudden; at night	Moderately progressive
Major symptoms	Dysphagia Stridor aggravated when supine Drooling High fever Toxic appearance Rapid pulse and respirations	URI Stridor Brassy cough Hoarseness Dyspnea Restlessness Irritability Low-grade fever Nontoxic appearance	URI Croupy cough Stridor Hoarseness Dyspnea Restlessness Symptoms waken child Symptoms disappear during day Tends to recur	URI Croupy cough Stridor Purulent secretions High fever No response to LTB therapy
Treatment	Antibiotics Airway protection	Humidity Racemic epinephrine	Humidity	Antibiotics

From Wong DL: *Essentials of pediatric nursing,* ed 4, St Louis, 1993, Mosby.

and the skin over bony prominences needs special care. Cleansing of the rectal area is essential. Rectal prolapse may be a complication. A soothing, local ointment may prevent irritation from the bulky stools. Any material soiled by feces should be removed immediately from the child's room. Stool size, color, consistency, and odor should be recorded.

The observation and report of respiratory distress is of paramount importance. Every effort should be made to protect the child from persons with any type of respiratory tract infection.

Because of the chronic nature of the disease, the severe strain it may place on family finances, and the psychological needs of the child and family, home care is recommended when possible. Parents may need counseling and practical assistance to help meet their child's social and emotional needs, as well as the child's physical needs. They also must be cautioned against becoming so preoccupied with the sick child that the needs of other family members are neglected.

Early diagnosis and improved methods of therapy have reduced the morbidity and greatly increased the longevity of children with cystic fibrosis. These children currently have a greater than 50% chance of living past the second decade.

Only rarely is a young man with cystic fibrosis fertile, since the same mechanisms that typically obstruct other glandular ducts of the body interfere with sperm transport. Female patients have borne children, but their ability to conceive seems to be below normal because cervical mucus is abnormal.

The nurse caring for the child with cystic fibrosis must realize the strain under which the parents may be operating and their feelings of fatigue and frustration. Many families have lost other children to this disease.

Toddler

Croup (laryngotracheobronchitis)

Acute obstructive subglottic laryngitis, or laryngotracheobronchitis (LTB), commonly known as *croup,* is a viral respiratory disease that involves the larynx, trachea, and bronchi. Mild to severe forms of LTB typically occur in children between 6 months and 3 years of age during cold weather. Croup is characterized by a sudden onset of crowing inspiratory stridor, hoarseness, and a barking seal cough following a 1- to 3-day history of a cold (see Table 34-2). These manifestations are the result of inflammatory edema of the vocal folds and subglottic area, causing varying de-

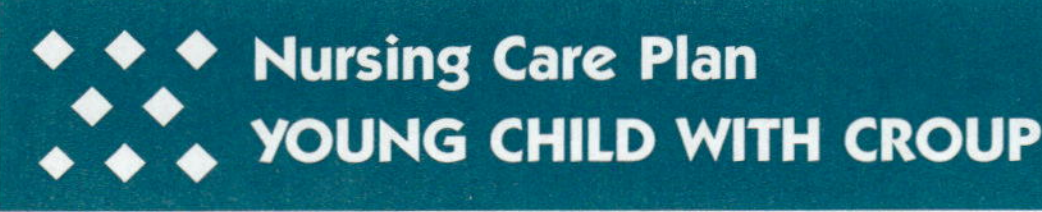

Nursing Care Plan
YOUNG CHILD WITH CROUP

	Selected Nursing Diagnoses	Expected Outcomes	Interventions
A	Potential for suffocation related to inflammation and obstruction of upper respiratory tract. Clinical manifestations: Barking cough, stridor, retractions, prolonged inspiration, pallor, cyanosis, nasal flaring, restlessness, or lethargy.	Child regains normal respiratory function.	Assess child for presence of barking cough, stridor, retractions, cyanosis, restlessness, lethargy, and disorientation and notify physician of worsening condition. Keep child in cool-mist tent and monitor mist and oxygen content every 2 hours. Assure respiratory treatments (racemic-epinephrine) are given as ordered and assess child's response. Keep child in upright position/helps ease motion of diaphragm in breathing. Maintain calm, quiet environment.
B	Anxiety related to respiratory distress, unfamiliar surroundings.		See Nursing Care Plan for The Hospitalized Child.
C	Fluid volume deficit related to respiratory distress.		See Nursing Care Plan for The Child with a Fluid Volume Deficit.

grees of laryngeal obstruction. Sometimes spasm accompanies the process. Most children are awakened without warning in the middle of the night by an acute attack. The child appears extremely anxious and frightened by this respiratory distress. Treatment is symptomatic. A cool-mist vaporizer near the head of the child's bed should be used throughout the night. Cool-mist nebulizers are preferred over steam vaporizers because the warm steam may have a drying effect and may raise the temperature of an already febrile child (Allen, 1991). If there is a spasm, it usually subsides in a few hours with high humidity therapy but may recur for 1 or 2 nights.

A more severe form of croup results when the inflammatory involvement of the trachea and bronchial tree produces a thick, viscous, purulent exudate. Edema and exudate lead to both inspiratory and expiratory difficulties. As the degree of severity of respiratory distress increases, suprasternal, intercostal, and substernal retractions occur. The child becomes hypoxic, restless, and extremely anxious. Impending suffocation is a real threat and a terrifying experience for both the child and the parents. This child needs immediate medical management and possible endotracheal intubation or tracheostomy.

Hospital admission

During the admission procedure, every effort should be made to prevent aggravation of respiratory distress. The parents should remain at the cribside as the child is gently and calmly placed in an atmosphere of high humidity with oxygen. Maximum humidification is best accomplished with cool mist in the tent. The moist vapor helps allay irritation of the mucosa and promote liquefaction of the thick secretions. Clear fluids are encouraged if the respiratory distress is not severe and are also important in mobilizing respiratory exudate. Refusal to take fluids orally or the presence of severe respiratory distress necessitates intravenous therapy.

Increased pulse rate, restlessness, severe stridor, and use of the accessory muscles for breathing must be reported immediately. If the signs and symptoms of acute airway obstruction increase, emergency airway intervention must be considered before the child is exhausted. This is achieved in most hospitals by the insertion of an endotracheal tube or tracheostomy. In recent years endotracheal intubation has become the preferred method. Arterial or arterialized capillary blood gases are helpful in assessing the clinical situation and determining the need for emergency airway intervention. Unfortunately, this procedure can

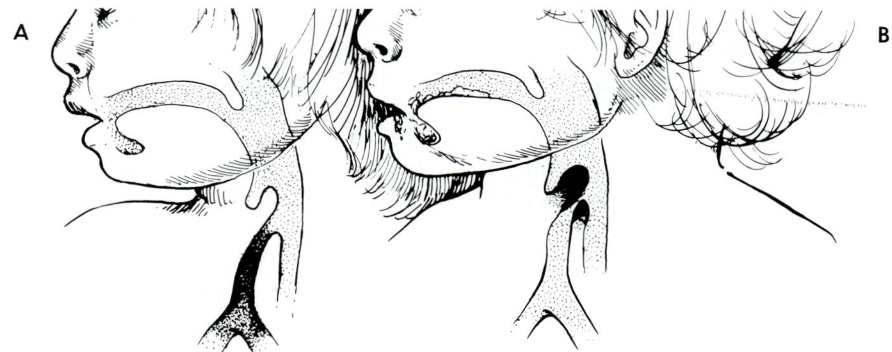

Fig. 34-4 Anatomical difference between acute subglottic and acute supraglottic obstruction. **A,** Laryngotracheobronchitis (LTB), an acute inflammation particularly involving subglottic area of larynx, trachea, and bronchial tree, most commonly occurring in toddlers. **B,** Epiglottitis, an acute inflammatory swelling involving structures above opening of trachea (glottis), most often seen in preschoolers.

upset the child to such a degree that the child may be more hypoxic during the blood drawing.

Nebulized racemic epinephrine (Vaponefrin) has been used with success in cases of severe LTB. At first the child struggles against the aerosol, but after a short time the child relaxes and the labored breathing subsides as the therapy is continued over 10 to 15 minutes. The procedure may be repeated at 3- to 4-hour intervals. Racemic epinephrine is used for its topical vasoconstrictive effect, resulting in decreased mucosal edema. This treatment is extremely helpful in providing immediate, temporary improvement in patients with croup. However, the obstruction can recur in 1 to 2 hours as a result of a rebound phenomenon in severe cases. Therefore severe cases should be observed closely for recurrence even after an improvement.

Acute LTB should not be confused with epiglottitis (acute supraglottic laryngitis), a more serious acute airway problem that can lead to complete respiratory obstruction (Fig. 34-4).

Foreign bodies in the nose or throat

Children frequently push objects into the nasal cavity. If the object is not dislodged by sneezing and the episode is not reported by the child, it may be indicated by a bloody or purulent, foul unilateral nasal discharge. A unilateral discharge suggests the presence of a foreign body. Removal of such an object should be attempted by a physician who has the necessary instruments.

If a child is choking but is conscious and able to cough, the child should be encouraged to cough. If the child develops complete obstruction, four short, controlled blows on the back with the hand may dislodge the object. If the problem still persists, CPR should be initiated. If respiratory distress continues, the child should be seen immediately by a physician who may schedule a chest x-ray examination and perform a bronchoscopy.

Bronchitis

Bronchitis is most often caused by the same virus that has invaded other areas of the respiratory tract. Bronchitis is usually preceded by an upper respiratory tract infection and is a common problem in toddlers. It may remain mild or become progressively severe, leading to pneumonia. A disturbing, productive cough appears as the disease develops. Paroxysms may occur, particularly when the position of the child is altered, such as in the morning on rising or when first lying in bed after sitting for a period. Vomiting as a result of gagging when the secretions are thick is not uncommon. Cool moisture is sometimes helpful. A generous intake of fluids thins bronchial secretions, and acetaminophen (Tylenol) may be necessary to lessen discomfort or fever. Unless the condition worsens, acute bronchitis is generally a self-limited infection that improves spontaneously in a few days.

Preschool-Age Child

Epiglottitis (Fig. 34-4)

Acute obstructive supraglottic laryngitis, commonly known as *epiglottitis,* is usually caused by the *H. influenzae* type b bacteria. It is characterized by acute respiratory distress, high temperature, drooling, difficulty in swallowing, and a "cherry red" epiglottis on physical examination. The signs and symptoms of supraglottic obstruction result from inflammatory edema of the epiglottis. Children between 3 and 7 years of age are most frequently affected. The condition is usually seen in the winter months, and the onset is sudden. The child first complains of a severe sore throat and difficulty in swallowing (dysphagia). Soon the child is anxious, unable to eat or drink, prostrated, in a toxic condition, and drooling. Rapidly increasing dyspnea and drooling are common manifestations. Once the diagnosis is made, children must have their airway maintained, either by endotracheal tube or tracheostomy. Endotracheal intubation or tracheostomy should not be deferred, as epiglottitis can lead to complete respiratory obstruction and death in just a few hours.

It is important not to disturb the child unduly or to separate the child from the parents. The diagnosis is confirmed by visualization of the inflamed epiglottis or by a lateral neck x-ray film, and the child is moved from the emergency room to the operating room, where an elective endotracheal intubation or tracheostomy can be performed in a controlled setting. One should be aware that physical examination to visualize the epiglottis can precipitate a sudden, complete obstruction of the upper airway. Intravenous therapy with ampicillin or cephalosporins should be initiated.

After the airway is secured, arterial blood gases are assessed to ensure adequate oxygenation. It is essential that warm mist with or without oxygen is administered through the artificial airways by a T-piece or tracheostomy collar. The child is then placed in a mist tent and returned to the pediatric intensive care unit, where an experienced staff can give constant care. No child should die from epiglottitis when it is diagnosed and treated promptly.

Epistaxis

Bleeding from the nose (epistaxis) is a common disorder of childhood, especially in boys from 4 to 10 years of age. On the anterior portion of the nasal septum, called Kiesselbach's area, a fragile network of capillaries subject to drying and multiple minor injuries is found. Trauma, such as nose picking and nose rubbing, forceful blowing, chronic allergies, and insertion of foreign bodies, all contribute to epistaxis.

Placing the child in a sitting position with the head tilted forward while compressing the nares with the thumb and forefinger is often sufficient to facilitate clot formation and stop the bleeding. This posture also prevents blood from dripping down the posterior pharynx, possibly leading to nausea and possible aspiration. Ice packs to the nasal area or to the back of the neck are of little or no value. If bleeding is persistent, an anterior nasal pack consisting of ½ inch of petrolatum-impregnated gauze or an application of agents such as aqueous epinephrine solution (1:1000) or thrombin may be beneficial.

Any condition that contributes to vascular congestion of the nasal mucosa, such as nasal allergy or sinusitis, increases the frequency of epistaxis. Bleeding from the posterior region of the nasal cavity is uncommon. Rarely nosebleeds are a symptom of underlying blood dyscrasias, such as purpura, leukemia, or conditions associated with a rise in blood pressure. Frequent nosebleeds may or may not be significant. Parental fears can best be allayed by not only stopping the bleeding but also by identifying and treating the underlying causes of the disorder.

Deviation of the septum

In some instances the cartilaginous and bony wall, or septum, that divides the nose into two lateral chambers does not occupy the midline. It may deviate toward one side or another as a result of natural development or, more commonly, as an aftermath of trauma. This may cause occlusion of a nostril and difficult breathing, particularly when the nose is inflamed. This structural anomaly can be corrected surgically by an operation called a *submucous resection.* To prevent external nasal deformity resulting from the surgery, it is usually not performed until adolescence.

Acute nasopharyngitis (acute coryza, common cold)

Preschool and young school-age children average approximately six colds a year. The common cold is caused by more than 156 different viral organisms that primarily attack the nose and throat. Symptoms include dry, scratchy, sore, inflamed pharynx, and an inflamed nasal mucosa, which produces a clear mucoid nasal discharge that later becomes thick and purulent. These local symptoms are often accompanied by headache, muscular pains, general malaise, and fever. As the viral infection continues, complications often arise from the intrusion of pathogenic bacteria, which may prolong the congestion and promote the extension of the inflammation to the middle ear, sinuses, larynx, trachea, and even to the bronchi and lungs. Complications make the common cold a potentially dangerous condition.

A common cold is contagious for a number of hours before symptoms are observed by the patient. Contamination by hand-to-hand contact spread of droplets is most common, thus thorough handwashing is the best preventive measure. It is very important to protect infants from exposure to colds because they are affected more seriously than older children. An infant may have a high temperature of 104° F (40° C), and febrile seizures are possible. Ears are always affected. Nasal congestion causes difficulties in breathing, nursing, breast-feeding, and eating.

Since nasopharyngitis is caused by many different viruses, no specific therapy is effective. Supportive treatment consists of rest, respiratory isolation, increased fluid intake, and a bland, soft diet. Nasal obstruction in infants can be partially relieved by humidification or instillation of 1 or 2 drops of physiological saline solution in each nostril, followed by gentle suction with an infant nasal (or ear) syringe. Phenylephrine (Neo-Synephrine) hydrochloride nose drops (1/8% for infants and 1/4% for older children) may also relieve nasal symptoms. Nasal vasoconstrictors should not be used for more than 3 days. If the use of vasoconstrictors has been prolonged, congestion greatly increases, or "rebounds."

Mild systemic symptoms and fever may be relieved by proper dosage of nonsalicylate acetaminophen (Tylenol or Tempra). Aspirin is not recommended for children or adolescents because of the complications of Reye syndrome.

To protect the nares or upper lip from excoriation caused by the fairly constant nasal discharge, a moisterizer or petrolatum is applied. Antibiotics are indicated if viral infections are complicated by secondary bacterial infection.

Sinusitis

Acute sinusitis is usually precipitated by an upper respiratory tract infection. Headache, congestion, and a mucopurulent discharge from one or both nostrils, cough, and a diffusely red pharynx with mucopurulent discharge clinging to the posterior wall are indications that bacteria have invaded the sinuses. Improved ventilation and drainage are primary goals of treatment. Hot compresses over the painful areas and increased humidification provide some comfort. Pain and fever are lessened by the use of acetaminophen. Instillation of nasal saline nose drops is beneficial. The use of nasal vasoconstrictors should be reserved for severe cases. Each nostril should be sprayed once while the child is in a sitting position. About 3 to 5 minutes later the spraying should be repeated to reach the posterior part of the nose. Oral decongestants, such as pseudoephedrine hydrochloride (Sudafed), are beneficial for some patients; however, their benefit in controlled studies has not been consistently demonstrated. The use of antihistamines, such as Dimetap or Actifed, may be helpful if allergies are suspected. Skin testing may be recommended in children over 3 years. Most acute sinus infections are self-limited; appropriate antibiotic therapy (culture-sensitive) shortens the course of illness and usually prevents any further complications. However, children are occasionally seen with the complication of periorbital cellulitis. This condition follows a severe bout of ethmoid sinusitis and must be treated vigorously to prevent ocular and central nervous system (CNS) complications.

Otitis media

Otitis media, or inflammation of the middle ear, is a common problem related to malfunction of the eustachian tube. Normally the eustachian tube protects the middle ear from nasopharyngeal secretions, provides drainage of secretions produced within the middle ear into the nasopharynx, and equalizes the air pressure in the middle ear with that of the atmosphere. Persistent obstruction of the eustachian tube caused by infection, allergy, and enlarged adenoids eventually leads to middle ear disease. Because the adenoids are located close to the opening of the eustachian or auditory tube, enlarged adenoids may be an underlying cause of frequent middle ear infections, or otitis media. The eustachian tube is more horizontal and is broader and shorter in infants and young children than it is in adults; thus ascending ear infections are fairly common in children. Bottle feeding in the supine position and parental smoking are contributing factors.

Acute otitis media is a common complication of upper respiratory tract infection in young children. Respiratory mucosa damaged by viral infection is readily colonized by pneumococci, *H. influenzae*, group A beta-hemolytic streptococci, and Branhamella catarrhalis. Bacteria usually gain access to the middle ear by way of the eustachian tube. Purulent fluid accumulates in the middle ear, causing severe pain, fever, and irritability. When the eustachian tube becomes inflamed, it may swell shut, and the purulent material produced by the infection builds up within the middle ear, causing ear pressure, ringing of the ears, elevated temperature, occasional vomiting, and ultimately spontaneous rupture of the tympanic membrane (eardrum).

Infants are especially susceptible to otitis media and may display discomfort by crying, fussy behavior, or pulling at the affected ear. Definitive diagnosis can be made only by visualization of the tympanic membrane and adjacent structures. Antibiotics are the mainstay of therapy. A successful outcome depends in large measure on early treatment. Parents should be encouraged to notify the health care provider promptly when the child has an earache. Acetaminophen and Auralgan ear drops may be given for pain, although it usually subsides in 12 to 24 hours after antibiotic therapy has been initiated.

Specific antibiotic therapy is usually effective in the prevention of such complications as mastoiditis, meningitis, and the incidence of eardrum perforation. Pediazole (erythromycin and sulfa), amoxicillin, trimethoprim with sulfamethoxazole (Septra), and the cephalosporins are effective against both gram-positive and gram-negative bacteria, and any of these drugs can be used alone. Therapy should be continued for at least 10 days. The nurse must forewarn parents that a follow-up visit to the health care provider is essential. The child's ear must be inspected and evaluated after 14 days of treatment, since the appearance of the eardrum dictates the duration of therapy. A follow-up hearing assessment is essential. No child is considered cured until the signs of middle ear disease have been resolved. Partially treated otitis media is a major cause of meningitis in young children.

In the past a myringotomy (surgical incision of the eardrum) with tubes was commonly performed to relieve pressure and evacuate fluid. Because most children respond well to antibiotic therapy, myringotomies currently are reserved for those patients whose improvement at follow-up examination has not been satisfactory.

Serous otitis media or otitis media with effusion (OME)

Recurrent attacks of acute otitis media characteristically precede serous, or "secretory," otitis media, a sterile middle ear effusion. The fluid varies greatly in its viscosity. When it is very thick, the condition is called *glue ear.* Serous otitis is the most common complication of acute otitis media, and since no significant symptoms are present, the development of a conductive hearing loss is a real possibility. Unless definitive measures are instituted to open the eustachian tube, permanent hearing loss can result. Learning difficulties often signal such a hearing loss in school-age children. Children with conductive hearing loss caused by chronic serous otitis media should be referred to an otologist. Surgical drainage (myringotomy) may be necessary. The aspirated fluid is cultured, and specific antibiotic therapy may be started. Placement of tiny middle-ear ventilating tubes through the eardrum may be necessary if antibiotic prophylaxis is unsuccessful and otitis media is recurrent (Fig. 34-5, *B*). The success of tympanostomy tubes is due to the artificial tubes providing equalization of air pressure on both sides of the tympanic membranes. Children with tympanostomy tubes must be protected when swimming or showering by wearing custom-made earplugs; otherwise, acute otitis media is a common sequela.

The most important aspect of long-term management is to relieve the underlying cause. Allergies must be investigated and treated, and hypertrophied adenoids must be removed if they are obstructing the eustachian tube. A significant advance in the identification of middle ear disease has resulted from the use of the electroacoustic impedance bridge. A small probe in a rubber cuff is placed in the external canal and attached to the impedance meter. A tympanogram, which reflects the dynamics of the entire tympanic membrane—middle ear and eustachian tube system—is produced. For detecting otitis media and common conductive defects in children, tympanometry is more reliable than otoscopic examination. Tympanometry is a simple procedure that can be easily administered.

Ear hygiene. Damage to the ear may be caused by probing of the external auditory canal with implements such as toothpicks. It is wise to follow the old saying, "Never put anything in your ear smaller than your elbow." The outer auditory canal should be cleaned by using a washcloth or a tightly rolled piece of cotton. If a collection of hardened wax, or cerumen, is suspected, the cerumen may be softened with an over-the-counter product. Then the ear should be examined, and a health care provider trained in irrigating technique should carry out the procedure.

Children occasionally push foreign bodies into the external ear canal. When foreign bodies are detected, they should be removed by a health care provider who has the knowledge, skill, and instruments. An irrigation should never be attempted before an otoscopic examination has been administered by the health care provider. If the object is made of vegetable matter, it can swell with the liquid and become more difficult to extract.

Adenoids and tonsils

Located in the nasopharynx are the nasopharyngeal tonsils, or adenoids. Farther down on the lateral walls of the oral pharynx are the palatine, or faucial tonsils. The tonsils are composed mainly of lymphoid tissue and play a role in the formation of immunoglobulins. In addition, they act as a respiratory tract defense mechanism by filtering microbes, thereby helping to prevent microbial invasion of the lower tract. This lymphoid tissue serves a useful purpose and should be preserved unless the problems caused by its presence outweigh its possible benefits. Tonsils and adenoids are present at birth and achieve their maximum size by the time the child is 5 years of age. At 2 years the tonsils are normally large, and the adenoids occupy one half of the nasopharyngeal cavity. The peak of adenoid size is reached by puberty, after which they cease to grow and begin to shrink. When adenoids are removed in very young children, they usually regrow. In the past

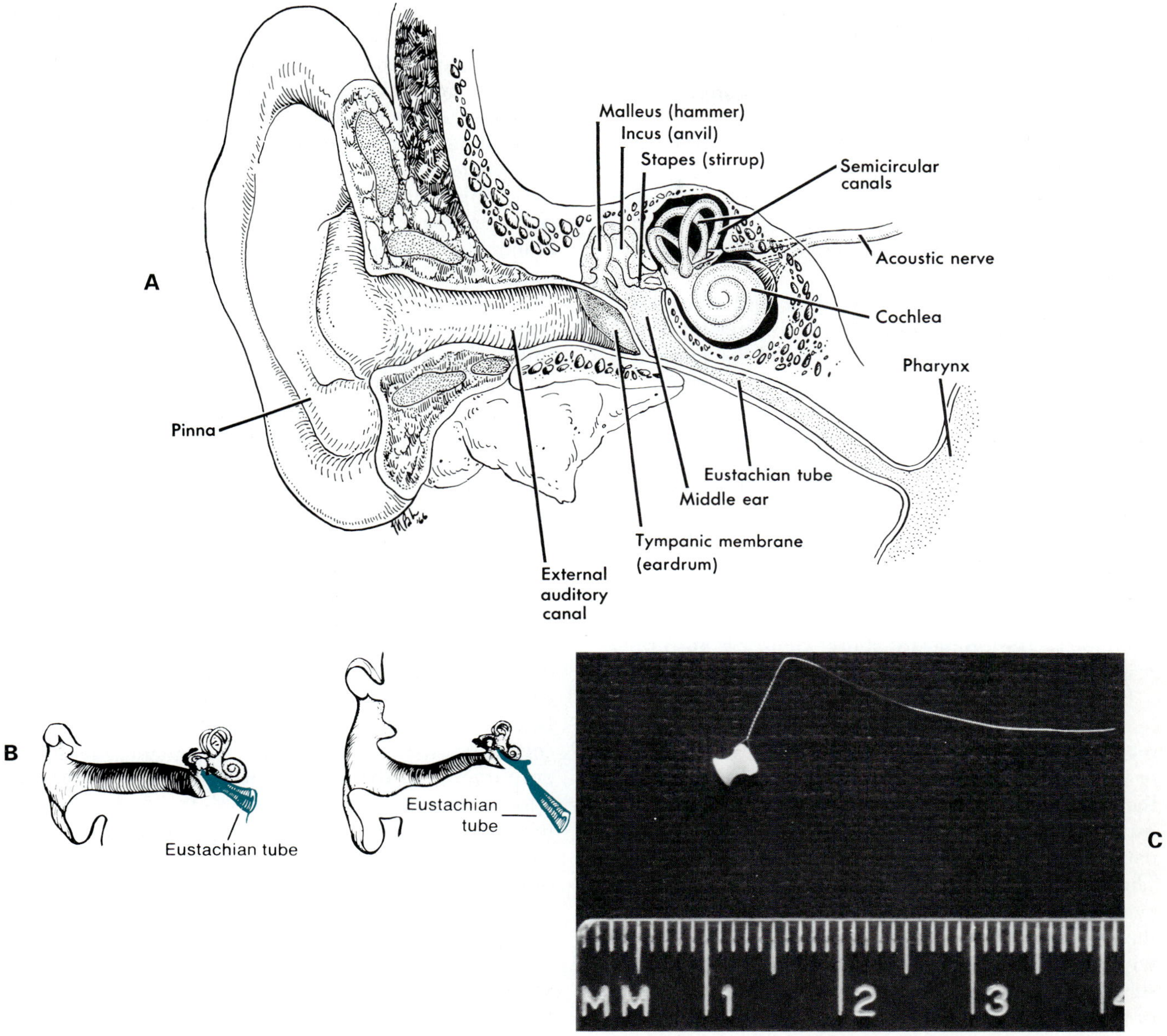

Fig. 34-5 **A,** Basic anatomy of ear. **B,** Comparison of anatomical position of the eustachian tube in (a) a child and (b) an adult. (**A** and **B** from Whaley and Wong: *Nursing care of infants and children,* ed 4, St Louis, 1991, Mosby.) **C,** Tympanostomy ventilating tube.

tonsils and adenoids were removed without much hesitation. However, much disillusionment has resulted from failure of surgery to achieve expected results. Moreover, this lightly regarded "minor" procedure has taken the lives of many children. In the United States alone reliable evidence shows that over 100 deaths a year result from cardiac arrest, hemorrhage, and infection that follow tonsillectomy. In addition to surgical risk the role that these immunological structures play is the subject of ongoing research.

Indications for removal. Indications for an adenoidectomy are obstructive adenoids with recurrent acute otitis media or chronic serous otitis media with conductive hearing loss. Children with the latter condition may require surgical drainage to remove the fluid and placement of tympanostomy tubes in the eardrum to promote ventilation and prevent reaccumulation of fluid.

A tonsillectomy need not be done with an adenoidectomy, since these are two independent procedures with very different indications. The best results from a tonsillectomy are obtained when the symptoms have been clearly referrable to the tonsils and not to problems such as frequent colds, sore throat, poor appetite, failure to gain weight, postnasal drip, or allergies. Definite indications for a tonsillectomy include a history of chronic airway obstruction, pulmonary hypertension, peritonsillar abscess (to prevent a second attack), chronic recurrent group A beta-hemolytic streptococcal tonsillitis (culture-proved), and hypertrophied tonsils.

Contraindications. Tonsillectomy and adenoidectomy (T and A) is contraindicated in children who have hematologic conditions, such as hemophilia, leukemia, aplastic anemia, or purpura. Routine laboratory screening of candidates for this surgery is particularly important to discover the potential postoperative "bleeder." Bleeding times (usually simplate method) and prothrombin levels may indicate the need for specific treatment or operative delay. Vitamin K is administered for prothrombin deficiencies. When systemic disorders, such as diabetes or cardiac or renal disease, are present, surgery can safely outweigh the risk. However, T and A surgery is always postponed if a child is beginning to show signs of an upper respiratory tract infection.

Because of the numerous blood vessels in the operative area and the character of the procedure, the most common complication of either a tonsillectomy or an adenoidectomy is hemorrhage. For this reason the nurse should carefully assess for symptoms of excessive bleeding and shock. If bleeding occurs, it usually occurs within the first 24 hours after surgery. The physician must be called to the bedside to evaluate the seriousness of the situation and to locate the source of bleeding. Minor bleeding usually stops when any associated clot, which inadequately obstructs a bleeding vessel yet impedes its constriction, is removed gently by suction. A sponge moistened with lidocaine (Xylocaine) and epinephrine is held firmly against the area for a few minutes. In the event of major hemorrhage from the tonsillar fossae, reanesthetizing and resuturing may be necessary. Bleeding from the adenoid area is more common. Again, any clot must first be removed, and if the bleeding does not stop, the patient must be returned to surgery for another general anesthetic and cauterization or laser therapy. If this treatment is not successful in curtailing bleeding, then a postnasal pack or Foley type of catheter with inflatable bag can be inserted and left in place until the next day (Fig. 34-6). Transfusions are rarely administered, but may be required if bleeding persists.

Postoperative care. Most children undergoing T and A will be cared for in an ambulatory day surgery center. The child is assessed for 2 to 3 hours of observation in a recovery room. Unless there are complications, the child will not be admitted to a pediatric unit. However, if a child is admitted to the unit, the best position is side-lying with the anterior chest at a 45-degree angle to facilitate oronasal drainage, prevent aspiration, and assist in observation. The nurse frequently assesses vital signs. With the advent of laser surgery, hemorrhage is rare; however, the color, amount, and consistency of drainage must be documented.

As soon as the patient is conscious and responding, sips of water are given to ascertain tolerance for oral fluids. The early introduction of clear, bland fluids helps prevent dehydration and fever. It also eventually helps to ease the sore throat. By the second day the child is ready for a soft, bland diet. More than 50% of children who have had their tonsils or adenoids removed are discharged the same evening as the surgery.

Discharge planning. Discharge planning should include written instructions for care. Parents and child should be told that throat pain may persist for several days. Complaints of earache (referred pain from the throat) are common. Acetaminophen with or without codeine may be prescribed for this discomfort. The child should be told not to blow his or her nose forcefully. A soft, bland diet should be continued for several days. The child should be encouraged to drink and eat and open the mouth widely. Fluids and food should be given at room temperature. Crisp or hard foods such as popcorn, chips, dry crackers, and acid foods such as pickles, oranges, grapefruit, and tomatoes should be avoided. About 10 days after surgery children may eat whatever they wish.

Children should rest for the first few days at home. They may go outside on the third or fourth day and resume their usual activities after 1 week, except for swimming, which should be avoided for 2 weeks. School-age children are allowed to return to school at the end of 1 week.

Signs and symptoms that should be reported promptly by the parents to the physician include fresh bleeding, fever over 101° F, chest pain, and persistent cough. As already stated, the most common postoperative complication is hemorrhage. Parents should understand that occasional blood-streaked nasal or oral mucus is normal during the first 2 days; but if increased bleeding should occur, the child must be promptly and calmly returned to the hospital. No surgery is without risk. T and A surgery is not a minor operation, nor is it the answer for all ear, nose, and throat problems. It is an effective therapeutic procedure for selected patients.

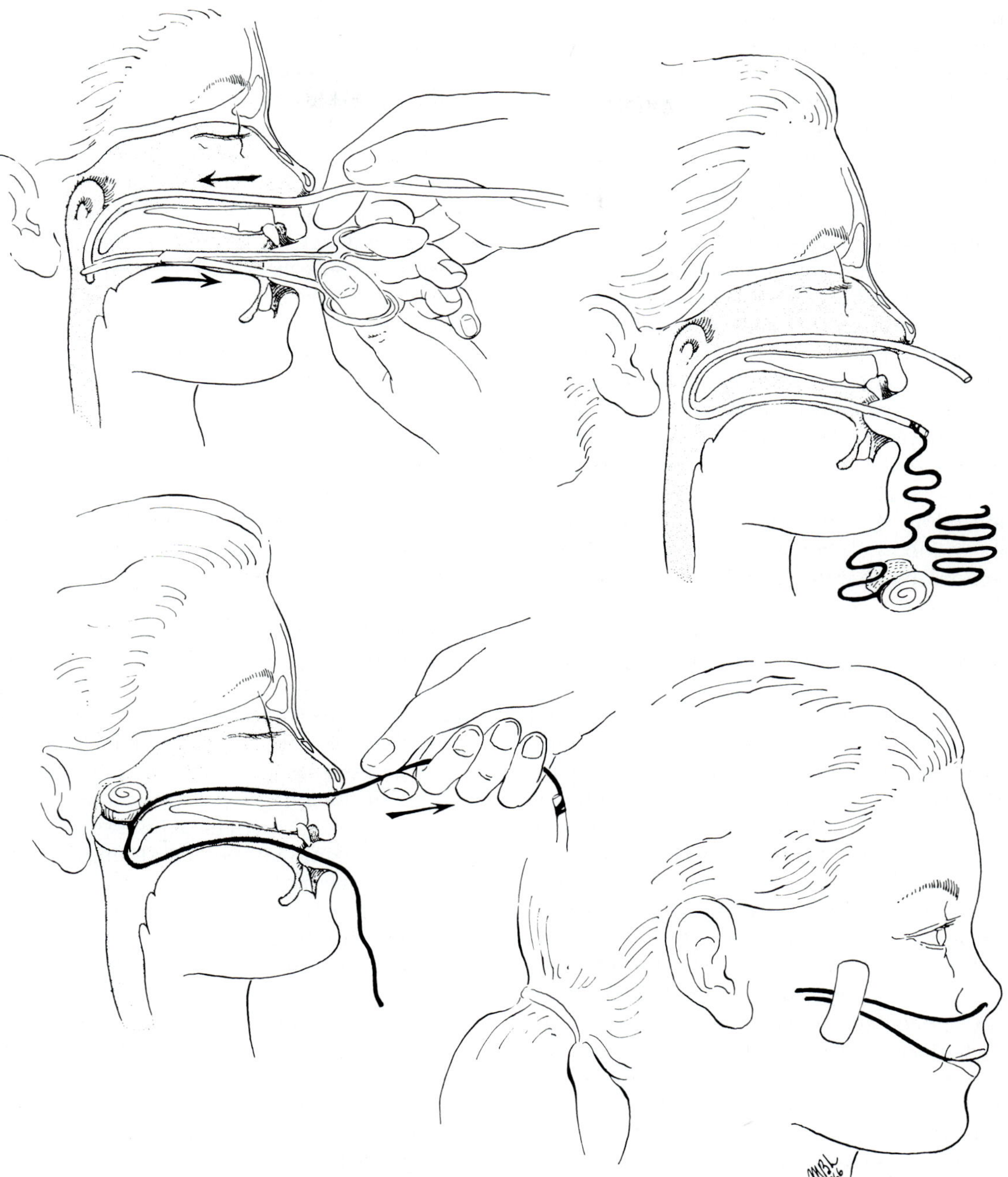

Fig. 34-6 Insertion of postnasal pack to stop bleeding from adenoid area.

School-Age Child

Streptococcal pharyngitis (strep throat)

A severe pharyngitis often develops from an infection by group A beta-hemolytic streptococcus. Such a condition is commonly called a *strep throat*. Streptococcal pharyngitis is uncommon before a child is 2 years of age and almost nonexistent in a child less than 1 year. Classically strep throat has sudden onset; the child has a high temperature, severe sore throat, tender cervical lymph nodes, exudate, a beefy, red pharynx, and petechiae on the soft palate.

Unfortunately strep throat cannot be diagnosed from clinical findings alone because the same clinical manifestations accompany viral infections. The demonstration of the group A beta-hemolytic streptococcal organism by means of a throat culture is therefore essential for an accurate diagnosis. Since rheumatic fever, heart disease, and glomerulonephritis follow untreated streptococcal infections in a significant number of children, patients coming to the health care provider with pharyngeal inflammations should have routine throat cultures taken. Initial a "quick strep" screen will be administered. The results will be available after 10 minutes. If the screen is administered correctly, it has a high correlation with throat culture. The patient's telephone number should be written on the laboratory slip, and those whose culture reveals a beta-hemolytic streptococcus should be notified and treated.

While awaiting culture results, patients can be treated symptomatically with saline gargles, lozenges, and or acetaminophen. The 48-hour delay in starting antibiotic therapy does not increase the incidence of rheumatic fever or glomerulonephritis but is thought to be beneficial in that it gives the patient time to develop an antibody response, which helps prevent future infections by that particular strain of streptococcus. If time is taken to explain this to the patient or the parents, they are most grateful. The patient who is in a toxic state and has physical findings suggesting streptococcal pharyngitis may be given antibiotics immediately, but controlled studies have shown that the speed at which the patient recovers is not appreciably influenced by such treatment. The reason for treating streptococcal pharyngitis with antibiotics is not for a more rapid recovery but for the prevention of complications. Numerous studies have shown that this can be done if the child is treated within 7 days of onset of the illness. The American Heart Association recommends that streptococcal infections be treated for a period of 10 days with penicillin (or erythromycin if the child is allergic to penicillin). Streptococcal organisms are extremely sensitive to an oral course of penicillin, but since many patients stop their medication prematurely, one intramuscular injection of benzathine penicillin G has been recommended by some health care providers as the treatment of choice. It is also advisable to take throat cultures of asymptomatic family contacts.

Respiratory disease resulting from allergy

About 24 million Americans (1 in 10) suffer from some type of allergy. Allergic conditions include respiratory problems such as "hay fever" (rhinitis) and asthma, as well as eczema, hives, and hypersensitivity to foods, venoms, and medications. Approximately 75% of these have hay fever, asthma, or both. Allergy is the leading chronic disease in children and a major cause of lost work days in adults. The word *allergy* describes an unfavorable reaction of the body to a normally harmless substance from the outside environment. These substances may be taken into the body through the nose and lungs (pollens, mold spores, animal danders, mites, and house dust), the mouth (foods and drugs), or the skin (insect bites or stings and injections). A substance that can produce an allergic reaction is called an *allergen,* but the reaction occurs only in a person sensitive to that substance.

The tendency to become sensitive, or allergic, to some otherwise harmless substance is usually inherited. People vary greatly not only in their susceptibility to allergic diseases but also in the kind of allergic diseases they have. The organs or tissues in which the allergic reactions occur (lungs, asthma; nose, rhinitis; eyes, conjunctivitis; skin, eczema, urticaria, or hives; gastrointestinal tract, diarrhea) may change during a person's lifetime. These organs are frequently referred to as *target organs.*

Although the tendency to become sensitive to a substance may be inherited, the allergic response develops only *after* exposure to that substance. This exposure can happen in utero, during childhood, or later in life. The development of a sensitivity to a particular substance depends on the *amount* and *frequency* of exposure to that substance. Sensitization may follow the first exposure or may not occur until after repeated exposures. Penicillin allergy is a well-known example of the latter phenomenon. A general outline of the allergic process follows:

1. A person contacts a substance and produces sensitizing antibodies (immunoglobulin E) to that material.
2. These antibodies are then deposited on special cells (mast cells and basophils) in the body.
3. The allergen (substance to which a person is sensitive or allergic) contacts the antibody E attached to these cells in a subsequent exposure.
4. A reaction occurs whereby chemicals, or "allergic mediators," such as histamine, are released from these cells and cause the symptoms of allergy. These symptoms may include nasal congestion, sneezing, wheezing, itching, hives, or, in the most serious reactions, anaphylactic shock.

Diagnosis of allergy. The best way to find the sources of allergic symptoms is by a carefully taken history of what exposures preceded symptoms and the seasonal occurrence of symptoms. Specific potentially sensitizing allergens can then be documented through skin tests. When the test allergen meets antibodies sensitive to that substance in the skin, the chemical mediators are released, resulting in a positive reaction that resembles a mosquito bite (hive). Tests that indicate inhaled allergens are reliable and commonly agree with the patient's symptoms. Although they can be helpful, skin tests cannot always determine a food allergy. Therefore different trial diets are sometimes suggested to further evaluate various foods as the source of the patient's symptoms.

Rhinitis. Rhinitis is one of the most common allergic manifestations in children. It is characterized by sneezing, a profuse, watery nasal discharge, swelling and itching of the nasal mucosa, and often conjunctivitis. Allergic nasal obstruction is unpleasant for the child, parents, and teacher. Frequently it leads to constant mouth breathing, snoring, abnormal midface development with associated orthodontic problems, and a nasal voice. Associated problems are sinusitis and otitis media. Allergic rhinitis is commonly classified as seasonal (hay fever) or nonseasonal (perennial). Seasonal allergic rhinitis results most often from plant pollen sensitivity. House dust, animal danders, mold spores, and foods, in addition, are causes of nonseasonal allergic rhinitis in children. A careful history, physical examination, laboratory aids (such as nasal cytology to identify increased eosinophil counts), and skin testing all are important etiological diagnostic measures. Treatment depends on the results of the diagnostic procedures. Most children with severe allergic rhinitis require specific treatment.

Treatment of allergic rhinitis. The best way to treat an allergy is avoidance of the allergen. For example, a fur-bearing pet should not be kept in a home with a person who has a history of allergic problems. Dust and mite exposure in a patient's bedroom can be minimized by removing cloth draperies, books, stuffed animals and fiber rugs and by using special hypoallergenic pillows and nonporous mattress encasements. A second method of treatment consists of desensitizing patients to their allergens by injections of these substances in gradually increasing amounts. This regimen is used when allergens (such as pollens) cannot be adequately avoided. The process is called *desensitization, hyposensitization,* or *immunotherapy.*

Medications of various types are also used for relief of symptoms. To be effective for this purpose, medication is often prescribed on a daily basis. Regular maintenance doses of medication should be taken as long as objective evidence exists of a symptomatic allergic state. Antihistamines, such as Dimetap, Actifed, Triaminic, or Chlor-Trimeton, are often effective for the control of allergic rhinitis. They may be combined with a decongestant, such as pseudoephedrine (Sudafed).The effectiveness of decongestants in the treatment of allergy is questionable. A new class of antihistamines appears to be effective without causing drowsiness. A representative of this group is terfenadine (Seldane) and Clasitine (Hismanal) for children over 12 years old. These medications should not be prescribed with erythromycin or Nizoral, since dangerous cardiac arrhythmias have occurred.

Another allergic rhinitis and asthma medication is cromolyn sodium (Nasalcrom, Intal). It is administered in nasal spray prophylactically and as an adjunct to the treatment and control of chronic symptoms. A number of nasal cortisone sprays (Nasalide, Beconase, Vancenase) are very effective in improving and controlling chronic nasal symptoms. Treatment with inhaled cromolyn sodium (Intal) or corticosteroids such as beclomethasone dipropionate (Vanceril, Beclovent) and triamcinolone (Azmacort) can offer prophylactic treatment for chronic symptoms of allergy.

In status asthmaticus, epinephrine is a rapid-acting, injectable bronchodilator and vasoconstrictor and is the most useful drug for the relief of anaphylactic shock, acute asthma, hives, and edema.

Improvements in allergic symptomatology can occur without significant side effects. Often, exercise ability and irritant tolerance are also increased. However, there may be a continued need for medication. Follow-up care is important with emphasis on prevention of emergency room visits.

Corticosteroids is the most potent group of respiratory medications. In addition, they are effective anti-inflammatory agents in all allergic diseases. Their main drawback is that they can produce multisystem, major adverse side effects when taken orally or parenterally over a prolonged period. These negative effects can be reduced by administering the total dose required for symptom control in the form of prednisone on alternate mornings rather than in a daily regimen. Substantial reduction in these untoward generalized responses occurs with the topical application of the steroid medication—using aerosols for asthma and rhinitis, and drops, creams, and ointments for conjunctivitis and eczema.

Asthma

Asthma is the most common major allergic manifestation in childhood. It affects 10% of all children with a rise in overall incidence over the past decade. Asthma accounts for 23% of school absenteeism and in the United States causes a growing number of deaths annually (Molfino, Nannini, Martelli, and Slutsky, 1991). It is characterized by difficulty in breathing as the result of spasm of the small bronchi, obstructive edema of the bronchial mucosa, and the production of tenacious secretions, all of which tend to obstruct air flow (Fig. 34-7). More difficulty is experienced in exhaling than inhaling. A pronounced expiratory wheeze is usually present. Rapid, shallow respirations are characteristic. Milder obstruction is frequently manifested by nocturnal or exertional coughing.

Asthma is the result of hyperreactivity of the bronchial airway. See Table 34-3 for a comparison of

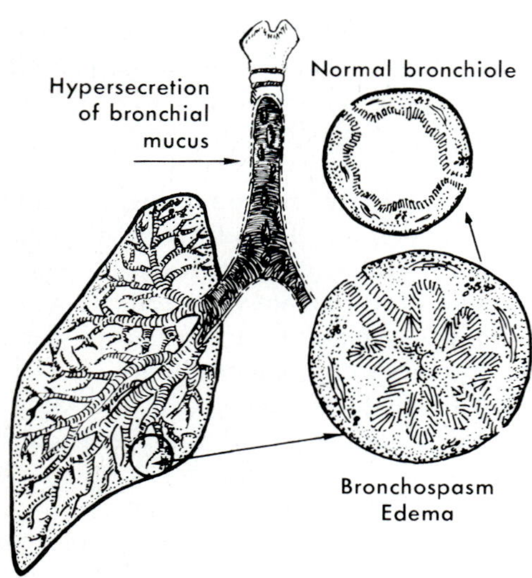

Fig. 34-7 Cardinal anatomic changes in asthma occur at bronchiole level. Bronchospasm, edema, and hypersecretions of mucus cause severe dyspnea and wheezing.

conditions affecting the bronchi. The lungs are clinically referred to as *twitchy.* Although often the spasm, edema, and mucus that create this reversible obstruction are caused by an allergic reaction, many nonimmunological precipitants can also initiate or compound the problem. These include viral, atypical, or bacterial infections, irritants, exercise, emotional stress, cold air, and weather changes. The clinical course of asthma therefore varies in different children as a result of its a multifactorial process.

Treatment of asthma. The treatment of asthma is usually divided into (1) specific measures, such as elimination of offending allergens and specific desensitization, and (2) nonspecific measures, which include medications, fluids, and supportive treatment. Acute attacks of asthma can occur at any time and are related to multiple factors. There may be no single cause. Children exhibit symptoms when they reach a certain level or threshold of exposure to certain offenders. The cardinal feature is airway obstruction; patients' shoulders are hunched, their thoracic soft tissues retract as they inspire, and their accessory muscles of respiration bulge with the effort of breathing. Their respiratory rates are initially increased but may be normal or decreased if the obstruction is severe, and their breathing is punctuated by spasms of coughing and audible wheezes. These children may be diaphoretic, restless, and fatigued. Difficulty in breathing produces anxiety, and the patients' anxiety and that of their parents tends to compound the respiratory problems.

Treatment of acute attacks of asthma usually includes the administration of epinephrine (Adrenalin) by injection and then inhalation therapy with isoetharine, metaproterenol, or albuterol. Epinephrine suspension (Sus-Phrine) is often used to achieve more lasting effects. Adequate fluid intake is extremely important.

A potentially life-threatening situation, *status asthmaticus,* exists when the patient's respirations do not clear after three consecutive doses of epinephrine 1:1000, given at 20-minute intervals or after a combination of epinephrine and inhalation therapy. This requires aggressive medical treatment and close follow-up. Most patients with status asthmaticus require hospitalization.

Children with status asthmaticus may be dehydrated because they have been too ill to eat or drink and have lost fluids by hyperventilating, coughing, and perspiring. Vomiting also adds to the child's dehydrated state. Intravenous administration of fluids should be started to correct any fluid imbalance, maintain liquefied bronchial secretions, and serve as a vehicle for important medications. The nurse should carefully check the amount and frequency prescribed to prevent overhydration.

Aminophylline, a compound of theophylline and a highly effective bronchodilator, may be given intravenously over a 15- to 30-minute period and then at 4- to 6-hour intervals or as a maintenance drip after a loading bolus. Signs of theophylline intoxication include headache, restlessness, irritability, vomiting, and abdominal pain and should not be confused with increased severity of the asthma attack. Theophylline levels should be monitored and kept within the therapeutic range of 10 to 20 μg/ml.

Isoetharine (Bronkosol), metaproterenol (Metaprel, Alupent), or albuterol (Ventolin, Proventil) by inhalation are effective in further relieving bronchospasm and dyspnea in children. They are generally given every 4 hours. The effectiveness of these medications in nebulized form may prevent the necessity for intravenous or oral forms of theophylline.

Hydrocortisone sodium succinate (Solu-Cortef) or methylprednisolone (Solu-Medrol) is given intravenously to children who do not respond to bronchodilators, who have recently had corticosteroids, or who are receiving maintenance doses of steroids. It is important to note that the therapeutic effect of hydrocortisone sodium succinate is often not seen until 8 to 12 hours after administration. If the patient improves, corticosteroids may be stopped abruptly after a short (less than 7 days) course. Although necessary for control of symptoms in severe cases, long-term use of steroids may have serious side effects, which include growth suppression, increased susceptibility to infection, and osteoporosis.

Antibiotics are indicated in the presence of bacterial infection. However, asthmatic flareups are more often

◆ **TABLE 34-3**
Comparison of Conditions Affecting the Bronchi

	Viral-Induced Asthma	Bronchitis	Bronchiolitis
Description	Exaggerated response of bronchi to infection Bronchospasm, exudation, and edema of bronchi	Usually occurs in association with URI Seldom an isolated entity	A more common infectious disease of lower airways Maximum obstructive impact at bronchiolar level
Age-group affected	Late infancy and early childhood	Affects children throughout childhood	Usually children 2 to 12 months of age; rare after age 2 Peak incidence at approximately age 6 months
Etiological agents	Most commonly viruses but may be any of a variety of URI pathogens	Usually viral Other agents (e.g., bacteria, fungi, allergic disorders, airborne irritants) can trigger symptoms	Viruses, predominantly respiratory syncytial viruses; also adenoviruses, parainfluenza viruses, and *M. pneumoniae*
Predominant characteristics	Wheezing, productive cough	Persistent dry, hacking cough (worse at night) becoming productive in 2 to 3 days	Dyspnea, paroxysmal nonproductive cough, tachypnea with retractions and flaring nares, emphysema, may be wheezing
Treatment	Bronchodilators	Cough suppressants, HS Antibiotics	Oxygen mist Ribavirin if severe

From Wong DL: *Essentials of pediatric nursing,* ed 4, St Louis, 1993, Mosby.

associated with viral infections; in these instances antibiotics are not helpful. Oxygen is given to relieve hypoxemia. Since cyanosis is an unreliable sign of hypoxia, pulse oximetry and arterial blood gas levels may need to be determined and observed carefully. Oxygen may be administered if blood arterial oxygen is not within normal range.

Parents should be encouraged to stay at the child's bedside to decrease the child's anxiety. A parent-health care provider partnership is optimal.

In patients with significant bronchitis or infection, chest physical therapy may be helpful. This consists of vibration, clapping, and coughing in various positions. Chest physical therapy and postural drainage are ordered as soon as the acute phase subsides. It is a significant therapeutic aid for children whose excessive mucus is a problem. It is most effectively performed after bronchodilation is obtained.

The nurse who is caring for the child with status asthmaticus must constantly but calmly evaluate the progress and changes that occur. Although most children demonstrate significant improvement after intravenous fluids, others may not respond for 12 to 24 hours. During this time, corticosteroids, antibiotics, and oxygen may be added to their therapeutic regimen. The foregoing measures are usually effective in time. Chest x-ray examination may be necessary when symptoms do not respond to therapy or when unusual signs are present, such as asymmetrical breath sounds. Atelectasis, with or without pneumonia, mucus plugs in the bronchi, and spontaneous pneumothorax account for the major complications and must be treated separately.

However, sometimes response is not satisfactory. Labored breathing may persist; the child becomes exhausted, incoherent, and no longer coughs or wheezes; and inspiratory retractions and cyanosis increase. These are the clinical signs of impending respiratory failure. Blood gas determinations exhibit a decreasing level of oxygen, rising carbon dioxide

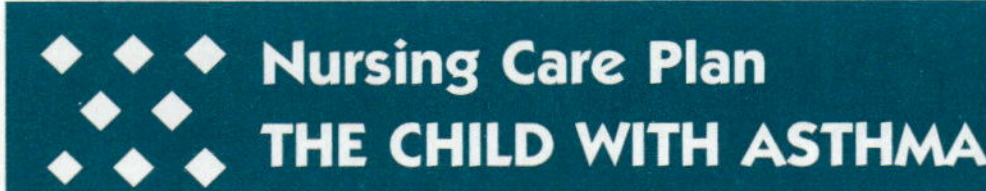

Nursing Care Plan
THE CHILD WITH ASTHMA

	Selected Nursing Diagnoses	Expected Outcomes	Interventions
A	Ineffective airway clearance related to edema, bronchospasms, and excess mucus. Clinical manifestations: Coughing, wheezing, increased RR and HR, retractions, moist breath sounds, nasal flaring, lethargy, and pallor.	Child maintains patent airway. Child regains normal respiratory pattern.	Assess child for signs of respiratory distress: increased respirations and pulse, wheezing, nasal flaring, and retractions. Elevate head of bed, place infant in infant seat. Assure aerosol treatments given as ordered and assess child's response. Administer medications as ordered and assess response, presence of side effects. Ensure adequate hydration. Check for significant allergies (i.e., food or medication).
B	Impaired gas exchange related to inadequate respiratory function. Clinical manifestations: Agitation, audible wheezing, lethargy, grunting, stridor, tachycardia, tachypnea, and cyanosis.	Child regains/maintains normal respiratory function.	Monitor respiratory rate, heart rate, blood pressure every 2 hours and prn. Anticipate change in intravenous medications. Assess child's response to therapy. Administer oxygen as needed. Obtain ABGs and blood work ordered. Be prepared for transfer to intensive care unit.
C	Anxiety related to respiratory distress and hospitalization.		See Planning Nursing Care, pp. 511-513.
D	Potential theophylline toxicity related to therapy. Clinical manifestations: Increased irritability, Increased HR, RR, and arrythmias. Nausea/vomiting/diarrhea Headache, restlessness, Insomnia, muscle twitching, Flushing, hypotension.	Child maintains theophylline level between 10 and 20 μg/L.	Assess for clinical manifestations of toxicity. Monitor carefully aminophylline intravenous drip and blood serum levels. Monitor vitals signs every 4 hours and prn. The effectiveness of albuterol in nebulized form may prevent the need for theophylline.

retention, and acidosis. This situation can be reversed if the danger is recognized and the child is moved to the intensive care unit where adequate equipment and personnel are available. Delivery of 100% humidified oxygen, continuous nebulization treatments, infusion of isoproterenol and sodium bicarbonate, and mechanical ventilation may be necessary.

CARDIOVASCULAR PROBLEMS

Before studying common cardiovascular problems, the nurse must review the structure and circulation of the normal heart (Fig. 34-8). Some of the more common pediatric problems involving the heart and blood vessels are illustrated in Fig. 34-9. Varied abnormalities

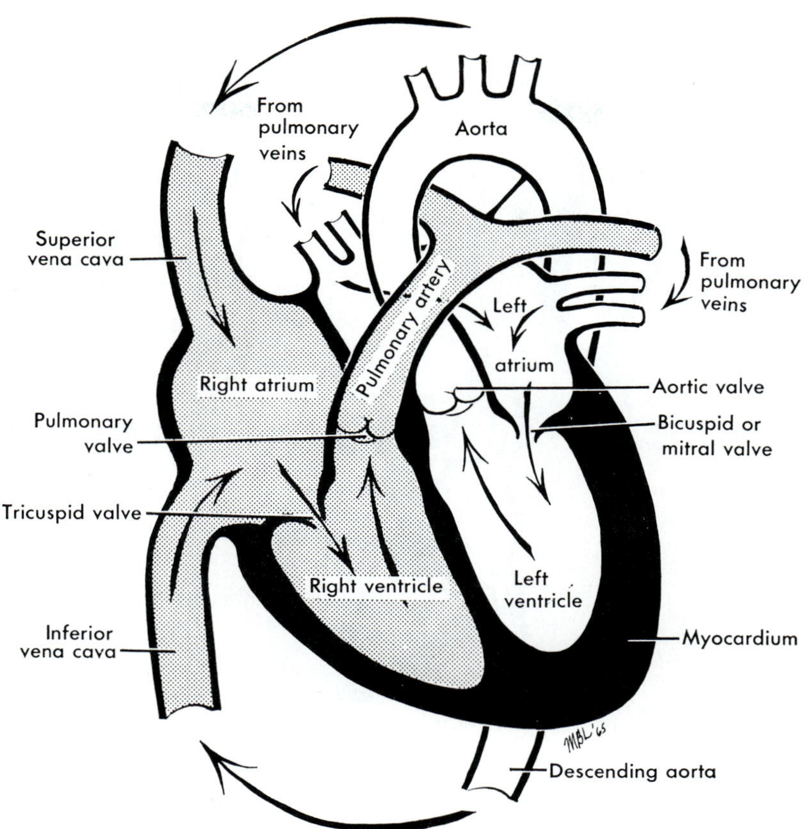

Fig. 34-8 Structure and circulation of normal heart. Shaded area represents blood with low oxygen content.

of the heart and large blood vessels may occur. Most are minor and do not affect activity or quality of life. Others produce several problems and are incompatible with life.

ASSESSMENT

To evaluate heart function and detect cardiac abnormalities, an accurate history of the patient's complaints is sought, a complete physical examination is carried out, and various tests and specialized procedures are ordered.

Common noninvasive tests include permanent recording of the size and shape of the heart by *x-ray examination,* external pulse and heart sound recordings by *phonocardiography,* tests of the activity of the heart by *electrocardiography,* and sonar recordings *(echocardiography),* which allow examination of human fetal cardiac development and when combined with *Doppler ultrasonography* techniques, provide diagnostic accuracy of most of the major congenital heart defects in infancy.

Laboratory tests of special significance include a complete blood cell count and hematocrit and hemoglobin determinations. Patients with a cyanotic type of heart disease may have an excessive amount of circulating red blood cells (polycythemia) manufactured in an attempt to deliver more oxygen to the deprived body cells, or they may suffer from anemia. If polycythemia is present, the blood thickens and circulation slows down, occasionally causing the development of abnormal clots in the bloodstream.

An *angiogram* may be warranted; however, because of its inherent risk, other less invasive tests may provide adequate diagnostic information. It involves the injection of a contrast medium into the circulation and observation of its flow by x-ray examination or fluoroscopy. When a contrast medium is injected directly into a heart chamber, it is termed *angiocardiography.* Such visualization of the aorta is termed *aortography.* Special procedures may also include right or left side of the heart catheterizations, which involve the introduction of a small catheter seen by fluoroscopy into a vein or artery and its gentle manipulation into various chambers of the heart and large associated vessels. This procedure is performed on an anesthetized or sedated patient and, although it is not without risk, yields considerable

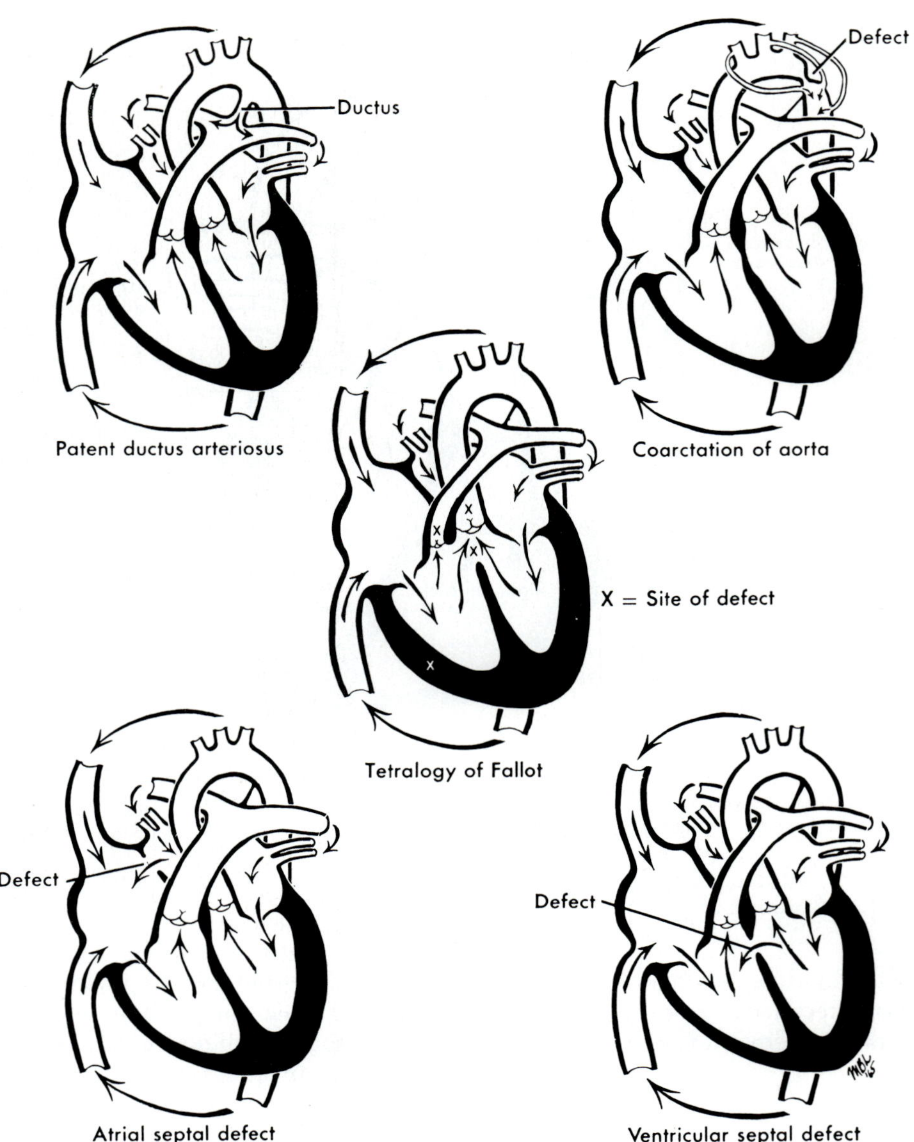

Fig. 34-9 Common congenital defects of heart and great vessels.

information. If possible, children are sedated, not anesthetized, so that they can cooperate during the procedure.

It is important for an anesthesiologist to be available in the catheterization laboratory for any possible need for anesthesia support. Heart catheterizations reveal the pressure in various areas of the cardiocirculatory system and the amount of oxygen in the blood at different sites. The presence of abnormal openings can be demonstrated by direct passage of the small catheter through the defects or by evaluation of oxygenation patterns.

Therapeutic catheterization is a term used to describe treatment approaches during the heart catheterization. These include balloon atrial septostomy to create a large interatrial communication and facilitate mixing of pulmonary and systemic venous blood in infants with a transposed aorta and pulmonary artery (transposition of the great vessels); balloon valvuloplasty to widen the obstructive and narrowed valve in patients with pulmonary stenosis; and balloon angioplasty to widen a narrowed blood vessel in patients with peripheral pulmonary stenosis or coarctation of the aorta.

Children returning to the nursing unit after cardiac catheterization should be treated as postoperative patients. Vital signs—pulse, respirations, and blood pressure—should be noted every 20 minutes until stable. Children should have blood pressure determinations on the opposite arm of the catheter insertion. A mist tent or oxygen mask should be in readiness as indicated. Dressing application should be recorded and evaluated. It is important to note skin color, temperature, and character of the pulse in the extremity catheterized, because this may detect blood vessel occlusion resulting from thrombus formation.

Infant

Congenital anomalies of the heart and great vessels

About 30,000 infants are born with heart disease every year in the United States. Before the advent of open heart surgery, about half of these infants died within 6 months. Currently, early diagnosis and treatment (through palliative or curative surgery) are effective in approximately 95% of cases.

Congenital heart disease refers to a structural abnormality present in the circulation at birth. These defects create at least three problems related to blood flow within the heart and circulatory system. A *volume overload* occurs when more blood than normal enters a ventricle. A *pressure overload* occurs when the outflow of blood is impeded or obstructed. Ventricular hypertrophy and finally congestive heart failure (CHF) can result. *Desaturation,* low oxygen content of circulating arterial blood, occurs when unoxygenated blood returning from the body mixes with the oxygenated blood returning from the lungs. Acidosis can occur as the result of poor oxygenation of the various organs. Acidosis leads to decreased cardiac performance and more severe acidosis. Some congenital anomalies of the heart illustrate all three types of blood flow problems. Early diagnosis and treatment are important (Fig. 34-9).

Clinical manifestations

Infants with serious congenital heart disease often manifest common signs and symptoms that reflect the underlying anomaly. *Cyanosis*—blueness of the lips, nail beds, and mucosal surfaces—may be caused by shunting of unoxygenated blood into the left side of the heart or may be associated with pulmonary edema. *Tachypnea* is defined as an excessive resting respiratory rate, 45 breaths per minute in the full-term infant or over 60 breaths per minute in the premature infant. Retractions and flaring of the nares occur with each breath. Rapid breathing is a response to heart failure or low oxygen content in the blood and is often precipitated by mild exercise. *Tachycardia,* an excessively rapid heart rate, can be difficult to evaluate in the infant, particularly if the child is moving and crying. A heart rate greater than 180 beats per minute when the infant is at rest is significant and should be reported at once, because infants quickly develop cardiac decompensation (inability to maintain the necessary blood flow). *Effort intolerance* is chiefly manifested by feeding problems. The infant usually starts feedings eagerly but soon becomes fussy and fatigued and stops feeding. The cycle is often repeated, but the infant seldom finishes a bottle. *Failure to thrive* is also common. Episodes of congestive heart failure and concurrent pulmonary infection are common causes of retarded growth. *Murmurs* occur when the flow of blood across a defect is turbulent or when valvular surfaces are irregular. They are the most commonly detected physical findings associated with congenital cardiac defects in infants. Murmurs are detected after careful auscultation of the first and second heart sound. The heart is auscultated over the entire precordium. (See Fig. 34-10.) Innocent murmurs (nonpathological) are noted in 30% of children.

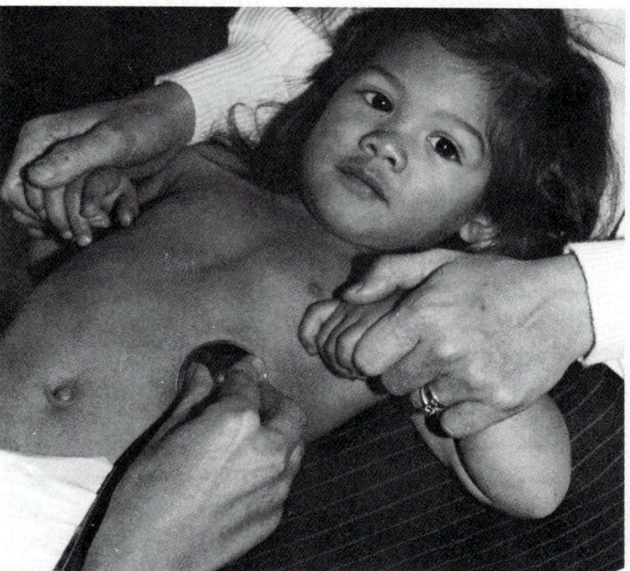

Fig. 34-10 Reclining position in parent's lap for auscultation of the heart. (From Whaley and Wong. *Nursing care of infants and children,* ed 4, St Louis, 1991, Mosby.)

Congestive heart failure occurs when the heart can no longer pump blood sufficiently to meet the body's needs. When infants develop CHF in the early months of life, it is usually secondary to structural defects, which produce a pressure or volume overload. In an effort to preserve cardiac output and accommodate the larger volume of residual blood, cardiac dilation occurs. CHF is typically recognized by a combination of tachypnea and tachycardia associated with hepatomegaly caused by circulatory congestion. The development of CHF warrants prompt cardiac consultation and diagnostic studies. Frequently surgery offers the only chance for survival.

Left-to-right shunts (acyanotic)

Patent Ductus Arteriosus (PDA). Patent means "open." The condition called *patent ductus arteriosus* refers to a holdover from the fetal circulation pattern. Review Fig. 34-9. The ductus arteriosus is a short blood vessel that connects the pulmonary artery with the aorta, making it unnecessary for the blood circulating through the pulmonary artery to continue on to the nonfunctioning lungs of the fetus. Normally this arterial duct closes soon after birth and within a few weeks becomes a ligament.

If the ductus arteriosus does not close, the higher blood pressure in the aorta, which results after birth, forces well-oxygenated blood from the aorta back into the pulmonary circulation for a return trip to the lungs. This puts an abnormal workload on the left ventricle and can cause a significant elevation of the blood pressure in the pulmonary circulation. Growth may be impaired if the duct remains large. Children may have dyspnea when they are active, and without appropriate treatment their life expectancy is reduced. The defect does not characteristically produce cyanosis unless pressures in the aorta and pulmonary artery are changed as the result of excessive pulmonary blood flow, which can increase pulmonary vascular resistance. Some premature infants with respiratory distress syndrome have delayed, spontaneous closure of the ductus or reopening of the ductus as a response to poor oxygenation in the lungs. Often this prevents weaning the infant from a mechanical ventilator unless the ductus is closed by medication or ligation.

Diagnosis is usually made on the basis of several findings. A continuous, machinery murmur or a thrill may be noted. *Thrill* refers to a vibration felt over the cardiac area. A bounding femoral pulse may also be noted. Blood pressure determinations may reveal a wide range between the systolic and diastolic readings—termed a *wide pulse pressure.* The patent duct may be visualized by echocardiography, aortography, or direct passage of a small catheter through the duct during fluoroscopy.

Medicines that inhibit the synthesis of prostaglandins by the body's tissues effectively close the duct in premature infants. This condition may also be treated surgically with excellent results. The duct is tied off (ligated).

Atrial septal defect (ASD). An abnormal opening in the wall, or septum, that separates the right and left atria may be the result of the persistence of the foramen ovale, which during fetal life shunts some of the blood from the right to the left side of the heart. It may also be caused by the presence of a septal opening unassociated with normal fetal circulation. Cyanosis does not characteristically occur, since the blood pressure is higher in the left side of the heart and unoxygenated blood does not enter the systemic circulation. However, if some other abnormality is present (e.g., pulmonary valve stenosis), right-to-left flow may occur, and cyanosis may result. Children with ASD usually have an overworked right side of the heart and congested pulmonary circulation because the extra flow through the defect reaches the lungs by way of the right ventricle. They may demonstrate cardiac enlargement, a systolic murmur, decreased resistance to respiratory tract infections, lowered exercise tolerance, and physical underdevelopment. A decision to attempt surgical correction is based on the condition of the individual child. If the shunt is small, patients do well without operative intervention. Surgery itself presents a minimum of risk. During surgery the defect is repaired either by direct closure with sutures only or by the incorporation of a plastic patch into the repair. The patch is eventually penetrated by growing heart fibers and becomes part of the septum.

Ventricular septal defect (VSD). The presence of an opening between the two ventricles is a common abnormality. Spontaneous closure will occur in 50% of children with this defect from 1 to 3 years of age. How seriously such an opening disturbs normal heart function depends on the position and size of the defect and the presence of other abnormalities in the heart or large vessels leaving the heart. If a large defect is found in the membranous portion of the septum, symptoms are usually severe. The blood generally travels through the opening from the left to the right ventricle. However, in some cases the shunt reverses as resistance in the pulmonary arterial bed increases, and the pressure in the right side of the heart mounts. Diagnosis is made on the basis of clinical symptoms, a characteristic harsh, holosystolic murmur, and the results of x-ray examination, electrocardiograms, echocardiography, and, when indicated, cardiac catheterization. Specific treatment may be recommended for the individual child and consists of surgical repair by open heart surgery similar to that employed for ASD. Surgical risk is somewhat increased with VSD repair.

Right-to-left shunts (cyanotic)

Tetralogy of Fallot. The word element *tetra* means *four.* Tetralogy of Fallot is a heart condition that is characterized by the presence of four classic features: a ventricular septal defect, a narrowing of the opening of the outflow tract of the right ventricle (pulmonary stenosis), an aorta situated above the septal defect (overriding aorta), and an enlarged, thickened right ventricular wall (right ventricular hypertrophy). Because the narrowed outflow of the right ventricle causes the pressure to rise in that chamber, hypertro-

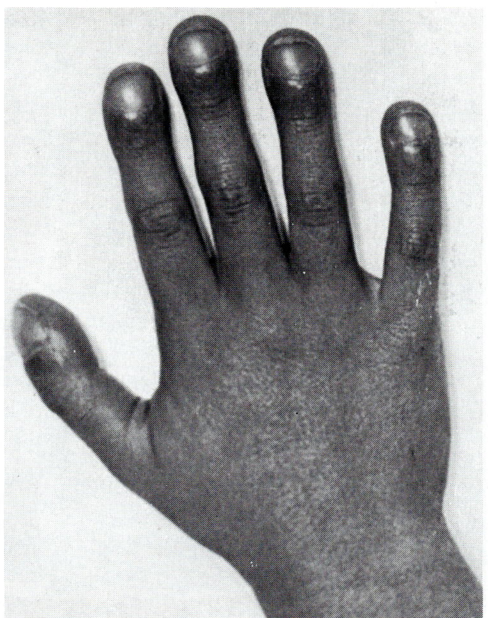

Fig. 34-11 When ends of fingers become wide and thick, they are termed *clubbed.* The fingers are also cyanotic. (Courtesy Naval Hospital, San Diego, Calif.)

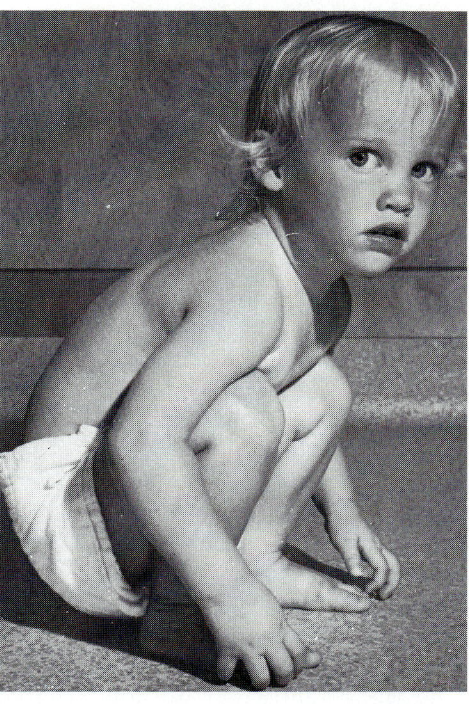

Fig. 34-12 Squatting position improves oxygenation in some children with congenital heart defects.

phy of the right heart wall results, and the shunt of blood through the septal defect goes from right to left, usually causing considerable cyanosis. The infant suffering from tetralogy of Fallot has been called a *blue baby.* The moderately to severely affected young child with this diagnosis typically has blue lips and nail beds and dusky-tinted skin, which becomes more cyanotic on exertion. Clubbing of the fingers and toes is often a feature (Fig. 34-11). A thrill and chest deformity may be noted. A child may have hypoxemic spells with respiratory distress, deep cyanosis, loss of consciousness, and a seizure. Affected children are small for their age.

When young children with cyanotic heart disease are fatigued, they often squat (Fig. 34-12). This position reduces the right-to-left flow of unoxygenated blood across the ventricular septal defect, traps desaturated blood in the lower extremities, and improves oxygenation.

Management of hypoxemic spells can be difficult and complex. Initially, when the infant is *excitable,* with respiratory distress, one can use a knee-chest position and administer oxygen. Morphine may be used for sedation. If the infant is flaccid or unconscious, morphine is contraindicated. If metabolic acidosis occurs, sodium bicarbonate is sometimes given intravenously.

Diagnosis depends on clinical manifestations, x-ray examination, electrocardiograms, echocardiograms, angiocardiograms, and cardiac catheterizations. Treatment can be medical or surgical, depending on the condition of the patient. In very blue newborns with tetralogy of Fallot, prostaglandin E_1 is given intravenously to dilate the ductus arteriosus, thereby increasing the flow of blood to the lungs and improving the supply of oxygen to the body's tissues. This medication can be life-saving and must be followed by surgery. Before open heart surgery was available, surgical techniques were devised to improve the pulmonary circulation by creating an artificial ductus arteriosus, which recirculated poorly oxygenated blood to the lungs for oxygen enrichment. The Blalock-Taussig operation and the Waterston operation are such techniques. This type of palliative surgery is still useful when the child is considered too small for total correction but is having life-threatening hypoxemic spells. Open heart surgery with total correction is preferable.

Transposition of the great vessels. Transposition of the great vessels is a serious cyanotic congenital heart defect. In this condition the pulmonary artery originates from the left ventricle, whereas the aorta arises from the right ventricle. Life is possible as long as the foramen ovale or ductus arteriosus remains open or a VSD exists. Prominent features are extreme cyanosis and CHF. Diagnosis is made on the basis of electrocardiogram, x-ray examination, echocardiogram, angiocardiogram, and cardiac catheterization. Usually a special balloon catheter (balloon septostomy) is used to create or enlarge an ASD without the risk of palliative surgery. Total correction is possible by switching the venous inflows to the heart. In the Mustard procedure, a "baffle," or partition made of pericardium, is placed in such a manner as to redirect the pulmonary venous return within the left atrium to the right ventricle and the systemic return to the left ventricle. Immediate results have been excellent, with an overall mortality of less than 10% in patients without additional complicating cardiac anomalies. Some centers advocate a switch of the great arteries and reimplantation of the coronary arteries in the aorta.

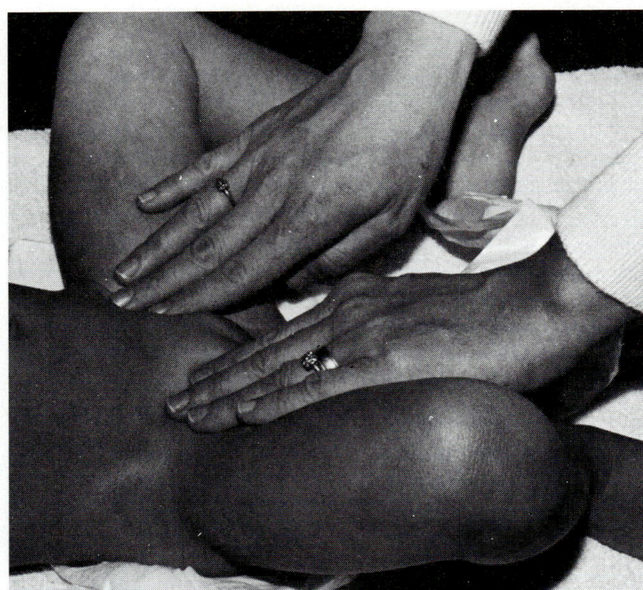

Fig. 34-13 Palpating for femoral pulses. (From Whaley and Wong: *Nursing care of infants and children,* ed 4, St Louis, 1991, Mosby.)

Obstructive lesions

Pulmonary stenosis. The pulmonary artery carries poorly oxygenated blood from the right ventricle through the pulmonary valve to the lungs, where it is reoxygenated. Narrowing of the valve itself or the areas immediately above or below it causes obstruction to the right ventricular outflow. The condition may be so mild that the infant has no symptoms, or it may be so severe that the infant is dyspneic and has effort intolerance, severe cyanosis, and CHF. A loud murmur is heard. The condition is diagnosed by electrocardiogram, x-ray film, and cardiac catheterization. Balloon valvuloplasty or open heart surgical repair is indicated if the right ventricular pressure is high. An incision in the pulmonary artery exposes the dome-shaped valvular stenosis, which is then incised (pulmonary valvotomy). If the primary obstruction is below the valve, the obstructing muscle can be resected. The results of this operation are usually excellent, and the risk is low, except in a small infant.

Nursing Alert

The presence of coarctation is suspected when a systolic murmur is heard in the pulmonic area with radiation of the murmur to the axillae and back. Forceful or bounding arterial pulses are present in the upper extremities, whereas diminished or absent pulses are assessed in the lower extremities (See Fig. 34-13).

Coarctation of the aorta. The aorta is the largest blood vessel in the body. As it leaves the heart, it normally arches to the left. The coronary arteries and three major vessels emerge from the aortic arch before it starts its descent into the lower thorax and abdomen. The innominate, left carotid, and left subclavian arteries are the three vessels that supply the head and upper extremities with oxygenated blood. The ductus arteriosus joins the aorta in the general area of the left subclavian artery before normal postnatal circulation develops. Sometimes the aorta is abnormally narrowed in the area of the arch, usually involving the segment just past the subclavian artery. Often smaller "collateral" vessels (usually branches of the subclavian and intercostal arteries) develop and bypass the narrowed portion to help supply circulation to the lower extremities. The narrowing of the aorta is often called *coarctation,* since a narrowed figure results when two arcs are drawn side by side, like two C's back to back. The resulting symptoms depend on the severity and location of the coarctation and whether any other cardiac or blood vessel abnormalities exist.

Severe coarctation in the infant, especially if associated with another congenital heart anomaly, may precipitate profound CHF and require surgical intervention. The older child may report headache, leg cramps, excessive fatigue, and frequent nosebleeds. Diagnosis is confirmed by blood pressure measurements, x-ray films, electrocardiogram, and echocardiogram.

Without intervention, the life span is often shortened because of the onset of complications, such as hypertension, cerebral hemorrhage, subacute bacterial endocarditis, or heart failure. Definitive treatment for coarctation is surgery. The narrowed portion may be cut out and the adjoining normal-sized segments sewn

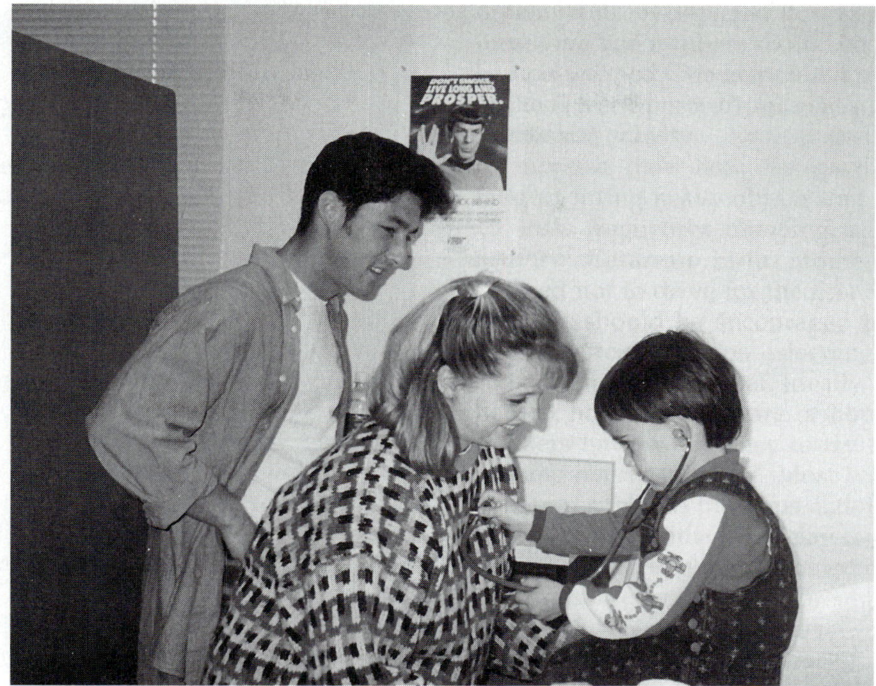

Fig. 34-14 Role-playing in preparation for surgery.

together. Occasionally the repair involves the insertion of a prosthesis or the use of the subclavian artery to widen the aorta. If stenosis occurs again after the operation, the preferred treatment is balloon angioplasty performed during cardiac catheterization.

Cardiac surgery

Assuming that facilities and a skilled team are available, surgical treatment of large blood vessel or heart defects depends on the extent of incapacity suffered by the patient, the possibility of a satisfactory repair, and the risk involved. Surgery on the aorta, pulmonary artery, or other associated blood vessels is extracardiac surgery. However, when the malformations exist in the interior of the heart and cardiac circulation must be interrupted, the difficulty of the procedure and the risk to the patient increase significantly.

The heart-lung machine was introduced in 1955. Before that time it was impossible to discontinue the beating of the heart long enough to make a lengthy repair without seriously depriving some vital organ, such as the brain or kidneys of carbon dioxide-oxygen exchange, thus causing tissue damage.

The heart-lung machine receives blood from the patient's venous circulation through tubes inserted into the inferior and superior venae cavae. It removes the carbon dioxide, instills oxygen, regulates blood temperature, and pumps the blood back into the systemic circulation in most cases by way of the aorta or femoral artery (called a *cardiopulmonary bypass*). This is a highly complex procedure, requiring a team of skilled physicians, nurses, and technicians.

Preparation for cardiac procedures. A patient with a congenital heart defect may undergo surgery as an infant, toddler, or child. The child undergoing surgery must be carefully prepared for the event. This is especially true in the case of scheduled chest surgery because of the seriousness of the operation and the many procedures that must be carried out that require the trust and cooperation of the child to achieve optimum results.

Play therapy techniques are often helpful in explaining anticipated events to the child (Fig. 34-14). Preparation of the child and family through the use of role playing with preoperative dolls, a tour of the facilities, and written materials including coloring books describing what will happen, have been shown to decrease anxiety and increase cooperation postoperatively. Explanations are tailored to the child's developmental level, questions and concerns, and cognitive abilities. The children can "practice" their breathing exercises with the intermittent positive-pressure machine or learn how to cough hugging a pillow and splinting the chest.

Children who are scheduled for heart surgery are usually admitted to the hospital the day before the procedure to enable them to become acquainted with some of the nurses who will be caring for them and to be introduced to some of the equipment and techniques that will be used after surgery. The preoperative period is also used as an opportunity to evaluate the child. It is a time when the child's general condition and nutritional needs are assessed. Weight and vital signs are recorded. Fever, signs of respiratory tract infection, or rash, are documented and reported immediately and may necessitate a postponement of surgery.

Treatment and nursing care

Postoperative nursing care. The postoperative nursing care of open heart surgery patients is a nursing specialty. A patient usually remains in the intensive care unit for several days. While the child is in the intensive care unit, the child's condition is monitored by machines that record heart action, arterial and venous blood pressures, respirations, and temperature. In some cases, heartbeat may be stimulated by the use of a pacemaker. The rate and quality of respirations are evaluated; the color, temperature, and moisture of the skin are noted. Chest suction is maintained to prevent a buildup of fluid or air in the thorax, which causes respiratory distress and atelectasis. Humidified oxygen is often administered by an oxygen tent or mask. The urinary catheter is checked frequently to determine kidney function. Intravenous fluids and blood transfusions are carefully calculated and maintained. Wound drainage and dressings are checked. Turning and encouraging the patient to cough are extremely important. Intermittent positive pressure may be prescribed. Tracheal and nasopharayngeal suctioning may be ordered. Initially the patient's temperature may be subnormal, but later, temperature-reducing procedures may be necessary, including the use of the hypothermia blanket. A relatively high temperature after open heart surgery is common. It may be a reaction to the blood transfusions received. However, the possibility of infection must not be discounted when a patient's temperature remains elevated.

Collaborative care. Frequent nursing assessments are made during this critical postoperative period. The vocational nurse collaborates with the registered nurse as a care partner in the immediate postoperative period. Carrying out routine orders including vital signs, assisting with position change, and care of chest tubes is essential.

Chest tubes are inserted into the mediastinal or pleural space during surgery or in the immediate postoperative period. The chest tube is attached to a disposable water seal drainage system. The purpose of the underwater drainage is to prevent air from traveling up the tube into the pleural space, causing a pneumothorax. Symptoms of pneumothorax include cyanosis, dyspnea, and chest pain.

> **Nursing Alert**
>
> Chest tube drainage greater than 3 ml/kg/hour for more than 3 consecutive hours may indicate postoperative hemmorrhage. Cardiac tamponade can develop rapidly; thus the surgeon must be notified immediately.

As the patient's condition improves, chest suction is discontinued and the tubes removed. If temporary heart pacing wires were attached to the heart during the operation, they are withdrawn if the heart rhythm is normal. The child is weighed while undressed each morning before breakfast to determine fluid retention. The child may be on a diet that limits sodium and carefully spaces a certain maximum oral fluid intake. The patient's pulse and respirations should be noted and recorded before and after any new activity. During periods of ambulation the child should be carefully evaluated for fatigue and given periods of rest as respirations, pulse, and color dictate. An apical pulse rate should be counted for 1 minute. This technique requires training, since there are two heart sounds (S_1 and S_2) in each cardiac cycle. The quality, as well as the rate, should be noted. Occasionally apical-radial pulse determinations are ordered. These pulse rates are taken simultaneously and then compared; for example, they may be written 110A/100R. This discrepancy signifies a pulse deficit. Blood pressure determinations are routinely made with the patient's pulse and respiration at scheduled intervals. The selection of cuff size is important. It should cover two thirds of the distance from the shoulder to the elbow or should be 20% wider than the diameter of the patient's arm.

Ambulation and activity level are gradually increased. Conferences are held with the parents and members of the health care team. Emotional and informational support is provided. Discharge planning, transition to the home environment, and optimal health maintenance are discussed.

Nonsurgical treatment and care. Sometimes cardiac problems cannot be corrected by surgery, or surgery is delayed until health status is stabilized or growth occurs. In these cases the children are treated by medication, special diets, and general health supervision. The nurse should be aware of the types of medication the child is receiving, the goals of therapy, and side effects. Sodium restriction is common. Patients with cardiac defects are weighed daily, and accurate intake and output records are maintained.

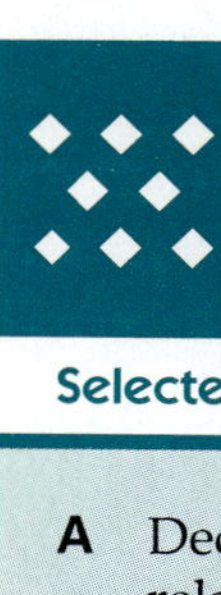

Nursing Care Plan
THE INFANT/CHILD WITH CONGESTIVE HEART FAILURE SECONDARY TO CONGENITAL HEART DEFECTS

	Selected Nursing Diagnosis	Expected Outcomes	Interventions
A	Decreased cardiac output related to structural defects and cardiac dysfunction. Clinical manifestations: Tachycardia, tachypnea, pallor, cyanosis, sudden weight gain associated with signs of dependent edema.	Child's heart rate will be within normal limits for age with strong and regular apical pulse. Child maintains normal serum K^+. Edema subsides, weight loss, increased voiding.	Assess heart rate 1 minute every 4 hours and before administration of digoxin. Administer digoxin as ordered (second nurse check dosage). Monitor serum K^+ daily. Adjust oral K^+ intake in diet as ordered. Assess child for presence of edema. Maintain strict intake and output. Obtain daily weights. Administer diuretics as ordered. Maintain fluid and diet restrictions. Check other serum electolytes as ordered.
B	Impaired gas exchange related to pulmonary congestion and anxiety. Clinical manifestations: Dyspnea, chest retractions, grunting, tachypnea, weak cry, restlessness.	Child maintains pink, warm skin. Child develops normal respiratory pattern.	Auscultate lungs every 4 hours and assess child for cyanosis, dyspnea, tachypnea. Position child in semi-Fowler's, position infant in cardiac chair to allow easier movement of diaphragm. Avoid restrictive clothing. Administer oxygen as ordered. Monitor oxygen saturation with pulse oximetry and blood gases as ordered.
C	Activity intolerance related to imbalance of oxygen supply and demand. Clinical manifestations: Tires with feedings and ADLs, fatigue, lethargy.	Child maintains balance between cardiac demands and oxygen consumption.	Provide quiet, restful environment. Include periods of rest in daily care. Offer child small, frequent feedings; low-salt formula (i.e., Lonalac or Similac PM). Use soft nipple with large hole. May need to gavage feed with supplementary oxygen source. Protect infant from sudden changes in temperature. Respond promptly to crying.
D	Anxiety related to perpetual dyspnea. Clinical manifestations: Restlessness, unhappiness, anxious face, perplexed frown, anorexia, breathlessness during feeding.	Evidence of peaceful, contented infant.	Feed early. Allow frequent rest periods. Limit sucking time to 45 minutes per bottle. Handle gently. Cuddle when possible. Consolidate nursing procedures. Provide uninterrupted sleep. Encourage parents to participate in care.

Signs of developing heart failure, cardiac irregularities, or possible respiratory tract infection should be promptly reported. Limitations of activity may be necessary, although many pediatric patients with congenital cardiac defects automatically limit themselves to only the activities they can tolerate. Quiet play is often more restful than enforced, "complete bed rest." The child who must be in an oxygen tent or who demonstrates susceptibility to fatigue should be disturbed as little as possible. When the child is disturbed, several procedures should be carried out at the same time to allow relatively long uninterrupted periods of sleep or rest. For example, temperature, pulse, respirations, and blood pressure determinations, offering fluids, changing the child's gown or diapers, and shifting position can all be accomplished during one interruption. Changes of position are important in preventing hypostatic pneumonia and skin breakdown. However, no *vigorous* back rubs should be performed on a patient with a cardiac defect. Proper positioning helps to prevent contractures and other deformities and assists proper body functions.

Complications of congenital cardiac defects

Cardiac decompensation—congestive heart failure (CHF). The most common complication is the failure of the heart to continue the circulation of the blood in sufficient volume to meet energy requirements and to prevent abnormal congestion of the blood. The heart may maintain an adequate blood flow by gradually increasing its size or altering its rate. If this occurs, the heart is said to be in *compensation*. If the heart cannot maintain the necessary blood flow, it is said to be in *decompensation*, or failure. Cardiac failure in infants, whatever the cause, is always a medical emergency.

Pulmonary congestion resulting from the inability of the left ventricle to pump effectively is characterized by pooling of blood in the lung capillaries, causing coughing, tachypnea, wheezing, and dyspnea. Blood-tinged froth may be expectorated. Acute pulmonary edema is a grave emergency. Immediate action is necessary. The following measures can be life-saving: placement of the infant in a sitting position and administration of oxygen by a ventilator and possibly parenteral morphine, digitalis, and diuretics.

Congestion of blood in the systemic venous system as the result of inefficient right ventricular contraction can cause nausea and vomiting, enlargement of the liver (hepatomegaly), and edema. In infants, edema is demonstrated by a weight gain. Cyanosis, tachypnea, dyspnea, and tachycardia warrant further diagnostic studies. Studies are performed after CHF is controlled, since the infant becomes fatigued by the work of breathing. The child may have an annoying cough and therefore difficulty with eating and sleeping. Prompt treatment with digoxin, oxygen, and diuretics decreases heart and respiratory rate and improves color, appetite, and disposition. Digoxin slows and strengthens the heartbeat and induces diuresis. A digitalizing dose (high dose) is given over a period of 16 hours, and a maintenance dose of 10% of the digitalizing dose is usually given every 12 hours. However, digoxin should be withheld and the physician notified if the apical pulse rate in the infant is less than 100 beats per minute. Signs and symptoms of toxicity include anorexia, vomiting, and excessive slowing or irregularity of the pulse rate. Diuretics help in relieving the pulmonary congestion that accompanies CHF if response to other forms of treatment is insufficient.

Nursing measures center around making infants more comfortable and conserving their energy. A sitting position in a cool, humidified oxygen tent is beneficial. Early feeding with soft nipples and allowing for frequent rest periods reduce fatigue. Uninterrupted sleep should be encouraged by bathing infants when they are awake and only when absolutely necessary. The recording of accurate, current vital signs, intake and output determinations, and weight is critical. As soon as the child's condition is stable, the preparation for surgery begins or the child is discharged until a surgical appointment can be made. The parents should be increasingly involved in care while their child is hospitalized so that they are well prepared when the child comes home. The assistance of a home health nurse is invaluable.

Subacute bacterial endocarditis. Any damage to cardiac tissue or a congenital heart or blood vessel anomaly can set the stage for inflammation of the lining of the heart (endocarditis) and arteries (endarteritis). The inflammation usually results from a blood-borne infection, originating at some other body site. It may have its onset after surgical procedures, such as dental extraction, tonsillectomy, or adenoidectomy, or it may be spread from an abscess or infection elsewhere in the body. Signs and symptoms include temperature elevation, weight loss, fatigue, anemia, leukocytosis, the presence of petechiae, an enlarged spleen, and perhaps even partial paralysis or other central nervous system symptoms caused by the presence of emboli in the brain that originated in the inflamed heart tissue. Prophylactic antibiotics must be prescribed before and during dental procedures or surgery since bacteria may be introduced into the bloodstream.

Cerebral thrombosis. Cerebral thrombosis may develop when an excess of circulating red blood cells is called into action to increase the oxygen-carrying

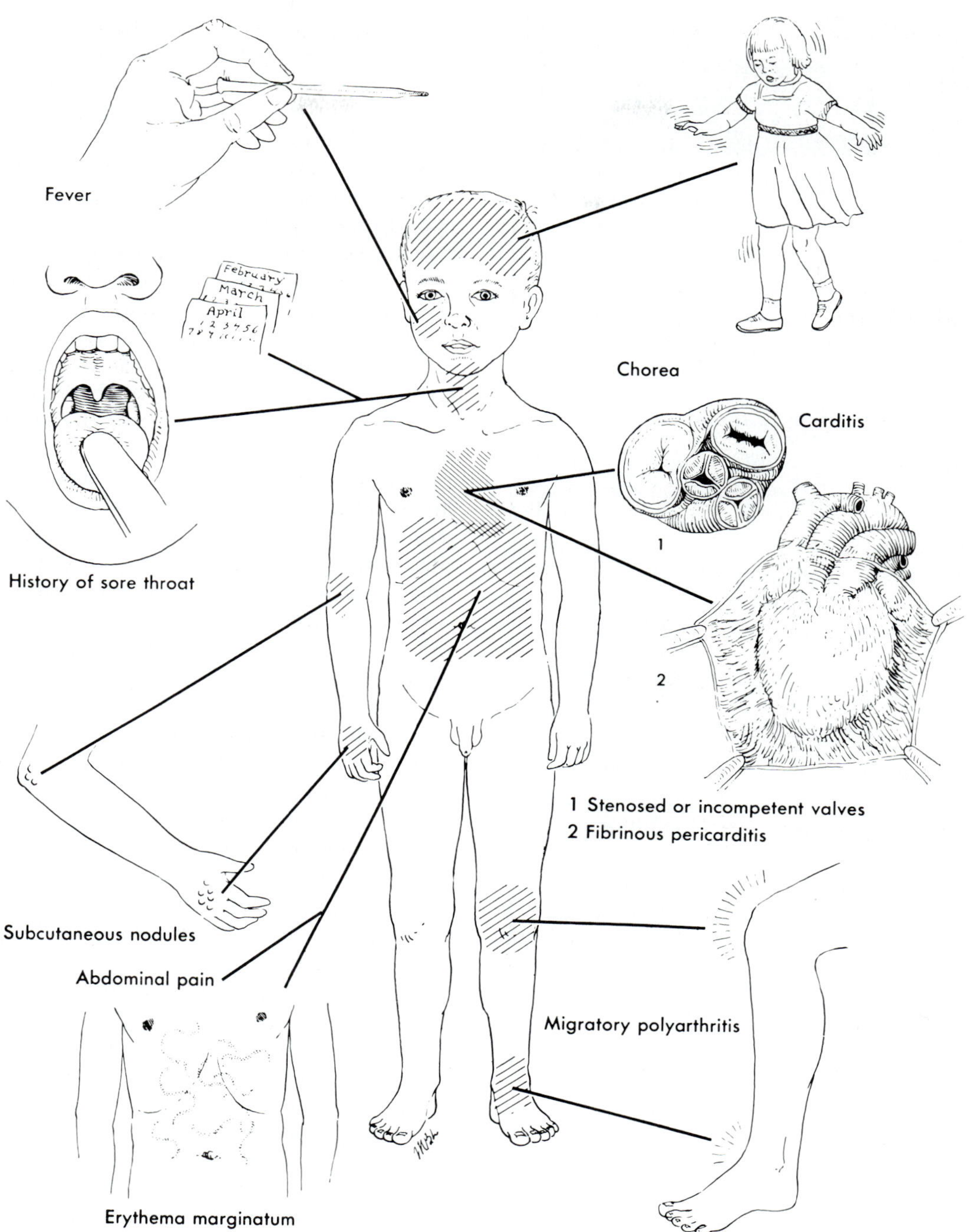

Fig. 34-15 Signs and symptoms of rheumatic fever.

capacity of the blood. Dehydration can result in a thicker, slower-moving fluid in the blood vessels. Clots, or thrombi, can form, and a cerebral vascular accident can take place. Maintenance of adequate fluid intake, the use of oxygen to relieve episodes of cyanosis, and possibly the cautious use of anticoagulants in patients likely to develop such a complication are suggested means of reducing the risk.

Rheumatic fever (Fig. 34-15). Rheumatic fever is a disorder of childhood or adolescence that can involve various organs of the body. However, because its most important complication is extensive cardiac damage, it is discussed here. There has been a resurgence of rheumatic fever in the United States in recent years. It is an important cause of acquired heart disease.

The mechanism of the disease is not completely

JONES CRITERIA (REVISED) FOR GUIDANCE IN THE DIAGNOSIS OF RHEUMATIC FEVER*

MAJOR MANIFESTATIONS
Carditis
Polyarthritis
Chorea
Erythema marginatum
Subcutaneous nodules

MINOR MANIFESTATIONS
Clinical
- Previous rheumatic fever or rheumatic heart disease
- Arthralgia
- Fever

Laboratory
- Acute phase reactions: erythrocyte sedimentation rate
- C-reactive protein, leukocytosis

Prolonged P-R interval

SUPPORTING EVIDENCE OF STREPTOCOCCAL INFECTION
Increased titer of streptococcal antibodies
- ASO (antistreptolysin O)
- Other antibodies

Positive throat culture for group A streptococcus
Recent scarlet fever

* The presence of two major criteria, or of one major and two minor criteria, indicates a high probability of the presence of rheumatic fever. Evidence of a preceding streptococcal infection greatly strengthens the possibility of acute rheumatic fever. Its absence should make the diagnosis doubtful (except in Sydenham's chorea or long-standing carditis).

known, but it is related to an abnormal immune response to a recent infection by group A beta-hemolytic streptococcus. This same organism causes the so-called strep throat, erysipelas, and scarlet fever. However, rheumatic fever itself is not communicable. It is not understood why some people develop rheumatic fever after group A beta-hemolytic streptococcus infections, whereas others do not. Rheumatic fever is most commonly found in the school-age child.

Clinical manifestations. The symptoms of rheumatic fever vary. However, a patient must exhibit certain minimal signs and symptoms for the diagnosis to be established (see Jones criteria in box above). Onset of the condition usually occurs about 2 weeks after the streptococcal infection. At times the infection is unapparent. The child may complain of leg aches and joint tenderness, which migrate from joint to joint—one time involving a knee, next an ankle, later a wrist (polyarthralgia). These pains occur during the day and the night. When the child begins to have hot, swollen, tender, enlarged joints (polyarthritis) and the symptoms migrate from joint to joint, the diagnosis is quickly suggested. The child may fatigue easily and have a fever. The extent of the fever varies considerably, depending on the severity of the illness.

Abdominal pain, caused by lymph node enlargement, is common. Epistaxis (nosebleed) may occur. *Carditis*, or inflammation of the heart, occurs in about 40% to 50% of cases during the initial attack of rheumatic fever. Assessment for rapid or irregular pulse, heart murmur, increased heart size, and signs and symptoms of cardiac failure is essential. Carditis is the most important feature of rheumatic fever with the prognosis of the patient largely resting on its severity. Over an extended period of time, small inflammatory nodules or growths can form in the heart. Often they interfere with the action of the mitral or aortic valves, making it difficult for the valves to close properly or open sufficiently.

A sign that occasionally accompanies rheumatic fever is the development of painless *subcutaneous nodules* near the occiput, knuckles, knees, elbows, and spine. These nodules appear late in the course of the disease and are usually associated with severe carditis.

Another common feature, especially in preadolescent girls, is Sydenham's *chorea* (St. Vitus' dance). Chorea may be described as involuntary muscular twitching or movement. It may manifest itself as grimacing. The child may seem exceptionally clumsy and may fail to accomplish muscle tasks involving concentration or fine control. The disorder is characterized by jerky, uncoordinated movements. It may be preceded by a period of emotional instability and behavior problems. It may be so mild as to escape the notice of the casual observer or so severe that it makes normal, daily activities dangerous or impossible. Speech may become slurred and handwriting difficult to decipher. Still another diagnostic sign of acute rheumatic fever is the appearance of a highly distinctive rash known as *erythema marginatum*. This red-line eruption forms irregular patterns on the trunk and extremities but not on the face. It is rarely seen.

Diagnosis is made on the evaluation of the signs and symptoms present plus the reports of several laboratory tests. None of the laboratory tests is specific for rheumatic fever, but when made in conjunction with a clinical evaluation of the patient, they are valuable aids. An increased *blood sedimentation rate* and presence of *C-reactive protein* in the blood indicate the presence of an inflammatory process in the body that may be rheumatic fever. One may also detect, with an *antistreptolysin o titer,* the presence of antibodies in the blood, formed in response to the invasion of streptococci. A nose or throat culture confirms a positive result for strep. Members of the patient's family should be checked for the presence of a streptococcal infection or the carrier state. Rheumatic fever has a tendency to run in families.

Treatment. Treatment of rheumatic fever includes the administration of penicillin to eliminate any lingering residual streptococci and prevention of reinfection. Penicillin does not cure the symptoms of rheumatic fever; it only helps prevent further attacks. If the patient is allergic to penicillin, erythromycin can be used to eradicate the streptococcus. Sulfonamides or penicillin are equally useful in preventing reinfections. Aspirin is helpful in controlling the pain of arthritis and lowering the temperature in older adolescents; however, its use is not recommended for young children. Prednisone is sometimes used in acute cases of carditis, with the goal of decreasing the possibility of permanent heart valve damage. Prednisone may be life-saving in cases of overwhelming inflammation of the structures of the heart.

Nursing care. The nursing care of the child with rheumatic fever depends on the severity of the disease and the symptoms present. When laboratory tests and clinical features indicate that the disease is active and perhaps progressive, every effort should be made to reduce the workload of the heart by providing emotional and physical rest. However, "doing nothing" is not very restful for most children, especially if they do not really feel sick. The nurse and the patient's family need a great deal of ingenuity to provide rest that is acceptable and therefore therapeutic for the child. Good observation, careful positioning, and skin care are essential.

The pulse rate is taken for a full minute to determine rate, rhythm, and character. The determination of the pulse while the patient is sleeping may be requested. The nurse should review the signs and symptoms of rheumatic fever and assess carefully for them. Signs of cardiac failure must be reported immediately. The child with symptoms of chorea needs special supportive care. Careful explanation of the condition to the child and family is a necessity. Chorea may appear as the sole symptom of rheumatic disease. In the event of moderate to severe disability, rest, prolonged warm baths under supervision, and tranquilizers may help. The condition usually subsides spontaneously in 2 to 3 months.

When the signs of inflammatory activity subside, the electrocardiogram results are favorable, and the pulse rate is within normal limits, the child may be allowed an increased activity level. However, the child must continue to be carefully evaluated to discover individual tolerance for increased exercise. Because recurrences of the disease are common and the possibility of permanent heart damage increases with each attack, it is imperative that the parents understand the importance of ongoing medical supervision. To prevent recurrences, the patient should avoid exposure to infections and receive either daily oral or, preferably, monthly intramuscular, long-acting penicillin therapy.

KEY CONCEPTS

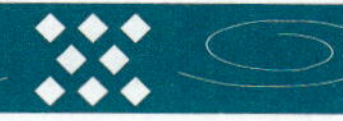

1. Respiratory disorders in infants include otitis media, bronchiolitis, pneumonia, and cystic fibrosis.
2. Pneumonia, whether primary or secondary, is a severe disease. In pediatrics, it is most commonly seen in infants and young children.
3. Cystic fibrosis is a hereditary, multisystem disorder in which generalized dysfunction of the exocrine glands occurs. It is usually characterized by chronic, severe pulmonary disease, pancreatic insufficiency, and abnormally high concentrations of sodium chloride in the sweat. Treatment is directed toward the organs involved and designed to meet the needs of the individual patient. Good nutrition has a positive effect on the overall prognosis.
4. Respiratory disorders in the toddler include otitis media, croup, foreign bodies in the nose or throat, bronchitis, and bronchiolitis.
5. Laryngotracheobronchitis (croup) is a viral respiratory disease characterized by a sudden onset of inspiratory stridor, hoarseness, and a barklike cough following a 1- to 3-day history of a "cold."
6. Respiratory disorders in the preschool child include otitis media, epiglottitis, epistaxis, deviation of the septum, acute nasopharyngitis, and sinusitis.
7. Symptoms of acute nasopharyngitis (common cold) are a dry, scratchy, sore, inflamed pharynx, an inflamed nasal mucosa resulting in nasal discharge, headache, muscular pains, general malaise, and fever. Supportive treatment consists of rest; increased fluid intake; a bland, soft diet; and

relief of nasal obstruction. Good handwashing is the best prevention.

8 Acute otitis media is a common complication of upper respiratory tract infection in young children. Symptoms include severe ear pain, fever, and irritability. Early administration of antibiotics is usually effective in preventing complications. Bottle-feeding in the supine position and parental smoking are contributing factors.

9 Respiratory disorders in the school-age child include problems with the adenoids and tonsils, streptococcal pharyngitis (strep throat), and respiratory disease resulting from allergy.

10 Postoperative nursing care of the T and A patient includes the following: position child on side, check pulse and respirations, assess level of consciousness, observe skin for color and moisture, and carefully evaluate the type and amount of oronasal drainage.

11 Strep throat is diagnosed by throat culture or a quick strep screen. Symptoms are often the same as those seen with viral infections. Diagnosis is important because rheumatic fever, heart disease, and glomerulonephritis follow untreated streptococcal infections in a significant number of children.

12 Allergies may be treated by separating the patient from the allergen, environmental control, immunizing the patient by the process of desensitization, or administering medications to relieve symptoms.

13 Asthma is the result of hyperreactivity of the bronchial airway. Although the spasm, edema, and mucus that create this reversible obstruction are often caused by an allergic reaction, nonimmunological precipitants can also initiate or compound the problem. The treatment of asthma includes specific measures to eliminate allergens or desensitize the patient and nonspecific measures to relieve symptoms.

14 Treatment of acute attacks of asthma is inhalation therapy with albuterol or metaproterenol. Status asthmaticus exists when this therapy does not improve respiration. This potentially life-threatening condition requires aggressive treatment with epinephrine, and the patient will need to be hospitalized.

15 Diagnostic procedures to evaluate heart function and detect cardiac abnormalities are noninvasive tests, such as electrocardiography and echocardiography, laboratory tests such as a complete blood cell count and hematocrit and hemoglobin determinations, and special procedures, such as angiography, angiocardiography, and cardiac catheterization. Children returning to the nursing unit after cardiac catheterization should be treated as postoperative patients.

16 Signs and symptoms commonly seen in infants with serious congenital heart disease are cyanosis, tachypnea, tachycardia, effort intolerance, failure to thrive, and heart murmurs.

17 Common congenital defects of the heart and great vessels include patent ductus arteriosus, coarctation of the aorta, tetralogy of Fallot, atrial septal defect, and ventricular septal defect.

18 A patient with a congenital heart defect may undergo surgery as an infant, toddler, or child. Preparation of these patients is particularly important because of the seriousness of the surgery and the many procedures that must be performed. Children and families who receive optimal preoperative preparation demonstrate decreased anxiety and increased cooperation postoperatively.

19 Complications that may develop in patients with congenital heart defects before, during, or after surgery include the following: pneumonia, congestive heart failure, subacute bacterial endocarditis, and cerebral thrombosis.

20 Signs and symptoms of rheumatic fever vary and usually occur about 2 weeks after a streptococcal infection. Treatment includes the administration of penicillin, aspirin, and sometimes prednisone. Nursing care depends on the severity of the disease and the symptoms present. Emotional and physical rest are essential.

CRITICAL THOUGHT QUESTIONS

1 What are the most common respiratory infections seen in infants and children? What symptoms are commonly seen with respiratory tract infections? What nursing interventions aid in the treatment of respiratory tract infections?

2 Why is the name mucoviscidosis very descriptive of the disease process seen with cystic fibrosis? Which body systems are involved in the disease process? What forms of therapy assist children afflicted with CF? What is the prognosis for children afflicted with

this disease? What can the nurse do to provide emotional and informational support to the child and family?

3 How are specific allergies identified? What types of treatment are available to persons with allergies? What is the nurse's role in care of persons with allergies? How are allergies significant in the administration of food and medication?

4 What is asthma? What is the relationship of asthma to allergies? Why is asthma very frightening to the child having an attack? How does caring for an asthmatic child affect the patients? What is the typical treatment for an acute asthmatic attack? Why is status asthmaticus a life-threatening condition? What are the nursing implications when providing care to an asthmatic child?

5 The fetal circulatory system differs from the postnatal circulatory system. Identify each of the circulatory changes that normally occur at birth. Which congenital heart defect occurs if fetal circulation persists?

6 Identify which cardiac conditions cause left-to-right shunts, right-to-left shunts, and obstruction. What nursing interventions are particularly important in caring for a child with cardiac conditions?

BIBLIOGRAPHY

Allen CL: Home management of the child with viral croup, *J Am Acad Nurse Practitioners* 3(2):59-63, 1991.

Bochner BS and Lichtenstein LM: Anaphlaxis, *N Engl J Med* 324(25):1785-1790, 1991.

Facione N: Otitis media: an overview of acute and chronic disease, *Nurse Practitioner* 15(10):11-22, 1990.

Hazinski MF: Cardiovascular disorders. In Hazinski MF, editor: *Nursing care of the critically ill child*, ed 2, St Louis, 1992, Mosby.

Hutton N et al: Effectiveness of an antihistamine decongestant combination for young children with the common cold, *J Pediatr* 118(1):125-130, 1991.

Molfino NA et al: Respiratory arrest in near-fatal asthma, *N Engl J Med* 324(5):285-288, 1991.

Martinez FD et al: Increased incidence of asthma in smoking mothers, *Pediatrics* 89(1):21-26, 1992.

Monett Z, Moynihan P: Cardiovascular assessment of the neonatal heart, *J Perinat Neonat Nurs* 5(2):50-59, 1991.

Sharkey AM and Clark BJ: Common complaints with cardiac implications in children, *Pediatr Clin North Am* 38(3):657-666, 1991.

Weitzman M et al: Racial, social, and environmental risks for childhood asthma, *Am J Dis Child* 144:1189-1194, 1990.

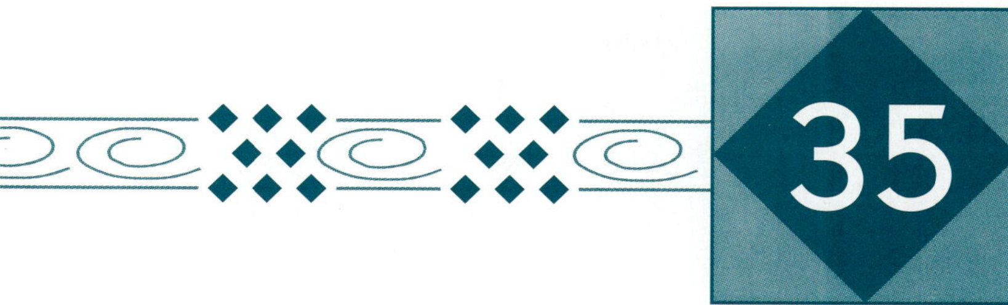
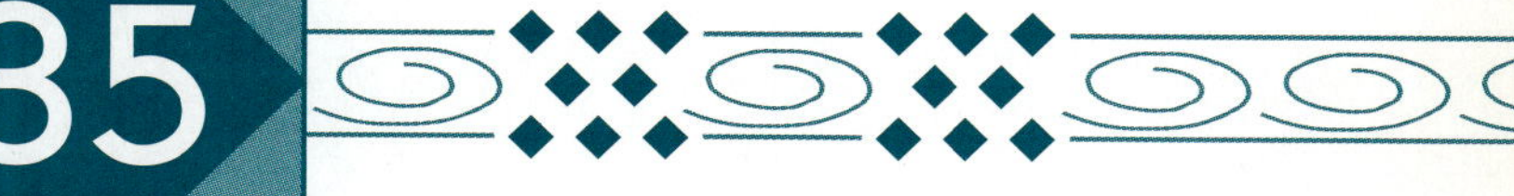

35

Digestive and Metabolic Problems

CHAPTER OBJECTIVES

After studying this chapter, the student should be able to:

1 Identify the causative organism for thrush, two ways that the problem may be acquired by an infant, and the usual treatment.
2 Describe pyloric stenosis; identify two possible signs of the condition and three important postoperative nursing considerations.
3 Discuss infant colic, including possible causes and nursing interventions.
4 Explain why *oral* intake is reduced and why hospitalization may be necessary for severe diarrhea.
5 Discuss four nursing considerations for the hospitalized child with diarrhea.
6 Describe the life cycle, diagnostic test, treatment, and health education for pinworm.
7 Describe umbilical hernia and indications for surgery when the condition persists beyond infancy.
8 Define the following pediatric digestive problems: Meckel's diverticulum, meconium ileus, intussusception, and congenital megacolon.
9 Describe how to construct a modified Stile's dressing, and explain why it is used.
10 Identify the basic endocrine problem faced by insulin-dependent diabetic patients (IDDM-1), and describe the clinical manifestations.
11 Describe four precipitating factors of diabetic ketoacidosis and four causes of insulin-induced hypoglycemia.
12 Outline the nursing interventions for hypoglycemic reaction.
13 Describe the administration of glucagon.
14 Explain administration of two different types of insulin in the same syringe.
15 Outline the daily nutritional requirements (calories, fat, carbohydrate, and protein) for a 7-year-old boy with insulin-dependent diabetes who weighs 50 pounds.
16 Explain the Somogyi phenomenon and its treatment.

Pediatric gastroenterology is the study of digestive diseases in children. This chapter presents the common malformations, infestations, infections, and foreign bodies found in the digestive tracts of children (Fig. 35-1). Although it is not primarily a digestive problem, a review of diabetes mellitus is included because it influences the metabolism of digested glucose and because dietary regulation is required. For the convenience of faculty and students, the material is presented according to the developmental group primarily affected.

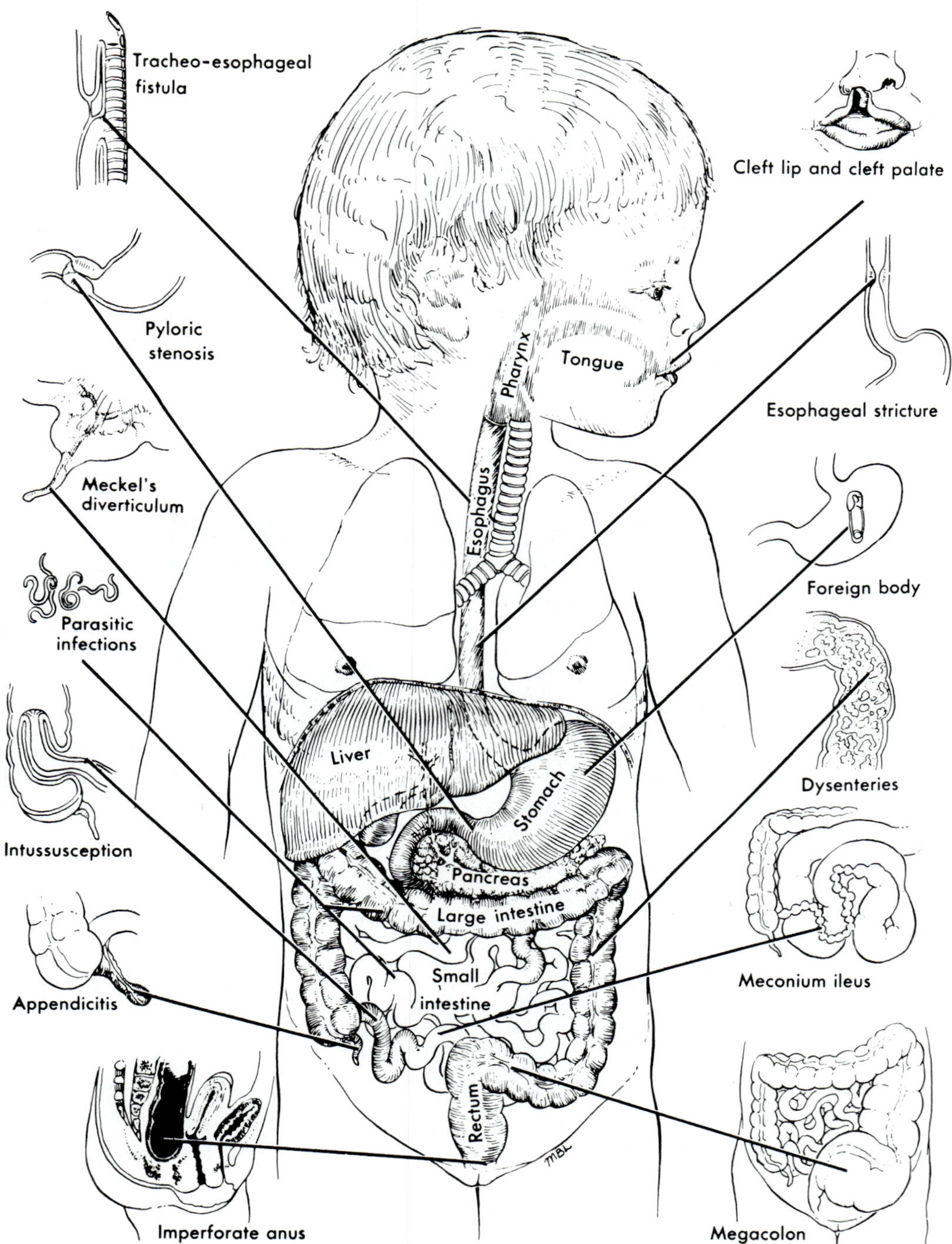

Fig. 35-1 Summary of common pediatric problems involving digestive system.

KEY VOCABULARY

digestion Process by which food is broken down mechanically and chemically in the gastrointestinal tract and converted into absorbable forms.

endocrine gland Structure producing a hormone that is discharged into the bloodstream.

exocrine gland Structure that produces a secretion deposited in a particular area of the body via a duct.

glycosuria Presence of glucose in the urine.

hyperglycemia Excess of glucose in the blood.

hypoglycemia Deficiency of glucose in the blood.

ileus Obstruction or paralysis of the small intestine.

metabolism All energy and material transformations that occur within living cells.

ANATOMY AND PHYSIOLOGY

The digestive system is formed by the mouth, esophagus, gastrointestinal tract, and related organs, such as the liver, gallbladder, and pancreas. The adult alimentary canal is an unsterile tract that, if stretched out for its entire length, reaches about 30 feet. The digestive tract and its accessory organs reduce foodstuffs (carbohydrates, proteins, and fats) to their smallest working chemical units. These chemical units are then absorbed through the mucous membrane of the intestinal walls and eventually reach the bloodstream to be distributed to the individual cells, providing the body with building materials, heat, and energy. To accomplish this, the digestive system works on food both *mechanically* (through the action of the teeth, tongue, cheeks, and muscular contractions of the tract, called *peristalsis*) and *chemically* (through the activity of various enzymes, emulsifiers, acids, and bacteria, which are normally active in different portions of the tract). Substances not absorbed by the body by way of the bloodstream or lymphatic system are removed normally by periodic defecation, or bowel movement. For additional review of the digestive process refer to Chapter 22.

Disorders of the digestive system reveal themselves in several predictable ways. Anorexia, nausea, vomiting, constipation, abdominal distention and pain, diarrhea, and weight loss are common manifestations. The observation of a child's stool is of great importance in pediatrics. The amount, color, consistency, general appearance, and odor of a child's bowel movements can be of real diagnostic significance and aid in evaluating the condition of the digestive tract.

DIGESTIVE AND METABOLIC PROBLEMS

Infant

For a discussion of cleft lip, cleft palate, and esophageal atresia with tracheoesophageal fistula see Chapter 18.

Oral moniliasis

Thrush, or oral moniliasis, results from contamination of the infant's oral cavity with vaginal secretion containing *Candida (Monilia) albicans* at the time of birth or from improper hygiene and feeding techniques after birth.

Clinical manifestations. White, curdlike plaques appear on the tongue and cheeks and adhere to the surface of the mucous membrane (Fig. 16-3). The mouth may be tender, and the desire to eat may be decreased.

Treatment. Thrush can be treated by nystatin (Mycostatin) oral suspension (1 ml) four times a day for 10 days. All objects that have entered the infant's mouth should be adequately sterilized. If breast-fed, the mother's breast should be assessed. If the nipple is erythematous, painful, or pruritic, treatment should be initiated for the mother also. This is not a contraindication for breast-feeding. Monilial or candidal diaper dermatitis should also be treated with nystatin or lotrimin cream. The condition usually responds well to therapy. Thrush is also a common condition among children receiving long-term, broad-spectrum antibiotic therapy. The antibiotics destroy the normal flora of the alimentary canal and allow the ubiquitous fungus to multiply without competition. Most cases of moniliasis associated with antibiotic therapy resolve when the drug is discontinued. If candidal infections persist beyond early infancy, an immune deficiency should be considered.

Esophageal stenosis

The narrowing of a child's esophagus, esophageal stenosis, can be congenital in origin or caused by incomplete development of the lumen (esophageal atresia). However, the condition can be acquired from prolonged peptic acid irritation, such as occurs with chronic reflux or vomiting. It can also be secondary to chemical burns from strong alkali or acid ingestion when inflammation and scar formation produces stenosis.

Treatment. Patients often require periodic esophageal dilations and may need a gastrostomy, or artificial opening into the stomach, because of difficulty in maintaining nutrition. Surgical excision of the narrowed area and joining together of the remaining parts (anastomosis), replacement of the area by a bowel transplant, or esophageal reconstruction using tissue from the greater curvature of the stomach may be undertaken.

Gastroesophageal reflux

Gastroesophageal reflux (GER) is one of the most common gastrointestinal problems in children. It produces a wide variety of symptoms and ranges in severity from mild regurgitation to a life-threatening disorder (Orenstein, 1993).

Clinical manifestations. A careful history is of utmost importance. Key questions related to GER include these: Spitting after feedings? Nonspecific fussiness? Perceived discomfort when passing stools? (Jonides, 1994). Infants and young children with GER can develop chronic bronchitis, recurrent pneumonia, bronchiectasis, atelectasis, or asthmalike symptoms as a result of the aspiration of gastric content, which is toxic to the airways and alveoli (Fig. 35-2). Other common complications of reflux include failure to thrive because of excessive regurgitation and esophagitis with possible stricture. A urine culture should always be done in an infant with feeding problems to rule out infection (Jonides et al, 1994).

Treatment. In most cases, effective treatment is attained through a medically conservative regimen, with thickening of the formula with rice cereal, maintenance of the child in an upright position at a 30- to 40-degree angle, and, in some instances, administration of medications, such as metoclopramide (Reglan) or bethanechol chloride (Urecholine). However, in severe or refractory cases a surgical intervention, such as a Nissen fundoplication (in which a valvelike mechanism is created by wrapping the fundus of the stomach around the distal esophagus, reducing reflux) is necessary. Aspiration of gastric content can also occur in tracheoesophageal fistula and in children with spastic neurological problems.

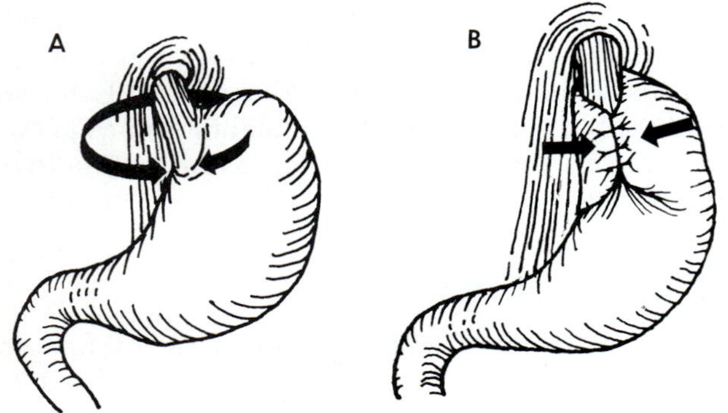

Fig. 35-2 **A,** Preoperative GER. **B,** Nissen fundoplication—fundus of the stomach is wrapped around the distal end of the esophagus.

Congenital pyloric stenosis

Abnormal narrowing of the pyloric sphincter, which forms the exit of the stomach, can cause progressive vomiting and malnutrition in the infant (Fig. 35-3). This narrowing is caused by spasm of the sphincter, local edema, and an overgrowth of the circular muscle fibers of the pylorus.

Clinical manifestations. The symptoms do not usually appear until the child is approximately 2 to 3 weeks old and rarely have their onset after 2 months of age. This disorder has an hereditary tendency and occurs more often in male infants.

At first the vomiting is only occasional. However, if the stenosis is unrelieved, vomiting becomes more frequent, forceful, and projectile. If this situation persists, the child loses weight and begins to show signs of dehydration, electrolyte imbalance, and malnutrition. The emesis contains no bile because the opening to the duodenum is too small to allow such staining. Despite the frequent vomiting, the infant continues to have a good appetite and takes fluids when they are offered. The primary care provider

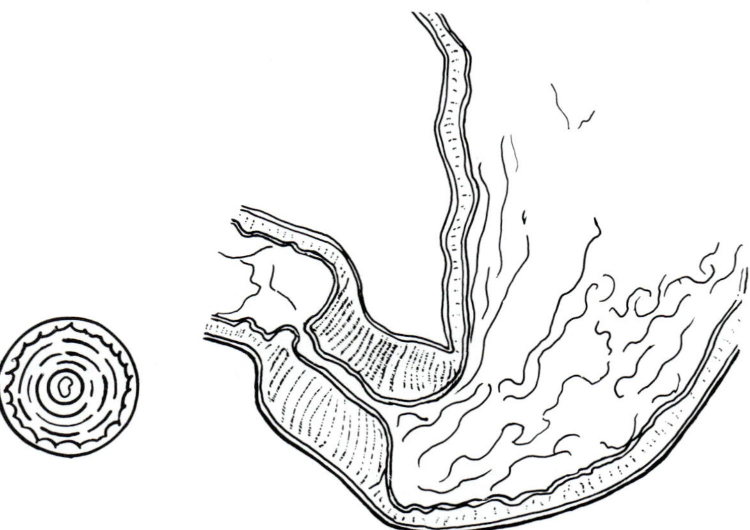

Fig. 35-3 Congenital hypertrophic pyloric stenosis. Abnormal narrowing of pyloric sphincter—sagittal and cross-sectional view.

makes a diagnosis on the basis of the history, the clinical examination, x-ray examination using a contrast medium, or ultrasound studies of the pylorus. An abnormal hypertrophy of the pylorus is noted. A hard, olive-shaped tumor (hypertrophied pylorus) may be palpated, and visible, left-to-right peristalsis may be noted as the stomach tries to force the swallowed milk or formula into the duodenum. When this effort proves ineffective, the peristaltic waves reverse themselves, and emesis results.

Treatment. In the United States, treatment of pyloric stenosis is usually surgical. A nasogastric tube is inserted before surgery to ensure that the stomach is empty and to prevent aspiration during the surgery. The procedure is called the *Fredet-Ramstedt operation.* The surgeon cuts through the enlarged muscle of the pylorus to the mucous membrane, relieving the constriction. This surgical procedure is highly successful in relieving the cause of the persistent vomiting.

Nursing care. Postoperative care consists of observation of the surgical site or dressing and careful introduction of glucose water in small amounts at fairly frequent intervals as ordered. The infant should be held at a steep incline while being fed; burped well before, during, and after a feeding; and placed in an infant seat or propped on his or her right side after feedings. When the child is in the infant seat, gravity aids the drainage of the offered fluid. Placing the infant on the right side also aids drainage and helps bubbles come to the top of the stomach, where they can be expelled with less formula loss. A side or upright position also helps prevent aspiration. After drinking, the infant should be disturbed as little as possible. It is important not to overfeed the child. This can lead to vomiting, which stresses the sutures. If three or four glucose-water feedings are well tolerated, the infant is given progressive amounts of diluted formula, beginning with 30 ml. When 75-ml feedings are reached, the child is started on the usual formula or begins monitored breast-feeding. If the feedings are retained and the infant's course is uncomplicated, discharge may occur on the same day of the surgery.

Meckel's diverticulum

A structural remnant from embryonic life is a pouch in the ileum called *Meckel's diverticulum.* During intrauterine life a duct joined the umbilicus with the intestine and led to the yolk sac, allowing temporary nourishment of the developing fetus. In the course of normal development this duct closes. However, remnants persist in a small percentage of people, and sometimes these remnants cause difficulty. An open tract, capable of discharging the contents of the small bowel onto the abdominal wall, can endure. More often a blind pouch with no connection or only a cord attachment to the umbilicus remains. Occasionally gastric mucosa is found within the pouch. Meckel's diverticulum can ulcerate and hemorrhage massively and painlessly or can act as the lead point for an intussusception. Symptoms similar to those of appendicitis or intestinal obstruction can occur. Frequently its presence is undiagnosed until exploratory surgery reveals the problem. Nursing care is similar to that involving any condition that necessitates exploration of the abdominal cavity.

Meconium ileus

Obstruction of the small intestine in the newborn infant caused by the presence of exceptionally thick, sticky meconium is called *meconium ileus.* The meconium is so viscous that it cannot pass normally through the bowel. Obstruction often occurs near the ileocecal junction. This condition virtually always indicates an exocrine disorder, cystic fibrosis of the pancreas, although it is not present in all cases of cystic fibrosis. Meconium ileus results because the pancreas fails to produce the enzymes that normally help liquefy the meconium. (See Chapter 34 for a discussion of cystic fibrosis.)

Clinical manifestations. Bile-stained emesis, abdominal distention, and absence of the normal meconium stool are symptoms of meconium ileus. This is a challenging pediatric problem because of the type of malfunction, the young age of the patient, and the disease process itself.

Treatment. In mild cases the treatment may be medical, with reliance on enemas that dissolve or mechanically clear the impaction. A therapeutic enema of diatrizoate meglumine (Gastrografin) is a successful nonoperative method of relieving the impaction. Oral administration of pancreatic enzymes is also undertaken. Intravenous fluid therapy is necessary during this procedure, because diatrizoate meglumine draws fluid and serum from the intravascular compartment into the lumen of the bowel in an effort to release the sticky meconium. Some cases require surgery to clear the obstruction. Resection of the intestine and a temporary ileostomy may be necessary. The child may be very ill, and the prognosis is guarded.

Intussusception

A telescoping of adjacent parts of the bowel is called *intussusception* (Fig. 35-4). Meckel's diverticulum or polyps can lead to intussusception. When intussusception occurs, it most frequently involves the area of the ileocecal valve. Circulation is disturbed to the affected

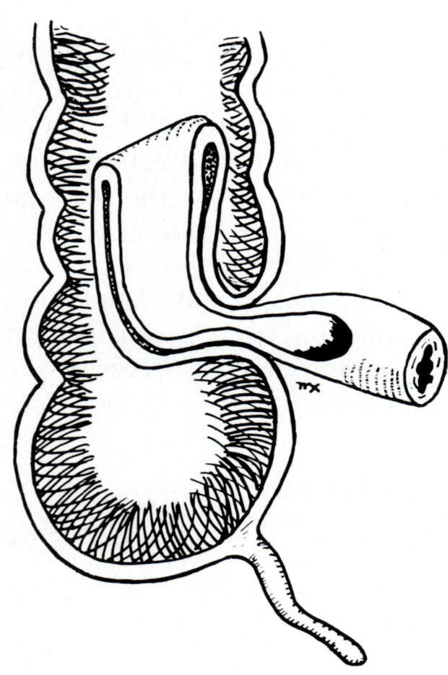

Fig. 35-4 Ileocecal intussusception—telescoping of adjacent parts of bowel.

portions of the intestine, which may result in gangrene, perforation, and bowel obstruction.

Clinical manifestations. This condition most often affects infants and toddlers. The onset is usually sudden. At first the child may draw up the legs and cry out intermittently. Later the discomfort is intensified by progressive vomiting of bile-stained and even fecal emesis. Stools, at first loose, become scanty and characteristically assume a color and consistency of currant jelly because they are formed largely of mucus and blood. If the condition is unrelieved, the child's condition rapidly deteriorates. A high temperature develops, and the child's life is endangered. A favorable prognosis depends on early detection and treatment of the condition.

Diagnosis. Diagnosis is made based on the history, physical examination, and plain survey films of the abdomen.

Treatment. Treatment of choice is barium enema if peritonitis or frank intestinal obstruction is suspected. The pressure of the inflowing enema can reduce an intussusception. In some cases, reduction comes only after raising the height of the barium or by giving repeated enemas after each evacuation. A small number of intussusceptions recur after primary barium enema treatment. When surgery is indicated, the intussusception is identified and usually "milked" gently backward until the telescoping is completely relieved. Resection of the damaged segment of intestine may be necessary.

Congenital megacolon (Hirschsprung's Disease or Aganglionic Megacolon)

Classic congenital megacolon, or Hirschsprung's disease, is characterized by lack of normal peristaltic activity in the distal segment of the colon, usually the sigmoid, because of improper *innervation* (lack of the necessary nerve ganglia in the musculature of the affected bowel or lack of coordination between the parasympathetic and sympathetic divisions of the nervous system). It is seen more often in males than in females.

Clinical manifestations. Symptoms appear early in infancy. Failure to pass a meconium stool within 24 hours in a term newborn should arouse suspicion. Constipation, interrupted by small amounts of stool, progressive abdominal distention (which may be sufficiently severe to cause respiratory embarrassment) anorexia, and occasional vomiting suggest the diagnosis. Pronounced abdominal distention can grossly distort the appearance of the child.

Diagnosis. Diagnosis is made after a review of the patient's history, palpation and auscultation of the abdomen, rectal examination, and x-ray examination. A rectal biopsy for microscopic examination of the tissue is mandatory for the definitive diagnosis. The biopsy is painless and is obtained surgically by securing three to four small fragments of tissue with a suction capsule 3 to 4 cm inside the rectum.

Treatment. Megacolon is treated surgically through resection of the aganglionic length of colon. In a small percentage of patients the entire colon can be involved, and, rarely, a portion of the small bowel needs inclusion in the resected intestine. The type of procedure performed depends on the age and individual needs of the child. The most satisfactory treatment appears to be an abdominoperineal removal of the abnormal section of bowel with an anastomosis of the remaining normal colon to the anal canal (Swenson's pull-through). A variation of this is the Soave procedure.

Nursing care. The child is fed parenterally. Gastric suction and an indwelling urinary catheter may be continued for an indefinite period. The anal sphincter may be dilated daily. The presence of bowel sounds and normal stool determine the success of the procedure. In some cases, this procedure is inadvisable, and a colostomy is performed.

Pseudo-Hirschsprung's disease

This disease is more common than Hirschsprung's or agangionic megacolon and has a psychogenic basis. Its onset is not in the newborn period. X-ray film and biopsy results are negative. A careful history of family living patterns and stressors is necessary with resultant referral for counseling.

Colic

Although colic is often spoken of as a disease entity, it is not a disease but a symptom.

Clinical manifestations. In the dictionary, colic is defined as "acute abdominal pain." However, when parents and nurses speak of colic they are usually referring to the intermittent abdominal distress in the newborn infant that is fairly common in the early months of life. Colic may last for 1 to 3 months. The time of peak incidence is in the late afternoon and early evening. Infants draw up their legs on their abdomens, clench their fists, become red in the face, and start to cry. This goes on intermittently as though they are troubled with periodic intestinal cramping. During these episodes they may pass gas by mouth or rectum.

Various explanations for the abdominal discomfort have been advanced. Probably there are multiple causes. Infants troubled with colic tend to have a low birth weight (5 to 7 pounds [2270 to 3180 g]). It may be caused by an immaturity of the gastrointestinal system. Most explanations of the pain experienced involve the presence of excessive gas in the digestive tract. Excessive air can result from the following:

1 Poor bottle-feeding techniques, including failure to tip the bottle sufficiently to ensure a full nipple at all times, too-rapid feeding, the use of nipples with very small holes, which necessitates considerable suction (and air swallowing) to obtain the formula, and failure to burp the infant often enough.
2 Excessive use of carbohydrate in the formula, which may cause increased fermentation and gas formation.
3 A tense, nervous infant fostered by a tense, nervous parent.

Nursing interventions are presented in the box at right.

Colic is not well understood; however, it is self-limited and rarely persists beyond the third month of life. Therefore reassurance is an essential part of treatment.

NURSING INTERVENTIONS FOR COLIC

1 Colic occurs more frequently in bottle-fed infants, thus breast-feeding should be encouraged.
2 Overfeeding should be avoided. Refer to Chapter 22 for a discussion of feeding techniques.
3 Frequent burping is helpful.
4 A small warm water bottle placed on the care provider's lap with the infant placed in prone position over the bottle may be soothing.
5 Avoid overstimulation. Gentle rocking, no bouncing.
6 A change from cow milk formula to soy formula may be helpful.
7 If colic is severe and other methods have not been helpful, the primary care provider may recommend an antispasmodic.

Diarrhea

Diarrhea results from digestive, absorptive, and secretory malfunction. Any diarrheal disease causing profuse fluid loss is a particular threat to a child. Subsequent dehydration and electrolyte imbalance is a significant danger. With the improvement in community sanitation and hygiene, the availability of refrigeration, and careful infant formula preparation, the incidence of infectious diarrhea has declined in the United States; however, it remains a serious problem in third world countries.

Diarrheal disease or gastroenteritis of early childhood is a syndrome, the course of which varies with age, severity, nutritional status, and cause.

Etiology. Some of the common causes of diarrhea include infection, anatomical abnormalities, malabsorption syndromes, and disease outside the gastrointestinal tract. Most acute diarrheas appear to have a viral cause with rotavirus being the most common viral organism. Diarrhea frequently accompanies acute upper respiratory tract infections. Bacterial causes of infectious diarrheas include the following: staphylococci most commonly from food poisoning, pathogenic *Escherichia coli, Shigella, Salmonella, Yersinia,* and *Campylobacter.* A common cause of diarrhea in toddlers and preschoolers is the parasite *Giardia lamblia. Hepatitis B* as a disease entity and as a cause of diarrhea is discussed in Chapter 31.

Clinical manifestations. With mild diarrhea, the child has a few loose, watery stools, often foul-smelling. With moderate diarrhea, the frequency of the stools increases and the child may also exhibit vomiting, fever, irritability, and slight weight loss. Severe diarrhea is comprised of numerous to continuous watery stools that may contain blood or mucus. Signs of dehydration are present, the child is irritable and weak, and the condition may progress to lethargy and coma.

Nursing care. Whatever the cause, acute diarrhea needs immediate treatment. The disturbance in intestinal motility and consequent malabsorption causes dehydration and fluid and electrolyte imbalances. Usually severe diarrhea subsides when fluid and electrolyte therapy is administered intravenously and oral intake is reduced. Oral intake is restricted initially to rest the gastrointestinal tract and make it less irritable.

For mild to moderate diarrhea with no clinical signs of dehydration, the child will be cared for in the home. Oral rehydration therapy (ORT) is administered for the first 6 to 24 hours in small amounts (5 to 10 ml) every 15 minutes. In the United States, Pedialyte, Resol, Ricelyte, and Lytren are used for oral rehydration. The breast-fed infant should continue to breast-feed in conjunction with ORT. Continued human milk feeding results in reduced severity and duration of the illness (Brown, 1991). If the child had been advanced to solid foods, a modified BRAT diet should be slowly introduced. BRAT is an acronym for *b*ananas, *r*ice, *a*pplesauce, and *t*oast. Modified refers to the addition of a protein source, such as pureed chicken. Dairy products, including full-strength cow's milk formula, should be avoided for 48 to 72 hours; however, soy formula may be offered in small amounts after the first 24 hours. By the fourth or fifth day the child may return to a regular diet if the diarrhea is resolved. Recent studies suggest that early reintroduction of normal nutrients is beneficial due to nutritional advantage, reduction in the number of stools, reduced weight loss, and shortened duration of illness (Brown, 1991).

The infant who becomes dehydrated because of diarrhea or vomiting and diarrhea may be admitted to the hospital. The infant should be weighed and a stool culture obtained on admission. Enteric precautions and antibiotic therapy may be indicated for treating diarrhea caused by pathogenic *E. coli* and staphylococci and for severe infections caused by *Salmonella* and *Shigella* type of organisms (see Chapter 31). Daily calculations of the child's fluid intake and output and weight must be accurately recorded. It may be necessary to weigh the infant's diaper to assess output. Because of the frequency of stools, a special medicated ointment may be prescribed for application after each cleansing of the perirectal area. The color, consistency, general appearance, and amount of stool should be regularly noted and recorded. Taking temperatures rectally is contraindicated to prevent stimulation and to reduce trauma to the rectum.

Abdominal hernias

A hernia is an abnormal protrusion of a portion of the contents of a body cavity through a defect in its surrounding wall, commonly causing abnormal swelling or pressure. Common in infancy and childhood are inguinal and umbilical hernias. They are usually congenital and often familial. Umbilical hernias are more common in African-American children.

Inguinal hernia. Inguinal hernias are found more often in males. They can be unilateral or bilateral and are usually on the right side when unilateral. When the testes originally descend into the scrotum from the abdominal cavity, they are surrounded by a small sac or tube of peritoneum that is continuous with the abdominal lining. Usually this sac soon closes off, making any further communication with the abdominal cavity impossible. Occasionally the closure is incomplete or does not take place, and the intestine can slip down the open inguinal canal, causing a swelling in the area. This prolapse of the intestine is not important in itself. However, a possibility exists that the misplaced loop of intestine can become trapped (incarcerated) in the inguinal canal or scrotum, and the circulation to the trapped segment can become impaired (strangulated), causing intestinal obstruction and gangrene of the bowel. Inguinal hernia also develops in girls. The anatomy is different but parallel. The inguinal canals, which are occupied by the round ligaments, can allow loops of intestine to enter the area of the groin. Only 10% of inguinal hernias involve females.

Clinical manifestations. Early clinical signs are vomiting and colicky abdominal pain, manifested as extreme irritability.

Treatment. To prevent incarceration, all inguinal hernias should be surgically corrected soon after diagnosis. In infants and small children up to 2 years of age the hernia is repaired in a simple procedure (herniotomy). In older children a slightly more complex procedure is used. A surgical incision is made in a natural skin crease where the scar will be less visible. The hernia sac is carefully tied off. For boys an abnormal collection of fluid may be found in the scrotal area surrounding the testes (hydrocele). This fluid is aspirated, and the abnormal peritoneal sac is excised. The child usually tolerates the procedure very well, and in most cases minimal postoperative analgesia is required. A protective spray dressing is applied over the new incision. This allows direct observation of the area. Diapers are usually not applied in a routine fashion until 24 hours after surgery. One approach to the diaper problem is the use of a modified Stile's dressing (Fig. 35-5). A small bed cradle is placed over the legs of the infant. A long infant gown, securely tied in back, is drawn tightly up over the frame and fastened with pins. The cradle is draped with a small blanket and a large absorbent pad is placed under the infant's buttocks. This keeps pressure off the incisional site and prevents the infant from touching the incisional site.

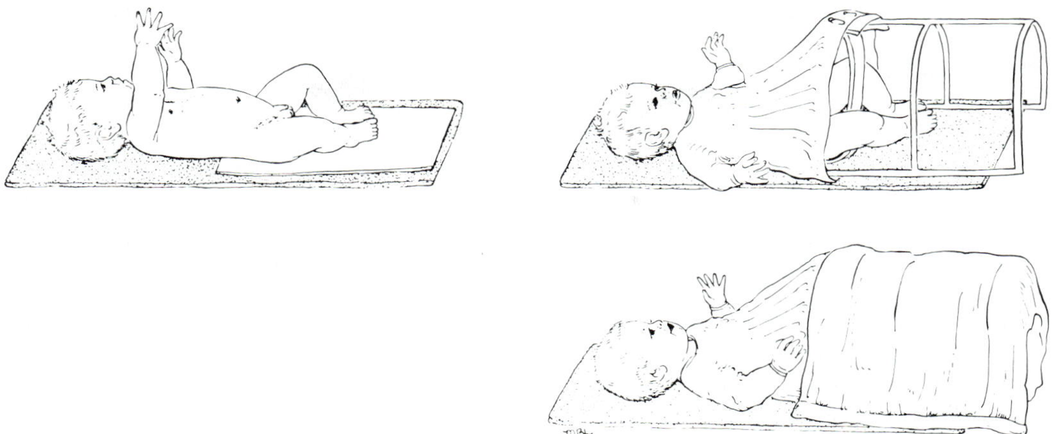

Fig. 35-5 Steps in constructing modified Stile's dressing. Be sure that gown is pulled tightly when attached to cradle. Cradle may need to be tied to crib.

A simple hernia repair is usually done as an outpatient procedure. Parents are instructed to bring the child to the hospital in a fasting state about 1 hour before the scheduled procedure. The parents remain until the child is taken to the operating room and are present when the child awakens. In 2 to 3 hours and when able to take fluids, the child may be discharged from the day surgery suite. Parents should be reminded to return in 4 days to have the sutures removed from the infant's incision. Older children's sutures may be removed six days after surgery.

Umbilical hernias. Umbilical hernias in infancy are thought to be caused by severe localized abdominal stress brought about by crying, coughing, and vomiting. Umbilical hernias often close spontaneously when the child learns to stand and walk and the abdominal muscles are strengthened through use. However, umbilical defects greater than 1.5 cm in diameter in children seldom close spontaneously. If an umbilical hernia is not closed during childhood, the defect often becomes more serious in pregnant women, and the multiparous woman is subject to the threat of incarceration. To prevent this serious problem in adulthood, a more aggressive approach is urged.

Treatment. Prophylactic umbilical hernia repair is recommended for all girls over 2 years and all boys over 4 years of age.

Imperforate anus

The problem of imperforate anus has already been mentioned in Chapter 18. Figure 18-15 depicts the common types of the malformation encountered.

Treatment. Surgery must be performed very early to prevent complications and ensure a better prognosis. If a male newborn infant has a rectourethral fistula, surgery must be prompt to prevent the development of serious ascending urinary tract infection. For infant girls with an associated posterior vaginal anus, corrective surgery can be delayed until the child is 4 to 6 months of age. Whether an abdominal or perineal surgical approach is necessary depends on the type of defect and the distance of the terminal end of the colon from the perineum. A temporary colostomy may be necessary. After creation or repair of the anorectal area, frequent dilation of the canal may be ordered.

Galactosemia

A metabolic defect that has dietary significance is *galactosemia.* If this congenital error in the metabolism of the sugar galactose is untreated, it may cause physical and mental retardation, cataracts, enlargement of the liver and spleen, and cirrhosis. The body is unable to change galactose to glucose, a chemical reaction that normally takes place primarily in the liver. An enzyme needed to accomplish the task is deficient or missing. Galactose builds up in the bloodstream and spills over into the urine, where it is identified by appropriate tests.

Clinical manifestations. Early signs of galactosemia in the infant are vomiting, listlessness, and failure to thrive. These signs are not apparent until 1 to 2 weeks after birth.

Treatment. Since galactose is present in milk sugar, it is important that the defect be diagnosed early and that a milk substitute, such as Nutramigen, or a meat-base formula be used. Like children with phenylketonuria (PKU), the diets of galactosemia patients must be closely supervised to prevent the ingestion of the offending food. Children with galactosemia may be able to expand their dietary horizons gradually after a period of several years on a carefully restricted regimen.

Toddler

Foreign body ingestion

Toddlers commonly ingest whatever they happen to find during this exploratory developmental phase. Most foreign bodies complete their journey through the intestinal tract without incident if they make it through the esophagus into the stomach.

Treatment. Most objects pass in 4 to 7 days but may be allowed 2 to 3 weeks if no symptoms such as pain or blood in the stools are present. Parents may carefully examine the stool for small round objects that have been ingested. Sharp or long, pointed objects can pose the threat of perforation. If the object is detectable by x-ray examination, it is viewed and periodically watched. If trauma to the tissue seems likely, an operation to retrieve it may be necessary. The abdomen of a child who has swallowed a foreign object should not be palpated. Care providers may advocate placing a small sign on the child, cautioning would-be examiners to avoid such maneuvers. Giving a child large amounts of bread or potato after ingestion of a foreign object is of doubtful value. A laxative should never be given in such circumstances. Objects obstructing the esophagus should be promptly treated as a medical emergency.

Toddler and Preschooler

Parasitic infestations

All bacteria are parasites; however, when one speaks of *parasitic infestations,* one is usually referring to organisms that are multicellular in their adult form and large enough to be seen with the naked eye. Many parasites are found in abundance in tropical areas of the world and represent tremendous public health problems. This text mentions only those found frequently in the United States: pinworms, roundworms, and *Giardia*.

Oxyuriasis (pinworm, threadworm, or seat-worm infestation). Although the official name of the pinworm is *Enterobius vermicularis,* the name of the disease this small, white, threadlike worm causes is known as oxyuriasis, or enterobiasis, an extremely common infestation. It does not always produce symptoms and often goes undiagnosed.

The pinworm eggs are ingested or possibly inhaled. Most often children introduce the eggs into their own mouths by their fingers, which have become contaminated by touching objects used by affected children. When the infestation becomes established, children can easily reinfect themselves. The eggs are swallowed and hatch in the intestine. They mature in and near the cecum. When the adult female worms are ready to lay their eggs, they migrate down the intestinal tract to the anus. During the night the female worms leave the anus and lay their eggs in the folds of the anal sphincter and the perineum. Occasionally the worms migrate to the vagina and cause a vaginitis in a little girl. All this activity usually causes considerable local irritation and itching. The child usually scratches the area, contaminating the fingers with the eggs laid in the region. In the course of time, fingers travel to the mouth again, and the cycle repeats (Fig. 35-6). The interval between the ingestion of an egg and the appearance of the female pinworm at the anus is approximately 6 to 8 weeks.

Clinical manifestations. Mild pinworm infestations cause few symptoms other than anal itching and secondary complications caused by scratching. However, sometimes pinworms cause sleep disturbances, restlessness, irritability, and occasionally secondary vaginal or periurethral irritation from scratching. Abdominal pain and grinding of teeth is not a part of the typical clinical picture. With large infestations inflammation of the appendix may occur.

Diagnosis. The child complains of anal itching, and the parent checks for small worms in the anal area 1 to 2 hours after the child is asleep. The eggs also may be observed on the surface of a stool, or microscopically. Since the female lays her eggs in the skin folds outside the body of the child, ova are rarely found in the stool. Usually a so-called Scotch tape test is ordered. The nurse or parent takes a piece of Scotch tape, which has been fastened sticky side out to a tongue blade, and presses it against the rectal area. Some microscopic eggs adhere to the tape. The tape is then carefully secured to a glass slide sticky side down and sent to the laboratory for examination.

Treatment. In the past when a child was affected, the entire family was treated. Currently, only the family members who have symptoms are treated. Mebendazole (Vermox), a single-dose, chewable tablet for all ages, is effective in most cases, or pyrvinium pamoate (Povan) can be given in one or two doses. The nurse and parents should know that pyrvinium pamoate colors the stools red, and if the child has an emesis while the medication is still present in the gastrointestinal tract, the emesis may also be reddish.

Other measures must be followed to help ensure a cure. Personal toilet hygiene should be stressed. The necessity for hand washing after using the toilet is not understood by children unless it is taught. Frequent cleansing of the rectogenital area is encouraged. The toilet seat must be cleaned often. Because of the intense itching that can occur at night, an affected child should have very short fingernails. Children may be infested without the nurse's or parent's knowledge; therefore it is important to refrain from shaking used bed linen. Bed linens should always be rolled.

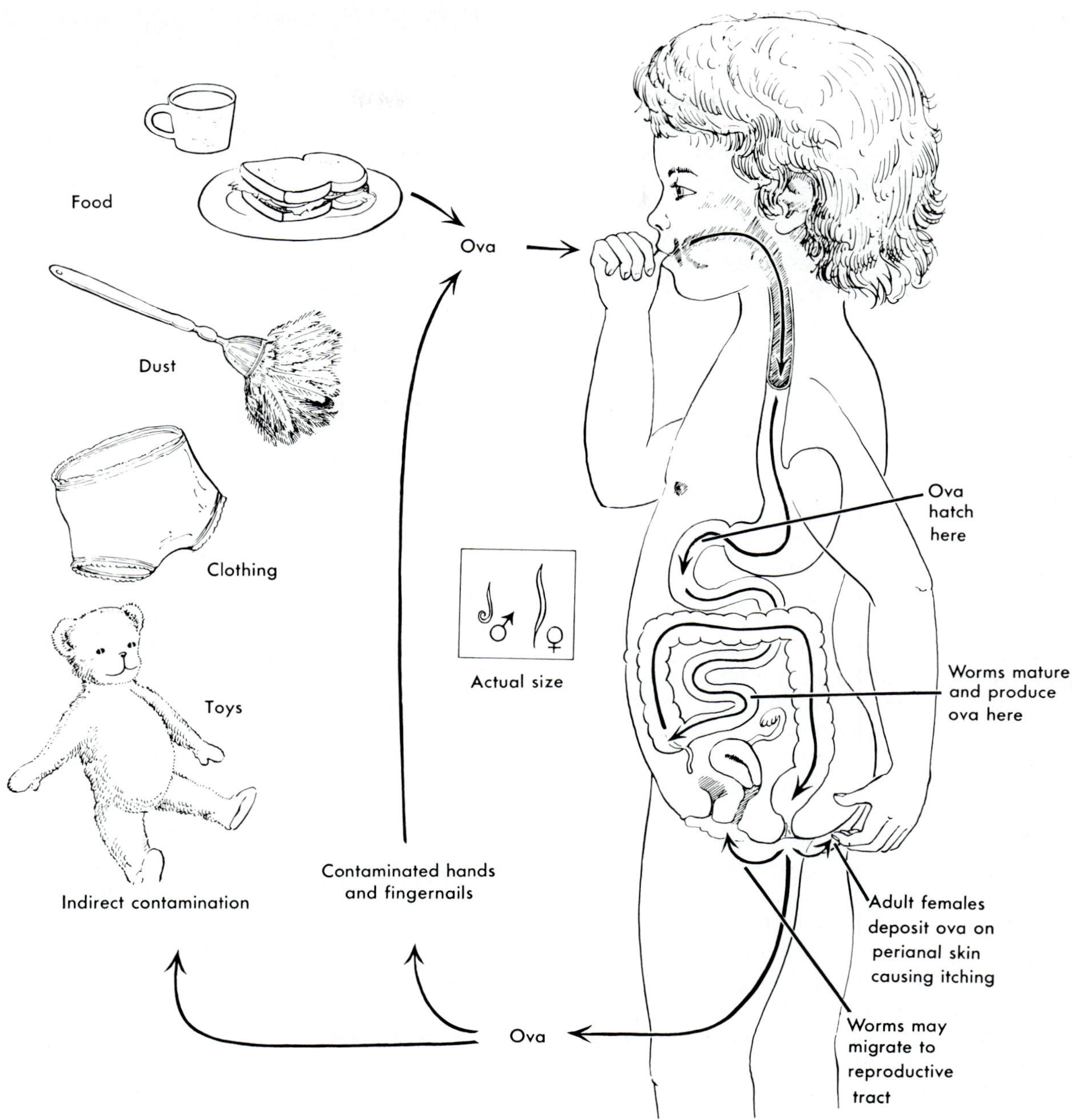

Fig. 35-6 Life cycle of pinworm *(Enterobius vermicularis).*

Giardiasis. *Giardia lamblia* is second most common parasite in the United States and the most common cause of chronic diarrhea in children in child care programs. It is predominantly spread by hand-to-mouth transmission, that is, poor hygiene; however, it can be spread by contaminated water or animals. The cysts are swallowed and develop in the duodenum as adult trophozoites with adherence to the intestinal mucosa.

Clinical manifestations. Diarrhea, weight loss, and failure to thrive are common presenting complaints. Suspected cases are diagnosed by collecting three stool specimens on separate days because the eggs (cysts) are shed intermittently. If the stools are negative and the diagnosis still highly suspected, fluid from the duodenum can be obtained by way of a swallowed string test (Entero-test) or a tube aspirate of duodenal fluid. The duodenal fluid samples are 95% accurate but obviously more invasive than stool testing, which is 40% to 60% accurate in good laboratories. Treatment for children is usually metronidazole (Flagyl) for 7 to 10 days or Furoxone.

Ascariasis (roundworm infestation). *Ascaris lumbricoides*, the worm that causes ascariasis, looks like a pink or white earthworm. It is usually 6 to 15 inches long. The eggs are found in the soil or on objects contaminated by soil containing involved feces. The disease is perpetuated by poor sanitary facilities and poor hygiene practices. The microscopic egg is swallowed and hatches in the duodenum. The small intermediate stages of the worm (larvae) pass through the wall of the intestine to penetrate the venules or lymphatics. They commonly migrate to the liver, the right side of the heart, and the lungs. The small larvae then penetrate the alveoli and ascend the bronchioles, bronchi, and trachea. On reaching the glottis they are swallowed. These same larvae develop into adult male and female forms in the small intestine. The adult male is approximately 6 to 10 inches long. The female is about 8 to 15 inches long and about the diameter of a pencil. The adult worms subsist on the semidigested food in the intestinal canal. Fertilized eggs expelled in feces must undergo a 2- to 3-week period of maturation in the soil before becoming capable of producing disease (Fig. 35-7).

Clinical manifestations. This parasite, because of its migratory habits, can cause a variety of symptoms if the infestation is intense. The larval migrations can cause nausea and vomiting or initiate symptoms of pneumonitis or intestinal obstruction. They may also produce perforation. Allergic reactions, skin rash, nervousness, and irritability are common.

Diagnosis. Positive diagnosis is made on the basis of finding the ova in the stool or seeing the worms emerge from the gastrointestinal tract.

Treatment. Treatment by piperazine citrate (Antepar) is effective for *Ascaris* infestation, provided that reinfection caused by poor hygiene practices does not occur. Mebendazole (Vermox) can also be used when ascariasis is associated with other worm species. All infected persons must be treated for successful control of the disease. Public education programs teaching general hygiene are extremely important. Turning infested topsoil under is also helpful. The prognosis is good unless secondary complications such as pneumonia, intestinal obstruction, or perforation develop. The outlook then becomes more guarded.

Appendicitis

Inflammation caused by local obstruction or infection of the vermiform appendix, located at the base of the cecum, is a common indication for abdominal surgery. Children who have appendicitis typically consume a low roughage diet; thus the condition is largely preventable.

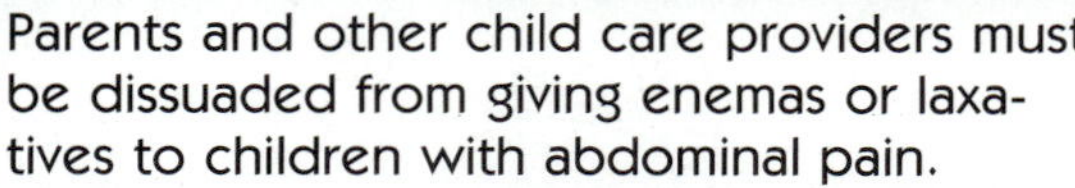

Nursing Alert

Parents and other child care providers must be dissuaded from giving enemas or laxatives to children with abdominal pain.

Clinical manifestations. Appendicitis is not easy to diagnose in young children. Other problems mimic the condition, and the young child is not often very descriptive regarding general discomfort. Pain may first be felt in the periumbilical area. Later it may be localized in the lower right abdominal quadrant. Restlessness, mild constipation or diarrhea, and anorexia followed by nausea and vomiting are often reported. A low grade fever is characteristic. The white blood cell count is usually elevated.

Treatment. If the inflamed appendix is removed before it has ruptured, recovery is usually prompt and uneventful. However, delay or the use of laxatives can result in the rupture of the appendix.

Peritonitis complicates appendicitis. Recovery is slower, and the risk to the patient increases. The patient with a ruptured appendix, related abscess, or peritonitis is very ill. This person usually cannot be sent to surgery immediately but must wait until the administration of antibiotics, intravenous fluids, and possible cooling measures are completed so that the patient is in the best condition possible for the appendectomy. A nasogastric tube is often passed to relieve flatus and prevent vomiting. At the time of surgery, a drain may be placed in the abdominal wound, and drainage may be significant. A high Fowler's position is maintained to prevent the spread of infection in the abdomen. Intravenous feedings are continued for several days postoperatively, and only ice chips or sips of water are allowed by mouth. Recording intake and output is important. Most patients have an uneventful postoperative course.

School-Age Child

Diabetes mellitus

Diabetes mellitus is the most common metabolic disorder of children. It is not a true digestive problem, since carbohydrates are reduced to glucose by the digestive system and the glucose is absorbed into the bloodstream. The difficulty arises because the islets of Langerhans in the pancreas fail to produce the hormone insulin. In the absence of sufficient insulin, utilization of glucose is impaired, and hyperglycemia with its acute and long-term manifestations results.

About 1 in 600 school-age children has a form of

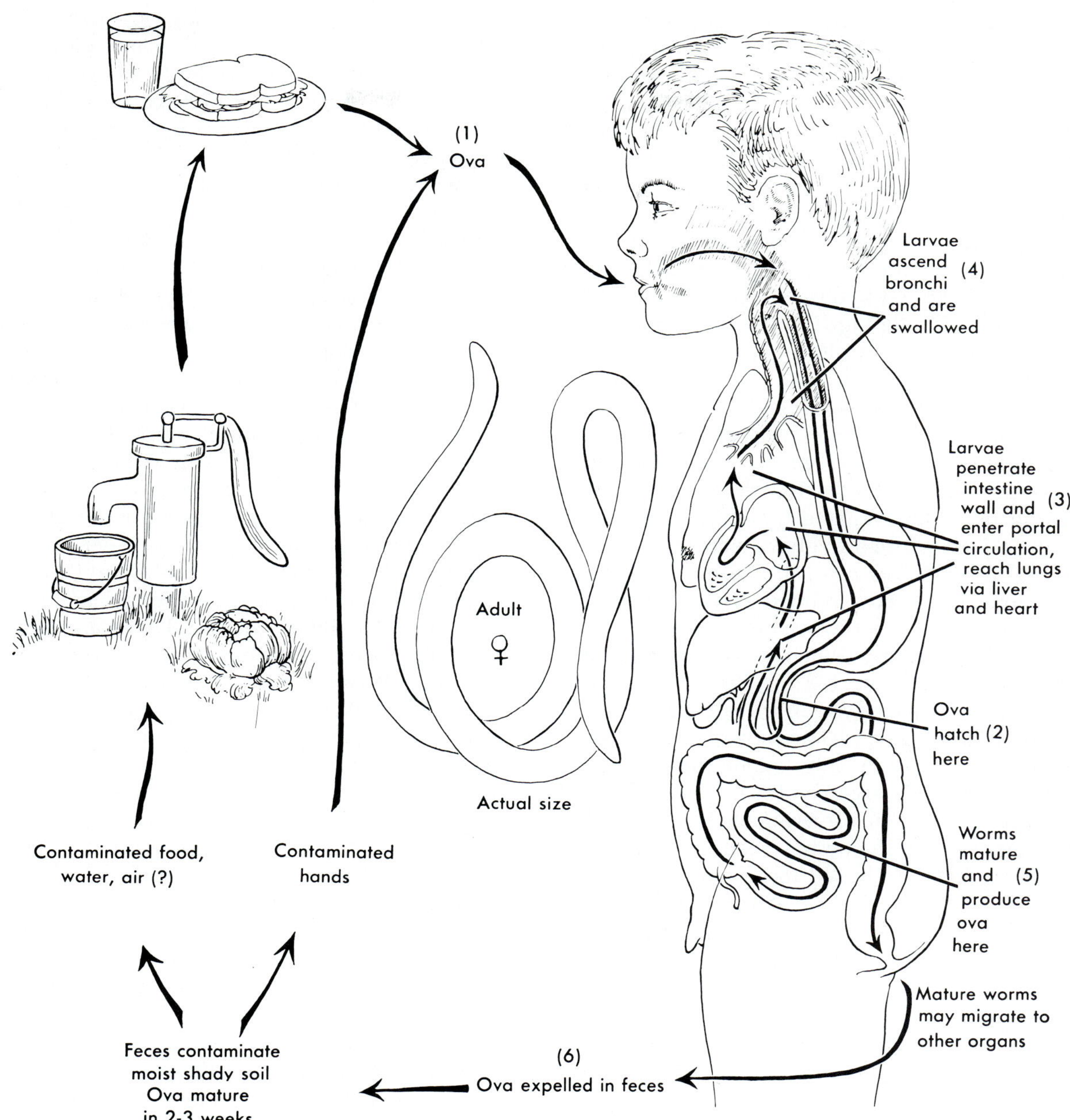

Fig. 35-7 Life cycle of *Ascaris lumbricoides.*

diabetes that requires insulin replacement throughout life. Males and females appear to be equally affected. No correlation with socioeconomic status has been found. Because varied etiological and pathological factors cause the different types of hyperglycemia, the term *insulin-dependent diabetes mellitus* (IDDM-1) is used most commonly to describe the disease exhibited by children and adolescents. In these patients diabetes usually begins before age 15. These children eventually demonstrate an absolute deficiency of insulin.

Although diabetes mellitus can manifest itself any time during a person's lifetime, the earlier the disease appears, the earlier that complications of the disease are encountered. During the first year after diagnosis of IDDM-1, the islets of Langerhans hypertrophy, causing an erratic production of insulin. As the condition progresses, the islets atrophy, finally becoming entirely incapable of insulin production. This is the main difference between IDDM-1, formerly termed *juvenile diabetes,* and maturity-onset diabetes

(IDDM-2), in which disturbed carbohydrate metabolism can be the result of many factors that together cause a relative decrease in the endogenous supply of needed insulin.

Etiological factors. The exact cause of diabetes mellitus is not known, but inheritance plays an important role. Evidence also indicates that certain environmental factors, such as toxins and viral infections, may precipitate the condition in susceptible persons through autoimmune destruction of the islet cells. Therefore it can be hypothesized that a genetic predisposition to developing IDDM-1 exists and that some unknown factor or insult can occur that precipitates the condition.

Pathophysiological factors. Insulin is important in the metabolism of carbohydrates, fats, and proteins. It is also required for efficient entry of glucose into skeletal muscle and fat cells. In insulin-dependent diabetes, glucose is unavailable for cellular metabolism. It cannot be converted to glycogen for storage in the liver and muscles nor can it be burned properly. Hyperglycemia and other compensatory symptoms occur as glucose utilization by tissue is impaired.

Clinical manifestations. When glucose concentration reaches approximately 180 mg/100 ml, glucose spills over into the urine (glycosuria), causing diuresis to occur (polyuria). Large amounts of water and electrolytes are lost, with subsequent dehydration. This is associated with excessive thirst (polydipsia).

When the amount of glucose available is insufficient to provide fuel to meet the body's needs, protein and fats are broken down and used to help furnish these necessities. However, metabolism of fat is not complete without the concurrent metabolism of carbohydrate. This incomplete fat metabolism produces ketone bodies (acetone, diacetic acid, and oxybutyric acid) that accumulate abnormally in the blood (ketonemia). Diacetic acid and oxybutyric acid must be neutralized in the body by bases, or alkalies. As the ketones are excreted, sodium, potassium, and neutralizing bases are also lost in the urine. The body's supply of base is depleted, the sensitive electrolyte balance is upset, and metabolic acidosis gradually develops (diabetic ketoacidosis).

Acute care. A serious complication of this disease is diabetic ketoacidosis (DKA). Severe dehydration, confusion, coma, and even death can occur unless the condition is reversed promptly by insulin and appropriate fluid replacement. DKA is truly a medical emergency requiring the close attention of a physician and a nurse at the bedside.

The goal of initial therapy is to improve circulation and then to correct the acidosis. Dehydration is often of the magnitude of 10%. An intravenous line is placed, and fluids are started immediately. Regular insulin is administered, usually as a bolus in normal saline, followed by an infusion to provide a constant steady insulin concentration in plasma. When acidosis is corrected (serum bicarbonate of 14 mEq/L or greater), insulin infusion is discontinued, and insulin is given subcutaneously. Blood glucose levels are monitored with a blood glucose monitor. Hypoglycemia must be prevented. When the blood sugar falls below 300 mg/dl, the intravenous fluids should contain enough glucose to keep up with the insulin. Since the urinary output is good, an acetest can be performed on a regular basis to give an indication that DKA is resolving. Intake and output are carefully plotted; vital signs should be monitored often; and any significant change should be reported promptly.

Treatment. Management during the period following control of DKA consists of establishing appropriate nutritional intake while discontinuing intravenous fluids and converting to subcutaneous insulin administration.

One of the essentials in the management of the child with diabetes is to provide a dosage of insulin that can effectively cover a 24-hour period. Approximately five types of insulin are available that are commonly used

Nursing Alert

The classic clinical symptoms of diabetes are polyuria, dehydration despite polydipsia, and weight loss despite polyphagia. Most children initially have a brief history of lethargy, weakness, and weight loss. Daily loss of water and glucose occur. Improper metabolism of fats and protein also occurs. Unexplained weight loss and polyuria or the resumption of nocturnal enuresis are indications for testing. Glycosuria, hyperglycemia, and ketonuria are diagnostic of insulin deficiency. No further tests are necessary to confirm the diagnosis.

Nursing Alert

Precipitating factors of diabetic ketoacidosis include trauma, infection, pregnancy, vomiting, or emotional stress. This life-threatening condition is relatively uncommon because of increased recognition of the classic symptoms of diabetes. However, a small number of children demonstrate repeated episodes of DKA, which can represent treatment failure or inadvertent or deliberate error by the patient in the administration of insulin.

in the management of the child with IDDM. Table 35-1 describes their activity. U-100 insulin is the standard concentration used. Special low-dose syringes are available to make doses more accurate. To maintain normal blood glucose levels, twice-a-day injections of a combination of short- and intermediate-acting insulins are often needed. For the prepubertal child, the total insulin dose generally does not exceed 1 unit per kilogram of body weight per day and is generally divided as follows: Two thirds of the dose is given before breakfast with longer-acting insulin and short-acting insulin in a 2-to-1 ratio; the predinner dose is composed of the remaining third of the total daily dose, with the longer- and short-acting insulins in equal doses. When both short-acting and intermediate-acting insulin are prescribed together, the two insulins should be drawn up in the same syringe and always in the same sequence, with the short-acting insulin drawn up first followed by the intermediate-acting preparation. This procedure ensures that any residual insulin in the "dead space" remains constant and that there is greater stability of the patient after a therapeutic dose has been established. The mixture should be injected within 5 minutes.

The "Honeymoon" period. During the initial presentation of IDDM-1, insulin requirements are 0.5 to 1.0 U insulin/kg/day, but after stabilization, insulin requirements decline as a result of partial recovery of the islet cells. This period, which lasts for up to 1 year, is characterized by easy control and general well being and is known as the *honeymoon period.* During the honeymoon period, normal blood sugar levels can usually be obtained with administration of a small daily dose of insulin.

> **Nursing Alert**
>
> Children most commonly have hypoglycemic episodes at 11 AM and 2 AM, when treated with split or mixed insulin dosing (combination short- and long-acting insulin morning and evening).

When children are regulated in the hospital, they are often placed on regular insulin coverage in addition to the two-dose schedule. Regular insulin has a rapid but relatively brief action. The amount of insulin that patients receive depends on the level of blood sugar and the presence or absence of urinary ketones. The sites of injection should be changed each day to prevent hypertrophy of subcutaneous fat. Children should be taught to keep a record of the daily placement of their insulin. Children 7 and 8 years of age express curiosity about the process of preparing the dosage, and many children are capable of giving their own injections (Fig. 35-8). Children must have considerable practice in preparing dosages with adequate supervision. They also should be taught about the actions of the different insulins to understand the relationship between regular, healthy dietary habits and insulin injections. Children and their parents need to know when the onset and the peak of action of the prescribed insulin occur, as well as its duration. Rotation of injection sites is essential.

At the onset of diabetes or after recovery from ketoacidosis, the total daily dose of insulin should range between 0.5 and 1 International Units (IU) of insulin per kilogram of body weight per day. The insulin dose can be adjusted at home so that the diet and exercise can be varied. This is done by adjusting the short-acting insulin, keeping in mind anticipated exercise and food.

Exercise. An integral component of growth and development is exercise, and children with diabetes should be encouraged to participate in any activity they like, including competitive sports. However, exercise decreases insulin requirements by increasing the sensitivity of skeletal muscle to insulin. Appropriate adjustments in food intake and insulin dosage must

♦ TABLE 35-1
Insulins Commonly Used in the Management of Children with Insulin-Dependent Diabetes Mellitus (IDDM-1)

Type of Insulin	Appearance	Onset (Hours)	Peak (Hours)	Duration (Hours)
Rapid action—short duration				
Regular	Clear	½-1	2-4	6-8
Semilente	Cloudy	½-1	2-4	8-10
Intermediate action—longer duration				
Globin	Clear	1-2	6-8	12-14
NPH	Cloudy	1-2	6-8+	12-14
Lente	Cloudy	1-2+	6-12	14-16

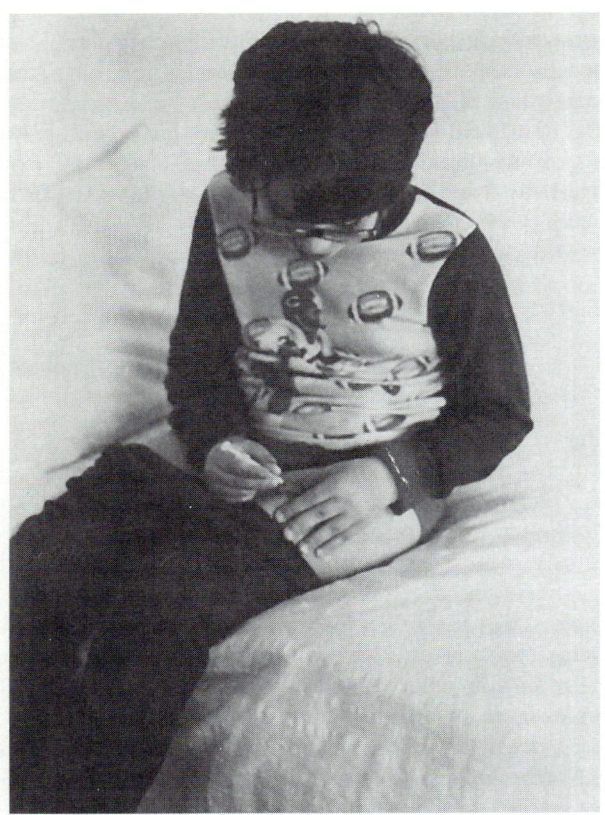

Fig. 35-8 School-age children are able to administer their own insulin. (From Wong D: *Essentials of pediatric nursing,* ed 4, St. Louis, 1993, Mosby.)

be considered. If exercise is increased or decreased, food intake must be adjusted accordingly.

Nutritional intake. The nutritional intake of a child with diabetes should be comparable to that of the healthy nondiabetic child of the same age, gender, weight, and level of activity. Since the amount and type of insulin prescribed depends on caloric intake, regularity of caloric intake for the fixed dose of insulin becomes vital.

Total calories should be adjusted to meet the individual child's needs relative to growth, activity, and appetite. Sensitivity to ethnicity, culture, and socioeconomic status is also important for meal planning. The American Diabetic Association has prepared a simplified method of calculating food intake based on the concept of food exchanges. Six basic exchanges are listed, and within each exchange a wide variety of foods can be substituted or exchanged. Common foods should be used that can be modified to meet the tastes and economic needs of the child and family. Emphasis should be placed on regularity of food intake and on the constancy of carbohydrate intake, avoiding simple sugars (see box above right).

DAILY NUTRITIONAL REQUIREMENTS THIS SUGGESTED GUIDE SHOULD BE MODIFIED IF ADDITIONAL EXERCISE IS PLANNED OR IF THE CHILD BECOMES ILL

PREPUBESCENT
65 kcal/kg
(30 kcal/lb)

PUBESCENT AND POSTPUBESCENT
35 kcal/kg
(16 kcal/lb)

COMPOSITION OF CALORIES
Should supply sufficient calories to meet the needs of exercise, growth, and appetite

Carbohydrate	50%-55%	(Avoid sucrose)
Fat	30%	(Use polyunsaturated fats)
Protein	15%-20%	

MEAL PLAN
Caloric intake should be divided into 3 meals and 2 or 3 snacks based on the individual's lifestyle and on the dynamics of insulin

Breakfast	4/18
Midmorning	1/18
Lunch	5/18
Midafternoon	2/18
Dinner	5/18
Bedtime	1/18

Nutritional intake should be evaluated annually to compensate for growth. Referral or consultation with the nutritionist should be made whenever necessary.

Insulin-food relationships. In the hospital the patient's nutritional intake is carefully measured to establish a baseline. Using the blood glucose patterns and the child's appetite, it is modified as needed. No food or liquids should be given, with the exception of water, without patient orders. The patient should be encouraged to eat all the food served on the tray on time. Before serving a tray, the nursing staff should determine whether the child has received any ordered insulin. The type of insulin the patient receives dictates when the meal should be served. The glucose content of any uneaten portion is calculated, and a liquid replacement is sent to the patient. An inability to eat or an emesis should be promptly reported. The way in which the child is adhering to the nutritional intake should be carefully reported and recorded. Conferences in which the nurse, physician, and nutritionist collaborate with the child and family are arranged.

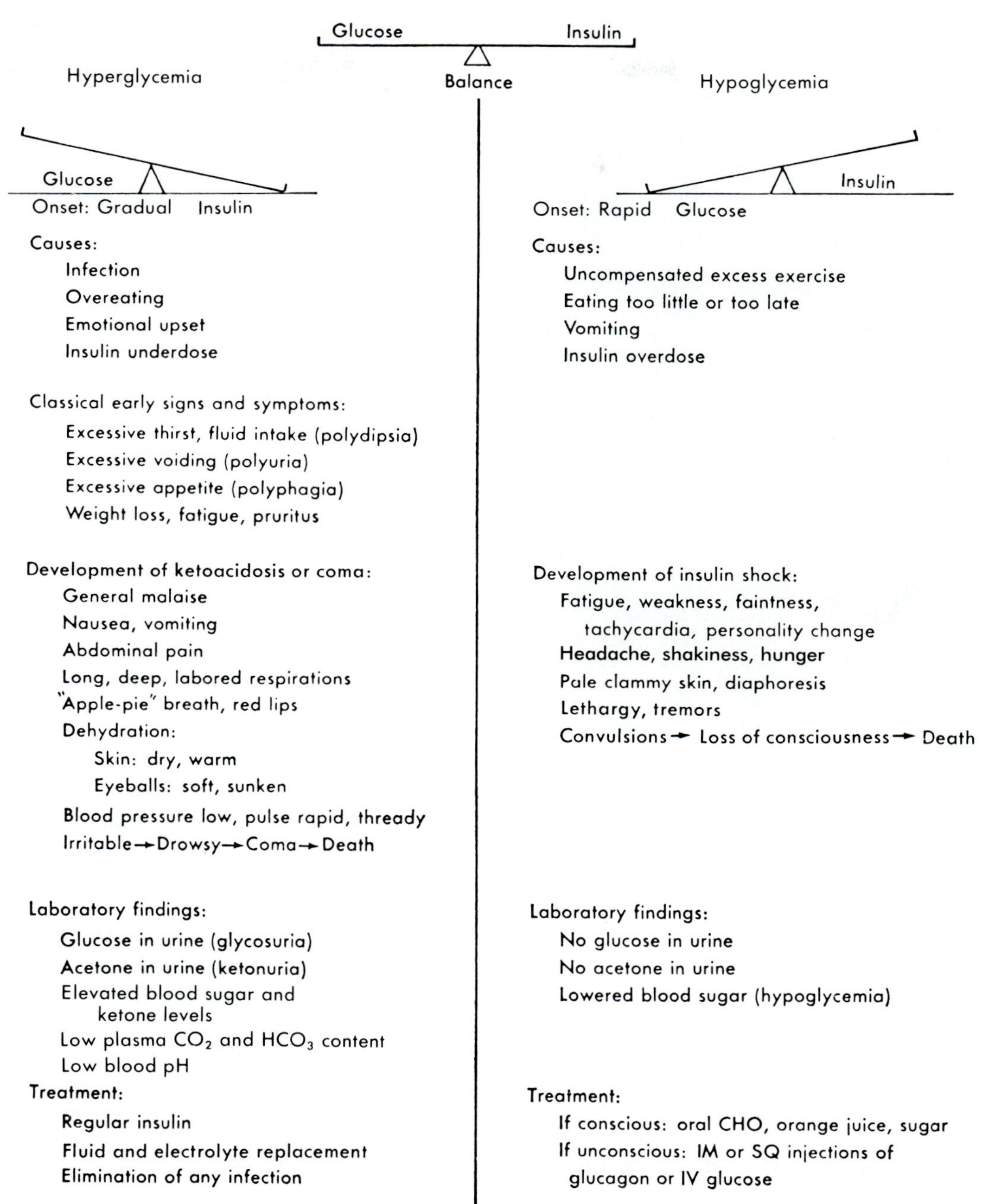

Fig. 35-9 Glucose-insulin balance chart.

When children contribute to the plan of care compliance is improved greatly.

Hypoglycemia (insulin-induced hypoglycemia). Insulin itself can cause problems. Too much insulin can be disastrous as the resultant hypoglycemia can cause severe neurological damage. A balance between the insulin needed and the insulin available must be maintained to prevent either hyperglycemia or hypoglycemia (Fig. 35-9).

Clinical manifestations. Nurses and patients and their families should be familiar with the early signs of hypoglycemia so that it can be easily counteracted Children learn to recognize their symptoms well. Unlike hyperglycemia, hypoglycemia can develop rapidly, within minutes or hours. The first signs of insulin-induced hypoglycemia are diaphoresis and personality change. This change can take various forms, depending on the patient; each person usually

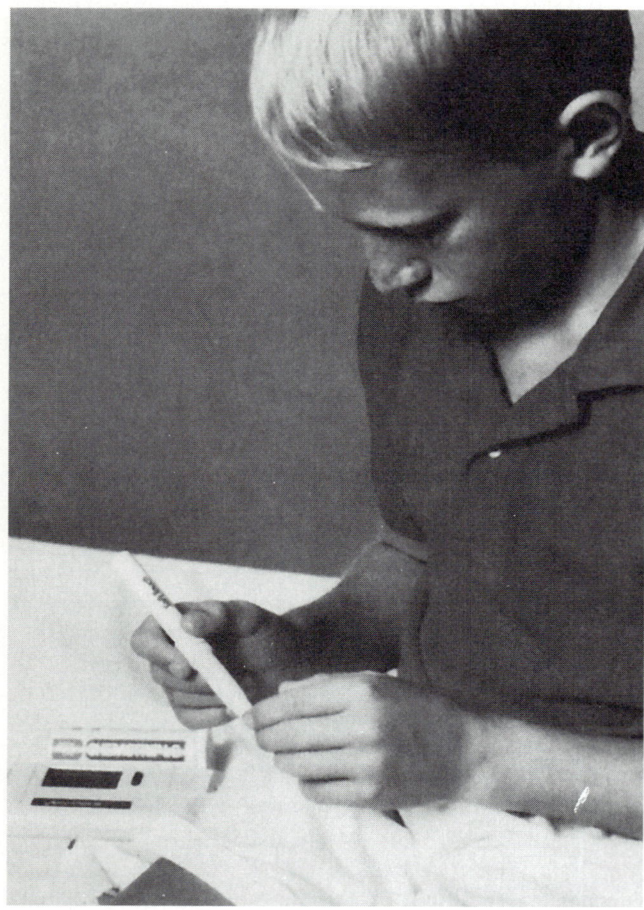

Fig. 35-10 Child using "finger stick" method to obtain blood sample with glucose monitor and reagent strips nearby. (From Wong D: *Essentials of pediatric nursing,* ed 4, St. Louis, 1993, Mosby.)

reacts in a way that is particularly characteristic for that individual. If the condition is not relieved, the patient can develop shock, become unconscious, and possibly have convulsions. Intractable hypoglycemia can cause severe brain damage.

Treatment. Nurses should be prepared to teach children and family members how to conduct home blood glucose monitoring (HBGM). This self-care technique provides a more accurate assessment of blood glucose levels than urine testing, thus the glucose-insulin balance can be maintained more effectively. A spring-loaded puncturing device is recommended for children (Fig. 35-10). However, the parents and children should also know how to use a lancet in the event of mechanical failure.

All persons with diabetes should carry some rapidly available source of glucose in the event they feel the beginning of an insulin reaction. Glucose tablets and gel are recommended. In the hospital a small glass of orange juice or crackers is usually given. If no improvement is obtained in 15 minutes, additional food should be given. If the child has difficulty taking the necessary oral glucose, an intramuscular or subcutaneous injection of glucagon is ordered. Glucagon activates liver enzymes that break down liver glycogen to produce glucose. It must be remembered that glucagon does not work in the glycogen-depleted child. However, when the hypoglycemia is caused by excess insulin, the liver glycogen stores should be generous, since such storage is enhanced by insulin. The family needs to know that glucagon should be given one time only for each episode and that the child should be fed immediately. Glucagon is available in 1-mg vials. The typical dose is 0.5 mg (or one-half vial) for children under 1 year of age and 1 mg for older children. The intramuscular route is preferred because of more rapid absorption. It usually takes 10 to 20 minutes for glucagon to work. Sometimes intravenous administration by the physician of a 20% to 50% solution of glucose is required. If the patient has been given a slow-acting, long-duration insulin, response to therapy for hypoglycemia can be slow and treatment more complex. The primary care provider and the child's endocrinologist should always be notified of the occurrence of insulin reactions. When a patient complains of symptoms of possible reaction or the nurse is suspicious that such a process is occurring, blood glucose should be evaluated immediately using one of the quick assays. At times it is difficult to determine clinically whether the complaints and appearance of the patient are caused by the lack of glucose or too much glucose in the blood. If no laboratory test is feasible, glucagon or intravenous glucose is often ordered. If the difficulty is caused by insulin reaction, the patient responds. If it is not, no real harm has been done. Hypoglycemia should be treated promptly. Prolonged, severe hypoglycemia can cause brain damage and subsequent mental deterioration, impaired motor coordination, and even death.

As can be seen from Fig. 35-9, a number of causes exist for insulin excess and resulting reactions. Probably the most common cause is uncompensated excessive exercise. Exercise causes sugar to be metabolized more effectively because of increased efficiency of insulin. Unless insulin dosage is reduced or glucose is increased, hypoglycemia is likely in the presence of unplanned exercise. Thus it is important for the child with diabetes to have periods of regular exercise suitably spaced after meals and to recognize the possibility of short-acting insulin adjustment to compensate for special activities.

Another cause of hypoglycemia is failure to eat, to eat enough, or to space the food intake appropriately.

Midmorning, midafternoon, and bedtime snacks are essential for small children but can be impractical for teen-aged children, who feel odd eating a snack at school. In a hospital setting the nurse should be sure snacks are given to and are consumed by the patient. If the child is nauseated or has an emesis, this should be immediately reported because this condition can also lead to hypoglycemia. Meals must be served on time. A long delay after the injection of regular insulin also sets the stage for an episode of hypoglycemia.

Difficulties in determining appropriate doses of insulin are also a source of glucose-insulin imbalance. The patient may not respond to the dosage as expected. Errors in insulin administration resulting in an overdose are also a real possibility. Great care must be taken in reading the orders and in preparing the injection. One strength (U-100) of insulin is available in both short-acting and intermediate-acting insulin.

The following technique must be followed to prevent the conversion of short-acting insulin into an intermediate-acting type by inadvertent injection of intermediate insulin into a vial of regular insulin:

1 Just enough replacement air must be injected into the bottle of cloudy (e.g., NPH) insulin without dipping the injecting needle into the insulin. The needle is then removed from the bottle.
2 The short-acting insulin should be withdrawn into the syringe, using the proper scale.
3 The intermediate insulin is then withdrawn into the syringe, using the proper scale.
4 An air bubble is put into the syringe and the syringe rocked back and forth to mix the two insulin types.

Hyperglycemia. Hyperglycemia occurs when the insulin available in the blood is insufficient to metabolize the glucose present. The most frequent cause of hyperglycemia is the onset of infection or illness. Infection greatly intensifies the body's need for insulin, and unless insulin dosage is adjusted, hyperglycemia can result. Prompt attention to even minor infections in the child with diabetes can prevent progression to a serious metabolic disturbance.

Failing to follow the prescribed meal pattern may be the source of the problem. It takes a great deal of self-discipline to refrain from eating some of the tempting but forbidden foods available. Development of self-control is of paramount importance for the young child and particularly for the adolescent. Nutritional discipline should be encouraged by allowing the child to participate in planning and making provisions for special occasions. The availability of so many 1-calorie soft drinks has made the social lives of teenagers with diabetes mellitus a bit less difficult. However, they should be cautioned that the label "dietetic foods" does not necessarily mean "foods for the diabetic." These foods are expensive, and children can have regular dessert items occasionally in moderate amounts.

Emotional upset also increases the possibility of hyperglycemia. The insulin requirement rises in periods of stress. The emotionally stable child is much easier to regulate with insulin than a child with multiple emotional stressors. Emotional problems are the most common cause of hyperglycemia in adolescents. Possible errors in the administration of insulin that can result in an underdose, as well as an overdose, must be prevented.

The need for insulin progressively increases as the child reaches sexual maturation and adolescence. Failure to increase insulin dosage leads to the development of hyperglycemia and ketosis. Under these circumstances, the daily dose of insulin may exceed 1.0 IU/kg/day. However, caution must be exercised in preventing rebound hyperglycemia, the Somogyi effect.

Somogyi phenomenon. Children receiving high doses of insulin, 1 to 2 IU/kg/day, are likely to have behavior changes, early morning sweating, restless sleep, or headaches. Other children may be asymptomatic but rapidly develop glycosuria and ketosis. This is the rebound phenomenon first described by Somogyi. The Somogyi phenomenon is comprised of repeated periods of unapparent hypoglycemia followed by rebound hyperglycemia. Treatment for the Somogyi phenomenon is frequent blood glucose checks and immediate reduction of insulin dosage.

Blood glucose self-monitoring. Before children are ready to give themselves insulin injections, they are able to test their own blood using reagent strips and a meter to determine the glucose level. Blood testing is accomplished by using specially designed lancets for obtaining fingerstick samples or by an automatic finger-pricking device. The drops of blood are placed on a reagent strip, and the resultant color change correlates with the blood sugar. This can be accomplished visually or by using a reflectance meter, such as the Accu-Chek II m (Fig. 35-11) or One Touch II. When using a blood glucose monitor, the instrument must be carefully programmed with the correct programming strip. The manufacturer's directions must be followed, especially the timing during the procedure. Blood glucose testing is one of the best ways to help control diabetes.

Testing should be done 30 minutes before eating and at least twice daily, before breakfast and the morning insulin and before dinner and the evening insulin. These results, when looked at in terms of 2- to 4-day trends, give enough information to justify or change the current insulin dosage. In addition, blood glucose levels should be done once per week before lunch to

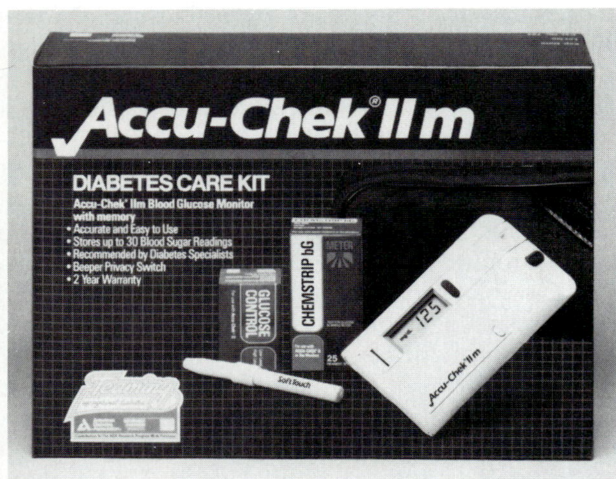

Fig. 35-11 AccuChek II-m is a battery-powered meter that uses test strips to measure blood sugar. It gives blood sugar results immediately, thus allowing home blood glucose monitoring and an accurate way to plan diet, exercise, and medication changes. (Courtesy Boehringer Mannheim Corporation, Indianapolis, Ind.)

ensure that the morning short-acting insulin is appropriate and at bedtime to evaluate the evening short-acting insulin. It is also important to measure the blood glucose at 2 AM or 3AM at least once a week because blood glucose concentration is lowest and insulin reactions may occur. Blood glucose measurements should not be less than 70 mg/dl to avoid hypoglycemia.

When the blood sugar exceeds 200 mg/dl on two successive occasions, the patient should check urine for ketones. If ketones are negative, the acute hyperglycemia should *not* be managed with more insulin. Only when the ketones are positive with a simultaneous elevation in blood sugar should extra insulin be given. The parents should contact the child's health care provider to get advice and to provide advance notice that DKA may be impending.

Long-term goals and prognosis. Long-term care begins immediately after the initial hospitalization and control of ketoacidosis. The goals of long-term care are these: (1) promotion of normal growth and development both physically and emotionally; (2) maintenance of a high level of metabolic control; (3) instruction of the child and family in the skills of self-care; and (4) healthy adaptation to chronic illness.

Advances in the therapeutic use of insulin have provided a reasonable approach to the treatment of children. Vascular disease follows within the second decade after diagnosis if control has not been well maintained. The vascular lesions are of two main types: (1) premature atherosclerosis leading to a high morbidity and mortality from cardiovascular, cerebrovascular, and renal disease and (2) microangiopathy or peripheral vascular insufficiency (caused by thickening of capillary basement membranes), leading to retinopathy and blindness, progressive renal failure, and various neuropathies. Poorly controlled IDDM-1 in children is associated with earlier vascular complications.

Recent advances in the care of children with IDDM-1 indicate that consistent improvement in life expectancy can be accomplished when plasma-glucose levels are maintained as close to normal as possible. To date this is approximated in most children by the split-dose insulin regimen and a multiple feeding plan.

Research efforts continue in the search for the exact cause and prevention of diabetes. In the meantime, technological advances in the monitoring of IDDM-1 continue to be sought in an effort to prevent or reduce the long-term complications. A portable insulin pump that is designed to mimic the release of insulin by the pancreas is now being used successfully with some children, after years of research trials with adults. This approach is costly and carries some degree of risk.

Review of nursing responsibility.

1. Take a careful history regarding the child's home environment, educational experience, activities, goals, and aspirations. Get to know the child and family.
2. Insulin requirement: know the type of insulin prescribed, when the patient receives injections, and when to rotate sites.
3. Nutrition: know the amount of calories prescribed, the diet ordered, what was actually consumed and replaced, if the patient is consuming other foods not on the diet, and if the patient has a scheduled interval nourishment.
4. Blood glucose testing: know the method used, how to collect the specimens properly, and where to record the results.
5. General hygiene: know how to balance exercise regimen with insulin, how to assess the condition of the skin, and how to assess for signs of infection.
6. Glucose-insulin imbalance: assess the signs and symptoms of hypoglycemia and hyperglycemia.
7. Patient-parent education and participation: assess the patient and parent's level of understanding of the disease and its treatment and control. Assess if self-care or overdependence is being promoted and whether records of insulin intake, blood glucose tests, and general health are being kept.

For diabetic patients to engage in self-care and

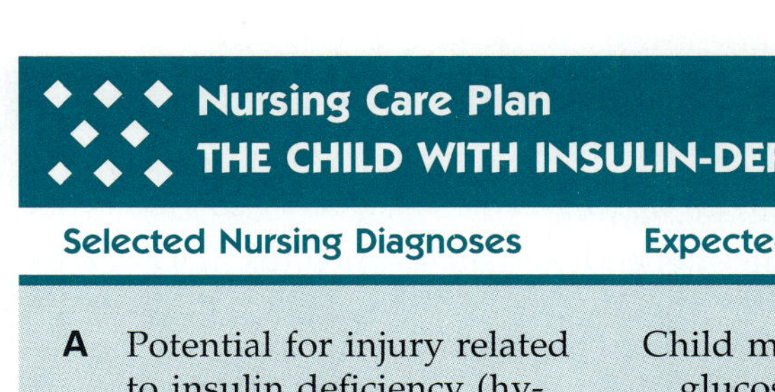

Nursing Care Plan
THE CHILD WITH INSULIN-DEPENDENT DIABETES MELLITUS I (IDDM-I)

Selected Nursing Diagnoses	Expected Outcomes	Interventions
A Potential for injury related to insulin deficiency (hyperglycemia). Clinical manifestations: Blood glucose elevated (180 mg/ml), glucosuria, polydipsia, polyphagia, polyuria, weight loss, dehydration, and dry skin.	Child maintains blood glucose level between 70 and 120.	Monitor blood glucose levels before meals and at bedtime. Administer/supervise child's administration of insulin as ordered by physician before breakfast and dinner. Monitor child's food intake and encourage child to eat planned meals. Offer snacks between meals and at bedtime, and encourage child to eat snack. Record foods not eaten and give replacement as needed. Encourage regularity of daily activity and exercise.
B Potential for injury related to insulin excess (hypoglycemia). Clinical manifestations: Blood glucose level below 70, fatigue, personality change, weakness, hunger, shakiness, drowsiness, pallor, and diaphoresis.	Child maintains blood glucose level between 70 and 120.	Check blood glucose level and report to physician. Administer orange juice or other sugar substitute or glucagon as ordered by physician. Evaluate feeding schedule and feed if appropriate. Evaluate insulin dosage. Evaluate activity.
C Knowledge deficit related to home management of child. Clinical manifestations: Need for information. Request for information.	Child/parent describes and demonstrates understanding of condition: dietary management; insulin injections; exercise needs and blood glucose monitoring.	Review/teach child and parents: a. Dietary exchange plan b. How to mix insulin c. How to administer injections d. Action and adverse side effects of insulin e. Exercise need to maintain physical fitness f. Use of blood glucose monitor and interpretation g. Signs of hyperglycemia and hypoglycemia Provide practice sessions to ensure understanding of lesson.

maintain an optimal quality of life, they must understand their disease, accept the limitations it imposes, and learn to function in a relatively independent setting. It is very helpful for patients with diabetes mellitus to be able to room together in the hospital. They usually are mutually supportive and learn from one another. Most of the time such learning is positive and beneficial. Children with this disorder should be encouraged to participate in school, religious, and community activities and to be open with teachers, peers, and employers regarding their diagnosis. Special summer camping experiences are available through the American Diabetes Association in most states.

KEY CONCEPTS

1 Thrush results from contamination of the infant's oral cavity with vaginal secretions containing *Candida albicans* at the time of birth, from improper hygiene and feeding techniques after birth, or as a sign of an immune deficiency. Thrush can be treated with nystatin oral suspension.

2 Congenital pyloric stenosis is the abnormal narrowing of the pyloric sphincter, caused by spasm of the sphincter, local edema, and an overgrowth of the circular muscle fibers of the pylorus. Symptoms include progressive vomiting and malnutrition. Treatment is usually surgical.

3 Most explanations of the pain associated with colic involve the presence of excessive gas in the digestive tract. Excessive air can result from poor bottle-feeding techniques, excessive use of carbohydrate in formula, or a tense, nervous infant and parent.

4 Dehydration and electrolyte imbalance are significant dangers when diarrheal disease causes profuse fluid loss in a young child. Severe diarrhea usually subsides when fluid and electrolyte therapy is administered intravenously and oral intake is reduced for a brief period.

5 Inguinal and umbilical hernias are common in infancy and childhood. About 90% of inguinal hernias are found in males. Repair is a common surgical procedure. Umbilical hernias often close spontaneously when the child learns to stand and walk. If this does not occur, repair is recommended for girls over 2 years and boys over 4 years of age.

6 Oxyuriasis, the disease caused by pinworms, causes few symptoms other than anal itching and secondary complications caused by scratching. Mebendazole is an effective treatment in most cases. Thorough cleansing and good personal hygiene must be stressed.

7 Round worm infestation causes ascariasis, which is perpetuated by poor sanitary facilities and poor hygiene practices. Treatment by piperazine citrate is effective. Public education programs teaching general hygiene are important.

8 Diabetes mellitus is the most common metabolic disorder of children. Insufficient insulin is produced, utilization of glucose is impaired, and hyperglycemia with its acute and long-term manifestations results.

9 Insulin-dependent diabetes mellitus (IDDM-1) describes the disease exhibited by children and adolescents. The classic clinical symptoms are polyuria, dehydration despite polydipsia, and weight loss despite polyphagia.

10 Diabetic ketoacidosis (DKA) is a serious complication of IDDM-1. Precipitating factors include trauma, infection, pregnancy, vomiting, and emotional stress.

11 Approximately five types of insulin may be used in the management of a child with IDDM-1. Action of these insulin types varies in onset, peak, and duration.

12 The amount of exercise and nutritional intake of a child with diabetes should be comparable to that of a healthy, nondiabetic child of the same age and gender. Exercise level, food intake, and insulin requirements are interdependent.

13 The first signs of insulin-induced hypoglycemia are diaphoresis and personality change. A source of glucose such as orange juice, a glucose tablet, or crackers should be given. If the child has difficulty taking oral glucose, an intramuscular or subcutaneous injection of glucagon is ordered.

14 Causes of hypoglycemia include uncompensated excessive exercise, failure to eat enough or to space food intake appropriately, and difficulties in determining appropriate doses of insulin.

15 Hyperglycemia occurs when the insulin available in the blood is insufficient to metabolize the glucose present. The most common cause is the onset of infection or illness. Other precipitating factors may include failure to follow the prescribed meal pattern, emotional upset, and errors in insulin administration.

16 The Somogyi phenomenon involves repeated periods of unapparent hypoglycemia followed by rebound hyperglycemia. Treatment includes frequent blood glucose checks and immediate reduction of insulin dosage.

17 Blood glucose testing is one of the best ways to help control diabetes. Children are able to test their own blood to determine the glucose level using reagent strips and a blood glucose monitor.

CRITICAL THOUGHT QUESTIONS

1 What clinical manifestations could indicate problems with the gastrointestinal tract? Why are vomiting and diarrhea particularly significant in an infant or young child? What nursing interventions are used in these situations?

2 What is a hernia? Compare and contrast the different types of hernias and the recommended interventions.

3 Discuss the significance of metabolic disorders such as galactosemia and phenylketonuria. When and how are these diagnosed? Discuss the dietary considerations related to these diseases. How can you help the child and the family to deal with the dietary restrictions?

4 Identify the most common parasitic and bacterial diseases of the intestine. How are these diseases most often acquired? How are they spread? How can they be recognized? What diagnostic tests are used? What is the typical treatment? How can the nurse reduce the spread of these parasites?

5 Describe the cause and pathophysiological conditions of diabetes mellitus. What are the signs and symptoms? Diagnostic tests? What is the current treatment? What are the nursing responsibilities when caring for a diabetic child?

6 Control of diabetes involves careful balance of diet, insulin, and exercise. Why is this particularly difficult in the child? Consider the developmental tasks of adolescence. Why might the adolescent diabetic rebel and deviate from the treatment plan? What can the nurse do to help?

REFERENCES

Brown K: Dietary management of acute childhood diarrhea:optimal time of feeding, *J Pediatr* 118(4)S92-S98, 1991.

Crowe L and Billingsley JI: The rowdy reactors: maintaining a support group for teenagers with diabetes, *Diabetes Educator* 16(1):39, 1990.

Jonides L: Infant with gastroesophageal reflux and fever, *J Pediatr Health Care* 8(1):41-48, 1994.

Orenstein S: Gastroesophageal reflux. In R Wylie and J Hyams, editors: *Pediatric gastrointestinal disease: pathopysiology, diagnosis, management,* Philadelphia, 1993, WB Saunders.

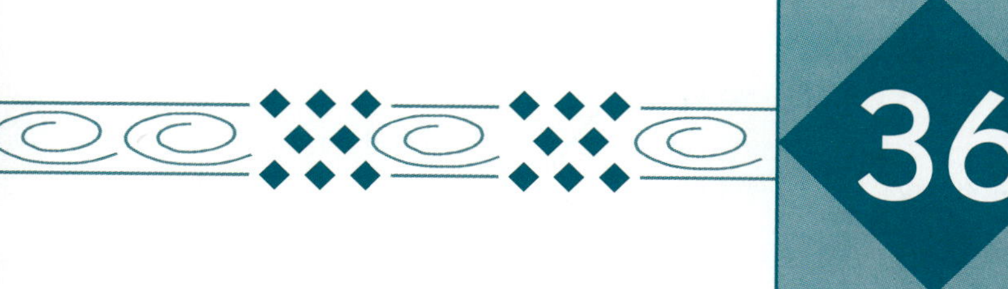
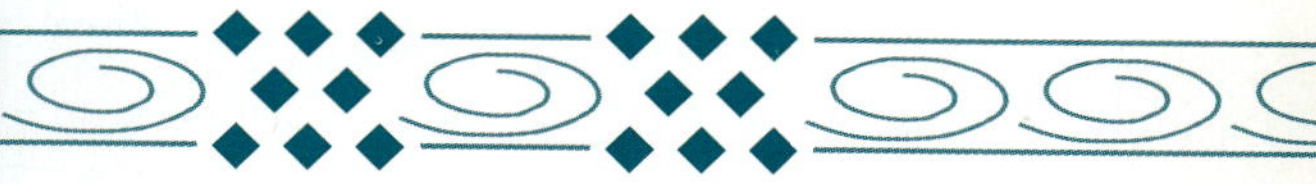

36

Conditions Involving the Genitourinary System

CHAPTER OBJECTIVES

After studying this chapter, the student should be able to:

1. Define the terms listed in the key vocabulary.
2. List three congenital abnormalities of the genitourinary tract and name three possible signs of internal structural genitourinary problems in the newborn.
3. Discuss the need for surgical correction of significant hypospadias and the postoperative observation and care required.
4. Discuss the need for correction of cryptorchidism and the methods of treatment.
5. Indicate three factors or conditions that may be associated with an increased incidence of urinary tract infections.
6. Identify four possible signs of urinary tract infection in the child under 3 years of age and three signs and symptoms characteristic of school-age children.
7. Emphasize the importance of treating pediatric urinary reflux and indicate three significant postoperative nursing considerations when ureteral reimplantation is performed.
8. Describe the common relationship between kidney disease and the potential development of hypertension in children.
9. Outline the nursing needs of the hospitalized child with generalized edema associated with childhood nephrotic syndrome.
10. Discuss enuresis, describing its incidence in the pediatric population, the physical, maturational, and psychological considerations that may be involved, and the therapies that can be used.

URINARY SYSTEM

The urinary system consists of two kidneys, two ureters, the bladder, and the urethra (Fig. 36-1). The primary function of these organs is to excrete metabolic waste products. The kidneys perform additional functions, such as the production of renin, which controls blood pressure, and erythropoietin, which stimulates red blood cell synthesis. To regulate the composition of blood, the kidneys perform the complex task of producing urine. The ureters, bladder, and urethra are involved in the transportation, storage, and elimination of the urine.

KEY VOCABULARY

agenesis Absence.
anuria Lack of urine formation.
albuminuria Presence of albumin in the urine.
bacteriuria Presence of bacteria in the urine.
enuresis Involuntary loss of urine in daytime or nighttime, after the age by which bladder control should have been established.
frequency Number of repetitions of a periodic process in a unit of time; when speaking of urinary func-

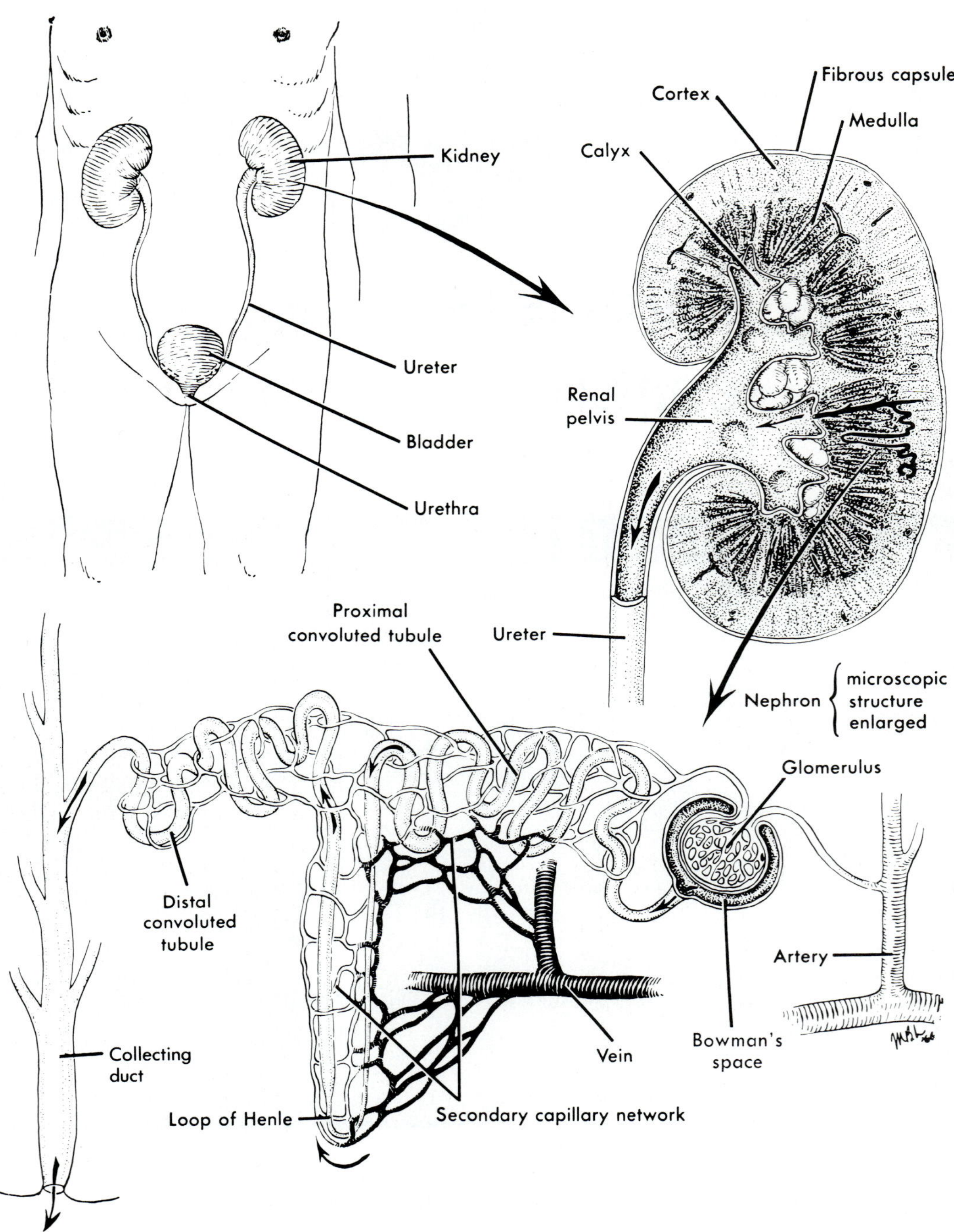

Fig. 36-1 Gross and microscopic structures of urinary system.

tion, the term implies an abnormal increase in the number of voidings.

hematuria Presence of blood in the urine.

hydronephrosis Collection of urine in the renal pelvis because of obstructed outflow producing distention and atrophy of the kidney.

nocturia Excessive urination during the night.

oliguria Diminished amount of urine production with subsequent scanty urination.

polyuria Abnormally increased urinary output.

proteinuria Presence of protein, usually albumin, in the urine.

pyuria Abnormal white blood cells in the urine.
uremia Toxic condition associated with renal insufficiency and the retention in the blood of nitrogenous substances normally excreted by the kidney.
urgency Patient cannot wait to void.
vesicoureteral reflux Regurgitation of urine from the bladder into the ureter.

Kidneys

The kidneys are paired organs located in the retroperitoneal cavity on each side of the vertebral column, just above the waistline. They lie outside the peritoneal cavity against the muscle of the posterior abdominal wall. In the adult the kidneys are about 4½ inches (11.5 cm) long and 2½ inches (6.4 cm) wide; they are somewhat bean-shaped. On the medial border of each kidney is a concave notch called the *hilus*. The renal artery, renal vein, nerves, and ureter join the kidney at the hilus.

When describing the internal structure of the organ, one may speak of two areas: the functioning portion, the *parenchyma*, and the collecting portion, the *pelvis*. A longitudinal section of the kidney reveals that the parenchyma in turn is composed of two parts: an outer portion called the *cortex* and an inner portion called the *medulla*. The pelvis is formed by the expansion of the upper end of the ureter. The pelvis subdivides to form the major and minor *calyces* (singular, calyx).

The parenchyma of each kidney consists of approximately 1 million functional units called *nephrons*. Each nephron has two parts: the glomerulus and the tubule. The glomerulus is a collection of specialized capillaries. Bowman's capsule is the outer layer of the glomerulus. It functions in the filtration of urine. The tubule has three main parts: the proximal convoluted tubule, the loop of Henle, and the distal convoluted tubule. Each nephron unit is linked by a connecting segment to the collecting duct, which drains urine into the renal pelvis. The glomeruli and the convoluted tubules are in the cortex. The medulla contains the loop of Henle. The collecting duct begins in the cortex and traverses the medulla.

The kidneys perform the complex task of removing toxic metabolic wastes, such as urea and uric acid, and excessive amounts of substances, such as water and electrolytes, from the blood. In this way the kidneys regulate the composition and volume of blood.

Three processes are involved in the production of urine: filtration, reabsorption, and secretion.

1 *Filtration* occurs in the glomerulus. As blood flows through the lumen of the glomerular capillary, some of the water, salts, and other small molecules are filtered through capillary walls and enter Bowman's space. Blood cells, platelets, and most plasma proteins are not filtered but remain in the capillary lumen because of their large size. The liquid that has passed into Bowman's space is called the *filtrate*. The filtrate flows down the lumen of the tubule, where it is modified by reabsorption and secretion. The modified filtrate eventually becomes urine.
2 *Reabsorption* occurs through the walls of the convoluted tubules, the loop of Henle, and the collecting duct. By means of a very complex process, the tubular cells reabsorb water, glucose, electrolytes, and other molecules from the filtrate. This reclamation process is vital to the maintenance of the fluid and electrolyte balance of the body.
3 *Secretion* takes place in the tubules. In the proximal convoluted tubules, medications such as penicillin, and dyes used to test renal function, iodopyracet, phenolsulfonphthalein, and hippuric acid, are among the substances secreted. In the distal convoluted tubule, hydrogen ions and ammonia are secreted in the varying amounts necessary to control and maintain the acid-base balance of the body. Sodium is exchanged for either potassium or hydrogen ion by a pump that is stimulated by the hormone aldosterone.

The modified filtrate first passes from the distal convoluted tubule into the straight collecting duct, where water is reabsorbed. From there it enters the renal pelvis as urine. In the normal adult the amount of filtrate is very great—generally 190 L per day. Large amounts of water and salt must be reabsorbed to keep the body fluids in balance. The tubules reclaim about 188.5 L, the remaining 1.5 L is excreted as urine. The average daily urinary output of urine varies greatly with the size of the child and the fluid intake. Urine output is approximatley 750 $ml/m^2/day$ or 1 to 2 ml/kg/hour.

Ureters

In the adult the ureters are small tubes about ⅕ inch (0.5 cm) in diameter and 12 inches (30 cm) in length. (The size varies with age.) The expanded upper end of the ureter collects the urine from the kidney, and peristaltic waves convey the urine down the ureters and into the bladder. The ureters lie behind the peritoneum and descend from the kidney to the posterior bladder wall. They enter the bladder in an oblique manner, preventing reflux, or backflow, of urine.

Bladder

The bladder is a dome-shaped, hollow, muscular sac that stores urine. It is located directly behind the symphysis pubis. Intertwining muscle bundles form the bladder wall. These muscular layers are collectively called the *detrusor muscle.* The internal sphincter is composed of smooth muscle bundles at the bladder outlet. The bladder outlet and the two ureteral openings outline a triangular area called the *trigone.*

The detrusor muscle is usually relaxed, allowing the bladder to expand as needed to accommodate urine storage. After a certain volume of urine is collected, the urge to void is felt. The desire to void is recorded by the sensory parasympathetic endings in the detrusor muscle. If the child decides to void, the detrusor muscle contracts, the internal sphincter opens, and urine enters the urethra. In the child who has developed neurological bladder control (2 to 3 years of age), voiding may be postponed, but when the bladder becomes very full, a point is reached at which even the most desperate efforts can no longer retain the urine.

Urethra

The urethra is a small tube that serves as a passageway for the elimination of urine from the bladder. The external outlet of the urethra is called the *urethral meatus.* The urethra is a comparatively short tube in the woman; it is about 1½ inches (3.8 cm) long. In the midportion of the female urethra is a circular striated muscle that forms the external sphincter.

The male urethra is about 8 inches (20 cm) long and also serves as part of the reproductive tract. It is divided into three sections: prostatic, membranous, and penile. The prostatic urethra is about 1 inch (2.54 cm) long and extends from the internal sphincter of the bladder through the prostate gland to the pelvic floor. The membranous urethra is about ½ inch (1.3 cm) long and lies between the prostatic and penile sections of the urethra; it is surrounded by the external sphincter. The penile urethra is about 6 inches (15 cm) long and extends through the penis, terminating at the urethral meatus.

Urine

Urine is a transparent, amber-colored liquid with a characteristic odor. It is usually acid in reaction. The specific gravity of urine ranges from 1.003 to 1.030. Approximately 95% of urine is water. The remaining 5% consists of wastes from protein metabolism and inorganic components, such as sodium and potassium chloride.

The examination of urine is the keystone in diagnosing disorders of the urinary system. A properly collected specimen can yield a wealth of information about renal function and the nature of kidney disorders. Urinalysis also reveals much information about infections and toxic and metabolic disorders. Proteinuria, hematuria, pyuria, bacteriuria, and casts are important clues to the presence of renal disease.

ANOMALIES OF THE GENITOURINARY TRACT

Infant

The embryological development of the urinary system is closely related to the development of the genital organs in both sexes. Because of this factor, genital and urinary tract deformities are discussed together. Genitourinary deformities comprise 30% to 40% of all congenital anomalies. A deformity of the genitalia may be accompanied by a deformity of the upper urinary tract. Deformities are multiple in approximately 20% of cases, and often they accompany anomalies in other systems (for example, imperforate anus). Improved prenatal ultrasound has identified many anomalies before birth, often allowing treatment to be instituted shortly after birth.

Malformations of the genitourinary tract may lead to death. When the anomaly can be recognized early, surgical correction or treatment may be life-saving. This is true because many anomalies are obstructive and lead to hydronephrosis, which, if bilateral, may ultimately result in renal failure.

External deformities are obvious and readily detected. However, there is little physical evidence of internal disease unless it is far advanced. The nurse should be aware of this and know the few signals demanding close observation. It is important to note the number and amount of voidings in the newborn infant. Failure to void within the first 24 hours after birth is a danger sign and should be reported to the physician immediately. Abdominal enlargement or swelling in the area of a kidney also warrants immediate attention. A poor urinary stream may be a sign of a pathological disorder in the genitourinary tract. Some neonates with nonspecific signs of illness (lethargy and failure to gain weight), have a urinary tract infection.

The signs and symptoms of urinary problems in older children are more easily detected. Crying on urination, urgent and frequent urination, straining to void, and dribbling all point to genitourinary system difficulties. Unexplained fever, lassitude, weight loss, and failure to thrive are nondescript symptoms but may relate to advanced disease. Serious kidney infections may run a silent course. It is always wise to investigate any of the preceding signals, since renal failure can be the result of a hidden anomaly.

Renal agenesis

Bilateral renal agenesis (absense) is incompatible with life. Autopsy studies have revealed that it is more common in males than in females. Lack of fetal urine causes a severe reduction in amniotic fluid (oligohydramnios). Since amniotic fluid is required for normal lung development, these patients have pulmonary hypoplasia. Oligohydramnios also causes the uterus to exert pressure on the fetus for prolonged periods of time, thus interfering with normal development. The combination of renal agenesis, pulmonary hypoplasia, and facial and limb abnormalities is called *Potter's syndrome.*

Unilateral renal agenesis is a survivable condition, but the single kidney is more likely to be diseased and associated with other malformations, especially of the ureter.

Double kidney

Duplication of the kidney and ureter is the most frequently encountered anomaly of the urinary tract and is more common in girls than boys. The ureters from each double kidney may enter the bladder at different points (complete duplication) or may unite to enter the bladder as one ureter (partial duplication). Sometimes the ureter from the upper kidney enters the genitourinary tract ectopically and causes incontinence. Duplication of the kidney and ureter is clinically significant only when other anomalies causing incontinence, obstruction, reflux, or infection exist.

Horseshoe kidney

A horseshoe kidney results when the lower ends of both kidneys fuse, forming a single mass shaped like a horseshoe. These kidneys lie closer to the spine and usually lower than does separate kidneys. A horseshoe kidney may be asymptomatic, but complications, especially obstruction, infection, and reflux, are common.

Polycystic kidney

True polycystic disease is always hereditary and always bilateral. Inheritance can be autosomal recessive or autosomal dominant (refer to Chapter 16 for a review of genetics). The autosomal-recessive form is associated with hepatic fibrosis. Polycystic kidneys are larger than normal and sometimes are huge, filling the entire abdomen. They contain innumerable cysts, compressing the parenchyma. Such kidneys are constantly susceptible to infection, obstruction, stone formation bleeding, and renal insufficiency. Treatment can only be palliative. The prognosis varies with the type of polycystic kidneys. Some patients survive only a few months, but others live into the third or fourth decade.

Ureterocele

A ureterocele is a ballooning of the lower end of the ureter because of an abnormally narrow ureteral orifice. Ureteroceles are usually unilateral. Double ureters are commonly associated with the anomaly. When an extra ureter is present, the one that enters the bladder normally is often distorted by the enormous ureterocele. As a result, it becomes obstructed, and kidney infection may ensue. Treatment consists of excising the redundant portion and reconstructing the opening so that obstruction is eliminated. The portion of kidney adjacent to the ureterocele is usually so destroyed as to require removal. If an obstruction does not exist, treatment is symptomatic.

Exstrophy of the bladder

Exstrophy of the bladder, fortunately, is a rare condition. It ranks with the most severe human anomalies. Because of a defect in midline closure associated with incomplete development of the pubic arch, the interior of the bladder lies completely exposed through an opening in the lower abdominal wall. A number of severe genital anomalies (for example, epispadias) usually accompany the defect.

Children who have exstrophy of the bladder become foul-smelling because they are constantly soaked in urine. Often the surrounding skin becomes excoriated, causing great pain. Early in life the exposed bladder mucosa becomes inflamed, bleeds readily, and is acutely sensitive. Infection is frequent but can usually be controlled by antibiotic therapy.

Treatment is surgical. An anatomical reconstruction of the bladder is the operation of choice. The most desirable time for this operation is at birth. After this operation the child is totally incontinent for a period of years, during which time the bladder grows sufficiently to make antireflux operations possible. When the bladder (vesicle) sphincters are made more complete and function somewhat normally, efforts can be directed to make the child continent. Dilation of the ureter, reflux, and chronic infection often occur when the child is rendered continent too early.

If the exstrophic bladder is deemed unsuitable for reconstruction or has failed prior attempts at closure,

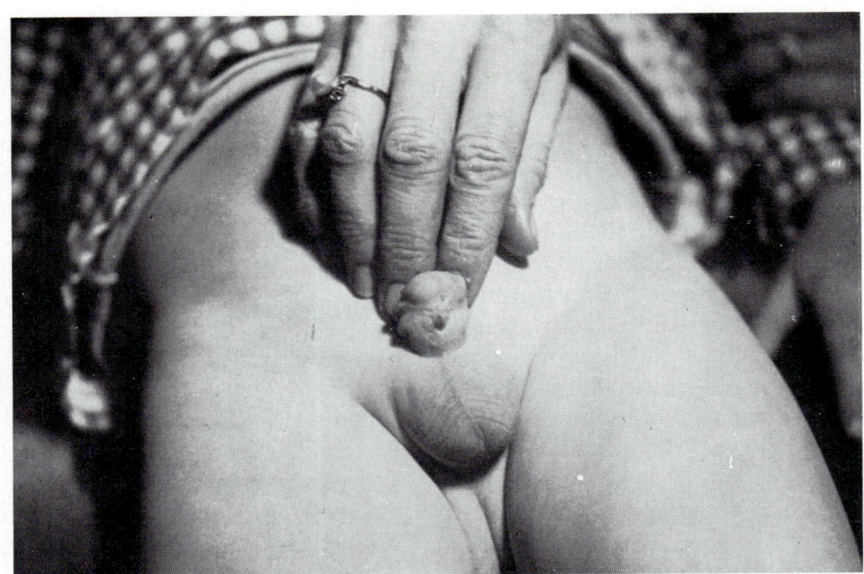

Fig. 36-2 Hypospadias (meatus located on undersurface of penis). (Courtesy Matthew Gleason, San Diego, Calif.)

other methods of draining, especially ileal bladder or conduit procedures, are employed. It is currently popular to "augment" small exstrophic bladders with intestinal segments to render them suitable for reconstruction.

Exstrophy of the bladder is a survivable condition; however, the prognosis depends in great measure on the extent of renal damage resulting from defective drainage and infection.

Hypospadias

Hypospadias is a common deformity in which the urethra terminates at some point on the ventral surface of the penis (Fig. 36-2). The position of the urethra on the penis or perineum determines the type of treatment. Because the prostatic urethra is never involved in hypospadias, the sphincters function normally, and the child has good urinary control. Often a meatal stricture is associated with varying degrees of hypospadias. When such a stricture is recognized, it is easily corrected by dilation or meatotomy.

In the more severe types a cordlike anomaly causes the penis to arc downward *(chordee)*. These more extensive deformities all require surgical repair to establish normal control of voiding and make normal reproduction possible later in life. Boys with hypospadias should not be circumcised without prior urological consultation, because the foreskin is needed in the repair.

Treatment. Operative repair is usually accomplished in one stage at about 1 year of age. In this way the child avoids teasing from peers and lasting psychological problems from genital surgery.

Various plastic techniques are employed to correct hypospadias, and the procedures are constantly being improved. The difficulties encountered in achieving a successful correction of hypospadias are considerable. The parents should be aware that more than one operation may be required. They should also know that after a successful urethroplasty the penis may be scarred, although appearing normal to the casual observer.

Postoperative care. When surgery is completed, the penis is wrapped in petroleum gauze and then covered with a dry gauze bandage. Some surgeons use a clear Tegaderm wrapping. This helps to prevent postoperative swelling, pain, and bleeding. Unless this precaution is taken, failure of the repair can occur. A catheter drains the bladder while the incision is healing. The nurse must observe the patient carefully to detect swelling, bleeding, or obstruction of the catheter. In many pediatric centers, hypospadias surgery is now performed on an outpatient day-surgery basis, thus parents must observe for signs of infection or obstruction. The child may be hospitalized for repair of more serious forms of hypospadias.

After the operation the child is kept on his back. A bed cradle helps to prevent pressure on the operative area. A Stile's dressing may be used (see Fig. 35-5).

On the second postoperative day the child may be allowed freedom of movement in his crib, provided the nurse can take time to sit, talk, and play with him. The nurse should attempt to keep his hands occupied lest he busy them with his dressing. Parents should be encouraged to stay with their children because they are best able to keep them constructively occupied.

Epispadias

When the urethra opens on the dorsal surface of the penis, the condition is called *epispadias.* Various degrees of epispadias can occur. However, the deformity is uncommon, except when associated with exstrophy of the bladder. Treatment is the same as that for hypospadias or exstrophy.

Intersexual anomalies

A semiemergency exists when simple inspection of the newborn infant's genitalia does not reveal the gender of the child. Chromosome and endocrine studies are usually helpful in these cases. Exploratory abdominal surgery for gonadal biopsy can also be undertaken to identify the gender of the sexually indeterminate child and decide on the most appropriate gender for rearing.

Pseudohermaphroditism. When a person possesses external genitalia resembling those of one gender and the gonads of the opposing gender, the condition resulting is termed *pseudohermaphroditism.* Sometimes a severe hypospadias with undescended testicles or a hypertrophied clitoris and malformed labia cause problems in gender identification. Female pseudohermaphrodites possess ovaries, but their external genitalia mimic those of the male. Such masculinization of the female infant results from an overdeveloped adrenal cortex (congenital adrenal hyperplasia) and subsequent increased production of male sex hormones (androgens) by the adrenal glands. Male pseudohermaphrodites are chromosomal males, but because of some testicular dysfunction or the existence of other problems, sexual ambiguity is present.

Whatever the condition, it should be corrected—but only after the true gender has been determined. Treatment usually consists of corrective plastic procedures on the external genitalia or the administration of appropriate missing hormones.

Mixed gonadal tissue and ambiguous genitalia. An extremely rare condition exists when a child possesses gonads of both genders. Prompt attention to this problem reduces the possibilities of serious emotional sequelae. Gender assignment should be performed as soon as possible so that the child has an opportunity for a normal, happy, and successful life. Treatment is not often an emergency, but gender assignment is crucial.

Hydrocele

As the testis descends through the inguinal canal to the scrotum, it is preceded by a fingerlike projection of the peritoneal cavity called the *processus vaginalis.* This processus obliterates shortly after birth in the majority of boys. If the processus persists, peritoneal fluid may travel to the scrotum causing a fluid collection or hydrocele around the testis (Fig. 36-3). Intestine may also pass into the processus as an indirect inguinal hernia. When an infantile hydrocele persists beyond 1 year of age, surgical correction is recommended to prevent hernia formation and correct the cosmetic abnormality. If a clinically detectable hernia develops, it is repaired as soon as it is diagnosed because of a tendency for bowel to become trapped and strangulated within the processus in infants.

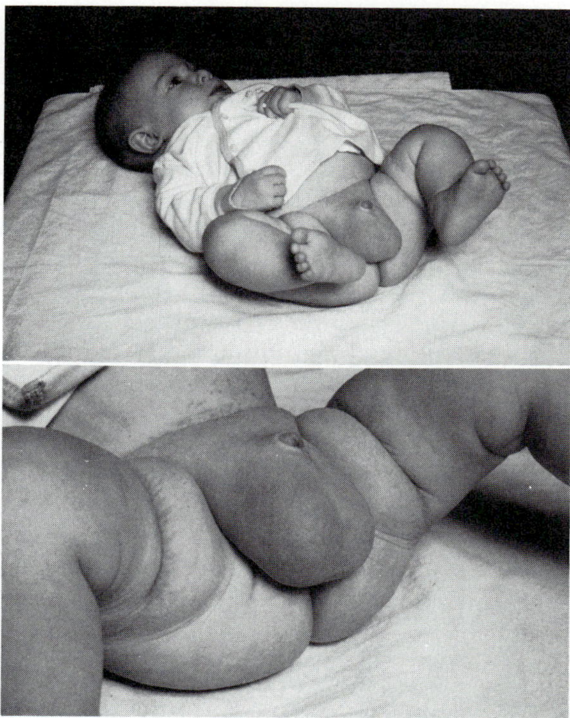

Fig. 36-3 Five-month-old infant with bilateral congenital hydroceles.

Cryptorchidism

Failure of the testes (singular, *testis*) to descend into the scrotum occurs in about 1% to 5% of full-term newborns and more frequently in premature infants. This cryptorchid condition is usually unilateral and frequently associated with an inguinal hernia.

Testicular maldescent is rarely associated with symptoms. It is associated with an increased incidence of testicular injury, torsion, and cancer. Other concerns are impaired fertility and a possible increased incidence of malignancy in the undescended testis. Although a predisposition to malignancy may exist with a nonscrotal testis, early surgical correction may prevent this.

If spontaneous descent is to occur for a cryptorchid testis, it is usually complete by 1 year of age. Human chorionic gonadotropin (HCG) can be a therapeutic aid in the management of bilateral cryptorchidism. Its use can aid descent, help differentiate between a retractile or a truly cryptorchid testis, or establish the presence or absence of bilateral intraabdominal testes.

If the testes do not descend spontaneously or in response to HCG, surgical correction, or orchiopexy, is indicated. Although an optimum age for this step is not agreed on universally, most pediatric urologists feel it should be performed between the ages of 1 and 2 years. Further delay accomplishes little and can result in impaired fertility in the individual or increased danger of eventual testicular malignancy. Early scrotal placement of the testes or placement of testicular prostheses for congenital absence is important for the child's healthy emotional and social development.

Toddler

Urinary tract infections (UTI)

The diagnosis of UTI requires significant bacteriuria, usually over 100,000 bacteria per milliliter of urine on a culture of a properly collected urine specimen. Infection may be confined to the bladder (cystitis) or may spread to the upper urinary tract (pyelonephritis). In patients with pyelonephritis the kidney can undergo irreversible damage as the result of bacterial invasion. Pyelonephritis can cause hypertension and chronic renal failure. UTIs are always considered serious and can be difficult to eradicate. Such infections are thought to rank second in frequency only to infections of the respiratory tract.

Etiological factors. There are many causes of UTI. Urinary stasis, which occurs when urine flow is obstructed, is associated with infection. Obstruction can occur at several sites: The ureteropelvic junction is one of the most common sites. Posterior urethral valves can cause obstruction in males. Kidney stones, vesicoureteral reflux, and urinary bladder dysfunction predispose to infection.

In most patients, bacteria enter the urine via the urethra. Because the female urethra is much shorter than the male's, females tend to have more UTIs than males. Prolonged tub bathing (greater than 20 minutes), inadequate hygiene (wiping from back to front), and irritants (nylon panties and bubble bath) contribute to the increased incidence of UTI in girls.

Incidence. UTI is relatively common in children. Uncircumcised male infants have a higher incidence of UTI than circumcised males. About 5% of all females have UTI during the school-age years.

Anatomical abnormalities of the urinary tract. Most children with proven infection should be screened for anatomical abnormalities of the urinary tract with sonographic or radiographic procedures. Both an intravenous pyelogram or renal ultrasound and a voiding cystourethrogram are necessary to assess the anatomy of the urinary tract. These studies detect a wide variety of urinary tract abnormalities, including reflux, obstruction, renal anomalies, and stones. Radiographic studies should be performed when the infected patient is male, regardless of the patient's age. All infected females under 3 years of age and older girls with repeated or febrile infections must also be screened.

Clinical symptoms. UTI symptoms vary considerably. In children under 3 years of age the onset is likely to be abrupt and severe, accompanied by a high temperature, which can reach 104° F (40° C). Pallor, anorexia, vomiting, diarrhea, and convulsions may occur. These *acute* symptoms usually disappear in a few days with appropriate treatment. Older children complain of sharp or dull pain in the flank. Gross hematuria or pyuria may be present. Bladder symptoms such as frequent, urgent, and burning urination are common complaints. Chills and fever may also be present. Occasionally UTI may be asymptomatic.

Some patients whose upper tract infections continue for a long period develop chronic pyelonephritis. Chronic pyelonephritis progresses slowly over many years. As the result of continuous low-grade infection, the patient characteristically has a history of recurrent bouts of nonspecific symptoms such as nausea, vomiting, diarrhea, fever, irritability, headache, and transitory urinary abnormalities. Poor general health, anemia, failure to grow, or failure to thrive are typical findings. The child may appear very pale or pasty looking. This condition suggests the late stages of renal damage and the development of uremia. Hypertension frequently appears as the end result of advanced renal scarring.

Treatment. Urinalysis and a culture of a properly collected specimen are the key to successful treatment. Therapy depends primarily on identification of the causative organism in a carefully collected urine culture. Detection and correction of anatomical abnormalities in the urinary tract are also essential to prevent progressive renal destruction.

A clean, midstream voided specimen is collected and sent to the laboratory for culture and sensitivity studies. If it is impossible to obtain an adequate specimen by such means, a catheterized specimen is ordered. Prompt therapy is indicated. Broad-spectrum antibiotics are administered until the laboratory studies are complete. Specific medications are ordered based on culture and sensitivity tests and continued for at least 10 days to 2 weeks.

The patient should be placed in bed in a cool, quiet environment until the fever has subsided. A tepid sponge bath may also be ordered. Fluids are encouraged to ensure adequate hydration and a good urine output. An accurate account of the fluid intake and urinary output is essential. Although it is not necessary to insert a catheter for accurate output, a simple check mark is not sufficient for the information needed. Weighing the diaper or an estimation of the amount of diaper saturation is far more valuable. After removing the diaper, the nurse should carefully wash and dry the child's genitalia before applying the clean diaper. This prevents further contamination and also protects the skin from becoming irritated and excoriated.

An adequate diet is important, and every attempt should be made to offer food that the child is able and willing to eat. A good milk intake supplies the needed protein, carbohydrate, fat, and most important, water. The parents should be encouraged to assist the child with meals. A daily check of weight, blood pressure, and vital signs offers valuable clues in the early detection of complications.

Reflux

In 20% to 30% of children with proven UTI, urine refluxes from the bladder into the ureters (vesicoureteral reflux) during voiding. This abnormality is detected by a radiographic procedure called a *voiding cystourethrogram* (VCUG). The persistence of reflux encourages infection. Vesicoureteral reflux is caused by anatomical defects in the urinary tract or by infection. The junction between the bladder and the ureter is only mildly abnormal when reflux is caused by infection. The abnormality improves if the patient's urine is kept sterile by administration of antibiotics for prolonged periods. Surgery is usually unnecessary when reflux is caused by infection alone, provided the infection can be controlled.

Anatomical defects in the connection between the ureter and the bladder or obstruction to urine flow in the urethra can also cause reflux. Patients with anatomical defects often require surgery. The functional anatomy of the vesicoureteral junction can be improved by surgically reimplanting the distal ureter into the bladder wall.

Nursing care. The general postoperative care of this patient is much the same as for any surgical patient. The nurse should recognize the importance of changing surgical dressings that have become saturated with urine. Urine is an excellent medium for the growth of bacteria. However, the nurse should be aware that some surgical drains can be purposely attached to the dressings, and special care is therefore required. Some physicians wish to change the dressings themselves for this reason. Drainage tubes must be carefully checked for patency. These postoperative patients can return to the nursing area with as many as three urinary catheters, depending on the extent of the surgery (one suprapubic cystotomy tube empties the bladder of any urine not drained via the ureteral tubes, and two ureteral catheters act as splints for the newly implanted ureters). Drainage from each of the tubes should be closely observed and recorded separately. These catheters are never clamped. When the patient is able to sit up in a wheelchair, the catheters should be arranged so that they do not kink. The collection bottles must hang below the level of the kidneys, draining freely. Water intake is always encouraged and recorded, particularly in young children, who quickly dehydrate. Dehydration promotes the growth of bacteria.

Pain is commonly associated with this type of surgery. Narcotics should be given as ordered on time. Antispasmodic drugs, such as oxybutynin chloride (Ditropan), propantheline bromide (Pro-Banthine), or methantheline bromide (Banthine bromide), are also ordered. These drugs usually relieve the immediate postoperative colicky pain.

Reflux associated with renal involvement is also caused by lower tract congenital obstructions. Unless the obstruction is corrected by reconstructive surgery when indicated, pyelonephritis can progress, leading to severe renal impairment. Reflux may be familial. If a new case of reflux is detected in a child, the siblings should be screened with a VCUG.

Prognosis. When the disease is recognized early and treated properly (long-term antibiotic therapy for infection or surgical removal of obstructions), the prognosis is excellent. Chronic infections present a much more serious and difficult problem because severe renal damage is the ultimate result.

Wilms' tumor

Wilms' tumor is one of the most common abdominal neoplasms of childhood. It is a congenital, mixed cell renal tumor that develops from abnormal embryonic tissue; occasionally (5% to 10%) occurs bilaterally. Composed of varying proportions of abnormal glomerulotubular structures, connective tissue, muscle, and blood vessels, the tumor initially grows within the renal capsule. As it grows larger it distorts the kidney in a bizarre manner and can occupy as much as one half of the abdominal cavity. Unfortunately, the tumor often invades the renal veins and metastasizes through the bloodstream to vital organs, especially to the lungs. Extension of the tumor through the renal capsule into surrounding tissues can occur and is associated with a poorer prognosis. Cure rates for even stage II or III tumors are excellent. (See Nursing Care Plan.)

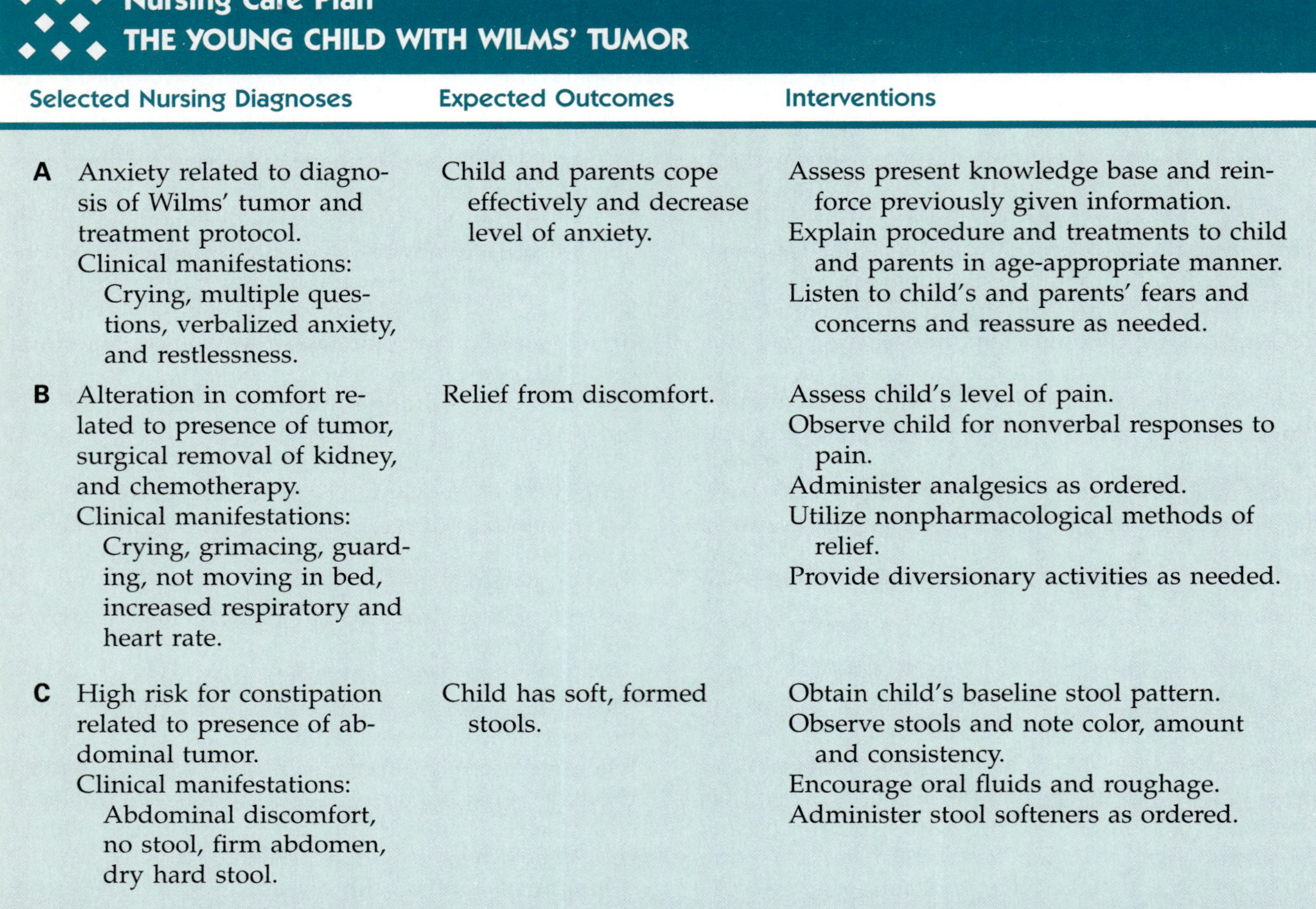

Nursing Care Plan
THE YOUNG CHILD WITH WILMS' TUMOR

	Selected Nursing Diagnoses	Expected Outcomes	Interventions
A	Anxiety related to diagnosis of Wilms' tumor and treatment protocol. Clinical manifestations: Crying, multiple questions, verbalized anxiety, and restlessness.	Child and parents cope effectively and decrease level of anxiety.	Assess present knowledge base and reinforce previously given information. Explain procedure and treatments to child and parents in age-appropriate manner. Listen to child's and parents' fears and concerns and reassure as needed.
B	Alteration in comfort related to presence of tumor, surgical removal of kidney, and chemotherapy. Clinical manifestations: Crying, grimacing, guarding, not moving in bed, increased respiratory and heart rate.	Relief from discomfort.	Assess child's level of pain. Observe child for nonverbal responses to pain. Administer analgesics as ordered. Utilize nonpharmacological methods of relief. Provide diversionary activities as needed.
C	High risk for constipation related to presence of abdominal tumor. Clinical manifestations: Abdominal discomfort, no stool, firm abdomen, dry hard stool.	Child has soft, formed stools.	Obtain child's baseline stool pattern. Observe stools and note color, amount and consistency. Encourage oral fluids and roughage. Administer stool softeners as ordered.

Etiological factors. Like other forms of cancer, the exact cause of Wilms' tumor is unknown. Recent evidence suggests that chromosomal abnormalities may play an important role.

Incidence. Wilms' tumor accounts for approximately 7% of all cancer in children. Boys and girls are equally affected. About two thirds of all children with Wilms' tumor are diagnosed before they are 3 years of age. The tumor can be present at birth and is rare after 7 years of age.

Clinical features. The initial manifestation of Wilms' tumor is a mass in the region of the kidney that is usually discovered by the parents in the course of daily care or accidentally during a routine examination. As the tumor grows, the child's abdomen becomes very large, and pressure symptoms arise. Constipation, vomiting, abdominal distention, and even dyspnea can occur. Weight loss, pallor, and anemia are common in the late stages. Pain, hematuria, and hypertension are uncommon, but, if present, they support the diagnosis of a renal tumor.

Treatment and nursing care. When Wilms' tumor is suspected, both parent and nurse must be careful not to feel or touch the child's abdomen because handling can cause rupture of the tumor through the renal capsule and metastasis via the bloodstream. Diagnosis is usually confirmed by intravenous pyelography and renal ultrasound. CT or MRI is used to evaluate the extent of the tumor. The choice of therapy is guided by the age of the child, extent of the tumor, and metastatic considerations at the time of diagnosis. Treatment usually consists of prompt radical nephrectomy. Radiation therapy has a limited role in treatment since the advent of more effective chemotherapy. The kidney, tumor, and perirenal fat are removed through a transabdominal approach. Blood transfusions may be given to replace blood lost during the surgical procedure and to correct preexisting anemia. Intravenous administration of fluids is continued for 24 hours. If bleeding occurs, it is easily detected when the child's pulse rate, respirations, blood pressure, and color are checked often. The dressings should be changed only if necessary, since little or no drainage occurs from the incision.

Actinomycin D has a significant antitumor effect and is particularly useful in the prevention of pulmonary metastases. Vincristine is also a highly effective drug in the treatment of Wilms' tumor. When both drugs are used in combination, the survival rate is significantly greater. Actinomycin D potentiates radiation. When indicated, courses of combination drug therapy are given at the time of resection, 6 weeks later, and then every 3 months. Length of treatment depends on the stage of the disease and "favorable" or "unfavorable" histology. Side effects from the administration of chemotherapy and radiation therapy include nausea, vomiting, anorexia, malaise, diarrhea, and loss of hair. During the interval between medication and radiation therapy, the child's hair usually grows back. Bone marrow depression, ulceration of the mucous membranes, and peripheral neuropathies are manifestations of acute toxicity associated with the administration of actinomycin D and vincristine. Drug therapy can be temporarily discontinued to allow the child to recover from the toxicity of the treatment.

Complications. The most serious complication in Wilms' tumor is metastasis. Characteristically, Wilms' tumor metastasizes through the bloodstream to the liver, lungs, brain, and other vital organs. The tumor can also spread by direct extension or by the lymphatics.

Prognosis. Wilms' tumor is always fatal if not treated and until recently has had a high mortality rate despite treatment. However, with major therapeutic advances in the last decade in surgery, radiation therapy, and combination chemotherapy, 90% of children with Wilms' tumor are currently expected to be cured of their disease. Although the prognosis is better when the tumor is discovered early, the use of combined therapy offers children with metastatic disease a good chance for cure. Follow-up care includes frequent x-ray examinations of the lungs and other areas of potential tumor involvement and close monitoring of the remaining normal kidney. As the child progresses favorably, less frequent examinations are required, but annual examinations are recommended to follow normal development and to detect any late effects of treatment.

Hypertension and renal disease

Measurement of blood pressure in children can be challenging. The patient should be as quiet as possible. The blood pressure cuff should cover at least two thirds of the upper arm. Repeated measurements should be done to establish an accurate average reading of the patient. Normal blood pressure is related to age and weight. Technically, high blood pressure, or hypertension, is defined as a blood pressure over 2 standard deviations above the mean for the age in question. For a child of 5 years of age, the upper limit of normal is 112/78.

The two basic categories of hypertension are borderline hypertension and definite hypertension. Patients with blood pressure over 140/90 are said to have definite hypertension. Patients with blood pressure elevated for age but less than 140/90 have borderline hypertension. Thus a 5-year-old with a blood pressure of 125/82 has borderline hypertension.

Investigators are currently collecting data on patients with borderline hypertension. From early studies it appears that these patients rarely have a known underlying cause for their hypertension. Borderline hypertension is thus "essential," or idiopathic, and a diagnostic workup is deemed unnecessary. Dietary salt restriction may be recommended for control of borderline hypertension. Use of antihypertensive drugs in these patients is controversial. Long-term followup is recommended.

Children with hypertension usually have an underlying disease causing the hypertension. The most common cause of hypertension in children is renal disease. Renal tumors, renal vascular disease, hydronephrosis, and glomerulonephritis can cause hypertension. Occasionally, excessive secretion of catecholamines or aldosterone by a tumor can cause hypertension in a child. Careful diagnostic workups are mandatory in children with hypertension. Obesity is also a contributing factor.

Children with hypertension tend to develop target organ disease. Congestive heart failure can occur. Blood vessels can also be damaged. Children with severe hypertension—blood pressure over 160/110—can suddenly develop hypertensive encephalopathy. Common signs and symptoms are headache, visual disturbance, tinnitus, seizures, and coma. In typical cases the neurological problem is reversible; occasionally, a stroke may occur. Sometimes hemorrhages, exudates, and arterial spasm can be viewed in the retinal vessels with an ophthalmoscope. These changes are called *hypertensive retinopathy*. Severe symptomatic hypertension is a medical emergency requiring prompt treatment.

Treatment of hypertension depends on its cause. Tumors should be surgically excised. Renal artery stenosis can be corrected by angioplasty or surgery. In other cases, medications are effective. Propranolol (Inderal), hydralazine (Apresoline), and diazoxide (Hyperstat) are commonly used. Diuretics also help lower blood pressure. Newer agents such as captopril (Capoten) and minoxidil (Loniten) and enalapril (Va-

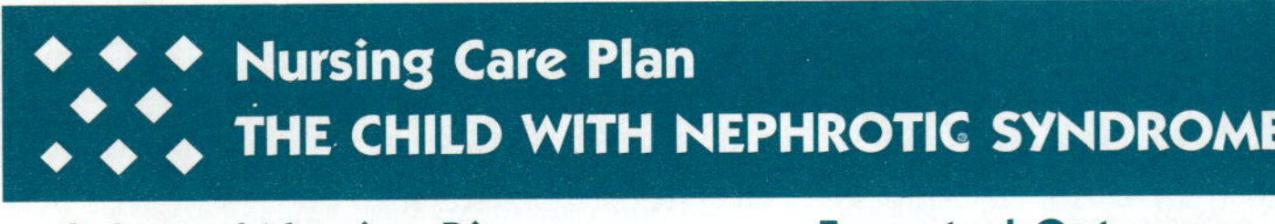

Nursing Care Plan
THE CHILD WITH NEPHROTIC SYNDROME

	Selected Nursing Diagnoses	Expected Outcomes	Interventions
A	Fluid volume excess (extravascular) related to depletion of serum protein. Clinical manifestations: Increased weight gain, pitting edema, firm and distended abdomen, edematous scrotum/labia, periorbital edema, respiratory distress.	Child regains and maintains fluid and electrolyte balance.	Assess child for presence of edema. Measure abdominal girth daily (same level and position). Maintain strict I & O (provide intake volume equal to output or as ordered by physician.) Weigh child daily (same time and scale). Check each void for specific gravity and for protein. Restrict salt and/or nutritional intake as ordered. Monitor BP and IV albumin and Lasix/diuretics as ordered and child's response to diuretic therapy. Monitor serum electrolytes daily.
B	High risk for infection related to bedrest, fluid excess; decreased immune response (from steroid therapy). Clinical manifestations: Fever, increase respiratory and heart rate, anorexia, abdominal pain, vomiting, diarrhea.	Child does not develop infection. Child shows no evidence of skin breakdown.	Promote good handwashing by care providers and visitors Place child in room with noninfectious children. Reposition child every 2 hours; cushion bony prominences and support edematous body parts (scrotum). Provide good oral hygiene and skin care. Utilize egg crate mattress. Bathe and dry skin carefully. Promote well-balanced "renal" diet. Observe child for signs of peritonitis (increased abdominal distention, pain, rigidity, vomiting and/or diarrhea). Monitor IV antibiotics.
C	Altered nutrition: less than body requirements related to anorexia, loss of protein in urine. Clinical manifestations: Poor appetite, proteinuria	Child has sufficient caloric intake to meet growth needs.	Offer nutritious diet. Restrict sodium. Allow child and family to assist with food selection. Offer small, frequent meals and snacks. Make mealtime pleasant and relaxed. Administer supplementary vitamins and iron as ordered.

sotec) are helpful in severe hypertension. The patient must be carefully monitored for adverse side effects. Aggressive medical management is important in an effort to lower the risk of stroke and other types of vascular injury.

Preschool Child

Nephrotic syndrome

Nephrotic syndrome is a chronic renal disease characterized by anasarca (severe generalized edema), heavy proteinuria, low serum albumin levels, and

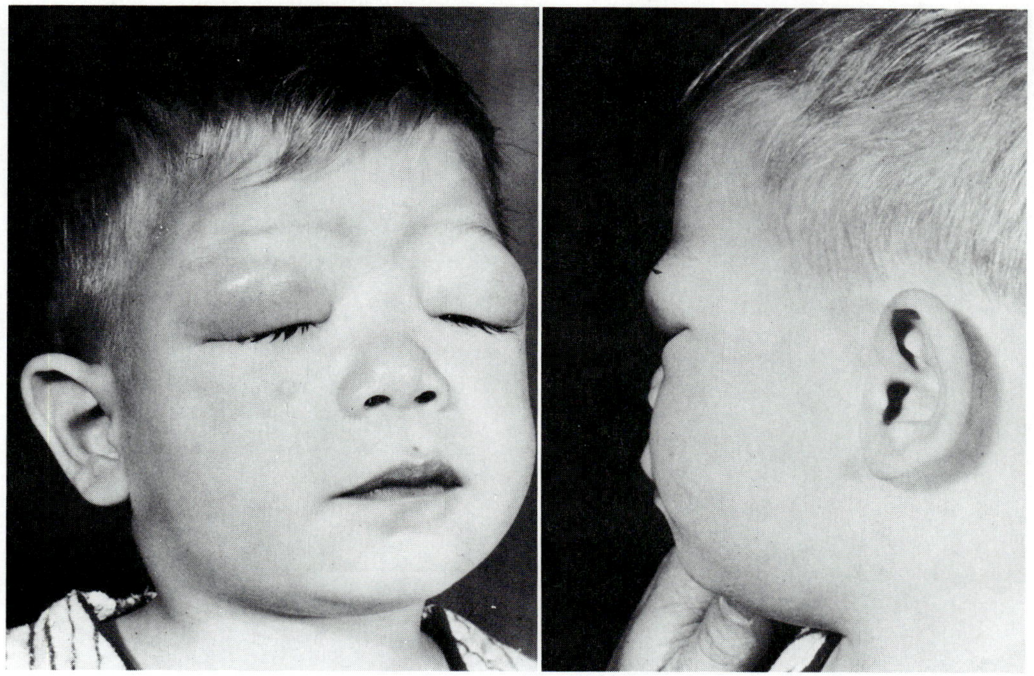

Fig. 36-4 Two-year-old child with nephrotic syndrome. Progressive periorbital edema. (Courtesy Naval Hospital, San Diego, Calif.)

high serum cholesterol values. (See Nursing Care Plan.)

Etiological factors. In 80% of children with nephrotic syndrome the renal biopsy shows only a minimum of abnormalities. This disease is also called *lipoid nephrosis, idiopathic nephrotic syndrome of childhood,* or *minimal change nephrotic syndrome.* In these patients the cause of nephrotic syndrome is unknown. In the remaining 20%, renal biopsies may show abnormalities such as glomerulonephritis.

Incidence. Minimal change nephrotic syndrome is more common in boys than in girls and occurs most frequently between 2 and 6 years of age. The incidence of nephrotic syndrome in childhood is 7 per 100,000.

Clinical symptoms. Onset of nephrotic syndrome is insidious. Periorbital edema may be the first sign. In severe cases, it progresses steadily until the eyes are closed (Fig. 36-4). As the edema increases, the arms, legs, and abdomen may reach massive proportions. At the peak of the edema, the child can weigh almost twice as much as normally (Fig. 36-5). Anorexia and varying degrees of diarrhea are commonly found. Discomfort from massive edema causes the child to be irritable and easily fatigued. Anasarca can lead to inadequate ventilation. Gross hematuria and hypertension are unusual in minimal change nephrotic syndrome and suggest the possibility of glomerulonephritis.

Nursing Alert

Nephrotic syndrome should be suspected if a child exhibits periorbital edema, excessive weight gain, decreased urine output, pallor, and fatigue.

Complications. The nephrotic child is vulnerable to infections, probably because of the loss of gamma globulin in the urine (proteinuria). Bacteremia associated with peritonitis is common. Encapsulated organisms, such as pneumococci, are frequently identified. Pneumococcal vaccine should be given when the patient is off steroids to prevent infection. Infections are the leading cause of death in patients with minimal change nephrotic syndrome. Hypercoagulability and vascular thrombosis may also occur.

Treatment and nursing care. The goal of treatment for nephrotic syndrome is a child in optimum health, judged by both clinical well-being and laboratory findings. The goals of nursing care include comforting the patient during the distress of massive edema, maintaining good nutrition, and preventing concurrent infection. Edema can be controlled in many patients with a low sodium, fluid-restricted diet. If the edema is severe, intravenous albumin and diuretics may be administered to increase urine production.

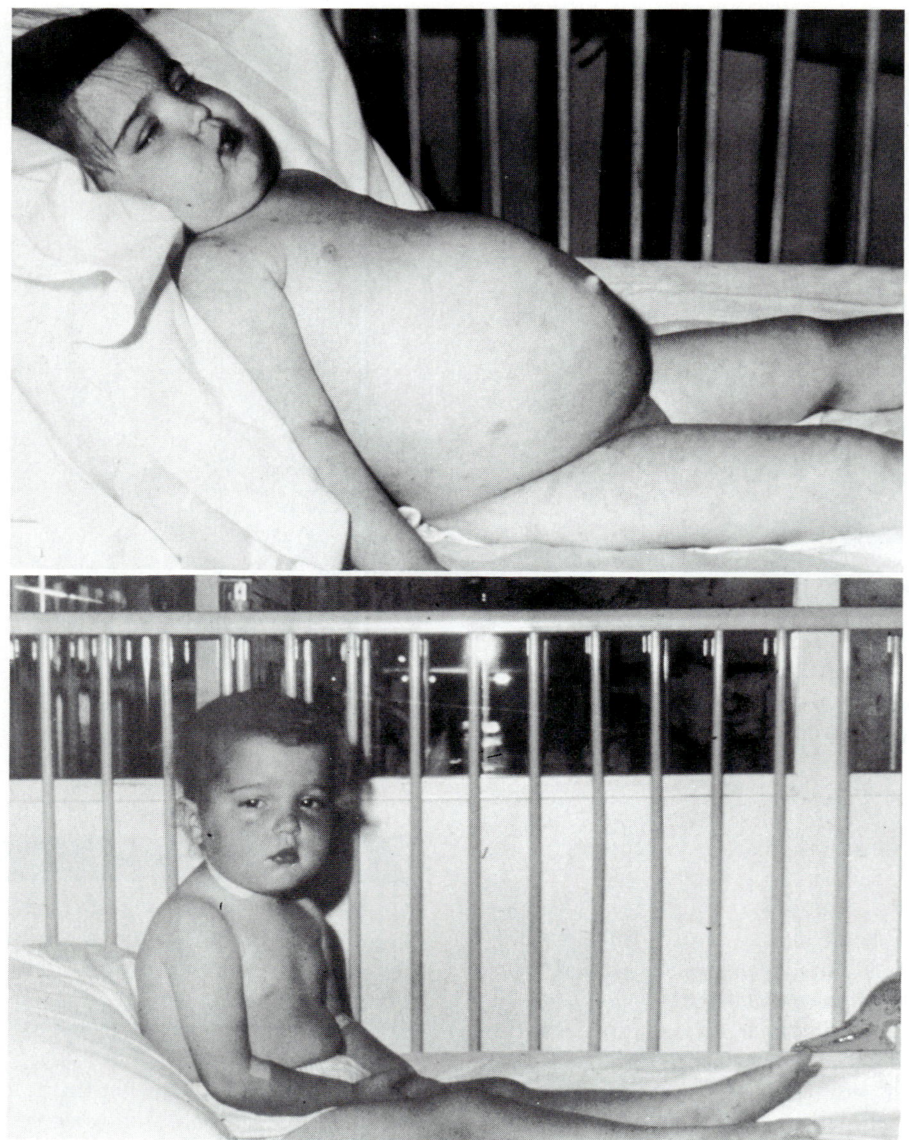

Fig. 36-5 2½-year-old child with nephrotic syndrome. **A,** Before therapy. **B,** After therapy. (Courtesy Naval Hospital, San Diego, Calif.)

Most patients with minimal change nephrotic syndrome respond to steroid therapy. Prednisone, 2 mg/kg/day, reverses the proteinuria, usually by 10 to 14 days. When proteinuria ceases, urine output improves, serum albumin normalizes, and edema disappears. During remission the steroid therapy is gradually withdrawn. Some patients stay in remission on no medication; other patients require maintenance therapy. Maintenance prednisone is usually given every other day to minimize side effects. Alkylating agents such as cyclophosphamide or chlorambucil can produce a prolonged remission in some patients but are not used routinely because of the risks of serious complications. Relapses of nephrotic syndrome are often associated with intercurrent infections, especially those involving the respiratory and urinary tracts. Immediate intensive antibiotic therapy is mandatory if infection arises.

In selecting a hospital room for the nephrotic child, the nurse must remember the child's increased susceptibility to infection. Placing the child in a double room with another child of the same age who also has nephrotic syndrome is most desirable.

Weighing the child on admission and each morning thereafter is one way of evaluating the amount of edema present. A daily abdominal girth measurement, taken in a flat position at the level of the umbilicus just after a breath is exhaled, is also helpful. If massive edema is present, the child's self-concept is likely to be greatly distorted. It is important for the parents to be reassured and to be given whatever information is necessary about the condition and its outcome so that they in turn can reassure their child. They should particularly realize the seriousness of the disorder, even though the prognosis is better than ever before. Fever or signs of respiratory distress should be reported to the physician.

Massive edema is uncomfortable. The skin is stretched thin and easily broken. Keeping the child's body dry and clean helps prevent skin infections. Application of powder between skin surfaces and in skin folds is soothing and protective. If the child is not toilet-trained, the nurse must take great care to prevent excoriation of the buttocks and genitalia. Medicines are given orally or intravenously but never intramuscularly or subcutaneously. Great care must be taken to protect the edematous skin from injury and subsequent secondary infection. Usually the child is most comfortable in a semi-Fowler's position to reduce respiratory distress. This position can also reduce periorbital edema.

Maintenance of good nutrition is essential because beneath the edema exists a thin, poorly nourished body. The child should be given a well-balanced, high-protein diet. Salty foods such as potato chips and pickles should be avoided. Restriction of fluid intake may be necessary to control edema. Allowing the child some choice encourages appetite and helps prevent severe nutritional depletion, which often readily occurs.

An accurate account of fluid intake is important when the output is scanty. Although the nurse may not be able to measure the exact output, she or he must record approximate amounts each time the child voids. Limited activity is recommended until diuresis begins. During the active phase of the disease, the child is usually sluggish and therefore satisfied to rest most of the time. When massive edema is present, the child is content to rest all the time.

After discharge from the hospital, the child is periodically examined until the prednisone is gradually discontinued. Although infection is a common complication in these children while they are receiving prednisone, it is not necessary to interfere with their normal home and school activities. If an outbreak of an infectious disease, such as chickenpox (varicella), should occur at school, it is wise to have the child remain at home. Varicella infection is very dangerous in immunosuppressed nephrotic children. Exposure should be avoided. If exposure occurs Zoster immune globulin (ZIG) should be given within 72 hours. Any sign of intercurrent infection must be reported to the physician and treated immediately.

Prognosis. By controlling infection, antibiotic therapy has greatly reduced the death rate of these patients to 1% to 2%. About 90% of the children respond to steroid therapy. Many of the children have recurrent episodes of nephrotic syndrome. Each episode usually resolves with steroid treatment. Eventually, after many years of intermittent treatment, these children usually fully enjoy healthful living with normal kidneys and absence of medication. Progression to end-stage renal disease is unusual in minimal change nephrotic syndrome.

School-age Child

Enuresis

Enuresis is defined as involuntary voiding of urine, occurring especially at night (nocturnal enuresis), after the child is 4 years of age. However, a wide age range is associated with the neuromuscular maturation of urinary sphincter control. Children with nocturnal enuresis usually have a normal urinary stream and good daytime bladder control. Enuresis can be primary or acquired. When bladder control has never been achieved, enuresis is said to be primary. If enuresis occurs after control has been achieved for at least 1 year, it is said to be acquired.

About 15% of pediatric patients are evaluated because of this disturbance. Enuresis is very common in childhood, and the condition is more prevalent in boys than in girls.

The exact cause of enuresis in most children is unknown. Psychological or developmental disorders are found in some patients, but enuresis is also caused by an anatomical defect or a systemic disease. The most significant step toward solving the problem is an attempt to find the correct cause. Before a psychological explanation is sought, anatomical abnormalities and organic disease must be ruled out.

Generally, daytime wetting (diurnal enuresis) and other urological symptoms are associated with organic disease. Diabetes mellitus, urinary tract infection, urinary tract anomalies, neurological defects, and obstructions such as meatal stenosis are often responsible for the condition. Psychological problems also account for some cases of enuresis. Improper toilet training, an unhappy environment, a poor parent-child relationship, immaturity associated with other infantile habits, and developmental disturbances such as jealousy and insecurity are examples of psychological causes of enuresis. Whatever the cause, the correction of enuresis is highly important to both these children and their parents. It enables children to develop normally and to be like their friends, and it offers the parents peace of mind and a healthy child.

Every enuretic patient should have a careful history and physical examination performed to determine if renal enlargements, a distended bladder, a constriction of the external urinary meatus, or a neurological change is present. An extremely careful urinalysis and urine culture are essential. Intravenous urography, cystography, and cystoscopy are sometimes necessary to diagnose organic causes. They are unnecessary if the child has simple nocturnal enuresis without daytime symptoms and if the history and physical examinations are otherwise within normal limits.

Imipramine hydrochloride (Tofranil) controls the condition completely in some patients. This drug, however, has some potential toxic manifestations. Therefore a physician or NP must carefully evaluate the problem before ordering imipramine hydrochloride, and if it is indicated, the child must be carefully watched for side effects such as facial tics, nightmares, and belligerent behavior. Large overdoses can prove fatal. Recently introduced for the treatment of nocturnal enuresis is DDAVP (Desmopressin) an antidiuretic hormone analogue administered as a nightly nasal spray. DDAVP reduces the volume of urine.

Enuresis may also diminish through the use of fairly simple techniques. Giving less fluids in the evening is helpful to a few children. Waking children and taking them to the toilet during the night saves embarrassment to school-age children.

Some children, principally those who have deep sleep patterns, benefit from the use of mechanical devices that wake them with lights or alarms when the bed becomes wet. Consistent use of these detectors and the associated behavioral programs encourage lighter sleep, more awareness of bladder filling, and fewer accidents.

Parents should not threaten or punish their children because they wet the bed. This only increases the child's sense of inferiority and failure and can even deter the will to improve. Instead, every effort should be made to assure children that they can overcome the condition. Encouragement comes in the form of rewards (for example, being allowed to go camping or sleep overnight at grandmother's house). Such rewards, together with the child's desire to stay dry, can achieve positive results. Enuretic children without any organic disease or severe psychologic problem usually gradually overcome the condition by age 10 to 12 years.

A condition often confused with enuresis is the presence in a girl of an ectopic ureter, which empties into the vagina or urethra beyond the sphincter. These children may void normally (from their normal ureters and bladder) but are always wet from constant drainage from the ectopic ureter. Surgery can correct this problem.

Torsion of the testicle

Contraction of the cremaster muscle not only elevates the testis but rotates it. Depending on the degree of twisting, torsion of the spermatic cord usually causes severe scrotal pain as the result of an interruption of the blood supply and ensuing necrosis of the testis. Torsion can occur at any age and is not uncommon in the adolescent. It can occur while sleeping, playing games, or jumping into cold water. Torsion of the testicle occurs in patients who have failure of fixation of the testicle to the bottom of the scrotum. The failure of fixation is usually bilateral.

Torsion is an acute emergency. Hope of saving the testicle depends on prompt diagnosis and immediate reduction by manipulative procedures or surgery. Isotope scans to determine blood flow to the testis are most useful diagnostic tools. Sonograms are very helpful in differential diagnosis to rule out acute epididymitis and tumor. If surgery is performed bilateral orchiopexy should be accomplished to prevent a future torsion of the opposite side.

Acute glomerulonephritis (Nephritis or Bright's disease)

Acute glomerulonephritis is an inflammatory disease of the glomeruli affecting both kidneys. The clinical manifestations include gross hematuria, often with cola-colored urine, edema, proteinuria, casts, hypertension, and elevated amounts of nitrogen products in the bloodstream (azotemia).

Etiological factors. Streptococcal infection is the most common cause of acute glomerulonephritis. The infection precedes the onset of glomerulonephritis by 1 to 3 weeks. Other infectious agents such as pneumococcus, hepatitis virus, or Epstein-Barr virus can also cause acute glomerulonephritis.

Patients with acute glomerulonephritis should be carefully studied to determine the infectious etiology. Since group A streptococcus is the most common cause, streptozyme titer test, antistreptolysin titer test, and direct culture of the pharynx or skin lesions are essential.

Incidence. Glomerulonephritis is common in children, especially between 5 and 10 years of age. It seems to be more common in boys than in girls and is most frequently observed in the late winter months or early spring. This seasonal pattern is related to the peak incidence of streptococcal infections of the upper respiratory tract.

Symptoms. Gross hematuria, proteinuria, edema, periorbital edema, hypertension, weakness, pallor, anorexia, headache, nausea, or vomiting may be present. Rarely, patients present with congestive heart failure or neurological problems from hypertension (hypertensive encephalopathy).

Nursing Alert

Acute glomerulonephritis should be suspected if the child exhibits periorbital edema that is worse in the morning, antecedent streptococcal infection, decreased urinary output, dark-colored urine, and anorexia.

Treatment and nursing care. Necessary bed rest is usually welcomed by the child during the acute phase of the disease. Activities can be resumed as soon as gross hematuria has cleared and signs of edema, hypertension, and other urinary abnormalities have subsided.

These children should be separated from other children who have infections (especially of the upper respiratory tract), but complete isolation is not indicated. They should be observed closely for any recurrences of upper respiratory tract infection. Exacerbations rarely occur with new strains of streptococcal organisms. Reinfection by the same nephritogenic strain is generally not possible by virtue of type-specific immunity after infection. Antibiotic therapy is indicated when evidence of infection is present. Long-term prophylactic use of penicillin in the prevention of recurrence of glomerulonephritis is not recommended. Treatment with furosemide diuretics controls edema in most patients. Antihypertensives such as hydralazine are frequently used. Dialysis is occasionally necessary for severe electrolyte imbalance resulting from renal failure.

Severe renal failure. Severe renal failure is uncommon in children but serious complications of acute glomerulonephritis may occur in some children. When an imbalance of fluids and electrolytes persists, peritoneal dialysis or hemodialysis may be needed to control the uremia.

Prognosis. Acute glomerulonephritis is usually a self-limited condition, and most children recover completely. A few children present a more complex entity with persistent urinary abnormalities and hypertension, which ultimately results in chronic glomerulonephritis.

Chronic glomerulonephritis

Chronic glomerulonephritis is a major cause of chronic kidney failure in children. There are many causes of chronic glomerulonephritis. Systemic infections, hereditary diseases, autoimmunity, immune complexes, drugs, and toxins are known causes. Renal biopsy can be helpful in defining the type and the prognosis of nephritis.

Gross hematuria, edema, severe hypertension, and anemia may be initial symptoms. The majority of untreated patients develop chronic renal failure and end-stage renal disease. The onset of end-stage renal disease varies in length from a few months to 10 to 20 years.

Treatment and nursing care. In general, chronic glomerulonephritis is difficult to treat; the nephrotic syndrome associated with chronic glomerulonephritis does not resolve with oral prednisone therapy. However, recent studies have shown that some forms of glomerulonephritis can be improved with new treatments. Removal of circulating immune complexes and autoantibodies, performed by an automated plasma exchange, can improve the conditions of certain patients. High-dose steroid therapy—methylprednisolone (Solu-Medrol) 30 mg/kg—given intravenously can also improve renal function. Sometimes treatments to reverse the destructive inflammation in the kidney are unsuccessful. These patients develop end-stage renal disease and require kidney transplants or dialysis.

Patients with chronic glomerulonephritis may be hospitalized for a course of treatment or for complications. They should be watched closely for hypertension. Daily weights are critical for estimating fluid balance. Frequently these children are anxious and benefit greatly from kind and understanding nursing care. Exposure to infectious illnesses should be avoided.

Acute renal failure

Acute, or temporary, renal failure can be caused by shock (acute tubular necrosis), toxins (such as aminoglycoside antibiotics or heavy metals), glomerulonephritis, or hemolytic uremic syndrome.

Hemolytic uremic syndrome is the most common form of acute renal failure to affect previously well children. Patients have a prodromal illness of vomiting and diarrhea, which is often bloody. The illness progresses quickly to severe hemolytic anemia, renal failure, thrombocytopenia, and neurological problems.

Recent studies have shown that most cases of hemolytic uremic syndrome are caused by the common bacteria *Escherichia coli*. *E. coli* can be found in the intestinal tract. Because of the short distance from the anus to the urethra, the organism may enter the urinary tract. *E. coli* also enters the bloodstream through the ingestion of undercooked, tainted meat. Some strains of this bacteria are capable of producing a powerful toxin, called *verotoxin,* which is thought to cause the disease. Young children are susceptible to the illness if they lack immunity to the toxin. The outlook for children with acute renal failure is good. In most cases renal failure will resolve if good supportive care is provided.

Treatment and nursing care. Treatment for acute renal failure consists in specific correction of electrolyte imbalances. Hyperkalemia, which can cause dangerous and even fatal arrhythmias, can be treated with Kayexalate. Infusion of sodium bicarbonate, glucose, and insulin can be used to control hyperkalemia in an emergency situation. Acidosis is treated with sodium bicarbonate. Hyperphosphatemia can be treated with oral phosphate-binding agents such as calcium carbonate. Hypocalcemia is corrected by oral and sometimes intravenous calcium administration. Supplemental vitamin D is frequently required.

Fluid overload can cause congestive heart failure. Dialysis can be used to correct fluid overload and electrolyte imbalance. Both peritoneal dialysis and hemodialysis can be safely performed in children.

Hypertension can be a serious problem in children with renal failure. Accurate measurement of the blood pressure should be performed frequently with an appropriate size cuff that covers at least two thirds of the upper arm. Oral and intravenous antihypertensive medications may be required.

Infection and neurological problems are common complications in renal patients. Fever should be promptly reported to the physician. Any changes in mental status should also be recorded and reported. Patients are at risk to have seizures from a variety of causes including hypocalcemia, hyponatremia, hypernatremia, hyperglycemia, hypoglycemia, and uremia. Hypertensive encephalopathy may also occur in these patients.

A restricted diet is frequently prescribed to help control hyperphosphatemia and hyperkalemia. Protein intake is adjusted on an individual basis depending on the particular needs of the patient. Sodium restriction is frequently prescribed.

End-stage renal disease

The term *end-stage renal disease* refers to patients with severe chronic failure of kidney function. This occurs when kidney function, as measured by creatinine clearance, is less than 10% of normal. It may be caused by congenital defects, toxins, glomerulonephritis, obstruction of the urinary tract, and pyelonephritis.

Patients with severe uremia are lethargic and anorexic. Confusion, seizures, and coma may also be observed. Pallor caused by anemia is often notable. Growth retardation is common. These complications can be controlled with treatment.

Treatment and nursing care. There are three treatments for patients with end-stage renal disease: renal transplantation, peritoneal dialysis, and hemodialysis. Renal transplantation is the best treatment for children. Although the child's immune system may try to reject the transplant, steroids and cyclosporine (Sandimmune) usually reverse rejection. Home peritoneal dialysis is successful when conscientious parents are involved. Erythropoietin is given to most patients to correct anemia. Special nutritional programs will help correct growth failure. Growth hormone is used in some patients. Children with severe renal failure can survive for many years. Almost all these patients attend school and participate in normal activities, with the possible exception of strenuous physical exercise. Nursing care for these patients is rewarding and challenging. Dialysis patients require special diets that are restricted in potassium, sodium, phosphorus, and protein.

KEY CONCEPTS

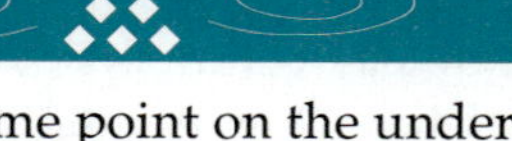

1 The urinary system consists of two kidneys, two ureters, the bladder, and the urethra. To regulate the composition of blood, the kidneys perform the complex task of producing urine. The ureters, bladder, and urethra are involved in the transportation, storage, and elimination of the urine.

2 Signs of genitourinary problems in infants include failure to void within 24 hours after birth, abdominal enlargement or swelling in the area of the kidney, and a scant urinary stream. In older children, signs include crying on urination, urgent and frequent urination, straining to void, and dribbling.

3 Hypospadias is a common deformity in which the urethra terminates at some point on the undersurface of the penis. Surgical repair is usually accomplished at about 1 year of age.

4 Cryptorchidism, testicular maldescent, is associated with an increased incidence of testicular injury and torsion. It may also be associated with infertility and possibly predispose the child to malignancies. If the testes do not descend spontaneously or in response to HCG, surgical correction is indicated.

5 Possible signs of a urinary tract infection in children under 3 years are high temperature, pallor, anorexia, vomiting, diarrhea, and convulsions. Older children experience sharp or dull

flank pain, gross hematuria, or pyuria. Frequent, urgent, and burning urination are common complaints.

6 Urinalysis and a culture of a properly collected specimen are the key to successful treatment of a urinary tract infection. Therapy depends primarily on identification of the causative organism.

7 Enuresis is defined as involuntary voiding of urine, and is very common in childhood. The condition may be caused by psychological or developmental disorders, an anatomical defect, or a systemic disease. Treatment depends on the cause.

8 Vesicoureteral reflux is caused by anatomical defects in the urinary tract or by infection. Patients with anatomical defects often require surgery. Long-term antibiotic therapy may be effective when the condition is caused by infection.

9 Wilms' tumor is one of the most common abdominal neoplasms of childhood. The initial manifestation is a mass in the region of the kidney. Constipation, vomiting, abdominal distention, and even dyspnea can occur. Treatment usually consists of prompt radical nephrectomy, followed by chemotherapy.

10 The most common cause of definite hypertension in children is renal disease. Renal tumors, renal vascular disease, hydronephrosis, and glomerulonephritis can cause hypertension. Treatment depends on the cause.

11 Nephrotic syndrome is a chronic renal disease characterized by anasarca, heavy proteinuria, low serum albumin levels, and high serum cholesterol values. The aims of nursing care include comforting the patient during the distress of massive edema, maintaining good nutrition, and preventing intercurrent infections.

12 Acute glomerulonephritis is an inflammatory disease of the glomeruli affecting both kidneys. Clinical manifestations include gross hematuria, often with cola-colored urine, edema, proteinuria, casts, hypertension, and azotemia. Antibiotic therapy is indicated when evidence of infection is present. Nursing care includes providing bed rest, limiting activities, and protecting the child from infection.

CRITICAL THOUGHT QUESTIONS

1 How do the structures and functions of the genitourinary tract of the infant and child differ from those of the adult? Identify some of the commonly occurring abnormalities of the genitourinary tract. What can be done in these conditions?

2 Why are urinary tract infections particularly common in infants and young children? Are they more common in boys or girls? Why is this the case? What can the nurse do to reduce the incidence of urinary tract infections?

3 Which renal diseases result in hypertension? How can you assess the blood pressure of an infant or young child? Discuss the two types of hypertension in children.

4 Streptococcal infections such as strep throat are common in childhood. What serious conditions can occur as a result of an untreated group A beta-hemolytic streptococcal infection? (You will also want to refer to Chapter 32.)

5 Nephritis and nephrotic syndromes affect the functioning of the kidneys. How do their clinical manifestations differ? What special nursing measures are instituted? What special precautions should you take in providing care to children with severe kidney involvement?

BIBLIOGRAPHY

Avner ED: Renal hypoplasia and dysplasia. In *Gellis and Kagan's Current pediatric therapy,* Philadelphia, 1993, WB Saunders.

Baer C: Acute renal failure: recognizing and reversing its deadly course, *Nursing 90* 20(6): 34-40, 1990.

Dabbagh S, Fleischmann LE, and Gruskin AB: Management of acute and chronic glomerulonephritis. In *Gellis and Kagan's Current pediatric therapy,* Philadelphia, 1993, WB Saunders.

Forest-Lalande L: Teaching nonsterile intermittent catheterization in a pediatric setting, *CAET J* 9(6):7-10, 1990.

Frauman A: Care of the family of the child with end stage renal disease, *ANNA J* 17(5):383-396, 1990.

Gibbs T: Genitourinary embryology and congenital malformations: the kidneys and ureters. I, *Urol Nurs* 10(3):16-24, 1990.

Gonzales R: Urologic disorders in infants and children. In Behrman RE, ed: *Nelson textbook of pediatrics,* ed 14, Philadelphia, 1992, WB Saunders.

Gutch CF, Stoner MH, and Corea AL: *Review of hemodialysis for nurses and dialysis personnel,* ed 5, St Louis, 1992, Mosby.

Herrin JT: Hydronephrosis and disorders of the ureter. In *Gellis and Kagan's Current pediatric therapy,* Philadelphia, 1993, WB Saunders.

Horton H: Hypospadius: when baby boys need surgery, *RN* 53(6):48-52, 1990.

Michell N and Stapleton FB: Routine admission urinalysis examination in pediatric patients: a poor value, *Pediatrics* 86, 345-349, 1990.

Nissen PD: Malignant tumors of the kidney. In *Gellis and Kagan's Current pediatric therapy,* Philadelphia, 1993, WB Saunders.

Sherbotie JR and Cornfeld D: Management of urinary tract infections in children, *Med Clin North Am* 75, 327-338, 1991.

Smoyer WE: Urinary tract obstruction in children, *Clin Pediatr* 31(2): 109-119, 1992.

Wingen A, Muller-Wiefel D, and Scharer K: Comparison of different regimens of prednisone therapy in frequently relapsing nephrotic syndrome, *Acta Pediatr Scand* 79:305-310, 1990.

37

Hematological Problems

CHAPTER OBJECTIVES

After studying this chapter, the student should be able to:

1. Differentiate the various types of anemia.
2. Describe iron-deficiency anemia: definition, prevention, importance, ages of peak incidence, and treatment.
3. Describe sickle cell anemia, sickle cell trait, and the circulation problems that can occur in children having the disease.
4. Describe nursing interventions for the child with sickle cell anemia.
5. Discuss the pathophysiology and clinical manifestations of hemophilia.
6. Identify four safety considerations for children with a diagnosis of hemophilia.
7. Describe five signs or symptoms associated with leukemia and how their appearance relates to the primary bone marrow abnormalities characteristically present.
8. Discuss the supportive care and needs of the child with leukemia and the family and how the nurse can provide informational and emotional support.
9. Discuss the general improvement in the prognosis of children currently diagnosed as having acute lymphoblastic leukemia (ALL), and list three factors that appear to aid in determining the individual child's prognosis.
10. Identify the diagnostic criteria for idiopathic thrombocytopenic purpura and the importance of parent education.

DISORDERS OF THE BLOOD AND BLOOD-FORMING ORGANS

The cardiovascular system (heart and blood vessels) is designed so that nutrients, hormones, and oxygen reach the individual body tissue cells and so that waste products from those cells are properly transported for elimination by the kidneys, lungs, or skin. To do this efficiently, the circulating fluid within the cardiovascular system—blood—contains many substances. Of particular interest are the three types of structures called the *formed elements.* The red blood cells, or erythrocytes, help transport oxygen and carbon dioxide in the blood to and from the lungs. The white blood cells, or *leukocytes,* and antibodies of various types help protect the bloodstream and surrounding body tissues from the intrusion of disease-producing microorganisms and foreign proteins. The platelets, or *thrombocytes,* assist in the formation of clots to repair any leak in a damaged blood vessel. Any lack or defect in the normal makeup of the blood is likely to cause symptoms of disease. This chapter focuses on four common pediatric hematological disorders including anemia, hemophilia, leukemia, and idiopathic thrombocytopenic purpura. For a review of acquired immune deficiency syndrome (AIDS) refer to Chapter 31.

KEY VOCABULARY

anemia	Reduction of red blood cells or hemoglobin concentration below normal.
CBC	Complete blood count.
coagulation	Process of clotting.
erythrocyte	Red blood cell.
hematocrit (Hct)	Percent of RBCs in total blood volume.
hemoglobin (Hgb)	Oxygen-carrying, iron-containing pigment in red blood cells.
hemolysis	The destruction of RBCs.
ITP	Idiopathic thrombocytopenic purpura.
lymphocyte	One of the major groups of WBCs.
platelet	Cellular fragment involved in coagulation.
reticulocyte	Immature RBC.
WBC	White blood cell.

Anemias

When the term *anemia* is used, it indicates a condition in which the total hemoglobin content of the blood is abnormally reduced, either because of lack of sufficient hemoglobin in the red blood cells or lack of red blood cells. Hemoglobin is the substance in red blood cells necessary for the normal transport of oxygen to the body cells. The most common cause of anemia in children is iron deficiency.

Iron-deficiency anemia

The most common type of anemia in the pediatric population is iron-deficiency anemia.

Etiology. The major cause of iron-deficiency anemia is insufficient dietary intake of iron to meet the demands of body growth (especially of low birth weight and premature infants and growing adolescents). Infants with iron deficiency commonly have a diet largely composed of cow's milk, which is low in iron. Causes of anemia other than dietary deficiency include (1) acute or chronic blood loss and (2) impaired absorption (severe prolonged diarrhea).

Clinical manifestations. Pallor of the mucous membranes, irritability, anorexia, and listlessness are signs of iron deficiency. The anemia is usually discovered on a routine screening during a well child visit. Hemoglobin concentrations of less than 11 g/100 ml and a hematocrit level of less than 33% in a healthy infant strongly suggest iron deficiency. Insufficient iron for synthesis of hemoglobin is the cause of this problem. Children under 3 years of age and adolescent girls have the highest incidence.

Treatment. Treatment consists of oral administration of iron preparations, preferably ferrous iron, and a revision of diet to include iron-rich foods (muscle meats, liver, eggs, wheat, green leafy vegetables). If the condition is particularly severe or unresponsive as a result of parental failure to provide iron-rich foods intramuscular injections of iron-dextran complex may be ordered. Packed red cells are rarely necessary. Since the highest incidence of iron-deficiency anemia is in infancy (6 to 18 months) the best and least expensive preventive measure against this form of anemia is the use of iron-fortified formulas during the entire first year of life in bottle-fed infants. Recent studies have shown that breast-fed infants are able to maintain adequate iron levels because more iron is absorbed from breast milk than from cow's milk. Premature, breast-fed infants require iron supplementation because of their greater growth requirements. The increased utilization of breast-feeding and iron-fortified formulas have led to significant reductions in iron-deficiency anemia in preschool children. Adequate iron intake promotes optimal growth, learning, and resistance to disease.

Sickle Cell Disease

Sickle cell disease is a collective term that includes several hereditary disorders whose clinical and laboratory features are related to the presence of sickle hemoglobin (Hb S) in red blood cells. Although a few cases have been reported in the caucasian race, sickle cell disease is found primarily in African-Americans. About 75,000 African-Americans have the disease. Hemolytic anemia with its intermittent crises leads to chronic illness of increasing severity and reduction of life expectancy.

The sickling abnormality is attributed to a mutant gene responsible for the synthesis of a type of hemoglobin different from the normal. The abnormal change in the shape of the red blood cell from a biconcave disk to a crescent, or sicklelike, shape becomes apparent following exposure to low oxygen tension or low pH. The basic defect in sickle hemoglobin is in the alteration of only one amino acid of the 574 that make up normal hemoglobin. This single change is responsible for all the clinical manifestations of sickle cell disease.

Sickle cell anemia (SCA)

Every person possesses a pair of genes that governs the synthesis of hemoglobin. One gene is inherited from each parent. Sickle cell anemia (SCA) is present in those persons who receive the mutant sickle cell gene from both parents (homozygous inheritance, SS) (Fig. 37-1).

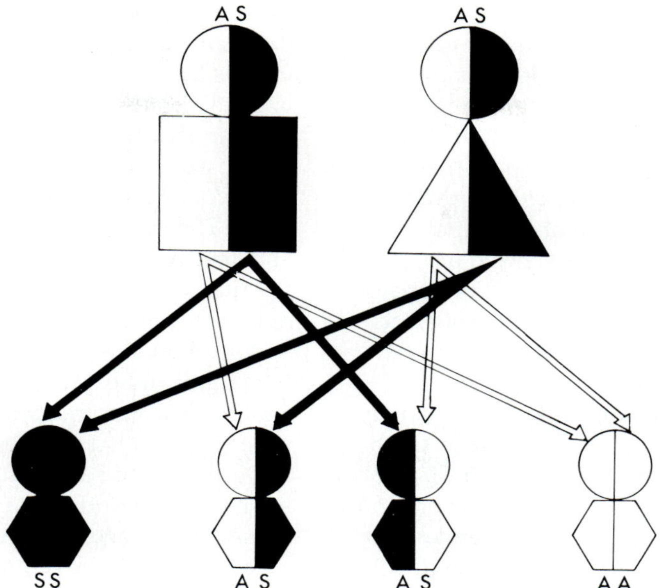

Fig. 37-1 Sickle cell anemia (homozygous inheritance). When both parents carry sickle cell gene *(AS)*, possibilities for inheritance in offspring are that one child in four will inherit sickle cell anemia *(SS)*; two children in four will inherit sickle cell trait *(AS)*; one child in four will be normal *(AA)*.

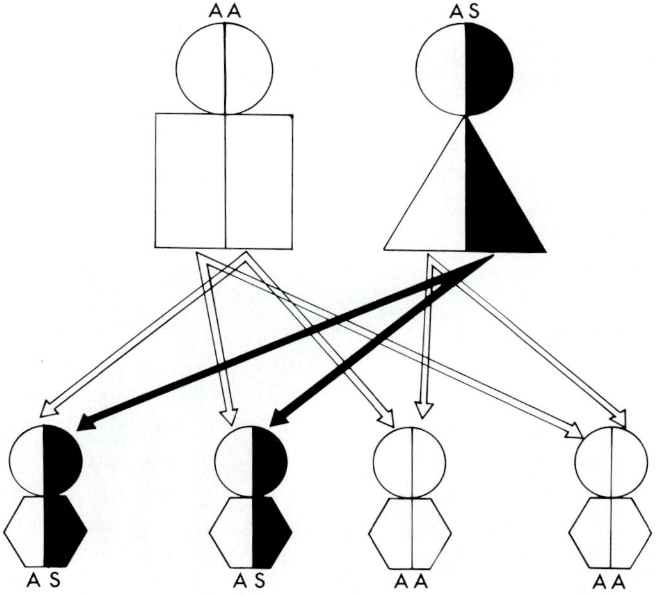

Fig. 37-2 Sickle cell trait (heterozygous inheritance). When only one parent is carrier of sickle cell gene *(AS)*, possibilities for inheritance in offspring are that two children in four will be normal *(AA)*; two children in four will carry sickle cell trait *(AS)*.

Sickle cell trait (SCT)

The sickle cell trait (SCT) is the most common defect in hemoglobin found in the United States. It is present in persons who have received a Hb S gene from one parent and a normal Hb A gene from the other parent (heterozygous inheritance, AS) (Fig. 37-2). The most important consideration in SCT is the genetic risk of SCA for the offspring. Although persons with SCT have as much as 40% Hb S under normal conditions, no clinical signs of disease or hemoglobin abnormalities are typically present. Rarely, someone with sickle cell trait manifests symptoms of stress when exercising excessively or traveling at high altitudes in nonpressurized airplanes. SCT confers some degree of protection against the lethal effects of malaria, which may account for the major distribution of Hb S in central Africa and the very fact that SCA exists. The presence of a gene for another abnormal type of hemoglobin, or the gene for thalassemia, should be suspected in a child with sickle cell disease when the blood of only one of the parents shows the sickle cell trait. These other sickle cell types (Hb SC and Hb SB thalassemia) cause the same problems as Hb SS disease.

Clinical manifestations. Young infants are usually spared the severe symptoms of SCA because of the temporary presence of fetal hemoglobin (Hb F). Hb F is gradually replaced with the Hb S. As the proportion of Hb S increases, the symptoms of anemia may appear—usually when the infant is between 6 and 12 months of age.

Hemolytic anemia. Hemolytic anemia is caused by intravascular sickling that occurs diffusely throughout the body. Sickling red cells often form spontaneously during venous circulation when the red blood cells give up oxygen to the tissues. They also form when there are changes in pH or electrolyte balance associated with infection, acidosis, or dehydration. The body acts quickly to remove these abnormal sickled cells from the bloodstream, and this causes the severe degree of anemia that occurs.

Vasoocclusive crisis. The exact events leading to the onset of painful crises are not clearly known. Many of these crises are preceded by infections. The basis of the painful crisis appears to be occlusion of blood vessels by sickled red blood cells. This interferes with normal tissue blood supply, resulting in subsequent cellular death and damage of the organs involved. Before an individual reaches 2 years of age, dactylitis, or the "hand-foot," syndrome commonly occurs (Fig. 37-3). The symmetrical, painful swelling of the hands and feet results from interference with circulation to the metacarpals and metatarsals. If the child's pain is not too severe, increased fluids, application of warmth, and acetaminophen relieves the pain. In other children the pain is unbearable and is relieved only by stronger analgesics. For hospitalized children, patient- or parent-controlled anesthesia (PCA) is beneficial.

Occlusive episodes after the first or second year of life most frequently occur during the preschool period. Episodes of acute abdominal pain can be severe, accompanied by fever, muscle spasm, nausea, vomiting, and leukocytosis.

Sequestration crisis. A crisis associated with shock is called "acute splenic sequestration crisis" (ASSC). The parent notes a rather sudden increase in pallor accompanied by abdominal distention and thirst. By the time these children arrive at the hospital, they have become notably dyspneic and weak. Left-sided abdominal (splenic) pain is present, and the pulse and respirations are elevated.

Treatment. Prompt diagnosis and treatment are essential to ensure survival. Transfusion of packed erythrocytes and plasma expanders should be started immediately on admission. The nurse who recognizes

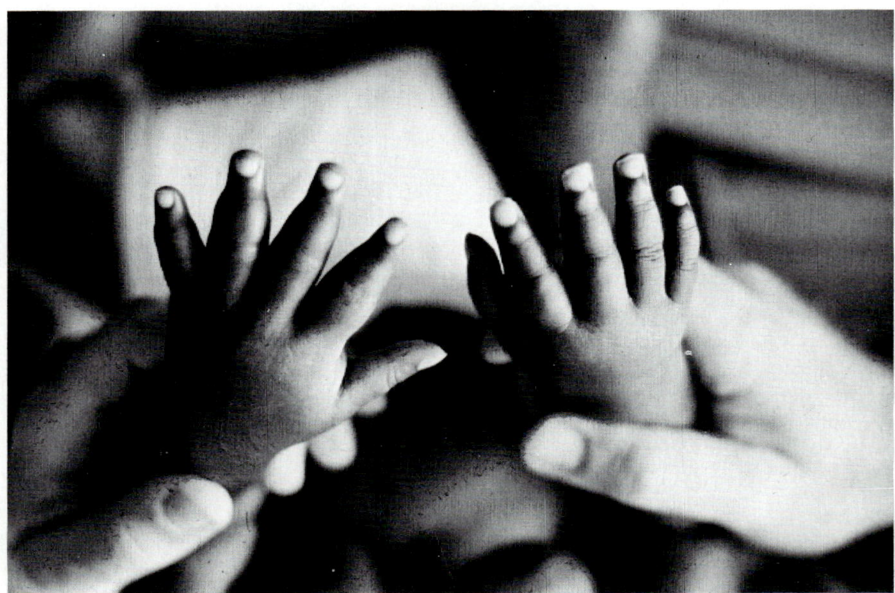

Fig. 37-3 Dactylitis—swelling of the hand—sickle cell interference in circulation. (Courtesy of CDR Alton L Lightsey, MC, USN, Naval Hospital, San Diego, Calif.)

the situation should hasten the admission procedure, but be sure to check the child's weight and height accurately. It is imperative to take blood specimens and urine samples immediately. Special equipment for transfusions is essential. A chest x-ray may also be ordered. Because reduced oxygenation increases sickling, an atmosphere of well-humidified oxygen by nasal cannula or mask is used. Pulse oximetry is essential for monitoring O_2 content of the blood. Because of the rapidity with which a sequestration crisis can occur (and even recur) and its threat of fatality, a splenectomy may be performed. A hyperbaric chamber may be utilized.

The nurse must recognize that parents may be experts on their child's disease and may offer important information regarding effective interventions. Common parental reactions include: fear, resentment, guilt, and anger. The nurse must give these parents every opportunity to explore their feelings. Active listening, encouragement, and a caring approach will assist the parents in coping and in providing support for their child.

Aplastic crisis. Since children with SCA have a continuing hemolytic anemia, they must produce increased numbers of new red blood cells each day. Conditions that suppress the bone marrow production of red blood cells can lead to a life-threatening anemia termed *aplastic crisis*. This commonly occurs after infections or as a result of a deficiency of materials needed to produce red blood cells (for example, iron or folic acid).

Treatment. Treatment for aplastic crisis involves transfusions of packed red cells until the cause of the decreased production can be determined and corrected.

Infections. Children with SCA develop irreversible damage to the spleen after numerous occlusive crises involving this organ. Since a normal spleen is needed to fight certain bacterial infections, children with SCA do not handle these infections well. Pneumococcal infection, which often complicates upper respiratory infections, has been a leading cause of death in children with SCA.

Treatment and prophylaxis. Prompt diagnosis and aggressive antibiotic therapy is essential. Parents should be instructed in the early signs and symptoms of infection, and children should have immediate access to medical care. All children with SCA should receive immunization with the pneumococcal vaccine, hepatitis B vaccine, and Hemophilus B (HbCV) vaccine, which are protective against the common strains of pneumococcus and hemophilus that can cause life-threatening infections in these children. The National Sickle Cell Care Study has demonstrated reduced mortality in children with sickle cell anemia who were given daily prophylactic penicillin. Currently, all children with sickle cell anemia should receive penicillin daily to prevent infection.

The therapy for SCA and frequent crises are major challenges in pediatric hematology. There is no cure for SCA or a completely satisfactory treatment for its crises. Optimal health maintenance is critical.

Detection and counseling

Screening programs for SCA or SCT should not be set up unless a genetic counseling service can be provided to those found to carry the trait. Otherwise, the benefits of the screening are lost, and anguish can be created over an essentially benign condition. Screening programs must incorporate meaningful education about the nature of SCA and its mode of inheritance, as well as individual counseling. In mass screening, Sickledex (sickle-turbidity tube test) or the sickle cell slide test is adequate, but positive reactions must be followed by hemoglobin electrophoresis to confirm results. Newborn infants can be screened in the hospital for both the condition and the trait. Such hospital programs facilitate optimum infant care and early diagnosis of crises and provide counseling for the parents.

Nursing care. The nursing care of children with anemia, whatever its basic cause, must take into account the excessive fatigue experienced by most of these children. Their energy must be conserved. They especially need help and encouragement to develop a healthy nutrition plan and to stay well-hydrated. Frequent small feedings are more healthful than large infrequent meals. The enlarged liver and spleen and tender muscles of some of these patients all demand gentle care. Attention to signs of bleeding (external or internal) is important. Signs of jaundice, increased pallor, increased lethargy, or irritability should be reported. Patients receiving blood transfusions should be carefully observed and protected against possible infiltration of the blood (a potentially serious event).

Nursing Alert

Nurses must immediately report signs of chest syndrome and stroke, which are potentially fatal complications of sickle cell anemia. Signs of chest syndrome include: a temperature of 102° F or higher, severe, radiating chest pain and cough, retractions, dyspnea, and tachypnea. Signs of stroke include twitching or jerking of the face, arms, or legs; severe headache and vomiting; slurred speech; vision changes; strange behavior; weakness or paralysis; unsteady gait; convulsions; or seizures.

PATIENT PERSPECTIVE BY SHERRIAN SIMPSON, AGE 29

After reading this chapter on hematological problems, I found that all of the technical facts were in order. When reading medical and nursing information involving "etiology," "clinical manifestations," and "treatment" my first question is, "OK, but how do the patients feel physically, emotionally, and psychologically?" This is where I enter in, because I know how a patient can feel. I am a patient—I have sickle cell disease (Fig. 37-4).

Looking back on my childhood, I cannot say that it was like that of most American children. I was happy and took things in stride, however, I always knew that I was different. Being different can mean many different things, but when you are a sick child, being different means not being able to stay out and play as long as your friends. I got extremely tired when I ran, and it would hurt when I would do simple things like jumping rope. Needless to say, I played a lot indoors—often alone. I have never once played in the rain, for fear of catching a cold, or worse, the dreaded pneumonia. Having sickle cell disease means the body doesn't have the defenses to fight infection, so the patient is highly susceptible. Thus the key is self-care and prevention. I have always had to protect myself—multivitamins, vitamin E, extra vitamin B, folic acid, eating nutritious foods, staying extremely well-hydrated (1.5 gallons/day), and avoiding people who have colds, flu, or other contagious maladies. Friends couldn't come over if they had the slightest inkling that they were ill. I remember my mother taking me out of elementary school several times, even though I was healthy, because there were epidemics of chicken pox and she was afraid that I would end up in the hospital. The irony is that at the age of 27 I finally contracted a mild case and there wasn't anything my mom could do except paint me with calamine lotion!

With all of this overprotection comes resentment, anger, and even hurt feelings. As a little girl, I didn't understand why I could not play with my best friend, Amy, when I wasn't sick and Amy was running around playing, even with a cold. My friend, David, who also has sickle cell disease, remembers not understanding why his parents did not want him to play football, and why they were so angry when he did it anyway, because he wanted to be with his friends. Being overprotected doesn't stop when a child becomes an adult—we are always children in the eyes of our parents.

The few times I had the opportunity to go to the mountains to play in the snow, I usually ended the return trip in the emergency room. Because of the lack of oxygen at higher elevations, my body would go into a sickle cell "crisis."

A crisis for me can be predictable and unpredictable at the same time. Unpredictable because I don't always know when I am getting sick and predictable in that a crisis can be triggered by any illness, including a common cold. A crisis can also be triggered by fatigue and stress. The ever-predictable thing for me is the pain and the instant lack of energy.

On admission to the hospital, the most important "nursing intervention" is effective communication. My greatest frustration is when care providers won't listen to me. If I explain that drawing blood from my portacath is easier for both of us, why must they insist on poking my already collapsed veins? I know that it takes 100 mg of Demerol to control my pain, yet less experienced nurses respond with shock and disbelief or insensitive comments like "she doesn't look that sick!"

My parents have also lived with this disease for the past 29 years, thus they are experts. They have taught me how to care for myself and to recognize my own limitations. Listen to parents' suggestions! We must all work together—the patient, parents, and the entire health care team for the best outcome. No one should be excluded from receiving accurate information and contributing to the plan of care.

I am fortunate in that I have always had the best medical and nursing care possible, thanks to my parents. It did not matter whether I was 5 years old or 25 years old, my parents have always been there for support and advocacy.

Finally, one of the hardest things for me now is regaining my independence after experiencing a stroke in 1988. I say regaining, because I was in remission during my high school and undergraduate years, thus I was moving through the normal tasks of adolescence. Although I've had nearly full recovery from the stroke, I have had to rely on my parent's support and advocacy daily for things that other young women take for granted. Nothing makes me angrier than seeing teens and young adults throw their lives away, or not take advantage of the wonderful things that life presents them. With a healthy lifestyle, inner strength, and the guidance, tolerance, and gift of hope that the health care team offers, I, too, look forward to the future and the wonderful gift of life.

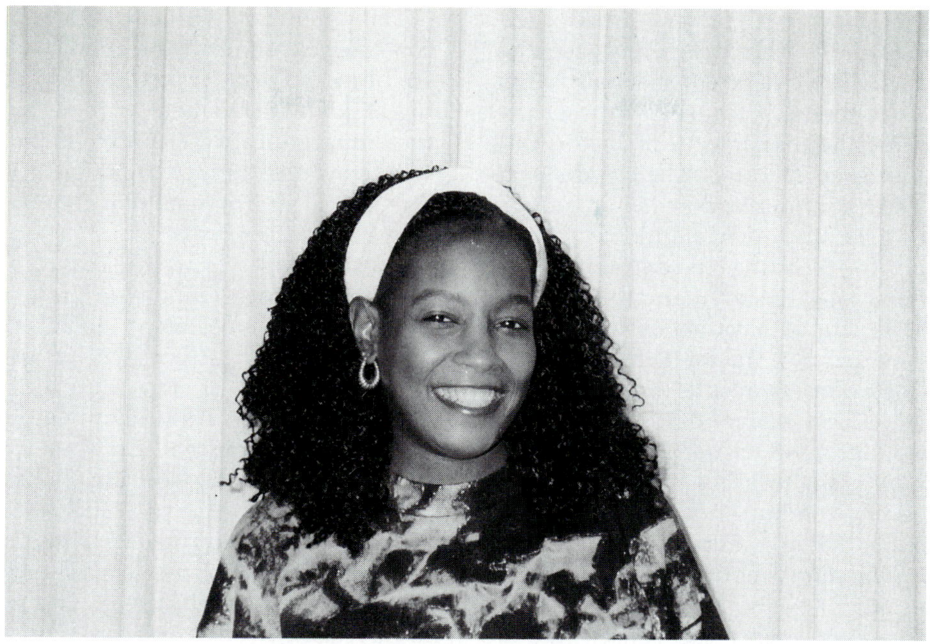

Fig. 37-4 Sherrian Simpson, age 29.

Signs of toxic reactions, complaints of chest or back pain, itching hives, or elevated temperature with or without chills should be noted and reported immediately. The rate of administration should be closely monitored to ensure that the circulatory system is not overloaded. For a patient perspective, see the box on p. 804.

Hemophilia

Hemophilia A-factor VIII deficiency. Classic hemophilia, antihemophilic globulin (AHG), or factor VIII deficiency, is a disorder involving a defect in the clotting mechanism of the blood. Hemophilia results from a defect in a gene on the X chromosome concerned with blood clotting (Table 37-1). It is a sex-linked, recessive condition confined almost exclusively to males and can pass from one generation to another from a carrier mother to her son. A male receives only one X, from his mother, which impairs his blood clotting process. Since the female receives two X chromosomes, one normal gene ensures normal blood clotting. A girl inherits the condition only if her father is a hemophiliac and her mother is a carrier. Because of its hereditary feature, it has figured prominently in the history of royal families and has been called the disease of kings.

◆ **TABLE 37-1**
Clotting Factors of the Blood

Factor Number	
I	Fibrinogen
II	Prothrombin
III	Thromboplastin
IV	Calcium
V	Labile factor
VII	Stable factor
VIII	Antihemophilic factor
	Antihemophilic globulin
IX	Christmas factor
X	Stuart-Prower factor
XI	Plasma thromboplastin antecedent
XI	Hageman factor
XIII	Fibrin stabilizing factor

The defect in clot formation is caused by the lack of antihemophilic globulin, or factor VIII, in the blood plasma. A wide range of factor VIII values (50% to 200%) exists, but in most healthy persons the average is 100%. A severe hemophiliac has less than 1% of factor VIII. Hemophiliac patients are susceptible to spontaneous, unprovoked hemorrhage. Moderate hemophiliacs have from 2% to 5% of factor VIII and may bleed excessively with minor trauma. Mild hemophiliacs have 10% to 20% of factor VIII and may, with care, live free from bleeding episodes. Surgical procedures, dental extractions, and even the normal rough-and-tumble existence of young children are especially hazardous for a hemophiliac patient.

Current treatment consists of administration of factor VIII concentrate in an amount necessary to control hemorrhage. However, protection afforded from one infusion rapidly disappears, because the concentration of factor VIII falls to one half of its original level in 8 to 10 hours. Because of this, it may be necessary to repeat administration of factor VIII within 10 hours if bleeding continues. The precise level of factor VIII needed to control bleeding is not known, but the amount of factor VIII given should be related to the seriousness of the bleeding. In central nervous system bleeding the goal is to maintain 100% factor VIII activity until the site of bleeding is completely healed. In joint bleeding, 50% factor VIII activity is usually sufficient for optimum results. The combination of immobilization and a level of 10% to 20% is usually adequate to control soft tissue bleeding. Efforts to control bleeding by using local measures (pressure, cold, or applications of thrombin) should be attempted if possible. Some cities have hemophilia centers that are prepared to render intravenous therapy to these patients on an outpatient basis. Many patients and families are taught to administer the concentrate at home. This allows faster therapy for bleeding episodes and the maintenance of a more normal lifestyle.

Factor VIII inhibitors. A small number (about 5%) of patients with classic hemophilia develop inhibitors (antibodies that block factor VIII). The presence of a circulating inhibitor is usually detected by the lack of response to a dose of factor VIII that normally would control the bleeding. Inhibitors may develop in young children after a few exposures to factor VIII, but no evidence shows that the inhibitors are related to the number of transfusions a patient receives. Without exposure to plasma products, the amount of inhibitor may gradually decrease, and factor VIII can then be given again with temporary benefit. Effective control of bleeding in patients is very difficult when the inhibitor is circulating.

Hemophilia B-factor IX deficiency (Christmas disease). Factor IX plasma thromboplastic component (PTC) deficiency accounts for about 15% of patients with hemophilia. The causes and symptoms are similar to those of hemophilia A. A factor IX concentrate has become available for treatment and is used in the same manner as factor VIII.

Hemophilia C-factor XI deficiency. Factor XI plasma thromboplastin antecedent (PTA) deficiency differs from hemophilias A and B. It is usually a mild disorder and may appear in either boys or girls as the result of an autosomal-recessive trait in which bleeding occurs only in the homozygote. Bleeding episodes in factor XI deficiency are best treated with infusions of fresh plasma. The nursing care of all patients with bleeding problems is similar except that the type of intravenous therapy ordered differs, depending on the kind of replacement needed.

The parents of a patient with hemophilia are under considerable strain. They must constantly observe the environment of their adventuresome toddler or growing child. With the help of their health care provider, they must educate the child to make choices in activity with consideration for the degree of hazard it entails. A creative, environment that allows exploration within safe limits is optimal.

Nursing care. The nursing care of children with hemophilia must emphasize prevention. The sides of infants' cribs should be padded. All toddlers should be denied toys and objects with sharp edges or objects that are easily broken, but they are particularly dangerous for the child with hemophilia. Rubber toys are satisfactory for play. Children learning to walk can be fitted with knee-pads. Bleeding into the joints may produce considerable pain and deformity. Every effort should be made to prevent stiffening of the joint and loss of function. The nurse must provide children with interesting but safe diversion and watch for any signs of increasing bruises or internal or external blood loss. The nurse must also observe the child for untoward reaction during transfusion and check whether the intravenous infusion is flowing as ordered.

Home care. Currently, patients are taught to self-administer replacement factors at home. It has been demonstrated and proved that prompt treatment at home can reduce the amount of factor needed and can save the patient time-consuming trips and hospital costs. In addition, early treatment of bleeding episodes has been shown to prevent the crippling complications caused by recurrent spontaneous bleeding into the joints.

In an effort to accomplish this goal, selected patients or their parents are instructed to administer cryoprecipitate and plasma concentrates as necessary at home. Whenever therapy becomes necessary to control minor bleeding episodes, the health care provider is contacted for advice about the proper dosage. Antihistamines and steroids are kept on hand to be taken by the patient if a transfusion reaction occurs.

Nurses often follow the progress of the patient at home, instructing the family about the importance of accurate records and emphasizing the need for periodic outpatient physical evaluations. The home care program spares patients the expense of frequent hospital visits and the burden of travel and waiting; most of all, it promotes a more normal life, utilizing the maximum intellectual and social potential of the hemophilic child.

Leukemia

Although cancer is the leading cause of death from disease in children, and leukemia is the most common

◆ TABLE 37-2
Pathology and Clinical Manifestations of Leukemia

Organ	Effect	Manifestations
Bone marrow dysfunction	Anemia Infection Bleeding tendency Bone weakness	Fatigue, pallor Fever Hemorrhage (petechiae) Tendency toward fracture Pain
Lymphatic system	Infiltration	Lymphadenopathy
Liver	Enlargement	Hepatomegaly
Spleen	Fibrosis	Splenomegaly
Central nervous system	Increased ICP Enlarged ventricles	Headache Vomiting Irritability Lethargy, coma
	Meningeal irritation	Stiff neck and back pain
Increased metabolism	Nutrient deprivation by invading cells	Anorexia Weight loss Muscle wasting Fatigue

childhood malignancy, the outlook can no longer be considered hopeless. Leukemia is a primary malignant disease of the bone marrow characterized by an abnormal increase of immature white blood cells or undifferentiated blast cells. This uncontrolled proliferation of leukemic cells prevents production and development of normal blood cells (hematopoiesis), which leads to infections, anemia, and bleeding. These abnormal white blood cells invade the various tissues of the body, causing pressure symptoms. (For example, infiltration of the bone marrow produces severe pain in bones and joints; mediastinal nodes can cause tracheal compression that in turn causes respiratory difficulty and cough.) The predominating symptoms depend on the area of the body invaded by the leukemic cells. Diagnosis is suspected on the basis of discovery of immature white blood cell forms in the circulating blood. An unequivocal diagnosis is confirmed by microscopic examination of the bone marrow, usually obtained from the posterior iliac crest. At times the number of circulating white blood cells is extremely elevated. Some cases demonstrate total white blood cell counts above 100,000 per mm^3. In some children the number of white blood cells in the peripheral circulation is relatively low, and proportionately few immature forms are seen; the disease is said to be *aleukemic*. However, at the same time the bone marrow can be packed with abnormal cells. (See Table 37-2).

Incidence. Leukemia is the most common form of cancer in children. The incidence is approximately 4 cases per 100,000 per year in children less than 15 years in the United States. A slightly increased incidence occurs in boys, and the peak age of onset in children is 3 to 4 years of age. Certain children have been clearly identified as being at increased risk for developing leukemia (Table 37-3). Although there seems to have been a decline over the past 15 years in the occurrence of acute leukemia, it accounts for almost 32% of the malignant diseases in children under 15 years of age.

Types. The different types of leukemia are classified according to the kind of white cells principally involved and the relative speed of the disease process. The most common leukemic cell observed in pediatric practice is the undifferentiated form called a *blast,* an immature form of white blood cell, usually of the lymphocytic cell line. Acute lymphoblastic leukemia (ALL) accounts for the majority of cases. Acute granulocytic or myelogenous leukemia (AML) accounts for about 20% of cases. This form, however, does not respond as favorably as ALL to the antileukemic agents currently available.

Clinical manifestations. The signs and symptoms of leukemia may be rather slow and insidious in onset or rapid in their development. These children may complain of fatigue and weakness, and lose weight. They may be pale and bruise easily. Fever, with a persistent respiratory tract infection, is a common complaint. The child's liver, spleen, and lymph nodes, (particularly cervical and inguinal) become infiltrated with abnormal cells and may be enlarged. Before the era of modern treatment—"Total Therapy" with central nervous system (CNS) prophylaxis—CNS involvement developed in approximately 50% of children during the course of their illness. A smaller number of children

◆ TABLE 37-3
Incidence of Leukemia*

Groups Affected	Number Affected
Nonwhite American children under 15 years of age	1 in 5500
White American children under 15 years of age	1 in 3000
Siblings of leukemic children	1 in 720
Children with Down syndrome	1 in 95
Children exposed to atomic irradiation	1 in 60
Monozygotic twin sibling (with one diagnosed in infancy)	1 in 5 (both will get it)

*Peak: white children, 3 to 4 years; nonwhite children, younger.

(8%) initially have central nervous system leukemia at the time of diagnosis. CNS leukemia causes increased intracranial pressure, which is typically manifested by headache, nausea and vomiting, slowed pulse, and elevated blood pressure. The child is highly irritable and tired. Spinal fluid examination confirms the physician's diagnosis.

The course of the disease usually involves several hospitalizations and many trips to the outpatient clinic to receive therapy or to be treated for complications of therapy. Complete remissions of the disease for extended periods have been induced with specific drug combinations (treatment protocol). The major objectives of chemotherapy are the induction of a complete remission and the maintenance of patients in a state of remission for the longest possible time, with the expectation that a significant percentage of children with ALL (50% to 80%) can be cured of their disease. A

◆ TABLE 37-4
Drugs Currently Used in the Treatment of Leukemia

Agent	Routes of Administration	Signs of Toxicity
Induction		
Prednisone	Oral	Moon-shaped face, osteoporosis, acne, fluid retention, ulcers, increased susceptibility to infection, personality changes, hyperglycemia
Vincristine (Oncovin)	IV	Peripheral neuropathy, alopecia
Daunomycin	IV	Bone marrow depression,* alopecia, nausea, vomiting, oral ulceration, congestive heart failure
L-Asparaginase	IV, IM	Hypersensitivity reactions, liver dysfunction, pancreatitis, hyperglycemia
Adriamycin	IV	Bone marrow depression,* alopecia, nausea, vomiting, oral ulceration, congestive heart failure
Cytarabine (Cytosar)	IV	Bone marrow depression, nausea, vomiting, fever, alopecia
Methotrexate	IV Intrathecal	Anorexia, abdominal pain, oral and gastrointestinal tract ulceration, bone marrow depression, alopecia (rare), hepatotoxicity
Maintenance		
6-Mercaptopurine	Oral	Bone marrow depression,* nausea, vomiting, oral and gastrointestinal tract ulceration, hepatotoxicity
Methotrexate	Oral IV Intrathecal	Anorexia, abdominal pain, oral and gastrointestinal tract ulceration, bone marrow depression,* alopecia (rare)
Cyclophosphamide (Cytoxan)	Oral IV	Bone marrow depression,* skin rashes, alopecia, hemorrhagic cystitis, oral ulceration, diarrhea
Cytosine arabinoside (Cytosar or ARA-C)	IV SQ Intrathecal	Bone marrow depression,* nausea, vomiting
Thioguanine	Oral	Bone marrow depression,* hepatotoxicity

*Bone marrow depression is characterized by leukopenia, thrombocytopenia, and anemia.

complete remission is defined as "restoration to normal health and clinical well-being." Physical and laboratory examinations are negative, blood and bone marrow are considered normal, and all evidence of disease is absent. Best results to date have been achieved with intensive courses of drug combinations and with optimum supportive care, including transfusions of platelets, red blood cells, and antibiotic therapy. Since 1947, when the first brief, temporary remission was induced with aminopterin, antileukemic drug therapy has greatly improved.

Treatment. Although intensive research continues in an attempt to unravel the origin and development of the disease, there is no doubt that the disease is treatable. In fact the word *cured* is being used to describe long-term survivors no longer receiving chemotherapy.

Modern treatment currently consists of intermittent administration of high doses of several drugs in combination (Table 37-4). The duration of remissions has been increased by the addition of prophylactic therapy to the central nervous system by radiation or spinal canal (intrathecal) injections of methotrexate. Use of this therapy has reduced the incidence of central nervous system leukemia from 50% to less than 5%. In an attempt to prevent the immunosuppressive effects of continuous chemotherapy the maintenance schedules currently used involve intermittent doses of multiple agents in combination, followed by rest periods without therapy or moderate daily dose schedules periodically reinforced with "induction" agents. Children with acute leukemia should be referred to specialized centers where the optimum opportunity for effective therapy is available (Fig. 37-5).

Complete remissions for long periods have been induced in almost all patients with acute lymphoblastic leukemia. Children in remission must have regular medical supervision, including frequent hematological studies. Relapse is marked by falling hemoglobin levels, thrombocytopenia, severe decreases in the white blood cells called *neutrophils,* and the reappearance of immature or "blast" cells in the blood and bone marrow.

Nursing care. Platelet transfusions have reduced the number of deaths caused by hemorrhage and increased the opportunity to use effective drugs that depress platelet production. Corticosteroids increase capillary resistance and are useful adjuncts in the control of bleeding. Bleeding from accessible areas is occasionally controlled by the local application of thromboplastin and Gel-Foam. Transfusion of packed red blood cells is frequently necessary due to anemia associated with bone marrow depression. The child generally feels better and has more energy when his hemoglobin is greater than 7.5 grams.

Infection poses the greatest threat to the life of the leukemic child. Although fever can result from the primary disease, it is important to search for infection in all patients with an elevated temperature. Cultures should be taken from blood, urine, and throat. Drugs used in the control of bacterial infection, until cultures are available, include oxacillin or a cephalosporin for staphylococci, streptococci, and pneumococci; ampicillin is used against *Haemophilus influenzae.* Amikacin or piperacillin or both are used against gram-negative organisms, such as *Pseudomonas, Escherichia coli,* and *Proteus.* Children who are in relapse are particularly at risk for fungal, viral, and protozoal infections. Oral moniliasis is seen frequently and is treated with oral nystatin (Mycostatin). A susceptible leukemic child who is exposed to chickenpox should receive zoster immune globulin Interstitial pneumonia caused by the protozoal organism *Pneumocystis carinii* is a major cause of illness and death. Trimethoprim-sulfameth-

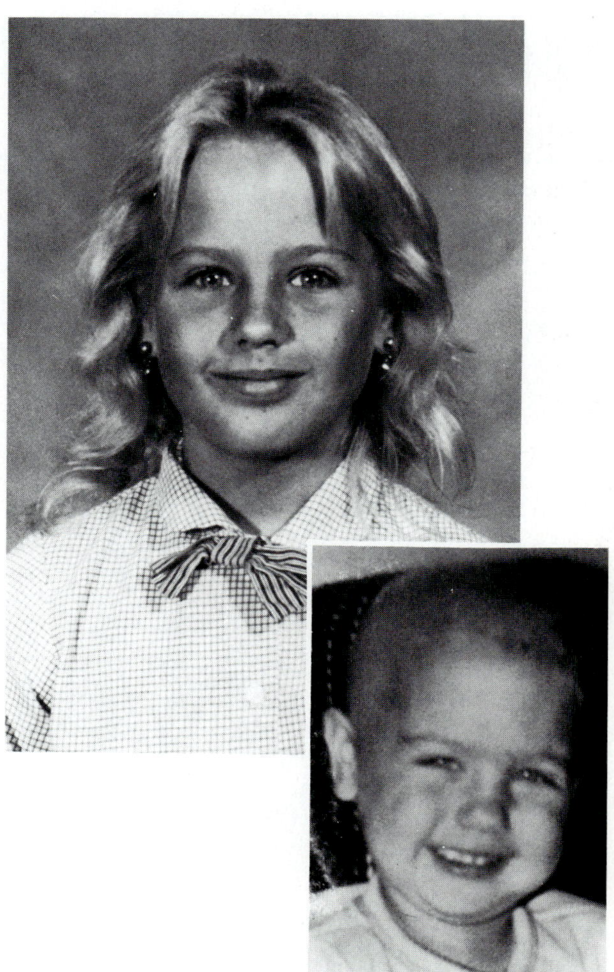

Fig. 37-5 Stephanie, age 11, was originally diagnosed with ALL at age 2 years *(insert).* Her chemotherapy was discontinued after 3 years.

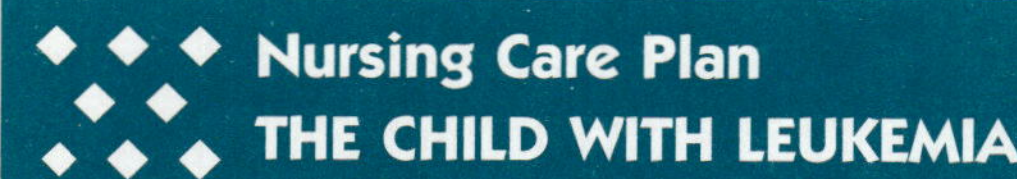

Nursing Care Plan
THE CHILD WITH LEUKEMIA

	Selected Nursing Diagnosis	Expected Outcomes	Interventions
A	Potential for infection related to immunosuppression. Clinical manifestations: Fever, increased respiratory and heart rate.	Child is free from infection.	Place child in room with noninfectious child. Screen visitors for illness. Provide good skin care and oral hygiene. Maintain aseptic technique with procedures. Monitor vital signs every 4 hours for signs of infection. Avoid rectal temps, suppositories, enemas and IM injections.
B	Potential for injury (hemorrhage) related to decreased platelet count chemotherapeutic agents. Clinical manifestations: Tachycardia, decreased blood pressure, pallor, diaphoresis.	No bleeding present.	Handle child gently; institute age-appropriate safety measures. Assess skin daily for petechiae and bruising. Provide meticulous but gentle oral hygiene and skin care. Test stool, urine, and emesis for presence of blood. Monitor platelet level daily and IV administration of platelets.
C	Altered nutrition: less than body requirements related to anorexia, nausea, vomiting, altered taste sensations. Clinical manifestations: Weight loss, decreased appetite, weakness/fatigue, delayed wound healing, nausea/vomiting.	Child has sufficient caloric intake to meet body needs.	Offer small, frequent high-caloric meals. Allow child to assist with food selection. Provide oral care before meals. Administer antiemetics before meals. Avoid hot, spicy, and rough foods and others that the child finds unpleasant. Monitor parenteral feedings as ordered.
D	Body image disturbance related to side effects of steroids and chemotherapeutic agents. Clinical manifestations: Verbalizes negative feelings toward self, decreased interest in self-care, withdrawal from peers.	Child will acknowledge and demonstrate positive coping with body changes.	Discuss with child what changes will occur. Be accepting of child's body changes. Provide opportunities for child to discuss concerns. Encourage early and consistent peer visits. Stress that hair will regrow in 3 to 6 months after therapy and hair loss will decrease with future therapy. Stress that "moon face" appearance is temporary. Discuss options for wigs, scarves, and hats. Reassure that appearance is temporary.

oxazole (Septra) is the drug of choice for this condition. Recent studies show that prophylactic Septra administration prevents the development of *P. carinii* pneumonia. Other methods that are currently available in some institutions to assist in the prevention and treatment of infection include granulocyte (white blood cell) transfusions and germ-free environments (laminar-flow rooms). These methods remain investigational, expensive, and not readily available to all patients.

Antileukemic drugs can cause a rapid breakdown in the malignant cells, which in turn raises the uric acid load that must be handled by the kidneys. This increased load, especially combined with a state of dehydration caused by poor fluid intake and vomiting, causes renal injury. Allopurinol helps accelerate the excretion of uric acid and reduces the risk of kidney stone formation. Patients are hyperhydrated with intravenous fluid containing sodium bicarbonate to prevent uric acid nephropathy.

Almost all patients on cancer chemotherapy experience moderate to severe nausea and vomiting. Recently the introduction of new antiemetic agents and a better understanding of dosages and scheduling has led to better control of chemotherapy-induced nausea and vomiting. Most institutions are now using Zofran (ondansetron) as antiemetic of choice. It has few side effects (headache) and has provided better antiemetic control of these unpleasant side effects than any other medication.

Another side effect of some of the antileukemic drugs is alopecia, or hair loss. For many patients (particularly teenagers) this is a very distressing problem, a visual reminder of their disease. The use of scarves, hats and/or wigs can help preserve a favorable body image. The child and the parent may be consoled by the fact that the hair will grow back.

Children with leukemia who are admitted to the hospital because of recurring symptoms are usually very uncomfortable and irritable. Pressure from the large number of white blood cells infiltrating the various body organs makes those organs tender. These children usually do not like to be moved, although changes in position are necessary to prevent respiratory tract infection and skin breakdown. The lowered platelet counts lead to easy bruising and spontaneous hemorrhages in many parts of their bodies. The anemia contributes to fatigue and pallor. Because of the frequent ulceration of the mucous membranes, oral hygiene must be gentle. Only soft toothbrushes, gauze, or sponge tipped swabs should be used. Mouthwashes of equal amounts of hydrogen peroxide and saline and the application of viscous lidocaine (Xylocaine) before meals are helpful local measures that often provide comfort. To maintain the child's nutritional needs during this difficult period and to lessen painful injections, a Hickman catheter is inserted. This catheter facilitates venous access and serves as a vehicle for intravenous medications and hyperalimentation.

Fever is often present, and measures to reduce temperature elevation (Chapter 29) frequently must be employed. Rectal temperatures are contraindicated because of the fear of inducing perirectal abscesses in children with low neutrophil counts. Tympanic thermometers are essential. The presence of a member of the family at the bedside at frequent intervals is a great help to the patient, and often the child responds by taking fluids offered by the parent when all other overtures are refused. The ability to minister to the needs of their child in these trying days is almost always a source of strength to the parents, who feel a need to do something for their child. Little routines and special ways of doing things that comfort the child are important to the parent and the patient. As much as possible, they should be followed. The nursing staff should not withdraw from the parents, thinking that there is little they can do. Nurses play a critical role in providing informational and emotional support throughout the illness.

Prognostic factors. The major prognostic determinants in children with ALL are age and white blood cell count at the time of diagnosis. Children between the ages of 2 and 10 years with white blood cell counts of less than 25,000 per mm^3 have the best prognosis. Young infants, older children, and children with white blood cell counts greater than 50,000 per mm^3 have a poorer prognosis. The length of the first remission is also considered to be a prognostic indicator of length of survival. The longer the remission continues, the more optimistic is the prognosis. In general, chemotherapy for acute lymphoblastic leukemia is discontinued after 3 years of continuous complete remission.

Subgroups of ALL with a poor prognosis have recently been identified. In infant ALL, which occurs in children 1 year of age or younger, patients more often have a high initial WBC, an increased incidence of extramedullary disease (CNS and renal), and a much lower 2-year, event-free survival rate (20%).

Children over 10 years of age, especially those with a high leukocyte count at diagnosis, have a poor prognosis. Many of these children have a mediastinal mass, organomegaly, and T-cell markers on their lymphoblasts. Similarly, children with Burkitt's (B-cell) leukemia have had a rapidly fatal course. Fortunately, newer intensive chemotherapy protocols appear to be improving the outlook for these children.

Various cytogenetic abnormalities of the leukemic cell have been associated with a poor prognosis. Patients whose lymphoblasts exhibit hypoploidy (less than 46 chromosomes) or those that possess a recipro-

◆ TABLE 37-5
Life Expectancy of the Child with Leukemia

Year	Treatment	Survival in Months
Acute lymphoblastic		
1937-1953	Supportive	3-5
1954-1962	Prednisone, 6-mercaptopurine, methotrexate	12
1963-1965	Prednisone, 6-mercaptopurine, vincristine, methotrexate, cyclophosphamide	24
1966-1968	Same drugs used in combination	33+
1969-1993	Total therapy Prednisone, vincristine, 6-mercaptopurine, methrotrexate, cyclophosphamide, L-asparaginase, cytarabine (Cytosar) Central nervous system prophylaxis	60+ (5 years +)
Acute myelogenous		
1993	Daunomycin, thioguanine, vincristine, cytosine, arabinoside, prednisone, cyclophosphamide	12-36+*

*Improved chemotherapy protocols and bone marrow transplantation offer hope for cure in 30% to 50% of children with acute myelogenous leukemia.

cal translocation of chromosome 4 and 11, 8 and 14, or 9 and 22 have had a poor outcome. These children should be treated aggressively in the hope of preventing relapse.

Intensive research ultimately designed to control completely the growth of leukemic cells continues. In the meantime a real effort is being made to develop a long-range therapeutic plan for each patient and family so that treatment can be largely conducted in cooperation with the primary care provider in the child's hometown.

In childhood, approximately 97% of the leukemias are acute rather than chronic. Before current methods of treatment were available, the survival time for children with acute leukemia from the time of diagnosis until death was sometimes as brief as 3 to 4 weeks and rarely spanned 6 months. Currently, 60% of children with ALL who get optimum treatment are in uninterrupted remission for at least 5 years. About 90% of these children will remain in remission indefinitely with only a rare relapse in the sixth or seventh year (Table 37-5).

Because most leukemic children experience long periods of remission and some indeed never suffer relapse, maintenance of the family's lifestyle is extremely important. Life should go on in as normal a fashion as possible. Discipline, consistent with developmental age, must be expected and maintained for the affected child just as it is for any sibling. Overly indulgent, permissive treatment usually leads to what becomes impossible demands, fails to make the child feel happier or more secure, and often creates resentment, jealousy, and increasing tension within the family.

The child should not be overprotected, and activity limits should be clearly spelled out by the health care team. The child should be encouraged to participate in desired activities as tolerated. Parents should emphasize what the child *can do.* Unless clarified, this one area may cause great dissension between parents. School is "where it's at" for this child. During the intense treatment periods the child will frequently be unable to attend school. It is essential that home tutoring and home study be encouraged to facilitate continued learning, to foster normalcy, and to assist the child in maintaining peer relationships. As soon as possible, the child should return to class. Through conferences with the school nurse and teachers, guidelines can be established. It is the parents' responsibility to make clear to the school staff from the beginning that special treatment is neither desired nor appreciated.

Idiopathic thrombocytopenic purpura

Idiopathic thrombocytopenic purpura (ITP) is an autoimmune response to disease related antigens. The disease is characterized by excessive destruction of platelets (thrombocytopenia) and purpura (a discoloration caused by petechiae beneath the skin). The acute form often follows an upper respiratory infection or a childhood disease, including varicella, measles, mumps, or rubella. It may also follow immunization for these diseases or ingestion of various medications.

ITP occurs in all age groups, with a peak incidence in the preschool group. In most younger patients the disease runs a benign, self-limited course, and most children experience a spontaneous remission within a period of 6 weeks to 4 months.

Children 10 years of age or over may have a more serious chronic type of ITP. In this age group, girls are affected more frequently than boys, and the condition is likely to be associated with bleeding and the presence of an antiplatelet factor in the plasma.

A normal circulating platelet count ranges from 150,000 to 400,000/mm^3. Each normal thrombocyte has a life span of 8 to 10 days. In ITP the platelet may survive for only hours. Seepage of blood into the mucous membranes, subcutaneous tissues, and skin occurs. A bone marrow sample reveals normal or increased thrombocyte formation, which rules out leukemia.

Clinical manifestations. ITP is characterized by the manifestations listed in the box at right.

Treatment and nursing care. Since the course of the disease is self-limited in the majority of cases, management is primarily supportive. While the platelet count is low, activity is restricted. Children with very low platelet counts should be kept in bed if possible. Cribs should be padded. Salicylates and other drugs that cause bleeding should be avoided because they may alter platelet function and trigger spontaneous hemorrhage. Other nursing measures include careful observation of the progress of skin lesions and assessment for any signs of internal bleeding. A major complication, and the most serious risk to the child in the early course of the condition, is intracranial hemorrhage.

CLINICAL MANIFESTATIONS OF ITP

BRUISING
- Common over bony prominences
- Petechiae
- Ecchymosis

BLEEDING FROM MUCOUS MEMBRANES
- Gingivitis (bleeding gums)
- Epistaxis
- Internal hemorrhage demonstrated by:
  - Hematemesis
  - Melena
  - Hemarthrosis
  - Hematuria
  - Menorrhagia

LOWER EXTREMITY HEMATOMAS

Corticosteroids have been used to help prevent bleeding and to suppress the synthesis of antiplatelet antibodies, but their use is not curative. Platelet transfusions have been given to control active bleeding, although platelet survival is short. Packed red blood cells may be given to replace blood loss. Large doses of intravenous immune globulin have been shown to increase platelet survival and increase platelet counts to safe levels. When treatments have failed and spontaneous recovery has not occurred within a year, splenectomy is done. This often results in a sustained restoration of platelet numbers.

KEY CONCEPTS

1 Anemia is a condition in which the total hemoglobin content of the blood is abnormally reduced. The most common cause of anemia in children is iron deficiency. Symptoms include pallor of the mucosa, irritability, anorexia, and listlessness. The primary cause is insufficient dietary intake of iron. Treatment consists in oral administration of iron preparations and increased dietary intake of iron-rich foods.

2 The sickling abnormality is attributed to a gene responsible for the synthesis of an abnormal type of hemoglobin. Children with this abnormality may experience hemolytic anemia, vasoocclusive crisis, sequestration crisis, aplastic crisis, and infections.

3 The nursing care of all patients with hemophilia is similar except that the type of intravenous therapy differs, depending on the kind of replacement needed. Prevention of bleeding is the primary goal.

4 Signs and symptoms of leukemia may be slow and insidious in onset or develop rapidly. They include fatigue and weakness, weight loss, pallor, easy bruising, and fever with a persistent respiratory tract infection. Current treatment consists of intermittent administration of high doses of several medications in combination.

5 Supportive care of the child with leukemia includes detection and treatment of infection, control of nausea and vomiting, careful positioning, gentle

oral hygiene, fever reduction, and emotional support of both the child and family.

6 Currently 60% of children with ALL who receive optimum treatment experience uninterrupted remission for at least 5 years. About 90% of these children remain in remission indefinitely.

7 Clinical manifestations of ITP include bruising, bleeding from mucous membranes, and lower extremity hematomas.

CRITICAL THOUGHT QUESTIONS

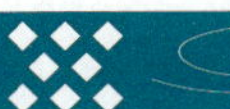

1 List three types of anemia observed in children. What is the most common cause of anemia in children? How does sickle cell anemia differ from other forms of anemia? Why is sickle cell disease a serious problem for the affected child?

2 Discuss the genetic nature of sickle cell anemia and hemophilia. What precautions must be taken when providing nursing care to children with these conditions? What special safety needs do these patients have?

3 What are the signs and symptoms of leukemia? How is it diagnosed? What treatments are currently used? What is the prognosis for children with leukemia? Develop a nursing plan for a 4-year-old boy whose family has just learned of his diagnosis of acute lymphoblastic leukemia.

4 Discuss the clinical manifestations and therapeutic management of ITP. How is nursing care altered while the platelet count is low?

REFERENCES

Behrman RE et al: *Nelson textbook of pediatrics*, Philadelphia, 1992, WB Saunders.

Dallman PR and Yip R: Changing characteristics of childhood anemias, *J Pediatr* 114(1):161-164, 1989.

Evans JP and Rogers DW: Sickle cell disease and thalassemia, *Curr Opin Pediatr* 2(1):121-123, 1990.

Milne RI: Assessment of care of children with sickle cell disease, *Br Med J* 300:371-374, 1990.

Pekrun A and Gratzer W: Disorders of the red cell membrane, *Curr Opin Pediatr* 2(1):116-120, 1990.

Ziegler EE et al: Cow milk feeding and GI blood loss, *J Pediatr* 116:11-18, 1990.

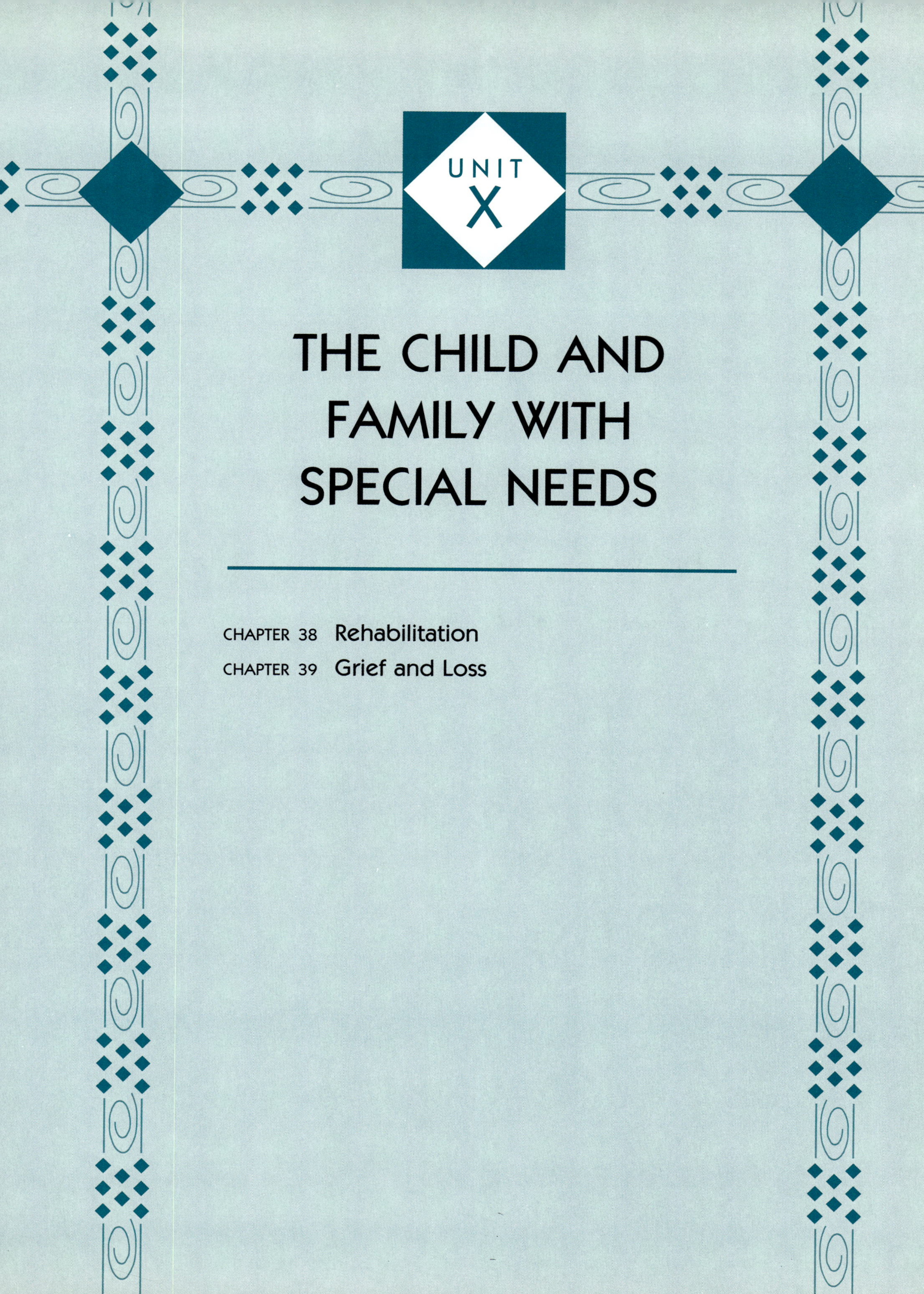

UNIT X

THE CHILD AND FAMILY WITH SPECIAL NEEDS

38

Rehabilitation

CHAPTER OBJECTIVES

After studying this chapter, the student should be able to:

1. Define rehabilitation and state how it differs from habilitation.
2. Discuss three recommendations related to psychological support, noted in the text, which are thought to be especially appropriate when nursing children and young people with long-term illnesses or disabilities.
3. Explain why the staffing pattern in a rehabilitation unit usually needs to be 30% to 60% above typical pediatric acute care unit ratios.
4. Indicate signs and symptoms of autonomic dysreflexia and the emergency treatment advised.
5. Explain the use of the Levels of Cognitive Functioning Scale developed at Rancho Los Amigos Hospital in Downey, California.
6. Point out six hazards of long-term bed rest.
7. Present a suggested schedule for a skin tolerance check.
8. List three ways that urinary control may be achieved by persons with neurogenic bladders.
9. Describe how a 10-year-old girl may safely perform a clean self-catheterization in the bathroom at home. What equipment will she need?
10. Identify three problems associated with the use of Foley catheters and state how their incidence may be reduced.
11. Emphasize five factors that influence bowel patterns, making regularity difficult.
12. Describe the process of behavior modification based on stimulus-response techniques, including the terms *intermittent reinforcement*, *shaping*, and *trapping*.

For most children the period of hospitalization is brief—a day to a week. The current trend is toward day surgery and home health care, resulting in even shorter hospital stays. This trend reflects cost-containment efforts and the psychological and social advantages for the child and the family if an adequate support system is in place.

For some patients, however, the period of hospitalization is prolonged. The severely ill child who has a long, complicated convalescence, the child undergoing orthopedic surgery, and the child with a spinal cord injury struggle to recapture skills once considered automatic and to adjust to new expectations and goals. Children with these diagnoses are considered long-term pediatric patients. The following is a brief discussion of the needs of these children who stay in the hospital for extended periods. This chapter emphasizes nursing perspectives, challenges, and skills related to the complex and challenging specialty of pediatric rehabilitation.

The term *habilitation* refers to the ability to perform those daily activities that are characteristic of the normal functions for one's age and culture. Some children for various reasons never become completely habilitated. In contrast, rehabilitation is "to restore to a functional state." The families of those patients who have suffered devastating physical disabilities need a coordinated multidisciplinary team that considers not only the physical but the sociological, emotional, vocational, and spiritual aspects of the whole patient. The rehabilitation of children is made more complex by their continuing need for normal growth and development in the face of disability.

Pediatric rehabilitation is based on two concepts: first, that each person is unique and has individual basic worth, and second, that the task involves a committed group of people working together as a team with a common goal. The overall goal of pediatric rehabilitation is to foster maximal growth, development, independence, and personal fulfillment within the limitations of the handicap. Many health care providers form the core rehabilitation team: nurses, physicians, physical and occupational therapists, speech pathologists and audiologists, social workers, dietitians, financial counselors, recreational therapists (child life specialists), teachers, and educational consultants. Vocational rehabilitation specialists assist older teens. Other specialty areas that may be utilized include: psychology, psychiatry, psychometric testing, and other community agencies. Team physicians representing each specialty, the primary care provider, home health nurse, and teacher are also important in achieving an optimal outcome for the child. Each team member evaluates the child, makes written recommendations, and participates in patient planning conferences. The patient and family are key members of the team and are included in conferences where current status and progress are discussed and new goals are set.

The needs of the area served by the rehabilitation center dictate the types of patients seen. Patients with various diagnoses who have functional, mobility, and cognitive problems usually make up the patient population. Generally speaking, any patient with a devastating injury or illness that produces lasting or permanent physical disabilities can and should be treated by the rehabilitation team. Nursing principles of rehabilitation must be initiated at the onset of illness or injury to prevent complications and further loss of function. Many of these children initially require specialized intensive care. Ideally, the principles of both acute and long-term care will be delivered simultaneously. When the patient's condition has stabilized and the youngster is no longer "ill," it is time to consider transfer to the rehabilitation unit. In both settings the nursing management is concerned with maintenance of function and prevention of complications.

In the best circumstances a rehabilitation program provides an inpatient unit, an outpatient clinic, and collaboration with supportive community agencies. The patient and the family progress more smoothly from onset of illness or injury to the home and community if each of these agencies is communicating effectively with one another. Some patients may continue to return to a rehabilitation program periodically as they grow older and their needs or level of function change. Coordination is essential for the patients' optimal transition from the initial care facility to the home and community. The patient, family, and team members must be kept informed of the patient's status, program, and goals. Continuity in care during and after transfer to the rehabilitation unit takes the coordinated effort and skills of all team members. One person must coordinate this process. The nurse's assessment skills, communication skills, and knowledge of community resources make the nurse an effective coordinator.

Staffing of a rehabilitation unit needs to be 30% to 60% above the typical acute care ratios. Caring, knowledgable nurses who enjoy teaching are requisite to an effective unit. Independence comes with patience, repetition, and allowing the patient or family member to "do" rather than the traditional "doing for."

Rehabilitation programs are expensive and the cost is passed on to the patient or third party payor (insurance companies or government agencies). The independence gained, however, may ultimately reduce the total financial burden.

Before contributing to the formation of an individualized care plan, each team member must assess the patient's current status. A logical, systematic approach will ensure the inclusion of all important facts in the nursing assessment. (See the box on p. 819 for a suggested initial assessment outline.) Using this evaluation of the patient's current status and pertinent history, one can formulate nursing interventions for existing and potential problems and identify teaching needs. Successful teaching also includes assessment of the cultural values, lifestyle, and learning capabilities of the child and family. Teaching needs and nursing interventions must always be planned with the patient in a developmentally appropriate manner. Assessment of the parent's emotional needs and learning readiness is also critical. Mutual strategies, goals, and target dates can then be incorporated into a written plan. Visual materials and demonstrations giving clear explanations of the treatment rationale and its importance to the patient enhance learning and the potential for success.

When the patient's progress on the unit is consistent or stabilized and progressive home passes have been successful, discharge plans are finalized. Discharge should be coordinated by one person. There should be a home visit by a member of the rehabilitation team before discharge to help plan for program needs or physical changes within the home environment. These will be evaluated during progressive pass experiences.

INITIAL NURSING ASSESSMENT OUTLINE

Introduction	Name, age, chief complaint or problem, circumstances of present injury or illness, referring physician
History	Past injuries, illnesses, hospitalizations
Vital signs	Temperature, pulse, respiration, blood pressure
Allergies	Reactions to drugs, food, airborne particles, contact agents
System check*	
Neurosensory	Level of consciousness, orientation, neurological checks, intellectual level, balance, coordination, sensory abnormalities, emotional stability
Integumentary (skin and mucous membranes)	Turgor, general condition, complete description of lesions, condition of mouth
Musculoskeletal	Muscle strength, range of motion, motor abnormalities, amputations (follow-up evaluation by PT), current therapy
Respiratory	Pattern and sound of respirations, URI? cough? Pulmonary function studies (follow-up evaluation by PT and RT)
Urinary	Vocabulary? Normal voiding or ostomy? (Continence? Urinary drainage devices, catheter size, catheterization program)
Gastrointestinal	Vocabulary? Schedule: time, frequency, bowel movement consistency, normal movement or ostomy? Effect of diet?
Diet	Type, likes and dislikes, time and amount; method: bottle, oral gavage, gastrostomy etc.
Health supervision	Dates of last dental, eye, and hearing examinations; performed by? Immunizations? Safety problems?
Growth and development (activities of daily living; motor skills)	Independent, with assistance; dependent: feeding, turning, transfer, bathing, dressing, toileting, standing, walking, grooming, dental hygiene (follow-up evaluation by OT and PT)
Equipment brought	Cane, crutches, walker, wheelchair, braces, appliances, scooterboards
Current medications and treatments	Medication: dosage, time, route, effects? Treatments: time, duration, specifics
Family composition	Parents, marital status, age, siblings, extended family, resources (follow-up evaluation by MSS)
Social and educational interests	Level of education, special friends, hobbies, security items, community contacts
Understanding of injury or illness	By patient, by family
Specialized care needs	

PT, physical therapy; *OT,* occupational therapy; *RT,* respiratory therapy; *MSS,* medical social service.
*In making this assessment, ascertain the status of the patient before his injury or illness.

Before discharge, arrangements must be made for the following: home health nurse follow-up, admission to a regular or special school, methods of obtaining supplies and medications, return appointments to the primary care provider, and sharing of phone numbers of team members with the family. After discharge, regular visits to a rehabilitation clinic enable the team to reevaluate each patient with feedback from the school, home health nurse, and other community agencies.

Because of improved health care over the last three decades, increasing numbers of people with various disabilities are contributing members of society. As a cohesive group, they are beginning to represent a political force. Through consumer awareness and pressure, legislation for the disabled has brought about improved wheelchair accessibility in many public buildings and businesses, leading to improved educational and employment opportunities. Additionally, the courts have begun to attack discrimination in the job market, making job performance the sole criterion for employment.

PSYCHOLOGICAL SUPPORT OF LONG-TERM PATIENTS AND THEIR FAMILIES

The character and severity of an injury or disease may be sources of considerable stress, but prolonged isolation from normal surroundings, the strange environment of the hospital, and frequent encounters with the many different people involved in patient care make hospitalization particularly difficult. The limited experience and development of the child increase the potential for emotional trauma at this time.

The three principles of nursing care—described as appropriate for all hospitalized children in Chapter 19 include (1) maintain a basic sense of trust, (2) protect from fear, frustration, and pain, and (3) facilitate social contacts and communication with the outside world—are particularly applicable to the long-term patient. A sense of trust is best fostered in children when their parents trust the child's caregivers. This trust is gradually developed as the parents and child learn that the staff, demonstrating forethought, accessibility, and reliability as well as technical skills, cares about them. It may be strengthened through the primary nursing concept or the consistent assignment of one or two nurses for each child's care. Trust also increases as the staff helps the family work through their grief. The grief experienced by the parents, family, and friends of these patients is similar to that encountered by those who mourn the death of a loved one.

Often the three-stage pattern of shock and denial, developing awareness, and restitution or resolution can be identified. The response of shock and disbelief is often still present on arrival at the rehabilitation unit. Statements such as "When will my child walk again?" and "When she is better, things will be like they were before," demonstrate denial. Each statement does not require refuting but should not be reinforced. The nurse should reinforce reality through an understanding but factual discussion of the patient's status, problems, and required nursing care. Involving the family in this care helps them feel useful, important, and needed.

The second stage of mourning is demonstrated by increasing awareness and feelings of guilt and anger. Laments of "Why me?" "It's all my fault," "If only I'd looked sooner," or "I shouldn't have let him go," poignantly demonstrate guilt. Anger is often directed toward the child for being careless or disobedient. One parent may accuse the other of being at fault. Often anger is directed at the hospital staff, since this outlet is "safer" than accusing a family member. Criticism of nursing care, the physician, or staff personalities is the most common manifestation. Understanding the causes of these feelings enables the staff to support the family. Reassurance that the accident was unpreventable (if, indeed, it was) will help. Giving the parents information about their child's condition and involving the family in care-giving and decision-making are essential. Nonjudgmental listening and prompt attention to problems help to smooth the way toward the third stage of grieving: restitution or resolution. This stage of grieving involves the sharing of grief with others and, it is hoped, the support of relatives and friends. When a loved one dies, a funeral may help a family to accept their loss. In the case of disability, the family frequently substitutes ritualistic behavior such as an exact time for visitation, weekly visits to a special physician, or daily trips to church. Some families seem to adjust to the changes imposed by disability better than others. Unfortunately, the stresses are great, and family dissolution all too often results. Trust helps ease these stresses. Trust through open communication helps the family work through the problems.

The parents and team members must realize that as children become aware of their disabilities and limitations, they too go through a grieving process. They may verbalize anger, quietly withdraw, or become overly cooperative. At times these children may show little motivation or may refuse to learn new skills. The goal during this period should be to assist the child to adjust to a new body image and activities of daily living rather than acceptance of the disability. Psychosocial support can help the child, parents, and team work through this normal process.

It is impossible and probably undesirable to protect a patient completely from fear, pain, or even frustration. However, these unpleasant feelings may be reduced. Preparation of the child and parents for procedures and brief, honest explanations are helpful. Opportunities to verbalize and to express themselves through drawings, play-acting, storytelling, or music should be made available. Feelings that cannot be put into words need to find an outlet before they, in turn, become symptoms. (See Chapters 19 and 25 for additional information.) The need for emotional release correlates with the need to facilitate social interaction and contact with the community. Maintaining friendships is sometimes difficult for a child with decreased energy and prolonged illness. Yet the knowledge that one still has such relationships encourages stability and incentive and usually makes return to the neighborhood after hospitalization less traumatic. Short, chaperoned trips to recreational areas, to cultural centers, or just to visit friends can also be a method of maintaining one's place in the world outside. These passes should begin as soon as the family has been given necessary instructions and has demonstrated competence in the child's care. Much support and encouragement are often needed, since the hospital often provides a safe, accepting environment of the child's disability, and this acceptance may not exist in the community. The child and parents must be prepared to respond to stares, handle avoidance, and answer questions.

The addition of a child life specialist to the staff of many hospitals is a welcome event. This specially prepared professional helps patients participate in a wide range of constructive activities either in groups or as individuals. A monthly newspaper planned by the patients, hobby fairs, and picnics on nearby lawns are sample activities. Whether in a rehabilitation unit or regular hospital area, convalescing long-term patients should be given the opportunity and responsibility of continuing their education. Ideally, a classroom for ambulatory patients will be available and provisions made for tutors from the public school system. Telephone or distance learning through two-way television is also available in some areas. It may be possible to maintain contact with the class and school attended before hospitalization and to work on assignments in the rehab unit. Although vocational choices may be somewhat limited due to the nature of the injury or illness, ongoing education is critical for optimal functioning and maintenance of self-esteem.

COMMON CONDITIONS

Common diagnoses found in rehabilitation units include spinal cord injuries, anomalies or diseases of the central nervous system, and brain injury caused by trauma, tumor, or disease.

Spinal Cord Injury

Children suffer spinal cord injury less frequently than adults. Spinal cord trauma in young children and teens occurs most often as a result of motor vehicle accidents or less frequently because of diving accidents and gunshot wounds. Although the spinal cord is partially protected by bone, shearing or torsion forces can destroy or severely damage the cord. The affected portion of the body is determined by the level of spinal injury. The higher the cord injury, the greater will be the resulting disability. Paraplegic patients (persons whose paralysis or functional loss involves lower extremities), even though they may experience loss of bowel and bladder control and perineal sensation, can be totally independent. Quadriplegic patients (persons whose paralysis or functional loss involves all four extremities) need supervision or assistance. The more hand function available, the more independent the patient will be. With improved emergency care and quicker retrieval, increased numbers of patients with high spinal cord injuries (C1, C2, and C3 levels) are surviving. These patients have no function below shoulder level. Their basic care remains the same as that required by other quadriplegic patients, but the nurse must become familiar with ventilatory equipment and be prepared for more intense psychological and adjustment problems. Eventual resocialization requires sophisticated electronic equipment such as electric wheelchairs with tongue switches, as well as environmental control systems to operate a television, radio, telephone, or intercom.

The application of lifesaving measures is of initial importance in the management of the patient with spinal cord injury. Immobilization and stabilization of the spine are critical. These are often accomplished with a "halo" apparatus that may be worn for a period of 10 to 12 weeks until the spine is stabilized. This apparatus consists of a halo ring to immobilize the head and metal bars that attach the ring to a vest that encompasses the chest and supports the apparatus weight. Plastic vests are often used, but a plaster vest may be needed for the irregularly shaped chest or back. The halo apparatus allows the child to have extra mobility to sit, stand, or lie prone, usually causing respiratory, circulatory, and muscular problems to improve. Orders for the child in a halo apparatus include administration of a mild analgesic for initial discomfort. The nurse should report swallowing problems, difficulty in opening the mouth, and loosened pins. The pins holding the halo barely penetrate the skull. Therefore these pin sites must be meticulously cleaned twice a day. Half-strength peroxide is commonly used. The use of povidone-iodine (Betadine) solution is discouraged for routine pin care because of allergic reactions and potential pin deterioration. Separate sterile applicators should be used for each pin. Some serosanguineous drainage is expected initially, but one must check for any change or increase in drainage, redness, swelling, or pain that would indicate the development of infection. Although the vests have a protective inner lining, pressure sores may develop over the scapulae and shoulders. These sores may be prevented with proper body positioning and frequent changes in position. The vest's resistance tends to inhibit respiratory function; therefore deep breathing and coughing exercises must be encouraged.

Assessment for spinal cord trauma by performance of daily upper extremity neurological evaluation is a standard of care. Any changes should be reported immediately to the physician. Finally, the nurse must teach the child some general safety rules to prevent falls that may inflict greater damage. During the time of bony healing the complications of bed rest must be prevented. The patient needs meticulous skin care, periodic range-of-motion exercises, adequate fluid intake, venous-support stockings (TED hose), bowel and bladder programs, and special respiratory care. The patient with injury at midtrunk level or above requires more than position changes and coughing. Because the respiratory muscles have been affected, incentive spirometers are valuable. An upper respiratory tract infection is a serious threat to this patient.

The higher the level of the cord injury, the less tolerance the patient displays for an upright position. The application of elastic hose from toes to groin or of a snug-fitting corset before the patient sits helps prevent pooling of blood in the lower extremities. Gradually, over a period of days, increasing the angle of the wheelchair back and lowering the legs help prevent dizziness, perspiration, fainting, and other signs of hypotension. When these symptoms occur, tipping the wheelchair back to lower the patient's head relieves the symptoms.

Below the level of injury, temperature regulation is affected in these patients, since nerve endings in the skin may not provide adequate temperature control. The skin does not perspire to aid cooling, nor do the muscles shiver to produce heat. Thus the skin may be injured by extremes of heat or cold that the patient cannot perceive, and the patient must be made aware of this possibility. In addition, the patient's response to an inflammatory process may register a higher body temperature than is typical for that type of problem. Control is usually obtained by uncovering the patient or using acetaminophen (Tylenol). In the patient with an injury above midtrunk, or T6, a complication known as *autonomic dysreflexia* or *hyperreflexia* may arise. This is a very serious rise in the blood pressure that can lead to a cerebrovascular accident (CVA) or seizures. Signs and symptoms include: flushing, headache, sweating, feelings of nasal stuffiness, goose bumps, bradycardia, and a rapid increase in blood pressure. These result from sympathetic nervous system activity and are usually related to physical stimuli such as bladder and bowel distention, severe pressure sores, and urinary tract infection. Less frequently, external stimuli may trigger autonomic dysreflexia. It should be treated by elevating the patient's head and removing the stimulus. A distended bladder is drained. If the patient does not improve hydralazine hydrochloride may be prescribed. Patients who are subject to such episodes and their family members should be fully instructed in self-care before discharge.

Brain Injury

A result of the fast-paced and highly technological society in which we live is an increase in traumatic injuries. Those children who survive severe head trauma resulting from motor vehicle or bicycle accidents, falls, or nonaccidental trauma caused by shaking, all are potential candidates for rehabilitation. Initial life-saving management seeks to prevent complications; consequently, tracheostomy and ventilator care become important aspects of the rehabilitation care plan. Children who have suffered cerebral vascular accidents, brain tumors, and anoxic insults caused by meningitis, near drowning, and status epilepticus may also benefit from rehabilitation services.

The physical needs of these children are considerable and in many ways not unlike those of the patient with spinal cord injury. The progress of the child varies according to the severity of the injury and the areas of the brain affected. The minimally injured child may completely recover or have one or more of the following disabilities: a limp, speech defect such as dysarthria (difficulty pronouncing words), a cognitive disorder (difficulty with sequencing thought), or a shortened attention span. These areas, however, must be addressed because they will affect the child's resocialization and academic progress. Another patient may suffer severe brain injury and may be left with multiple deficits or may be totally nonfunctional.

The brain-injured patient typically regains awareness and orientation slowly. Eight helpful levels of cognitive function and behavioral response developed at Rancho Los Amigos Medical Center in Downey, California have been identified in the recovery process. Table 38-1 describes these eight Levels of Cognitive Functioning and corresponding strategies for nursing intervention. Stimuli should be presented in a manner that matches the patient's present functioning level yet offers a challenge of advancement to the next level.

Sensory stimulation must be carefully planned by the team and introduced slowly. The physical and occupational therapists work with the patient in developing both fine and gross motor coordination. Although strong, such patients may be unable to feed or dress themselves. Activities of daily living (ADLs) are introduced early in the rehabilitation program so that the patient can begin to achieve some degree of independence. Speech, intellect, and emotional stability are typically affected. Since the healing process of the

◆ TABLE 38-1
Levels of Cognitive Functioning

Level	Patient Behavior	Nursing Intervention
I No response	Patient appears to be in deep sleep and is unresponsive to visual, auditory, or painful stimuli.	Be calm and soothing in manner of speech and physical manipulation of the patient.
II Generalized response	Patient reacts inconsistently and nonpurposefully to stimuli in a nonspecific manner. Responses may be physiological changes, gross body movements, and vocalization.	Do not talk with others when working with the patient. Assume that the patient can understand what is being said.
III Localized response	Patient reacts specifically but inconsistently to stimuli. He can track and focus on objects and turn toward or away from auditory stimuli. The patient may withdraw from painful stimuli. Simple commands may be followed in an inconsistent or delayed manner. The patient may show vague awareness of self and body by responding to discomfort by pulling at a nasogastric tube or restraints.	Talk to the patient about things he or she is doing or about family members and friends. Do not overwhelm the patient with talking. Control environmental stimuli. Activation of patient's behavioral responses at these levels depends on external stimuli; too much can suppress movement toward awareness of the environment. Encourage the family to follow the same pattern of care.
IV Confused-agitated	Patient is in a heightened state of activity with severely decreased ability to process information. The patient may scream, cry, pull at tubes, verbalize inappropriately, confabulate, or become euphoric or hostile. Inability to discriminate among persons or objects is common. Patients at this level are often unable to cooperate with treatment efforts.	Be calm and soothing when working with the patient. Describe what you are going to do with the patient before beginning the activity. Talk in a slow soft voice. Loudness may be startling. Multiple stimuli within the environment may be more than the patient can handle. If the patient becomes upset, allow him or her time to adjust or remove the patient from the situation.
V Confused inappropriate nonagitated	Patient appears alert and is able to follow simple commands. More complex commands produce responses that are nonpurposeful or fragmented. The patient may show some agitated behavior but at this level, only in response to external stimuli. The patient is highly distractible, verbalizes inappropriately, and demonstrates severe memory impairment. Self-care activities and feeding can be managed with assistance. Mobile patients often wander randomly.	Create an environment for the patient that can produce purposeful and appropriate responses to internal and external stimuli with greater frequency and duration. Present only one task at a time and allow the patient to complete the task or a great portion of it before presenting another task. Tell the patient what you are going to do several minutes before you begin. Explain again just before working with the patient. Demonstrate instructions or use gestures whenever possible.

Continued.

◆ **TABLE 38-1**
Levels of Cognitive Functioning—cont'd.

Level	Patient Behavior	Nursing Intervention
VI Confused-appropriate	Patient shows goal-directed behavior but depends on input for direction; is able to relearn old skills such as self-care but requires maximum assistance with learning new skills. Selective attention to difficult tasks may be impaired; has increased awareness of self and family members.	Maintain a structured quiet environment for the patient. Describe the daily routine to him or her on a daily basis. Keep him or her mentally challenged by reading and playing games with him or her.
VII Automatic-appropriate	Patient appears appropriate and oriented. He goes through daily routine in an automatic, robotlike fashion; has recall of activities and increased awareness of self and family. There is superficial awareness of, but lack of insight into, his or her condition. He or she has decreased judgment and problem-solving abilities and a lack of realistic planning. At this level the patient demonstrates poor safety awareness.	Provide structure through the use of an orientation board or a daily schedule. Place a clock and a large calendar in the patient's room. Instruction should be used only for those activities or times when he or she becomes confused. Have the patient keep a written daily log of his or her activities to assist in orientation.
VIII Purposeful and appropriate	Patient is alert and oriented and is able to recall and integrate past and recent events. Carryover for new learning is now evident. Patient needs no supervision once activities are learned; is independent at home but has difficulty in abstract reasoning and stress intolerance may persist.	

Adapted from Hagen C, Malkmus D, and Durham P: Levels of cognitive functioning. In *Rehabilitation of the head injured adult: comprehensive physical management*, Downey, Calif, 1979, Staff Association of Rancho Los Amigos Medical Center.

brain is measured in months to years in these children, ongoing psychological testing and educational counseling are helpful. The more severely affected children attend special schools or they may be mainstreamed.

A child with an impaired intellect and a functional body may ultimately be happy and satisfied. A child with a normal intellect and severe physical disability, such as aphasia (loss of normal speech) or ataxia (lack of coordination of voluntary muscles producing a characteristic abnormal staggering gait and/or uncontrolled upper extremity movement) understands his or her condition and often has a great deal of difficulty adjusting.

At puberty the brain-injured person also has awakened sexual interest. If the brain injury occurs during this time, the patient may be difficult to manage in the rehabilitation unit, since the individual may have little or no control over his inhibitions. Parents must be cautioned that the child may be overly friendly and invite unwanted sexual encounters.

PHYSICAL ASPECTS OF REHABILITATION

The complications of prolonged bed rest and immobility represent the greatest dangers to the longevity of the rehab patient (Fig. 38-1). Examples of such complications are as follows:

1 Motor and sensory loss involving superficial nerves, skin ulcers, and skeletal deformities
2 Muscle wasting and shortening (contractures),

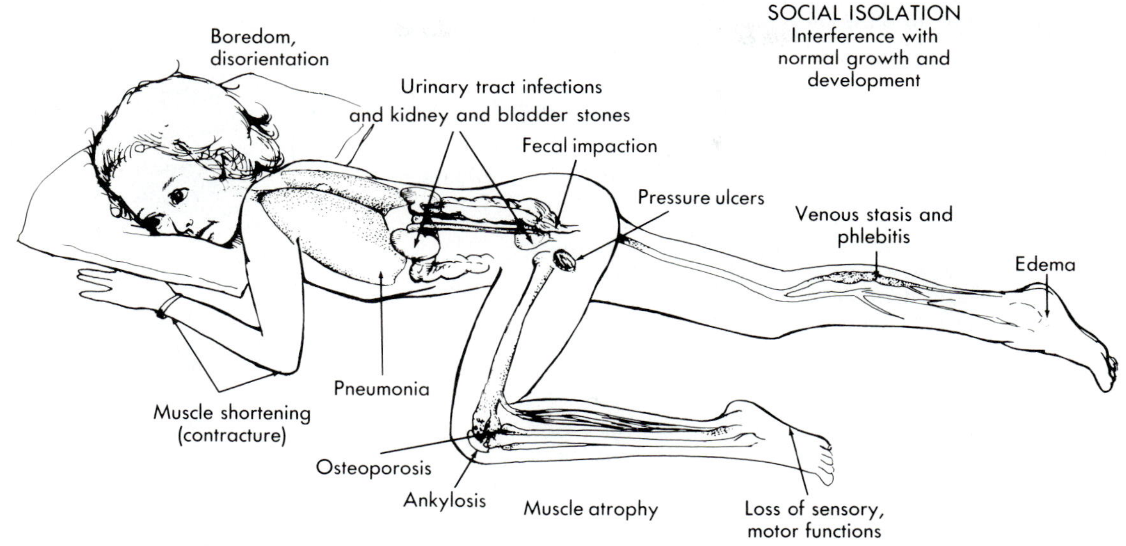

Fig. 38-1 Complications of prolonged bed rest. These complications may not be seen in every patient.

bone calcium loss, ankylosis of joints, edema, venous stasis, and thrombosis from disuse atrophy

3 Urinary tract infection, stones, constipation, and fecal impaction related to poor fluid intake and lack of mobility
4 Hypostatic pneumonia from pooling of secretions in the lungs
5 Depression and psychological disorders resulting from isolation and interference in normal activities
6 Disturbance in normal growth and development

The meticulous application of basic nursing principles can prevent many of these complications from occurring. These principles are discussed in the following sections.

Routine Skin Care

An adequate blood supply maintains integumentary function and repair. Conversely, decreased blood supply to an area will cause cell death. The small vessels in the skin form a network that supplies oxygenated blood. Any pressure, such as that from sitting, standing, lying, braces, shoes, or appliances, causes compression of these small vessels and does not allow blood to reach the cells. Where bony prominences (such as hips, sacrum, and knees) are close to the surface, there is no muscle tissue to pad or distribute the pressure evenly, and considerable pressure develops, which can cause skin damage. The sequence of events leading to skin breakdown and the sores or lesions that result are described in Fig. 38-2. When red marks are seen, the child must not bear pressure on that area until the skin has returned to normal. Any surface that comes into contact with the skin must be suspect. Soft, moldable surfaces distribute pressure over a larger area, and any one spot receives less pressure, with less damage resulting. If you recall the difference between sitting on a concrete step and a well-upholstered chair, you will appreciate why items such as foam rubber mattresses, wheelchair cushions, and soft leather shoes are encouraged.

For the patient who is wheelchair-bound and who lacks sensation over the buttocks area, it is imperative that pressure be relieved over the bony ischial prominences. The method for relieving pressure is called a *chair raise*. For the paraplegic patient it consists of lifting the buttocks by using the arms of the wheelchair to raise oneself or alternately shifting from side to side. Recommended frequency for the paraplegic patient is every 20 or 30 minutes for 30 seconds. This activity should soon become automatic so that the patient does it without having to think about it. The quadriplegic patient must have assistance to relieve this ischial pressure.

The use of new braces, shoes, or different positions or postures must be introduced gradually and evaluated frequently. (See box on p. 827 for suggested schedule.) In addition to pressure-caused skin problems, one must be aware of the danger of burns, bumps, scratches, and pustules (pimples). Burns can be caused by hot car upholstery, electric blankets, sunburn, hot sand at the beach, spilled hot drinks, and other accidents. Although they may appear to be minor, these can be very serious and must be evaluated

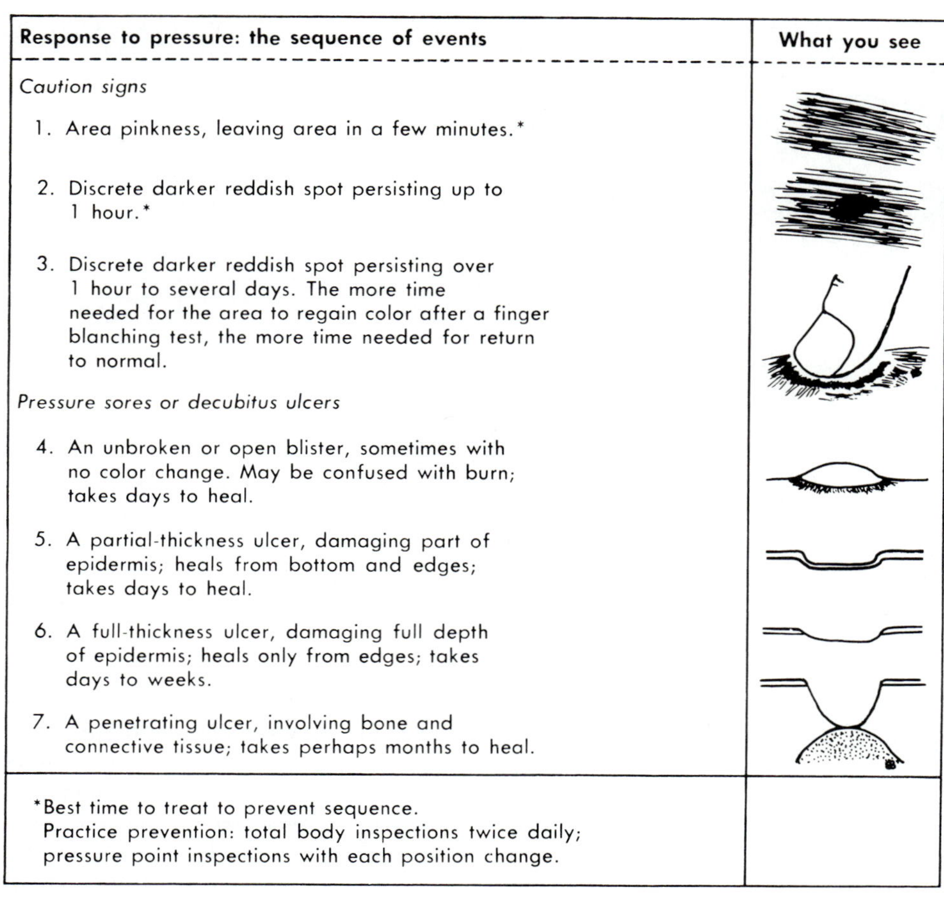

Response to pressure: the sequence of events	What you see
Caution signs	
1. Area pinkness, leaving area in a few minutes.*	
2. Discrete darker reddish spot persisting up to 1 hour.*	
3. Discrete darker reddish spot persisting over 1 hour to several days. The more time needed for the area to regain color after a finger blanching test, the more time needed for return to normal.	
Pressure sores or decubitus ulcers	
4. An unbroken or open blister, sometimes with no color change. May be confused with burn; takes days to heal.	
5. A partial-thickness ulcer, damaging part of epidermis; heals from bottom and edges; takes days to heal.	
6. A full-thickness ulcer, damaging full depth of epidermis; heals only from edges; takes days to weeks.	
7. A penetrating ulcer, involving bone and connective tissue; takes perhaps months to heal.	
*Best time to treat to prevent sequence. Practice prevention: total body inspections twice daily; pressure point inspections with each position change.	

Fig. 38-2 Sequence of events leading to skin breakdown.

by the health care provider. Any abrasion or scratch that involves a pressure-bearing surface must be completely healed before pressure bearing is resumed. Diaper rashes and irritations that do not quickly respond to the application of Desitin ointment or zinc oxide paste should be examined immediately before a severe problem results. Pustules or abrasions on weight-bearing surfaces should be cleaned gently with mild soap and water and observed closely for increasing size and inflammation.

Because of poor blood supply to scar tissue, healed lesions may leave scars that are susceptible to future breakdown. A small amount of time spent daily in prevention will save a great deal of time, trouble, and money later. Remember the following: (1) never permit any pressure on reddened areas, blisters, or sores; (2) increase positioning times according to the guidelines; and (3) regularly check total body skin, using mirrors as necessary. Teach the child and the family these precautions. By the age of 10 or 11 years a child, with supervision, should be assuming responsibility for his own skin care.

If a patient with an existing decubitus ulcer (pressure sore) is admitted, treatment must be initiated. Many theories exist regarding optimal care of pressure sores. No weight bearing should be allowed. It may be possible to avoid the one position that causes pressure; however, if there are ulcers in several different places, the nurse may have no alternative but to position the patient carefully on an affected side. If this must be done, pressure must be relieved from the ulcer by bridging either side of the ulcer with foam rubber pads or pillows, thus freeing the lesion itself from pressure. Circular or doughnut-shaped supports are not recommended because they may further decrease circulation.

Pressure sores must be kept clean. Whatever agent is used, cleaning must be done gently to preserve the new delicate epithelium being formed. Physiological saline or half-strength hydrogen peroxide on applicator sticks have been used to clean away drainage. If the ulcer is infected, a topical enzyme, such as Travase or Elase, and hydrotherapy will debride the sore. A small pressure sore may be left open to the air to dry. Covered sores should be taped loosely to allow air circulation. Op-Site is effective in areas where incontinence is a problem because it prevents moisture from entering the wound, but allows passage of air and gases. Debrisan (hydrophilic wound-cleaning beads) absorbs

SUGGESTED SCHEDULE FOR SKIN TOLERANCE CHECK

TRIAL PERIODS

1. Beginning periods—15 minutes
   Increase by 15-minute periods according to tolerance until 2-hour level is reached
2. After 2-hour level is reached, trial periods may be increased to 30 minutes

OBSERVATIONS OF PRESSURE AREAS (RED MARKS)

Clearing in 15 minutes or no pressure area seen, increase trial period by 15 minutes
Clearing in 30 minutes, repeat trial period
Clearing in 45 minutes, reduce trial by 15 minutes
Persists 60 minutes or more, keep patient off area
Use same clearing time evaluation, but substitute 30-minute trial periods

NOTE: Any interruption in the use of a brace, appliance, or position may require a reevaluation period. Prolonged intervals between their use may mean starting again at the beginning of the schedule. When any pressure area is detected, check methods of positioning. Cocoa butter or lotion applied daily to bony prominences helps keep skin supple.

excess drainage from clean sores, however, it should not be used in tracts.

Positioning

In the discussion of skin care we underlined the importance of relieving pressure by turning and changing position. Proper anatomical positioning can help prevent skeletal deformities, muscle shortening (contractures), and venous stasis. Six basic positions may be used: back (supine), abdominal (prone), lying on either side (lateral recumbent), sitting, or standing. These all can be modified to a certain degree. Positioning problems vary according to the diagnosis and individual needs of the patient. Fig. 38-3 illustrates good prone positioning to prevent pressure areas and contractures and to protect catheter drainage when necessary.

Another positioning device is the splint. Resting splints are designed to maintain the position of an extremity. There are also splints designed to improve alignment or support the extremity so that improved mobility can be achieved.

Venous pooling and the danger of thrombosis can be decreased by thigh-high, closed-toe support stockings to help collapse the superficial leg veins. To further

Nursing Alert

Large ulcers are better managed by moist dressings. A sterile, fine-mesh gauze pad, such as any eye pad, is cut the exact size of the ulcer and moistened with physiological saline solution. This should be covered with a dry dressing taped down with paper tape to prevent drying. The dressing is changed every 4 to 6 hours, depending on the drainage present and how long it stays moist. If it is allowed to dry, the gauze should be soaked off to preserve the new epithelium. As the ulcer heals, the gauze is reduced in size until finally one can leave the small ulcer open to the air.

prevent venous stasis, as well as muscle shortening and contractures, a full range of motion should be carried out. The nurse is responsible for joint range of motion (ROM) *without* stretching muscles. Gentleness and patience are essential. The hands and fingers are exceptionally delicate, and specific instructions about appropriate range should be obtained from the physician, physical or occupational therapist. Overzealous ROM of the fingers can make the hand less functional later.

Position changes also lessen stasis of fluid in the lungs. With regular deep breathing, an incentive spirometer, and coughing, pneumonia may be prevented. Changing position and forcing fluids will also help prevent urinary stones and constipation.

As soon as patients are physically able to tolerate a wheelchair, they should be placed in a more normal sitting position, even if they are still comatose. These wheelchairs have special supports and/or belts to facilitate a more upright position while maintaining safe body alignment. This maneuver adds a position to the patient's repertoire and lets them see people and their environment from the more customary vertical perspective, which helps to prevent disorientation.

Another technique is the use of a tilt table designed to bring the supine patient to a more upright position. Here, the patient is safely restrained with belts placed at chest, hips, and knees. The position of the tilt table is gradually elevated; the child usually "tilts" for about 30 minutes, for a total of 2 to 3 times per day (see Fig. 31-16).

Depression, disorientation, and hallucinations can result from prolonged horizontal positioning and social isolation of the normal individual. This, added to the physical and emotional trauma of an injury, is a tremendous problem. Anything that stimulates and orients the mind—people, predictable routines, a clock

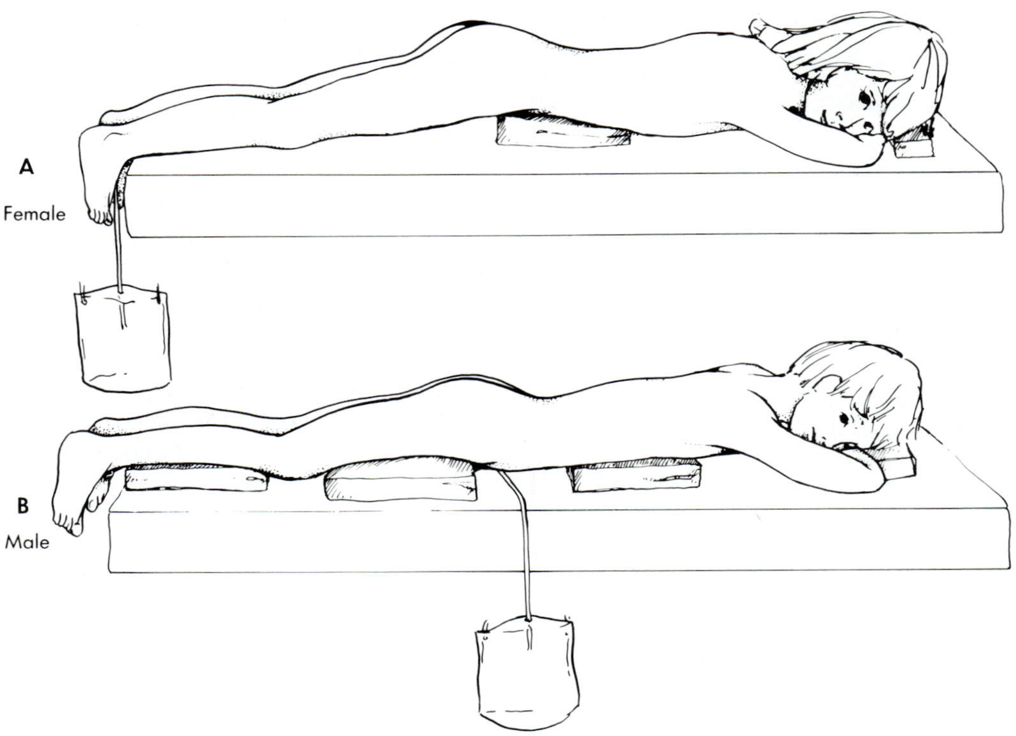

Fig. 38-3 **A,** Prone position with pillow below breast level and small foam rubber support under forehead. Note position of Foley catheter between legs. **B,** Prone position with pillows under chest, thighs, and shins to leave hips, knees, and feet free from pressure. Note position of Foley catheter.

or calendar—is helpful. Frequent visits by the nurse just to say hello are helpful. Conversation with the patient while in the room or delivering care is essential. The presence of parents and siblings and the friendship of another patient who has experienced a similar injury and made progress helps tremendously.

Interference with growth and development, manifested by disrupted bone growth, delay in reaching skill or functional milestones, or inability to play normally, occurs frequently in young disabled children. They must have the chance to explore and move about the floor and, if possible, achieve the vertical position. Their environment should be as home-like as possible and include increasing independence and responsibility appropriate for their age, developmental level, abilities, and general condition.

Urinary Bladder Care

Neurogenic bladder disease

Neurogenic bladder disease (NGB) refers to bladder dysfunction resulting from lesions of the central or peripheral nervous system. The goals are (1) preservation of normal urinary tract anatomy and renal function, (2) prevention of significant urinary infection, and (3) attainment of urinary continence.

The lower urinary tract (bladder and urethra) has two basic functions—the storage and evacuation of urine. The bladder is capable of expanding in response to increasing intravesical volumes without a significant rise in intravesical pressure. When a person with normal bladder control desires to void, intravesical pressure is raised as bladder outlet resistance falls. When intravesical pressure is higher than outlet resistance, urine flows. Urination is a highly complex, coordinated activity under the control of the parasympathetic and sympathetic nervous systems. The parasympathetic system promotes bladder emptying; the sympathetic system promotes storage. A balance between these two systems provides for reliable low pressure storage and controllable emptying. Disorders of the central or peripheral nervous systems can lead to an imbalance, resulting in inability to store urine reliably, or in the storage of urine at high intravesical pressures, or the inability to empty the bladder effectively. High intravesical pressures can lead to upper tract dilatation, infection, and renal damage. Loss of storage ability leads to incontinence and danger of skin inflammation. NGB can occur from injury to or disease in the brain, spinal cord, or peripheral nerves. Historically NGB has been classified according to the level of the lesion, as patterns of dysfunction vary with

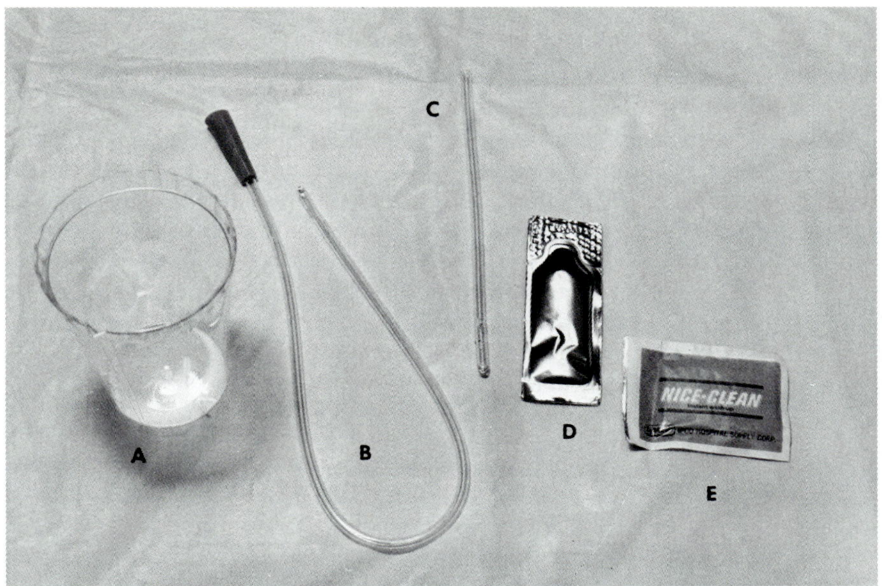

Fig. 38-4 Supplies for clean catheterization technique. **A,** Calibrated plastic container; **B,** catheter for male; **C,** catheter for female; **D,** lubricant; and **E,** cleansing wipe.

the level. The *uninhibited neurological bladder* results from damage to the brain center that controls voluntary voiding. A typical patient is one who has suffered a stroke. They recognize that the bladder is about to contract and empty but are unable to inhibit this activity. Voiding commences in a low pressure, coordinated fashion but without voluntary control. This pattern is normal in infants and young children before they are toilet trained.

The *reflex neurological bladder* is the result of spinal cord injury or disease that occurs above the voiding reflex arc located in the lower cord. Traumatic spinal cord injury is the most common cause. The bladder works automatically, without the patient's awareness or controllability. The relaxation of the bladder outlet may not be coordinated with bladder contractions. Bladder contractions against contracted sphincters cause intermittent high intravesical pressures and renal damage is likely. Since reflex voiding is not controllable the patient is not reliably dry. Occasionally a *balanced bladder* can be attained by reflex emptying elicited by stimulation of the pubic genital area with massaging or stroking. This prompts voiding at controllable intervals. Unfortunately, reflex bladder contractions may occur in response to other motions (chair transfers, coughing, etc.) with resultant incontinence.

An *autonomic neurogenic bladder* results from injury to the voiding reflex arc in the area of the sacral spine (S2-4) or to the peripheral sensory or motor nerves that lead to and from this area. In these patients the bladder is relatively atonic and does not contract. Urine leaks out of the bladder in an overflow fashion. If the sensory nerves are the only ones involved (as in diabetes), the patient may be able to void voluntarily but will never have the urge to void, and the bladder is gradually enlarged and damaged. If the motor nerves only are involved (as in a herniated disk), the sensation of a need to void and even pain from overdistention may occur, but the patient is not able to generate a bladder contraction.

The most common cause of neurogenic bladder in a child is spina bifida (myelomeningocele), in which the posterior elements of the spine fail to close during development leaving the underlying spinal cord exposed. The classification of neurogenic bladder above does not apply to this disorder because unpredictable, mixed abnormalities of bladder and sphincter dysfunction occur. These children are best classified by the abnormality of function they exhibit, failure to store or failure to empty.

Clean intermittent catheterization (CIC)

With failure-to-empty problems, programs of clean intermittent catheterization (CIC) have been very beneficial (Fig. 38-4). Every bladder has a point at which passive filling causes intravesical pressure to be higher than outlet resistance. If the bladder is emptied by catheterization before this point is reached, an individual can theoretically remain dry between catheterizations. In addition to providing a means of continence, CIC offers a method of keeping intravesical pressure at a lower level, thus protecting the kidneys.

Catheterization is generally performed every 4 hours during the day, using a clean rather than a sterile technique. The parent or patient is advised to lubricate the catheter with a water-soluble lubricant, and cleanse the perineal area with soap and water. Thorough handwashing is essential. Infants are generally catheterized in the supine position, whereas older children may catheterize while sitting on a toilet. Females are taught to separate the labia with the index and ring finger of their nondominant hand while inserting the catheter with the dominant hand. Males hold the penis erect, taking care not to pinch off the urethra. The parent or patient is instructed to insert the catheter until a stream of urine is obtained, then advance the catheter about 1 inch farther. It is sometimes helpful to slowly rotate the catheter while applying gentle pressure as the catheter passes through the external sphincter and prostatic urethra. A slight "give" may be encountered as the catheter passes through the sphincter area in males. The catheter is held in place until the stream of urine stops at which time the catheter is slowly withdrawn. The patient stops withdrawal any time that a stream is again encountered.

After the catheter has been removed, it is washed with soap and water, dried with a clean paper towel and stored in a clean plastic bag or container until the next use. At the initiation of the CIC program the parent is instructed to keep accurate records of the child's intake and output and to note whether the child remains dry between catheterizations.

There are times when CIC may not be possible or appropriate. CIC is unsatisfactory for patients with intermittent reflex bladder contractions, poor stretchability of their bladder muscle, or incompetent bladder outlets. Urodynamic studies better define these problems for more specific management. Anticholinergic drugs (probanthine, ditropan, etc.) are used to control or lessen reflex contractions. Adrengenic drugs (ephedrine, propadrine, etc.) improve bladder neck competence. Surgical enlargement of the bladder using segments of intestine (augmentation enterocystoplasty) is useful in treating poor compliance or low capacity bladders. Surgical reconstruction or compression procedures can improve incompetent bladder necks, not controlled by adrenergic drugs. If the above pharmacological and/or surgical measures are successful in converting storage or control problems to a failure to empty status, then CIC can be initiated. Children who develop upper urinary tract damage because of high intravesical pressures either from uncoordinated reflex bladder contractions occurring against a closed bladder outlet or from poor bladder compliance are managed in a similar way to the failure to empty group of children. However, close medical management of all children with spina bifida together with early urodynamic evaluation in infancy identifies those children at risk for upper urinary tract deterioration and allows for preventive rather than salvage therapy.

Children who are on a program of CIC often have asymptomatic positive urine cultures. These are generally not a matter of concern and are not treated unless symptoms develop or the child has associated vesicoureteral reflux. Unexplained fevers or the sudden onset of wetting between catheterizations in a previously dry child, are symptoms of a urinary tract infection.

External urinary collection devices

For the child who does not use intermittent catheterization an external device may be desirable. Many collection devices are available for boys. Some new female external collection devices are now on the market for adolescents and adults, but no successful device exists for young girls. Regular diapers are frequently used for young children and as the child grows, custom-fitted diapers may be purchased or made from patterns. Since urine may contribute to skin breakdown, a protective ointment should be applied with each diaper change. Meticulous skin observation and care are needed to protect the vulnerable perineal areas.

Catheter care

In the past, indwelling urinary catheters were used frequently in rehabilitation areas. Now with the increased utilization of clean intermittent catheterization and various triggering mechanisms to stimulate planned voiding, Foley catheters are rarely used. However, in certain situations a child or youth may not meet the criteria for a successful CIC program. In this event, indwelling catheters may be employed.

Proper catheter care can help prevent abscesses and periuretheral fistulas and can reduce infections. The male patient with a Foley catheter usually has more problems. The smaller catheter that will drain without clogging is desired. The catheter should be taped to the abdomen so that the penis and catheter are directed toward the upper body. This helps prevent the catheter from being accidentally pulled, causing damage to the sphincter or urethra. It also eliminates the constant movement of the catheter and penis and irritation and destruction of urethral mucosa. This position prevents excessive pressure against the urethra by the elimination of the normal curve from the penis to the bladder. Foley catheters in girls should be taped to the thigh. The patient should be taught the importance of maintaining straight gravity drainage. Maintaining a sterile closed system, and forcing fluids is important. The use of Foley catheters is associated with infection, stone formation, and periuretheral abscesses and fistulas.

Neurogenic Bowel

Bowel care

Neurogenic bowel may be classified in the same way as neurogenic bladder. Uninhibited neurogenic bowel results in defecation without volitional control when the rectum fills. The reflex, or spastic, bowel exhibits above-normal rectal sphincter tone. When the rectum fills, frequent automatic, partial emptying results. In autonomous neurogenic bowel the rectal sphincter is flaccid and frequent small stools may result.

When the patient has lost normal control, a bowel program should be established early. This helps protect already vulnerable skin from rashes and breakdown. Then, too, the socialization of the older child can be drastically affected by soiling, obnoxious odors, and diapers.

An adequate program consists in (1) keeping the stool normal or slightly firmer than normal as soiling is more likely to occur if it is soft or liquid, and (2) scheduling evacuation time. All children are individuals, and their programs must be tailored precisely to their needs. Therefore one child's program may not be identical with that of another child with a similar problem. Many factors influence bowel patterns. Diet has a very great effect; disruption of eating patterns—skipping meals, eating extra meals, or changing meal times, amounts, or types of food eaten—may disturb the program by causing constipation or diarrhea. By trial and error one learns exactly what foods constipate or loosen the stool for each patient. Generally, citrus juices, prune juice, and bulk or roughage items, such as raw vegetables and nuts, tend to loosen the stool. Inadequate fluid intake and foods such as bananas and cheese constipate. Gas-forming items, such as beans and cabbage, may cause diarrhea. Most of these foods are not a problem unless eaten in large quantities. A normal, stable diet with sufficient fluid intake usually maintains the stool consistency. If possible, any changes in factors affecting bowel habits should be added singly so that the effect of each change will be known.

Bowel patterns are also affected by physical activity

Inactivity usually causes constipation, whereas exercise speeds the movement of food through the digestive system and may cause loose stools. Aging, a change of climate or community, altered living patterns, anxiety, and stress may also affect bowel patterns.

A number of reflexes, techniques, and agents can be employed to assist in establishing a sound bowel program free of accidents. These include the gastrocolic reflex, digital stimulation, abdominal straining, stool softeners, and bisacodyl (Dulcolax) suppositories. The gastrocolic reflex is an increase in the peristaltic muscle activity of the large bowel after the stomach has distended from ingestion of food or warm liquids. It is strongest with the entrance of food in a fasting stomach (e.g., breakfast). Therefore about 30 minutes after a meal is a logical time to carry out a bowel program. If the stool is too hard in spite of fluid and dietary measures, stool softeners, such as dioctyl calcium sulfosuccinate (Colace) or dioctyl sodium sulfosuccinate (Surfak), which retain water in the stool, may be used. Bisacodyl is a safe means of chemically inducing peristaltic movement of the large bowel. It is more predictable and safer than irritating laxatives or mineral oils that could decrease vitamin absorption. An appropriately sized bisacodyl suppository is inserted high up in the rectum, against the side of the bowel wall so that it will dissolve and be absorbed easily. Bisacodyl usually dissolves in 10 to 15 minutes, reaching peak action in another 10 or 15 minutes. Bisacodyl small-volume enemas may be effective for the paraplegic or meningomyelocele patient.

Digital stimulation does not refer to the digital removal of stool from the rectum. It is a gentle circular motion made by the gloved finger inserted ½ inch (1.25 cm) against the rectal sphincter muscle. The patient may be positioned on the left side or may sit on a raised toilet seat. This gentle motion both relaxes and dilates the rectal sphincter and causes peristaltic muscle contractions of the large bowel. The procedure should be continued for 10 to 15 minutes. It can be used in conjunction with suppositories or by itself. As evacuation occurs, one should gently pull the rectum to one side and allow the stool to be eliminated.

Although any combination of these techniques and agents may be used in the child's bowel training, the program should start with the least and the simplest. The time of day for evacuation should be chosen with regard to previous bowel habits, daily schedules, time limitations, and personal preferences. A reasonable time seems to be about 30 minutes after the morning or evening meal. Once a time is selected, it must remain consistent within 30 minutes. For a child with a spinal cord injury, one possible routine might be as follows:

1. Immediately after breakfast, insert one half of a Dulcolax suppository as high as possible into the rectum. (The amount depends on age and size of the child. Too much causes abdominal cramping; too little, no action.)
2. Wait 10 to 15 minutes, continuing personal care.

3 Place the child on a "potty chair" or toilet with the feet touching the floor so that the hips are flexed into the squat position.
4 Have the child lean forward against the thighs (to increase intraabdominal pressure), and massage the abdominal muscles. Encourage the child to strain at the same time. (Have children who do not understand this blow on a toy balloon.) If diarrhea should occur, it is wise to check for impaction because liquid feces can seep around impaction, resulting in false diarrhea.

Consistency in the program is essential. Some children may require the program twice a day. A bowel program takes time, patience, and attention to detail but in most instances is successful.

BEHAVIORAL ASPECTS OF REHABILITATION

Many problems that are encountered in rehabilitation, although based on physiological disability, are psychological in content. If undesirable behavior can be changed, the long-term outlook for the patient improves. One method of behavioral change, based on the work of BF Skinner and his stimulus response (S-R) techniques, is called *behavioral modification.* A behavior is an action—something a person does. It may be desirable or undesirable. To be changed, using this technique, it must be observable, describable, and measurable. An action can be made to occur more often by following it with a favorable consequence—a *positive reinforcer.* A behavior may be reduced or eliminated by withdrawing its reinforcer or influenced less effectively by punishment.

Case Presentation: While recovering from head trauma, 4-year-old Joseph became incontinent of urine. By positive reinforcement of an observable, describable target behavior that can be counted, he again learned to void in the toilet. After recording the number and frequency of his voidings, his primary nurse established a toileting schedule. The nurses explained what behavior was expected, then remained with him quietly. When Joseph voided into the toilet, he was immediately reinforced with praise, a smile, and a few minutes of attention. In a short time, Joseph was voiding in the toilet, and, as his physical and mental condition improved, by further reinforcement he was able to summon the nurse for assistance to the bathroom. In examining Joseph's problem, his nurse discovered that busy staff members had nagged and cajoled him when he voided incontinently. Because Joseph had valued their attention, their actions had reinforced incontinent voiding. During the modification program, if he voided incontinently, his nurse would change him in a matter-of-fact manner, withholding both positive and negative attention.

A reinforcer must affect the frequency of the behavior. If the rate of behavior does not change, no reinforcement has taken place and a true reinforcer must be found. For Joseph praise was appropriate, although a toy or food might have been successful in another situation. A reinforcer must be delivered promptly only when the target behavior occurs. Joseph was reinforced with praise immediately on voiding in the toilet; otherwise, he was matter-of-factly returned to bed. Early in a program, reinforcement may occur after each desired behavior (continuous). Later, it may be intermittent—a more effective and efficient technique. At times it is inconvenient to deliver reinforcers at the time of target behavior. In this instance a token may be delivered after each desired behavior to be exchanged later for a desired reinforcer. This makes it possible to use a variety of reinforcers for single or multiple behaviors. Adults use this system when they work for money.

As Joseph progressed, he learned to dress himself. Each time he completed a dressing behavior he was praised and a poker chip was placed in a glass by his bed. Each chip was worth 5 minutes of evening television time. When establishing a token-trade rate, one should aim for a high rate of success. As the patient progresses, trade rates should be revised to require increased performance for a given amount of reinforcement.

A large task achieved through a series of small, planned successes is called *shaping.* When Joseph learned to dress himself, he began with putting on his socks. In the beginning he was reinforced when he picked up his socks to prepare to put them on. Later he received reinforcement only when he placed his socks over his toes. Finally, his reward was given only after he pulled his socks over his heels.

Generalization occurs when a behavior learned in one situation occurs in another environment or time, or as a broadened scope of behavior (for example, patients who learn to walk in the hospital, then return home where they walk, dress, and brush their hair). They have generalized in all three aspects. This can be accomplished by direct methods using a trained family member or visiting nurse to reinforce the behavior. An indirect approach is called *trapping,* which ties the desired behavior to a naturally occurring reinforcer. Assuming that the previous patient enjoyed the socialization of school, attendance would involve dressing, grooming, and walking. These target behaviors are reinforced by attending school. Trapping increases the chance that the behavior will continue.

In behavioral terms, punishment is either the withdrawal of a reinforcer or application of an aversive stimulus. The latter method is rarely appropriate for the health professional. In some instances, isolation or loss of privileges may apply; however, aversive stimuli are more often used to reinforce the adult's feelings of power and control. The effect of punishment is relatively temporary and produces reactions of fear, anxiety, frustration, and hostility. Alternative approaches are (1) changing the circumstances that evoke undesirable behavior, (2) reinforcing an incompatible behavior, (3) permitting the behavior in a safe place until the desire is satiated, and (4) extinguishing the behavior through lack of reinforcement. Family and staff attention is perhaps the strongest reinforcer of behavior.

The goals of pediatric rehabilitation are to foster growth and development, to improve function, independence, and personal fulfillment, and to prevent complications. This complex and challenging specialty requires the collaboration of the child, family, and rehabilitation team.

KEY CONCEPTS

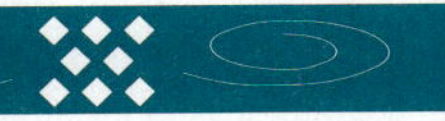

1 Pediatric rehabilitation is based on two concepts: (1) each person is unique and has individual basic worth and (2) the task involves a committed group of people working together as a team with a common goal. The overall goal is to foster maximal growth, development, independence, and personal fulfillment within the limitations of the handicap.

2 A rehabilitation unit requires 30% to 60% more staff than the typical pediatric acute care unit to provide expert nursing care, ongoing teaching, and reinforcement.

3 Three principles of nursing care that are particularly applicable to the long-term patient are (1) maintain a basic sense of trust; (2) protect from fear, frustration, and pain; and (3) facilitate social contacts and communication with the outside world.

4 The child who is injured or has been impaired by disease, as well as his or her family and friends, experiences grief similar to that encountered by those mourning the death of a loved one. A three-stage pattern of shock and denial, developing awareness, and restitution or resolution is observed.

5 Psychosocial support of these children includes providing opportunities to express their feelings, facilitating social contact and interaction, and assisting them to continue their education.

6 Common diagnoses found in rehabilitation units include: spinal cord injuries, anomalies, or diseases of the central nervous system, and brain injury caused by trauma, tumor, or disease.

7 In the patient with an injury above midtrunk, autonomic dysreflexia may arise. Symptoms include: flushing, headache, sweating, feelings of nasal stuffiness, goose bumps, bradycardia, and a rapid increase in blood pressure. Treatment includes elevating the patient's head and removing the stimulus.

8 The brain-injured patient typically regains awareness and orientation slowly. Eight helpful levels of cognitive function and behavioral response have been identified in the recovery process.

9 The complications of prolonged bed rest and immobility represent the greatest dangers to the longevity of the rehab patient. Such complications include motor and sensory loss, contractures, edema, thrombosis, urinary tract infection, fecal impaction, hypostatic pneumonia, psychological disorders, and disturbances in normal growth and development.

10 Routine skin care should include the following: prevent pressure on reddened areas, blisters, or sores; increase positioning times according to the guidelines; and regularly assess the skin.

11 Proper anatomical positioning can help prevent skeletal deformities, muscle shortening, and venous stasis.

12 The primary goals of management of the pediatric neurogenic bladder are preservation of normal urinary tract anatomy and renal function, prevention of significant urinary infection, and attainment of social urinary continence.

13 Clean intermittent catheterization provides a means of continence and offers a method of keeping intravesical pressure at a lower level, protecting the kidneys.

14 Factors that influence bowel patterns include: diet, physical activity, aging, change of climate or community, altered living patterns, anxiety, and stress.

15 Behavior modification can be accomplished by positively reinforcing desirable actions. A behavior may be reduced or eliminated by withdrawing its reinforcer or, less effectively, by punishment.

CRITICAL THOUGHT QUESTIONS

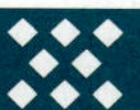

1. In childhood rehabilitation the team includes teachers and educational consultants. Why are these team members especially important for the child?
2. Nursing in rehabilitation focuses on teaching the parents and child to "do" as much as possible. Why is this better than "doing for" the family and child? How would you respond if the mother says, "You can do it so much better than I can?"
3. Severe illness or injury causes stress in the family. What indications might you observe that indicates high stress level? What can you as the nurse do to help families cope with this stress? How should the nurse redirect parental anger regarding their child's loss of function?
4. Identify specific injuries and illnesses that require specialized long-term rehabilitative care. In what setting would individuals with these problems receive the best care?
5. With the trend toward home care when possible, what teaching regarding physical and emotional care should be provided to the parents? Should parents perform"nursing skills" such as catheterization and suctioning in the home?

REFERENCES

American Association of Neuroscience Nurses: *Core curriculum for neuroscience nursing,* Des Plaines, Ill, 1990, The Association.

Behrman R: *Nelson textbook of pediatrics,* ed 14, Philadelphia, 1992, WB Saunders.

Burkett KW: Trends in pediatric rehabilitation, *Nurs Clin North Am* 24(1)239, 1989.

Deatrick J and Knafl K: Management behaviors: day to day adjustments to childhood chronic conditions, *J Pediatr Nurs* 5(1)15-22, 1990.

Editorial: Acute care nursing shortens stays for patients with brain injuries, *Am J Nurs* 6:795, 1989.

Krier J: Involvement of educational staff in the health care of medically fragile children, *Pediatr Nurs* 19(3) 251-259, 1993.

Loughrey L: Avoiding the pitfalls of rehabilitation at home, *Nursing '89* 19(10):63, 1989.

Olson E et al: Hazards of immobility: effects on cardiovascular and respiratory function, *Am J Nurs* 90(3):43, 1990.

Warda M: The family and chronic sorrow: role theory approach, *J Pediatr Nurs* 7(3)205-210, 1992.

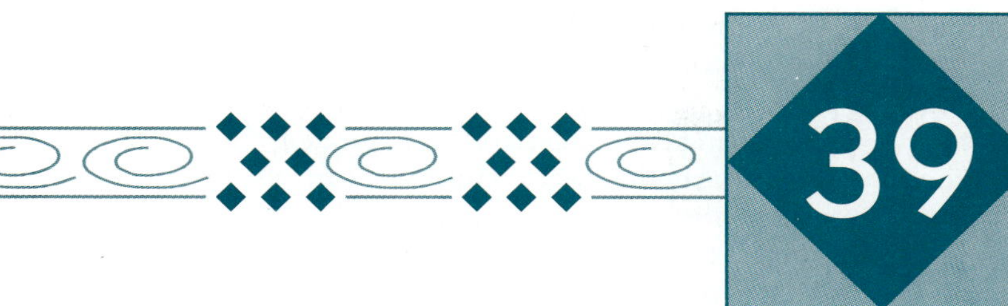

39

Grief and Loss

CHAPTER OBJECTIVES

After studying this chapter, the student should be able to:

1. Identify nursing interventions that reflect sensitive, nonjudgmental support for families coping with the life-threatening illness of their child.
2. Discuss four factors that contribute to a child's concept of death.
3. Describe the typical progression in the growth of a child's understanding of the nature of death, based on age at less than 3 years; 5 to 6 years; 7 years; 10 to 11 years.
4. Discuss four ways in which children who are unable to verbalize their fears may express themselves.
5. Discuss the need for usual behavioral expectations and discipline for the child who has a life-threatening illness.
6. Describe effective communication techniques that impart active listening, honesty, and hope when interacting with an ill child and his or her family.
7. Explain three stresses that all hospitalized children experience but that may be a particular challenge for the terminally ill child and his or her family.
8. Describe Bowlby's four phases of mourning and interpret their importance for providing nonjudgmental nursing care.

CHALLENGE OF UNCERTAINTY

The emotional, social, and spiritual concerns of the child and family who are experiencing grief and loss is a challenging assignment for the nurse. This chapter focuses on the nurse's role in the provision of informational and emotional support of the child and family coping with the terminal phase of illness.

Today, because of great medical and technological advances, children with terminal illnesses typically live longer than ever before. Helping such a child reach his or her developmental potential, physically, intellectually, psychologically, and socially, has become a multidisciplinary challenge. The short-term and long-term prognoses are often unclear. This burden of uncertainty is challenging for the child, the family, and caregivers.

Culturally sensitive informational and emotional support are very important if the child and family adaptation to the stressor of chronic and terminal illness is to be sustained during this period of instability. The nurse can promote effective coping with honest, knowledgable, and understanding care. Health care providers must not only have a working knowledge of the ongoing medical treatment and nursing care, but equally important, its psychosocial implications for the child and family. The nurse must recognize that the impact of impending death is influenced by the child's developmental age and the child's experience with life-threatening illness.

It is extremely important that the child's optimal quality of life be maintained without pain, with dignity and respect, and with family support. Communicating this concept to the child's family, teachers, and other significant persons is essential. For example, the school-age child with a life-threatening illness frequently experiences scholastic difficulties because of absences, psychological problems and fears, and differences caused by amputation, chemotherapy, and other treatment or disease sequelae. These problems must be recognized and addressed as quickly as possible to maintain the child's own psychological well-being and rapport with his peer group. To face the overwhelming demands of a long-term, life-threatening illness, the child, parents, and health care providers need to identify and utilize supportive resources.

The nurse must realize the child's reactions are influenced by his developmental level and concept of death. An understanding of typical parental reactions and the nurse's own personal feelings and philosophy concerning death helps the nurse to provide culturally sensitive informational and emotional support.

Reactions of the Child

A child's concept of death parallels their psychosocial and cognitive development and is influenced by past experience and cultural background. Children under the age of 3 years experience loss and grief through separation anxiety once parent-infant attachment and trust have been well established. They fear being separated from people who are an integral part of their lives, such as parents or other consistent caregivers. If these significant people detach themselves physically or emotionally from the dying child, the child senses this and becomes fearful at first, then extremely withdrawn. Young children typically do not perceive death as final or terminal. For children 3 to 5 years of age death may be perceived as a kind of sleep. It is only a change of some kind, a departure, and is not viewed as permanent. Children 5 to 6 years of age have a better understanding of death in the concrete sense. They begin to recognize the permanence of death, but cannot conceive of it as resulting from chance or a natural happening. Causation is personified as a ghost, the devil, God, or a hostile act on the part of the person who died. In the child's mind the event may be perceived as deprivation and personal abandonment.

From approximately 6 years of age onward, children seem to understand that death is final. Many 6- and 7-year-old children suspect that their parents will die someday and that they too may die, but they are comforted by the thought that the death of their parents (and their own death) is still a long time away.

Children 9 to 10 years of age and older achieve an adult concept of death as a permanent biological process. A child over 10 years of age is capable of integrating the concept of "not being" if the parents can do so. At this age, children can understand the universality and permanence of death.

As children approach adolescence, they are equipped with the intellectual tools necessary to comprehend time, space, life, and death in a more logical manner. In spite of the common depiction of violence in the media, children in the United States are often shielded from any real involvement with or explanation of death. Many families do not perceive death as a normal part of the life cycle. Studies indicate that children often fear their own death or those of their loved ones in terms of separation and loss of security. Since death is a part of life, deliberate, thoughtful education about death in the observation of nature and daily life is appropriate for children and families.

Children who are terminally ill may not manifest an *overt* concern about death, probably because they attempt to repress their anxiety concerning the outcome of their illness. Nevertheless, children should be allowed and encouraged to express their fears verbally through play (drawing pictures, relating to puppets, playing with dollhouse or doll families, and handling, pounding, and shaping clay). Highly susceptible to the attitudes of their parents, terminally ill children will likely sense the gravity of the situation and will need to vent their feelings. They pick up many cues from their families and surroundings that something has changed, that something different, important, and probably bad is happening or will occur. These cues may include a change in expectations, less emphasis on discipline, unnatural silences or forced chatter, and unusual gifts. These children should not be deprived of the security of usual behavioral expectations, and they should be allowed to participate in their normal activities as much as possible.

What to Tell the Child

Children should be reassured that their illness is not their fault and is not a punishment for anything they did. If a child with a life-threatening illness asks about dying, a statement such as, "You have a serious illness but no illness is without hope," may be reassuring. To deprive a person of hope even when the outcome is clouded is unrealistic and unkind. One must also individualize responses according to the child's developmental age, illness experience, and cultural background. If the child sees or asks about the death of another child, you might say, "Johnny was very sick and died." Answer questions simply and honestly. Keep in mind the child's level of comprehension. Opportunities to talk should be given. Many times older children select one staff member who appears open and accepting of what they say for sharing their fears and concerns. Most important is the maintenance of an atmosphere that allows patients to ask as much or as little as they wish. Nurses, social workers, psychiatrists, or chaplains may coordinate the care of the grieving family.

The majority of parents say they believe that when the terminally ill child asks, the child needs to be told honestly that he is dying. To hold out false hope or to deny the imminence of death is very confusing to the child who senses the gravity of the illness. The child knows from the behavior of those close to him that he or she is going to die. Being honest with the child allows him or her to express his fears and concerns and ask questions about what happens when a person dies and what will await him or her after death; this can be answered in terms of the family's religious beliefs. Many children take comfort in knowing that relatives or friends who have died will be "waiting" for them. Terminally ill children sometimes express guilt about leaving their parents and families. It is important to talk with families about giving their child "permission to die." They can reassure the child that he or she has worked hard, fought his disease as best he or she could, and now it is permissible to stop fighting. It helps for parents to let their child know that he or she will be missed greatly and never forgotten, but the parents and siblings will be all right.

Three Stresses of Terminal Illness

The child who is facing impending death experiences three stressors common to all hospitalized children: separation from parents, traumatic procedures, and isolation. Modification of hospital routine and procedure must be considered.

Separation from parents

For the child who is terminal, there is no greater comfort than the security and closeness of a parent. Allowing unnecessary separation is unacceptable. Children want their parents with them particularly during stressful experiences. Nurses should encourage parents to touch and hold their child. The warmth of physical contact is the most primitive and basic nonverbal comforting technique human's possess. Touch can communicate a solace or comfort to the frightened child that words cannot achieve.

Traumatic procedures

When parents understand the reasons why tubes are inserted, intravenous feedings are ordered, blood is withdrawn, and other treatments are initiated, their comfort level is increased. Parents are better able to provide emotional support to their child if consistent informational support is provided by the health care team. The nurse is able to help children allay their fears through their parents. Allowing the child as much control as possible over the necessary procedures and routines is vitally important. The child should be able to make choices among appropriate alternatives and participate in decisions relative to the plan of care.

Older children may be assisted by diverting their attention and concern from their illness to comfort measures that make a difference. The nurse who listens with interest and attentiveness will help the child and family to make the best of an extremely stressful situation. Treating and eliminating intercurrent infections, such as rashes, gives the child reassurance and relief. Children perceive these measures as evidence that care providers have not given up, that they are not being deserted.

Pain should be well-controlled on a preventive schedule. Whenever possible the oral route is preferable. Injections are avoided. Continuous intravenous or subcutaneous infusions may provide the greatest relief. Patient controlled anesthesia (PCA) is used with older children and teens. See Chapter 24 and pp. 553-557 for further information on pharmacological and nonpharmacological pain control.

Isolation

The most dreaded fear does not seem to be that of dying but of dying alone. Children feel secure with other children, and they believe that nothing too terrible can happen when parents are present. The child who is terminal should not be isolated from his or her parents, siblings, friends, other relatives, or staff. The nurse cannot conceal a child's impending death from other children in the unit. Parents and relatives should be encouraged to say when they will come back. It implies a promise: "I will see you again, and you will have nothing to fear in the interim." Although relatives and staff are encouraged not to isolate the child, the nurse should not permit constant or prolonged visits that the child may interpret as a "death watch." Parents also need respite to attend to other responsibilities, to care for well siblings, to rest, and to reorganize. They should not be encouraged to stay continually. Arrangements can usually be made for someone to stay with the child, allowing parents a well-deserved break.

Most children are very concerned about their special

possessions and what will happen to them when they are gone. Many children, even in the younger age groups, find it comforting to make a "will" in which they designate who is to have their favorite toys or treasured books. Older children, particularly those who have spent much time in the hospital, frequently want to be sure they are not forgotten and may take comfort in planning for the donation in their memory of a plaque, a television, video game, or toys to the hospital. Patients may choose to donate a treatment device such as a Serojet, used for numbing the site before bone marrow aspiration or lumbar puncture. Other children request the donation of a refrigerator to an individual room so that other children can have their favorite foods close at hand.

Dying at Home

Increasingly, if the family desires, terminally ill children spend their last weeks or months at home. Home health care must be adapted to the family and to the facilities available. Although home care for the terminally ill child is a change from recent methods, it has been the norm during most of human history. With the advent of specialized diagnostic and emergency services available only in hospitals, this significant event was often moved outside the home. Yet for many sick children who can no longer benefit from the sophisticated facilities offered in a hospital, the home may be more comfortable and secure if the family is willing and able to provide the care needed.

The impetus for home care of the terminally ill child has been influenced by cost-containment and the ongoing study of Ida Marie Martinson. The shared experiences of nursing and medical personnel and parents who participated in the Home Care for the Dying Child Project, first developed as a research study at the University of Minnesota, have been extremely valuable. The nurse should refer to Martinson, Spinetta, Craft, and others for more detailed perspectives.

Another recent trend has been the organization of volunteer nurses who reside near the affected family and can more easily provide the on-call support essential to the family. Decreased costs associated with this type of support are an important factor. The consulting home care nurse should be prepared to refer the family to financial and other community resources as part of the total care plan. One should bear in mind that financial demands on the family added to the loss of the child can have a devastating effect on the entire family unit.

Many families have found home care preferable and fulfilling. It helps decrease the parents' feelings of helplessness, although the final result may be unchanged. The child's emotional well-being and comfort are much enhanced by the familiar surroundings and association with family members (Miles, 1990). Even if a medical emergency requires rehospitalization, the survivors have expressed great satisfaction in the home health care experience.

Hospice, a specialized center for care of the terminally ill, was first developed in Europe and has flourished in the United States. Centers devoted to pediatric patients are growing partly in response to the increasing numbers of children who are diagnosed with pediatric AIDS. Hospice is intended for the child who has no reasonable expectation of cure to live life to the fullest without pain, with choices and dignity, and with family support (Armstrong-Dailey, 1990). The team approach that this concept offers is highly valued by patients and families.

PARENTAL REACTIONS

One of the nurse's most important roles in the care of the child with a terminal illness is helping the grieving parents cope with their impending loss in a nonjudgmental manner. Integrating the tragic event of death into their life experience is most difficult. The parents' reactions to the impending death of the child is similar to extreme separation anxiety.

Mourning Process

In recent years much has been written regarding the reactions of patients who face a terminal illness and of the behaviors of parents and close family members or friends when they mourn the impending death of a child. The descriptions and analyses offer guidelines for the interpretation and anticipation of events that will be helpful to all concerned.

John Bowlby was one of the earliest writers in the field to describe the mourning process. He identified four phases in the natural mourning process: (1) numbness, (2) yearning and searching, (3) despair and disorganization, and (4) hope and rebuilding. Bowlby's work covers the phases of mourning in the period following death. However, anticipatory mourning often begins before death occurs, and Bowlby's phases have been helpful in describing parental reactions before the death of the child.

Mourning is the process of healing that helps people face and recover from loss. The normal healing process takes a year or more. The clearest evidence of recovery is the ability to remember comfortably and realistically both the pleasures and disappointments of the lost relationship. Most persons progress through four phases whether the child's death occurs before, after, or during the mourning process. It is very important for nurses to be aware of and sensitive to the different interactions that may occur among family members and health care providers.

Numbness

The first phase is characterized by a state of shock at the news of the loss or of the impending loss. Denial also occurs during this phase. For some parents their denial may be a positive response allowing them time to adapt to the loss. Denial may range from extreme to slight and will come and go throughout all of the stages. The overriding need of this phase is for protection from the pain of the loss, and this need is met by refusal to recognize the diagnosis or loss.

Yearning and searching

The second phase involves an intense desire to find the lost loved one. Many strong emotions are brought into play—anxiety, yearning, anger, and guilt. Parents cannot believe that this could happen to their child. Often a parent's attitude is one of hostility, and constant criticism. Hope for the child is stressed but in a nonspecific way. Parents tell themselves, "Something will be discovered." They want to try anything that might offer hope for a cure no matter how irrational it may seem.

Anxiety is manifested by an intense need to weep, an empty feeling in the abdomen, loss of appetite, and other somatic complaints. With anxiety there is yearning, longing for a sign that a cure will be found and that the child will get well. Guilt feelings are constantly expressed in tears: "If only I had done this or that, if only I had notified the physician sooner." It is natural and necessary to cry, to be angry, and to feel guilty. These are all healthy signs of normal grief. It is a stage in the gradual process of accepting a great loss.

Involvement of parents when possible in the physical care of the child is extremely important in facilitating parental adaptation. However, although parental participation in the care of the sick child is desirable, it should not be at the expense of the emotional and physical well-being of the rest of the family. Parents usually want to be with their sick child and need to feel that they personally have done everything possible for the child. Feelings of guilt are somewhat relieved by the expenditure of personal effort in the care of the child. Parents are encouraged to participate in the physical care of their children by bathing, feeding, or entertaining them and accompanying them to the laboratory and x-ray departments. Thus parents become integrated into the hospital routine, and communication with personnel is enhanced.

During the initial period in the hospital, parents physically cling to their children. They are involved solely in their care. In time, parents want to help with the care of other children. Assisting children to the playroom and reading to a group rather than just their own child are examples of this desire. Manifestations of the capacity to help other children mark a turning point in parental adjustment that reflects acceptance of the child's illness and impending death.

Actually, the second phase of the mourning process as described by Bowlby is very similar to the stages noted by Elizabeth Kubler-Ross in which she describes the ill patient's reaction as "No, not me!" (shock and denial) and "Why me? Why now?" (anger, rage, and envy). The parent's mourning, however, also typically includes a destructive guilt factor.

Despair and disorganization

The third phase in Bowlby's mourning process parallels the observations of Kubler-Ross. It is similar to her "Yes, me, but . . ." (bargaining) and "Yes, me" (depression) stages. Facing and accepting the reality of the fatal illness, parents feel helpless. Life is stripped of meaning. Active, realistic efforts to prolong life typify the early part of this phase.

Often the mother is the parent who spends the most time ministering to the needs of the sick child, although in some families fathers may play a more nurturant role. When possible the child's father should be incorporated into the plan of care as a source of support for the mother and child and to promote his healthy grieving process. During this phase the nurse must be aware that the parent's attempts to cope with the situation may fluctuate from gentle, assured bedside care to inappropriate, exhausting activity. At one moment parents may express exaggerated gratitude to the health care providers; in the next they may be overly critical. Emotions may range from philosophic resignation to sentimentality. Parents are emotionally fragile and inconsistent. The staff must avoid reacting to the criticism and maintain a nonjudgmental, supportive approach recognizing the emotional roller coaster that the parents are experiencing.

The reality of the terminal illness and its meaning begins to penetrate the parent's consciousness during this phase. Denial of the illness may disappear but hope of a cure persists. Hope is more specific now, often related to particular scientific efforts. Parents cling less to their children and encourage them to participate in hospital activities. Parents should be encouraged to express their grief and loss during moments away from the child. This helps them move beyond the initial shock and recognize some of the specific things they still have to offer their child. Every attempt must be made to enable parents to see the continuing value of their function as parents, despite their feelings of despair and helplessness in the face of death.

As the child's physical energy begins to diminish, preoccupation with measures that involve treatment of the disease begins to subside, and parents are interested in relieving the child's discomfort and pain. Although they continue to hope that their efforts will save the child, the intensity of the expectation is gradually reduced. They are separating themselves emotionally from the child.

Hope and rebuilding

The fourth phase is characterized by a calm acceptance of the child's impending death. Separation from the child is no longer an adaptive problem for the parents. The mother or father remains with the child whenever possible but with adequate consideration for the remainder of the family. For the first time the parents express a wish that the child could die so that the suffering would end.

Many parents never reach this fourth phase of mourning during their child's illness. It may not be until after the child dies that this phase begins. With the loss acknowledged and the depth of pain plumbed, new people, relationships, and activities become meaningful. Some parents take interest in organizations such as the American Cancer Society and the Cystic Fibrosis Association. By so doing, the parent is able to reduce preoccupation with self and loss. This allows the parents to reinvest feelings in other love objects—spouse, remaining children, or close relatives. Again, the last stage of "yes", described by Kubler-Ross as acceptance or resignation appears appropriate.

SIBLING REACTIONS

Nursing care for the family must include assessment of the siblings adaptation to the situation. Siblings are usually distressed by the continuing illness and may require considerable support from parents, extended family members, friends, and health care providers. Parents should be encouraged to divide their time among the various members of the family as the situation warrants. The importance of communication with siblings must always be borne in mind by the parents, extended family and friends during this difficult period (Hogan et al, 1990). Siblings need developmentally appropriate ongoing open, honest communication and emotional support. Martinson (1976) in her classic study found that home care for dying children did not have an adverse effect on siblings, even when they actually witness the death. In fact the experience of participating in terminal care seems to remove many of the false anxieties and fantasies experienced by siblings who could not participate in the hospital experience. For additional content on sibling reactions refer to pp. 507-508.

NURSE'S REACTIONS

Awareness of one's feelings about death is essential to giving comprehensive nursing care to dying children and their families. Information about children's concepts of death and their parents' fears is not enough. To give sensitive and supportive care to the dying child, the nurse needs help in understanding personal fears regarding death. The nurse may experience frustration and a sense of failure because cure or rehabilitation is an unrealistic goal for the child. Helping the family cope with their stress gives the nurse a sense of purpose at a difficult time for all concerned.

Fear of death is the most inescapable and realistic of human fears. Fear and anxiety lead to convictions of immortality on a conscious or unconscious level that are universal to all humans. Each individual recognizes that other people must die but may not acknowledge their own mortality.

Every person feels or reacts differently to the death experience. If the reality of death is so painful that one handles it by either immersing oneself in it or utterly denying it, it will be difficult to fulfill one's role as a nurse. Nurses ought to let themselves recognize, at least to a limited degree, the awe and fear that everyone experiences in the face of death. Fear of death is managed in several ways: (1) by a religious belief in immortality, (2) by a denial of the awe felt for death, (3) by withdrawal from the dying child, and (4) by the formation of various phobias or compulsions. Nurses are involuntarily influenced by illogical but protective defenses in the presence of impending death. However, if they are to help parents who are experiencing grief and loss, nurses must avoid reacting in a nonjudgmental manner. Nurses must become aware of their own feelings.

The entire health care team should be offered access to support groups, patient conferences, and access to information regarding helpful techniques and approaches. Nurses who care for dying children frequently find it difficult to admit to themselves or to others that they need support (Fig. 39-1). Ongoing open communication among staff members can be encouraged by the provision of regularly scheduled meetings that give permission to caregivers to grieve (Small et al, 1991). To cope successfully with the loss of a child, nurses must recognize that although the outcome was inevitable, the professional care and support they provided for the patient and family were the very best possible. They have given comfort to those who need it most and, in turn, can take comfort in this knowledge.

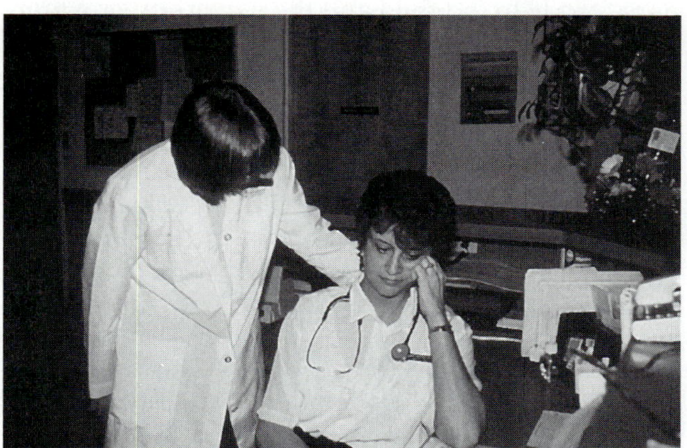

Fig. 39-1 Mutual nurturance among members of the health care team is of critical importance. (Courtesy of Michael Clement, Mesa, Ariz.)

Nursing the dying child requires courage. The nurse must remember that courage is not the absence of fear but the willingness and ability to function in its presence. Nurses who care for dying children and counsel their parents must be sympathetic and empathetic, while preserving their own emotional well-being.

PARENT/STAFF SUPPORT GROUPS

There has been a trend in university centers to set aside special times for the staff to meet with the parents of children with life-threatening diseases. Common problems are shared in these small mutual support groups. Discussions center around the nature of the disease and its treatment, as well as the emotional distress faced by parents, siblings, friends, and health care providers. It is normal for primary caregivers to openly share their own sense of loss with parents and one another. Parents appreciate when the staff sincerely care about the child. Support groups are usually facilitated by clinical nursing specialists, physicians, social workers, or chaplains. Through an open, nonjudgmental approach and active listening parents and staff members develop a mutual understanding. These meetings provide an opportunity for parents to meet the staff in a more relaxed setting and with ample time for discussion. Specific benefits from these meetings include mutual support during times of stress and uncertainty, the realization that discipline of the child is still desirable, and the possibility for sharing feelings about loss and grief. Perhaps the most important benefit is the opportunity for parents to share and identify with one another.

Nursing Alert

The American Academy of Pediatrics (1992) recommends the supine or side-lying position for healthy infants. Infants with breathing problems or excessive vomiting may continue to sleep in the prone position.

Although, these infants are not hospitalized, the nurse may encounter a family who has lost a child under these circumstances in clinics or emergency rooms. The intensity or duration of mourning must not be underestimated. The shock of their sudden loss renders them incapable of making even simple decision. The nurse serves as a compassionate listener and provider of information. The National Sudden Infant Death Syndrome Foundation and the SIDS Information and Counseling Centers have been established by Public Law 92-270 and are excellent resources for parents and family members.

Sudden Infant Death Syndrome

The sudden death of a child from unknown causes is particularly tragic. In the United States sudden infant death syndrome (SIDS) is the *second leading cause* of infant with an incidence of 1.4 per 1000 live births and a peak age of 2 to 4 months. SIDS, defined as the unexpected death of a previously healthy infant between 1 month and 1 year of age, is usually a diagnosis of exclusion, dependent on the postmortem findings. The etiology of SIDS is unclear, although several risk factors are known. Siblings of SIDS victims have a tenfold increased risk of SIDS. African Americans and Native Americans have a rate of SIDS two to three times that of whites. Preterm and low–birth-weight infants who continue to have pathological apnea at the time of hospital discharge, infants who have required CPR or vigorous stimulation, and infants with certain diseases such as central hypoventilation are also at greater risk for SIDS.

Recent studies link sleep habits with an increased risk of SIDS. The infant's positioning during sleep is a critical factor. Infants who sleep in a prone position are at greater risk of dying of SIDS, than infants who are positioned on their back or side. The prone position may cause oropharyngeal obstruction, affect thermoregulation causing overheating of the infant, or affect arousal state (Dwyer et al, 1991; Fleming et al, 1990).

Basic Concepts of Religion

Understanding a family's religious beliefs concerning death is extremely important. The nurse may observe that parents with deep faith in God find genuine comfort in their religious beliefs. For Catholics and Protestants who believe in personal immortality, great solace and comfort can be found in the conviction that they will one day rejoin their loved ones.

In the Jewish faith the concept of immortality is not clearly defined. Judaism teaches that perhaps there is a life after death, but the only immortality of which man is certain is the immortality he or she may achieve while still alive or through his or her descendants.

Knowing the basic concepts of the various religious faiths concerning death may be of great assistance to the nurse. The nurse is not expected to be a theologian nor should he or she attempt to share his or her religious beliefs concerning death unless asked, but the nurse can help the child and the parents by providing physical care, emotional support, and the comfort of spiritual counsel by contacting the parent's clergy. A spiritual advisor who has counseling skills may be a major source of support and comfort for the parent, thus facilitating the grief process.

Just as it may be the nurse's privilege to help parents and their infant at the event of birth, the nurse may also be privileged to ease and comfort the child and family who are experiencing grief and loss. The nurse's supportive, nonjudgmental acceptance and understanding fosters healthy grieving. This is a most challenging yet growth-promoting aspect of the nursing role.

KEY CONCEPTS

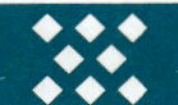

1. When caring for the family of a terminally ill child, the nurse must have both a working knowledge of the ongoing medical treatment and nursing care and an understanding of the psychosocial implications for the child and family.
2. A child's concept of death is influenced by psychosocial and cognitive developmental, past experience, and cultural background.
3. Children who are terminally ill should be encouraged to express their fears verbally or through play.
4. When caring for the terminally ill child, the nurse should answer questions simply and honestly, keeping in mind the child's level of comprehension.
5. Children suffering from terminal illnesses are subjected to three stresses common to other hospitalized children: separation from parents, traumatic procedures, and isolation.
6. For many terminally ill children who can no longer benefit from hospital facilities, the home may be the most comfortable and secure place to spend their final weeks or months. Nursing care must be adapted to the family and to the facilities available.
7. Bowlby identified four phases in the natural mourning process: (1) numbness, (2) yearning and searching, (3) despair and disorganization, and (4) hope and rebuilding. Although these phases are not to be construed as undeviating or applicable to all persons and situations, they provide guidelines for interpretation and anticipation of events.
8. The importance of open, honest communication with siblings is critical for parents, extended family members, friends, and health care providers.
9. To give sensitive and supportive care to the child facing impending death and the child's family the nurse must come to terms with personal feelings about death.
10. Knowing the basic concepts of the various religious faiths concerning death may be of great assistance to the nurse caring for the family of a dying child.

CRITICAL THOUGHT QUESTIONS

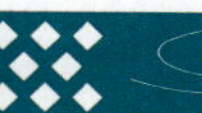

1 How does a child's concept of death change at various ages? How can the nurse help a child express his feelings regarding death?
2 Children are very sensitive to the attitudes and emotions of the adults around them. How do adults respond to death and dying? What impact does or should this have on the parents and health care providers?
3 Terminal illness is stressful to the child, the parents, and the health care providers. What are the greatest stressors? What can be done to reduce these?
4 Do you think that the death of a child is more difficult to cope with than the death of an adult? If so, why? If not, why not? What can be done to help parents through the grieving process?
5 Sudden infant death syndrome (SIDS) can result in the death of an apparently normal infant. What feelings might the parents experience in this situation? What resources are available in your community for families who experienced SIDS? Discuss the relationship of positioning to SIDS.

REFERENCES

Armstrong-Dailey A: Children's hospice care, *Pediatr Nurs* 16(4):337-339, 409, 1990.

Bowlby J: *Attachment and loss: loss, sadness and depression*, vol 4, New York, 1980, Basic Books.

Craft M and Denehy J: *Nursing interventions with infants and children*, Philadelphia, 1991, WB Saunders.

Dwyer T et al: Prospective cohort study of prone sleeping position and sudden infant death syndrome, *Lancet* 337(8752):1244-1247, 1991.

Fleming PJ et al: Interaction between bedding and sleeping position in the sudden infant death syndrome, *Br Med J* 301:85-89, 1990.

Hogan N and Balk D: Adolescent reaction to sibling death: perceptions of mothers, fathers, and teenagers, *Nurs Res* 39(2):103-106, 1990.

Kubler-Ross E: *On death and dying*, New York, 1969, Macmillan.

Lawson L: Culturally sensitive support for grieving parents, *MCN* (15):76-79, 1990.

Martinson IM: *Home care for the dying child: professional and family perspectives*, New York, 1976, Appleton-Century-Crofts.

Miles A: Caring for families when a child dies, *Pediatr Nurs* 16(4):346-9, 1990.

Small M, Engler A, and Rushton C: Saying goodbye in the intensive care unit: helping caregivers grieve, *Pediatr Nurs* 17(1):103-5, 1991.

COMMUNITY SUPPORT GROUPS

Candlelighters
Childhood Cancer Foundation
Suite 200
1312 18th St NW
Washington, DC 20036
(202) 659-5136
(for families of children with cancer)

Compassionate Friends
P.O. Box 1347
Oak Brook, IL 60421
(for parents who have lost children of all ages)

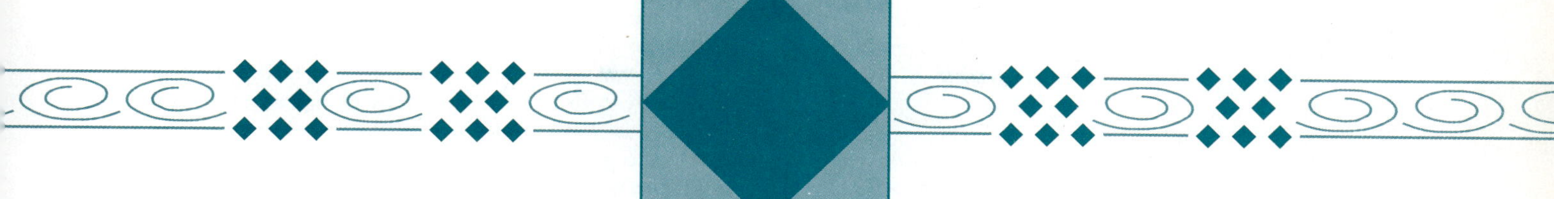

Glossary

KEY TO PRONUNCIATION

ā	āte	ȧ	sofȧ
ē	ēat	ī	"eye"
ō	ōh	ü	boot
ă	ăs	ä	ärm
ĕ	bĕt	ĭ	ĭt
ŏ	nŏt	ū	"you"
ȧ́	ȧ́h	er	(ur)her
ȯ	saw	ŭ	bŭt

abduction (ăb-dŭk′shŭn) Movement away from the midline.

abortion (ȧ-bŏr′shŭn) Termination of a pregnancy before the fetus is sufficiently developed to live; may be spontaneous or induced.

abortus (ȧ-bŏr-tŭs) An aborted fetus (expelled from the uterus before sufficiently developed to live).

abrasion (ă-brā′zhŭn) Loss of superficial tissue, skin, or mucous membrane because of friction.

abruptio (ăb-rŭp′shē-ō) A tearing away from.

abruptio placentae (plȧ-sĕn′tē) Premature separation of a normally implanted placenta.

abscess (ăb′sĕs) Focus of suppuration within a tissue; pocket of pus.

abstinence (ab′stĭ-nents) Going without voluntarily; refraining from sexual intercourse.

acetabulum (ăs-ĕ-tăb′ū-lŭm) Rounded cavity on the external surface of the innominate bone that receives the head of the femur.

acidosis (as-ĭ-dō′sis) Abnormal increase in acidity of the blood and tissues.

acinus (ăs′ĭ-nŭs) (pl. acini) Smallest division of a gland, often referring to the mammary glands.

adenoids (ăd′ĕ-noyds) Grouping of lymphoid tissue located on the posterior wall of the nasopharynx (the pharyngeal tonsils).

adnexa (ăd-nĕx′ȧ) Accessory parts of a structure; uterine adnexa—oviducts and ovaries.

afebrile (ā-fĕb′ril) Without fever.

afibrinogenemia (ā-fĭ″brĭn-ō-jĕ-ne′mĭ-ȧ) Lack of the protein fibrinogen in the blood, causing problems in coagulation.

agenesis (ā-jĕn′ĕsĭs) Absence.

aggregate (ăg′grē-gāt) Total substances making up a mass.

agonist (ă′gō- nĭst) A drug that stimulates a cell receptor site and produces physiological activity.

airway Normal passageway for respired air or a device used to prevent or correct respiratory obstruction.

albinism (ăl′bĭn-ĭsm) Abnormal but nonpathogenic absence of pigment in skin, hair, and eyes.

albumin (ăl-bū′mĭn) One kind of protein.

albuminuria (ăl-bū′-mĭ-nū′rĭ-ȧ) Presence of albumin in the urine.

alignment (ă-līn′ment) Arranging in a line.

alimentation (ăl-ĭ-mĕn-tā′shŭn) General process of nourishing the body.

alkalosis (ăl″kȧ-lō′sĭs) Abnormal increase of alkalinity of the blood and tissues.

allergen (ăl′er-jĕn) Any substance that produces an allergic response.

alveolus (ăl-vē′ō-lŭs) (pl. alve′oli) Little hollow or cavity; the air sac or cell of the lung tissue.

ambient (ăm′bē-ȧnt) Surrounding.

ambivalence (ăm-bĭv′ȧ-lĕnts) Simultaneous feelings of attraction and repulsion, love and hate for a person, object, or action.

amblyopia (ăm-blĭ-ō′pē-ȧ) Reduction or dimness of vision in one eye without apparent associated organic abnormality.

amenorrhea (ā-mĕn-ō-rē′ȧ) Absence of menstruation.

amnesic (ăm-nē′sĭk) Capable of producing amnesia, or loss of memory.

amniocentesis (ăm′nē-ō-sĕn-tē′sĭs) Puncture of the intrauterine amniotic sac usually through the abdominal wall to obtain a sample of amniotic fluid.

amniotic (ăm-nē-ŏt′ĭk) Pertaining to the amnion, the innermost of the fetal membranes that secretes the fluid inside the bag of waters.

analgesic (ăn′ăl-jē′sĭk) Capable of producing analgesia, or relief from pain.

analogue (ăn′ă-lȯg) One of two organs in different sexes or species that are similar in function but different in structure.

anaphylactic shock (ăn″ȧ-fĭ-lăk′tĭk) Syndrome that occasionally occurs after the reintroduction of a substance (antigen) into a person or animal previously sensitized to it; characterized by circulatory collapse and shock.

anasarca (ăn-ȧ-sär′ka) Severe generalized edema.
anastomosis (ă-năs′tō-mō′sĭs) Natural or surgical joining of blood or lymph vessels, or a surgically created communication between different hollow organs or parts of the same organs.
ancillary (ăn′sĭ-ler-ē) Subordinate or auxiliary.
android (ăn′droyd) Manlike; adjective used to describe a male type of pelvis.
anemia (an-ē′mē-ȧ) Condition in which there is a reduction below normal of hemoglobin in the blood.
anencephalic (ăn-ĕn-sĕf′ȧ-lĭk) Lacking a cerebrum, cerebellum, and part of the cranium.
anesthetic (ăn′ĕs-thĕt′ĭk) Capable of producing anesthesia, that is, complete or partial loss of feeling.
angiocardiography (ăn″jē-ō-cär-dē-ŏg′ră-fē) Injection of contrast material into the pulmonary circulation and observation of its flow by radiography or fluoroscopy.
anion (ăn′ī-ȧn) Particle of matter (ion) carrying a negative electrical charge.
ankylosis (ăn-kĭ-lō′sĭs) Abnormal immobility and consolidation of a joint.
anomalies (ă-nŏm′ă-lēz) Deviations from the normal.
anorexia (ăn-ȧ-rĕk′sē-ȧ) Loss of appetite.
anovulatory (ăn-ov′ū-lă-tō″rē) Not accompanied by production and discharge of an ovum.
anoxia (ăn-ŏk′sē-ȧ) Lack of oxygen.
antagonist (ăn-tag′ō-nĭst) A drug that stimulates a cell receptor site and prevents or reverses a specific physiological activity.
antagonistic (ăn-tăg-ȧ-nĭs′tĭk) Acting with antagonism, that is, in opposition to an agent or principle; counteracting; hostile.
antenatal (ăn-tē-nā′tȧl) Before birth; prenatal.
antepartal (ăn-tē-pär′tȧl) Before delivery.
anteroposterior (ăn′tĕr-ō-pŏs-tĭr′ē-ur) From front to back.
antiarrhythmic (ăn″tē-ȧ-rĭth′mĭk) Preventing (or effective against) arrhythmia, or irregular cardiac contractions.
antibody (ăn′tĭ-bŏd-ē) Protective protein substance formed by the body in the presence of pathogenic organisms or foreign materials.
antipyretic (ăn″tĭ-pī-rĕt′ĭk) A substance or procedure which reduces fever usually by lowering the thermoregulating set point in the hypothalamus.
antisepsis (ăn″tĭ-sĕp′sĭs) Literally "against infection or decay"; the use of procedures usually involving chemicals (antiseptics) that hinder the growth of microorganisms without necessarily destroying them.
antitoxin (ăn-tĭ-tŏk′sĭn) Protective protein formed by the body in response to the presence of a toxin; a preparation containing antibodies designed to produce passive immunization.
anuria (ȧ-nyur′ē-ȧ) Failure of kidney function; lack of urine formation.
AOM Acute otitis media, inflammation of the middle ear.
apnea (ăp′nē-ȧ) Absence of respiration, temporary or permanent.
areola (ȧ-rē′ō-lȧ) (pl. areolae) Ring of pigment on the breast surrounding the nipple.
arteriogram (är-tĭr′ē-ō-grăm) X-ray procedure that reveals arterial pathways injected with special contrast materials.
artery (är′ter-ē) Blood vessel that carries blood away from the heart.
arthralgia (ar-thrăl′jĭ-ă) Pain in a joint.
arthritis (är-thrī′tis) Inflammation of a joint, usually accompanied by pain and frequently by changes in structure.
arthrodesis (är″thrŏd-ē′sĭs) Surgical fusion of a joint performed to gain stability for weight bearing.
arthroplasty (är′thrō-plăs-tē) Surgical formation or reconstruction of a joint.
asepsis (ȧ-sĕp′sĭs) Literally "without infection or decay;" refers to the absence of living disease-producing microorganisms or to procedures that produce such an absence.
asphyxia (ăs-fik′sē-ȧ) Lack of oxygen and excessive carbon dioxide buildup in the body resulting from an abnormal gaseous environment, disease, aspiration etc.; leads to death if uncorrected.
aspirate (also see aspiration.) That which is obtained by aspiration.
aspiration (ăs-pĭ-rā′shun) Process of drawing in or out as by suction.
assimilation (a-sĭm-ĕ-lā′shun) Processes whereby the products of digestion change to resemble the chemical substances of the body tissues, first passing through the lacteals and blood vessels.
astrocytoma (ăs-trō-sī-tō′ma) Tumor of the brain tissue.
ataxic (ȧ-tăk′sĭk) Pertaining to ataxia, or the incoordination of the voluntary muscles; one possible result of brain damage.
atelectasis (ăt-ĕ-lĕk′tȧ-sĭs) Lack of proper lung expansion; collapsed or airless segment of lung.
athetoid (ăth′ĕ-toyd) Pertaining to athetosis, or the presence of involuntary, purposeless weaving motions of the body or its extremities; one possible result of brain damage to the basal ganglia of the brain.
atopic (ā-tŏp′ĭk) Pertaining to allergic responses, particularly those having a hereditary tendency such as asthma.
atresia (ȧ-trē′zhuh) Lack of a normal opening or canal.
atrium (ā′trē-ŭm) (pl. atria) Cavity or sinus; one of two upper chambers of the heart.
atrophy (ăt′rȧ-fē) Lack of nourishment; wasting or reduction of size of cells, tissues, organs, or regions of the body.
attenuate (ȧ-tĕn′yoo-āt) To weaken the virulence of; to reduce in force; to make thin.
attitude (ăt′ĭ-tüd) In speaking of fetal position, refers to the degree of flexion of the baby's head and extremities in the uterus.
aura (är′ȧ) Subjective warning of an impending epileptic seizure.
auscultation (aws-kŭl-tā′shŭn) Process of listening for sounds produced in some body cavity.
autoclave (aw-tŏ-clāv) Appliance used to sterilize objects by steam under pressure.
autoimmune (ah′tōh-ĭ-mū′n) Production in an organism of antibodies that react against its own tissues, with appearance of certain clinical and laboratory manifestations.
autonomy (aw-tŏn′ȧ-mē) State of self-government or self-direction.
autosomal (aw′tō-sōhm-ŭl) Having the character of a non-sex-determining chromosome.

autosome (äw'tō-sōhm) Any chromosome except sex-determining X and Y.

bacteriuria (băk-tē"rē-ū'rē-ȧh) Presence of bacteria in the urine.
bacillus (bȧ-sĭl'ŭs) (pl. bacilli) Rod-shaped bacterium.
ballottement (bah-lŏt'mȧw) A maneuver used to detect pregnancy by inserting two fingers into the vagina and pushing the fetal head or breech, causing the fetus to move away, then rebound to touch the examiner's fingers; a probable sign of pregnancy.
barrier techniques Various forms of ways of preventing the spread of infection from one person to another.
basophil (bā'so-fĭl) One type of white blood cell.
bilirubin (bĭl-ĭ-rū'bĭn) Orange or yellow pigment in bile; a product of red blood cell destruction; elevated levels in the blood may cause jaundice.
biopsy (bī'ŏp-sē) Procurement of a specimen of tissue for microscopic examination.
birth rate The number of live births per 1000 population.
blastocyst (blăs'tō-sĭst) Spherical mass consisting of a central cavity surrounded by a single layer of cells produced by the cleavage of the ovum.
body substances A general term used to describe body products that are characteristically moist and that support the growth of organisms. Examples are feces, urine, emesis, wound drainage, pus, saliva sputum, genital secretions, blood, serum, and cerebral spinal fluid.
bolus (bō-lŭs) A lump of food ready to be swallowed; a relatively large dose of medication or contrast material given at one time, usually intravenously.
booster injection Substance or dose used to renew or increase the effect of a drug or immunizing agent.
bossing Rounded protuberance, particularly on the skull, in the area of the forehead; one possible manifestation of rickets.
bradycardia (brăd"ē-kär'dē-ȧ) Slowness of the heartbeat; in adults, usually a rate of fewer than 60 beats per minute.
Braxton Hicks (brăx'ton hĭks) contractions Uterine contractions that occur throughout pregnancy and help enlarge the uterus to accommodate the growing fetus; during the last weeks of pregnancy they may become very noticeable; false labor contractions.
breech birth (brēch) Delivery of the child, feet or buttocks first.
bronchiectasis (brŏn-kē-ĕk'tȧ-sĭs) Abnormal dilatation of the bronchi in response to inflammation, which may lead to structural changes and chronic cough.
bronchiolitis (brŏng"kē-ō-lī-tĭs) Inflammation of the bronchioles caused by RSV (respiratory syncytial virus).
buffer Apparatus or substance serving to neutralize the shock of opposing forces.
bulbar (bul'bär) Pertaining to the "bulb," or medulla, of the brain and the cranial nerves.
bulbourethral (bŭl"bō-ū-rē'thrȧl) Referring to the bulb of the urethra.

calcaneus (kăl-kā'nē-ŭs) Heel bone, or os calcis; type of clubfoot in which only the heel touches the ground; patient may walk on inner side of heel.
callus (kăl'ŭs) New bone formation at the site of a healing fracture; also a thickening of the epidermis at sites of pressure or friction.
calyx (ka'lĭks) (pl. calyces) Small subdivision of the pelvis of the kidney.
Candida albicans (kăn'dĭ-dȧ ăl'bĭ-kănz) Formerly called *Monilia albicans*; a yeastlike fungus that may infect various portions of the body, causing a variety of symptoms (e.g., leukorrhea, dermatitis, stomatitis).
cannula (kăn'ū-lȧ) (pl. cannulae) Small tube; large needle sheath used for insertion into a body cavity or tube.
canthus (kăn-thŭs) (pl. canthi) Corner at each side of the eye where the eyelids meet.
caput succedaneum (kă'pŭt sŭk-sē-dā'nē-ŭm) Abnormal collection of fluid under the scalp.
carbohydrate (kăr"bō-hī'drāt) A compound of carbon combined with H_2 and O_2 that supplies heat and energy to the body.
cardiac cycle Sequential contraction (systole) and dilatation (diastole) of the heart chambers.
cardiac output Blood volume ejected by heart in one cardiac cycle.
cardiovascular (kär-dē-ō-văs'kūl-är) Pertaining to the heart and blood vessels.
caries (kăr'ēz) Dental decay.
carrier Person or animal capable of transmitting a contagious or hereditary disease but showing no outward sign of the disease.
cast Solid mold usually made of plaster to help protect, position, or immobilize a part; microscopic sediment that has been partially shaped by the kidney tubules; any other body discharge or excretion retaining the shape of a body part that held it.
catalyst (kăt'ȧ-lĭst) Substance that speeds the rate of a chemical reaction without itself being permanently altered by the reaction.
catamenia (kăt-ȧ-mē'nē-ȧ) Menses, or menstruation.
cataract (kăt'ȧ-răkt) Abnormal opacity of the crystalline lens of the eye.
catecholamines (kăt-ĕ-kōl'ȧ-mēnz) Group of similar compounds that includes dopamine, norepinephrine, and epinephrine.
catheter (kăth'ĕ-ter) Hollow tube for insertion into a cavity or a canal for the purpose of discharging fluid contents or introducing other substances.
cation (kăt'ī-ȧn) Particle of matter (ion) carrying a positive electrical charge.
CBC Complete blood count.
cecum (sē'kŭm) Blind pouch that forms the first portion of the large intestine or colon; the attachment for the appendix.
celiac (sē'lē-ăk) disease Chronic intestinal indigestion.
cellulitis (sĕl-ū-lī'tŭs) Inflammation of the body tissues, most commonly the skin.
cephalhematoma (sĕf-ȧl-hē-mȧ-tō'mȧ) Swelling on the head caused by a collection of bloody fluid under the periosteum of the skull as the result of trauma.
cephalic (sē-făl'ĭk) Pertaining to the head.
cephalocaudal (sĕf-ȧ-lō-cawd'ȧl) Moving from the head toward the base of the spine.

cephalopelvic (sĕf′-ȧ-lŏ-pĕl′vĭk) The relationship of the fetal head to the maternal pelvis.
cerumen (sĕ-rü′mĕn) Ear wax.
cervical (sĕr′vĭ-kȧl) Pertaining to the neck or cervix.
cesarean birth (sĕz-ăr′ē-ăn) Abdominal delivery made possible by incising the uterine and abdominal walls.
Chadwick's sign (chăd′wĭks) Violet tinge of the cervical and vaginal mucous membranes; a presumptive sign of pregnancy.
chancre (shăng′ker) Craterlike lesion seen in first-stage syphilis.
chemotherapy (kē′mō-thĕr″ă-pē) Use of chemical agents in the treatment of disease.
Cheyne-Stokes respiration (chān′stōks) Irregular, cyclic-type breathing characterized by a period of increasing respiratory action followed by an interval of apnea.
childhood mortality The number of deaths from birth to 19 years of age per 100,000 population.
chlamydia (klȧh-mĭd′dē-ȧh) A contagious bacterial infection of the genitourinary system. It may be transmitted to the infant during the birth process.
chloasma gravidarum (klō-ăz′mȧ grăv-ĭ-dā′rŭm) Deepening pigmentation of skin during pregnancy, especially of the face; "mask of pregnancy."
chordee (kŏr-dē′) Abnormal downward curvature of the penis.
chorea (kō-rē′a) Involuntary muscular twitching or movement.
chorioamnionitis (kȯ″rē-ō-ăm″nē-ō-nī′tĭs) Inflammation of the amniotic membranes (amnion and chorion).
choriocarcinoma (kō-rĭ-ō-kär-sĭ-nō′mȧ) Rare malignancy associated with hydatidiform mole of pregnancy.
chorion (kō′rĭ-ŏn) Outermost membrane of the growing fertilized egg; one of two membranes that later form the "bag of waters."
chorionic gonadotropin (kō′rē-ŏn-ĭk gŏ-năd′ō-trō′pĭn) Gonad-regulating hormone produced by the chorionic villi (human chorionic gonadotropin [hCG]).
chorionic villi (vĭl′ī) Fingerlike tissue projections of chorion on the outer wall of the fertilized egg.
chromosomes (krō′mȧ-sōmz) Microscopic structures seen fairly easily in the nucleus of a cell during its reproduction, which contain the genes or determiners of heredity.
chronicity (krŏn-ĭs′ĭt-ē) State of being chronic.
cisternal puncture (sĭs-tĕr′nȧl) Puncture with a hollow needle between the cervical vertebrae, through the dura mater, into the cisterna at the base of the brain.
clavicle (klăv′ĭ-kȧl) Collarbone.
clitoris (klĭ′tȧ-rĭs) Small, sensitive erectile structure located at the anterior junction of the labia minora.
coagulation (ko-ăg-ye-lā′shun) Process of clotting.
coccus (kŏk′ŭs) (pl. cocci) Spherical bacterium.
coitus (kō′ĭ-tŭs) Sexual intercourse.
colic (kŏl′ĭk) Intermittent pain caused by spasm of any hollow or tubular soft organ; abdominal cramping fairly common in first 3 months of infancy.
collagen (kŏl′ȧ-jĕn) Protein substance existing in many of the body's connective tissues.
collateral (kȧ-lăt′er-ȧl) Situated at the sides; supplementary, reinforcing.
colonization (kȯl′ĭ-nī-zā′shun) Presence and multiplication of organisms without tissue invasion or damage.
colostrum (kōl-ŏs′trŭm) Breast secretion produced by the mother the first few days after childbirth.
colporrhaphy (kŏl-pōr′ă-fē) Surgical repair of the walls of the vagina.
comatose (kō′mȧ-tōs) In a coma, or abnormally deep sleep, caused by illness or injury.
comedo (kŏm′ē-dō) (pl. comedones) Discolored, dried, oily secretion plugging the pores of the skin; blackhead.
comminuted (kŏm′ĭ-nŭt-ĕd) Broken into many pieces; comminuted fracture, a crushed bone.
compatible Able to work together; not in opposition; able to be mixed without destructive changes.
compression (kom-presh′un) Squeezing together; state of being pressed together.
conception (kon-sĕp′shŭn) Union of the male sex cell, spermatozoon, and the female sex cell, ovum; fertilization; beginning of a new being.
conduit (kŏn′dü-ĭt) Tube or other device conveying water or other fluid from one region to another.
condyloma (kŏn-dĭ-lō′ma) Wartlike growth usually found near the anus or vulva; the broad, flat form (c. latum) is characteristic of syphilis in its secondary stage.
congenital (kon-jĕn′ĭ-tȧl) Existing at birth.
conjugate (kŏn′jū-gāt) Anteroposterior diameter of the pelvis.
conjunctiva (kŏn-jŭnk-tī′vȧ) Mucous membrane that lines the inner surface of the eyelid and covers the anterior portion of the eye.
contagious disease (communicable or transmissible) Illness caused by living microorganisms or their toxins, which may be transmitted to susceptible persons by contact with persons carrying the organisms, their infected body substances, or other reservoirs. Transmission may occur by direct, indirect, or droplet contact or by airborne route.
contaminated Soiled, stained, touched, or exposed in such a manner that the article in question becomes unsafe to use as intended or without barrier techniques.
continence (kŏnt′ĭ-nĕnts) Control of bladder or bowel function, or self-restraint, especially in regard to sexual intercourse.
contraception (kŏn-trȧ-sĕp′shun) Prevention of the fertilization of an egg or ovum.
contracture (kon-trăk′chur) Permanent contraction of a muscle resulting from spasm or paralysis causing limitation of motion; high resistance to the passive stretch of a muscle.
contusion (kŏn-tū′zhŭn) Injury that does not result in breaking the skin; black and blue area; bruise.
convulsion (kon-vŭl′shŭn) Violent, involuntary contraction or series of contractions of muscles; seizure.
corium (kō′rĭ-ŭm) Dermis layer of the skin; "true skin."
cor pulmonale (kōr pŭl-mŏn-al′ē) Cardiac enlargement or failure secondary to respiratory disease.
cortex (kōr′tĕks) Outer or more superficial part of an organ.
coryza (kōrī′zȧ) "Common" head cold.
crepitus (krĕp′ĭ-tŭs) Grating sensation sometimes heard or felt at the site of a fracture; crackling sound heard in certain diseases.

cretinism (krē'tĭn-ĭzm) Infantile hypothyroidism characterized by mental retardation and other disturbances in mental and physical development.
crust (crustation) External protective layer; scab.
cryptorchidism (krĭpt-or'kĭd-ĭzm) Failure of the testicles to descend into the scrotum.
cul-de-sac of Douglas Blind pouch formed by the peritoneal lining of the abdominal cavity located between the uterus and rectum.
culture The learned patterns of behavior shared by a particular group.
curettage (kä-ret'aj) (uterine) Scraping with a curette to remove uterine contents (as in inevitable, incomplete, or early abortion), to obtain specimens for use in diagnosis, or to remove growths (e.g., polyps).
CVA Cerebrovascular accident.
cyanosis (sī-ăn-ō'sĭs) Bluish or grayish coloration of the skin caused by poor oxygenation of the blood.
cystitis (sĭs-tī'tĭs) Inflammation of the urinary bladder.
cystocele (sĭs'tō-sēl) Prolapse of the urinary bladder caused by the weakened tissue wall between the bladder and vagina.
cystourethrogram (sĭs"tō-ū-rĕth'rō-gram) X-ray film of the bladder and urethra.
cytology (sī"tŏl'ō-jē) Study of cells.
cytomegalovirus (CMV) (sī"tō-mĕg"ȧh-lō-vī'rŭs) A herpesvirus that may cause illness in the fetus or infant if the mother is infected.
cytoplasm (sī'tō-plăz-ŭm) Portion of a cell inside the cell membrane but outside the nucleus.

debilitate (dē-bĭl'ĭ-tāt) To produce weakness; enfeeble.
debridement (dā-brēd-mŏn') Surgical removal of dead, damaged, or contaminated tissue.
debris (dȧ-brē) Rubbish; ruins.
decalcification (dē-kăl-sĭ-fĭ-kā'shŭn) Removal or withdrawal of lime salts from bone.
decidua (dĭ-sĭd'ŭ-ä) Pertaining to endometrium of pregnancy, which is cast off at parturition.
deciduous teeth (dē-sĭd'ū-ŭs) Primary or baby teeth.
decubitus (dĕ-kū'bĭ-tŭs) Bedsore.
dehydration (dē-hī-drā'shŭn) Condition in which the body tissues lack normal fluid content.
dentition (dĕn-tĭsh'ŭn) Process or time of teething.
dermatitis venenata (dĕr-mȧ-tī'tĭs) Skin disturbance caused by external irritants.
deterioration (di-tir"ē-ȧ-rā'shun) Gradually worsening.
detrusor muscle (dē-trü'sor) Smooth muscle of the bladder wall.
developmental stages Periods of relative stability that are distinct from periods that precede or succeed them.
developmental tasks Physical and psychosocial growth work that must be achieved during a developmental stage.
diaphoresis (dī-ă-fō-rē'sĭs) Profuse sweating.
diaphragmatic hernia (dī-ȧ-frăg-măt'ĭk) Protrusion of abdominal contents through an abnormal opening in the diaphragm.
diaphysis (dī-ăf'ĭ-sĭs) Shaft or middle part of a long bone.
diastolic (dī-ăs-tŏl'ĭk) Pertaining to diastole—the blood pressure at the time of greatest cardiac relaxation.
digestion (dĭ'jĕs'chĕn) Process by which food is broken down mechanically and chemically in the gastrointestinal tract and converted into absorbable forms.
digital (dĭj'ĭ-tȧl) Pertaining to the digits; that is, the fingers or toes.
digitalization (dij'ĭ-täl-ĭ-zā'shŭn) Administration of digitalis to slow and strengthen the heartbeat (particularly the initial administration of the drug).
dilation (dĭl-ȧ-'shŭn) Expansion of an organ or orifice; dilation.
diploid (dĭp'loyd) Having double the number of chromosomes found in the ova or sperm, the normal chromosome number for body cells.
disorientation (dĭs-ō-rē-ĕn-tā'shŭn) Inability to evaluate properly direction, location, time, surroundings, or personal role.
disseminated intravascular coagulation (DIC) (dĭ-sĕm'-ĭ-nāt" ĕd) An abnormal form of rapid coagulation in which clotting factors are consumed and depleted, resulting in generalized bleeding.
distal (dĭs'tȧl) Farthest from the trunk of the body or from a specific point of reference.
distention (dĭs-tĕn'shŭn) (also distension) Inflation, stretching, ballooning.
diuresis (dī"ū-rē'sĭs) Increased urine output.
diuretic (dī-ū-rĕt'ĭk) Agent that increases the secretion of urine.
diverticulum (dī-ver-tĭk'ū-lŭm) (p. diverticula) Sac or pouch in the walls of a canal or organ, especially the colon.
ductus arteriosus (duk'tŭs är-tĕr-ē-ō'sŭs) Short blood vessel located between the pulmonary artery and aorta in the fetus.
ductus deferens (dŭk'tŭs dĕf'ĕr-ĕnz) Excretory duct of the testicle; vas deferens.
dyscrasia (dĭs-krā'zhē-ȧ) Undefined disease, malfunction, or abnormal condition, often used when speaking of abnormalities of the blood.
dysentery (dĭs'ĕn-tĕr-ē) Inflammation of the intestines, especially of the colon, usually characterized by mild to severe diarrhea.
dysmenorrhea (dĭs-mĕn-ō-rē'ȧ) Painful or difficult menstruation.
dyspnea (dĭsp-nē'ȧ) Difficult breathing.
dystocia (dĭs-tō'shȧ) Difficult labor, particularly difficulty in the mechanics of childbirth.

ecchymosis (ĕk-ĭ-mō'sĭs) Black-and-blue mark caused by hemorrhage into the skin, usually a relatively large area.
eclampsia (ĕ-klămp'sē-ȧ) Toxemia of pregnancy also known as preeclampsia or pregnancy-induced hypertension (PIH) may involve the serious complications of convulsion or coma. If it does, the condition is then called eclampsia.
ecology (i-kŏl aji) Interrelationships of organisms and their environment as manifested by natural cycles and rhythms.
ectopic pregnancy (ĕk-tŏp-ĭk) Pregnancy that develops in an abnormal place (e.g., in the uterine tube, abdomen, or ovary).
edema (ē-dē'ma) Abnormal, excessive amount of fluid within the body tissues.
edematous (ĕ-dĕm'ăt-ŭs) Characterized by the presence of edema, that is, an abnormal amount of fluid in the tissues.

effacement (ĕf-ās′mĕnt) (of the cervix) Shortening and thinning of the cervix or neck of the uterus.
efficacious (ef″ȧ-kā′shus) Capable of producing an intended effect.
effleurage (ĕf-lü-rahzh′) Stroking movement used in massage.
effusion (ē-fū′shun) Escape of fluid into an area.
EIA Exercise induced asthma.
ejaculation (ē-jăk-ū-lā′shŭn) Ejection of the seminal fluid from the male urethra.
electroencephalogram (ē-lĕk-trō-ĕn-sĕf′ȧ-lō-grăm) Tracing made by an apparatus designed to detect and record brain waves.
electrolyte (ē-lĕk′trō-līt) Substance that, in solution, conducts electric current.
embolus (ĕm′bō-lŭs) (pl. emboli) Foreign substance traveling in the circulatory system (e.g., a blood clot or air).
embryo (ĕm′brē-ō) Unborn young of any creature in an early stage of development when specific identification is difficult with the naked eye.
emesis (ĕm′ĕ-sĭs) Referring to vomiting or the substance vomited.
emission (ē-mĭsh′ŭn) Discharge (e.g., discharge of semen), especially involuntary.
emphysema (ĕm-fĭ-sē′mȧ) Abnormal dilation and loss of elasticity of the alveoli or air sacs of the lungs.
empyema (ĕm-pī-ē′mȧ) Collection of pus in a body cavity, especially the pleural cavity.
encephalitis (ĕn-sĕf-a-lī′tĭs) Inflammation of the encephalon within the brain.
encephalopathy (ĕn-sĕf″ȧ-lŏp′ȧ-thē) Any dysfunction of the brain.
endarteritis (ĕnd-är-tĕr-ī′tĭs) Inflammation of the lining of the arteries.
endocarditis (ĕn-dō-kär-dī′tĭs) Inflammation of the lining of the heart.
endocrine (ĕn′dō-krĭn) Pertaining to ductless glands that discharge their secretions (hormones) directly into the bloodstream.
endocrine gland Structure producing a hormone that is discharged into the bloodstream.
endogenous (ĕn-dŏj′ĕ-nŭs) Originating or growing from within.
endometritis (ĕn-dō-mē-trī′tĭs) Inflammation of the endometrium, or lining of the uterus.
endometrium (ĕn″dō-mē′trē-ŭm) The innermost mucous membrane lining the uterus.
endorphin (ĕn-dor′fĭn) Morphinelike hormonal substances produced by the body. They raise the pain threshold and produce sedation and euphoria.
endotracheal (ĕn′dō-trā′kē-ȧl) Within the trachea.
engagement (ĕn-gāj′mĕnt) In obstetrics, refers to the entrance of the presenting part of the fetus into the true pelvis; the passage of the largest diameter of the presenting part into the true pelvis.
engorgement (ĕn-gōrj′mĕnt) In obstetrics, refers to the swelling of the breasts because of local congestion of the veins and lymphatics associated with lactation.
enteric (en-tĕr′ĭk) Pertaining to the small intestine.
enterobiasis (ĕn″tĕr-ō-bī′a-sĭs) Disease caused by pinworm infestation.
enterostomy (ĕn-tĕr-ŏs′to-mi) The surgical creation of an opening into the small intestine through the abdominal wall.
enuresis (ĕn-ū-rē′sĭs) Bed-wetting at an age when urinary control should be present.
epicanthus (ĕ-pĭ-kăn′thŭs) Fold of skin extending from the nose to the median end of the eyebrow, characteristic of the Mongolian race.
epidemiologic (ep′ĭ-dē″mē-o-loj′ĭk) Pertaining to the study of epidemics, their origin, and prevention or, more broadly, the origins of any condition.
epididymis (ĕp-ĭ-dĭd′ĭ-mĭs) (pl. epididymides) Small oblong organ, situated on the testis, containing a coiled extension of the tubules of the testis, which eventually joins the vas deferens.
epiglottitis (ĕp″ĭ-glŏt′tĭs) Inflammation of the epiglottis.
epiphysis (ĕ-pĭf′ĭ-sĭs) (pl. epiphyses) End of a long bone.
episiotomy (ĭ-pĭz-ē-ŏt′ȧ-mē) Surgical incision extending from the soft tissue of the vaginal opening into the true perineum, performed to protect the perineum from laceration or help hasten the delivery of an infant.
epispadias (ĕp-ĭ-spā′dē-ȧs) Abnormal condition in which the urethral opening is located on the upper (dorsal) surface of the penis.
epistaxis (ĕp-ĭ-stăk′sĭs) Nosebleed.
epithelial (ĕp″ĭ-thē′lē-al) Pertaining to the outermost layer of the skin and/or the lining tissue of hollow organs and inner passages of the body.
equilibrium (ē-kwĭ-lĭb′rē-um) Equal balance, between powers; mental balance; equality of effect.
equinus (ē-kwī′nŭs) Condition characterized by a tiptoe walk affecting one or both feet, often associated with clubfoot.
Erbs' palsy (erbz pawl′zē) Injury to the brachial plexus causing partial paralysis of the arm.
erectile (ē-rĕk′tĭl) Capable of becoming erect.
erysipelas (ĕr-ĭ-sĭp′ĕ-lŭs) Acute febrile disease, with localized inflammation and swelling of the skin and subcutaneous tissue accompanied by a systemic disturbance of a variable degree, caused by a streptococcus.
erythema (ăr-ĭ-thē′mȧ) Redness of the skin; characteristic red blotches on the skin of the newborn infant.
erythema marginatum (märj-ĭ-nȧ′tŭm) Rash occasionally seen in cases of rheumatic fever.
erythroblast (ĕ-rĭth′rō-blăst) Immature, inadequate form of red blood cell normally found only in the bone marrow.
erythroblastosis fetalis (ĕ-rith″rō-blăst-ō-sĭs fĕ-tă′lĭs) Hemolytic disease of the newborn characterized by anemia, jaundice, enlarged liver and spleen, and the presence of erythroblasts circulating in the blood stream.
erythrocyte (ĕ-rĭth′rō-sīt) Red blood corpuscle or cell.
eschar (ĕs′kär) Thick crusts that may form over burned areas on the body, composed of hardened drainage.
esophageal (ĕ-sŏf″a-jē-ȧl) Pertaining to the esophagus, or food tube, leading from the throat to the stomach.
estrogen (ĕs′trō-jĕn) Class name for a female sex hormone; more particularly, the hormonal secretion of the ovary that builds up the lining of the uterus and promotes feminine characteristics.

ethnicity Ethnicity refers to membership, usually through birth, in a cultural group based on traits such as religion, language, or racial characteristics.
ethnocentrism The belief that the values and practices of one's own culture are superior to those of other cultural groups.
etiology (ē″tē-ŏl′ō-jē) Cause of a disease or any other phenomena.
euglycemia (ŭ-glī-sēm-ia) Normal or acceptable blood glucose levels.
eupnea (ūp-nē′ȧ) Normal breathing.
excoriation (ĕks-kō-rĭ-ā′shŭn) A raw exposed area on the body without skin cover as a result of injury.
excrete (ek-skrēt) To separate and eliminate from an organic body.
exocrine (ĕks′ō-krĭn) Term applied to glands whose secretion reaches an epithelial surface either directly or through a duct.
exocrine gland Structure that produces a secretion deposited in a particular area of the body via a duct.
exogenous (ĕks-ŏj′-ĕ-nŭs) Originating or growing from without; resulting from external causes.
exstrophy (ĕks′trō-fē) Eversion or the turning inside out of a part with or without the abnormal exposure of the part.
exudate (ĕks′ū-dāt) Accumulation of a fluid in a cavity; drainage flowing from one body area to another; drainage from wounds.

fallopian tubes (fă-lō′pī-on) Uterine tubes, or oviducts, leading from the uterine cavity toward each ovary.
familial (fȧ-mĭl′ēȧl) Pertaining to or characteristic of a family.
family-centered care Health care based on the philosophy that quality care can be provided in an environment that supports family integrity and promotes the psychological and physiological health of both the individual and the family.
fascia (făsh′ē-ȧ) Fibrous connective tissue found under the skin or covering, supporting, and separating muscles and other organs.
febrile (fēb′rĕl or fĕb′rĭl) State of being feverish.
fertility (fertile) (fĕr-tĭl′ĭ-tē) Quality of being productive; capable of bearing children.
fertilization (fĕr-tĭ-lĭ-za′shŭn) Union of male and female sex cells; conception.
fetus (fē′tŭs) Later stages of the developing young within the uterus or egg when the species is distinguishable by the naked eye.
FHR Fetal heart rate.
fibrinogen (fī-brĭn′ō-jĕn) Protein in the blood plasma necessary for coagulation.
fissure Ulcer or cracklike lesion.
fistula (fĭs′tū-lȧ) (pl. fistulae) Abnormal tubelike passageway from a normal body cavity or canal to another body cavity or to the outside of the body.
flaccid (flă′sĭd) Soft, flabby, relaxed; lacking normal tension or tone.
flexion (flĕk′shŭn) Act of being bent.
follicle (fŏl′ĭ-kȧl) Small secretory sac or cavity; protective tissue envelope of the female sex cell, or ovum.
fontanel (fŏn′tȧ-nĕl) Soft spot found between the cranial bones of the skull of an infant, formed where sutures meet or cross.
foramen (fō-rā′mĕn) Small opening.
foramen ovale (ō-vā′lē) Normal opening between the atria in the heart of the fetus.
foreskin (fōr′skĭn) Prepuce, or fold of skin covering the glans penis.
fornix (fō′nĭx) (pl. fornices) Arch or fold.
fourchette (fŭr-shĕt′) Tense band of mucous membrane connecting the posterior ends of the labia minora.
fraternal twins (fra′tern-al) The result of two simultaneous pregnancies developing from the fertilization of two separate ova by two distinct spermatozoa.
frenulum (frĕn′ū-lŭm) (pl. frenula) Any small fold of mucous membrane or tissue that acts like a bridle; fold of mucous membrane extending from the underside of the tongue to the floor of the mouth at the midline; lower fold of the labia minora that surrounds the clitoris.
frequency (frē′kwĕn-sē) Number of repetitions of a periodic process in a unit of time; when speaking of urinary function, the term implies an abnormal increase in the number of voidings.
FSH Follicle-stimulating hormone.
fulminating (fŭl′mĭ-nā-tĭng) Occurring with great rapidity.
fundus (fŭn′dŭs) (pl. fundi) Part of an organ opposite its opening; top of the uterus.
furuncle (fū′rŭng-kȧl) Infected hair follicle; a boil.
fusion (fū′shŭn) Process of uniting.

galactosemia (gă-lăk″tō-sē′mē-a) Metabolic condition involving the metabolism of galactose, which may produce mental retardation and other symptoms.
gamete (găm′ēt) Male or female reproductive cell capable of entering into union with each other in the process of fertilization.
gamma globulin (găm′mȧ glŏb′ū-lĭn) Blood protein fraction containing most of the protective immune antibodies (immune globulin [IG]).
gastroenteritis (găs″trō-ĕn-ter-ī-tĭs) Inflammation of the mucosa of the stomach and intestines.
gastrostomy (găs-trŏ′sta-mē) Intentional establishment of an opening into the stomach through the abdominal wall, usually for artificial feeding.
gavage (gȧ-vazh′) Feeding through a stomach tube passed either nasally or orally.
gene (jēn) Hereditary determiner located on the chromosomes.
genetics (jĕ-nĕt′ĭks) Study of inheritance or genes.
genitalia (jĕn-ĭ-tal′ē-ȧ) Organs of generation, or reproduction.
gestation (jĕs-tā′shŭn) Period of intrauterine fetal development; pregnancy.
gingivitis (jĭn″jĭ-vī′tĭs) Inflammation of the gums.
glans penis (glănz pē′nĭs) Sensitive portion (tip) of the penis.
glioma (glī-ō′mȧ) Tumor involving the supportive tissue of the brain or glial cells.
glomerulus (glō-măr′ū-lŭs) (pl. glomeruli) Cluster or coil of connecting capillaries located at the top of the expanded

end (Bowman's capsule) of the urinary tubules in the kidney.

glottis (glŏt′ĭs) Opening of the larynx including the associated vocal cords.

gluten (glü′tĕn) Protein found in wheat, rye, and oats.

gluteus (glü-tē′us) Any of the three muscles that form the buttocks.

glycosuria (glī-kō-sü′rē-ȧ) Presence of glucose in the urine.

gonadotropic (gō-năd-ō-trō′pĭk) Relating to stimulation of the gonads, that is, the ovaries or testes.

gonorrhea (gŏn″ō-re′āh) A highly contagious, sexually transmitted bacterial infection of the genitourinary system. It may be transmitted to the infant during the birth process.

Goodell's sign (güd′ĕlz) Softening of the uterine cervix; a probable sign of pregnancy.

gravida (grăv′ĭ-dȧ) Pertaining to the number of pregnancies a woman has had; a pregnant woman.

gumma (gŭm′mȧ) Soft gummy tumor that may develop during the third stage of syphilis.

gynecoid (gī′nĕ-coyd or jĭn′ĕ-coyd) Womanlike; typical female pelvis.

gynecomastia (gī-nĕ-kō-măs′tĭ-ȧ or jĭn-ĕ-kō-măs′tĭ′ȧ) Swelling of the newborn or adult male breast tissue.

habilitate (hă-bĭl′ĭ-tāt) To teach skills needed for everyday living or prepare for a specific job or task.

hallucination (hă-lŭ-sĭ-nā′shŭn) False perception having no relation to reality and not accounted for by any external stimuli; may be visual, auditory, olfactory, etc.

Hegar's sign (hā′gärz) Softening of the uterine isthmus, the area between the cervix and body of the uterus; a probable sign of pregnancy.

helix (hē′-lĭks) A spiral or coil-like formation.

hemangioma (hē-măn-jē-ō′mȧ) Blood vessel tumor.

hematocrit reading (hē-măt′ȧ-krĭt) The percentage of whole blood volume occupied by red blood cells after they have been separated through use of a centrifuge.

hematoma (hē-mă-tō′mȧ) Tumor composed of blood cells, resulting from tissue injury.

hematuria (hē-mă-tü′rĭ-ȧ) Presence of blood in the urine.

hemoglobin (hē-mō-glō′bĭn) Oxygen-carrying protein pigment found in the red blood cells.

hemolysis (hē-mŏl′ĭ-sĭs) The destruction of RBCs.

hemolytic (hē-mō-lĭt′ĭk) Pertaining to or causing the breakdown of red blood cells.

hemoptysis (hē-mŏp′tĭ-sĭs) Presence of blood-stained sputum.

hemorrhoid (hĕm′ō-royd) Rectal varicosity; "pile."

heparinized (hĕp′er-rĭn-ĭzed) Containing heparin employed as an anticoagulant.

hermaphroditism (her-măf′rō-dīt-ĭsm) Possession by one individual of the gonads and external genitalia of both sexes.

hernia (hĕr′nĭ-ȧ) Rupture; an abnormal protrusion of a portion of the contents of a body cavity because of a defect in its surrounding walls, frequently causing swelling, pressure symptoms, or other complications.

herpes simplex (hĕr′pēz) Viral infection characteristically causing an eruption of small, clustered blisters on the skin or mucous membranes.

heterozygous (hĕt″er-ō-zī′gŭs) Having the two members of one or more pairs of genes dissimilar.

homozygous (hō″mō-zī′gŭs) Having both of a given pair of genes alike.

hordeolum (hŏr-dē′ō-lŭm) Sty or infection involving the eyelash follicle.

hormone (hōr′mōn) Internal secretions of thyroid gland, pancreas, etc.; chemical substance originating in an organ, gland, or part that is conveyed through the blood to another part of the body, helping to regulate body processes.

Hutchinson's teeth (hŭch′ĭn-sŭnz) Notched teeth characteristic of congenital syphilis.

hydatidiform mole (hī″da-tĭdĭ-fōrm) Condition in which the fertilized ovum becomes altered and an abnormal tissue develops instead of an infant and normal placenta.

hydrocele (hī′drō-sēl) Abnormal collection of fluid in the lining tissue (tunica vaginalis) of the testis.

hydrocephalus (hī-drō-sĕf′ȧ-lŭs) Collection of abnormal amounts of cerebrospinal fluid within the cranium, causing enlargement of the immature skull.

hydronephrosis (hī″drō-nĕ-frō′sĭs) Collection of urine in the renal pelvis because of obstructed outflow producing distention and atrophy of the kidney.

hydrophobia (hī-drō-fō′bē-ȧ) Rabies; fear of water.

hydrotherapy (hī-drō-thĕr′ă-pē) Scientific application of water to treat diseases (e.g., hot baths).

hymen (hī′mĕn) Membrane partially covering the vaginal opening; "the maidenhead."

hyperalimentation (hī″per-ăl′ĭ-mĕn-tā′shŭn) Term typically used to describe total parenteral nutrition (TPN) by vein.

hyperbilirubinemia (hī″pĕr-bĭl″ĭ-rü″bĭ-nē′mē-ȧh) An excess of bilirubin in the blood; classified as conjugated or unconjugated according to the form of bilirubin present.

hypercalcemia (hī-per-kăl-sē′mē-ă) Excessive amount of calcium in the blood.

hypercapnia (hī″per-kăp′nē-ȧ) (increased PCO_2) Excessive amount of carbon dioxide in the blood.

hyperemesis gravidarum (hī-pĕr-ĕm′ĕ-sĭs grăv-ĭ-dā′rŭm) Persistent, exaggerated nausea and vomiting during pregnancy.

hyperextension (hī″pŭr-ĕck-stĕn′shŭn) Maximum extension or overextension of a limb or part.

hyperglycemia (hī-pĕr-glī-sē′mē-ȧ) Excessive amount of glucose in the bloodstream.

hyperkalemia (hī-per-kȧ-lē′mē-ă) Excessive amount of potassium in the blood.

hypernatremia (hī-per-nȧ-trē′mē-ă) Excessive amount of sodium in the blood.

hypertension (hī-per-tĕn′shŭn) Abnormal elevation of the blood pressure, especially the diastolic pressure.

hyperthermia (hī-per-ther′-mē-ȧ) Abnormally elevated body temperature caused by a breakdown of normal thermoregulating processes (such as in heat stroke) or, rarely, artificially induced in an effort to combat disease.

hypertonic (hī″per-tŏn′ĭk) Excessive or above normal in tone or tension; a solution containing excessive amounts of salts.

hypertrophy (hī-per′trō-fē) Increase in size or bulk; excessive development.

hyperventilation (hī-per-vĕn-tĭl-ā′shŭn) Overbreathing accompanied by a carbon dioxide deficit commonly causing dizziness as well as tingling and numbness in the hands.
hypnotic (hĭp-nŏt′ĭk) Medication that causes sleep.
hypocalcemia (hī-pō-kăl-sē′mē-ă) Abnormally low-blood-calcium level.
hypogastric (hī-pō-găs′trĭk) Pertaining to lower middle area of the abdomen.
hypoglycemia (hī-pō-glī-sē′mē-ȧ) Deficiency of glucose in the blood.
hypokalemia (hī-pō-kȧ-lē′mē-ȧ) Deficiency of potassium in the blood.
hyponatremia (hī-pō-nā-trē′mē-ȧ) Deficiency of sodium in the blood.
hypospadias (hī-pō-spā′dē-ȧs) Condition characterized by the abnormal opening of the urethra on the under-surface of the penis.
hypostatic (hī-pō-stăt′ĭk) Pertaining to the settling of a deposit or congestion in an area, caused by lack of proper activity.
hypotension (hī-pō-tĕn′shun) Abnormal decrease of systolic and diastolic blood pressure.
hypothalamus (hī-pō-thăl′ȧ-mŭs) Area of heat control and other body regulation located near the base of the brain.
hypothermia (hī″pō-thur′mē-ȧ) Pertaining to subnormal temperature of the body.
hypotonic (hī″pō-tŏn′ik) An abnormally reduced tone or tension; a solution having an osmotic pressure lower than that of the solution with which it is compared.
hypovolemia (hī″pō-vō-lē′mē-ȧ) Diminished blood volume.
hypoxia (hī-pŏks′ē-ă) Lack of adequate amount of oxygen.
hysterotomy (hĭs-tĕr-ŏt′ō-mē) Opening of the uterus; cesarean birth.

icterus (ĭk′tĕr-ŭs) Jaundice; a yellow tint to the skin.
identical twins The result of the division of one fertilized ovum into two identical halves that develop into two individuals of the same appearance and the same gender.
idiopathic (ĭd-ē-ō-păth′ĭk) Adjective meaning that the cause of a condition is unknown.
ileostomy (ĭl″ē-ŏs′tȧ-mē) Surgical formation of a fistula or artificial anus through the abdominal wall into the ileum, or an ileal pouch created as a part of the Bricker procedure.
ileum (ĭl′ē-ŭm) Lower portion of small intestine.
ileus (il′ē-ŭs) Obstruction or paralysis in the intestines.
iliopectineal line (ĭl″ē-ō-pĕk-tĭnē-al) Imaginary line dividing the upper or false pelvis from the lower or true pelvis; the linea terminalis forming the brim or inlet of the pelvis.
immunity (ĭ-mū′nĭ-tē) Ability to protect oneself against the development of infectious disease.
immunofluorescent antibody technique (ĭm″mŭ-nō-floo-ō-rĕs′ĕnt) Detection of antibodies using special proteins labeled with fluorescein to illuminate with fluorescent light source.
immunosuppressive (ĭm″yo̍o̍-nō-sŭh-prĕs′ĭv) Capable of interfering with a normal immune response.
impaction (ĭm-păk′shŭn) State of being lodged and retained abnormally in a part or strait; a large accumulation of relatively hard stool in the rectum or colon, difficult to move.
imperforate (ĭm-pĕr′fōr-āt) Without an opening.
impetigo (ĭm-pĕ-tī′gō) Contagious skin infection caused by coagulase-positive *staphylococci* or group A beta-hemolytic *streptococci*.
implantation (ĭm-plăn-tā′shŭn) Nesting of the fertilized ovum in the wall of the uterus; artificial placement of a substance in the body.
incarcerated (ĭn-kär′sĕr-ā-tĕd) Trapped; confined.
incest (ĭn′sĕst) Sexual intercourse between close relatives.
incontinence (ĭn-kŏn′tĭ-nĕnts) Inability to retain urine or feces because of loss of sphincter control.
incubation period (ĭn-kū-bā′shun) Period of time that must elapse from the infection of an individual at the time of exposure until the appearance of signs and symptoms of the disease.
inertia (ĭn-ĕr′shȧ) Sluggishness; absence of activity; resistance to movement or change.
infanticide (ĭn-făn′tĭs-ī d) Killing of an infant.
infant mortality The number of deaths in the first year of life per 1000 live births.
infectious disease (ĭn-fĕk′shŭs) Disorders caused by organisms that invade tissue and cause symptoms of illness.
infecund (ĭn′fĕk-ŭnd) Unfruitful; infertile; unable to conceive.
infertile (ĭn-fer′til) Unable to conceive; may refer to a man or woman.
infusion (ĭn-fŭ′zhun) Introduction of a solution into a vein.
inguinal (ĭn-gwĭ-nal) Pertaining to the region of the groin.
inhibitor (ĭn-hĭb-ĭt-er) Agent that curtails or stops certain activity.
insemination (ĭn′sĕm-ĭ-nā-shŭn) (artificial) Injection of semen into the uterine canal by a process unrelated to intercourse.
integumentary (ĭn-tĕg-ū-mĕn′tȧ-rē) Referring to the integument, that is, the skin, including the hair, nails, oil and sweat glands, and superficial sensory nerve endings.
interstitial fluid (ĭn-tĕr-stĭsh′al) Body fluid found outside the bloodstream in the spaces between the tissue cells.
intertrigo (ĭn″ter-trē′gō) Reddened skin eruption produced by friction of adjacent parts; chafing.
intractable (ĭn-trăk′tĕbl) Not easily controlled, difficult to treat.
intrauterine device (IUD) Object placed into the uterus to avoid pregnancy by perhaps preventing or disrupting implantation or fertilization.
intravesical (in″truh-vĕs′ĭ-kul) Inside the urinary bladder.
intubation (ĭn″tŭ-bā′shŭn) Introduction of a tube into a hollow organ or passageway to keep it open.
intussusception (ĭn-tŭs-sŭs-sĕp′shŭn) Telescoping of adjacent parts of the bowel, usually in the ileocecal region.
in utero (ū′tĕr-ō) Inside the uterus.
inversion (ĭn-vĕr′shŭn or ĭn-vĕr′zhŭn) A turning upside down, inside out, or end to end.
involution (ĭn-vō-lū′shŭn) A turning or rolling inward; the reverse of evolution, a term especially used to describe the return of the uterus to approximately its prepregnant size and position after childbirth.

iodophor (ī-ō′dȧ-fōr) Antiseptic containing iodine combined with detergent or an agent or carrier that enhances its solubility.
ion (ī′ȧn) One or more atoms carrying an electrical charge.
irrigation (irr″ĭ-gā′shŭn) Act of cleansing by a stream of water or other solution.
ischemia (ĭs-kē′-mē-ȧ) Deficiency of blood in a body part due to constriction or obstruction of a blood vessel resulting in localized tissue anemia.
ischial spines (ĭs′kē-al) Two relatively sharp bony projections protruding into the pelvic outlet from the ischial bones that form the lower lateral border of the pelvis; used in determining the progress of the fetus down the birth canal.
ITP Idiopathic thrombocytopenic purpura.

jaundice (jawn′dĭs) Yellow tinge to the skin or sclerae; icterus.

karyotype (kăr′ē-ō-tīp) Total characteristics of the chromosomes of a cell nucleus including number, form, size, and grouping, usually photographed, cut out, and arranged on a card for study.
kernicterus (ker-nĭk′ter-ŭs) Yellow staining of the basal ganglia of the brain in the jaundiced newborn infant; a complication of severe hyperbilirubinemia.
ketoacidosis (kē″tō-ăh″sĭ-dō′sĭs) The accumulation of ketone bodies in the blood, which results in metabolic acidosis.
ketogenic diet (kē-tō-jĕn′ĭk) High-fat, low-carbohydrate diet.
ketone bodies (kē′tōn) Group of compounds produced during the oxidation of fatty acids; one example is acetone.
kwashiorkor (kwash-ĭ-ōr′kōr) Disease resulting from protein deprivation in infancy and childhood, common in certain parts of Africa.
kyphosis (kī-fō′sĭs) Humpback.

labia majora (lā′bē-ȧ mȧ-jō-ra) (sing. labium) Two fleshy, hair-covered folds located on both sides of the perineal midline, extending from the mons veneris almost to the anus in women.
labia minora (mĭ-nō′ra) Two small folds of tissue covering the vestibule located just under the labia majora in women.
laceration (lăs-er-ā′shŭn) Jagged cut or tear.
lacrimal glands (lăk′rĭm-al) Tear glands.
lactation (lăk-tā′shŭn) Process of milk production or the period of breast-feeding in mammals.
lactogenic (lăk-tō-jĕn′ĭk) Inducing the secretion of milk (e.g., the lactogenic hormone prolactin [LTH]).
lanugo (lȧ-nü′gō) Soft, fine hair on the body of the fetus or newborn.
laparotomy (lăp-a-rŏt′ō-mē) Abdominal operation; surgical opening of the abdomen.
laryngospasm (lăr-ĭng′gō-spă-zŭm) Spasm of the muscles of the larynx.
larynx (lăr′ĭnks) Voice box.
lesion (lē′zhŭn) Any change or irregularity in tissue resulting from disease or injury.
lethargic (lĕth-är′jĭk) Drowsy; sluggish.
leukemia (lū-kē′mē-a) Disease characterized by overproduction of abnormal, immature, white blood cells; "cancer of the blood."
leukocyte (lü′kō-sīt) White blood cell.
leukocytosis (lü-kō-sī-tō′sĭs) Excessive increase in the number of white blood cells circulating in the blood.
leukopenia (lü-kō-pē′nē-ȧ) Abnormal decrease of circulating white blood cells.
leukorrhea (lü-kō-rē′ȧ) White or yellowish cervical or vaginal discharge.
levator ani (lĕ-vā′tōr ā′nē) Major muscle that helps form the pelvic diaphragm or floor.
lie (lī) The relationship of the long axis of the fetus to the long axis of the mother.
ligament (lĭg′ȧ-mĕnt) Strong, fibrous tissue that serves to connect bone to bone or to support an organ.
ligation (lī-gā′shŭn) Closing off by tying, especially arteries, veins, tubes, or ducts.
lightening (līt′ĕn-ĭng) Descent of the fetus into the true pelvis, which lessens pressure on the maternal thorax and abdomen.
linea nigra (lĭn′ē-ȧ nī′gra) Dark line that develops during pregnancy extending from the pubis to the umbilicus.
lipoids (lĭp′oydz) Fatty type of substances.
lipoprotein (lĭp″ō-prō′tēn) Simple protein combined with a lipid or fatlike substance.
lithotomy (lĭth-ŏt′a-mē) Cutting operation for removal of a calculus, usually a urinary tract stone.
lochia (lō′kē-ȧ) Vaginal drainage after childbirth.
lordosis (lōr-dō′sĭs) Exaggerated lumbar curvature; swayback.
lues (lū′ēz) Syphilis.
lumbar puncture Needle insertion into the subarachnoid space of the spinal cord between the lumbar vertebrae for diagnosis or therapy.
luteal hormone (lü′tē-ȧl) Progesterone.
lymphocyte (lĭm′fō-sīt) One kind of white blood cell.

macule (măk′ūl) Flat spot or stain.
magnetic resonance imaging (MRI) A noninvasive method of viewing the internal structures of certain body parts combining a strong magnetic field and radiofrequency waves plus computer technology to produce diagnostic images; the preferred technique to discover and evaluate CNS abnormalities.
malaise (ma-lāz′) General discomfort, uneasiness.
mandible (măn′dĭ-bŭl) Jawbone.
mastitis (măs-tī′tĭs) Inflammation of the breast.
maternal mortality The number of maternal deaths during pregnancy or within 42 days of the end of pregnancy per 100,000 live births.
maternicity (mă-tern-ĭs′ĭtē) Emotional attachment of mother to infant with bonds of affection.
maturation (măt-ū-rā′shŭn) Process of developing, ripening, or becoming more adult.
meatotomy (mē-ā-tŏt′ō-mē) Incision of the urinary meatus or opening to enlarge the passage.
meatus (mē-ā′tŭs) Passage or opening.

mechanism of labor The series of passive position adjustments the fetus makes as it accomodates to the pelvic space.
meconium (mĕ-kō′nē-ŭm) First feces of the fetus or newborn.
medium-chain triglyceride (MCT) (trī-glĭs′ŭr-id) A glycerine ester combined with an acid and distinguished from other triglycerides by having 8 to 10 carbon atoms; easily digested, high-caloric in nature.
medulla (mĕ-dŭl′ȧ) Inner portion of an organ (e.g., the medulla of the kidney or adrenal gland).
megacolon (mĕg-ȧ-kō′lŏn) Abnormally large colon.
megaloblast (mĕg′ȧ-lō-blăst) Large, early form of red blood cell with a characteristic nuclear pattern, found in the blood where there is vitamin B_{12} or folic acid deficiency.
menarche (mĕ-när′kē) First menses, or menstruation, experienced by a girl.
meningitis (mĕn-ĭn-jī′tĭs) Inflammation of the meninges covering the spinal cord or brain.
meningococcemia (mĕ-nĭn-gō-kŏk-sē′mĭ-ă) Presence of meningococci in the blood.
meningococcic meningitis (mĕ-nĭn-gō-kŏksik) Cerebrospinal fever.
meningomyelocele See myelomeningocele.
menopause (mĕn′ō-pawz) Period that marks the permanent cessation of menstrual activity.
menorrhagia (mĕn-ō-rā′jē-ȧ) Excessive bleeding at time of the menstrual period.
menses (mĕn′sēz) Menstruation.
menstruation (mĕn-strū-ā′shŭn) Monthly elimination of a bloody vaginal discharge, the portion of the lining of the uterus that had been prepared for the fertilized egg in the event of pregnancy.
mentum (mĕn′tŭm) Chin.
metabolic (mĕt-ȧ-bŏl′ĭk) Pertaining to the physical and chemical changes that take place within a living organism.
metabolism (mĕ-tăb′ȧ-lĭz-ĕm) All energy and material transformations that occur within living cells.
metacarpal (mĕt″ȧ-kă′pȧl) Pertaining to one of the five bones of the palm of the hand.
metastasis (mĕ-tăs′tȧ-sĭs) Spread of disease (e.g., cancer) from its primary location to secondary locations; the colonizing element.
metrorrhagia (mĕ-trō-rā′jē-ȧ) Presence of bloody vaginal discharge between menstrual periods.
microcephaly (mī-krō-sĕf′ȧ-lē) Failure of the brain to develop to a normal size.
microgram (μg) One millionth of a gram (μ = mu; used for the prefix micro, which stands for multiplication of a gram by 10^{-6}).
microorganism (mī-krō-or′gȧn-ĭzm) Minute living body not perceptible to the naked eye (e.g., bacterium, protozoon).
milia (mĭl′ē-a) (sing. milium) Pinpoint white or yellow dots commonly found on the nose, forehead, and cheeks of newborn babies resulting from nonfunctioning or clogged sebaceous glands.
miliaria rubra (mĭl-ē-ā′rĭ-ȧ rü′brȧ) Heat rash; prickly heat.
miscarriage Spontaneous abortion.
mitosis (mī-tō′sis) Cellular division in which the chromosomes split longitudinally to reproduce an identical tissue cell.
mohel (moy′ĭl) Ordained Jewish circumciser.
molding Shaping of the infant's head as it travels through the birth canal.
Monilia (mō-nĭl′ē-ȧ) See moniliasis.
moniliasis (mō-nī-lī′ȧ-sĭs) Yeast infection of the skin or mucous membranes caused by *Candida albicans*, formerly called *Monilia albicans*; commonly found in the vagina; infection of the mouth is termed thrush.
monitrice (mŏn′ȧ-trĭs) A monitor or adviser of a patient, especially during labor and birth.
monocyte (mŏn′ō-sīt) Type of white blood cell.
mons pubis (mŏns pū′bĭs) A fatty pad over the symphysis pubis which, after puberty, is covered with pubic hair.
mortality (mōr-tăl′ĭ-tē) State of being mortal, subject to death or destined to die; the death rate.
morula (mŏr′ü-lȧ) Mass of dividing cells resembling a mulberry, resulting from the fertilization of an ovum; an early stage of life.
mosaicism (mō-zā′ĭ-cĭzm) Presence of body cells with different genetic contents in the same individual.
motile (mō′tĭl) Capability of spontaneous movement.
mucosa (mū-kō′sȧ) Mucous membrane.
mucous (mū′kŭs) (adj.) Secreting or containing mucus; slimy.
mucoviscidosis (mū-cō-vĭs-ĭd-ō′sĭs) Another name for cystic fibrosis, a genetic disease affecting the exocrine glands involving primarily the respiratory and digestive systems.
mucus (mū′kŭs) (n.) Slippery secretion produced by the mucous membranes.
multifactorial Caused by many factors; involving many genes or combinations of genes.
multiform (mŭl′tĭ-form) Having many forms or shapes.
multigravida (mŭl-tĭ-grăv′ĭ-dȧ) Woman who has had two or more pregnancies.
multipara (mŭl-tĭp′ȧ-ra) Technically, a woman who has completed two or more viable pregnancies.
musculature (mŭs′kū-lȧ-tūr) Arrangement and condition of the muscles in the body or its parts.
mutation (myoo-tā′shŭn) Process of change or alteration particularly involving hereditary potential (genes, chromosomes).
myelin (mi′lĭn) The white fatty sheath that covers some nerves.
myelinization (mī′lĭn-ī-zā′shŭn) Process of supplying or accumulating myelin during development, or repair, of nerves.
myelitis (mī-ĕl-ī′tĭs) Inflammation of the spinal cord or bone marrow (osteomyelitis).
myelomeningocele (mī″ĕl-ō-mĕ-nĭng′ō-sēl) Herniation of elements of the spinal cord and the meninges through an abnormal opening in the spine.
myocarditis (mī″ō-kär-dī′tĭs) Inflammation of the muscular tissue of the heart.
myomectomy (mī-ō-mĕk′tō-mē) Removal of a portion of muscle or muscular tissue.

myometrium (mī″ō-mē′trē-ŭm) Muscular layer of the uterus.
myopia (mī-ō′pē-ȧ) Nearsightedness.
myringotomy (mĭr-ĭn-gŏt′ō-mē) Incision into the eardrum.

nebulization (nĕb′ū-lȧ-zā′shŭn) Producing spray or mist-like particles from a liquid.
necrosis (nĕk-rō′sĭs) Death of tissue.
neonatal (nē-ō-nā′tȧl) Concerning the newborn infant or the first 4 weeks of life after birth.
neonatal mortality The number of deaths under 28 days of life per 1000 live births.
neoplasm (nē′ō-plă-zŭm) Tumor.
nephron (nĕf′rŏn) Working unit of the kidney; the renal corpuscle and its tubule.
nephrosis (nĕf-rō′sĭs) Renal disease of unknown cause seen in children, characterized by massive edema and albuminuria.
neuropathy (nū-rŏp′ă-thē) Any disease of the nerves.
neutrophil (nū′trō-fĭl) One kind of white blood cell.
nevus (nē′vŭs) (pl. nevi) Mole, pigmented area, or vascular tumor on the skin.
nitrous oxide (nī′trŭs ŏk′sīd) Laughing gas (N_2O).
nocturia (nŏk-tū′rĭ-a) Excessive urination during the night.
nodule (nŏd′ūl) Small aggregate of cells.
nosocomial (nō′so-ko-mĭ-ȧl) Of or pertaining to a hospital; an infection associated with hospitalization.
nuchal (nū′kȧl) Pertaining to the neck.
nucleotide (nū′-klē-ō-tīd) The basic structural unit of nucleic acid.
nucleus (nū′klē-ŭs) Central point about which matter is gathered; controlling portion of a cell regulating metabolism and reproduction of the cell.
nulligravida (nŭl-ĭ-grăv′ĭ-dȧ) Woman who has never been pregnant.
nullipara (nŭl-ĭp′ȧ-rȧ) A woman who has never completed a pregnancy of viable age.
nurture (ner′cher) To feed, rear, foster, care for; nourishment, care, and training of growing children or things.
nystagmus (nĭs-tăg′mŭs) Constant, involuntary movement of the eyeballs.

oblique (ō-blēk′) Slanting; inclined.
obturator (ŏb′tū-rā″tōr) Small, curved rod with an olive-shaped tip that fits inside a tracheostomy tube to aid in its insertion.
occiput (ŏk′sĭ-pŭt) Occipital bone or back part of the skull.
occlude (ŏ-klūd′) To close or plug.
occluded (ŏ-klūd′ĕd) Closed up; obstructed.
occult (ŏ-kŭlt′) Obscure, hidden.
oligo (ŏl-ĭ-gō) Combining form meaning few, diminished, or scanty amount.
oligohydramnios (ŏl′-ĭ-gō-hī-drăm-nē-ōs) Deficiency of amniotic fluid during pregnancy.
oliguria (ŏl-ĭ-gū′rē-ȧ) Diminished amount of urine production with subsequent scanty urination.
omphalocele (ŏm′făl-ō-sēl) Absence of the normal abdominal wall in the region of the umbilicus creating defects of varying sizes.
opaque (ō-pāk′) Lacking transparency.
ophthalmia neonatorum (ŏf-thăl′mē-ȧ nē-ō-nă-tōr′ŭm) Infection of the eyes of the newborn infant, particularly that caused by gonorrheal organisms.
opisthotonos (ŏ-pĭs-thŏt′ō-nŏs) Involuntary arching of the back because of irritation of the brain or spinal cord.
orchiopexy (or″kē-ō-pĕk′sē) Surgical fixation of a testis or testicle in the scrotum to correct undescent.
orthopnea (ŏr-thŏp-nē′ȧ) Condition in which breathing is difficult except when the patient is in a standing or sitting position.
orthostatic (ŏr-thō-stăk′ĭk) Concerning an erect position or related to a standing position.
osmosis (ŏs-mō′sĭs) Passage of a liquid (solvent), usually water, through a semipermeable partition separating solutions of different concentrations to equalize the concentration of any substance dissolved in the solutions.
ossification (ŏs-ĭ-fĭ-kā′shŭn) Process of bone formation.
osteomalacia (ŏs″tē-ō-mȧ-lā′shē-ȧ) Adult rickets or softening of the bone.
osteomyelitis (ŏs″tē-ō-mī-ĕ-lī′tĭs) Inflammation of the bone marrow and surrounding cells.
osteoporosis (ŏs″tē-ō-po-rō′sĭs) Deossification with decrease in bone tissue resulting in structural weakness.
otitis media (ō-tī′tĭs mē′dē-ȧ) Middle ear infection.
ovary (ō′vȧ-rē) Paired, almond-shaped gland that produces female hormones and female sex cells, or ova.
oviduct (ō′vĭ-dŭkt) Fallopian, or uterine, tube.
ovulation (ŏ-vŭ-lā′shŭn) Rupture of an ovarian follicle and the expulsion of the ovum.
oximeter (ŏks-ĭ′-mĕtr) Instrument used to measure O_2 concentrations (percentages).
oxytocic (ŏk-sē-tō′sĭk) Medication that stimulates the uterus to contract.

palliative (păl′ē-ā-tĭv) Alleviates without curing.
palpation (păl-pā′shŭn) Examination by touch or feel.
papule (păp′ūl) Small, solid elevation on the skin; the typical early stage of a pimple.
papulovesiculopustular (păp-ū-lō-vĕ-sĭk″ū-lō-pŭs′tū-lar) Adjective used to describe a rash; characterized by papules, vesicles, and pustules.
para (păr′ȧ) The number of pregnancies a woman has completed that have resulted in viable births.
paracentesis (păr-ă-sĕn-tē′sĭs) Artificial withdrawal of fluid by puncture of a body cavity, especially the abdominal cavity.
paralytic (păr-ȧ-lĭt′ĭk) Describes person suffering from loss of the ability to move a part or parts of his body.
parametrium (păr″ȧ-mē′trē-ŭm) Outermost covering of the uterus formed in part by a portion of the peritoneum.
paraplegia (păr′ȧ-plē″jȧ) Paralysis of legs and lower part of the body; both motion and sensation are affected.
parenchyma (pȧ-reng′kĭ-mȧ) Functioning portion of an organ as distinguished from supportive cells forming its framework.
parenteral (pȧ-rĕn′ter-ȧl) Pertaining to methods of drug or food administration other than through the use of the gastrointestinal tract (e.g., intravenous or subcutaneous routes).
paresis (pȧ-rē′sĭs) Partial or incomplete paralysis; term also used to describe neurologic deterioration associated with late stage syphilis (incoordination, paralysis, seizures).

paroxysmal (păr″ok-sĭz′mȧl) Of the nature of a sudden attack.

parturient (pär-tū′rē-ĕnt) Laboring or mother of a newly delivered child.

parturition (păr-tū-rĭsh′ŭn) Childbirth; delivery.

patency (pā′tĕn-sē) State of being freely open.

pathogen (păth′ō-jĕn) Microorganism or substance capable of producing a disease.

pathologic (păth′ȧ-lŏj′ĭ-kȧl) Caused by or involving disease; concerning disease.

pediculosis (pĕ-dik-ū-lō′sĭs) Infestation of an individual by head, body, or pubic lice.

pelvimeter (pĕl-vĭm′ĕ-ter) Device used to measure the pelvis.

pendulous (pĕn′dū-lŭs) Hanging; lacking proper support.

percussion (per-kush′ŭn) Tapping the body lightly but sharply for diagnosis or therapy.

perimetrium (pĕr″ĭ-mē′trē-ŭm) The outermost serous membrane enveloping the uterus.

perinatal (pĕr-ĭ-nāt′ȧl) The period from 28 weeks of pregnancy through the first 28 days after birth.

perinatal (pĕr-ĭ-nāt′ȧl) Associated with the period before or after birth.

perineum (per-ĭ-nē′ŭm) Area of the external genitalia in both male and female; specifically, the area between the vagina and the anus or the scrotum and the anus.

periorbital (pĕr′ē-or′bĭt′ȧl) Surrounding the socket of the eye.

periosteum (pĕr-ĭ-ŏs′tē-ŭm) Fibrous membrane that forms the covering of bones except at their articular surfaces.

peripheral (per-ĭf′er-al) Located at the surface or away from the center of the body.

peristalsis (pĕr-ĭs-tăl′sĭs) Progressive, wavelike movement that occurs involuntarily in hollow tubes of the body, especially the alimentary canal.

peritoneum (pĕr″ĭt-o-nē′ŭm) Serous membrane lining the interior of the abdominal cavity and surrounding the contained internal organs.

peritonitis (pĕr-ĭ-tō-nī′tĭs) Inflammation of the peritoneum.

permeable (pur′mē-ȧ-bȧl) Capable of being penetrated.

per se (per sā) Essentially; by itself; of itself.

pertussis (per-tŭs′ĭs) Whooping cough.

petechiae (pȧ-tē′kē-ī) Small, bluish purple dots on the skin resulting from capillary hemorrhages.

petrification (pĕt″rĭ-fĭ-kā′shŭn) Process of turning into stone.

phagocytosis (făg″ō-sī-tō′sĭs) Ingestion and digestion of bacteria and microscopic particles by phagocytes, certain white blood cells.

pharynx (făr′ĭnks) Musculomembranous passageway at the back of the nose and mouth partially shared by both the respiratory and digestive systems.

phlebitis (flĕ-bī′tĭs) Inflammation of a vein.

phlebotomy (flĕ-bŏt′ō-mē) Withdrawal of blood from a vein.

photophobia (fō-tō-fō′bē-ȧ) Unusual intolerance to light.

pica (pī′kȧ) Abnormal craving for substances not meant for consumption.

pigmentation (pĭg-mĕn-tā′shŭn) Coloration resulting from the deposit of certain substances in the skin.

pipette (pī-pĕt′) Narrow calibrated glass tube with both ends open, used to measure and transfer liquids from one container to another by application of oral suction.

pituitary gland (pĭ-tū′ĭ-tăr-ē) Endocrine gland located at the base of the brain involved in many body functions; the "master gland."

placenta (plȧ-sĕn′tȧ) Flattened, circular mass of spongy vascular tissue attached to the inside of the uterine wall that serves as the metabolic link between the fetus and the mother; from its surface protrudes the umbilical cord that carries food and oxygen to the fetus and waste away from the fetus; also serves as a point of attachment for the bag of waters that encloses the fetus.

placenta previa (prē′vēȧ) Low implantation of the placenta near or over the cervix within the uterine cavity causing hemorrhage late in pregnancy.

placentae abruptio See abruptio placentae.

plantar (plăn′tăr) Concerning the sole of the foot.

platelet (plā′lĕt) (blood platelet) Thrombocyte, a necessary element for blood clot formation.

platypelloid (plăt″ē-pĕl′oyd) Abnormal type of female pelvis, flattened from front to back.

pneumatocele (nū-mă′tō-sēl) Herniation of lung tissue; a sac or tumor containing gas.

pneumomediastinum (nū″mō-mē-dē-ăs-tī′nŭm) Air or gas in the mediastinal tissues located between the lungs.

pneumonia (nū-mō′nē-ȧ) Inflammation of the lung tissue.

pneumothorax (nū-mō-thō′răks) Collection of air or gas in the pleural cavity (the potential space between the two coverings of the lungs).

polyarthritis (pŏl″ē-ăr-thrī′tĭs) Inflammation that involves more than one joint, often migratory in character.

polycystic (pŏl-ē-sĭs′tĭk) Composed of many cysts, that is, little sacs usually containing fluid.

polycythemia (pŏl″ē-sī-thē′mē-ȧ) Abnormal condition characterized by an excess of red blood cells.

polydactylism (pŏl-ē-dăk′tĭl-ĭzm) Presence of extra fingers or toes.

polydipsia (pŏl-ē-dĭp′sē-ȧ) Excessive thirst and fluid intake.

polyhydramnios (pŏl″ē-hī-drăm′nē-ōs) Excessive volume of amniotic fluid.

polymorphonuclear (pŏl″ē-mor-fō-nū′klē-er) Leukocyte having a lobated or segmented nucleus.

polyphagia (pŏl-ē-fā′jē-ȧ) Excessive appetite.

polyuria (pŏl-ē-ū′rē-ȧ) Excessive urinary output.

portal of entry Avenue by which an infectious agent gains entrance into the body.

position The relationship of a reference point on the presenting part of the fetus to the pelvic quadrants of the mother.

postneonatal mortality The number of deaths from 28 days of life to the first birthday per 1000 live births.

precipitate (prē-sĭp′ĭ-tāt) delivery Birth that occurs with such rapidity that proper preparation and medical supervision are lacking.

preeclampsia (prē-ĕk-lamp′sē-a) Toxemia of pregnancy uncomplicated by convulsion or coma; pregnancy-induced hypertension (see eclampsia).

pregnancy-induced hypertension A hypertensive disorder of pregnancy or early postpartum that includes the condi-

tions known as preeclampsia and eclampsia; characterized by hypertension, edema, and proteinuria.
prehension (prē-hĕn′shŭn) Use of the hands to pick up small objects; grasping.
prepuce (prē′pŭs) Foreskin of the penis or hood of the clitoris.
presenting part Part of the baby that comes through or attempts to come through the pelvic canal first; often synonymous with "obstetric presentation."
Primary or Initial Lesions:
bleb or bullae (adj., bullous) Blister.
macule (adj., macular) Flat lesion; a freckle.
papule (adj., papular) Small, solid elevation on the skin; the early state of a pimple.
pustule (adj., pustular) Pus-filled vesicle; a superficial cutaneous abscess.
primigravida (prĭ-mĭ-grăv′ĭ-dȧ) Woman who is having or has had one pregnancy.
primipara (prī-mĭp′ȧ-rȧ) A woman who has carried one pregnancy to a viable age.
progesterone (prō-jĕs′tĕr-ōn) Female sex hormone manufactured by the corpus luteum of the ovary and, during pregnancy, by the placenta; aids in preparing the lining of the uterus for pregnancy and maintaining a pregnancy once established.
progestin (prō-jĕs′tĭn) Any progestational hormone; a synonym for progesterone.
prognosis (prog-nō′sĭs) Prediction regarding the course of a disease and the likelihood of recovery.
prolapse (prō-lăps′) Falling out of place (e.g., a rectocele).
prophylactic (prō-fĭ-lăk′tĭk) That which prevents disease.
prophylaxis (prō-fĭ-lăk′sĭs) Preventive treatment.
proptosis (prŏp-tō′sĭs) Forward displacement.
prostaglandin (prŏs′tă-glănd-ĭn) Group of fatty acid derivatives present in many tissues, including the prostate, involved in regulating many body processes.
prostate (prŏs′tāt) Exocrine gland found at the base of the male bladder that secretes an alkaline fluid stimulating sperm motility.
prosthesis (prŏ-thē′sĭs) Artificial body part.
proteinuria (prō-tē-ĭn-ū′rē-ȧ) Finding of protein, usually albumin, in the urine.
prothrombin (prō-thrŏm′bĭn) Chemical substance found in the blood, necessary to coagulation.
protozoa (prō-tō-zō′ȧ) (sing. protozoon) Simple microscopic animals, usually single celled.
protrusion (prō-trü′zhŭn) State or condition of being forward or projecting.
protuberant (prō-too′ber-ȧnt) Bulging.
pruritus (prü-rī′tŭs) Itching.
pseudohermaphroditism (sū″dō-hĕr-măf′rō-dīt-ĭzm) Condition in which an individual possesses external genitalia resembling those of one sex and the internal sex organs, or gonads, of the opposite sex.
psychosis (sī-kō′sĭs) Mental disturbance involving personality disintegration and loss of contact with reality.
psychosocial (sī″kō-sō′shȧl) Involving both psychological and social factors.
ptyalism (tī′ȧ-lĭzm) Excessive salivation.
puberty (pū′ber-tē) Period in life when one becomes capable of reproduction.
puerperium (pū-er-pĭr′ē-ŭm) Six-week period after childbirth; the postpartal period.
purpura (pur′pū-rȧ) Purple discoloration that occurs as a result of spontaneous bleeding into the skin or mucous membranes.
pustule (pŭs′tŭl) Pus-filled papule; a superficial cutaneous abscess.
pyelogram (pī′ĕl-ō-grăm) Radiograph of the ureters and renal pelves.
pyelonephritis (pī″ĕl-ō-nĕf-rī′tĭs) Infection of the renal pelvis and the working units of the kidney, the nephrons.
pyogenic (pī-ō-jĕn′ĭk) Producing pus.
pyrosis (pī-rō′sĭs) Heartburn.
pyuria (pī-ū-rē′ȧ) Abnormal white blood cells in the urine.

quickening (kwĭk′ĕn-ĭng) Maternal identification of fetal motion; felt by multiparas at about the sixteenth week of pregnancy and by primiparas 2 weeks later.

radiograph (rā′dĭ-ō-grăf) X-ray film.
rationale (răsh-ŭn-ăl′) Logical reason for a course of action or procedure.
rectocele (rĕk′tō-sēl) Prolapse or displacement of the rectum because of weakening of the rectovaginal wall.
reduction (rē-dŭk′shŭn) In orthopedics, refers to realignment of a broken bone or the correct placement of a dislocation.
reflux (rē′flŭks) Return or backward flow (e.g., regurgitation of urine from the bladder into the ureter).
regurgitation (rē-gŭr-jĭ-tā′shŭn) Return of solids or fluids to the mouth from the stomach; any abnormal backflow of fluid within the body.
remission (rē-mĭsh′un) Lessening of severity or abatement of symptoms.
reservoir (rĕz′er-vwȧr) Chamber or receptacle for holding fluid; store; reserve.
resorption (rē-sōrp′shŭn) Disappearance of all or part of a process, tissue, or exudate by biochemical reactions.
reticulocyte Immature red blood cell.
retinoblastoma (rĕt-ĭn-ō-blăs-tō′mȧ) Malignant tumor of the eye.
retinopathy (rĕt″ĭn-ŏp′a-thē) Any disorder of the retina.
retraction (rē-trăk′shŭn) State of being drawn back.
retroflexion (rĕt-rō-flĕk′shŭn) Bending or flexing backward; an abnormal position of the uterus bent backward toward the rectum, forming an angle between the cervix and the body of the organ.
retrograde (rĕt′rō-grād) Moving backward; degenerating from better to worse.
retrolental fibroplasia (rĕ″tro-lĕn′tȧl fī″brō-plā′zē-ȧ) Oxygen-induced separation of the retina of the eye behind the lens; characteristic of premature infants.
retroversion (rĕt-rō-ver′shŭn) Turning or state of being turned back; backward displacement of the body of the uterus so that the cervix points toward the symphysis pubis instead of toward the sacrum.
Reye syndrome A potentially life-threatening disease possibly associated with recent viral illness such as chicken pox

or influenza and salicylate use, although its cause is unclear. It is characterized by nausea, vomiting, rash, liver function changes with typical fatty degeneration, and progressive brain dysfunction, coma, and seizures.

Rh blood factor Blood protein found in approximately 85% of the American population; those persons who possess it are termed Rh positive.

rheumatism (rü'mȧ-tĭzm) Any of numerous conditions characterized by inflammation or pain in muscles, joints, or fibrous tissue.

rhinitis (rī-nī'tĭs) Inflammation of the nasal mucosa.

rickets (rĭk'ĕts) Disturbance in skeletal development because of poor nutritional intake or absorption of vitamin D and/or calcium or phosphorus; characterized by abnormal softening of the bones.

rubella (rü-bĕl'ȧ) German, or 3-day, measles.

rubeola (rü-bē'ō-lȧ) Red, or 2-week, measles.

sacrum (sā'krŭm) Fused bone that, with the coccyx, forms the lower portion of the spine and posterior surface of the pelvis.

salmonellosis (săl"mō-nĕl-ō'sĭs) Infection (including typhoid) caused by ingesting foods containing species of the genus *Salmonella.*

salpingitis (sal"-pĭn-jī'-tĭs) Inflammation of the oviduct or uterine tube.

sarcoma (sär-kō'mȧ) Malignant tumor originating in connective tissue.

scabies (skā'bēz) Infestation of the skin by the itch mite *Sarcoptes scabiei*; "7-year itch."

sclera (sklĕ'rȧ) (pl. sclerae) White outercoating of the eyeball extending from the optic nerve to include the cornea.

scoliosis (skō-lĭ-ō'sĭs) Abnormal lateral spinal curvature.

scrotum (skrō'tŭm) Pouch forming part of the male external genitalia and containing the testicles and part of the spermatic cord.

scultetus binder (skŭl-tē'tŭs) Many-tailed abdominal binder.

seborrhea (sĕb-ōr-ē'ȧ) Functional disorder of the sebaceous (oil) glands of the skin and/or scalp causing crusting and scaling; on the scalp it may be called dandruff, milk crust, or cradle cap, depending on the location and density of the scaling.

sedative (sĕd'ȧ-tĭv) Medication that quiets and reduces tension.

semen (sē'mĕn) Fluid discharge from the male reproductive organs that contains the sperm to fertilize the female ovum.

sensitization (sĕn-sĭ-tĭ-zā'shŭn) Process of making a person reactive to a substance such as a drug, plant, fiber, or serum.

sepsis (sĕp'sĭs) Presence or state of contamination, putrefaction, or infection (adj., septic).

septicemia (sĕp-tĭ-sē'mē-ȧ) Disease condition resulting from the absorption of pathogenic microorganisms and/or the poisons resulting from infectious processes into the blood.

sequela(e) (sē-kwē'lă) Condition following and resulting from a disease.

sequestrum (sē-kwĕs'trŭm) (pl. sequestra) Fragment of a diseased, decaying bone that has become separated from surrounding tissue.

serology (ser-ŏl'ō-jĭ) Study of blood serum.

serosanguineous (sē"rō-săn-gwĭn'ē-ŭs) Containing both serum and blood.

show In obstetrics, the blood-tinged mucoid vaginal discharge that becomes more pronounced and red as cervical dilation increases during labor.

shunt (shŭnt) To turn away from; to divert; a normal or artificially constructed passage that diverts a flow from one main route to another.

sibling (sĭb'lĭng) One of two or more children of the same parents.

smegma (smĕg'mȧ) Cheesy secretion of the sebaceous glands found in the area of the labia minora and the clitoris of the female or the prepuce in the male.

souffle (soo'fl) A soft, blowing sound heard through a stethoscope.

spastic (spăs-tĭk) Type of muscular action characterized by stiff, uncoordinated movement.

spasticity (spăs-tĭs'ĭ-tē) Stiff, awkward, uncoordinated movements caused by hypertension of the muscles, usually caused by brain damage.

sperm Male sex cell, spermatozoon, carrying the male hereditary potential.

spermatozoon (sper"ma-tō-zō'on) (pl. spermatozoa) Male sex cell.

spermicide (sper'mĭ-sīd) Agent that kills spermatozoa.

sphincter (sfĭngk'ter) Circular muscle constricting or closing an opening.

spinnbarkeit (spĭn'bähr-kīt) Cervical mucus forms a thread when spread onto a glass slide and drawn out by a cover glass.

spore (spōr) Protective form assumed by some bacilli (usage in bacteriology).

stasis (stā'sĭs) Cessation of flow in blood or other body fluids.

station (stā'shŭn) Depth of the presenting part in the pelvic canal as measured by the relationship of the presenting part to the ischial spines of the pelvis.

status asthmaticus (stăt'ŭs ăz-măt'ĭ-kŭs) Severe asthmatic condition that does not respond to usual treatment with epinephrine.

steatorrhea (stē-ăt-ōr-rē'ȧ) Presence of excessive fat in the stool.

stenosis (stĕn-ō'sĭs) Abnormal narrowing of a passage or opening.

sterile (stĕr'ĭl) Free of living microorganisms, including spore forms.

stoma (stō'mȧ) Mouth or opening of a pore; a body opening, natural or artificial; term usually applied to a colostomy, ileostomy, or ileobladder opening.

strabismus (stră-bĭz'mŭs) Crossed or crooked eyes; squint.

streptococcus (strĕp-tō-kŏk'ŭs) (pl. streptococci) Spherical microorganism that forms a pattern resembling beads on a string.

striae (strī'ē) Stretch marks often seen on the skin of pregnant women.

stridor (strī'dōr) Harsh-sounding respirations.

subcostal (sŭb-kŏs′tál) Lying beneath a rib or ribs or just below the last rib adjacent to the abdomen.
subinvolution (sub-ĭn-vō-lū′shŭn) Incomplete return of a part to its normal position or dimensions; term usually applied to an abnormal, incomplete return of the uterus to its prepregnant state after childbirth.
subluxation (sŭb″lŭk-sā′shŭn) Incomplete dislocation of a bone.
supine (sü-pīn′) Positioned on the back or palm up.
suprapubic (sü″prá-pū′bĭk) Above the pubis.
suprasternal (sü″prá-stur′nál) Above the sternum, adjacent to the neck.
surfactant (ser-făk-tănt) A secretion of lipoproteins produced in the lungs which reduces the surface tension of pulmonary fluids allowing more efficient respiration. Its absence is a key factor in the incidence of infant respiratory distress syndrome.
suture (soo′cher) The line at which adjoining bones of the skull meet.
syndactylism (sĭn-dăk′tĭl-ĭzm) Fusion or webbing of two or more fingers or toes.
syndrome (sĭn′drōm) Complete picture of a disease; all the symptoms of a disease considered as a whole.
synthetic (sĭn-thĕt′ĭk) Artifically prepared.
syphilis (sĭf′ĭlĭs) A contagious, primarily sexually transmitted disease characterized by structural and skin lesions. It may be transmitted to the fetus in utero.
systolic pressure (sĭs-tŏl′ĭk) pressure Pertaining to systole; blood pressure at the time of greatest cardiac contraction.

tachycardia (tăk″ē-kär′dē-á) Excessive rapidity of the heart's action.
tachypnea (tăk″ĭp-nē′á) Rapid rate of breathing.
talipes (tăl′ĭ-pēz) Any of a number of deformities of the ankle or foot, usually congenital; clubfoot.
telangiectasia (tel-ăn″jē-ĕk-tā′zē-á) Small reddened areas often found on the eyelids, midforehead, and nape of the neck of newborn infants, caused by superficial dilation of capillaries.
tendon (tĕn′dŭn) Fibrous tissue that connects muscle to bone or other structures.
teratogenic (tĕr″á-tō-gĕn′ĭk) Capable of causing a major or minor deviation from normal structure or function in the developing embryo or fetus.
testis (tĕs′tĭs) (pl. testes) Paired, oval, male sex gland that produces a male sex hormone and spermatozoa.
testosterone (tĕs-tŏs′tĕr-ōn) Male hormone produced by the testes.
tetanus (tĕt′ă-nŭs) Lockjaw; an acute potentially fatal infectious CNS disease caused by *Clostridium tetani* often found in the soil; immunization is critical.
tetany (tĕt′a-nē) Nervous disorder characterized by intermittent tonic spasms of the muscles that may be caused by inadequate calcium levels in the bloodstream.
therapeutic (thĕr′á-pū′tĭk) Having medicinal or healing properties; a healing agent.
thermal (ther′măl) Pertaining to heat.
thoracentesis (thō-răs-ĕn-tē′sĭs) Removal of fluids through the chest wall by the insertion of a special needle.
thrombocyte (thrŏm′bō-sīt) Blood platelet necessary for coagulation.
thrombocytopenia (thrŏm″bō-sī″tō-pēn′ĭ-á) An abnormal decrease in the number of platelets in the blood.
thrombophlebitis (thrŏm″bō-flē-bī′tŭs) Inflammation of a vein in conjunction with the development of a blood clot.
thrombosis (thrŏm′bō′sĭs) Formation of a blood clot.
thrombus (thrŏm′bŭs) Blood clot formed in a blood vessel or cavity of the heart.
thrush (thrŭsh) Fungous infection caused by *Candida albicans* in the mouth or throat, especially in infants; characterized by white patches that adhere to the mucous membranes.
tincture (tĭngk′tūr) Substance that, in solution, is diluted with alcohol.
tinea capitis (tĭn′ē-á kăp′ĭ-tĭs) Ringworm of the scalp.
tinea corporis (kōr′por-ĭs) Any fungous skin disease, especially ringworm of the body.
tinea pedis (pĕd′ĭs) Fungous skin disease or ringworm of the foot; commonly called athlete's foot.
tocolytic (tō-kō-lĭ′-tĭk) Medication or regimen designed to stop labor.
torsion (tōr′shŭn) Act or condition of being twisted.
torticollis (tŏr-tĭ-kŏl′ĭs) Wryneck or tilting of the head caused by the abnormal shortening of either sternocleidomastoid muscle.
toxemia (tŏk-sē′mē-á) Presence of poisonous products in the blood and body; disease of unknown etiology suffered by some pregnant women, characterized by high blood pressure, albumin in the urine, and edema (see eclampsia and preeclampsia [pregnancy-induced hypertension]).
toxoid (tŏks′oyd) Preparation that contains a toxin or poison produced by pathogenic organisms capable of producing active immunity against a disease but too weak to produce the disease itself.
toxoplasmosis (tŏk-sō-plăz-mō′sĭs) A parasitic disease resulting from the organism *Toxoplasma gondii*.
tracheostomy (trā-kē-ŏst′ō-mē) Surgical opening of the trachea through the neck to help ensure an airway; a planned intervention usually of some duration or permanence.
traction (trăk′shŭn) Process of pulling.
tranquilizer (trăn′kwĭ-lī-zĕr) A technique or medication that relieves anxiety and quiets an anxious person.
transcutaneous (trăn″kū-tā′nē-ŭs) Performed through the skin.
transilluminated (trăns-ĭl-lū mĭ-nā′tĕd) Inspection of cavity or organ by passing light through its walls.
translocation (trănz″lō-kā′shŭn) Displacement of part or all of one chromosome onto another.
transverse (trăns-vĕrs′) Lying at right angles to the long axis of the body; crosswise.
transverse presentation Presentation in which the fetus lies crosswise in the pelvis and cannot be delivered vaginally unless turned.
trauma (träw′má) Injury or wound; a painful emotional experience.
treponemal (trĕp″ō-nē′mál) Pertaining to a genus of spiral organisms, parasitic to man, with undulating or rigid bodies.
trichomonas vaginitis (trĭ-kŏm′ō′nás vă-jĭ-nī′tĭs) Inflammation of the vagina caused by the parasitic protozoan

Trichomonas vaginalis that results in itching and a profuse, bubbly, yellow discharge.
trigone (trī'gōn) Triangular space; triangular area in the urinary bladder formed by the urethral outlet and the two ureteral openings.
trimester (trī-mĕs'tĕr) Three-month period of time.
trisomy (trī'sō-mē) Occurrence of three of a given chromosome in a cell rather than the normal diploid number of two.
trophozoite (trŏf-ō-zō'īt) Animal spore during its developmental stage; motile form of the ameba.
tuberculosis (tū-ber″kū-lō'sĭs) An infectious, inflammatory disease that is chronic in nature and commonly affects the lungs.
turbidity (tûr-bĭd'ȧ-tē) Cloudy or dense state; like a fog.
turgor (tur'gur) Normal tension in living cells; distention or swelling.

ubiquitous (ū-bĭk'wėt-ŭs) Existing or seeming to exist everywhere.
µg See microgram.
ulcer (ŭl'ser) Raw area often depressed or forming a cavity by loss of normal covering tissue.
ultrasonography (ŭl″trȧ-sō-nŏg'rȧ-fē) Pulse echo diagnosis or technique using high-frequency, inaudible sound waves.
umbilicus (ŭm-bĭl'ĭkŭs or ŭm-bĭ-lī'kŭs) Site of the umbilical cord attachment; the navel.
uremia (ū-rē'mē-ȧ) Toxic condition associated with renal insufficiency and the retention in the blood of nitrogenous substances normally excreted by the kidney.
ureter (ū-rē'tur/ūr'ĕ-ter) Long tubes conveying the urine from the kidneys to the urinary bladder.
ureterocele (ū-rē'ter-ō-sēl) Ballooning of the lower end of the ureter.
urethra (ū-rē'thra) Canal through which the urine is discharged.
urethroplasty (ū-rē'thrō-plăs-tē) Operation to correct hypospadias; surgical repair of the urethra.
urgency Patient cannot wait to void.
urogram (ū'rō-gram) X-ray photograph of any part of the urinary tract.
urticaria (ur-tĭ-kā'rē-ȧ) Wheals; hives; large, slightly raised, reddened or blanched areas often accompanied by intense itching; hives.
uterine inertia (ū'ter-ĭn ĭn-er'shȧ) Abnormal relaxation of the uterus either during labor, causing lack of obstetric progress, or after childbirth, causing uterine hemorrhage.
uterus (ū'ter-ŭs) Hollow, muscular organ that serves as a protector and nourisher of the developing fetus and aids in his expulsion from the body; the womb.

vaccine (văk'sēn) Preparation containing killed or weakened living microorganisms that, when introduced into the body, cause the formation of antibodies against that type of organism, thereby protecting the individual from the disease.
vagina (vȧ-jī'nȧ) Canal opening between the urethra and anus in the female that extends back to the cervix of the uterus.
varicella (văr-ĭ-sĕl'ȧ) Chicken pox; acute contagious disease, commonly of childhood, characterized by a body rash seen simultaneously in all stages of development.
varicosity (văr-ĭ-kŏs'ĭ-tē) Abnormal swollen vein, the walls of which are thinned and weakened.
vas deferens (văs dĕf'er-ĕnz) Excretory duct of the testis.
vasodilator (văs-ō-dī-lī'tŏr) Drug that dilates the blood vessels.
vein (vān) Blood vessel that carries blood to the heart.
venereal (ven-ĭr'-ēȧl) Pertaining to or caused by genital contact or sexual intercourse.
ventricle (vĕn'trĭk-ŭl) Small cavity or chamber; one of two lower chambers of the heart; one of several cavities in the brain where cerebrospinal fluid is formed or drains.
vernix caseosa (vĕr'nĭks cāz-ē-ō'sȧ) Yellowish, creamy protective substance on the fetus caused by the secretion of the sebaceous glands of the skin.
version (ver'shŭn) In obstetrics, the changing of the fetal presentation by internal or external manual maneuvers.
vertex (ver'teks) The top of the head.
vertigo (ver'tĭ-gō) Dizziness.
vesicle (vĕs'ĭ-kĕl) Elevation of the skin, obviously containing fluid; a blister; or referring to the urinary bladder.
vesicoureteral reflux Regurgitation of urine from the bladder into the ureter.
vesicular (vĕs-ĭk'ū-lar) Blisterlike.
vestibule (vĕs'tĭ-būl) Triangular space between the labia minora in which the openings of the urethra, vagina, and Bartholin's glands are located.
viable (vī'ȧ-bŭl) Capable of life; capable of living outside the uterus; subject to legal definition.
virulent (vĭr'ū-lĕnt) Highly poisonous; infectious.
virus (vī'rŭs) Submicroscopic infective agent.
viscid (vĭs'ĭd) Sticky.
viscosity (vĭs-kŏs'ĭ-tē) State of being thick, gummy, or sticky.
vulnerable Susceptible to being wounded; in an unfavorable condition.
vulva (vŭl'vȧ) External female genitalia.

WBC White blood cell.
wheal (wēl) Large, slightly raised, reddened or blanched area, often accompanied by intense itching.

zygote (zī'gōt) Fertilized egg.

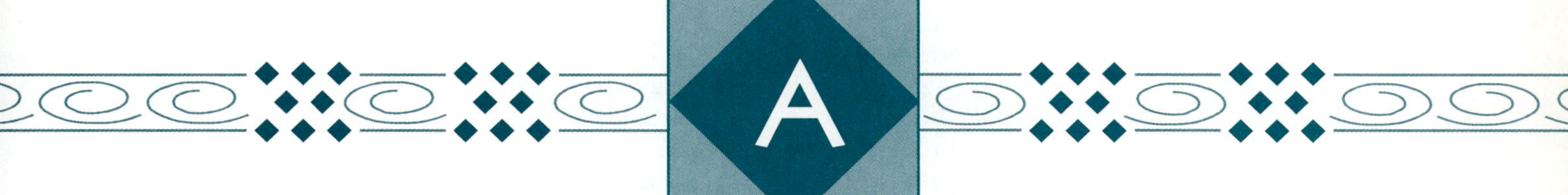

The Pregnant Patient's Bill of Rights

The Pregnant Patient has the right to participate in decisions involving her well-being and that of her unborn child, unless there is a clear-cut medical emergency that prevents her participation. In addition to the rights set forth in the American Hospital Association's "Patient's Bill of Rights," the Pregnant Patient, because she represents TWO patients rather than one, should be recognized as having the following additional rights*:

1. *The Pregnant Patient has the right,* prior to the administration of any drug or procedure, to be informed by the health professional caring for her of any potential direct or indirect effects, risks or hazards to herself or her unborn or newborn infant which may result from the use of a drug or procedure prescribed for or administered to her during pregnancy, labor, birth or lactation.
2. *The Pregnant Patient has the right,* prior to the proposed therapy, to be informed, not only of the benefits, risks and hazards of the proposed therapy but also of known alternative therapy, such as available childbirth education classes which could help to prepare the Pregnant Patient physically and mentally to cope with the discomfort or stress of pregnancy and the experience of childbirth, thereby reducing or eliminating her need for drugs and obstetric intervention. She should be offered such information early in her pregnancy in order that she may make a reasoned decision.
3. *The Pregnant Patient has the right,* prior to the administration of any drug, to be informed by the health professional who is prescribing or administering the drug to her that any drug which she receives during pregnancy, labor and birth, no matter how or when the drug is taken or administered, may adversely affect her unborn baby, directly or indirectly, and that there is no drug or chemical which has been proven safe for the unborn child.
4. *The Pregnant Patient has the right* if cesarean birth is anticipated, to be informed prior to the administration of any drug, and preferably prior to her hospitalization, that minimizing her and, in turn, her baby's intake of nonessential preoperative medicine will benefit her baby.
5. *The Pregnant Patient has the right,* prior to the administration of a drug or procedure, to be informed of the areas of uncertainty if there is *no* properly controlled follow-up research which has established the safety of the drug or procedure with regard to its direct and/or indirect effects on the physiological, mental and neurological development of the child exposed, via the mother, to the drug or procedure during pregnancy, labor, birth or lactation—(this would apply to virtually all drugs and the vast majority of obstetric procedures).
6. *The Pregnant Patient has the right,* prior to the administration of any drug, to be informed on the brand name and generic name of the drug in order that she may advise the health professional of any past adverse reaction to the drug.
7. *The Pregnant Patient has the right* to determine for herself, without pressure from her attendant, whether she will accept the risks inherent in the proposed therapy or refuse a drug or procedure.

* From *The Pregnant Patient Bill of Rights.* Published and distributed by the International Childbirth Educational Association, Inc (ICEA), P.O. Box 20048, Minneapolis, MN 55420. Reprinted with permission.

8 *The Pregnant Patient has the right* to know the name and qualifications of the individual administering a medication or procedure to her during labor or birth.

9 *The Pregnant Patient has the right* to be informed, prior to the administration of any procedure, whether that procedure is being administered to her for her or her baby's benefit (medically indicated) or as an elective procedure (for convenience, teaching purposes or research).

10 *The Pregnant Patient has the right* to be accompanied during the stress of labor and birth by someone she cares for, and to whom she looks for emotional comfort and encouragement.

11 *The Pregnant Patient has the right* after appropriate medical consultation to choose a position for labor and for birth which is least stressful to her baby and to herself.

12 *The Obstetric Patient has the right* to have her baby cared for at her bedside if her baby is normal, and to feed her baby according to her baby's needs rather than according to the hospital regimen.

13 *The Obstetric Patient has the right* to be informed in writing of the name of the person who actually delivered her baby and the professional qualifications of that person. This information should also be on the birth certificate.

14 *The Obstetric Patient has the right* to be informed if there is any known or indicated aspect of her or her baby's care or condition which may cause her or her baby later difficulty or problems.

15 *The Obstetric Patient has the right* to have her and her baby's hospital medical records complete, accurate and legible and to have their records, including Nurses' Notes, retained by the hospital until the child reaches at least the age of majority, or to have the records offered to her before they are destroyed.

16 *The Obstetric Patient,* both during and after her hospital stay, *has the right* to have access to her complete hospital medical records, including Nurses' Notes, and to receive a copy upon payment of a reasonable fee and without incurring the expense of retaining an attorney.

It is the obstetric patient and her baby, not the health professional, who must sustain any trauma or injury resulting from the use of a drug or obstetric procedure. The observation of the rights listed above will not only permit the obstetric patient to participate in the decisions involving her and her baby's health care, but will help to protect the health professional and the hospital against litigation arising from resentment or misunderstanding on the part of the mother.

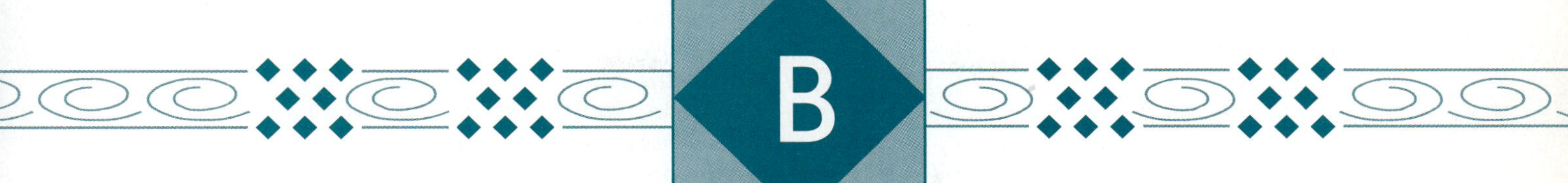

United Nations Declaration of the Rights of the Child

Preamble

Whereas the peoples of the United Nations have, in the Charter, reaffirmed their faith in fundamental human rights, and in the dignity and worth of the human person, and have determined to promote social progress and better standards of life in larger freedom,

Whereas the United Nations has, in the Universal Declaration of Human Rights, proclaimed that everyone is entitled to all the rights and freedoms set forth therein, without distinction of any kind, such as race, color, sex, language, religion, political or other opinion, national or social origin, property, birth or other status,

Whereas the child, by reason of his physical and mental immaturity, needs special safeguards and care, including appropriate legal protection, before as well as after birth,

Whereas the need for such special safeguards has been stated in the Geneva Declaration of the Rights of the Child of 1924, and recognized in the Universal Declaration of Human Rights and in the statutes of specialized agencies and international organizations concerned with welfare of children,

Whereas mankind owes to the child the best it has to give

Now Therefore the General Assembly Proclaims

This Declaration of the Rights of the Child to the end that he may have a happy childhood and enjoy for his own good and for the good of society the rights and freedoms herein set forth, and calls upon parents, upon men and women as individuals and upon voluntary organizations, local authorities and national governments to recognize these rights and strive for their observance by legislative and other measures progressively taken in accordance with the following principles:

Principle 1

The child shall enjoy all the rights set forth in this Declaration. All children, without any exception whatsoever, shall be entitled to these rights, without distinction or discrimination on account of race, color, sex, language, religion, political or other opinion, national or social origin, property, birth or other status, whether of himself or his family.

Principle 2

The child shall enjoy special protection, and shall be given opportunities and facilities, by law and by other means, to enable him to develop physically, mentally, morally, spiritually and socially in a healthy and normal manner and in conditions of freedom and dignity. In the enactment of laws for this purpose the best interests of the child shall be the paramount consideration.

Principle 3

The child shall be entitled from his birth to a name and a nationality.

Principle 4

The child shall enjoy the benefits of social security. He shall be entitled to grow and develop in health; to this end special care and protection shall be provided both to him and to his mother, including adequate pre-natal and post-natal care. The child shall have the right to adequate nutrition, housing, recreation and medical services.

Principle 5

The child who is physically, mentally or socially handicapped shall be given the special treatment, education and care required by his particular condition.

Principle 6

The child, for the full and harmonious development of his personality, needs love and understanding. He shall, wherever possible, grow up in the care and under the responsibility of his parents, and in any case in an atmosphere of affection and of moral and maternal security; a child of tender years shall not, save in exceptional circumstances, be separated from his mother. Society and the public authorities shall have the duty to extend particular care to children without a family and to those without adequate means of support. Payment of state and other assistance toward the maintenance of children of large families is desirable.

Principle 7

The child is entitled to receive education, which shall be free and compulsory, at least in the elementary stages. He shall be given an education which will promote his general culture, and enable him on a basis of equal opportunity to develop his abilities, his individual judgment, and his sense of moral and social responsibility, and to become a useful member of society.

The best interests of the child shall be the building principle of those responsible for his education and guidance; that responsibility lies in the first place with his parents.

The child shall have full opportunity for play and recreation, which shall be directed to the same purposes as education; society and the public authorities shall endeavor to promote the enjoyment of this right.

Principle 8

The child shall in all circumstances be among the first to receive protection and relief.

Principle 9

The child shall be protected against all forms of neglect, cruelty and exploitation. He shall not be the subject of traffic, in any form. The child shall not be admitted to employment before an appropriate minimum age; he shall in no case be caused or permitted to engage in any occupation or employment which would prejudice his health or education, or interfere with his physical, mental or moral development.

Principle 10

The child shall be protected from practices which may foster racial, religious and any other form of discrimination. He shall be brought up in a spirit of understanding, tolerance, friendship among peoples, peace and universal brotherhood and in full consciousness that his energy and talents should be devoted to the service of his fellow men.

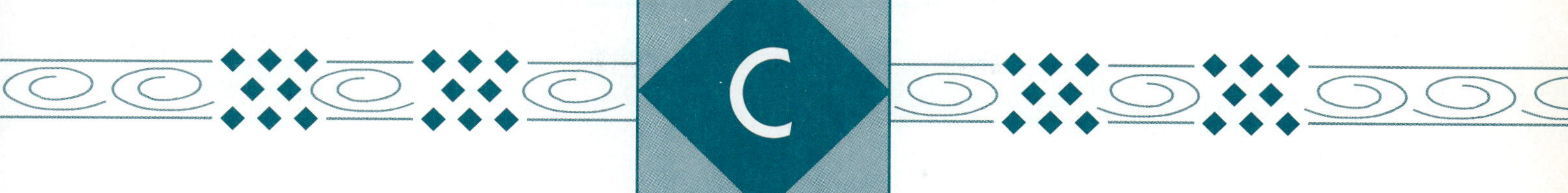

Standard Laboratory Values: Pregnant and Nonpregnant Women

	Nonpregnant	Pregnant
HEMATOLOGICAL VALUES		
Complete Blood Count (CBC)		
Hemoglobin, g/dL	12-16*	11.5-14*
Hematocrit, PCV, %	37-47	32-42
Red cell volume, mL	1600	1900
Plasma volume, mL	2400	3700
Red blood cell count, million/mm^3	4-5.5	4-5.5
White blood cells, total per mm^3	4500-10,000	5000-15,000
Polymorphonuclear cells, %	54-62	60-85
Lymphocytes, %	38-46	15-40
Erythrocyte sedimentation rate, mm/h	≤	30-90
MCHC, g/dL packed RBCs (mean corpuscular hemoglobin concentration)	30-36	No change
MCH/(mean corpuscular hemoglobin per picogram [less than a nanogram])	29-32	No change
MCV/μm^3 (mean corpuscular volume per cubic micrometer)	82-96	No change
Blood coagulation and fibrinolytic activity†		
Factors VII, VIII, IX, X		Increase in pregnancy, return to normal in early puerperium; factor VIII increases during and immediately after birth
Factors XI, XIII		Decrease in pregnancy
Prothrombin time (PT)	12-14 sec	Slight decrease in pregnancy
Partial thromboplastin time (PTT)	60-70 sec	Slight decrease in pregnancy and again decrease during second and third stage of labor (indicates clotting at placental site)
Bleeding time	1-3 min (Duke) 2-4 min (Ivy)	No appreciable change
Coagulation time	6-10 min (Lee/White)	No appreciable change

*At sea level. Permanent residents of higher levels (e.g., Denver) require higher levels of hemoglobin.
†Pregnancy represents a hypercoagulable state.

	Nonpregnant	Pregnant
Platelets	150,000 to 350,000/mm^3	No significant change until 3 to 5 days after birth, then marked increase (may predispose woman to thrombosis) and gradual return to normal
Fibrinolytic activity		Decreases in pregnancy, then abrupt return to normal (protection against thromboembolism)
Fibrinogen	250 mg/dL	400 mg/dL
Mineral/vitamin concentrations		
Vitamin B_{12}, folic acid, ascorbic acid	Normal	Moderate decrease
Serum proteins		
Total, g/dL	6.7-8.3	5.5-7.5
Albumin, g/dL	3.5-5.5	3.0-5.0
Globulin, total, g/dL	2.3-3.5	3.0-4.0
Blood sugar		
Fasting, mg/dL	70-80	65
2-hour postprandial, mg/dL	60-110	Under 140 after a 100 g carbohydrate meal is considered normal
CARDIOVASCULAR DETERMINATIONS		
Blood pressure, mm Hg	120/80*	114/65 during midtrimester, then return to usual value by end of third trimester
Pulse, rate/min	70	80
Stroke volume, mL	65	75
Cardiac output, L/min	4.5	6
Circulation time (arm-tongue), sec	15-16	12-14
Blood volume, mL		
Whole blood	4000	5600
Plasma	2400	3700
Red blood cells	1600	1900
Chest x-ray studies		
Transverse diameter of heart	—	1-2 cm increase
Left border of heart	—	Straightened
Cardiac volume	—	70 mL increase
HEPATIC VALUES		
Bilirubin total	Not more than 1 mg/dL	Unchanged
Serum cholesterol	110-300 mg/dL	↑ 60% from 16-32 weeks of pregnancy; remains at this level until after birth
Serum alkaline phosphatase	2-4.5 units (Bodansky)	↑ from week 12 of pregnancy to 6 weeks after birth
Serum globulin albumin	1.5-3.0 g/dL 4.5-5.3 g/dL	↑ slight ↓ 3.0 g by late pregnancy
RENAL VALUES		
Bladder capacity	1300 mL	1500 mL
Renal plasma flow (RPF), mL/min	490-700	Increase by 25%, to 612-875
Glomerular filtration rate (GFR), mL/min	105-132	Increase by 50%, to 160-198
Nonprotein nitrogen (NPN), mg/dL	25-40	Decreases
Blood urea nitrogen (BUN), mg/dL	20-25	Decreases
Serum creatinine, mg/kg/24 hr	20-22	Decreases
Serum uric acid, mg/kg/24 hr	257-750	Decreases
Urine glucose	Negative	Present in 20% of pregnant women
Intravenous pyelogram (IVP)	Normal	Slight-to-moderate hydroureter and hydronephrosis; right kidney larger than left kidney

*For the woman about 20 years of age; 10 years of age: 103/70; 30 years of age: 123/82; 40 years of age: 126/84.
Modified from Bobak IM and Jensen MD: *Maternity and gynecologic care,* ed 5, St. Louis, 1993, Mosby.

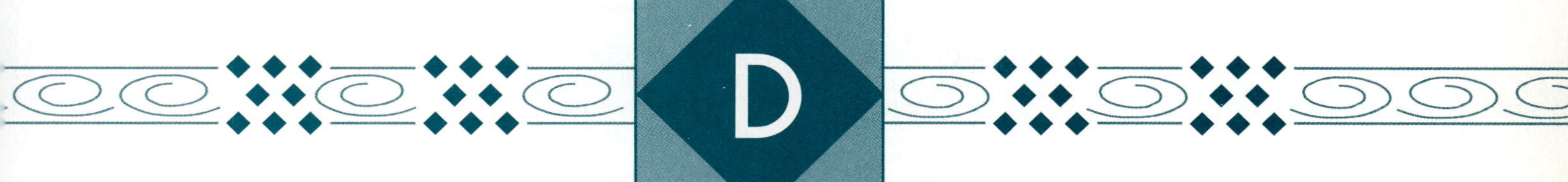

COMMUNITY, NATIONAL, AND INTERNATIONAL RESOURCES

AIDS Information Clearinghouse
P.O. Box 6003
Rockville, MD 20849-6003
(800) 458-5231 (English and Spanish)

AMEND
Aiding a Mother Experiencing Neo-Natal Death
4324 Berrywick Terrace
St. Louis, MO 63141
(314) 487-7582

American Academy of Husband-Coached Childbirth (The Bradley Method)
P.O. Box 5224
Sherman Oaks, CA 91413
(818) 788-6662

American Academy of Pediatrics
Publications Department
P.O. Box 927
141 Northwest Point Blvd.
Elk Grove Village, IL 60007
(708) 228-5005
(800) 433-9016

American Cancer Society, Inc.
1599 Clifton Road, NE
Atlanta, GA 30329
1-800-ACS-2345

American Cleft Palate Craniofacial Association
National Office
1218 Grandview Ave.
Pittsburgh, PA 15211
(412) 481-1376

American Diabetes Association
Diabetes Information Service Center
1660 Duke Street
Alexandria, VA 22314
1-800-ADA-DISC

American Dietetic Association
216 W. Jackson Blvd., Suite 800
Chicago, IL 60606
(312) 899-0040

American Fertility Society
1209 Montgomery Highway
Birmingham, AL 35216-2809
(205) 978-5000

American Foundation for Maternal and Child Health, Inc.
439 E. 51st St., #4A
New York, NY 10022-5473
(212) 759-5510

American Hospital Association
840 N. Lake Shore Drive
Chicago, IL 60611
(312) 280-6000

American Red Cross
National Headquarters
431 18th Street, NW
Washington, DC 20006
(202) 737-8300

American Society for Psychoprophylaxis in Obstetrics (ASPO)
1200 19th Street, NW
Suite 300
Washington, DC 20036-2401
(202) 857-1128

Association of Birth Defects in Children
Orlando Executive Park
5400 Diplomat Cir.
Suite 270
Orlando, FL 32810
(407) 629-1466

Association for Neuro-Metabolic Disorders
5223 Brookfield Lane
Sylvania, OH 43560
(419) 885-1497

Association for the Care of Children's Health
7910 Woodmont Avenue, Suite 300
Bethesda, MD 20814
(301) 654-6549

Boys Town
The Boys Town Press
Father Flanagan's Boys' Home
Boys Town, NE 68010
(402) 498-3200, (800) 448-3000 (crisis calls only)

Cancer Information Service
National Cancer Institute
Building 31, Room 10 A 07
Bethesda, MD 20892
(800) 422-6237, (800) 4-CANCER (hotline)

Centers for Disease Control and Prevention
1600 Clifton Rd, N.E.
Atlanta, GA 30333
(404) 329-1819, (404) 329-3286

Children's Defense Fund
25 E Street, NW
Washington, DC 20001
(202) 628-8787

Child Welfare League of America
440 First St., N.W., Suite 310
Washington, DC 20001
(201) 638-2952

Cleft Palate Foundation
1218 Grandview Avenue
Pittsburgh, PA 15211
1-800-24-CLEFT

C/SEC, Inc. (Cesarean/Support Education and Concern)
22 Forest Road
Framingham, MA 01701
(508) 877-8266

DES Action USA
National Office
1615 Broadway, #510
Oakland, CA 94612
(510) 465-4011

Empty Cradle
11793 Lake Grove Court
San Diego, CA 92116
(619) 692-2144

Endometriosis Association
8585 N. 76th Place
Milwaukee, WI 53223
(414) 355-2200

Food and Drug Administration (FDA)
Office of Consumer Affairs
Public Inquiries
5600 Fishers Lane (HFE-88)
Rockville, MD 20857
(301) 443-3170

International Childbirth Education Association (ICEA)
P.O. Box 20048
Minneapolis, MN 55420

La Leche League
P.O. Box 1209
Franklin Park, IL 60131-8209
(708) 519-7730, (800) LA-LECHE

March of Dimes See *National Foundation/March of Dimes*

Maternity Center Association
48 East 92nd Street
New York, NY 10128
(212) 369-7300

Medic-Alert Foundation U.S.
P.O. Box 1009
Turlock, CA 95381
(209) 668-3333, (800) 344-3226

National AIDS Information Clearinghouse
1-800-458-5231 (English and Spanish)
(See AIDS)

National Association for Sickle Cell Disease
3345 Wilshire Blvd., Suite 1106
Los Angeles, CA 90010-1880
(213) 736-5455, 1-800-421-8453

National Center for Education in Maternal and Child Health
2000 15th Street North
Suite 701
Arlington, VA 22201
(703) 524-7802

National Coalition Against Domestic Violence
P.O. Box 34103
Washington, DC 20043-4103
(202) 638-6388

National Down Syndrome Congress
1605 Chantilly Dr.
Suite 250
Atlanta, GA 30324
1-800-232-6372

National Down Syndrome Society
666 Broadway
New York, NY 10012
(212) 460-9330

National Easter Seal Society
230 West Monroe, Suite 1800
Chicago, IL 60606
(312) 726-6200, (312) 726-4258 (TDD)
(800) 221-6827

National Foundation/March of Dimes
1275 Mamaroneck Avenue
White Plains, NY 10605
(914) 428-7100

National Information Center for Children and Youth with Handicaps (NICHCY)
P.O. Box 1492
Washington, DC 20013-1492
(800) 695-0285 (Voice/TT)

National Information Clearinghouse for Infants with Disabilities and Life Threatening Conditions
Center for Developmental Disabilities
School of Medicine, Dept. of Pediatrics
University of South Carolina
Columbia, SC 29208
(800) 922-9234, Ext. 201 (Voice/TT)

National Institutes of Child Health and Human Development
Building 31, Room 2A-32
9000 Rockville Pike
Bethesda, MD 20892
(301) 496-5133

National Institute of Mental Health
"Plain Talk" Series
Information Resources and Inquiries Branch
Room 7C-02
5600 Fishers Lane
Rockville, MD 20857

National Maternal and Child Health Clearinghouse
8201 Greensboro Drive
Suite 600
McLean, VA 22102

National Mental Health Association
1021 Prince St.
Alexandria, VA 22314
(703) 684-7722

National Organization of Mothers of Twins Clubs, Inc.
P.O. Box 23188
Albuquerque, NM 87192-1188
(505) 275-0955

National Rehabilitation Association
633 S. Washington St.
Alexandria, VA 22314
(703) 836-0850

National Safety Council
1121 Spring Lake Drive
Itasca, IL 60143-3201
(708) 285-1121, (800) 621-7615 or 7619

Parents Without Partners
401 N. Michigan Ave.
Chicago, IL 60611-4267
(312) 644-6610

Patient Counseling Library
Budlong Press Co.
5428 N. Virginia Avenue
Chicago, IL 60625
(312) 631-6484

Planned Parenthood Federation of America, Inc.
810 Seventh Avenue
New York, NY 10019

Pregnancy and Infant Loss
1421 East Wayzata Boulevard
Suite 30
Wayzata, MN 55391
(612) 473-9372

RESOLVE, Inc.
5 Water Street
Arlington, MA 02174-4814
(617) 643-2424

RTS Bereavement Services
Formerly known as: Resolve Through Sharing
1910 South Ave.
La Crosse, WI 54601
(608) 791-4747, (800) 362-9567, Ext. 4747

SIDELINES NATIONAL SUPPORT NETWORK
P.O. Box 1808
Laguna Beach, CA 92652
(714) 497-2265

SKIP (Sick Kids Need Involved People) of New York, Inc.
545 Madison Ave., 13th Floor
New York, NY 10022
(212) 421-9160

Spina Bifida Association of America
4590 MacArthur Blvd., NW
Suite 250
Washington, DC 20007
800-621-3141, (202) 944-3285

Sudden Infant Death Syndrome Resource Center
8201 Greensboro Dr., Suite 600
McLean, VA 22102
(703) 821-8955, Ext. 474 or 249

Twins Magazine
P.O. Box 12045
Overland Park, KS 66212
1-800-821-5533

VBAC (Vaginal Birth After Cesarean)
10 Great Plain Terrace
Needham, MA 01292
(617) 449-2490

Wyeth-Ayerst Laboratories
P.O. Box 8299
Philadelphia, PA 19101
(610) 688-4400

Women Against Rape
P.O. Box 02084
Columbus, OH 43202
(614) 291-9751, (614) 221-4447 (crisis line)

World Health Organization
Organization Mondiale de la Sante
20 Avenue Appia, CH-1211
Geneva 27, SWITZERLAND

U.S. Committee for the World Health Organization
1129 20th Street, NW
Suite 400
Washington, DC 20036
(202) 466-5883

NURSING ORGANIZATIONS

American College of Nurse Midwives
1522 K Street, NW
Suite 1000
Washington, DC 20005
(202) 289-0171

American Nurses Association (ANA)
Head Office
600 Maryland Ave. SW
Suite 100 West
Washington, DC 20024-2571
(202) 554-4444

AWHONN: The Association of Women's Health, Obstetric, and Neonatal Nurses
Formerly: NAACOG
c/o Communications Department
409 12th St. SW
Suite 300
Washington, DC 20024
(202) 638-0026

Canadian Nurses Association
50 The Driveway
Ottawa, Ontario, Canada K2P 1E2

Licensed Vocational Nurses League (LVNL)
451 Waller Street
San Francisco, CA 94117
(415) 558-8501

NAPNAP: National Association of Pediatric Nurse Associates and Practitioners
1101 Kings Hwy. N., No. 206
Cherry Hill, NJ 08034
(609) 667-1773

National Association for Practical Nurse Education and Service (NAPNES)
1400 Spring St., #310
Silver Springs, MD 20910
(301) 588-2491

National Federation of Licensed Practical Nurses (NFLPN)
1418 Aversboro Rd.
Garner, NC 27529
(919) 779-0046

National League for Nursing (NLN)
350 Hudson St.
New York, NY 10014
(212) 989-9393

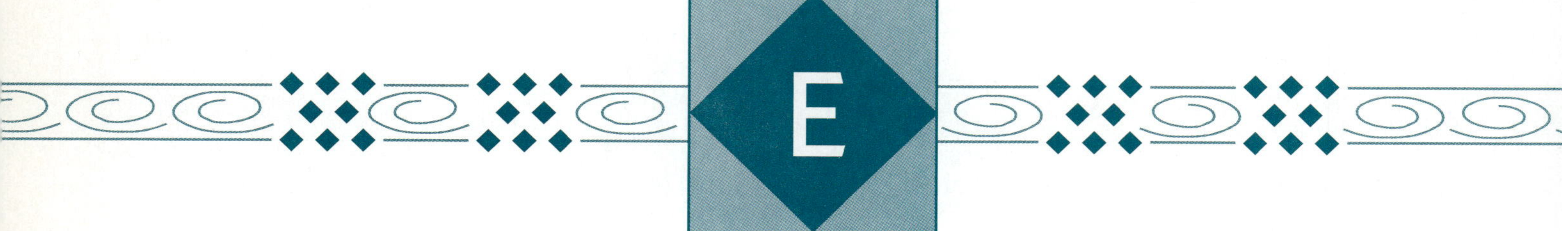

Growth Charts

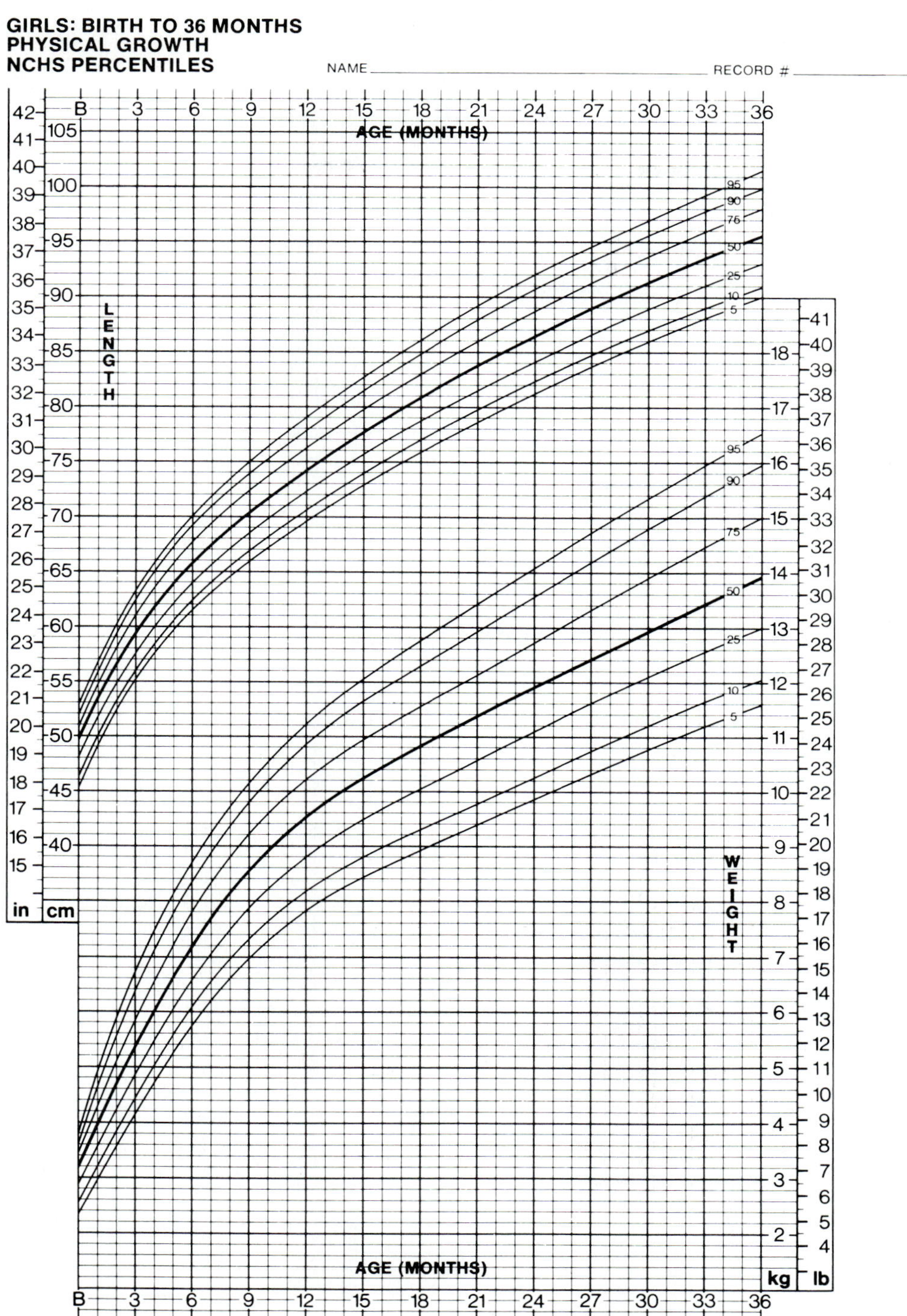

Girls: birth to 36 months. Length and weight. These charts were constructed with data from the National Center for Health Statistics, United States Public Health Service. The data on these charts are considered representative of the general United States population. *(Reproduced with permission from Ross Laboratories.)*

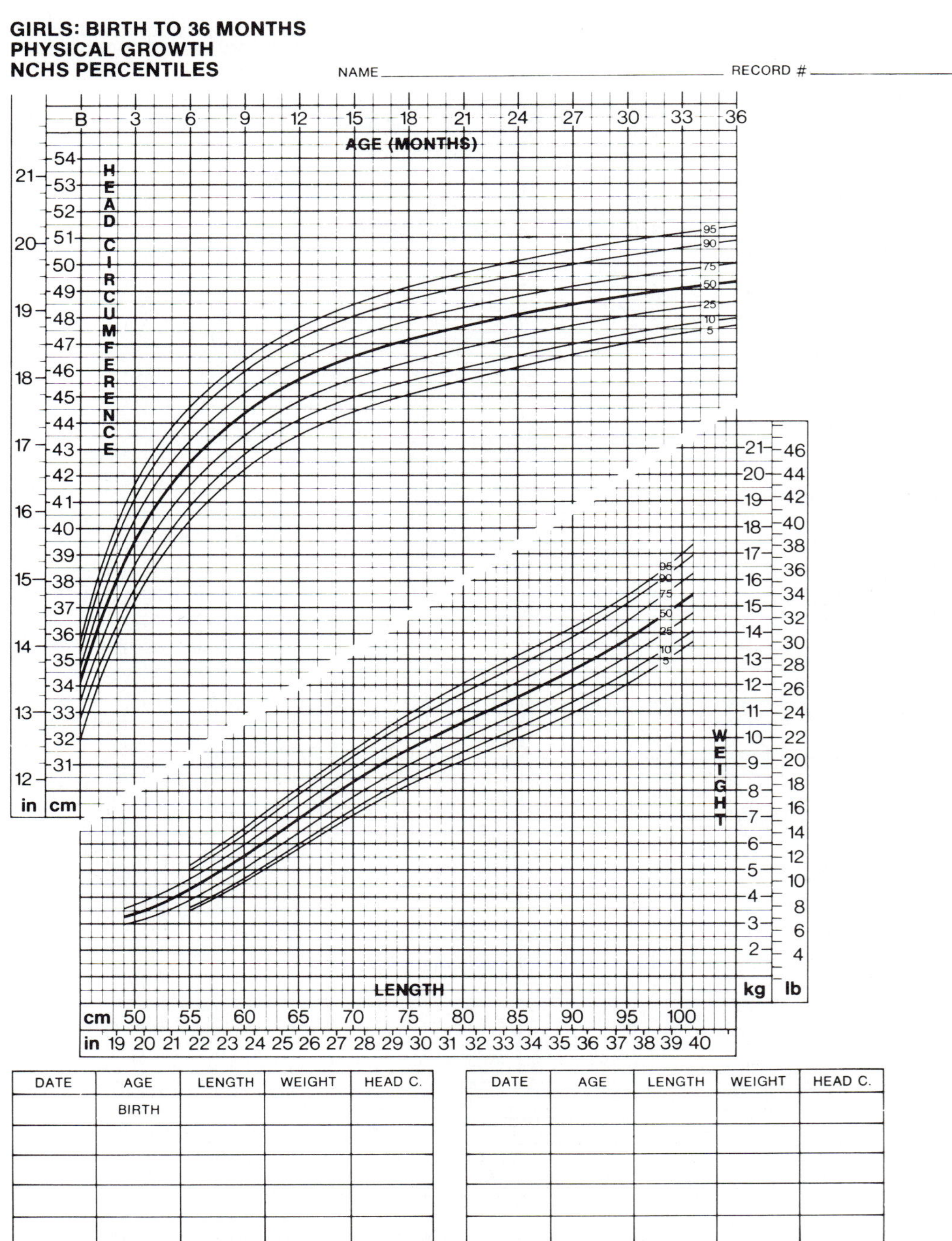

Girls: birth to 36 months. Head circumference, length, and weight.

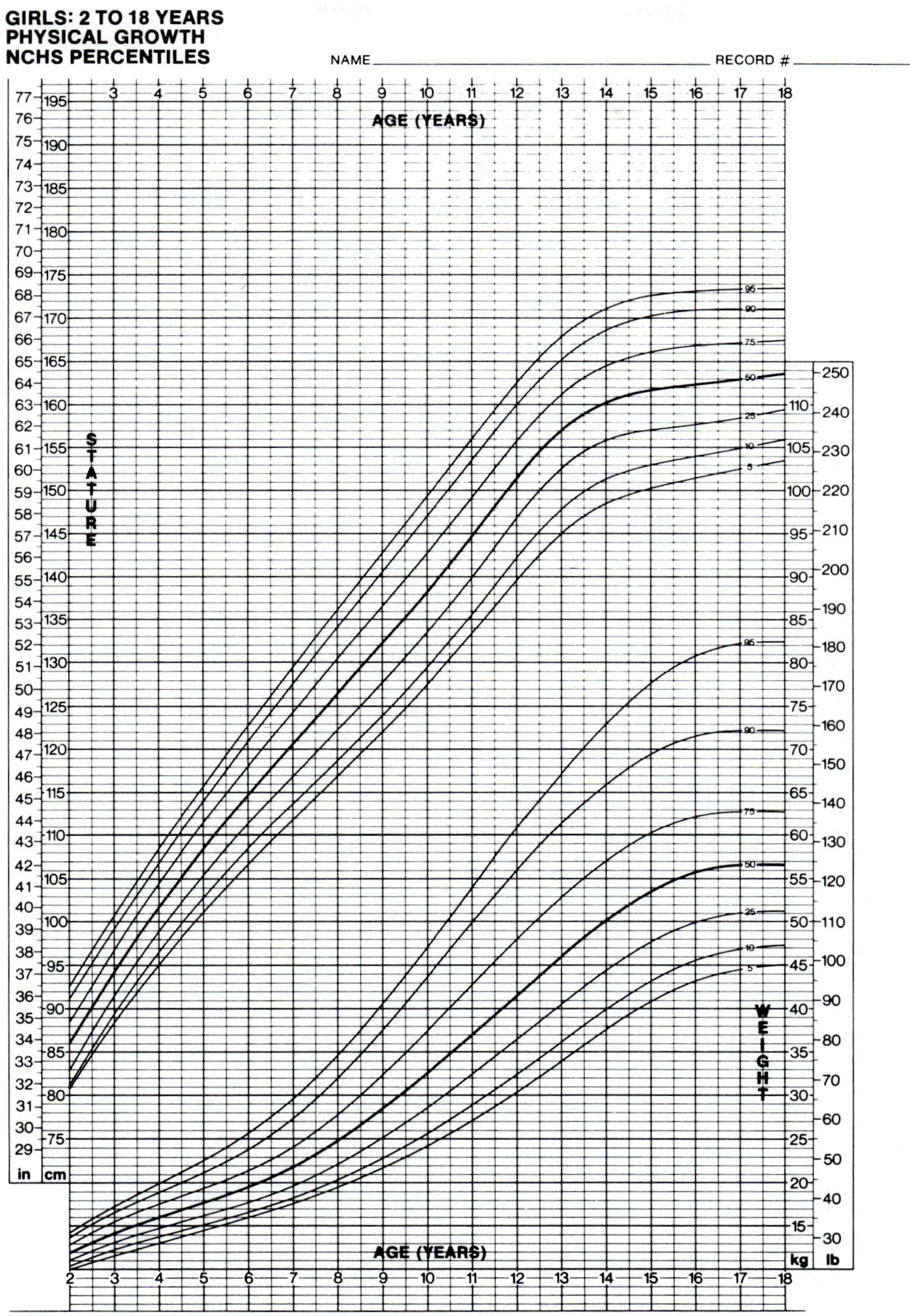

Girls: 2 to 18 years. Stature and weight.

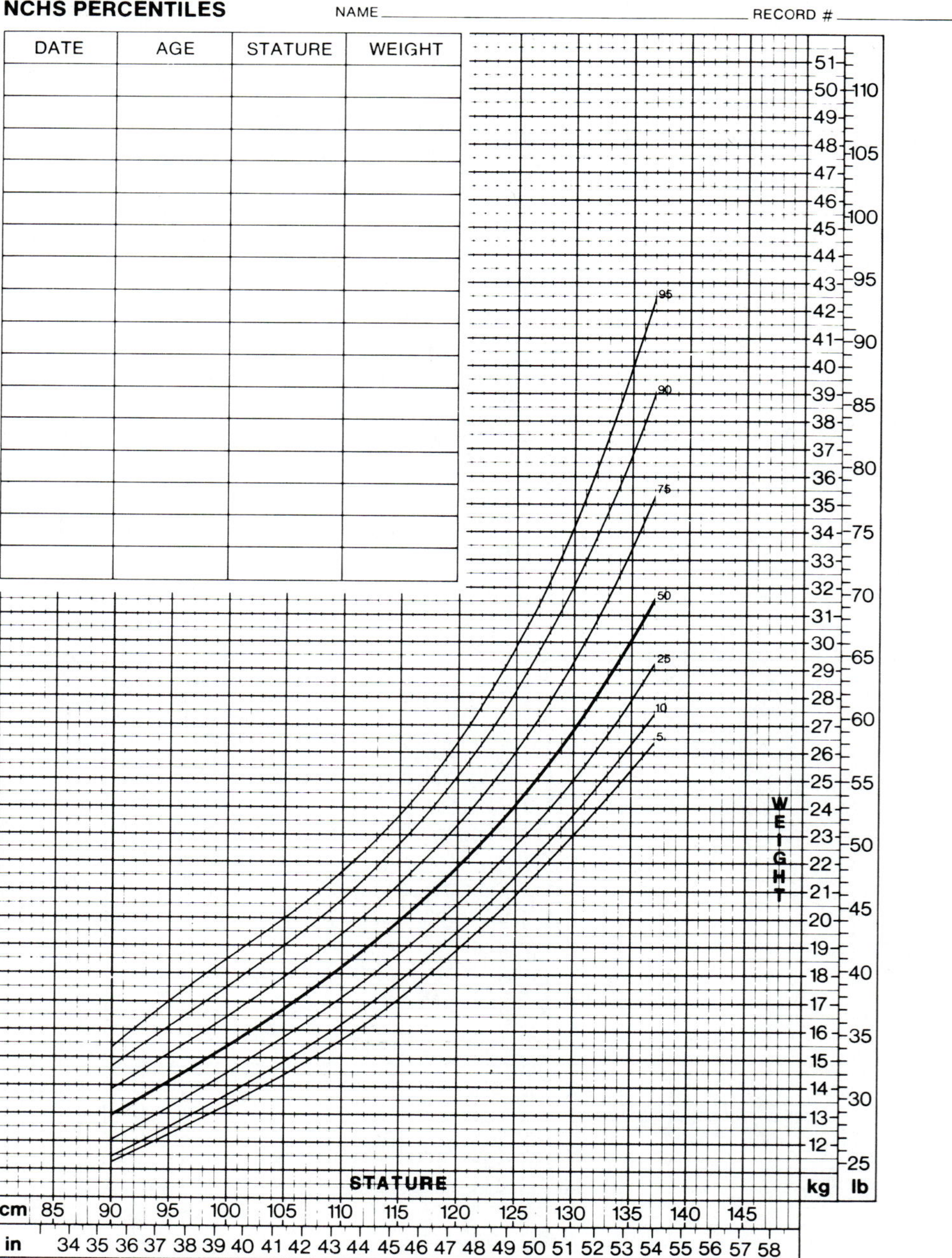

Girls: prepubescent. Physical growth.

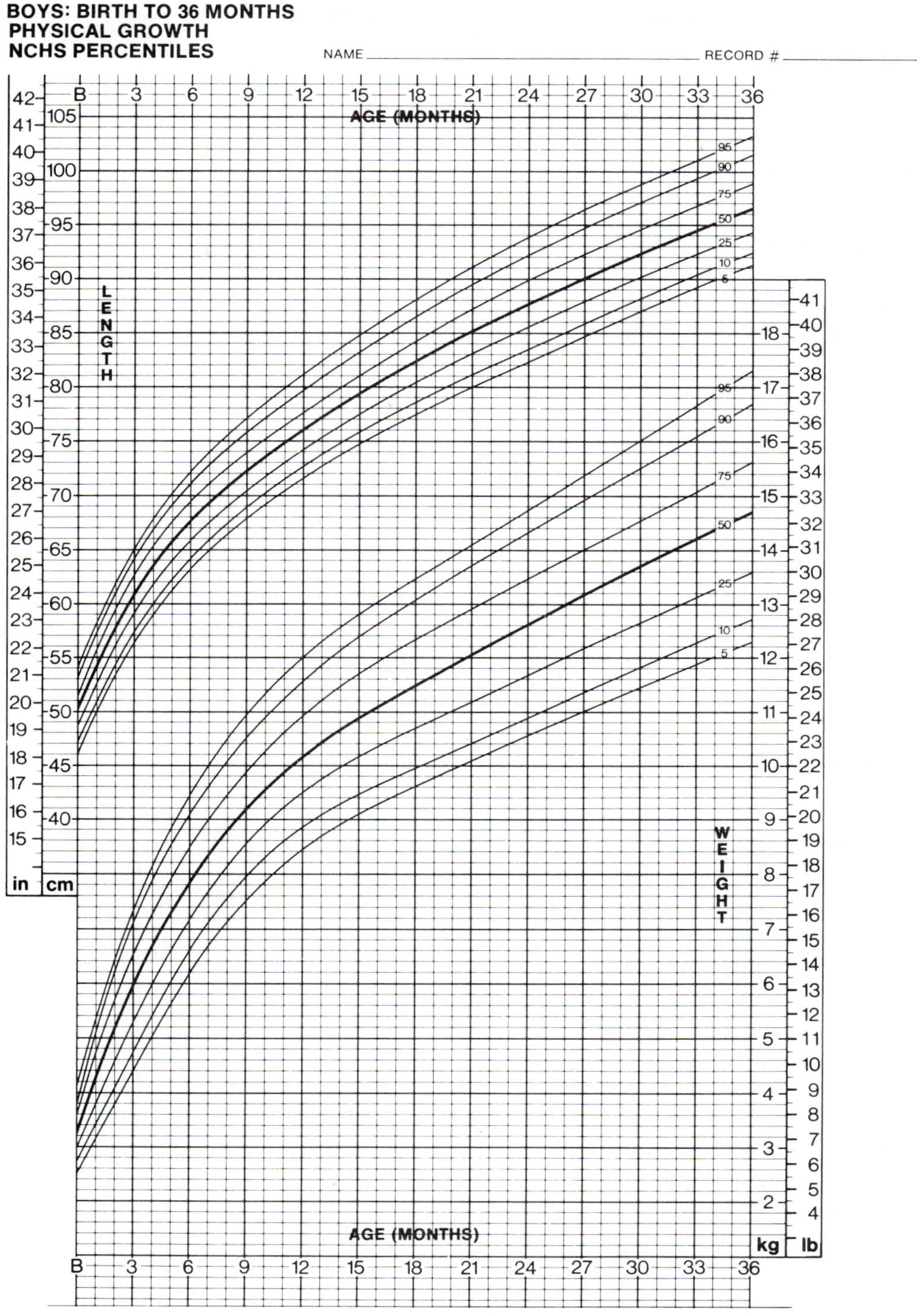

Boys: birth to 36 months. Length and weight.

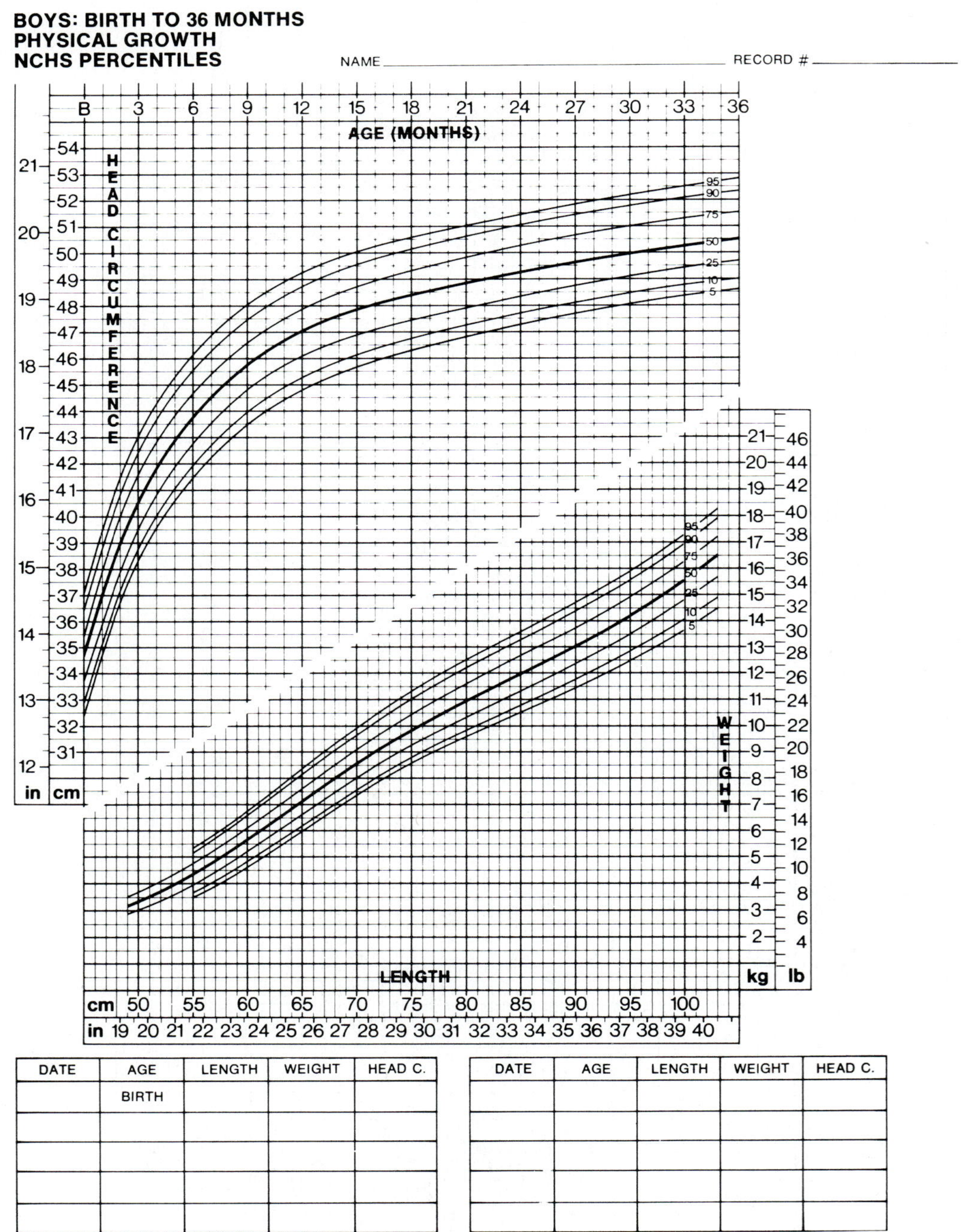

DATE	AGE	LENGTH	WEIGHT	HEAD C.
	BIRTH			

DATE	AGE	LENGTH	WEIGHT	HEAD C.

Boys: birth to 36 months. Head circumference, length, and weight.

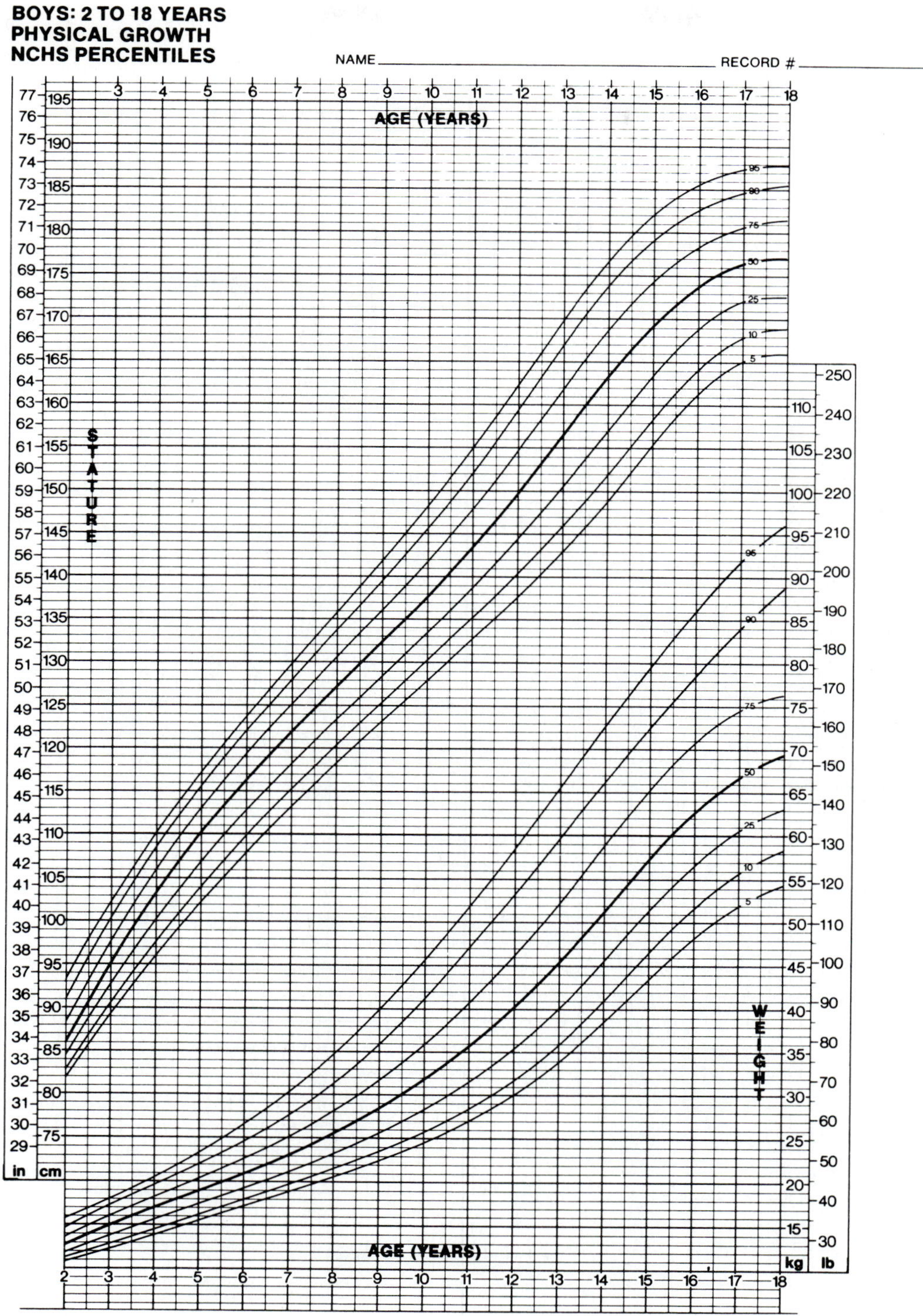

Boys: 2 to 18 years. Stature and weight.

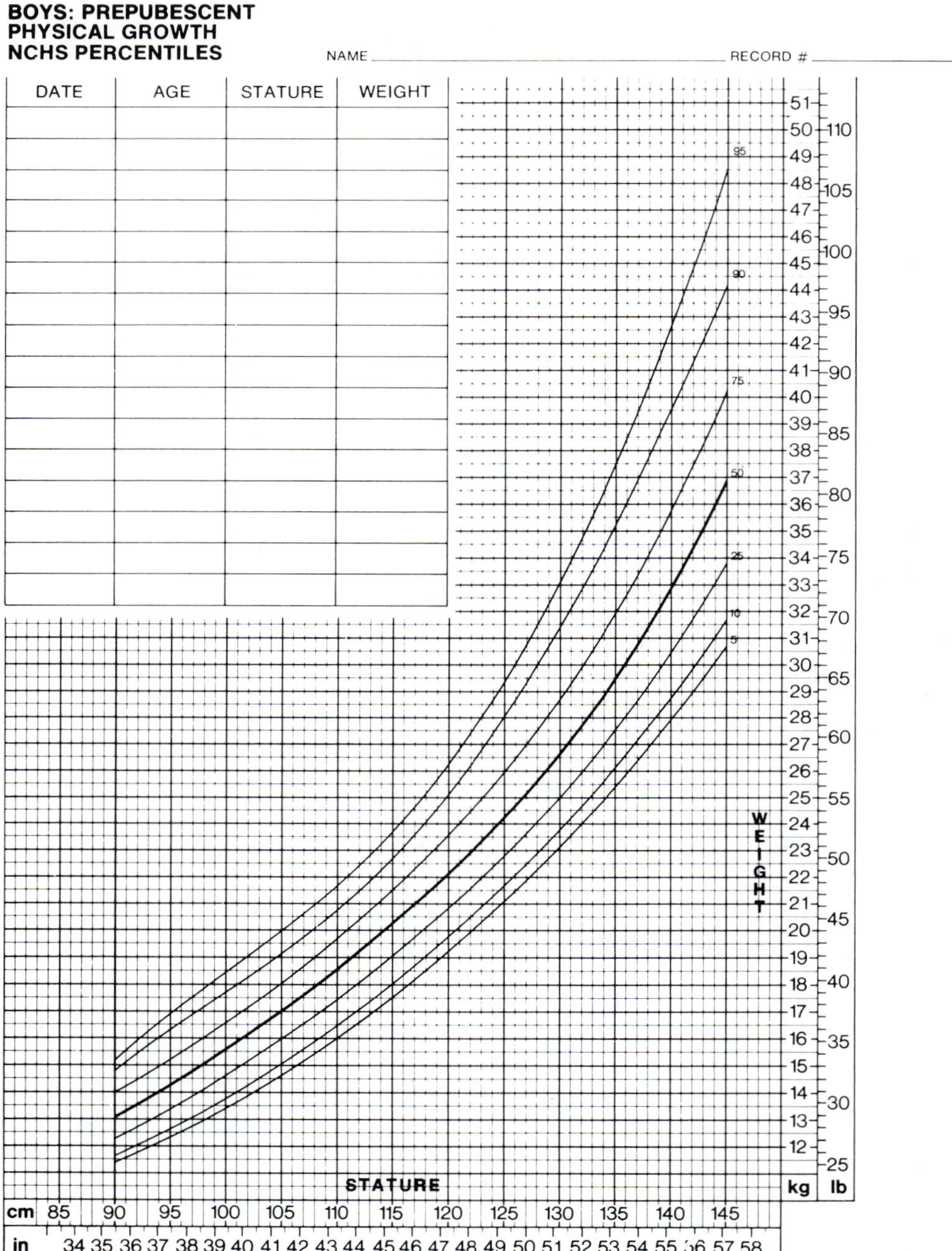

Boys: prepubescent. Physical growth.

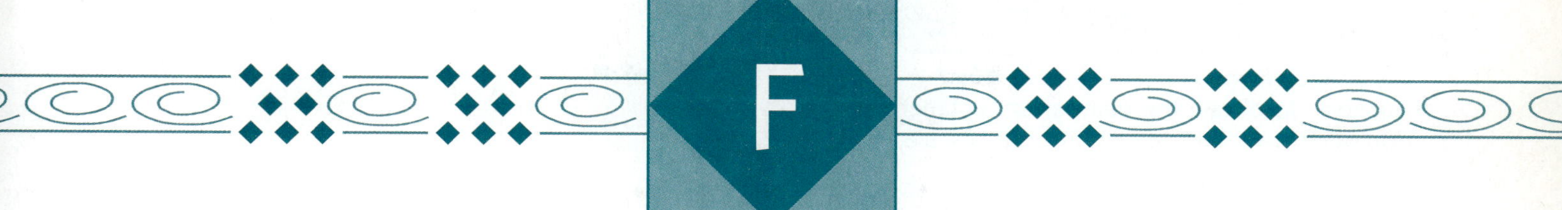

Newborn Metric Conversion Tables

◆ Weight (Mass): Pounds and Ounces to Grams

Example: To obtain grams equivalent to 6 lb 8 oz, read "6" on top scale, "8" on side scale; equivalent is 2948 gm.

OUNCES (OZ)	POUNDS (lb) 0	1	2	3	4	5	6	7	8	9	10	11	12	13	14
0	0	454	907	1361	1814	2268	2722	3175	3629	4082	4536	4990	5443	5897	6350
1	28	482	936	1389	1843	2296	2750	3203	3657	4111	4564	5018	5471	5925	6379
2	57	510	964	1417	1871	2325	2778	3232	3685	4139	4593	5046	5500	5953	6407
3	85	539	992	1446	1899	2353	2807	3260	3714	4167	4621	5075	5528	5982	6435
4	113	567	1021	1474	1928	2381	2835	3289	3742	4196	4649	5103	5557	6010	6464
5	142	595	1049	1503	1956	2410	2863	3317	3770	4224	4678	5131	5585	6038	6492
6	170	624	1077	1531	1984	2438	2892	3345	3799	4252	4706	5160	5613	6067	6520
7	198	652	1106	1559	2013	2466	2920	3374	3827	4281	4734	5188	5642	6095	6549
8	227	680	1134	1588	2041	2495	2948	3402	3856	4309	4763	5216	5670	6123	6577
9	255	709	1162	1616	2070	2523	2977	3430	3884	4337	4791	5245	5698	6152	6605
10	283	737	1191	1644	2098	2551	3005	3459	3912	4366	4819	5273	5727	6180	6634
11	312	765	1219	1673	2126	2580	3033	3487	3941	4394	4848	5301	5755	6209	6662
12	340	794	1247	1701	2155	2608	3062	3515	3969	4423	4876	5330	5783	6237	6690
13	369	822	1276	1729	2183	2637	3090	3544	3997	4451	4904	5358	5812	6265	6719
14	397	850	1304	1758	2211	2665	3118	3572	4026	4479	4933	5386	5840	6294	6747
15	425	879	1332	1786	2240	2693	3147	3600	4054	4508	4961	5415	5868	6322	6776

From Newborn Metric Conversion Tables, Clinical Education Aid No. 3, Ross Laboratories, Columbus, OH. Note: 1 lb = 453.59237 gm; 1 oz = 28.349523 gm; 1000 gm = 1 kg. Gram equivalents have been rounded to whole numbers by adding 1 when the first decimal place is 5 or greater.

◆ Length: Inches to Centimeters

1-inch increments
Example: To obtain the number of centimeters equivalent to 22 in, read "20" on top scale, "2" on side scale, equivalent is 55.9 cm.

INCHES	0	10	20	30	40
0	0	25.4	50.8	76.2	101.6
1	2.5	27.9	53.3	78.7	104.1
2	5.1	30.5	55.9	81.3	106.7
3	7.6	33.0	58.4	83.8	109.2
4	10.2	35.6	61.0	86.4	111.8
5	12.7	38.1	63.5	88.9	114.3
6	15.2	40.6	66.0	91.4	116.8
7	17.8	43.2	68.6	94.0	119.4
8	20.3	45.7	71.1	96.5	121.9
9	22.9	48.3	73.7	99.1	124.5

From Newborn Metric Conversion Tables, Clinical Education Aid No. 3, Ross Laboratories, Columbus, OH.

◆ Conversion Factors for Temperature*

CELSIUS	FAHRENHEIT	CELSIUS	FAHRENHEIT	CELSIUS	FAHRENHEIT	CELSIUS	FAHRENHEIT
34.0	93.2	36.4	97.5	38.6	101.5	41.0	105.9
34.2	93.6	36.6	97.9	38.8	101.8	41.2	106.1
34.4	93.9	36.8	98.2	39.0	102.2	41.4	106.5
34.6	94.3	37.0	98.6	39.2	102.6	41.6	106.8
34.8	94.6	37.2	99.0	39.4	102.9	41.8	107.2
35.0	95.0	37.4	99.3	39.6	103.3	42.0	107.6
35.2	95.4	37.6	99.7	39.8	103.6	42.2	108.0
35.4	95.7	37.8	100.0	40.0	104.0	42.4	108.3
35.6	96.1	38.0	100.4	40.2	104.4	42.6	108.7
35.8	96.4	38.2	100.8	40.4	104.7	42.8	109.0
36.0	96.8	38.4	101.1	40.6	105.2	43.0	109.4
36.2	97.2			40.8	105.4		

*(°C × 9/5) + 32 = °F; °C = Temperature in Celsius (centigrade) degrees. (°F − 32) × 5/9 = °C; °F = Temperature in Fahrenheit degrees.

Index

A

NOTE: References followed by *t* or *f* indicate tables or figures, respectively.

C

S

T

U

V